NUTRITION

An Integrated Approach

NUTRITION

An Integrated Approach
Third Edition

RUTH L. PIKE
The Pennsylvania State University

MYRTLE L. BROWN
Virginia Polytechnic Institute
and State University

MACMILLAN PUBLISHING COMPANY
New York

COLLIER MACMILLAN PUBLISHERS
London

Copyright © 1984 by Macmillan Publishing Company
a division of Macmillan, Inc.
Copyright © 1967, 1975, by John Wiley & Sons, Inc.

Macmillan Publishing Company
866 Third Avenue, New York, New York 10022
Collier Macmillan Canada, Inc.

Library of Congress Cataloging in Publication Data:

Main entry under title:
Nutrition, an integrated approach.

   Bibliography: p
   Includes index.
   1. Nutrition   I. Pike, Ruth L.   II. Brown,
   Myrtle L. (Myrtle Laurestine), 1926-

QP141.N776   1984   613.2   83-16766
ISBN 0-02-395780-8

Printed in the United States of America

Printing   6 7 8   Year   8 9 0

ISBN 0-02-395780-8

preface to the third edition

The enormous task of bringing so large and so broad a volume up to date before it, too, becomes dated led us to seek the assistance of others. We asked some of the contributors to revise chapters and some to revise sections of chapters. We retained complete editorial responsibility, which in a number of instances, entailed rewriting contributions to conform to the style, purpose, and spirit of the book.

The format remains essentially the same as the second edition, and we still subscribe to one of our original and expressed purposes: to show how present knowledge evolved from previous findings through a step-by-step procedure over long years of study. To further the appreciation of this concept, we have stressed historical development of the science of nutrition throughout this volume as in the two editions that have preceded it. We believe that it is necessary to know where one has been in order to understand where one is going. In examining the past, ideas often arise that have remained buried in the literature waiting to be rediscovered and reinterpreted in the context of current scientific knowledge.

We are grateful to all our contributors and especially acknowledge the outstanding contribution of Dr. Carol V. Gay who provided an excellent revision of eight chapters in the style and spirit established by the authors.

We wish to thank Dr. Howerde E. Sauberlich for his careful review of the material sent to him, and Dr. J. Elizabeth Miles for her helpful suggestions.

For the preparation of the index, we extend thanks to Sylvia MacKinnon Carson.

For this edition, as for the previous two, we are indebted to Dr. Helen G. Oldham for her counsel and help in the writing and preparation of the manuscript and for her assistance in the tedious work of proofreading the entire book.

Ruth L. Pike
Myrtle L. Brown

preface to the second edition

What started out to be a revision has become almost a completely rewritten book. In addition to bringing the subject matter in this rapidly changing field up to date, we have reorganized it and presented it in a more logical fashion.

The book is now divided into five parts. Part I, "The Nutrients," is essentially the same as it was in the previous edition but it has been expanded. Part II, "Physiological Aspects of Nutrition," includes a new chapter on digestion and an enlarged section on absorption. Another new chapter is devoted to exchange and transport as well as mechanisms of homeostatic control. Since the nutrients must go through the intestinal mucosa and be transported to the cells to participate in metabolism, it seemed logical to place this material before the section on the cell. Part III, "The Cell," presents the basic biochemical cytology that is important to the nutritionist. As in the first edition, the nutrients are brought to the organelles within the cell, the locus of physiological and biochemical action. Where possible, basic reactions in cellular metabolism are discussed in terms of the complex multicellular organism. Each of these chapters has been rewritten and expanded. Two new chapters have been added: an introductory one on the methods used in studying cellular structure and mechanisms, and a chapter on the Golgi apparatus. Part IV, "Specialized Cells," is a new section that replaces the single chapter in the previous edition. The cells discussed are the ones that we think are of special interest to the nutritionist. Parts III and IV may contain more detail than some nutritionists believe is essential; others, however, will agree that the nutritionist must understand cell structure to understand how the nutrients participate as part of the dynamic complex of the cell. Part V, "The Complex Organism," includes a new chapter presenting the fundamental concepts underlying growth and development. Two chapters in the previous edition have been omitted. "Nutrients in Foods" was primarily a discussion of methodology; this material now has been incorporated into other parts of the book. Instead of the chapter on "Interrelationships of Nutrients," we have shown the interrelationships throughout the book because, indeed, they are interrelated on metabolism.

Our purpose is the same: to integrate the contributions of related scientific disciplines with the study of nutrition; to foster a questioning attitude; and to emphasize the depth and limitations of present knowledge.

We thank Dr. Helen G. Oldham for counsel and help in the preparation of the manuscript; Dr. Marian E. Swendseid for carefully reading the manuscript and making suggestions; and Dr. Lawrence M. Marshall for critically reading portions of the material.

Again we are indebted to Dr. Harald Schraer, who prepared many of the electron micrographs for our use.

If there are errors in the text, we assume full responsibility for them.

Ruth L. Pike
Myrtle L. Brown

preface to the
first edition

"He that publishes a book runs a very great hazard, since nothing can be more impossible than to compose one that may secure the approbation of every reader."

Don Quixote, Book III

Advanced study in nutrition presupposes basic knowledge of biochemistry, physiology and, of course, nutrition. This previously acquired knowledge too often tends to be separated in time and in the students' thinking, whereas, in fact, the biochemical, physiological, and nutritional aspects of living matter are inseparable. The disciplines that we have thought of as nutrition, physiology, biochemistry, and genetics have converged at the cellular level and, because the approach of each has been from a different perspective, the convergence has been to mutual advantage.

The nutritionist who understands how the coordination of structure and function is related to the metabolic needs of the cell and its response to its environment has at his disposal the fundamental knowledge for evaluating the nutrient needs of the whole man. The plan of this book and the philosophy that we hope pervades it are based upon this premise.

The book is divided into three parts. Part I briefly presents the historical development of nutritional science and basic information on the nutrients. This section is not intended as a substitute for fundamental biochemistry but includes relevant material applying specifically to mammalian metabolism, which will be drawn upon in later chapters. Part II presents basic biochemical cytology from the viewpoint of the nutritionist, bringing the nutrients to their locus of physiological and biochemical action and indicating, where possible, how basic reactions in cellular metabolism become meaningful in terms of the complex multicellular organism. Part III presents fundamental concepts underlying applied human nutrition. We have concentrated upon the development of these concepts in the belief that *how* and *why* are ultimately of greatest value to the student.

The purpose of this book has been to integrate, as far as possible, the contributions of related scientific disciplines to the study of nutrition. We have tried throughout to foster a questioning attitude and a recognition of both the depth and the limitations of present knowledge. The book is not all-inclusive nor was it intended to be, and we take seriously Don Quixote's warning. We are fully aware that our directions, interests, prejudices, and concerns show and, indeed, we believe that they should. Any nutrition text, to be a complete treatise and to cover the broad areas of concern to all nutritionists in today's world, would have to delve in depth not only into those disciplines we have included but also into public health, sociology, psychology, economics, and perhaps still other areas. Choices therefore are inevitable. It is our belief that a nutritionist must understand the biological aspects of the subject before venturing into the sociological or psychological arenas and, whereas we are convinced of their importance, these are areas that are outside our province. If we have been able to impart an enthusiasm and insight into the study of nutrition, we will have accomplished what we set out to do.

We wish to express our gratitude to Dr. Helen G. Oldham for her counsel in the preparation of the manuscript and for her active participation in the chores associated with the checking of galleys and preparation of the index.

We are sincerely grateful for the helpful suggestions and criticisms we received from Dr. Rosemary Schraer, Dr. Max Kleiber, Dr. Terence A. Rogers, Dr. Lawrence M. Marshall, and Dr. Augustus C. Jennings. However, we assume full responsibility for any errors that may appear in the text.

We are greatly indebted to Dr. Harald Schraer for the preparation of the majority of electron micrographs that appear in the text.

Thanks are due to Dr. Janet M. Wardlaw and to Mrs. Helen A. Guthrie for testing our approach in the teaching of courses in advanced nutrition; and to our own students who were, in fact, most helpful in the development of this manuscript.

We also wish to thank Mrs. Lois Smith and Mrs. Elizabeth Isenberg for their help in the preparation of the manuscript; and Mrs. Carol Winkler for her help in reading proof.

Ruth L. Pike
University Park, Pennsylvania

Myrtle L. Brown
Honolulu, Hawaii

January, 1967

contributors

John G. Bieri, Ph.D.
Scientist Emeritus
National Institutes of Health
Bethesda, Maryland

Elsworth R. Buskirk, Ph.D.
Laboratory for Human Performance
  Research
The Pennsylvania State University
University Park, Pennsylvania

Margot P. Cleary, Ph.D.
The Hormel Institute
University of Minnesota
Austin, Minnesota

Gary J. Fosmire, Ph.D.
Department of Nutrition
The Pennsylvania State University
University Park, Pennsylvania

Carol V. Gay, Ph.D.
Molecular and Cell Biology Program
The Pennsylvania State University
University Park, Pennsylvania

June L. Kelsay, Ph.D.
Carbohydrate Nutrition Laboratory
Agricultural Research Service
U.S. Department of Agriculture
Beltsville, Maryland

Frank W. Lowenstein, M.D. D.P.H.
Nutrition Consultant
U.S. Public Health Service (retired)
Washington, D.C.

Mary W. Marshall, M.S.
Lipid Nutrition Laboratory
Agricultural Research Service
U.S. Department of Agriculture
Beltsville, Maryland

Peter L. Pellett, Ph.D.
Department of Food Science and Nutrition
University of Massachusetts
Amherst, Massachusetts

Harald Schraer, Ph.D.
Molecular and Cell Biology Program
The Pennsylvania State University
University Park, Pennsylvania

John Edgar Smith, Ph.D.
Department of Nutrition
The Pennsylvania State University
University Park, Pennsylvania

Noel W. Solomons, M.D.
Department of Nutrition and Food Science
Massachusetts Institute of Technology
Cambridge, Massachusetts
Institute of Nutrition of Central
  America and Panama
Guatemala City

contents

part one

the nutrients

Much of the material in Chapters 2 through 5 should be familiar to the student, but since it is fundamental to the integrated study that follows and since memories sometimes falter, it is included either for surreptitious reading or careful study, whatever the need may be.

Nutrition is the science that interprets the relationship of food to the functioning of the living organism. It includes the intake of food, liberation of energy, elimination of wastes, and all the syntheses that are essential for maintenance, growth, and reproduction. These fundamental activities are characteristic of all living organisms from the simplest to the most complex plants and animals.

Nutrition is a relatively new science that evolved from chemistry and physiology just as biophysics has more recently evolved from biology and physics. Recognition of nutrition as an independent field of study came only after the beginning of this century following a developmental period that stemmed from the experiments of Antoine Lavoisier almost 200 years earlier. Lavoisier's work formed the basis for the studies on respiratory exchange and calorimetry, the beginnings of scientific nutrition. Almost 100 years elapsed before carbohydrates, fats, and proteins were identified as the sources of energy for the animal body. By the end of the nineteenth century the significance of protein as a source of nitrogen and the necessity for certain minerals in the diet were established. During the early part of this century conclusive evidence was obtained indicating that proteins varied in their ability to support growth and maintenance. Furthermore it was established that purified diets containing only the major foodstuffs (including suitable protein sources) and minerals were inadequate to maintain life. It was therefore obvious that foods carried other substances yet to be identified.

Investigations with laboratory animals led to the crude separation of fat-soluble and water-soluble fractions from foods that contained the essential factors, but it was not until the 1930s that the majority of the vitamins were identified, isolated from foods, and synthesized in the laboratory. The development of methods for synthesizing the vitamins was a crucial step in the future of nutritional research. It then became possible to develop a completely synthetic diet that could support the life of laboratory animals, and research could be directed toward elucidating the functional roles of individual nutrients.

However crude the early work appears from the vantage point of current methodology and instrumentation, much of it was sophisticated, elegant in design, and carefully executed; this work provided the basic information that is the core of the science of nutrition.

chapter 1

historical perspective

"What little we know, what little power we possess, we owe to the accumulated endeavors of our ancestors. Mere gratefulness would already oblige us to study the history of the endeavors, our most precious heirlooms. But we are not to remain idle spectators. It is not enough to appreciate and admire what our ancestors did, we must take up their best traditions, and that implies expert knowledge and craftsmanship, science and practice."

George Sarton, The History of Science and the New Humanism, 1956

Ancient and Medieval Ideas

Before the eighteenth century little of a truly scientific nature was accomplished in the development of nutrition or, in fact, of any science. The ancient Greek philosophers apparently were interested in science, but logical reasoning, rather than experimentation, was the Greek way.

Hippocrates (460–364 B.C.) wrote the following passage that is accurate in essence although somewhat imprecise in detail.

Growing bodies have the most innate heat; they therefore require the most food, for otherwise their bodies are wasted. In old persons, the heat is feeble and therefore they require little fuel as it were to the flame, for it would be extinguished by much . . .

For nearly 1500 years after Hippocrates' time, little was accomplished in the development of science. The alchemists of the Middle Ages were devoted to the task of transforming common metals into gold, and medical knowledge had advanced little beyond the knowledge possessed by the ancient civilizations. It was not until the sixteenth century that the intellectual climate again became conducive to scientific development; interest revived in the relation of man to his environment and particularly to the air surrounding him. It was in the seventeenth century that van Helmont (1577–1644), a Belgian nobleman, discovered the lethal effect of carbon dioxide. In the same period, Sanctorius (1561–1636) published the results of experiments on himself clearly indicating that a major pathway of excretion from the human body was the "insensible perspiration," a loss of body weight not accountable by measurements of urine and feces and thus presumed to be expelled into the surrounding air. The sketch of Sanctorius sitting in his chair-scale has escaped few students of nutrition.

The Phlogiston Theory of Combustion

A major contribution to scientific thought at the beginning of the eighteenth century, unfortunately, was a misconception, the phlogiston theory of combustion that was promoted by Stahl (1660–1734), a German chemist. Although the theory was accepted by a majority of scientists of the period, it was based apparently on no more than a lively flight of imagination. Stahl maintained that all combustible materials contained phlogiston, which passed from them into the atmosphere when the substances were burned. The phlogiston theory, along with the generally held misconception that air was an elemental substance, profoundly influenced scientific thinking and interpretation of new discoveries for almost a century. Consequently, Black (1728–1799) termed carbon dioxide "fixed air"; Cavendish (1731–1810) called hydrogen "inflammable air" and believed it to be phlogiston. Rutherford's (1749–1810) "residual air" was what we now know as nitrogen. Two independent discoverers of oxygen, Priestley (1733–1804) and Scheele (1742–1786), used the terms "dephlogisticated air" and "fire air."

It was in a scientific climate dominated by misconception that Lavoisier began his experiments on combustion that led to studies on animal respiration and paved the way for the development of modern calorimetry.

Studies of Respiration: Development of Calorimetry

The truly great scientist not only observes phenomena (which anyone can do) but has the genius to interpret his findings and the strength to bear the consequences of possible failure. As Szent-Györgyi (1957) stated:

There is but one safe way to avoid mistakes; to do nothing, or, at least, to avoid doing something new . . . The unknown lends an insecure foothold and venturing out into it, one can hope for no more than that the possible failure will be a honorable one.

Antoine Lavoisier (1743–1794) was one of the first to repudiate Stahl's theory of phlogiston.[1] By repeating experiments previously performed by some of his contemporaries of the late eighteenth century, for example, heating mercury oxide with carbon, Lavoisier concluded that "fixed air" (carbon dioxide) was formed by the combination of carbon and "air eminently respirable" (oxygen). In his *Reflections upon Phlogiston* he stated, "All the phenomena of combustion and calcination are much more readily explained without phlogiston than with phlogiston." (See Lusk, 1928.)

Thus without the impediment of the phlogiston theory, Lavoisier went on to apply his theory of combustion to the problem of the origin of animal heat. Experimenting with guinea pigs and later with his assistant, Seguin, as subjects, Lavoisier measured body heat loss, oxygen consumed, and carbon dioxide expired and concluded that respiration is a combustion process similar to what happens when substances are burned outside the body. Furthermore, he was able to show that heat production in the animal body is directly related to oxygen consumption.

Respiration is only a slow combustion of carbon and hydrogen which is entirely similar to that which obtains in a lamp or lighted candle and from this point of view, animals which respire are truly combustible bodies which burn and consume themselves. In respiration as in combustion it is the air which furnishes the heat—if animals do not repair constantly the losses of respiration, the lamp soon lacks oil, and the animal dies, as a lamp goes out when it lacks food. (See Lusk, 1928.)

Measurements taken in the fasting and resting state, as initially performed by Lavoisier, represent essentially the basal metabolism. In another series of experiments in which Seguin was the subject, Lavoisier showed that oxygen consumption and therefore heat production was increased above the basal state by a decrease in environmental temperature, ingestion of food, and by physical exercise. The following table indicates the relative increases in oxygen consumption under the conditions of his experiment.

There were some technical inaccuracies in Lavoisier's work and in his interpretation of the data. His figures for oxygen consumption were too high, and he erroneously believed that carbon dioxide and water were formed in the lungs. However, in spite of these errors, refinements in instrumentation and in scientific thought have added little to the general concepts derived from his experiments. The increase in oxygen consumption following ingestion of food was later described by Rubner (1854–1932) as the *specific dynamic effect* of food (Rubner, 1902). The effects of temperature and exercise on oxygen consumption and body

---

[1]As the result of a long series of experiments, Lavoisier established the law of the conservation of mass, a concept later refined by Einstein. For this reason Lavoisier is known as the father of modern chemistry as well as the father of nutrition.

Condition	Environmental Temperature	Liters Oxygen Absorbed per Hour
Without food	26	24
Without food	12	27
With food		38
Work (9.195 foot pounds—without food)		65
Work (9.195 foot pounds—with food)		91

Source: From G. Lusk, *The Elements of the Science of Nutrition*, 4th ed., W. B. Saunders Co., Philadelphia, 1928, p. 19.

heat production have been confirmed repeatedly and are basic tenets of modern calorimetry.

Lavoisier, however, did not recognize the nature of the foodstuffs and believed that elemental carbon and hydrogen were oxidized in the body. François Magendie (1783–1855), an early nineteenth century physiologist, was the first to distinguish between the different kinds of foodstuffs (carbohydrate, fat, and protein). Even so, this information was not applied to studies of respiratory exchange for many years. Regnault (1810–1878), however, showed that the ratio of carbon dioxide to oxygen consumed varied with kind of food (Regnault and Reiset, 1849). This ratio is now called the *respiratory quotient* (RQ).

Later Calorimetric Studies

Liebig (1803–1873), of the nineteenth century German school, apparently recognized that proteins, carbohydrates, and fats were oxidized in the body, and he then calculated energy values for some foodstuffs. He proposed that since only proteins contain nitrogen, the nitrogen of the urine must arise from protein in the body (Liebig, 1842). He erroneously believed that muscular work caused the metabolism of protein and that oxygen caused the destruction of carbohydrate and fat.

The first report of a balance-type experiment is credited to Boussingault (1802–1887), a Frenchman and contemporary of Liebig. He measured carbon, hydrogen, oxygen, nitrogen, and salts of a cow's food and excreta. During the same period in Germany, Bidder (1810–1894) and Schmidt (1822–1894) performed a similar experiment but also related their balance data to the animal's respiratory exchange, a closer approximation to modern calorimetric method (Bidder and Schmidt, 1852). In their writings, they described a *typical minimum* of necessary metabolism which is apparent in experiments when no food is given. This typical minimum is now referred to as the *resting metabolism.*

Voit (1831–1908) was a particularly gifted student of Liebig and was distinguished not only by his own work but also by that of his students: Rubner (1854–1932), Atwater (1844–1907), Lusk (1866–1932), and many others. In the late nineteenth century the laboratory at Munich was the center for calorimetric studies; researchers from many countries went there to learn the most advanced techniques. From a series of calorimetric and balance experiments, Voit was able to disprove two theories proposed by his former professor, Liebig. He demonstrated first that protein metabolism is *not* affected by muscular work and second that oxygen consumption is not the cause of metabolism but, instead, that oxygen consumption is the result of cellular metabolism (Voit, 1881). Voit said, in what appears to be advanced thinking for his day:

> The life of the body is the sum of the action of all the thousands of minute workshops. A combination with oxygen is not first necessary, but there is a breaking up into various constituents which, under certain circumstances may remain unoxidized . . . What the eye of the layman regards as rest is in reality an interminable movement to and from of the finest cellular particles, the most complicated of all processes.

Obviously Voit suspected that even the apparently inert constituents of body tissues existed in a dynamic state (proved many years later by Schoenheimer, 1942) and, furthermore, that the balance experiments that scientists then performed were but a first step in unraveling the mysteries of cellular metabolism.

Rubner was one of Voit's most outstanding students. While still an assistant in Voit's laboratory, he determined caloric values of urine and feces under varying conditions of dietary intake; these figures formed the basis for later calorimetric work. Rubner proved conclusively that for the resting animal, heat production is equivalent to heat elimination, thus confirming that the law of conservation of energy [proposed in 1845 by Mayer (1814–1878) and in 1847 by Helmholz (1821–1894) and implied in Lavoisier's experiments] was applicable to the living organism as well as to inanimate matter. Furthermore, Rubner related heat production in the basal state to surface area, which also had been implied by experiments conducted previously by Regnault in France. The caloric values for different kinds of foodstuffs were determined by Rubner, and average values were calculated for carbohydrates, proteins, and fats. Rubner's computed caloric values are very nearly the same as those now used in dietary calculations.

Studies on the Physiology of Digestion

At the same time that chemists were delving into the composition of foods and the mysteries of metabolism, physiologists were attempting to elucidate the mechanisms involved in digestion, the means by which food becomes available to the body for oxidation.

Some of the first experimental work on the digestive process was done by Reaumur in 1752. When he administered perforated metallic tubes containing food to birds that normally regurgitate indigestible residues remaining at the completion of digestion, he found that the regurgitated tubes were empty. This was obvious proof that something had occurred in the stomach other than grinding or crushing. A fascinating review of his and other early experiments is presented by Rose (1959) in an essay introducing a facsimile reprint of a dissertation presented to the University of Pennsylvania by John R. Young (1782–1804) entitled *An Experimental Inquiry into the Principles of Nutrition and the Digestive Process, 1803* (Young, 1959).

In the following century and a half, the physiological and biochemical aspects of the digestive process were studied and fairly well clarified through the work of many investigators and the dedication of several subjects with fistulas. First came the published work of Beaumont (1785–1853) in 1833 reporting observations on his patient, Alexis St. Martin, who had the misfortune of receiving a gunshot wound that, after healing, left him with an opening, or fistula, directly into the stomach. Beaumont not only treated but immortalized his patient by using him as the subject for a series of studies on digestive processes. By introducing specific foods into the stomach through the fistula (always with a string attached), Beaumont was able to ascertain the relative rates of digestion for different kinds of foodstuffs. He also described gastric juice and identified the acid as hydrochloric. He noted the movements of the stomach and was probably the first to report the effects of the emotions on gastric motility and secretion. This work suggested to Claude Bernard (1813–1878) the use of artificial fistulas in laboratory animals for the study of gastrointestinal function.

At the beginning of this century, W. B. Cannon (1871–1945) at Harvard University did much definitive work on motility and secretion of the gastrointestinal tract and trained a generation of physiologists. Through happenstance, other investigators and subjects with fistulas teamed together: Fred, at the University of Chicago, served as laboratory worker and experimental subject for Carlson (1875–1956), Luckhardt (1885–1957), and their associates who did much to advance the work started by Cannon; and Tom, at Cornell University Medical School, who had a long association with Wolf and Wolff as helper and subject in the laboratory and was the true subject of their now-classic volume, *Human Gastric Function: An Experimental Study of a Man and His Stomach* (1943) and its sequel, *The Stomach* (Wolf, 1965).

Nutrition in Early Twentieth-Century America

Up until the late nineteenth century most of the outstanding laboratories for physiological research were in the great European universities. Americans who wished to work with the leaders in these areas were obliged to go to the centers abroad to further their studies. Atwater (1844–1907) was among the first to make an outstanding contribution to the development of nutritional science in this country. After spending a year in Voit's laboratory he returned in 1888 to become chief of the newly organized Office of Experiment Stations of the U.S. Department of Agriculture. With the physicist, Rosa, he was responsible for the construction of the first calorimeter, which could be used for studying the energy exchange of man. Atwater and Bryant (1899), also of the Department of Agriculture, published a compilation of the composition of a large number of foods and forerunner of the classic tables of food composition known as *Handbook 8* (Watt and Merrill, 1963). These tables are currently under extensive revision.

Lusk, who also studied with Voit and Rubner at Munich, upon returning to this country began work on intermediary metabolism and on the specific dynamic effect of foods. He built a small calorimeter at the Cornell Medical College for use with small animals and babies and was instrumental in promoting the construction of a calorimeter at Bellevue Hospital in New York. Lusk's book, *The Science of Nutrition*, which went through four editions between 1906 and 1928, is a classic work and should be familiar to every serious student of nutrition.

A second large calorimeter was built in this country by Armsby (1853–1921) at The Pennsylvania State University. It was originally used for the study of energy exchange of large farm animals. Later this calorimeter was used for studies with human subjects (Swift et al., 1957). The calorimeter still remains in perfect working condition, and the building housing it has become the Armsby Museum (Fig. 1.1).

At the beginning of the twentieth century considerable work had been done on energy exchange and on the nature of the major foodstuffs. The proximate composition (carbohydrate, fat, protein, fiber, water, and ash) and the energy

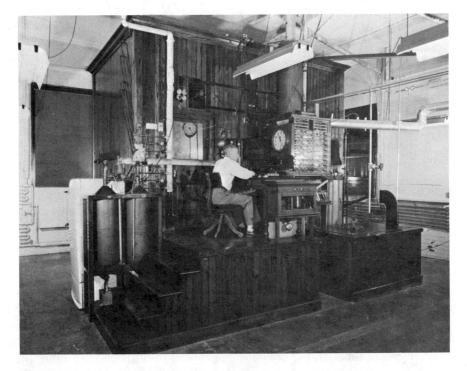

Figure 1.1
The Armsby respiration calorimeter at The Pennsylvania State University. Seated at the controls is Raymond W. Swift (1895–1975).

value of a large number of foods was known. Nutritional science was coming of age, however, as evidenced by the *Laws of Nutrition*, summarized by C. F. Langworthy (1864–1932), an associate of Atwater in the U.S. Department of Agriculture (Langworthy, 1897–1898).

LAWS OF NUTRITION

1. All nitrogen is supplied by food, that is, none from atmosphere.
2. All nitrogen is excreted in urine and feces, none as gaseous nitrogen.
3. The animal adjusts itself to its nitrogen intake and comes into N-balance, in which state the intake and output are equal.
4. A certain amount of food material, that is, protein, fat, and carbohydrate, is required for maintenance. Mineral is also essential, but very little is known regarding the kind and amount necessary.
5. A more abundant ration is required for muscular work, fattening, and milk production.
6. Food supplied in excess of all needs is stored, in part at least, as reserve material, principally as fat and glycogen.
7. The body comes into nitrogen equilibrium at different levels of protein intake.
8. Body fat may be formed from food fat (precipitated as such), or from carbohydrate, and doubtless from protein also.
9. As furnishers of energy the different nutrients may replace each other in approximately the following ratios: protein:fat:carbohydrates as 1:2.5:1. That is, having the requisite amount of nitrogen for repair or some vital process not understood, or both, it is theoretically and within certain limits, unimportant which nutrient supplies the necessary energy.
10. The nutrients of the food combine within the body with oxygen of the air and undergo combustion, thus liberating energy for the body.

No argument can be raised against Langworthy's laws. Fundamentally, they are as valid today as when he stated them. The vitamins remained to be discovered and it was within the next ten years that these essential food factors also were recognized.

Recognition of Mineral Requirements

Knowledge of mineral needs grew as data accumulated on the composition of body tissues and fluids. The mineral structure of bone and teeth was recognized by early workers although the element calcium was not discovered until 1808. In the latter part of the nineteenth century, however, the necessity for small amounts of calcium for blood coagulation had been demonstrated by the addition of calcium precipitants, such as oxalate and citrate, to blood.

The iron content of blood and various tissues was known well before the beginning of this century. Boussingault (1802–1887), for example, published data on the iron content of animals and believed iron to be an essential nutrient. Liebig suggested that oxygen was carried in blood by iron in the corpuscles. From Grecian times iron compounds had been used therapeutically, but the significance of the element in the treatment of anemia was not discovered until about 1840. Even with this knowledge available, however, the necessity of iron as a dietary constituent appears generally to have been ignored.

Liebig was aware of the differences in the distribution of sodium and potassium in the animal, and Boussingault had observed the deleterious effects of salt-free diets on animals. It was the observation that dogs deprived of sodium chloride died earlier than animals given no food, however, that led to the conclusion that certain mineral constituents of animal tissues are essential to life and consequently must be necessary in the diet (Forster, 1873).

The significance of electrolyte concentrations in body fluids received most attention from the work of Ringer (1835–1910). Ringer (1895) found that solutions containing a combination of the chlorides of sodium, potassium, and calcium were satisfactory in maintaining the functional integrity of isolated animal tissues. Individually any one of these compounds was detrimental to isolated muscle activity, but the antagonistic effect could be removed by addition of the other salts (Locke, 1895). Early in this century Loeb (1859–1924) continued the work on salt antagonism and observed the effect of various concentrations of salts on living tissues. No combination tested was more favorable than the equivalent of the concentrations found in blood. Thus it was firmly established that the presence of certain salts in living tissues was not the result of incidental contamination, but that mineral elements were, indeed, nutrients essential to animal functioning and therefore they must be supplied in the diet.

The general belief at the beginning of the twentieth century was that sodium chloride, calcium, phosphorus, and probably iron were the minerals significant in animal nutrition. Little attention was given to other elements known to be present in tissues in relatively small amounts. The importance of the trace elements in animal nutrition was accepted more readily following the discovery of other essential micronutrients: the vitamins.

Development of the Vitamin Theory

Recognition of the existence of organic compounds present in minute amounts in foods came less than 15 years after the beginning of this century. Dietary deficiency diseases, however, had been known for many years. Lind's (1716–1794) famous *Treatise on Scurvy* (Lind, 1753) was published just ten years after the birth of Lavoisier. A syndrome described as beriberi, which could be prevented by dietary means, was reported to occur among Japanese sailors (Takaki, 1887). Three years later in the Dutch East Indies Eijkman (1858–1930) produced beriberi in birds (see Williams, 1961). Holst (1860–1931), working in Sweden, produced scurvy in guinea pigs and was able to cure the disease by feeding fresh fruits and cabbage (Holst and Frölich, 1907). Except for the realization that the diseases were of dietary origin, however, none of these investigators was aware that specific nutrients were involved in their etiology.

Near the end of the nineteenth century chemical methodology had progressed considerably so that relatively purified foodstuffs could be isolated from foods. Purified foodstuffs provided the tool needed for studying the physiological effects of various combinations of the nutrients then believed to be essential and thus for determining the function of individual foodstuffs in biological systems. Animal feeding experiments, however, produced unexpected results.

One of the first recorded studies was that of Lunin (1853–1937), who found that mice fed a purified diet simulating milk died within one month, but others fed fluid milk survived and were healthy for twice as long (Lunin, 1880). Purified diets supplemented with small doses of whey were found to be as effective as milk in experiments conducted by Pekelharing (1848–1922). He concluded that the active substance was not one of the major foodstuffs and, moreover, stated,

> If this substance is absent, the organism loses its power properly to assimilate the well-known principal parts of food, the appetite is lost and with apparent abundance the animals die of want. (See van Leersum, 1926.)

Frederick G. Hopkins (1861–1947) in England performed similar experiments with purified diets and independently reached a similar conclusion. However, Hopkins also clearly recognized the relationship between the *accessory food factors* (vitamins) and the dietary deficiency syndromes that had been observed for centuries (Hopkins, 1912). The theory that certain disease syndromes were the result of a dietary lack of specific substances present in foods was proposed also by Casimir Funk (1884–1967) in his classical paper, *The Etiology of the Deficiency Diseases* (Funk, 1912), which reviews much of the early history of beriberi and scurvy. Funk's outstanding contribution was to propose a name for the unknown accessory food factors. He chose *vitamines,* inspired by the knowledge that the factors were essential for life (vita) and that the antiberiberi factor that he was attempting to isolate was an amine. Vitamine thus was a misnomer and was modified to *vitamin* at the suggestion of Sir Jack Drummond (1891–1952) who proposed at the same time the alphabetical nomenclature for the vitamins (Drummond, 1920). Acceptance of the vitamin theory was not immediate in all circles of thought (new ideas rarely are!), but with the discovery of vitamin A by McCollum (1879–1967), the vitamin era in nutrition investigations was securely launched (cCollum and Davis, 1913).

Details of the discovery, isolation, and synthesis of each of the vitamins are too voluminous to record at this point and will be discussed in the chapters on the vitamins. The furor created by the discovery of the minute factors in food reached a peak between 1930 and 1940. The literature of this period is crowded with new discoveries, wrong turns, and rediscoveries. In the excitement attending the discovery of the vitamins, many nutritionists tended toward overenthusiasm rather than the restraint more typical of new ideas. This overenthusiasm probably helped to encourage the development of the multimillion dollar vitamin business now supported by our population; the money spent on vitamins could best be spent at the local food market.

Significance of Protein Source: Identification of the Essential Amino Acids

At about the same time that the existence of minute quantities of accessory food factors was emerging, evidence also began to accumulate suggesting that dietary proteins varied widely in their ability to support growth and life in laboratory animals. The essential nature of protein as a source of nitrogen had been suggested by the work of Magendie (1816) and later was confirmed by Mulder (1802–1880), who coined the term protein from the Greek word *proteus*, which roughly may be translated as "first." It was clearly recognized then that protein was necessary for life in a more fundamental way than could be attributed to either carbohydrate or fat. Liebig also recognized the nitrogen-containing components of food as necessary for tissue building and suggested that urinary nitrogen could serve as a measure of protein destruction in the body (Liebig, 1842). Later, Voit established the principle of nitrogen equilibrium (Bischoff and Voit, 1860). This method remains the most widely used criterion for evaluating protein metabolism and requirements.

By 1900, 16 different amino acids had been isolated from hydrolysates of various biological materials (see McCollum, 1957), but the nature of protein composition was poorly understood. Mulder (1839; 1848) had proposed that only one protein was present in any one food although the proteins differed among different foods; this view was accepted by Liebig. It was not until the beginning of this century that T. B. Osborne (1859–1929) in work begun in the 1890s with R. H. Chittenden (1856–1943) at Yale was able to demonstrate conclusively that foods (and thus other biological materials) contained not one, but a mixture of several different proteins. (See Osborne, 1924.) The availability of the isolated proteins enabled Osborne in the classic animal feeding experiments performed with L. B. Mendel (1872–1935), also at Yale, to demonstrate differences in the capability of individual proteins to promote growth and to maintain life (Osborne and Mendel, 1911). This work, along with the studies of Hopkins on the essential nature of tryptophan, provided the framework for the basic understanding of proteins and amino acids in nutrition (Willcock and Hopkins, 1906–1907). This work was carried further by W. C. Rose (1887–), a former student of Mendel at Yale, and culminated in the identification and isolation of the final essential amino acid, threonine. For the first time it was demonstrated by Rose and his associates at the University of Illinois that rats could be reared to maximum growth on mixtures of purified amino acids (McCoy et al., 1935–1936). The isolation of the essential amino acids made possible the later studies on amino acid requirements of experimental animals and humans and provided the fundamental information necessary for exploring the intermediary metabolism of proteins.

Conclusion

This chapter was intended to reveal the general development of nutrition as a field of scientific study. Much of significance has, of necessity, been omitted as, for example, the discovery of the essential fatty acids (Burr and Burr, 1929). These and other historical developments will be discussed in later chapters, but much still remains for the interested student to search out individually.

chapter 2

carbohydrates, lipids, proteins, nucleotides, and nucleic acids

"I, too, dislike it: there are things that are important beyond all
  this fiddle.
Reading it however with a perfect contempt for it, one discovers in
it after all, a place for the genuine.
  Hands that can grasp, eyes
  that can dilate, hair that can rise
    if it must, these things are important not because a
high-sounding interpretation can be put upon them but because
  they are
  useful . . ."

Marianne Moore, Poetry

Carbohydrates

Carbohydrates are defined as polyhydroxy aldehydes and ketones and their derivatives and vary from simple three-carbon sugars to complex polymers. Most carbohydrates conform to the general formula $(CH_2O)_n$, but the classification of carbohydrates includes compounds that are not true hydrates as the name implies. For example, deoxyribose contains 5 carbon atoms, 10 hydrogens, but only 4 oxygens rather than 5 as is customary for a pentose. Moreover, some compounds that are properly classified as carbohydrates in terms of chemical properties contain nitrogen or sulfur in addition to carbon, hydrogen, and oxygen.

Carbohydrates are classified into three main groups: monosaccharides, or simple sugars; oligosaccharides, of which the most prevalent in nature are the disaccharides; and polysaccharides, the most complex of the carbohydrates. Many of the compounds to be discussed in this chapter are of biological importance. Only three, however, are significant as dietary sources of carbohydrate. Starch is by far the most important source of carbohydrate in the human diet amounting to approximately 50 percent of total carbohydrate in the American diet, but often as much as 75 percent of total carbohydrate in the diets in some of the developing countries. Sucrose ranks next in importance comprising about 25 percent of total carbohydrate intake. In the last 70 years the intake of complex carbohydrate in the diet of Americans has decreased, and the intake of sucrose has markedly increased (Friend, 1967). Lactose or milk sugar comprises approximately 10 percent of the total carbohydrate intake in the United States but, of course, is of little significance in nonmilk-drinking populations. For a comprehensive listing of the carbohydrates present in a large variety of foods see Hardinge et al. (1965).

Biologically the carbohydrates are a significant source of energy for cellular metabolism, but they also serve functional and structural roles in the animal body.

MONOSACCHARIDES

Monosaccharides are, as the name implies, the simplest of the carbohydrates. This classification includes a series of aldehydes (aldoses) and ketones (ketoses) grouped according to the number of carbon atoms in the chain: trioses, tetroses, pentoses, hexoses, and heptoses (Table 2.1). These sugars may be more definitively described according to structure and number of carbon atoms as aldotrioses, ketotrioses, and so on.

With the possible exception of the hexoses, monosaccharides are of little dietary significance. Both glucose and fructose have long been known to occur in free form in certain fruits and in honey. Small amounts of mannose have also been detected in a few fruits. (See Herman, 1971.) However, it appears at present that only the pentoses and hexoses play fundamental roles in cellular metabolism although trioses, tetroses, and sedoheptulose are important intermediates in the metabolism of carbohydrate in animal cells. Indeed, the simple triose, glyceraldehyde, is potentially the building block of all cell carbohydrates as will be seen in the later discussion of carbohydrate metabolism (Chapter 13).

TABLE 2.1
Monosaccharides

Classification	Aldoses	Ketoses
Trioses ($C_3H_6O_3$)	Glyceraldehyde	Dihydroxyacetone
Tetroses ($C_4H_8O_4$)	Erythrose	Erythrulose
	Threose	
Pentoses ($C_5H_{10}O_5$)	Xylose	Xylulose
	Ribose	Ribulose
	Arabinose	
Hexoses ($C_6H_{12}O_6$)	Glucose (dextrose)	Fructose (levulose)
	Galactose	Sorbose
	Mannose	
Heptoses ($C_7H_{14}O_7$)		Sedoheptulose

Pentoses

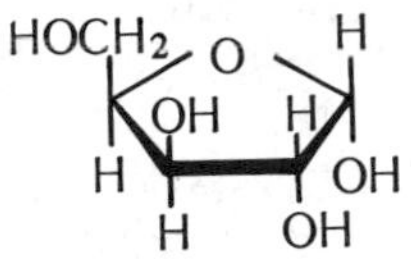

D-Xylose

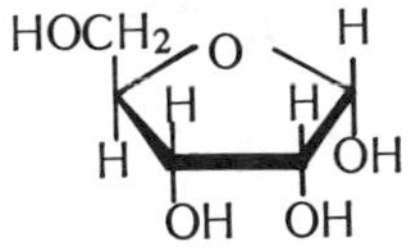

D-Ribose

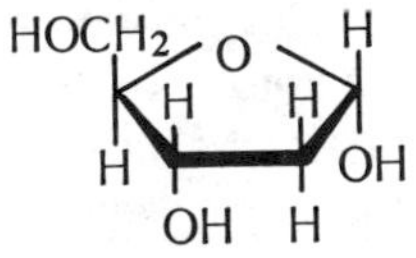

2-Deoxy-D-ribose

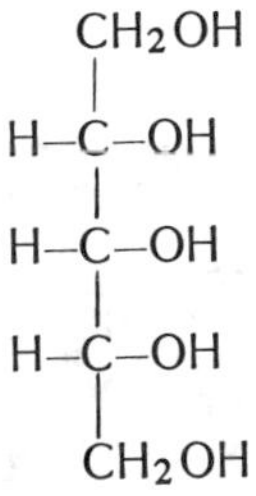

Ribitol

Pentose sugars are readily synthesized in the cell. Ribose is the most important of the pentoses in biological systems and can be converted to deoxyribose and ribitol, neither of which can be classified strictly as a carbohydrate. Deoxyribose has two hydrogen atoms attached to carbon atom 2, instead of one hydrogen atom and one hydroxyl group. Both ribose and deoxyribose are constituents of a nucleic acid that bears their name: ribonucleic acid (RNA) and deoxyribonucleic acid (DNA). Ribose also is a constituent of many other nucleotides including the adenosine phosphates (ATP, ADP, AMP) and the nicotinamide adenine dinucleotides (NAD, NADP). Deoxyribose is encountered less frequently as a nucleotide constituent.

Ribitol, a reduction product of ribose, is a component of the vitamin, riboflavin, and therefore, like ribose and deoxyribose, performs a functional role in cell metabolism.

Hexoses

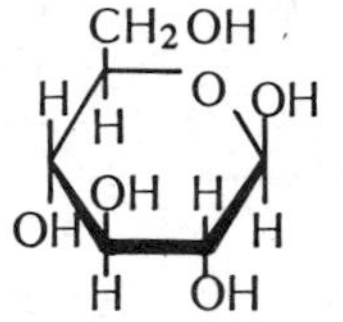

CH_2OH

β-D-Glucose

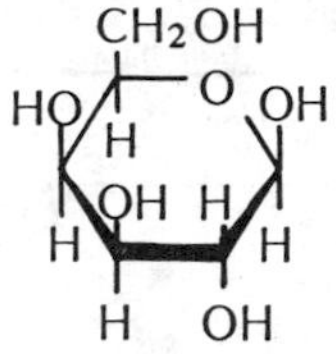

CH_2OH

β-D-Galactose

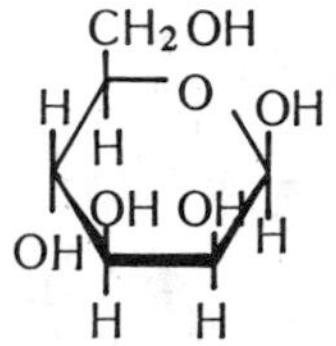

CH_2OH

β-D-Mannose

CH_2OH

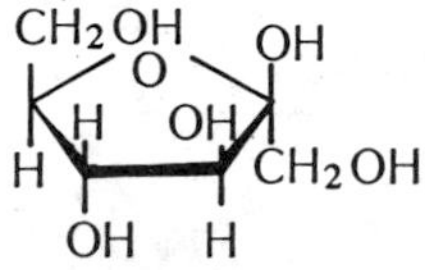

β-D-Fructose

The principal hexoses are glucose, galactose, mannose, and fructose. The first three are aldohexoses; fructose is a ketohexose. Glucose is the central compound in the catabolism and synthesis of carbohydrates and is the form in which carbohydrate is supplied to the cell from body fluids. Glucose concentration in the blood is closely regulated. (See Chapter 15.) The sugar is a metabolic substrate for all cells, but cells of nerve tissue and lens of the eye are normally entirely dependent on glucose as a source of energy. However in starvation or other conditions of excessive lipolysis, brain tissue switches to ketone bodies as the primary source of energy. (See Chapter 15.) Fructose and galactose are converted to the storage carbohydrate, glycogen, in the liver and thus may give rise to glucose and contribute to the cell energy supply.

The hexoses and their derivatives also are constituents of a large number of complex substances that are synthesized by the cell as structural components and secretions. These substances generally consist of combinations with proteins or lipids and hence are known as glycoproteins, mucopolysaccharides, or glycolipids. Mannose, for example, is of little significance as a direct energy source for the cell, but it is an important constituent of both glycoproteins and glycolipids. Two six-carbon deoxy sugars, L-rhamnose (6-deoxy-L-mannose) and L-fucose (6-deoxy-L-galactose) also are components of the glycoproteins of cell membranes.

MONOSACCHARIDE DERIVATIVES

Like all monosaccharides, the metabolically active forms of the hexoses are the phosphorylated derivatives. For example, it is glucose-6-phosphate, shown below, and not the free sugar that holds the central position in the metabolism of carbohydrate. All of the phosphorylated sugars involved in carbohydrate degra-

TABLE 2.2
Monosaccharide Derivatives

Derivative	Characteristic Grouping	Structure
Amino sugars	Hydroxyl group is replaced by an amino group.	β-D-Glucosamine
Acetyl amino sugars	Acetyl group is attached to the nitrogen of an amino sugar.	N-Acetyl-β-D-glucosamine
Uronic acids	Primary alcohol group is oxidized to a carboxyl group.	β-D-Glucuronic acid
Glyconic acids	Aldehyde group is oxidized to a carboxyl group.	D-Gluconic acid (glyconic acid)
Sugar alcohols	Aldehyde or ketone group is reduced to an alcohol group.	D-Glucitol (sorbitol)

dation and synthesis exist as fleeting intermediaries and thus are active metabolites that do not accumulate within the cell to any great extent. Indeed, the bulk of carbohydrates within the cell exists in the form of the complex polysaccharides.

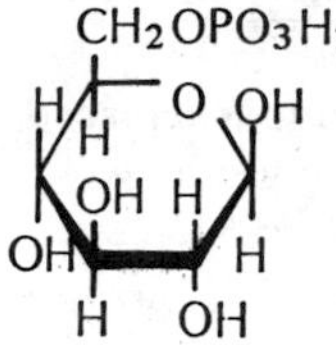

β-D-Glucose-6-phosphate

Certain of the other commonly occurring sugar derivatives are shown in Table 2.2; for simplicity, derivatives of glucose are used to illustrate structural characteristics. Of these compounds, the amino and acetyl amino sugars are significant components of the complex structural carbohydrates.

OLIGOSACCHARIDES

Of the oligosaccharides the most common are the disaccharides: sucrose, lactose, and maltose. The general class of oligosaccharides, however, includes sugars containing any number from 2 to as many as 10 monosaccharide units joined together through the hydroxyl groups of each sugar with the loss of one molecule

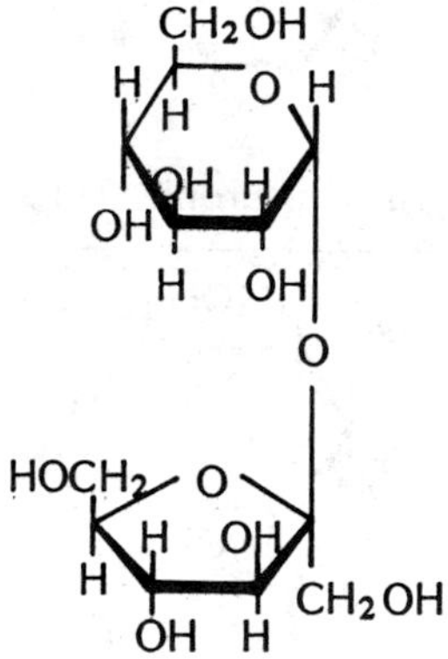

Sucrose

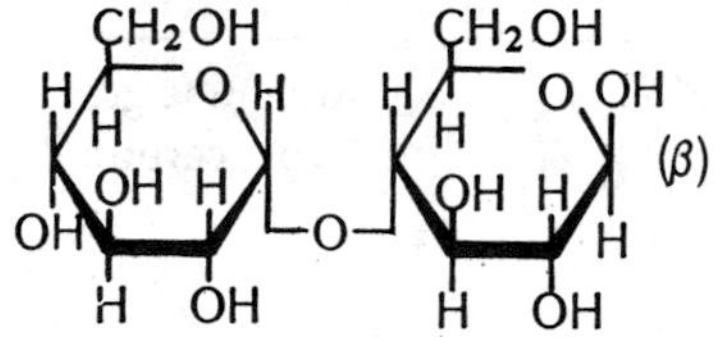

Maltose

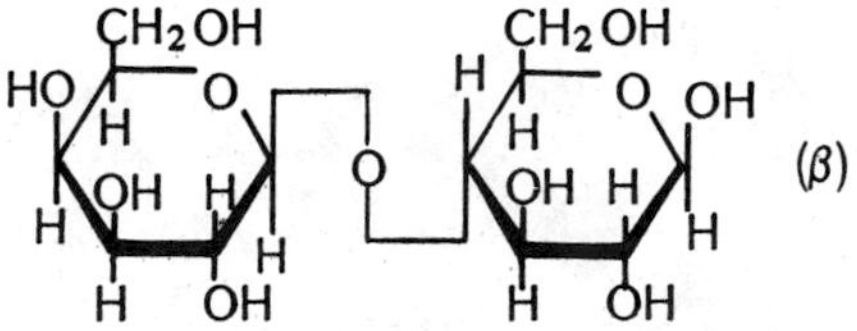

Lactose

of water. This type of bonding, or glycosidic linkage, is common to the disaccharides and other more complex carbohydrates. Most generally, it is the 1,4- or 1,6-linkage, the hydroxyl group on C-1 of the molecule in a glycosidic bond to the hydroxyl on C-4 or C-6 of another monosaccharide unit.

Sucrose, the most widely distributed of the disaccharides, on hydrolysis yields glucose and fructose. Lactose is found only in milk and is composed of glucose and galactose. Maltose contains two molecules of glucose and is formed by the partial hydrolysis of starch. It is found in beer and in high-maltose corn syrups that are often used in industrially prepared foods (Strickler, 1982).

The disaccharides are unimportant in the metabolism of the animal cell and contribute to body function solely through their products of digestion, the monosaccharides. Sucrose, if injected into the blood stream of an animal, for example, cannot be metabolized and is rapidly excreted intact. Synthesis of lactose is a highly specialized function both in terms of site (cells of the mammary glands) and period of the life cycle (lactation).

POLYSACCHARIDES

Polysaccharides are complex polymers containing only one monosaccharide, *homopolysaccharides*, or several different monosaccharides or monosaccharide derivatives, *heteropolysaccharides*. Many polysaccharides exist in the plant and animal kingdoms. However, only a few of these are known to be significant in mammalian nutrition, either as dietary constituents or as animal cell metabolites.

The most common digestible polysaccharide in plants is *starch*, a polymer of glucose. Starch is present primarily in the cells of grains, fruits, and tubers in the form of granules that, under microscopic examination, appear to be typical for each starch. The composition of starches also differs somewhat, but all types contain both *amylose*, a straight chain polymer of glucose, and *amylopectin*, a branched-chain polymer. The average chain contains 20 to 25 glucose units with approximately 5 to 8 glucose molecules between branching points within the chain. On hydrolysis in the intestinal tract, starch yields dextrins and maltose and, eventually, glucose.

Glycogen is the only homopolysaccharide of importance in animal metabolism. Its presence in liver was first detected in 1856 by Claude Bernard, who recognized the relationship between the glycogen of liver and the sugar present in the blood. Subsequently Voit proved that the common monosaccharides give rise to liver glycogen. Although the total quantity of glycogen in the animal body is low, considerably less than one-tenth percent of the total body weight, its role is primarily that of a storage carbohydrate, similar to the role of starch in plant cells. It occurs predominantly in the liver where it is important in the homeostatic mechanism regulating glucose level of the blood. (See Chapter 15.) In skeletal muscle, glycogen serves as a source of energy for muscle contraction. (See Chapter 18.)

Glycogen is a branched-chain polymer of 6,000 to 30,000 glucose units. It is similar to amylopectin in structure but is more highly branched. The average chain length is only 10 to 14 glucose units with 3 to 4 glucose units between branching points. The size of the molecule varies with its source and with the metabolic state of the animal. Muscle glycogen is estimated to have a molecular weight of about 10^6 whereas the liver glycogen molecule is much larger, approximately 5×10^6. Both molecules, however, constantly change in size as glucose molecules are added or removed.

Glycogen is of no importance as a dietary source of carbohydrate. When animals are slaughtered, the small amount of glycogen in the body is quickly degraded and has practically disappeared by the time the meat reaches the consumer's table.

Cellulose is a straight chain polymer of glucose. It is a constituent of the cell walls of plants and gives rigidity to the plant structure much as the skeleton supports the animal body. It is not attacked by digestive enzymes of the human, and although it provides bulk to the diet it does not contribute significantly to the nutrition of body cells. Cellulose tends to be affected little by usual acid hydrolysis and requires the action of strong mineral acids.

Some partially digestible polysaccharides also occur in foods and together comprise roughly 2 percent of the total carbohydrate intake. Inulin, galactogens, mannosans, and pentosans are homopolymers of fructose, galactose, mannose, and pentoses, respectively. Raffinose, a heteropolymer, contains glucose, fructose, and galactose.

Hemicellulose is also present in the plant cell wall and along with lignin gives toughness to the cell wall. It is a mixture of linear and highly branched polysaccharides containing pentoses, hexoses, and uronic acids and is extractable with acids and alkalis. It is more susceptible to bacterial breakdown than is cellulose.

Pectin substances are found in the primary cell wall and intercellular layers of plant cells and serve as intercellular cementing materials. They include protopectin, pectinic acids, pectic acids, and pectin. Pectin is a polyuronic acid polymer which forms a gel. It is water-soluble and is almost completely broken down by colonic bacteria.

Gums are highly branched polymers of uronic acids with neutral sugars. They are exudates that give protection at the site of injury to plants. *Mucilages* are found in the endosperm of seeds, not in cell walls. They hold water and prevent dehydration of the plant. They are generally branched molecules containing a variety of sugars and varying amounts of uronic acids.

Cellulose, hemicellulose, pectic substances, gums, and mucilages belong to a group of polysaccharides which is also classified as "fiber." Fiber is generally defined as those components of plant material that are resistant to digestion by enzymes of the human gastrointestinal tract. These components occur in different combinations and quantities which vary from plant to plant. For more information on fiber components, see Kay and Strasberg (1978).

The physiological effects of the polysaccharides classed as fiber differ considerably due to their varying chemical and physical properties. Because of its high water-holding capacity, hemicellulose appears to be the most effective polysaccharide in increasing stool bulk. Certain of the gel-forming and mucilaginous types of polysaccharides found in fruits, legumes, and vegetables (e.g., pectin and guar gum) have been shown to lower serum cholesterol levels, probably by decreasing fat and cholesterol absorption. In contrast, wheat bran has little or no effect on blood lipids or on lipid absorption (See Vahouny, 1982). Pectin and other gel-forming fibers also tend to reduce glucose and insulin responses to a test meal, a property that is of importance in diabetic diets (Anderson, 1980).

Cellulose, hemicellulose, pectin, and guar gum have been shown to bind minerals *in vitro* (Thompson and Weber, 1979). The effect of fiber on mineral absorption *in vivo*, however, is controversial. In some studies, increased dietary fiber appeared to decrease mineral availability; in others it did not (Kelsay, 1981; 1982). For further information on the physiological effects of the various types of fiber, see Kimura (1977), Kay and Strasburg (1978), Spiller and Kay (1980), Kay (1982), and Kelsay (1982).

MUCOPOLYSACCHARIDES

The mucopolysaccharides (sometimes called acidic glycoaminoglycans) are heteropolysaccharides and occur in combination with protein in both body secretions and structures. Many mucopolysaccharides tend to be highly viscous and are responsible for the viscosity of body mucous secretions. They are generally components of the extracellular, amorphous ground substance that surrounds the collagen and elastin fibers and the cells of connective tissue and may be involved in the induction of calcification, control of metabolites, ions, and water, and the healing of wounds. Mucopolysaccharides, along with glycoproteins and glycolipids, also form the cell coat that is present in most animal cells. The cell coat is visible by electron microscopy but is not a well-defined structure as is the cell wall of plant cells. For this reason the cell coat permits more intimate interaction between the cells and between the cell and its environment. (See Chapter 9.)

Mucopolysaccharides contain amino sugars, either D-glucosamine or D-galactosamine together with uronic acids, either D-glucuronic acid or L-iduronic acid; in addition they may contain acetyl or sulfate groups. Two compounds that are generally included in the mucopolysaccharide classification do not follow the usual pattern of composition. Keratan sulfate, which is found in connective tissues, contains D-galactose instead of a uronic acid component. Heparin is similar in composition and is synthesized and stored in the mast cells of connective tissue.

Hyaluronic acid is a typical mucopolysaccharide. It is a component of the ground substance of intercellular material; the human umbilical cord and cattle synovial and vitreous fluids are the most common sources of hyaluronic acid, but it is widely distributed and is found in most connective tissues. Its name is derived from hyaloid (vitreous) and uronic acid. Hyaluronic acid is composed of equimolar proportions of D-glucuronic acid and acetyl glucosamine occupying alternating positions in the molecule. The structure is shown as follows.

**Repeating Unit of
Hyaluronic Acid**

The molecular weight varies depending on the source with reported values ranging from a few hundred thousand to well over a million. Large polymers of hyaluronic acid form a mesh that enables it to bind a large amount of water. In loose connective tissue such binding of tissue fluid forms a jellylike matrix filling the space between capillaries and cells. The large amount of fluid that is held by the polymers permits diffusion of solutes between capillaries and cells. In the synovial cavity, the viscosity of the synovial fluid assists in the lubrication of joints.

Chondroitin and *chondroitin sulfates* are polysaccharides containing D-glucuronic acid and acetyl galactosamine. Their general structure is similar, but they differ in the content and location of sulfate ester groups in the molecule. Chondroitin contains only a small number of sulfate ester groups, whereas both chondroitin 4- and chondroitin 6-sulfates (previously known as chondroitin sulfates A and C) contain one sulfate group for each disaccharide grouping. Their structures are shown as follows.

Chondroitin 4-sulfate   **Chondroitin 6-sulfate**

Chondroitin sulfates have a high viscosity and a capability for binding water and, in connective tissue, apparently play a role similar to that of hyaluronic acid. In addition, these compounds are distinguished by the ion-binding capacity of the sulfate groups. Chondroitin is a component of the cell coat (see Chapter 9), and chondroitin 4-sulfate is the principal organic component of the ground substance of cartilage and bone. (See Chapter 17.)

Dermatan sulfate (formerly chondroitin sulfate B or β-heparin) contains largely L-iduronic acid in place of D-glucuronic acid; iduronic acid is a derivative of the obscure hexose, idose. It has been suggested, however, that dermatan sulfate is a hybrid molecule containing both iduronic acid and glucuronic acid (Fransson, 1970). Dermatan sulfate generally occurs in tissues that are rich in collagen (Meyer et al., 1956). Its biological role appears to be different from the chondroitin sulfates, and it is present mainly in the skin.

Keratan sulfate (keratosulfate) is composed of D-galactose, N-acetyl-D-glucosamine and sulfate groups in a molar ratio of 1:1:1. Certain sources also have been found to contain 6-deoxyhexose (which is presumed to be L-fucose), sialic acid, and amino acids (Jeanloz, 1970). The function of keratan sulfate is not known. Apparently it is related to the blood group substances; it is degraded by enzymes that also degrade blood group substances, but not by hyaluronidases and chondrosulfatases. In addition, after removal of the sulfate groups, the de-sulfated keratan sulfate strongly cross-reacts with antibodies that also cross react with blood group substance A (Hirano et al., 1961). The basic structure of keratan sulfate is as follows.

Keratan sulfate

Heparin (or α-heparin), the naturally occurring anticoagulant in blood and other tissues contains glucosamine, glucuronic acid, and varying proportions of sulfate and acetyl groups. Its structure is not entirely clear. It is produced by mast cells of the connective tissue and is stored as granules within the cells. The heparin content of tissues correlates with the number of mast cells present. These cells are particularly numerous in the loose connective tissue along the path of small blood vessels. Heparin is secreted into the intercellular substance and functions there to prevent the fibrinogen that escapes from capillaries from forming fibrin clots. It also functions in the formation or activation of lipoprotein lipase, which clears chylomicrons from the plasma. (See Chapter 20.) There is an insufficient amount of heparin in the bloodstream to perform these functions, but the mast cells along the capillaries supply additional amounts.

For detailed information concerning the structure and function of the muco-polysaccharides, see Balazs (1970) and Jeanloz (1970).

Lipids

Lipids include all substances that are extractable from biological materials with the usual fat solvents (ether, chloroform, benzene, carbon tetrachloride, acetone, etc.). Certain lipids are an energy source for the cell, others are structural com-pounds (particularly important are the lipid constituents of cell and organelle membranes), and still others function as hormones. This diversity of function recalls the not-too-remote past when lipids were considered to be inert constit-uents of adipose cells. The work of Schoenheimer (1942) established the concept of the dynamic state of lipid metabolism and led to a new appreciation of adipose tissue as an active participant in the metabolic scheme.

Of the many compounds classified as lipids, only a fraction is significant in the diet, or in the structure and function of the animal cell. The following classification is limited to lipids of importance in animal nutrition and excludes the fat-soluble vitamins which, although properly classified as lipids, will be discussed in a separate section on the vitamins, following the classic practice of nutritionists. Glycolipids and lipoproteins also will be discussed in a later section.

A. Simple Lipids
    1. Fatty acids
    2. Neutral fats (mono-, di-, and triacyl glycerols)
    3. Waxes (esters of fatty acids with higher alcohols)
       a. Sterol esters (i.e., cholesterol esters with fatty acids)
       b. Nonsterol esters (i.e., vitamin A esters, etc.)
B. Compound Lipids
    1. Phospholipids
       a. Phosphatidic acids, lecithins, cephalins, etc.
       b. Plasmalogens
       c. Sphingomyelins
    2. Glycolipids (carbohydrate-containing)
    3. Lipoproteins (lipids in combination with protein)
C. Derived lipids, alcohols (including sterols and hydrocarbons)

FATTY ACIDS

The fatty acids, the simplest of the lipids, are defined as monocarboxylic acids that tend to be more soluble in organic solvents than in water. The molecule consists of a polar carboxyl group that is soluble in water and a nonpolar hydro-carbon chain that is insoluble in water but soluble in the common organic solvents. The solubility of fatty acids in water therefore is fairly high for those of low chain length but decreases markedly as chain length increases.

The names and structures of some common fatty acids are shown in Tables 2.3

TABLE 2.3
Some Naturally Occurring Saturated Fatty Acids

Common Name	Chemical Name	Formula	Abbreviation[a]	Source
Butyric	Butanoic	$CH_3(CH_2)_2COOH$	C4:0	Butterfat
Caproic	Hexanoic	$CH_3(CH_2)_4COOH$	C6:0	Butterfat, coconut, and palm nut oils
Caprylic	Octanoic	$CH_3(CH_2)_6COOH$	C8:0	Coconut and palm nut oils, butterfat
Capric	Decanoic	$CH_3(CH_2)_8COOH$	C10:0	Coconut and palm nut oils, butterfat
Lauric	Dodecanoic	$CH_3(CH_2)_{10}COOH$	C12:0	Coconut and palm nut oils, butterfat
Myristic	Tetradecanoic	$CH_3(CH_2)_{12}COOH$	C14:0	Coconut and palm nut oils, most animal and plant fats
Palmitic	Hexadecanoic	$CH_3(CH_2)_{14}COOH$	C16:0	Almost all animal and plant fats
Stearic	Octadecanoic	$CH_3(CH_2)_{16}COOH$	C18:0	Animal fats and some plant fats
Arachidic	Eicosanoic	$CH_3(CH_2)_{18}COOH$	C20:0	Peanut oil
Behenic	Docosanoic	$CH_3(CH_2)_{20}COOH$	C22:0	Peanut, mustard seed, and rapeseed oil
Lignoceric	Tetracosanoic	$CH_3(CH_2)_{22}COOH$	C24:0	Most natural fats and peanut oil in small amounts
Cerotic	Hexacosanoic	$CH_3(CH_2)_{24}COOH$	C26:0	Wool fat

[a]Abbreviated formulas indicate the number of carbon atoms, followed by a colon and 0 denoting no double bonds in the molecule.

TABLE 2.4
Some Naturally Occurring Unsaturated Fatty Acids

Common Name	Chemical Name	Formula	Family[a]	Abbreviations[b] (n series)	Source
Monoenoic					
Palmitoleic	Cis-9-hexadecenoic	$CH_3(CH_2)_5CH=CH(CH_2)_7COOH$	n7	C16:1n7 (Δ^9)[c]	Marine animal oils, small amounts in plant and animal fats
Oleic	Cis-9-octadecenoic	$CH_3(CH_2)_7CH=CH(CH_2)_7COOH$	n9	C18:1n9 (Δ^9)	Plant and animal fats
Elaidic	Trans-9-octadecenoic	$CH_3(CH_2)_7CH=CH(CH_2)_7COOH$	n9	C18:1n9	Animal fats
Erucic	Cis-13-docosenoic	$CH_3(CH_2)_7CH=CH(CH_2)_{11}COOH$	n9	C22:1n9	Rapeseed and mustard oils
Dienoic					
Linoleic	All cis-9,12 Octadecadienoic	$CH_3(CH_2)_3(CH_2CH=CH)_2(CH_2)_7COOH$	n6	C18:2n6 ($\Delta^{9,12}$)	Corn, safflower, soybean, cottonseed, sunflower seed, and peanut oils
Trienoic					
Linolenic	All cis-9,12,15 Octadecatrienoic	$CH_3(CH_2CH=CH)_3(CH_2)_7COOH$	n3	C18:3n3 ($\Delta^{9,12,15}$)	Linseed, soybean, and other seed oils
Tetraenoic					
Arachidonic	All cis-5,8,11,14 Eicosatetraenoic	$CH_3(CH_2)_3(CH_2CH=CH)_4(CH_2)_3COOH$	n6	C20:4n6 ($\Delta^{5,8,11,14}$)	Major polyunsaturated fatty acid in animal fats—in small amounts
Polyenoic					
Timnodonic	All cis-5,8,11,14,17 Eicosapentaenoic	$CH_3(CH_2)(CH=CH-CH_2)_5(CH_2)_2COOH$	n3	C20:5n3 ($\Delta^{5,8,11,14,17}$)	Fish and marine animal oils
Monohydroxy					
Ricinoleic	12-Hydroxy-cis-9 Octadecenoic	$CH_3(CH_2)_5CHOHCH_2CH=CH(CH_2)_7COOH$	—	C18:2	Castor and peanut seed oils
Cyclopropenoic					
Sterculic	ω-(2-n-octyl)-cyclo-prop-1-enyl Octanoic	$CH_3(CH_2)_7C{=}C(CH_2)_7COOH$ (cyclopropene CH_2 bridge)	—	C19:1	Cottonseed meal and some plant oils

[a] Different "families" of unsaturated fatty acids have been designated as n families. Using palmitoleic as an example, n7 denotes the position of the double bond from the terminal methyl carbon.

[b] Shorthand abbreviation for unsaturated fatty acids. C16: = Carbon chain length; the number following colon is the number of double bonds.

[c] Δ notation in parentheses is followed by a number that also represents the position of the double bond from the carboxyl carbon.

and 2.4. Note that for the unsaturated fatty acids (Table 2.4) two different systems for abbreviated formulas are given, one based on the position of double bonds from the carboxyl carbon, the other on the position of the first double bond from the terminal methyl group of the fatty acid molecule.

Most naturally occurring fatty acids are straight-chain saturated or unsaturated acids containing an even number of carbon atoms. Those in animal products generally contain 16 to 26 carbon atoms. Fatty acids of greater than 20 carbon atoms occur infrequently. Palmitic acid (C16:0) and stearic acid (C18:0) are by far the most commonly occurring and widely distributed of the saturated fatty acids; oleic acid (C18:1) and linoleic acid (C18:2) are the most prevalent of the unsaturated. These four fatty acids account for over 90 percent of the fatty acids in the average American diet. Fatty acids of shorter chain length are for the most part minor constituents of plant and animal fats. However, butyric acid (C4:0) and myristic acid (C14:0) occur in milk fat in large amounts, and about 60 percent of the fatty acid in coconut oil consists of lauric acid (C12:0) and fatty acids of shorter chain length.

Odd-numbered and branched-chain fatty acids occur in some cells (Kingsbury et al., 1961). Certain fish and bacteria contain fairly high amounts of odd-numbered fatty acids; the occurrence of these compounds in some common sources is shown in Table 2.5.

The polyunsaturated acids—linoleic, linolenic, and arachidonic—have often been designated the *essential fatty acids* (EFA). Of these three, linoleic acid is most abundant in human diets. Essential fatty acid activity, however, is shared by other unsaturated acids having the 9,12 double bond (counting from the carboxyl group) of the C_{18} acids or the 11,14 bond of the C_{20} acids. Some synthetic odd-numbered fatty acids also have EFA activity (Schlenk, 1972). The

TABLE 2.5
Occurrence of Odd-numbered Fatty Acids

Source	Percent Odd of Total Fatty Acids
Olive oil	<0.4
Chicken fat	0.4–1.5
Lard	0.8
Menhaden	2.4, 3.0
Mullet	19.1, 20.4
Tuna	4.2
Rat liver	2.9, 0.5
Human (depot fat)	1.1
Human (erythrocytes)	0.8
Euglena gracilis	33.4
Ochromonas danica	<1

Source: Adapted from H. Schlenk, *Fed. Proc.*, *31*: 1431 (1972).

essentiality of linoleic acid in the diet of the rat was first demonstrated by Burr and Burr (1929) who found that the acid would prevent or cure a characteristic dermatitis observed in rats fed a fat-free diet. Other effects of EFA deficiency in the rat are shown in Table 2.6. Later Wiese et al. (1958) demonstrated a requirement for linoleic acid in human infants. The dietary requirement for the human adult, however, appears to be variable. Collins (1971) found that linoleic acid at a level of 4 to 6 percent of energy intake satisfies the needs of adults. Symptoms of EFA deficiency have been observed with total parenteral feeding (Steglink et al., 1977), and the occurrences have been frequent enough to warrant the practice of adding EFA to the parenteral mixtures after five days of feeding.

The animal cell is capable of forming certain unsaturated fatty acids but not linoleate nor linolenate which must be supplied in the diet. Linoleate, linolenate, and oleate are all precursors for the biosynthesis of individual "families" of polyunsaturated fatty acids (Fig. 2.1). In the interconversions of unsaturated fatty acids new double bonds are introduced between the carboxyl group and the first double bond of the fatty acid molecule. Therefore, in this type of conversion, the terminal double bond remains fixed. Thus, linoleate ($18:2n6$) may be converted to arach-

TABLE 2.6
Major Effects of EFA Deficiency in the Rat

1. Skin symptoms	Dermatosis; increased water permeability; drop in sebum secretion; epithelial hyperplasia.
2. Weight	Decrease.
3. Circulation	Heart enlargement; decreased capillary resistance; increased permeability.
4. Kidney	Enlargement; intertubular hemorrhage.
5. Lung	Cholesterol accumulation.
6. Endocrine glands	(a) *Adrenals.* Weight decreased in females and increased in males.
	(b) *Thyroid.* Reduced weight.
7. Reproduction	(a) *Females.* Irregular estrus and impaired reproduction and lactation.
	(b) *Males.* Degeneration of seminiferous tubules.
8. Metabolism	(a) Changes in fatty acid composition of most organs.
	(b) Increase in cholesterol levels in liver, adrenals, and skin.
	(c) Decrease in plasma cholesterol.
	(d) Changes in swelling of heart and liver mitochondria and uncoupling of oxidative phosphorylation.
	(e) Increased triglyceride synthesis and release by the liver.

Source: From M. I. Gurr and A. T. James, *Lipid Biochemistry: An Introduction,* Cornell University Press, Ithaca, 1971, p. 56.

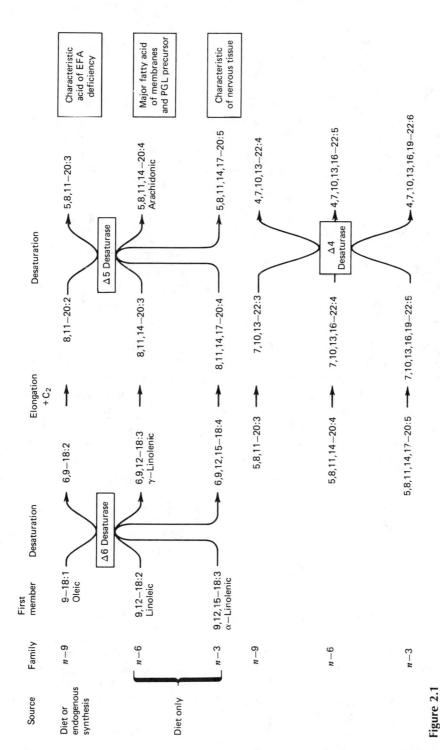

Figure 2.1

Metabolic transformations, by desaturation and elongation, of the three major unsaturated fatty acid families. (From M. I. Gurr and A. T. James, *Lipid Biochemistry: An Introduction*, 3rd ed., Chapman and Hall, New York, 1980, p. 48.)

idonate (20:4n6), but no conversion of other acids to linoleate occurs and no interconversion of fatty acids occurs between families. In contrast, plant cells are able to introduce a second double bond between carbon atoms 12 and 13 of oleic form linoleic acid.

Because of the double bonds in the molecule, unsaturated fatty acids may exist as isomers. This type of isomerism is known as *cis-trans* isomerism and involves changes in the geometrical configuration of the molecule. *Cis* isomerism results in a doubling back of the molecule in a horseshoelike configuration whereas *trans* isomerism has the effect of extending the molecule. As an illustration, the *cis* and *trans* forms of the C_{18} monounsaturated acid are shown as follows.

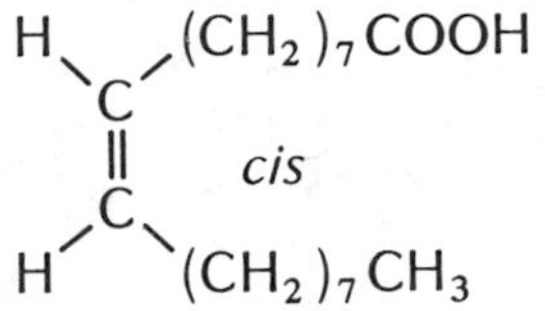

Oleic Acid 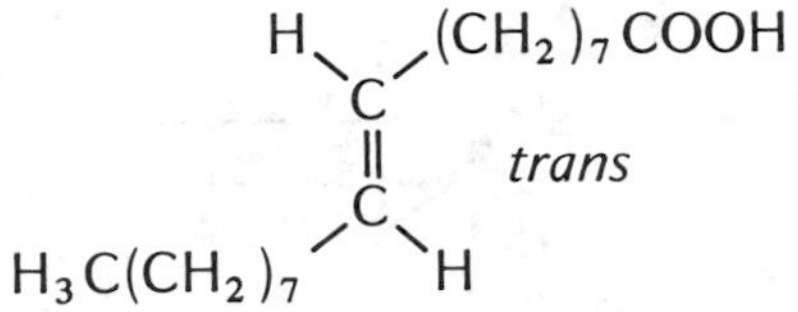   **Elaidic Acid**

In either case, however, the hydrocarbon chain of a fatty acid does not exist as a long straight chain but, instead, in a zigzag conformation. When a *cis* double bond is present the molecule becomes bent, and the bending is more drastic as the number of double bonds increases as shown below. The zigzagging along with the bending of the molecule makes for a bulky structure instead of the tidy straight chain suggested by the formula. The molecular configuration of the fatty acids play an important role in both the structure and function of membranes. (See Chapter 9.)

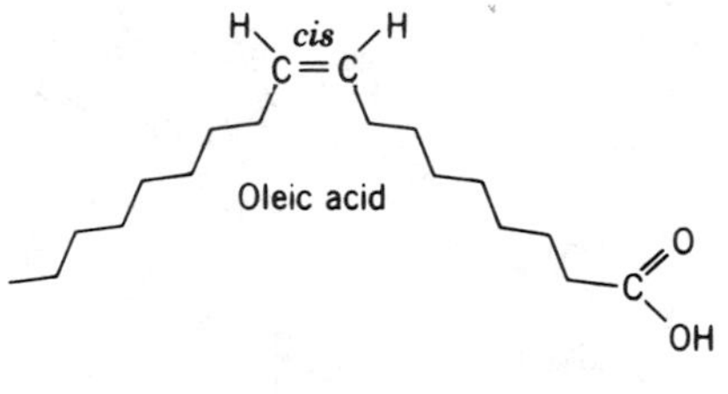

Oleic Acid (one *cis* bond) 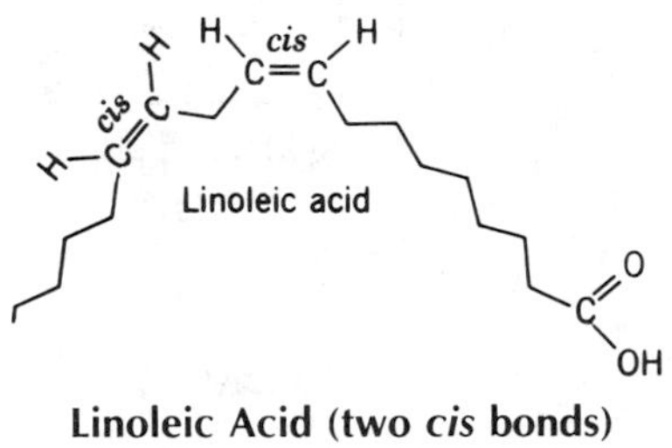   **Linoleic Acid (two *cis* bonds)**

Most naturally occurring fatty acids are largely of the *cis* configuration although conversion to the *trans* form results from heating or hydrogenation. However, *trans* fatty acids also exist in natural fats and oils. In cow's milk, for example, *trans* unsaturated fatty acids comprise about 8 percent of total fat and about 20 percent of total unsaturated fatty acids (Woodrow and de Man, 1968). The role of *trans* fatty acids in the metabolism of essential fatty acids is being actively investigated (Kinsella et al., 1981).

PROSTAGLANDINS

Essential fatty acids are precursors of a ubiquitious family of lipids—the prosta-glandins. These compounds have hormonelike activity and are among the most potent biological substances known. The first indication of the existence of this new family of compounds came when Kurzrok and Lieb (1930) reported that human seminal fluid produced both relaxation and strong contractions when applied to isolated strips of human uterine tissue. Subsequently both Euler (1934) and Goldblatt (1933; 1935) independently observed similar effects of seminal fluid on smooth muscle. Shortly thereafter, Euler (1935) reported that the activity was due to an acidic lipid fraction that he named prostaglandin. More than 25 years passed, however, before the structure was determined by Bergström et al. (1962) using a variety of techniques including mass spectrometry, X-ray crystal-lography, and nuclear magnetic resonance. Two years later the essential fatty acids were found to be precursors (Bergström et al., 1964; Van Dorp, 1964).

Work on the prostaglandins then mushroomed. As of the end of 1981, a large number of different compounds has been identified and classified in general as eicosanoids having 20 carbon atoms and the same basic molecule of prostanoic acid (see Fig. 2.2a and 2.2b). The carbon chains are bonded in the middle by a five-member ring. They are synthesized in membranes from C20 fatty acids that contain at least three double bonds.

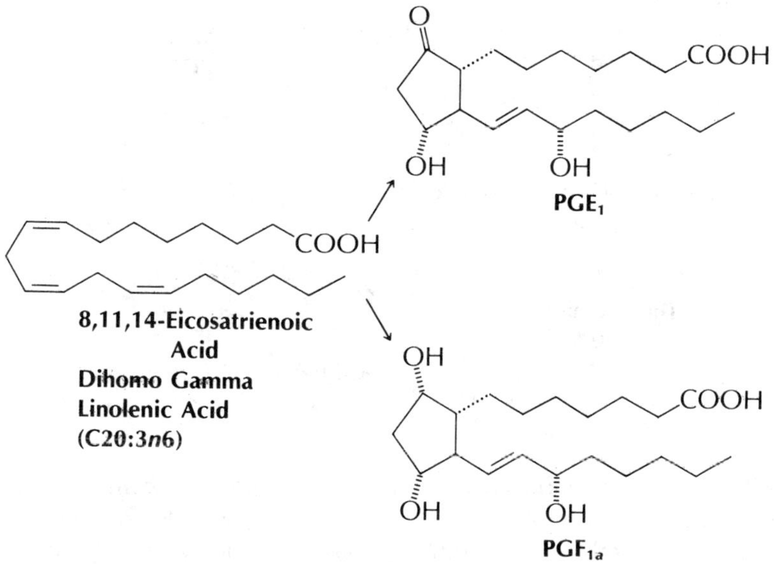

8,11,14-Eicosatrienoic
Acid
Dihomo Gamma
Linolenic Acid
(C20:3n6)

PGE$_1$

PGF$_{1a}$

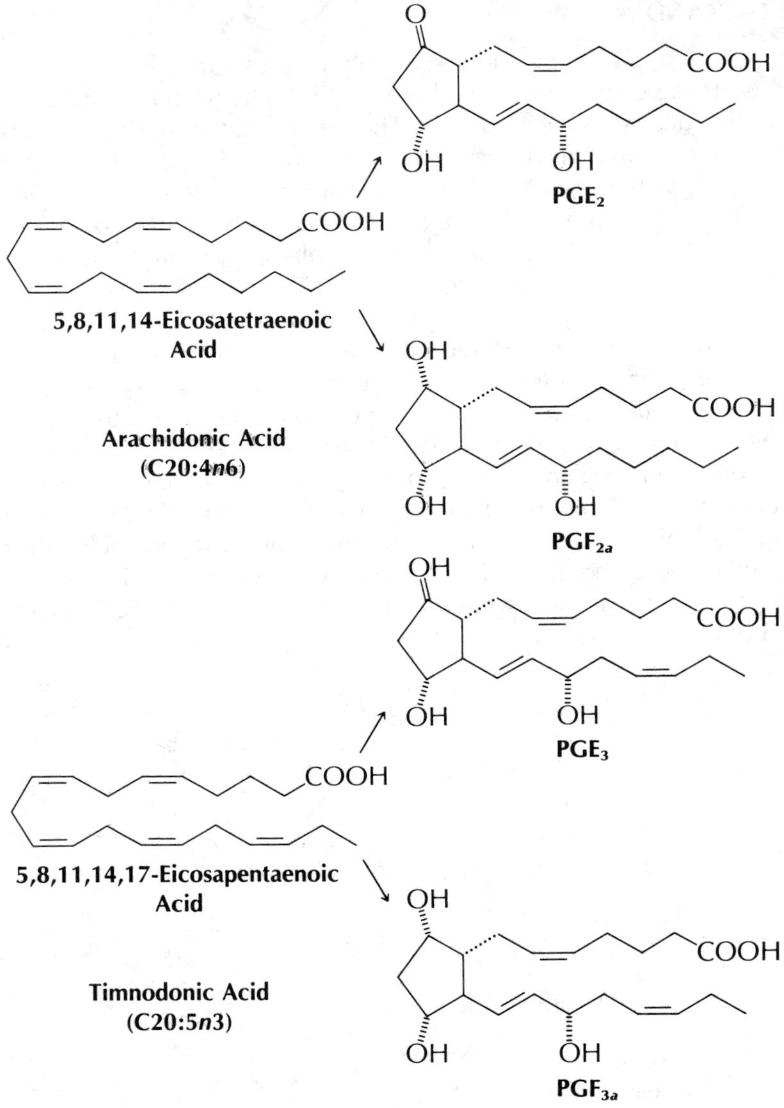

COOH

PGE$_2$

OH   OH

5,8,11,14-Eicosatetraenoic
Acid

COOH

Arachidonic Acid
(C20:4*n*6)

OH

COOH

OH   OH

PGF$_{2a}$

OH

COOH

OH   OH

PGE$_3$

COOH

5,8,11,14,17-Eicosapentaenoic
Acid

Timnodonic Acid
(C20:5*n*3)

OH

COOH

OH   OH

PGF$_{3a}$

Six primary prostaglandins occur in most cells and arise from eicosatri-, tetra-, and pentaenoic acids as shown above. These compounds are converted to the six secondary natural prostaglandins that have been identified. It is probable that yet other of these compounds will be discovered. The rapid growth in the knowledge of the eicosanoids and their biosynthesis, as elucidated from the large number of these compounds derived from arachidonic acid (the "arachidonic acid cascade"), and their role in many aspects of health and disease have been the subject of several reviews (Chase and Dupont, 1978; McGiff, 1981; Willis, 1981; and Hammarstrom, 1982). See Fig. 2.2*a* and 2.2*b*.

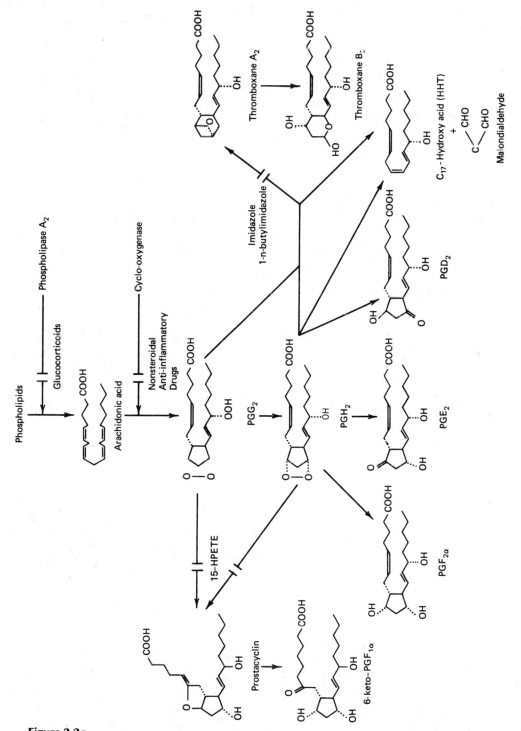

Figure 2.2a
Conversion of arachidonic acid to prostaglandins by the cyclooxygenase pathway. (HPETE = hydroperoxy eicosatetraenoic). (From A.G. Herman, *Cardiovascular Pharmacology of the Lipids,* A.G. Herman, P.M. Vanhoutte, H. Denolin and A. Goosens, eds., Raven Press, New York, 1982, p.3.).

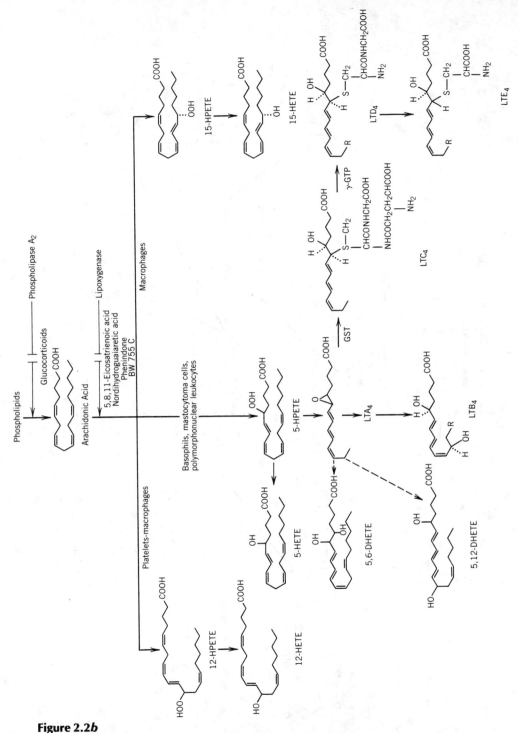

Figure 2.2b
Conversion of arachdonic acid to leukotrienes by the lipoxygenase pathway. (HETE = hydroxy eicosatetraenoic; DHETE = dihydroxy eicosatetraenoic; HPETE = hydroperoxy eicosatetraenoic; GST = glutathione-S-transferase; α-GTP = α-Glutamyl transpeptidase; R = C₇H₁₃, (n-6). (From A.G. Herman, *Cardiovascular Pharmacology of the Prostaglandins*, A.G. Herman, P.M. Vanhoutte, H. Denolin and A. Goosens, eds., Raven Press, New York, 1982, p. 4.).

Prostaglandins produce a variety of physiological effects including the effect on smooth muscle already mentioned, reduction of blood pressure, inhibition of gastric secretions, antagonism to some hormones, and activation of others. Thus prostaglandins are one of the most exciting discoveries of this century in the fields of clinical medicine and pharmacology as well as in cell biochemistry.

The first unstable endoperoxide, PGH$_2$ formed from PGG$_2$, was isolated in 1973 (Samuelsson et al., 1975). These endoperoxides were found to have biological effects on platelet aggregation and on contraction of smooth muscle in the vascular and respiratory systems, and in the stomach, heart, and uterus. Another platelet aggregating factor derived from arachidonic acid, different from the prostaglandins and the endoperoxides, is the unstable thromboxane A$_2$ that has been identified in a number of tissues (Samuelsson et al., 1978). Subsequently, it was found that the endoperoxide, PGG$_2$, was converted to a prostaglandin with potent vasodilator and antiaggregating properties. This prostaglandin, originally referred to as PGX, a more potent antiaggregating factor than PGE$_1$ or PGD$_2$, was later identified as prostacyclin or PGI$_2$ (Moncada et al., 1976a; 1976b). Prostacyclin is synthesized in endothelial cells of the blood vessel walls, whereas the thromboxanes are synthesized by the platelets. It is believed that an imbalance in the formation of these two potent substances may be responsible for some disease states. PGI$_2$ is measured as its stable metabolite, 6-keto-PGF$_{1a}$, whereas the thromboxane A$_2$ is measured as its stable metabolite, thromboxane B$_2$. For further discussion on the metabolism and importance of these substances see Moncada and Vane (1980; 1981) and McGiff (1981).

Prostaglandins of the D, E, and I series stimulate cyclic AMP formation in several tissues (Samuelsson, 1978). It is by this mechanism that they produce hormonelike or neurohormonal responses. Prostacyclin inhibits platelet aggregation through the stimulation of platelet adenyl cyclase, leading to an increase in platelet cAMP which acts as a second messenger (Moncada and Vane, 1981).

The role of prostaglandins in the regulation of blood pressure and their interaction with vasoconstrictor pressor hormones, angiotensin II and norepinephrine, is not entirely clear. Whether the rate of conversion of linoleic acid to arachidonic acid and thence to prostaglandins (which counteract the vasoconstrictor action of the pressor hormones) or the natriuretic effect is more important is being intensively investigated (McGiff, 1981).

The most recent research in the prostaglandin field has focused on the products of another pathway of arachidonic acid metabolism, the lipoxygenase pathway (Samuelsson et al., 1980; see also Fig. 2.2b). Samuelsson and his coworkers demonstrated the formation of several substances resembling the slow reacting substance (SRS), a compound associated with the production of anaphylactic shock in rabbits. These compounds, which are produced by way of the lipoxygenase pathway, have been designated "leukotrienes." They are produced in leucocytes and have been associated with the production of inflammatory responses and the impairment of immune responses. For more detailed information, see Samuelsson et al. (1980), Kuehl and Egan (1980), Gemsa (1981), Morley (1981), and Samuelsson (1983).

Because essential fatty acids are the precursors of the prostaglandins it has been speculated that some effects of EFA deficiency may be due to inhibition of prostaglandin synthesis. Indeed Guanieri and Johnson (1970) suggested that pros- have been shown to be involved in the endogenous regulation of free fatty acid release from adipose tissue of EFA-deficient animals (Bizzi et al., 1967).

Studies of the effects of dietary essential fatty acids and indirectly, the prostaglandins, on blood pressure, thrombogenesis, and platelet function have been reviewed (Marcus, 1978; Galli et al., 1980; Horton et al., 1981; Iacono et al., 1981; Vergroesen et al., 1981; Dyerberg, 1982; Goodnight et al., 1982; Nasjletti and Malik, 1982).

ACYLGLYCEROLS (GLYCERIDES)

Fatty acids are consumed in the diet and stored in tissues largely as triacylglycerols (triglycerides). Monoacylglycerols and diacylglycerols occur in negligible amounts in tissues but are important intermediates in a number of degradative and biosynthetic reactions.

The acylglycerols are esters of one, two, or three fatty acids with the trihydroxy alcohol, glycerol, and are designated as simple or mixed acylglycerols depending on the number of different fatty acids present in the molecule. (The location of the fatty acids in the molecule is shown by the system designated below.) Tristearin, for example, indicates a simple triacylglycerol containing only stearic acid in the molecule, whereas 1-oleo-2-stearo-3-palmitin is a triglyceride containing oleic, stearic, and palmitic acids. As mentioned before, these acids along with linoleic acid are the most widely distributed of the fatty acids. Generally, triacylglycerols in biological systems contain different fatty acyl groups.

$$
\begin{array}{ll}
1 \text{ or } a & CH_2OH \\
2 & \beta\ CHOH \\
3 & a'\ CH_2OH
\end{array}
$$

Glycerol

$$
\begin{array}{l}
CH_2-O-C{\overset{\displaystyle O}{\underset{\displaystyle}{\parallel}}}R \\
CHOH \\
CH_2OH
\end{array}
$$

**Monoacylglycerol
(monoglyceride)**

$$
\begin{array}{l}
CH_2-O-C{\overset{O}{\parallel}}R \\
CH-O-C{\overset{O}{\parallel}}R \\
CH_2OH
\end{array}
$$

**Diacylglycerol
(diglyceride)**

$$
\begin{array}{l}
CH_2-O-C{\overset{O}{\parallel}}R \\
CH-O-C{\overset{O}{\parallel}}R \\
CH_2-O-C{\overset{O}{\parallel}}R
\end{array}
$$

**Triacylglycerol
(triglyceride)**

Triacylglycerols are classed as fats or oils depending on the state of the acyl-glycerol at room temperature, which varies with the fatty acid composition. In general, acylglycerols containing a high proportion of short chain (less than eight carbon atoms) or unsaturated acids have a low melting point and are liquid (oils) at room temperature. The longer chain saturated fatty acids produce a fat of higher melting point that is solid at room temperature.

Triacylglycerols are a form of stored energy in animal tissues (adipose cells) and are commonly referred to as neutral fat. The capacity to store fat in the animal body unfortunately appears to be unlimited. Fatty acids are released from adipose cells in free form. These are designated both as FFA (free fatty acids) and NEFA (nonesterified fatty acids). Once released from neutral fat the FFA are transported in the blood bound to serum albumin (Goodman, 1957).

Although triacylglycerols containing exclusively fatty acids with chain length of 6 to 12 carbon atoms are rare or nonexistent in nature, such compounds, called medium chain triglycerides or MCT, have been synthesized. The synthetic MCT contain approximately 75 percent caprylic acid (C_8), 22 to 23 percent capric (C_{10}), 1 percent each of caproic (C_6) and lauric (C_{12}), and traces of other fatty acids such as palmitic, stearic, and linoleic (Greenberger and Skillman, 1969). These compounds are liquid at room temperature due to the low melting points of the shorter chain fatty acids.

Because of the shorter hydrocarbon chain the MCT are also more soluble in water than the naturally occurring triacylglycerols containing the long chain fatty acids. They are readily absorbed from the gastrointestinal tract and do not require bile salts for absorption. For these reasons the MCT appear to have therapeutic value in the treatment of a number of diseases including tropical and nontropical sprue, pancreatic insufficiency, and other conditions affecting lipid absorption. For a comprehensive review of the nutritional and medical uses of MCT, see Bach and Babayan (1982).

PHOSPHOLIPIDS

$$
\begin{array}{l}
CH_2-O-C \overset{\displaystyle O}{} R_1 \\
CH-O-C \overset{\displaystyle O}{} R_2 \\
CH_2-O-P \overset{\displaystyle OH}{=} O \\
OH
\end{array}
$$

Phosphatidic acid

Phosphatidic acids are compounds consisting of glycerol, two fatty acids, and a phosphate group and, as the structure suggests, they easily give rise to triacyl-glycerols or to phospholipids. Because they are active intermediates in the biosynthesis of other lipid compounds, the phosphatidic acids do not accumulate in tissues in significant amounts.

Phospholipids differ chiefly in the specific compound attached to the phosphate group of the phosphatidic acid core. The fatty acids present in the molecule are usually saturated in the α-position (palmitic or stearic) and unsaturated in the β-position (oleic or linolenic). The phospholipid structures are shown in Table 2.7.

Phospholipids have the useful property of attracting both water-soluble and fat-soluble substances due to the hydrophilic (water-attracting) phosphoryl grouping and the hydrophobic (water-repelling) fatty acids in the molecule. In combination with protein, they are constituents of cell membranes and membranes of sub-cellular particles where they serve as a liaison between fat-soluble and water-soluble materials that must penetrate the membrane and interact once they have gained entry. In this structural role, phospholipids are not generally available as an energy source. Even a starved animal will retain the phospholipid necessary to maintain the integrity of cells.

SPHINGOLIPIDS

$$CH_3(CH_2)_{12}CH=CH$$
$$HO-CH \qquad \text{From palmitic acid}$$
$$\text{-----------} | \text{-----------}$$
$$H_2N-CH \qquad \text{From serine}$$
$$CH_2OH$$

4-Sphingenine (sphingosine)

Sphingolipids are classed as phospholipids but, in place of the glycerol characteristic of the glycerophospholipids, they contain 4-sphingenine (sphingosine), an 18-carbon monounsaturated alcohol derived from palmitic acid and the amino acid serine. Carbon atoms 1-3 form the glycerol-type part of the molecule; the structure differs from glycerol principally in that an amino group (from serine) is attached to the second carbon.

Sphingomyelins

Sphingomyelins occur in large amounts in the myelin sheath of nerve tissue and derive their name from this structure. The sphingomyelins contain phosphorylcholine attached to the terminal carbon atom of sphingosine and a fatty acid attached in amide linkage to the nitrogen of carbon 2.

$$OH$$
$$|$$
$$\overset{O}{\underset{\parallel}{}} \quad CH-CH=CH(CH_2)_{12}CH_3$$
$$R-C-N-CH$$
$$| \quad | \qquad \overset{O}{\underset{\parallel}{}}$$
$$H \quad CH_2-O-P-O-CH_2CH_2N^+(CH_3)_3$$
$$|$$
$$OH$$

Sphingomyelin

TABLE 2.7
Glycerol Phospholipids

Name	Characteristic Group	Structure
Phosphatidyl cholines (lecithins)	Choline	CH_2OCOR^1 R^2COOCH $CH_2-O-\overset{\overset{O}{\|\|}}{\underset{\underset{O^-}{\|}}{P}}-OCH_2CH_2\overset{+}{N}(CH_3)_3$
Phosphatidyl ethanolamines (cephalins)	Ethanolamine (aminoethanol)	CH_2OCOR^1 R^2COOCH $CH_2-O-\overset{\overset{O}{\|\|}}{\underset{\underset{O^-}{\|}}{P}}-OCH_2CH_2\overset{+}{N}H_3$
Phosphatidyl serines (cephalinlike compounds)	Serine	CH_2OCOR^1 R^2COOCH $CH_2-O-\overset{\overset{O}{\|\|}}{\underset{\underset{OH}{\|}}{P}}-OCH_2\underset{\underset{COO^-}{\|}}{CH}CH_2\overset{+}{N}H_3$
Phosphatidyl inositols (inositides or lipositols)	Myo-inositol	CH_2OCOR^1 R^2COOCH $CH_2-O-\overset{\overset{O}{\|\|}}{\underset{\underset{OH}{\|}}{P}}-O-$ (inositol ring with OH groups)
Plasmalogens	Ethanolamine One fatty acid replaced by a long-chain unsaturated ether	$\alpha CH_2OCH=CHR^1$ $R^2COOCH\beta$ $CH_2-O-\overset{\overset{O}{\|\|}}{\underset{\underset{O^-}{\|}}{P}}-OCH_2CH_2\overset{+}{N}H_3$

A rare inherited disease, Niemann-Pick disease, is due to the lack of sphingo-myelinase, the enzyme responsible for sphingomyelin cleavage. The disease is characterized by deposition of sphingomyelin in almost every organ and tissue of the body and is usually fatal before the third year of life.

STEROIDS AND STEROLS

Cyclopentanoperhydrophen-
anthrene nucleus

Cholesterol

Steroid compounds are derivatives of a ring structure with the formidable name of the cyclopentanoperhydrophenanthrene nucleus. Certain steroids are charac-terized by a free hydroxyl group and thus behave chemically like alcohols. These alcohollike steroids do not contain carbonyl or carboxy groups common to other steroids and are generally referred to as *sterols*. The most common sterol in animal tissues is cholesterol, which occurs in the free form or combined in ester formation with fatty acids. The proportion of free cholesterol to cholesterol esters varies considerably among different tissues. Sterol esters predominate in plasma and adrenals although nearly all cholesterol in brain and nerve tissue is in the free form. Cholesterol is present only in animals. Egg yolk, dairy products, and meats, for example, contain fairly high amounts. Many other sterols are found in plant tissues, the most important being β-sitosterol.

Cholesterol is readily synthesized from acetate in all animal tissues. (See Chapter 15.) It is a normal component of all body cells and occurs in large concentration in nerve tissue. Cholesterol is the precursor of cholic acid, a constituent of the bile acids (taurocholic and glycocholic), and its 7-dehydro derivative is a precursor of the vitamin D of animal tissues, cholecalciferol. Estrogens, androgens, pro-gesterone, and most of the adrenocortical hormones are derived from cholesterol. The relationships among these compounds are shown in Fig. 2.3. It is interesting and significant that the adrenal gland contains a fairly high concentration of cholesterol that is rapidly depleted under stress when cortical activity is high.

Proteins

Nearly half of the dry weight of a typical animal cell is protein. Structural com-ponents of the cell, antibodies, and many of the hormones are proteins, but as much as 90 percent of cellular proteins are the enzymes on which fundamental

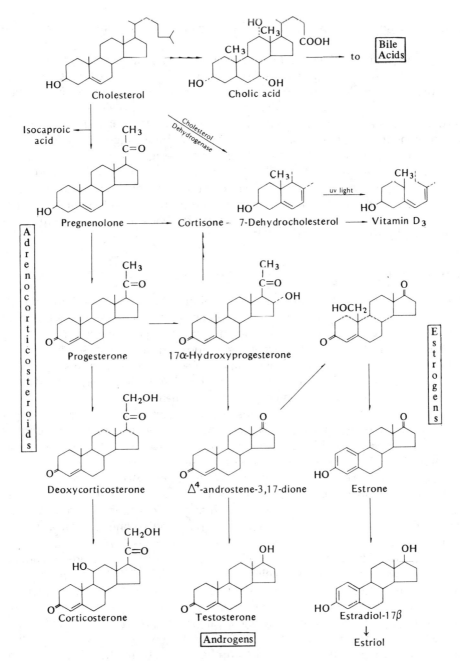

Figure 2.3
Metabolic relationships among the steroids.

43

cellular function depends. There may be as many as 1,000 different enzymes in a single cell.

The protein molecule is a polymer of amino acids joined in peptide linkages. Although the molecular weight is usually high, there is a vast range in both structure and complexity of protein molecules. Hemoglobin, for example, has a molecular weight of about 64,500; myosin, a muscle protein, is estimated to have a molecular weight of about 468,000 (Klotz and Darnall, 1969). It is not uncommon for peptide structures of fairly low molecular weight (less than 10,000 and containing less than 100 amino acids) to be designated polypeptides rather than proteins. On the average, about 20 different amino acids occur in most proteins. The amino acids present, their position in the molecule, and the spatial arrangement of the molecule all determine the properties and characteristics of the protein. In turn, the function of a protein depends in large measure on its structure. (See Hess and Rupley, 1971.)

AMINO ACIDS

The amino acids are the fundamental units of protein structure. All amino acids contain at least one amino group in the alpha position and one carboxyl, and all (except glycine) contain an asymmetric carbon atom. For this reason, they may exist as isomers. Most naturally occurring amino acids are of the L-configuration, although D-amino acids are not uncommon in some microorganisms. The presence of a D-amino acid oxidase in mammalian tissues, however, suggests that the D-forms may play some yet unrecognized role in mammalian protein metabolism.

The common amino acids in proteins and their chemical structures are shown in Table 2.8 together with their systematic names, one and three letter abbreviations and molecular weights. They are classified according to their chemical structure, but other classifications are also possible.

The amino acid composition of proteins varies greatly. However, certain amino acids, such as methionine and tryptophan, generally are present in small amounts; others, such as alanine, are present in much larger proportions. All amino acids occurring in proteins are of the α-type and have the L-configuration at the α-carbon atom.

Although only 20 amino acids are coded for, some 140 amino acids and amino acid derivatives can occur in proteins (Uy and Wold, 1977). These amino acids are formed posttranslationally or after the primary synthesis. (See Chapter 11.) The majority of these compounds occur rarely, but some more commonly found amino acids formed posttranslationally are shown in Table 2.8. These include hydroxylysine and hydroxyproline found primarily in collagen, formed by hydroxylation (See Chapter 17); 3-methyl-histidine in muscle, formed by methylation (see Chapter 18); and cystine present in many proteins, formed from two cysteine residues by cross linking.

A summary of posttranslational modification reactions that result in the formation of new amino acids and derivatives is shown in Table 2.9. Proteolysis as a means of converting inactive precursors to active enzymes has been known for

TABLE 2.8
Classification of the L-α-Amino Acids Found in Proteins

Name	Abbreviations		Structural Formula	Molecular Weight

ALIPHATIC MONOAMINOMONOCARBOXYLIC ACIDS

Name	Abbr.		Structural Formula	Mol. Wt.
Glycine[a] (Amino acetic acid)	Gly	G	$H-\begin{array}{c} NH_2 \\ | \\ CH-COOH \end{array}$	75
Alanine (2-amino propanoic acid)	Ala	A	$CH_3-\begin{array}{c} NH_2 \\ | \\ CH-COOH \end{array}$	89
Valine (2-amino-3-methyl-butanoic acid)	Val	V	$CH_3-CH-\begin{array}{c} CH_3 \\ \\ \end{array}\begin{array}{c} NH_2 \\ | \\ CH-COOH \end{array}$	117
Leucine (2-amino-4-methyl-pentanoic acid)	Leu	L	$CH_3-CH-CH_2-\begin{array}{c} CH_3 \\ \\ \end{array}\begin{array}{c} NH_2 \\ | \\ CH-COOH \end{array}$	131
Isoleucine (2-amino-3-methyl-pentanoic acid)	Ile	I	$CH_3-CH_2-CH-\begin{array}{c} CH_3 \\ \\ \end{array}\begin{array}{c} NH_2 \\ | \\ CH-COOH \end{array}$	131
Serine (2-amino-3-hydroxy-propanoic acid)	Ser	S	$CH_2-\begin{array}{c} OH \\ \\ \end{array}\begin{array}{c} NH_2 \\ | \\ CH-COOH \end{array}$	105
Threonine (2-amino-3-hydroxy-butanoic acid)	Thr	T	$CH_3-CH-\begin{array}{c} OH \\ \\ \end{array}\begin{array}{c} NH_2 \\ | \\ CH-COOH \end{array}$	119

TABLE 2.8 (continued)

Name	Abbreviations	Structural Formula	Molecular Weight
AROMATIC AMINO ACIDS			
Phenylalanine (2-amino-3-phenyl propanoic acid)	Phe F		165
Tyrosine (2-amino-3-(4 hydroxyphenyl) propanoic acid)	Tyr Y		181
Tryptophan (2-amino-3-(3 indoyl) propanoic acid)	Try W		204
ACIDIC AMINO ACIDS AND THEIR AMIDES[b]			
Aspartic Acid (2-amino-butane-1,4 dioic acid)	Asp D (B)		133
Asparagine (2-amino-butane-1,4 dioic acid-4-amide)	Asn N (B)		132

Name	Abbr.	Code	MW	Structure
Glutamic Acid (2-amino-pentane-1,5-dioic acid)	Glu	E (Z)	147	$HOOC-CH_2-CH_2-\underset{\underset{NH_2}{\vert}}{CH}-COOH$
Glutamine (2-amino-pentane-1,5-dioic acid-5-amide)	Gln	Q (Z)	146	$H_2N-\underset{\underset{O}{\Vert}}{C}-CH_2-CH_2-\underset{\underset{NH_2}{\vert}}{CH}-COOH$

BASIC AMINO ACIDS

Name	Abbr.	Code	MW	Structure
Lysine (2,6-diamino-hexanoic acid)	Lys	K	146	$\underset{\underset{NH_2}{\vert}}{CH_2}-CH_2-CH_2-CH_2-\underset{\underset{NH_2}{\vert}}{CH}-COOH$
Arginine (2-amino-5-guanido-pentanoic acid)	Arg	R	174	$H_2N-\underset{\underset{NH}{\Vert}}{C}-NHCH_2-CH_2-CH_2-\underset{\underset{NH_2}{\vert}}{CH}-COOH$
Histidine [2-amino-3(imidazole)-propanoic acid]	His	H	155	imidazole$-CH_2-\underset{\underset{NH_2}{\vert}}{CH}-COOH$
Cysteine (2-amino-3-mercatopropanoic acid)	Cys	C	121	$HS-CH_2-\underset{\underset{NH_2}{\vert}}{CH}-COOH$
Methionine [2-amino-4(methylthio)-butanoic acid]	Met	M	149	$CH_3-S-CH_2-CH_2-\underset{\underset{NH_2}{\vert}}{CH}-COOH$

TABLE 2.8 (continued)

Name	Abbreviations	Structural Formula	Molecular Weight
IMINO ACID			
Proline (2-pyrrolidine-carboxylic acid)	Pro	P	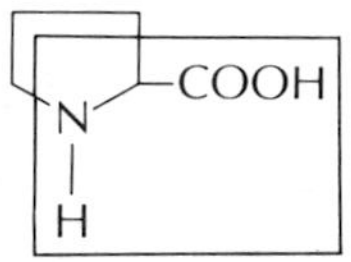	115
AMINO ACIDS FORMED POST TRANSLATION[c]			
Cystine 3-3-dithiobis-(2-amino propionic acid)	Cys-S-S-Cys	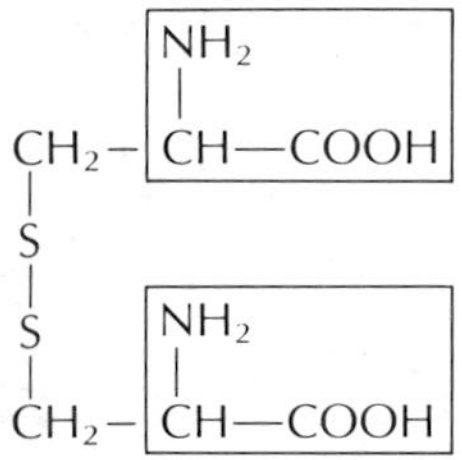	240
δ-Hydroxylysine (2,6-diamino-5-hydroxy-hexanoic acid)	Hyl	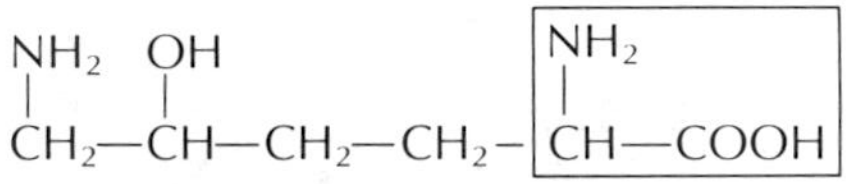	162
Hydroxyproline (4-hydroxy-2-pyrrolidine-carboxylic acid)	Hyp	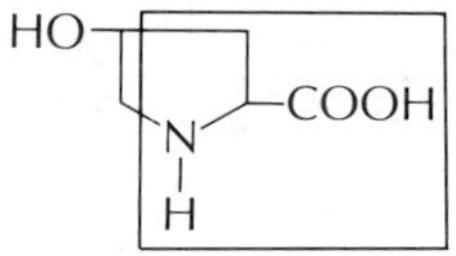	131

Structural formulas:

Proline:

Cystine:
$$NH_2-CH-COOH$$
$$|$$
$$CH_2-S-S-CH_2$$
$$NH_2-CH-COOH$$

δ-Hydroxylysine:
$$NH_2 \quad OH$$
$$|\qquad\;|$$
$$CH_2-CH-CH_2-CH_2-CH-COOH$$

Hydroxyproline:

3-Monoidotyrosine
[2-amino-3(3-iodo-4-hydroxy phenyl) propanoic acid]

307

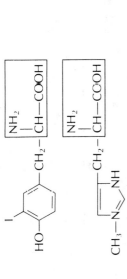

3-Methyl histidine
[2-amino-3(2 methyl-4-imidazole) propanoic acid]

169

[a] No asymmetric carbon atom.

[b] Single-letter abbreviation in brackets is used when amino acid can be acid or amide.

[c] Some 140 have been described (Uy and Wold, 1977) which include glycosylated amino acids and cross-linked amino acids. Those included here are those found most commonly in proteins.

49

TABLE 2.9
Posttranslational Modification Reactions of Proteins[a]

	Posttranslational Modification	
		Covalent	
Noncovalent	Peptide bond	Amino Acid side chain

Conformation of tertiary structure
Polymer formation
Holoenzyme assembly
	A. Breakage
	  Activation of zymogen and hormones
	  Synthesis of immunoglobulins
	  Blood coagulation
	  Collagen synthesis
	  Conversion of secretory protein from precursor
	  Virus assembly
	
	B. Formation
	  Addition of arginine or phenylalanine to -NH$_2$ end of proteins
	  Amide bond
	  Cross linkages
		A. Addition
		  Methylation
		  Acetylation
		  Phosphorylation
		  Thiolation
		  Hydroxylation
		  Carboxylation
		  ADP—ribosylation
		  Nucleotidylation
		  Glycosylation
		  Iodination
		B. Removal
		  Dehydration
		  Deguanidation

[a] Simplified from Paik and Kim (1980).

many years. More recently, posttranslational proteolytic processing of polypeptides has been recognized as a widespread phenomenon involving a large number
of important protein hormones and other active proteins such as the immuno-
globulins (Dean and Judah, 1980).

Functions of Protein and Individual Amino Acids

It would be impossible to discuss in detail the specific functions of all of the
amino acids in the limited space that can be devoted to this subject. Certain
reactions, however, will be mentioned briefly. It should not be assumed that these
reactions are necessarily the most important of the many metabolic reactions in
which the amino acids take part. Instead, they are merely examples intended to
refresh memories and to stimulate further study.

Traditionally amino acids have been described as *ketogenic* and *glucogenic*,
that is, they tend to give rise to acetoacetate or to carbohydrate intermediates. In
light of the present knowledge of interrelated metabolic pathways, these terms
are obsolete. Nonetheless, it is perhaps useful to remember that phenylalanine,
tyrosine, leucine, and isoleucine are degraded in part to acetoacetate whereas
other amino acids are degraded chiefly to pyruvate, oxaloacetate, α-ketoglutarate,
succinate, and fumarate.

The dietary requirements of certain of the amino acids are influenced by the
intake of other nutrients. For example, phenylalanine is converted to tyrosine in
the animal cell. The dietary requirement for phenylalanine, therefore, is a function
of the total aromatic amino acid content of the diet. Similarly, methionine may
function metabolically as a precursor of other sulfur-containing amino acids so
that both the dietary methionine and cystine determine the requirement for methionine. The relationship between tryptophan and nicotinic acid is another important example. Tryptophan can be metabolized to form nicotinic acid and,
therefore, contributes to the total amount of the vitamin available for cellular
metabolism. (See Chapter 3.)

Many of the amino acids are precursors of other significant compounds required
in metabolic processes. For example, tyrosine and, therefore, phenylalanine give
rise to the hormones thyroxine and epinephrine. Glutamic acid, cysteine, and
glycine are components of a tripeptide glutathione, which functions in cellular
oxidation-reduction reactions and in amino acid transport. Sulfur-containing amino
acids give rise to taurine, a bile acid component. Tryptophan can be metabolized
to form serotonin (5-hydroxytryptamine), a tissue hormone that is found predominantly in serum, blood platelets, gastrointestinal mucosa, and nerve tissue. Methionine provides methyl groups for synthesis of choline, creatine, and methylation
of nicotinamide to its major excretion product N'-methylnicotinamide. Glycine
contributes to the porphyrin ring of hemoglobin and, along with serine, provides
part of the structure of the purines and pyrimidines of the nucleic acids. Two
hydroxylated amino acids—hydroxyproline and hydroxylysine—are important
constituents of collagen; approximately 12 percent of the total amino acid content
of collagen is hydroxyproline.

Two diamino acids—ornithine and citrulline—probably do not occur as con-

TABLE 2.10
Other Functions of Some Amino Acids

Amino Acid	Precursor of	Role
Alanine	Pyruvate	Amino transport
		Gluconeogenesis
Arginine	Creatine	Energy metabolism
	Ornithine	Urea formation
	Polyamines	Cell division?
	Oxaloacetic acid	Gluconeogenesis
Aspartic acid	Aparagine	Ammonia transport
	Purine, pyrimidines	Nucleic acids
Cysteine	Glutathione	Oxidation/reduction
		Amino acid transport
	Taurocholic acid	Fat absorption
Glutamic acid	α-Ketoglutarate	Gluconeogenesis, transamination
	Glutamine	Ammonia transport
	Glutathione	Oxidation/reduction
	γ-Amino butyric acid	Neurotransmitter
Glutamine	Purines, pyrimidines	Nucleic acids
	Amino sugars	Glycoproteins
	Citrulline	Ammonia transport
Histidine	Histamine	Biological amine
Lysine	Carnitine	Lipid transport
Methionine	S-adenosylmethionine	Methylation reactions
Phenylalanine	Tyrosine	Hormone synthesis
Serine	Ethanolamine, phosphoserine	Phospholipid synthesis
	4-Sphingenine	Cerebroside synthesis
Tryptophan	Serotonin	Neurotransmitter
	Niacin	Vitamin
Tyrosine	Melanin	Pigment
	Catecholamines	Hormones
	Thyroxin	

Note: All amino acids have additional roles as energy sources that are important in high-protein diets. See Chapter 23.

stituents of protein molecules, but they are important intermediates in the formation of urea and thus contribute to the synthesis of arginine (see Chapter 15).

The roles of some amino acids, including those not found in proteins, is summarized in Tables 2.10 and 2.11.

PROTEIN STRUCTURE

The basic structure common to all proteins is the *peptide bond,* which is formed by condensation of the carboxyl group of one amino acid with the amino group of another. In this way chains are created; these chains range from the smallest

TABLE 2.11
A Selected List of Amino Acids That Are Important Metabolites but Do Not Occur in Proteins

Name	Molecular Weight	Formula	Function
Ornithine	132	$\underset{\displaystyle |}{\text{NH}_2}$ $\underset{\displaystyle |}{\text{NH}_2}$ CH$_2$—CH$_2$—CH$_2$—CH—COOH	Urea synthesis Citrulline synthesis
Citrulline	175	NH$_2$ | C=O | NH $\quad$ NH$_2$ |$\qquad\quad$| CH$_2$—CH$_2$—CH$_2$—CH—COOH	Urea synthesis Glutamine metabolism
Argininosuccinic acid	290	COOH | NH—CH—CH$_2$—COOH | C=NH | NH $\qquad$ NH$_2$ |$\qquad\qquad$| CH$_2$—CH$_2$—CH$_2$—CH—COOH	Urea synthesis
Homocysteine	135	SH $\qquad$ NH$_2$ |$\qquad\quad$| CH$_2$—CH$_2$—CH—COOH	Methionine metabolism
Cysteinesulfinic acid	153	O || SOH $\;$ NH$_2$ |$\qquad$| CH$_2$—CH—COOH	Cysteine catabolism

TABLE 2.11 (continued)

Name	Molecular Weight	Formula	Function
Cystathionine	222	NH_2—CH—COOH, —CH$_2$—, S—CH$_2$—CH$_2$—CH(NH_2)—COOH	Methionine metabolism Cysteine synthesis
Homoserine	119	OH—CH$_2$—CH$_2$—CH(NH_2)—COOH	Methionine metabolism
Saccharopine	276	COOH—CH(NH_2)—CH$_2$—CH$_2$—COOH, NH—CH$_2$—CH$_2$—CH$_2$—CH$_2$—CH(NH_2)—COOH	Lysine metabolism
Dihydroxyphenylalanine	197	HO, HO—C$_6$H$_3$—CH$_2$—CH(NH_2)—COOH	Melanin synthesis Phenylalanine/tyrosine metabolism
Thyroxine	777	(diiodophenol)—O—(diiodophenol)—CH$_2$—CH(NH_2)—COOH	Thyroid hormone precursor

TABLE 2.11 (continued)

Name	Molecular Weight	Formula	Function
Other Amino Acids			
β-Alanine	89	$\underset{\displaystyle |}{NH_2}$ CH_2-CH_2-COOH	Part of coenzyme A. Part of carnosine. Formed from aspartate and also in pyrimidine metabolism
β-Amino isobutyric acid	103	$\underset{\displaystyle |}{NH_2}$ $\underset{\displaystyle |}{CH_3}$ $CH_2-CH-COOH$	Pyrimidine metabolism
γ-Amino butyric acid (GABA)	103	$\underset{\displaystyle |}{NH_2}$ $CH_2-CH_2-CH_2-COOH$	Neurotransmitter formed from glutamate
Taurine	125	$\underset{\displaystyle |}{NH_2}$ $CH_2-CH_2-SO_3H$	Bile acid constituent. Possible neurotransmitter
δ-Aminolevulinic acid	131	$\underset{\displaystyle |}{NH_2}$ $\overset{\displaystyle O}{\|}$ $CH_2-C-CH_2-CH_2-COOH$	Porphyrin synthesis

55

peptide units, such as glutathione which contains only 3 amino acids, to complex polymers of 1,000 or more.

Peptide bond

$$H_3N^+ -CH-COO^- + H_3N^+ -CH-COO^- \longrightarrow H_3N^+ -CH \overset{O}{\underset{C}{||}} -N-CH-COO^- + H_2O$$

R	R′	R H R′
Amino acid	**Amino acid**	**Dipeptide**

Naming of compounds formed by peptide bonds follows the convention that a compound with two residues is a *dipeptide,* with three a *tripeptide* and so on. Relatively short chains of several residues are called *oligopeptides* and longer chains are called *polypeptides*. With more than 100 residues, they are called *proteins*. The cut-off points are not sharp and polypeptides with less than 100 residues can be described as proteins if their conformations are well defined.

The chain direction of a polypeptide coincides with the chain synthesis *in vivo* which is from the amino end (N terminus) to the carboxyl end (C terminus). The geometry and dimensions of the peptide bond were derived by Pauling (1951).

The sequence in which amino acids are arranged in the peptide chain is known as the *primary structure* of the molecule (Fig. 2.4a). The proper sequence of amino acids tends to be a critical factor in protein function. In some heritable diseases, such as sickle cell anemia, the defect is due to the genetic substitution of only one amino acid for another in the hemoglobin molecule. (See Chapter 16.)

Biological activity of a protein, however, depends not only on the sequence of the amino acids but also on the spatial arrangement of the long peptide chain. Although the peptide bond is the primary and also the strongest linkage in the protein polymer, other types of bonding occur. These additional linkages or *secondary bonds* are partly responsible for the arrangement of the molecule (see Fig. 2.4b).

A very important linkage in the protein molecule is the hydrogen bond, a weak attachment between the hydrogen atom of an amino group and the oxygen of a carboxyl group (Fig. 2.5). A peptide chain may be held in a coiled or helical form by a series of hydrogen bonds that, although individually weak, are cumulatively strong enough to stabilize the structure. The uncharged polar amino acids are the sites of hydrogen bonding.

Another type of secondary bonding occurs by means of the disulfide linkage of two cysteine residues in a single polypeptide or in different peptide chains (see Fig. 2.5). Disulfide bonds appear to form spontaneously *in vitro* and can occur both between and within polypeptide chains. Disulfide bonds give extra stability to proteins but sometimes can be broken without loss of the protein's function.

The structure of proteins is dependent on the patterns of folding and association of polypeptide chains. Four levels of organization are recognized. Although the

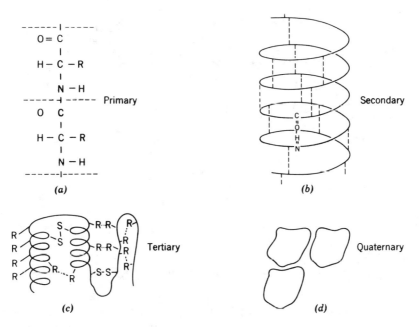

Figure 2.4
Schematic representation of the structural levels in proteins. Amino acid chains are denoted by R, noncovalent interactions by . . . (From E. D. P. DeRobertis et al., *Cell Biology*, 5th ed., W. B. Saunders Co., Philadelphia, 1970, p. 53.)

concepts cannot be defined with precision, the IUPAC-IUB has recommended the following definitions:

1. The *primary structure* of a protein is the amino acid sequence of the polypeptide chain(s) without regard to spatial arrangement. Since this definition does not include the positions of disulfide bonds, it is not identical with "covalent structure."
2. The *secondary structure* of a segment of polypeptide chain is the local spatial arrangement of its main chain atoms without regard to the conformation of its side chains or to its relationship with other segments.
3. The *tertiary structure* of a protein molecule, or of a subunit of a protein molecule, is the arrangement of all its atoms in space, without regard to its relationship with neighboring molecules or subunits.
4. The *quaternary structure* of a protein molecule is the arrangement of its subunits in space and ensemble of its intersubunit contacts and interactions, without regard to the internal geometry of the subunits. A protein molecule that is not made up of at least potentially separable subunits (not connected by covalent bonds) possesses no quaternary structure. Examples of proteins without quaternary structure are ribonuclease (1 chain) and chymotrypsin (3 chains).

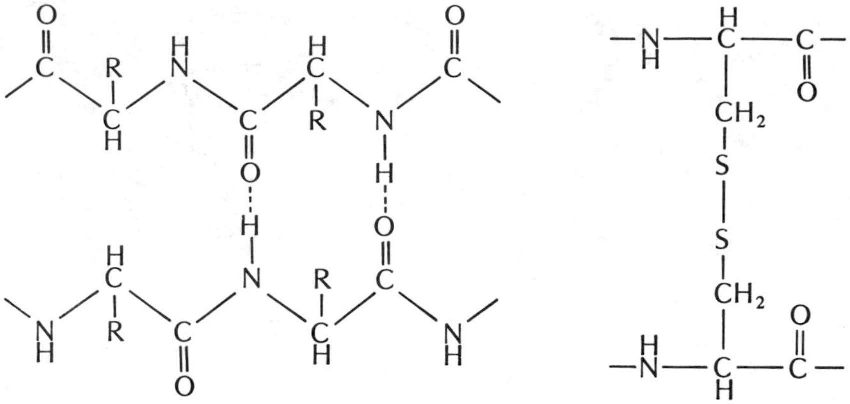

Hydrogen bonding
(dotted lines)

Disulfide bonding

Figure 2.5
Hydrogen and disulfide bonding between amino acids in a peptide chain.

Two further levels of structural organization have been suggested: *supersecon-dary structures* that denote aggregates of secondary structure and *domains* that refer to those parts of a protein that form well-separated globular regions.

Although all the levels of organization are important in understanding the functions of proteins, the primary level, that is, the amino acid sequence, is fundamental and it alone determines the resulting protein structure. Secondary structures are regular arrangements of the polypeptide chain which are stabilized by hydrogen bonds between peptide, amide, and carboxyl groups. Like any long repeating polymer, polypeptide chains tend to form coils. The most common coil is the α-helix. The α-helix is formed by hydrogen bonding of the —NH of each amino acid residue to the —C=O groups of the fourth following residue on an adjacent turn of the helix (see Fig. 2.6). There are 3.6 amino acid residues in each complete turn of the helix. Other types of helix are possible but are less common.

Collagen is also helical in structure, but it is a superhelix (Fig. 2.6) formed by three parallel left-handed helices. It also contains some hexose molecules attached to hydroxylysine residues. (See Chapter 17.) Collagen is one of the most abundant proteins in nature. Its extended polypeptide chain allows it to withstand strong mechanical tension along its axis and makes it suitable as a force transmitter in tendons (Bailey and Etherington, 1980).

Polypeptide chains can also form folded sheetlike structures. Pleated sheets are divided into two categories, parallel and antiparallel. In the former, carboxyl and amino terminal ends are in the same direction whereas in the latter they are in opposite directions. An example of a pleated sheet is shown in Fig. 2.7.

The tertiary structure involves the arrangement and interrelationship of the folded chains (secondary structure) of a protein into a specific shape which is maintained by salt bonds, hydrogen bonds, —S—S bridges, Van der Walls' forces, and hydrophobic interactions (Fig. 2.4c).

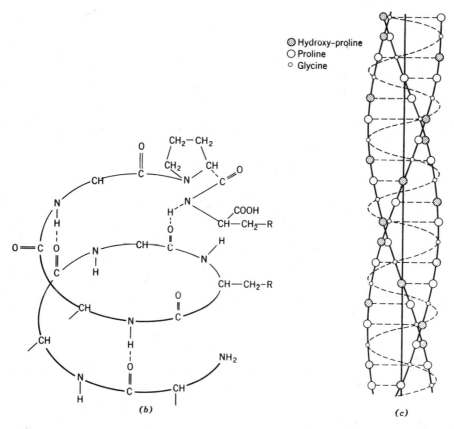

Figure 2.6
(a) Alpha-helix (From I. H. Page, *Arch. Int. Med.*, 111:112, 1963. (b) Superhelix. (From F. O. Schmitt, *Biophysical Science*, F. L. Oncley, ed., Wiley, New York, 1959, p. 352.)

Quaternary structures are the association of protein subunits into oligomers with some degree of symmetry. Because weaker noncovalent forces hold the subunits together, they can be dissociated under relatively mild conditions. Combination of subunits in this manner is essential for the aggregate structures to function (e.g., hemoglobin, actomyosin). The function of isozymes (isoenzymes) is the result of varying proportions of several subunits that produce different kinetic properties to the enzyme.

The ultimate goal of studies of protein structure is the explanation of biological function. In general, a protein has a special structure and, hence, a special function. However it is now clear that multifunctional proteins exist (see Bisswanger and Schimcke-Ott, 1980). These proteins combine several autonomous functions that exist independently at different domains on the polypeptide chain.

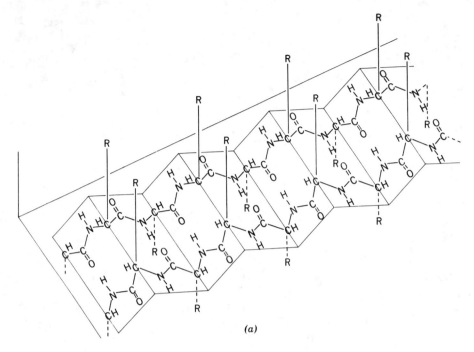

(a)

Figure 2.7
(a) Pleated sheet structure of β-protein chains. (See the description in the text.) (From P. Karlson, 1963.)

PROTEIN CLASSIFICATION

Early systems devised for classification of proteins were based on solubility and chemical properties but such properties, determined on isolated proteins under laboratory conditions, are of only limited value when applied to living systems. As more data on protein structure become available it should be possible to establish a more precise system of classification with the ultimate aim of correlating structural characteristics with biochemical function. (See Hess and Ruply, 1971.)

Present information on structure and solubility may nevertheless be coordinated to provide a useful although likely an artificial and ill-defined system (Table 2.12). The problem of classification is further complicated by the realization that protein is usually present in the cell in combination with nonprotein substances, such as lipids, nucleic acids, carbohydrates, and various metals; these conjugated proteins perform specific functions that neither constituent could properly perform alone. For example, neither the lipid nor protein moiety of a lipoprotein provides the requisite selectivity of a cell membrane; neither could riboflavin nor its associated protein individually perform the enzymatic function of a flavin nucleotide. In other words, neither protein nor any other cell constituents are apt to occur and function as single entities.

Although the classifications shown in Table 2.12 are crude they are widely used and are the best available at this time. Glycoproteins and lipoproteins will be discussed in more detail later in this chapter. Further details on the properties of some other proteins can be found in a number of books and reviews, for example, phosphoproteins (Weller, 1979; Rosen and Krebs, 1981), metalloproteins (Brown et al., 1977), nucleoproteins (Delange and Smith, 1979), and protein fibers (Asquith, 1977; Bornstein and Traub, 1979). In addition, a large body of data on physical and chemical properties (amino acid composition, sequence, molecular weight, molar extinction coefficients, etc.) of proteins of all types can be found in the three volumes of the *Handbook of Biochemistry and Molecular Biology* (Fasman, 1976).

PROTEIN-ENERGY MALNUTRITION (P-EM)

Uncomplicated protein or amino acid deficiency probably never occurs in humans. The disease syndrome of kwashiorkor first described by Williams (1933) is believed to be due to protein deficiency, but it occurs to varying degrees in conjunction with energy deficiency. For this reason the term protein energy malnutrition or protein-calorie malnutrition is preferred to the more limiting terms, kwashiorkor or marasmus (Behar et al., 1959) although the latter have not yet been discarded. Indeed, the degree of severity of P-EM ranges in a graded fashion. The two distinct syndromes, marasmus and kwashiorkor, occur at either end of the spectrum; in between there is a continuum that is termed marasmic-kwashiorkor.

The disease syndrome is variable since the degree of both energy and protein malnutrition, as well as other nutrients, will influence the biochemical and clinical changes. (See Scrimshaw and Behar, 1959; McCance and Widdowson, 1968.) In uncomplicated protein deficiency, for example, protein catabolism should be minimal; when total energy is the limiting factor, however, protein catabolism must increase to cover energy needs. (See Chapter 23.) Severe marasmus, or chronic starvation, is characterized by growth retardation, loss of body fat, and muscle wasting. When total caloric intake has been adequate or nearly adequate, as is possible when starchy low-protein foods are dietary staples, the symptoms are more toward changes associated with protein deficiency: pellagra-type dermatitis, fatty liver, changes in texture and pigmentation of hair, gastrointestinal disturbances, and diarrhea with resulting loss of electrolytes. The lesion appears to be the result of a deficiency of amino acids for protein synthesis and, indeed, most of the symptoms can be attributed to reduced synthesis. Analyses of liver biopsy samples suggest that approximately one-third of liver protein may be lost (Waterlow and Weisz, 1956). Enzyme changes are highly variable and depend both on the degree of deficiency and the tissue examined (Waterlow, 1959). Some differences and similarities in response to predominately protein deficiency (kwashiorkor) and energy deficiency (marasmus) are shown in Table 2.13.

Adaptation to a lack of food allows maintenance of homeostasis for prolonged periods. This adaptation is an efficient protective response. The breakdown of

TABLE 2.12
Protein Classification Based on Solubility and on Composition

Classification Type	Protein	Characteristics	Examples	Nonprotein Components
SOLUBILITY				
	Albumin	Soluble in water and in dilute acid, base, and salt solutions. Precipitated by saturation with $(NH_4)_2SO_4$	Lactalbumin Ovalbumin Serum albumin	
	Globulin	Soluble in salt solutions, insoluble in water	Immunoglobulin Fibrinogen Myosin	Carbohydrate
	Histones	Basic; soluble in water, dilute acids and alkalis, insoluble in dilute ammonia	Thymus histone Nucleoproteins	Nucleic acids
	Protamines	Soluble in water, dilute acids, alkalis, and ammonia. High arginine content	Sperm protamine	Nucleic acids
	Collagens	Insoluble, resistant to digestive enzymes, high in hydroxyproline, low in sulfur-containing amino acids.	Skin, tendon, bone proteins	
	Elastins	Insoluble, partially resistant to digestive enzymes	Artery, tendon, and elastic tissue protein	
	Keratins	Highly insoluble, very resistant to digestive enzymes; many S-S bridges	Skin, hair, and nail protein	

COMPOSITION

Class	Description	Examples	Composition
Nucleoproteins	Often histones present that stabilize DNA in a compact form	Viruses, chromosomes	Nucleic acids
Glycoproteins, Mucoproteins	Many or few carbohydrate chains but CHO present in short, highly branched chains. Level of hexosamine distinguishes glycoproteins and mucoproteins	Immunoglobulins Serum and globulins. Blood group specificity proteins	Carbohydrate: (mucopolysaccharide hexosamines)
Lipoproteins, Proteolipids	May have solubility characteristics of proteins or lipids depending on proportions present. Present in cell and organelle membranes and nerve sheaths	Chylomicrons, HDL, LDL, and VLDL's. Myelin	Lipids (triglycerides, cholesterol, cholesterol esters)
Phosphoproteins	Present in proteins for nutrition of the young (e.g., eggs and milk). Calcium present by chelation	Phosphovitin (egg) Casein	Ester-linked phosphoric acid
Metalloproteins	Metals attached directly to protein, i.e., not part of a nonprotein prosthetic group	Cerruloplasmin Ferritin Carboxypeptidase Transferrin Xanthine oxidase (metalloenzyme)	Copper Iron Zinc Iron Molybdenum, iron FAD
Chromoproteins	Proteins in association with a nonprotein pigment. Frequently involved in oxidation and reduction reactions	Flavoproteins Myoglobin Hemoglobin Cytochromes	Riboflavin (FAD) Heme (iron containing porphyrin) Hemin-Heme

TABLE 2.13
Some Comparisons Between Marasmus and Kwashiorkor

Feature	Marasmus	Kwashiorkor
GENERAL		
Incidence	Worldwide	Regional
Age	Less than 1 year	1–2 years
CLINICAL SIGNS		
Edema	Absent	Present
Dermatosis	Rare	Common
Enlarged liver	Common	Very common
Muscle and fat wasting	Severe	Mild
Stunting	Severe	Moderate
Anemia	Common and severe	Mild
BIOCHEMICAL SIGNS		
Total body water	High	High
Extracellular water	Moderate	High
Body potassium	Some depletion	Much depletion
Fatty liver	Absent	Common and severe
Serum proteins	Slightly low	Very low
Serum albumin	Slightly low	Very low
Essential amino acids/ nonessential amino acids	Normal	Reduced
LDL	Normal	Low
Nonesterified fatty acids	Normal	High

Source: Adapted from D. S. McLaren, *Nutrition and its Disorders*, 110–111 (1981).

muscle allows transamination to occur thus providing alanine to the liver for gluconeogenesis. Muscle breakdown also supplies amino acids for synthesis of serum proteins, especially albumin and lipoproteins. Edema is not present in marasmus and few metabolic abnormalities other than wasting occur (Table 2.13; Fig. 2.8).

In contrast, human adaptation to diets that are low in protein and high in carbohydrate is much less efficient and results in a number of metabolic derangements. (Table 2.13; Fig. 2.8). In kwashiorkor, the serum amino acid pool is distorted (Whitehead and Alleyne, 1972). This response may be due to insulin-induced movement of amino acids into muscle accompanied by continued high activity of branched-chain amino acid transaminases in muscle. As a result the ratio of the amino acids glycine, serine, and glutamic acid to branched-chain amino acids in serum is markedly increased and has been used as a means of diagnosing kwashiorkor (Whitehead and Alleyne, 1972). The distorted serum

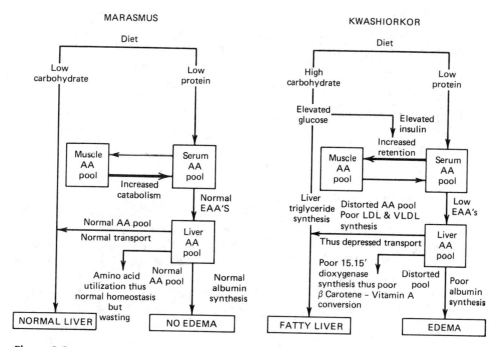

Figure 2.8
Contrasted adaptations to diet in marasmus and kwashiorkor. (From R. G. Whitehead and G. A. O. Alleyne, *Brit. Med. Bull.* 28:72, 1972.)

amino acid pool, thus produced, results in a similarly distorted pool in liver and in reduced synthesis of albumin. Hypoalbuminemia often is related to increased levels of extracellular fluid and frank edema although it is not the sole causative factor.

The distorted liver amino acid pool also interferes with adequate synthesis of lipoprotein fractions necessary for the transport of triglycerides and other lipids from the liver. Thus, lipid accumulates in the liver and in extreme cases of kwashiorkor, fat may account for as much as half of liver weight.

In addition to these metabolic adaptations there are other interrelationships between malnutrition and infection (Keusch and Katz, 1978), and hormonal changes (McLaren, 1981) that occur simultaneously. For additional information on the biochemical and clinical manifestations of P-EM, see Waterlow and Alleyne (1971), Whitehead and Alleyne (1972), and Olson (1975).

Complexes of Carbohydrates, Proteins, and Lipids

As mentioned earlier in this chapter, few nutrients occur or function alone in biological systems. The combinations are innumerable and many such unions will be discussed in later chapters. The following section is devoted to some of the better defined and identifiable complexes of carbohydrates, proteins, and lipids. These include the glycoconjugates and the lipoproteins. The term glycoconjugates includes glycoproteins, proteoglycans, and glycolipids.

GLYCOPROTEINS

The *glycoproteins* contain protein cores to which oligosaccharide chains are attached. The chains vary in length from very few units, as in ribonuclease, to several hundred units, as in the mucus glycoproteins. Two major types of linkage are common: (1) N-acetylgalactosamine linked glycosidically to the hydroxyl groups of serine or threonine residues of the polypeptide, and (2) N-acetylglucosamine linked to asparagine residues.

An important derivative of N-acetylgalactosamine is N-acetylneuraminic acid (sialic acid). The structure of this compound is shown in Fig. 2.9. Several types of sialic acids exist; they differ from each other in the degree of O-acetylation and N-glycolylation. These acids are major carbohydrate components in the human salivary glycoproteins.

Proteoglycans contain mucopolysaccharides attached to a protein. (See Horowitz and Pigman, 1977.) The attachment is often by means of a triad of one D-xylose and two D-galactose units. Typical mucopolysaccharides are the sulfates of chondroitin, dermatin, and heparin. Despite the theoretical distinction between glycoproteins and proteoglycans, they often are referred to simply as glycoproteins. The nomenclature tends to vary and often is confusing.

Glycoproteins and proteoglycans occur in only a limited number of sites (plasma membranes, lysosomes, and extracellular fluid) but include a wide variety of compounds such as enzymes, hormones, antibodies, structural proteins, and

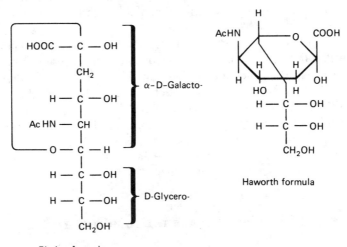

Figure 2.9
Structure of N-acetylneuraminic acid.

plasma membrane components. They also include other important compounds such as the blood group substances, hormone receptors, viral envelopes, and even the antiviral compound, interferon. The distribution and function of some glycoproteins are shown in Table 2.14. The structures of many of the glycoproteins are well identified. (See Horowitz and Pigman, 1977.)

The routes for biosynthesis of several glycoconjugates are outlined in Fig. 2.10. Note that glucosamine-6-phosphate is central to several of the biosynthetic routes.

GLYCOLIPIDS

Glycolipids are compounds that have the solubility properties of a lipid and contain one or more molecules of a sugar. They are often associated with protein in biological systems. The classification of glycolipids is difficult and confusing

TABLE 2.14
Distribution and Function of Some Glycoproteins

Presumed Function	Name
Structural	Bacterial cell wall
	Collagen
	Mucopolysaccharides
Food reserve	Casein
	Endosperm glycoproteins
	Ovalbumin, ovomucoid
	Pollen allergens
Enzyme	Bromelin
	Fungal glucoamylase
	Prothrombin
	Ribonuclease B
	Taka-amylase A
Transport	Ceruloplasmin
	Thyroglobulin
	Transferrin
Hormone	Erythropoietin
	Interstitial cell-stimulating hormone
	Thyroglobulin
Plasma and body fluids	Fetuin
	Fibrinogen
	α-, β-, and γ-Glycoproteins
	Plasminogen
"Protective"	Blood-group substances
	Epithelial mucins
	Fibrin
	γ-Globulins

Source: From R. Montgomery, "Glycoproteins," *The Carbohydrates,* Vol. IIB, Acad. Press, N. Y., 1970, pp. 627–709.

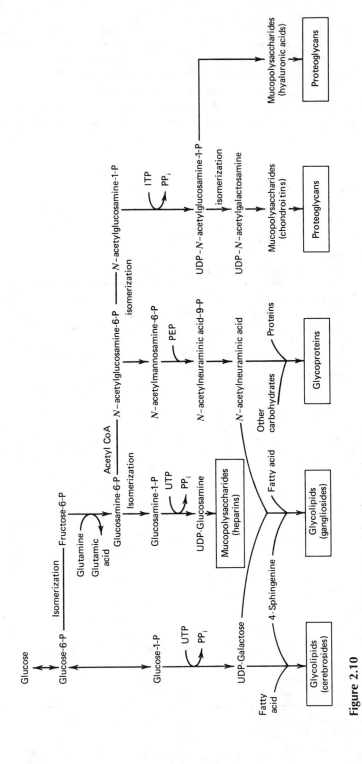

Figure 2.10
Some biosynthetic relationships of the glycoconjugates.

68

as different terms are often used by different workers. For the purpose of this discussion we will follow the nomenclature developed by the IUPAC-IUB Commission on Biochemical Nomenclature (1967). Further, we will be concerned only with those glycolipids of animal origin. The generic terms used are shown in Table 2.15.

Many animal glycolipids are derivatives of a class of compounds known as *ceramides*. These compounds are formed from 4-sphingenine (sphingosine) in which the hydrogen of the amino group attached to carbon 2 is replaced by a long-chain acyl group. The fatty acids vary depending on the tissue source, but they usually contain 16 to 24 carbons and generally are saturated. Fatty acids from some tissue ceramides may contain hydroxyl groups at the carbon-2 position or they may contain an odd number of carbon atoms. (See McKibbon, 1970.) The sugars present in glycolipids are D-glucose, D-galactose, D-galactose-3-sulfate, L-fucose, 2-acylamido-2-deoxy-D-galactose, 2-acylamido-2-deoxy-D-glucose, and sialic acid. The carbohydrate components contain from one to seven monosaccharides linked in straight or branched chains and glycosidically linked to the primary alcohol group (C-1) of the sphingenine base.

The relationship of these principal glycolipids—the cerebrosides, sulfatides, and gangliosides—to the ceramides and the sphingenine molecule is shown in Fig. 2.11 and their biosynthetic relationships are shown in Fig. 2.10 and Fig. 2.12. Note that UDP-galactose is the most important carbohydrate in the initial synthesis of the glycolipids.

Cerebrosides (and sulfatides) are present in a large amount in the white matter of brain. The myelin cerebrosides are 1-O-β-D-galactopyranosylceramides. The fatty acids of brain cerebrosides generally contain 18 to 24 carbons; they may be even or odd numbered and often contain carbon-2 hydroxyl groups (Kishimoto and Radin, 1966). Cerebrosides are also found in other tissues including blood serum, erythrocytes, liver, spleen, and kidney, but the amounts present are usually considerably less than that found in brain myelin.

Gangliosides also are present in high amounts in brain tissue and in lesser

TABLE 2.15
Generic Terms for the Mammalian Glycolipids

Sphingolipid	Any lipid containing a long chain base
Glycosphingolipid	Any lipid containing a long-chain base and one or more sugars
Glycoglycerolipid	Any lipid containing glycerol fatty acid (or fatty ether) and carbohydrate
Ceramide	A N-acyl long-chain base
Cerebroside	A galactose-substituted ceramide
Ganglioside	A glycosphingolipid containing neuraminic acid

Source: Adapted from Sweeley and Sidduqui (1977).

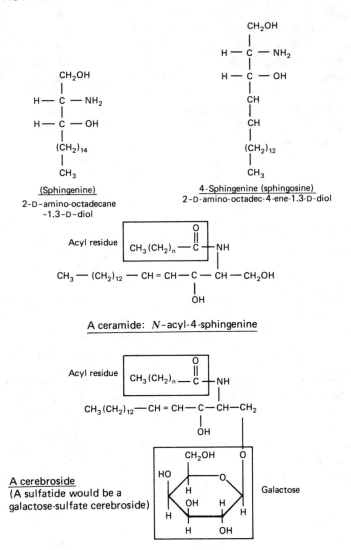

Figure 2.11
Chemical structures of the cerebrosides and related compounds.

amounts in other tissues. In many animal species 79 to 96 percent of the fatty acid in brain gangliosides is stearic acid (Trams et al., 1962).

A number of heritable diseases are due to enzyme deficiencies that result in the abnormal accumulation of glycolipids in various tissues. These include ganglioside accumulation in Tay-Sachs disease and neurovisceral gangliosidosis and cerebroside accumulation in Gaucher's disease, Fabry's syndrome, and metachromatic leucodystrophy. These diseases are usually fatal in early childhood. Victims of Fabry's syndrome, however, often survive well into adulthood.

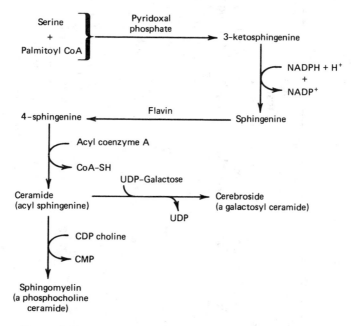

Figure 2.12
The biosynthetic routes for sphingomyelin and the cerebrosides.

The function of the glycolipids as components of the plasma membrane will be discussed in Chapter 9. For more detailed information concerning these compounds see McKibbin (1970), Gurr and James (1971), and Sweeley and Siddiqui (1977).

LIPOPROTEINS

Lipids and proteins are associated in a wide variety of complexes that are significant in both the structure and function of cells. The exact nature of the lipid-protein bond is not well defined. Indeed much remains to be learned about these complex entities. Lipoproteins appear to be of two types. Those that exist as relatively discrete and identifiable macromolecules are called *soluble types*. Those that are aggregates of the complex membrane structure are called *membrane types or structural lipoproteins*. The latter type, also known as proteolipids, are the most difficult to characterize precisely.

Lipoproteins are synthesized in the intestinal mucosa and the liver. They are generally large complexes with a micellar structure that contains triacylglycerols and cholesteryl esters surrounded by a hydrophilic envelope containing phosphatidyl choline and protein. The protein appears to be aligned with the hydrophobic regions on the inside and the hydrophilic areas on the outside of the micelle (Smith et al., 1978). The combination of lipid and protein is advantageous because it permits the transport of a host of water-insoluble lipid compounds.

TABLE 2.16
Classification and Functions of Human Serum Lipoproteins

Fraction	Abbreviation	Electrophoretic Mobility	Flotation Units (SF)	Density Range g/ml	Diameter nm	Approximate Molecular Weight	Amount Present In Normal Plasma mg/dl	Transport Function
Chylomicra			>400	<0.95	>100	500	100–250	Triglyceride from GI tract
Very low density	VLDL	Pre-β	20–400	0.95–1.006	30–80	5–100	130–200	Triglyceride from liver
Intermediate density[a]	IDL	β	12–20	1.006–1.019	25–30	3–5	210–400	Triglyceride cholesterol
Low density	LDL	β	6–12	1.019–1.063	20–25	2–3	?	Cholesterol triglyceride
High density	HDL$_2$	α	0–6	1.063–1.12	10–20	0.3	50–130	Cholesterol
High density	HDL$_3$	α	?	1.12–1.21	7–10	0.2	290–400	Cholesterol

Source: Based on the original classification by DeLalla and Gofman (1954) and Gofman et al. (1954) with additional information from White et al. (1978) and Scanu and Landsberger (1980).

[a]IDL appears to be formed in the plasma during the conversion of VLDL to LDL (Eisenberg, 1980).

TABLE 2.17
Composition of the Major Human Serum Lipoproteins

	Approximate Composition—Percent					
	Protein	Triglyceride	Phospholipid	Cholesterol Ester	Cholesterol	Major Apoproteins
Chlylomicra	2	83	7	6	2	B,C-I,C-II
VLDL	9	50	18	15	7	B,C-I,C-II,C-III,E[a]
LDL	21	10	22	38	8	B
HDL_2[b]	33	8	29	23	7	A-I,A-II
HDL_3	57	5	21	14	3	A-I,A-II

Source: Based on the original classification by DeLalla and Gofman (1954) and Gofman et al. (1954) with additional information from White et al. (1978) and Scanu and Landsberger (1980). (IDL are not well characterized but apparently contain triglyceride and cholesterol in amounts that are intermediate between those of VLDL and LDL.)

[a]Apoprotein E is also known as arginine-rich protein.

[b]HDL_1 exists but is present in very small quantities.

Two major methods of chemical separation of the lipoproteins have been developed: one based on ultracentrifugation and the other on electrophoresis. (See Lingren, 1980.) Thus, two systems of terminology have arisen. The high density lipoproteins, for example, are known as HDL when separated by ultracentrifugation or as α-lipoproteins when separated by electrophoresis.

As analytical procedures have become more discriminating, the number of definitive fractions has increased. However, the known fractions are heterogeneous and contain a range of molecules that vary in size and composition. The physical properties of the six major classes, their abbreviations, the relative amounts present in normal plasma, and their major transport roles are shown in Table 2.16.

The lipid and protein components of the major serum lipoproteins are shown in Table 2.17. The proteins comprise several classes and subclasses designated as Apo-A, Apo-B, Apo A-I, Apo A-II and so on. (See Scanu et al., 1980.) Several of these proteins have been sequenced and vary in length from 57 amino acid residues in Apo C-I to 245 residues in Apo A-I (Osborne and Brewer, 1977). It has been suggested that the apoproteins contain helical segments with one part primarily hydrophilic and the other hydrophobic. Such a structure could account for their lipid-binding capacity. The term "amphipathic helix" has been coined to describe this structure. Evidence to support the structure is based on the *in vitro* synthesis of peptide fragments capable of forming lecithin complexes that have some of the characteristics of lipoproteins. (See Smith et al., 1978.)

Nucleotides and Nucleic Acids

NUCLEOTIDES

Nucleotides consist of three parts: a nonprotein heterocyclic nitrogen base, ribose (or deoxyribose), and a phosphate group (or groups). In most cases the base is a purine or pyrimidine, but one important nucleotide contains niacinamide. The latter will be discussed in Chapter 3. The structures of the purines and pyrimidines are shown in Fig. 2.13.

The nitrogen base is attached to carbon 1 of the pentose sugar that in turn is attached to the phosphate group at carbon 5. The basic structure of the nucleotides is as follows.

A ribose nucleotide

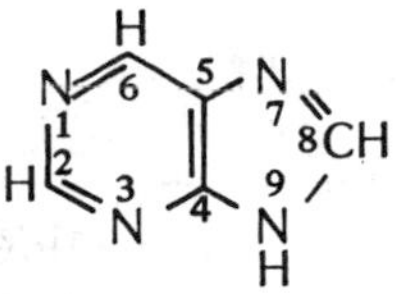

Purine

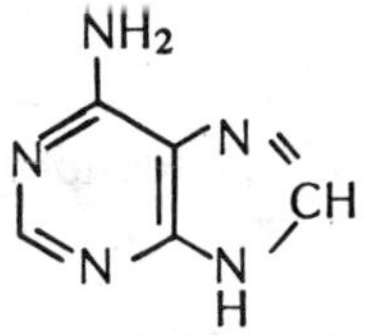

Adenine
(6-aminopurine)

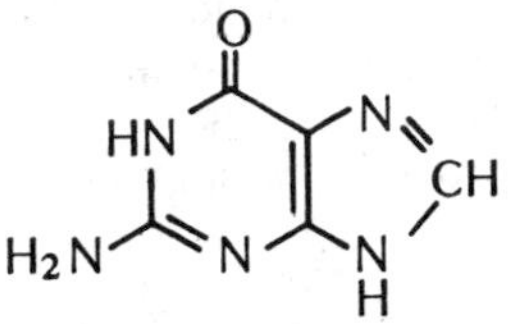

Guanine
(2-amino-6-oxypurine)

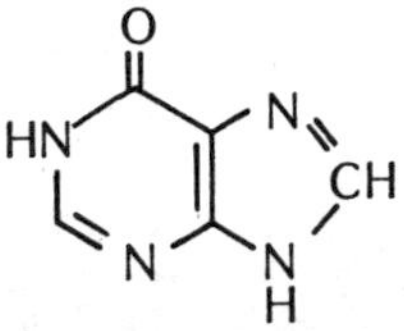

Hypoxanthine
(6-oxypurine)

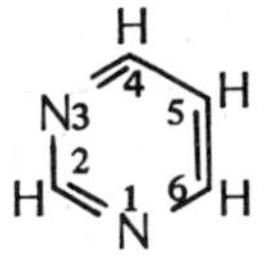

Pyrimidine

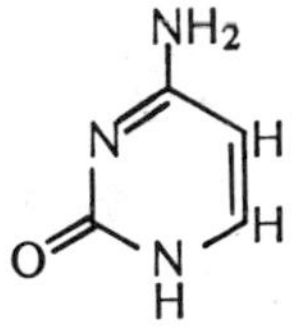

Cytosine
(2-oxy-4-aminopyrimidine)

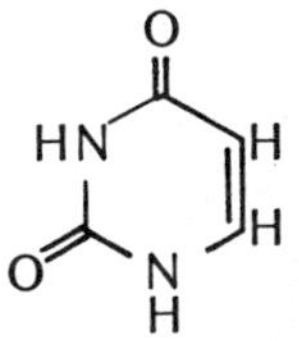

Uracil
(2,4-dioxypyrimidine)

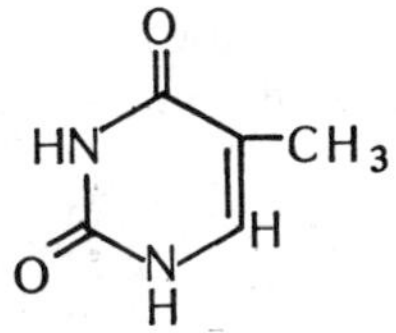

Thymine
(5-methyl-2,4-dioxypyrimidine)

Figure 2.13
Structure of the purines and pyrimidines.

Nucleotides without the phosphate group are called nucleosides. Both take their names from the nitrogen base present in the formula. The purines and pyrimidines and their corresponding nucleosides and nucleotides are shown in Table 2.18.

The nucleotides are important in cellular metabolism. Nucleosides, as such, rarely are involved in metabolic reactions and are significant chiefly as components of the nucleotides.

TABLE 2.18
The Major Purines and Pyrimidines and Their Corresponding Nucleosides and Nucleotides

Nitrogen Base	Nucleoside	Nucleotide
PURINES		
Adenine (6-amino purine)	Adenosine	Adenosine monophosphate (AMP) or adenylic acid
Guanine (2-amino-6-oxypurine)	Guanosine	Guanosine monophosphate (GMP) or guanylic acid
Hypoxanthine (6-oxypurine)	Inosine	Inosine monophosphate (IMP) or inosinic acid
PYRIMIDINES		
Uracil (2,6-dioxypyrimidine)	Uridine	Uridine monophosphate (UMP) or uridylic acid
Cytosine (2-oxy-6-amino pyrimidine)	Cytidine	Cytidine monophosphate (CMP) or cytidylic acid
Thymine (5-methyl uracil)	Thymidine	Thymidine monophosphate (TMP) or thymidylic acid

AMP and ATP

Adenosine-5'-monophosphate (AMP) is one of the most important of the nucleotides. It is a part of the nucleic acids (as are several other nucleotides) and of the niacinamide nucleotides. It is also the precursor of adenosine diphosphate (ADP) and adenosine triphosphate (ATP), which are involved in cellular energy transfer. The participation of these compounds in energy metabolism will be discussed in Chapter 13. The structure of ATP is shown as follows.

Adenosine triphosphate (ATP)

The other nucleotides shown in Table 2.18 also form di- and triphosphates. These compounds also are involved in energy transfer in a minor way but are most significant in the metabolism of carbohydrates (see Chapter 11) and as components of the nucleic acids (see below).

Cyclic AMP

Adenosine-3',5'-monophosphate or cyclic AMP (cAMP) was among the most exciting discoveries of the past 25 years. This compound is produced from ATP through the action of an enzyme—adenyl cyclase—which is stimulated by a vast number of hormones including catecholamines, glucagon, luteinizing hormone, vasopressin, parathyroid hormone, prostaglandins, and thyrocalcitonin as well as other biologically active agents such as histamine and serotonin. Cyclic AMP in fact was discovered as a result of studies aimed at delineating the mechanism of the hyperglycemic action of epinephrine and glucagon. (See Robison et al., 1971.) The structure of cAMP is shown below.

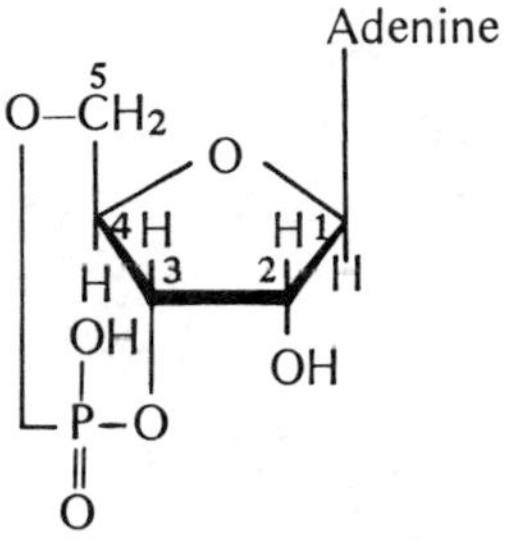

Adenine

O–CH_2 (5)
O
4H H1
H 3 2 1'I
OH
OH
P–O
O

Adenosine-3',5' -monophosphate (cAMP)

Cyclic AMP was described by Sutherland (see Robison et al., 1968) as a *second messenger* indicating that cAMP mediates the effects of hormones and other active agents. The number and variety of agents stimulating cAMP synthesis suggests that the reactions influenced by this cyclic nucleotide are extremely varied. Indeed cAMP plays a regulatory role in cellular metabolism and controls the rate of a number of cellular reactions as varied as the synthesis and activity of proteins, glycogenolysis, lipolysis, steroidogenesis, and active transport. This ubiquitious compound will be discussed further in Parts III and IV. For excellent reviews on this subject see Robison et al. (1971), Hardman et al. (1971), Jost and Rickenberg (1971), and Pastan et al. (1975).

NUCLEIC ACIDS

Nucleic acids are polynucleotides formed by the joining together of many mononucleotides. Two types of nucleic acids exist: deoxyribonucleic acid (DNA) and ribonucleic acid (RNA). They are distinguished by differences in the pentose in the molecule and by the structure of one of the four nucleotide bases present in the molecule.

DNA

Deoxyribonucleic acid is made up of four nucleotides: AMP, TMP, CMP, and GMP that contain, respectively, the bases adenine, thymine, cytosine, and guanine. Deoxyribose is the pentose component. These four nucleotides are linked

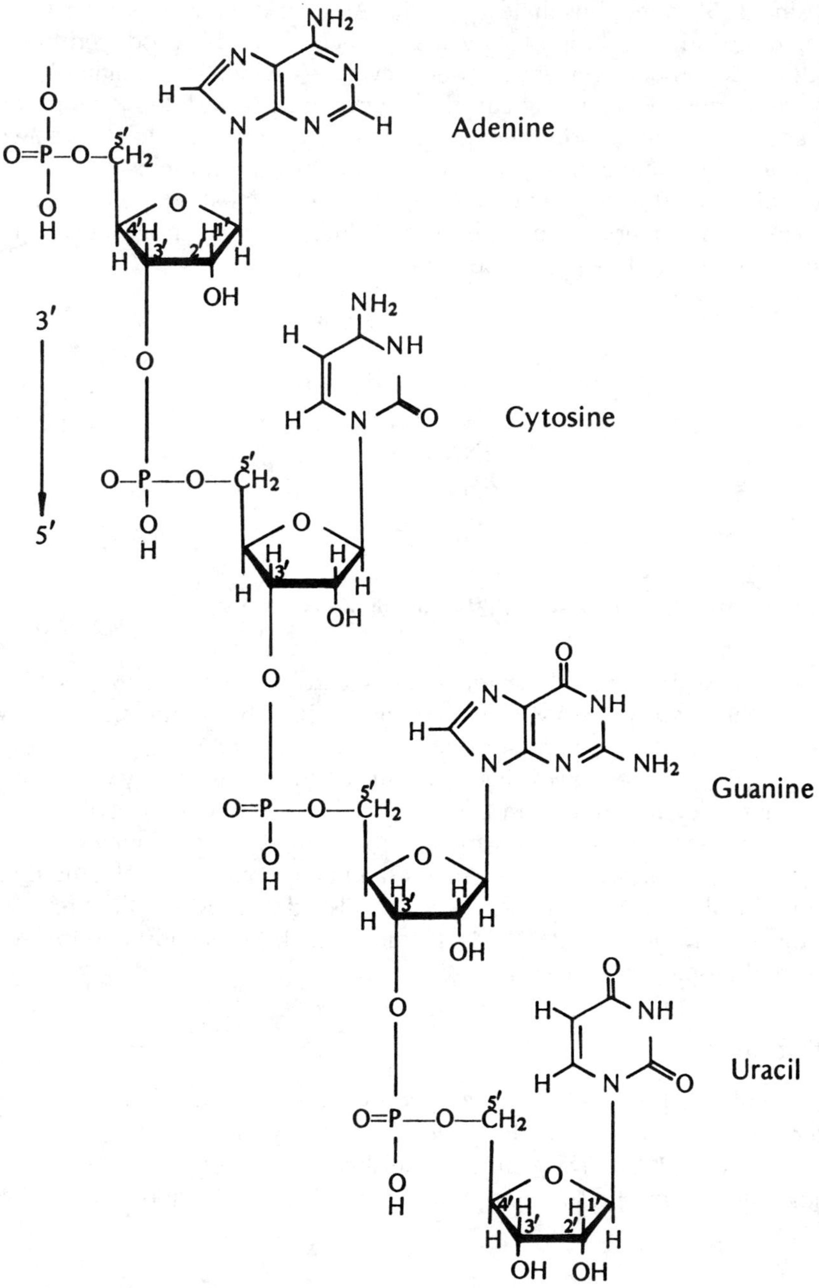

Figure 2.14
Section of chain of nucleotides in DNA.

together in long polymeric chains, the 3-hydroxyl of the pentose joined to the phosphate of the adjacent nucleotide (Fig. 2.14). The pairing of the two strands always occurs by the sharing of three hydrogen bonds by cytosine and guanine and the sharing of two hydrogen bonds by adenine and thymine (Fig. 2.15). The pairing of bases and the double helical structure of the molecule discovered and described by Watson and Crick (1953) is characteristic of all DNA from the simplest one-celled organism to the most specialized cell of the largest mammals. The differences in the DNA, and therefore the differences in the genes and characteristics of species, are due to the order of the nucleotides in the strand and to the length of the strand which can vary from several thousand angstroms (Å) to several millimeters (1 mm = 10^7 Å). The sequence of the nucleotides in the strand provides the code for genetic information. (See Chapter 10.)

The established sequence of the nucleotides in one DNA strand will always determine the sequence in the paired strand. This provides the means whereby DNA can replicate itself and, barring error, transmit the exact code to a daughter

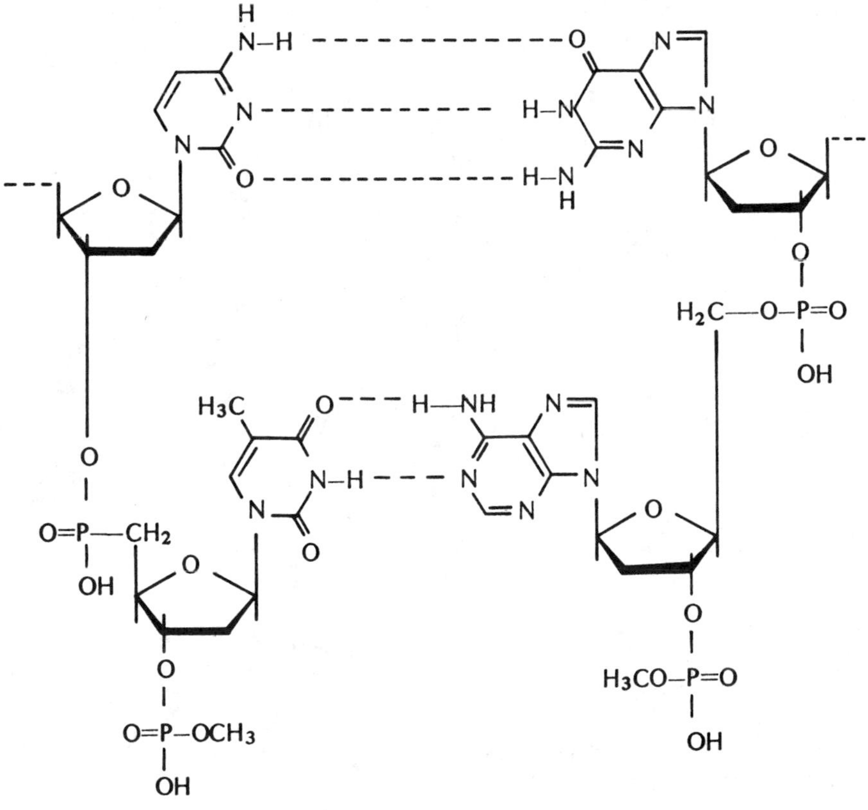

Figure 2.15
Section of helix showing details of base pairing.

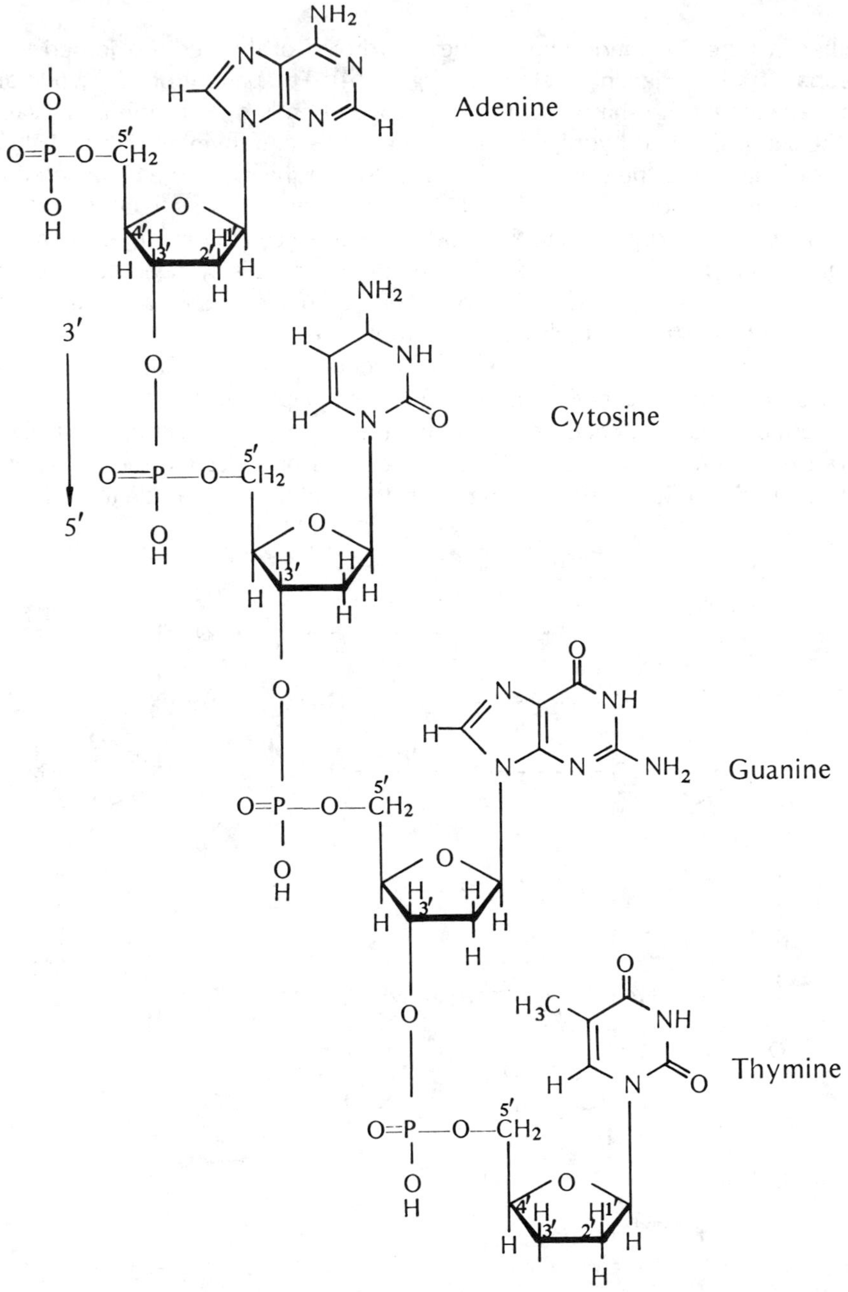

Figure 2.16
Section of nucleotide chain of RNA showing substitution of ribose for deoxyribose and uracil for thymine.

cell. Replication takes place under the influence of the enzyme DNA polymerase. Kornberg (1960) purified DNA polymerase from *Escherichia coli* and found that with the enzyme, a strand of DNA as a template, and a supply of nucleotides the synthesis of DNA could proceed *in vitro*. The enzyme produced long chains of nucleotides by base-pairing to produce a macromolecule with most of the properties associated with DNA isolated from nature.

RNA

The chemical constituents of RNA differ from those in DNA in two respects: the pentose is ribose instead of deoxyribose, and uracil is substituted for thymine, making the base content cytosine, guanine, adenine, and uracil (Fig. 2.16). The structure of RNA differs from DNA in that it is a single strand containing less than a hundred subunits, whereas DNA is a double helical structure with many thousands of subunits. The two, RNA and DNA, also differ in some other features; these are summarized in Table 2.19. Ribonucleic acid exists in three forms which can be distinguished by size, function, composition, and location. These are transfer RNA (tRNA), messenger RNA (mRNA), and ribosomal RNA (rRNA).

TABLE 2.19
Major Features of DNA and RNA

Characteristics	DNA	RNA
Sugar		
Major Bases	Deoxy-D-Ribose	D-Ribose
	Adenine	Adenine
Purines	Guanine	Guanine
Pyrimidines	Cytosine	Cytosine
	Thymine	Uracil
Varieties		Transfer RNA (tRNA)
		Messenger RNA (mRNA)
		Ribosomal RNA (rRNA)
Stability to weak alkali	Stable	Hydrolyzed tomononucleotides
Shape	Base paired, double stranded	Single stranded, some basepairing in tRNA
Number of bases	Many, up to 5.5×10^9 base pairs	Relatively few, 80–5,000 depending onvariety and on the proteinbeing synthesized
Associated proteins	Histones in chromatin	Ribosomal protein (enzymes and structural) with rRNA
Where found	Nucleus, mitochondria	Ribosomes, cytoplasm
Role	Information storage	Bridge between genetic information of DNA and specific protein synthesis

Transfer RNA is a single chain polymer with between 75 to 93 subunits. It consist of relatively small molecules and comprises less than 20 percent of cellular RNA. Although tRNA is composed largely of the four main ribonucleotides, it also contains smaller quantities of other nucleotides. Two of these nucleotides, pseudouridine and dihydrouridine, are universally distributed, and various methyl and thio substituted adenines, guanines, and cytosines are common constituents (Fig. 2.17). How these modified nucleotides affect function of tRNA is not clear.

Messenger RNA is the form of RNA that contains the linear sequence of coding for protein synthesis. Like the other types of RNA it is a single strand. Its size and molecular weight vary depending on the size of the polypeptide it encodes.

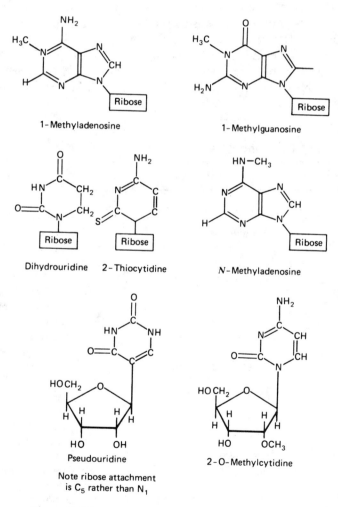

1-Methyladenosine   1-Methylguanosine

Dihydrouridine   2-Thiocytidine   N-Methyladenosine

Pseudouridine   2-O-Methylcytidine

Note ribose attachment is C_5 rather than N_1

Figure 2.17
Structures of some modified bases found in tRNA.

Ribosomal RNA, like tRNA, contains a series of methylated bases and pseudouridine in addition to the major bases adenine, guanine, cytosine, and uracil. It is the most abundant form of RNA in cells and is associated with proteins in the ribosomes.

These forms of RNA collaborate in the transfer and assembly of specific amino acids for protein synthesis and will be discussed in greater detail in Chapter 11.

chapter 3

water-soluble vitamins

The goal of vitamin research is to establish (1) the abnormalities that result when a vitamin is absent from the diet and therefore from cellular metabolism, (2) the metabolic functions that depend on the presence of the vitamin, and (3) the ways that utilization, functions, and, therefore, requirements are modified by physiological and environmental factors. The last goal is the most difficult to attain and, by far, the area in which least is known. In historical perspective and investigational procedure, knowledge of the deficiency disease syndromes must come first. For the modern nutritionist, however, it is clearly more important to think in terms of what vitamins *do* rather than the diseases they prevent.

Vitamins are chemically unrelated organic substances that are grouped together because each is essential in the diet in minute amounts and is required for specific metabolic reactions within the cell. Traditionally they are classified according to their solubility in water or fat and fat solvents and, from a physiological standpoint, this property determines the patterns of transport, excretion, and storage within the animal body. Several of the vitamins, while conveniently considered as a single substance, actually are a group of structurally related compounds that tend to behave alike physiologically. In general, however, physiological function tends to be limited to one active form to which the related forms are converted.

Whether a substance must be supplied intact to the cell or can be synthesized by the cell depends on the assortment of enzymes peculiar to the cell species. A substance, therefore, may be a vitamin for one species but not for another. The difference lies in whether the substance is required in the diet or whether it can be synthesized by the animal. The number of substances supplied by cellular synthesis tends to vary inversely with the complexity of the organism and appears to reflect an evolutionary adaptation as more complex organisms evolved from a simple one cell origin. Thus people depend on their environment for some nutrients that microorganisms and other lower forms of life can synthesize for themselves.

All of the vitamins of the B-complex are known to function as coenzymes. Vitamins, like the hormones, play fundamental catalytic roles in specific metabolic reactions although some vitamins (e.g., ascorbic acid and vitamin E) function in a more general fashion. It is conceivable that the apparent general function may be a secondary effect elicited by a single specific, yet unknown, biochemical action at a variety of sites.

A *coenzyme* may be defined as a small molecule loosely bound to an enzyme protein, or apoenzyme, and easily separated from the protein moiety by dialysis. A *prosthetic* group refers to a molecule that is firmly bound to the enzyme protein and that, on dialysis, remains bound to the enzyme protein. The distinction between the two is of little functional significance and, most often, the two terms are used interchangeably. Both serve as cofactors in enzymatic reactions and contain one of the active sites of the enzyme complex to which the substrate is attached. For most enzyme systems that require coenzymes, the coenzyme (i.e., the vitamin) is part of the active site.

Certain compounds similar in structure to the vitamin molecule (or to the portion of the molecule containing the active site) can replace the vitamin by attaching themselves to the enzyme. These substances are called *antimetabolites* or *metabolic antagonists*. They block the normal action of the coenzyme and, in effect, result in a functional deficiency through competitive inhibition of its actions. Certain other antimetabolites exhibit antivitamin activity because they are capable of blocking biosynthesis of the coenzyme molecule; such compounds may or may not resemble the vitamin in structure. In either case, a condition similar to true vitamin deficiency is produced. Antimetabolites are useful in producing experimental vitamin deficiencies, especially those deficiencies that develop slowly from dietary restriction alone. Antimetabolites are also useful adjuncts in delineating the biochemical pathways in which the vitamin is involved and in relating metabolic disturbances to symptoms of deficiency. (For discussions of antimetabolites see Woolley, 1944a; 1963; and Somogyi, 1973.)

Significantly, the vitamins were discovered not by their presence in the diet but because of their absence. A lack of most of the vitamins known to be required by the human results in typical clinical syndromes or symptoms that can be prevented or cured by adding the necessary vitamin to the diet. This negative approach to the function of the vitamins is a useful tool in research. The investigator obtains some clues to the metabolic role of nutrients when functional failures are observed when the nutrient is absent from the diet.

Carefully controlled studies with many species of animals thus have helped to elucidate the role of vitamins in humans since most nonruminant mammals tend to metabolize most vitamins similarly. Even microorganisms, however, have contributed to knowledge of human nutrition and are useful as test organisms for nutrient analyses. The microbiological assay and the rat and chick bioassays all take advantage of the requirements of these species for specific nutrients since growth or some other response due to an unknown amount of vitamin in food may be measured directly against response to a known amount of pure vitamin.

The clinical course of deficiency, however, may vary widely among species; symptoms observed in a rat, for example, often are quite different from those observed in chicks or in humans. Biochemical lesions tend to be more similar.

To establish that vitamin deficiency results in growth failure or dermatitis or any other symptom establishes a nutrient as essential in the diet and defines the deficiency syndrome so that it can be recognized when it occurs naturally (Table 3.1). It does not, however, establish the function of the nutrient. Only by careful and often tedious experimentation to determine the specific metabolic reactions affected by nutrient deficiency have the basic functions of many of the vitamins been delineated. If we think of cellular metabolism as a series of reactions that

TABLE 3.1
Water-soluble Vitamin Deficiency Symptoms in Humans

Vitamin	Symptoms
Thiamin	Beriberi: chiefly nervous and cardiovascular systems affected; mental confusion, muscular weakness, loss of ankle and knee jerks, painful calf muscles, peripheral paralysis, edema (wet beriberi), muscle wasting (dry beriberi), enlarged heart. Infantile beriberi: cyanosis, dyspnea, tachycardia, aphonia (soundless crying), eventual cardiac failure.
Riboflavin	Ariboflavinosis: cheilosis, angular stomatitis (fissures at the corners of the mouth), nasolabial dermatitis, photophobia, corneal vascularization (not specific).
Nicotinic acid	Pellagra: bilateral dermatitis particularly in areas exposed to sunlight, glossitis, diarrhea, irritability, mental confusion, eventually delirium or psychotic symptoms.
Vitamin B_6	Convulsions in infants. Experimental deficiency in humans: seborrheic dermatitis, glossitis, angular stomatitis, abnormal EEG, hypochromic microcytic anemia, hyperirritability.
Folacin	Glossitis, gastrointestinal disturbances, diarrhea, megaloblastic anemia.
Vitamin B_{12}	Megaloblastic anemia (pernicious anemia when due to intrinsic factor deficiency), severe neurological disorders. Dietary deficiency occasionally seen in strict vegetarians.
Ascorbic acid	Scurvy: red, swollen, bleeding gums; perifolliculosis, poor wound healing, subcutaneous hemorrhage, swelling of joints.

eventually lead to the complete oxidation of foodstuffs, or the synthesis of a phospholipid or of an enzyme protein, it is not difficult to visualize the havoc that could result if any *one* reaction in the sequence is blocked. The experimental nutritionist plays the role of detective who follows a long list of clues before the motive and the culprit of a committed crime are identified. The path is often long and arduous.

Thiamin

The disease beriberi had been known for several centuries before its dietary origin was recognized. Beriberi is characterized by extensive damage to the nervous and cardiovascular systems and may be accompanied by severe muscle wasting (dry beriberi) or edema (wet beriberi). In the late nineteenth century, Takaki, a surgeon in the Japanese navy, demonstrated that addition of meat and whole grains to the customary naval ration resulted in a marked decrease in the incidence of what was then known as "shipboard beriberi." Some 15 years after Takaki's finding, Eijkmann made his famous observations of a beriberi-type syndrome (characterized by a peculiar head retraction of neurological origin) in birds maintained on a diet of highly polished rice. He was able to cure the disease with rice bran. The proper interpretation of Eijkmann's work, however, was left to Grijns, another Dutch physician, who theorized that the disease was due to the lack of a dietary constituent in polished rice that was present in the whole grain. It was not until 1926 that the vitamin was isolated by another group in the Dutch East Indies, Jansen and Donath. Ten years later Williams and Cline (1936) won the race to develop a successful method for synthesis of thiamin; this discovery led to large-scale commercial production of the vitamin.

   Prior to the commercial synthesis of the vitamin, research on thiamin had been limited to a few laboratories. The yield of thiamin isolated from rice bran, for example, was in the order of 5 grams of the vitamin for every ton of bran. Availability of the synthetic vitamin permitted rapid treatment of patients known to be suffering from beriberi; only a few milligrams of the vitamin are necessary to promote dramatic improvement. The early history of thiamin and the drive to eradicate beriberi as a serious threat to the public health was recorded by Williams (1961).

Thiamin

CHEMISTRY

Thiamin is a relatively simple chemical compound composed of linked pyrimidine and thiazole rings; pure thiamin is a base and is very hygroscopic but it is available commercially as the hydrochloride and other stable salts. Thiamin hydrochloride is highly soluble in water and slightly soluble in 95 percent alcohol and absolute ethyl alcohol. In acid solution the vitamin is quite stable at temperatures up to 120°C. In alkaline solution the vitamin decomposes rapidly; decomposition is hastened by heat. Thiamin mononitrate is a white crystalline substance. It is quite soluble in water and is more stable to heat than the hydrochloride. For this reason, thiamin mononitrate often is preferred for fortification of cereal products that have to be cooked. Sulfur dioxide is not allowed as a preservative in foods recognized as major sources of thiamin because sulfite, formed by reaction of SO_2 with water, splits the molecule into its pyrimidine and thiazole moieties, thus destroying the activity of the vitamin. This chemical reaction was used as one of the characterizing reactions in the early determination of the structure of thiamin.

When treated with potassium ferricyanide in alkaline solution, thiamin is converted to a fluorescent compound called thiochrome. This reaction is the basis for the most commonly used chemical determination for the vitamin. (See *Association of Official Agricultural Chemists*, 1960; Association of Vitamin Chemists, 1966; Association of Official Analytical Chemists, 1980.) Several modifications of this method have been described; a most recent one is that of McBride and Wyatt (1983). Thiamin also reacts with diazotized para-aminoacetophenone to form a red-colored complex that can be measured spectrophotometrically. Various microbiological techniques also have been described (Pearson, 1967; Baker et al., 1964; Baker and Frank, 1968). The method of using *Lactobacillus viridescens* as assay organism is more sensitive and more accurate than the thiochrome procedure in analyzing for thiamin in urine (Sauberlich et al., 1979). More recently, an assay using high performance liquid chromatography (HPLC) was described (Walker et al., 1981).

BIOCHEMICAL FUNCTION

As early as 1911 the decarboxylation of pyruvic acid by yeast cells was known to depend on an enzyme—carboxylase. This reaction was shown to require Mg^{++}. Twenty-five years later Peters (1936) reported that thiamin was necessary for carbohydrate metabolism in pigeons and that pyruvate accumulated in tissues of thiamin-deficient birds. This discovery marked the first time that the action of a vitamin had been defined in terms of intermediary metabolism. (See Thompson, 1971.) In the following year the coenzyme of the carboxylase enzyme was isolated from yeast by Lohmann and Schuster (1937) and shown to be thiamin pyrophosphate (TPP). The coenzyme was originally called cocarboxylase and later was known as diphosphothiamin.

Thiamin Pyrophosphate (TPP)

Phosphorylation of free thiamin to the coenzyme requires ATP. The active site of the coenzyme at which combination with substrate takes place is carbon 2 of the thiazole ring, indicated in the formula for TPP by an asterisk. The yeast carboxylase system is a mixture of thiamin, Mg^{++} or Mn^{++}, and the apoenzyme protein.

In mammalian cells TPP functions in several critical metabolic reactions.

1. Oxidative decarboxylation of α-keto acids to carboxylic acids.
   a. Pyruvate → acetyl CoA
   b. α-Ketoglutarate → succinyl CoA
2. Transketolase reaction of the pentose phosphate shunt: transfer of an α-keto group from xylulose-5-phosphate to ribose-5-phosphate to form sedoheptu-lose-7-phosphate and glyceraldehyde-3-phosphate (Fig. 3.1)

These reactions are discussed in detail in Chapters 11 and 13.

The thiamin-dependent decarboxylation reactions catalyzed by the dehydro-genase complexes are necessary for the entry of pyruvate into the citric acid cycle as acetyl CoA and for the production of succinyl CoA from α-ketoglutarate. The reactions catalyzed by transketolase are not directly in the main glycolytic pathway for carbohydrate metabolism. Transketolase is essential in the pentose phosphate pathway, which is the chief source of pentoses for the cell and a major source of NADPH for fatty acid and other biosyntheses. (See Chapter 11.) The stimulation of erythrocyte transketolase by *in vitro* addition of thiamin pyrophosphate may be used to determine thiamin nutritional status (Brin, 1962; see Chapter 24).

TPP, or the closely related thiamin triphosphate, is essential for peripheral nervous system functioning. These forms of the vitamin occur in nerve tissue and appear to play an essential role in transmission of nerve impulses (Pincus et al., 1973). This function correlates closely with the impaired neurological function observed in beriberi. Thiamin may be localized in the synaptosomal membranes (Matsuda and Cooper, 1981).

Although the clinical syndrome of thiamin deficiency (see Table 3.1) and bio-chemical function of the vitamin are well defined, very little is known of how disturbances in metabolic function caused by thiamin deficiency lead to the pathology so characteristic of the disease. One of the first symptoms of thiamin deficiency in experimental animals, for example, is anorexia and subsequent loss of weight. Bai et al. (1971) reported that a decrease in transketolase activity of

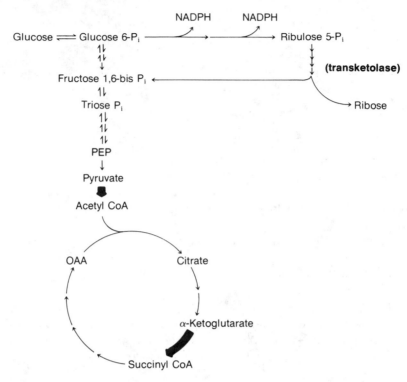

Figure 3.1
Summary of important reactions involving thiamin pyrophosphate. The reactions involving thiamin pyrophosphate are indicated in boldface type. (From Devlin, *Textbook of Biochemistry*, John Wiley, New York, 1982, p. 1213.)

intestinal mucosa correlated more closely with the development of anorexia than did decrease in pyruvate dehydrogenase activity. This evidence, however, does not establish that anorexia is the result of decreased mucosal transketolase activity. Transketolase activity is known to be affected early in thiamin deficiency (Brin, 1962) and simply may coincide with the development of anorexia (Chong, 1970). In contrast to anorexia, the central nervous system is affected late in thiamin deficiency (Truswell et al., 1972).

Moderately severe thiamin deficiency in humans contributes to a group of symptoms known as the Wernicke-Korsakoff syndrome. This syndrome is characterized by mental confusion, memory disturbances, ataxia, opthalmoplegia, and nystagmus. It is most commonly observed in alcoholics (Victor et al., 1971). Thiamin-deficient rats also exhibit polyneuritis, ataxia, and behavioral deficits that persist after recovery from physical signs of the deficiency (Vorhees et al., 1975). It has been suggested that neurological symptoms observed in thiamin deficiency might be due to decreased acetylcholine synthesis as a result of diminished acetyl CoA production accompanying lessened activity of the thiamin-dependent enzyme pyruvate dehydrogenase. Vorhees et al. (1977) report moderate decreases in acetylcholine in certain sections of thiamin-deficient rat brain, but significant decreases only in the midbrain. These data are not strong support for the suggestion that the neurotransmitter acetylcholine is a major factor influencing the development of neurological deficits in thiamin deficiency. Both a mono- and triphosphate of thiamin are known to be present in peripheral nerves and blood of rats (Rindi et al., 1968). Whether these compounds exert a specific effect in nerve tissue is not known.

Similarly, although biochemical defects in heart tissue of thiamin-deficient rats have been studied extensively (Gubler, 1969; McCandless et al., 1970), the mechanism by which thiamin deficiency results in bradycardia and ultimately in heart failure are not resolved. Studies by Phornplutkul et al. (1974) suggest that the primary effect of thiamin deficiency on the cardiovascular system of the rat is the result of an increase in cardiac output caused by an increase in blood flow to the various organs deprived of the vitamin. However, because myocardial oxygen consumption was increased in hearts from thiamin-deficient animals, it is possible that the myocardium is affected directly (ibid.). Clearly, the problem of relating deficiency symptoms to biochemical lesions is a perplexing one; this problem exists not only for thiamin deficiency, however, but for other vitamin and mineral deficiencies as well.

THIAMIN METABOLITES

A large number of thiamin metabolites have been identified in mammalian urine. Ziporin (1965) demonstrated that both pyrimidine and thiazole were excreted in the urine. Excretion of these two compounds remained at high levels even after thiamin excretion ceased on a thiamin-deficient diet. Thiamin, thus, is degraded by cleavage of the molecule to produce the pyrimidine and thiazole moieties. It is further degraded by splitting the thiazole ring so that carbon-2 is released as carbon dioxide (Balaghi and Pearson, 1966). Studies utilizing thiamin labeled with ^{14}C in both the pyrimidine and thiazole rings indicated at least 22 breakdown products from ^{14}C-labeled pyrimidine (Neal and Pearson, 1964) and 29 different products from ^{14}C-labeled thiazole (Balaghi and Pearson, 1966). A refined procedure for isolation of thiamin metabolites from urine was described by Neal (1970) and with this procedure several additional degradation products have been identified. Two major metabolites, 4-methyl-thiazole-5-acetic acid and 2-methyl-4-amino-5-pyrimidine were identified in urine of humans and rats (Amos and Neal, 1970; Ariaey-Nejad et al., 1970).

THIAMIN ANTAGONISTS

Although several thiamin antagonists are known (see Cerecedo, 1955; Rogers, 1970), the two most commonly used in experimental studies are oxythiamine and pyrithiamine. Oxythiamine is formed by substitution of an hydroxyl group for the amino group of the pyrimidine moiety of the thiamin molecule. Pyrithiamine results from the substitution of a pyridine ring for the thiazole ring of thiamin. It appears that, in general, thiamin activity is impaired when the number 2 position of the pyridine ring is changed. However, both the 2-ethyl and 2-propyl compounds possess thiamin activity to some degree.

Both oxythiamine and pyrithiamine possess potent antithiamin activity, but the mechanism by which they oppose thiamin function differs. Oxythiamine is readily converted to the pyrophosphate and competes with thiamin for its place in the TPP-enzyme systems. It markedly depresses appetite, growth, and weight gain and produces bradycardia, heart enlargement, and an increase in blood pyruvate. However, it does not produce neurological symptoms. Pyrithiamine exerts its antithiamin activity chiefly through its effect on thiamin kinase, the enzyme involved in formation of TPP. Thus pyrithiamine is not converted to the pyrophosphate but rather prevents conversion of thiamin to TPP. It has a specific and marked effect on the central nervous system and quickly produces the neurological symptoms of thiamin deficiency. Treatment with pyrithiamine results in loss of thiamin from tissues, bradycardia, and heart enlargement but does not produce an increase in blood pyruvate. In addition its effect on weight gain is considerably less than that of oxythiamine. The comparative physiological and biochemical effects of these two thiamin antagonists were detailed by Steyn-Parvé (1967) and Gubler (1968).

Amprolium, the 2-*n*-propyl pyrimidine analog of thiamin, is used in the treatment of coccidiosis in chickens. When fed at high levels, this compound has antithiamin activity and has been used experimentally to some extent. (See Brin, 1964; Rindi et al., 1966.)

Substances with antithiamin activity also occur naturally in some foods. Originally the antithiamin factor was referred to as thiaminase and was presumed to be an enzyme that splits the thiamin molecule thus rendering the vitamin inactive. It is now known that two types of thiaminase exist in foods. (See Murata, 1982.) Thiaminase I catalyzes the cleavage of the vitamin by reacting with an organic base and a sulfhydryl compound whereby the methylene group of the pyrimidine moiety of thiamin is displaced, thus inactivating the vitamin. Thiaminase II acts as originally presumed by catalyzing the hydrolysis of the thiamin molecule into its pyrimidine and thiazole components. Thiaminase was discovered as the result of an outbreak of a paralyzing disease in silver foxes raised on a farm owned by one J. S. Chastek. The disease, called "Chastek paralysis," was traced to raw fish fed to the animals and was later characterized by Green et al. (1942) as a thiamin deficiency. Heating or cooking destroyed antithiamin activity. Thiaminase has been found in both fresh- and salt-water fish, and more recently in various plant sources including tea, coffee, blueberries, Brussels sprouts, and red cabbage (Grossman et al., 1973; also Hilker and Somogyi, 1982).

Riboflavin

In the early days of vitamin research it was believed that the antiberiberi factor represented a single vitamin. After thiamin was isolated, however, it became clear that at least two factors were involved, a heat-labile fraction that was the true antiberiberi vitamin and a heat-stable fraction essential for growth (Emmett and Luros, 1920). The latter fraction for some time was thought to be only one substance and was named vitamin B_2 in Great Britain and vitamin G in the United States. Subsequently the heat-stable fraction was shown to be not one vitamin but a mixture of several vitamins (later identified as riboflavin, vitamin B_6, niacin, and pantothenic acid). The orange-yellow color of riboflavin and its natural fluorescence in solution undoubtedly aided in its discovery since its presence in extracts from foods and other biological materials could be confirmed with the naked eye.

Riboflavin

The vitamin was first isolated from egg white and called "ovoflavin". (See György, 1954.) Compounds later isolated by other groups from milk and liver were designated "lactoflavin" and "hepatoflavin." The name riboflavin was adopted only after the compound was shown to contain the sugar alcohol, ribitol, in the molecule. The name was changed to riboflavine, and then back to riboflavin (IUPAC, 1966).

Riboflavin was synthesized independently by Kuhn et al. (1935) and Karrer et al. (1935).

CHEMISTRY

The chemical name for riboflavin is 6,7-dimethyl-9 (D-1'-ribityl) isoalloxazine. It is an orange-yellow crystalline substance that is very slightly soluble in water or acid solution. In neutral or acid media it is stable to heat. It is highly soluble in alkaline solution but is not stable to heat under alkaline conditions. In solution at any pH riboflavin is unstable to both visible and ultraviolet light. Hence special precautions must be taken when riboflavin is analyzed in the laboratory to avoid exposure of solutions to light. Analyses usually are carried out in a darkened room; as further precaution dark red glassware, which filters out the blue portion of the spectrum, should be used. The natural yellow-green fluorescence characteristic of riboflavin in solution is the basis for the fluorometric assay for the vitamin. (See AOAC, 1960; Koziol, 1970.) Riboflavin and its derivatives also may be determined by spectrophotometric and polarographic methods (see McCormick and Wright, 1971a) as well as microbiologically (Snell and Strong, 1939;

Baker and Frank, 1968). For additional information on riboflavin assay, see Association of Official Analytical Chemists (1980).

The vitamin is easily reduced to a colorless compound, leucoriboflavin, by hydrogen in the presence of a catalyst and sodium hydrosulfite or other reducing agents. In the analysis of riboflavin by the fluorometric technique, fluorescence is measured before and after reduction of riboflavin by sodium hydrosulfite in order to correct for fluorescence produced by interfering substances. The reversible reduction takes place by a shifting of bonds in the isoalloxazine ring as shown below. The ease with which riboflavin can be reversibly reduced and oxidized is the basis for its function in cellular respiration.

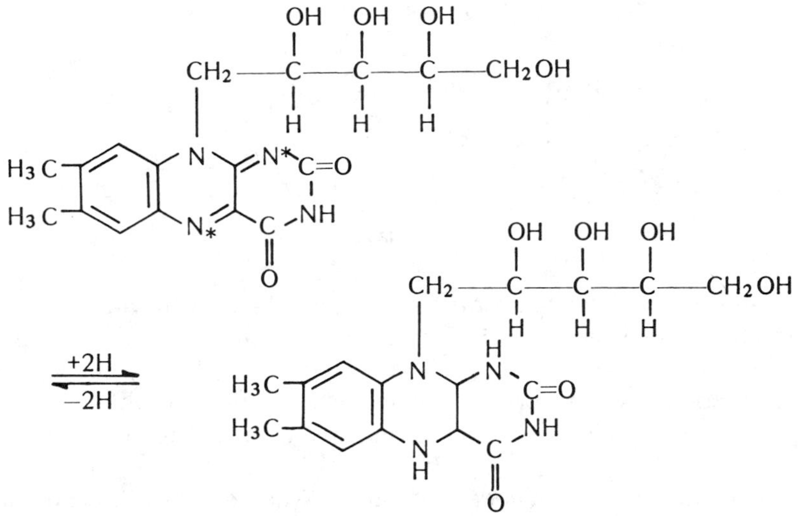

BIOCHEMICAL FUNCTION

Riboflavin is a constituent of two coenzymes: flavin mononucleotide (FMN) and flavin adenine dinucleotide (FAD). For the most part the vitamin is present in mammalian tissues as these two compounds. The identification of the flavin coenzymes dates back to the early 1930s when Warburg and Christian (1932) isolated a fluorescent oxidative enzyme from yeast and were able to separate the enzyme into a protein and a yellow-pigmented component. Two years later, Theorell (1934) showed that the active component of the yellow enzyme was flavin phosphate. FAD was identified from a group of enzymes known as diaphorases, and its structure was determined by cleavage to riboflavin-5'-phosphate and adenosine-5'-phosphate (Abraham, 1939). The formulas for the two coenzymes are as follows.

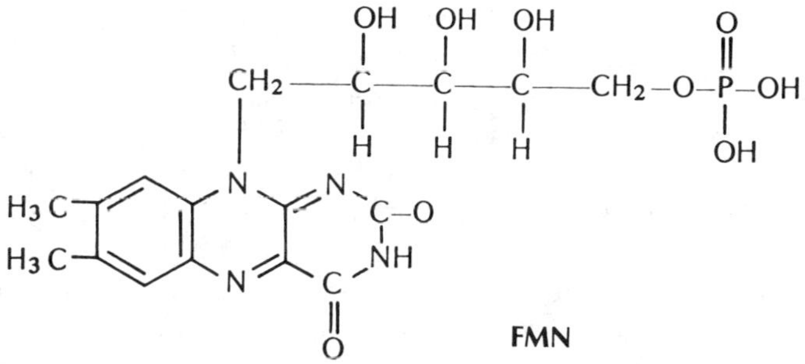

OH   OH   OH   O
  | | | ‖
CH₂——C——C——C——CH₂—O—P—OH
  | | | |
  H   H   H   OH

H₃C   N   N   C—O
H₃C   N   C   NH
                          ‖
                          O   **FMN**

OH   OH   OH
  | | |
CH₂——C——C——C——CH₂
  | | | |
  H   H   H   O
                            |
H₃C   N   N   C=O   O=P—OH
H₃C   N   NH |
                      C   O
                      ‖ |
                      O   O=P—OH   NH₂
                                       |
                                       O   N
                                       | CH
                                     CH₂   N   N
                                         O

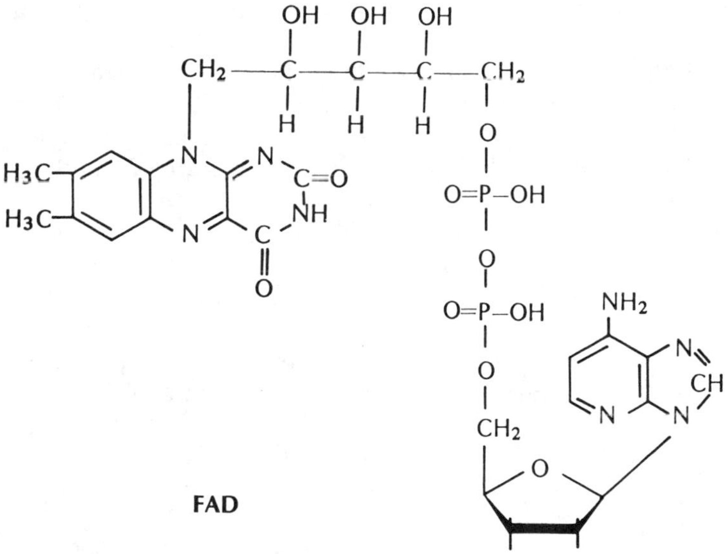

FAD

The riboflavin coenzymes function in a large number of enzyme systems and serve as carriers in the electron transport system leading to the formation of the high-energy compound ATP. (See Chapter 13.) Essentially these coenzymes function in dehydrogenations in the course of which the coenzyme is reduced. In turn, the flavin enzymes become substrates for reactions involving other electron acceptors resulting in the regeneration of the oxidized form of the coenzyme.

FMN is a part of the L-amino acid oxidase that participates in enzyme systems that oxidize L-α-amino acids and L-α-hydroxy acids to α-keto acids. FAD is a part of many enzyme systems including succinic dehydrogenase, xanthine oxidase, glycine oxidase, lipoyl dehydrogenase, NAD^+-cytochrome c reductase, and D-amino acid oxidase. Flavin enzymes also are involved in the specific dehydrogenation of adjacent carbon atoms resulting in the introduction of double bonds into certain molecules such as butyryl CoA and other acyl CoA compounds in the metabolism of fatty acids. Some of the flavoproteins contain a metal as, for example, xanthine oxidase that contains molybdenum and cytochrome c reductase that contains iron. Both FAD and FMN participate in the mixed-function oxidase system; the specific coenzyme requirement depends on the organ and the species. In this system the flavin coenzyme serves as the redox center for the NADPH:cytochrome P_{450} reductase enzyme that transfers electrons from NADPH to the iron of the cytochrome, a necessary step before binding and oxidation of the substrate (Coon, 1978). FAD is the coenzyme for glutathione reductase, an enzyme essential for maintenance of reduced glutathione levels needed in detoxification of peroxides, some organic compounds, and some heavy metals as well as in the λ-glutamyl cycle for amino acid transport. Glutathione reductase is the enzyme most commonly used to determine riboflavin status. (See Sauberlich et al., 1974; Chapter 24.)

The classic symptoms of riboflavin deficiency in humans include cheilosis, glossitis, and scaly dermatitis especially of the face and scrotum. (See Sebrell, 1979.) In contrast, riboflavin deficiency in the young growing rat has much more severe consequences: growth ceases and death ensues. Clearly, the rat is more susceptible to a lack of dietary riboflavin than the human. One might theorize that in the human alternative pathways exist for performing the vital functions normally mediated through the flavoproteins, but it seems more likely that the human is not readily depleted of the vitamin. The fact that riboflavin is tightly bound to the enzyme protein, that is, it is technically a prosthetic group, may impart a stability that the more loosely bound coenzyme vitamins do not have. Because riboflavin is associated with protein in metabolic systems and, therefore, in foods it seems possible that a riboflavin deficiency that is severe enough to result in debilitation or death does not occur except in conjunction with severe protein deficiency. In such a case the symptoms might merge into a variable syndrome such as that observed in protein-energy deficiency and might well be obscured by the devastating effects of this syndrome. Such speculation is interesting, but it is only speculation.

RIBOFLAVIN METABOLITES

Apparently little degradation of riboflavin occurs in mammalian tissues. Following injection of 2-^{14}C-riboflavin to rats, the vitamin is excreted rapidly in the urine (Yagi et al., 1966; Yang and McCormick, 1967). Only a trace of the radioactive riboflavin is converted to radioactive carbon dioxide (Yang and McCormick, ibid.). In studies with humans given oral doses of riboflavin, however, West and Owen (1969) reported the occurrence in the urine of at least three fluorescent compounds that were identified as degradative products of the vitamin: hydroxyethylflavin, formylmethylflavin, and an unknown compound designated as "Compound A." The amount of the compounds excreted represented considerably less than 1 percent of the dose of riboflavin fed to the subjects. Hydroxyethylflavin and formylmethylflavin were shown to be identical to riboflavin breakdown products that were isolated from the rumen and cecum of goats, and it was presumed that these metabolites originated from bacterial action in the intestinal tract and were absorbed as such.

Further breakdown of formylmethylflavin apparently occurs in animal tissues. This compound has been shown to be reduced by liver and kidney homogenates from goats, sheep, and cattle to hydroxymethylflavin (West and Owen, 1973). The enzyme responsible for the conversion has been found in tissues from other species including the rat, chicken, mouse, rabbit, and guinea pig (ibid.).

Thus, there is yet no clear evidence of tissue breakdown of riboflavin. The continuous need for a dietary source of riboflavin appears, therefore, to be the result of a continuous loss of the vitamin via the urine rather than to any extensive tissue degradation.

RIBOFLAVIN ANTAGONISTS

Among the riboflavin antagonists galactoflavin (Emerson et al., 1945) in which the ribitol moiety is replaced by galactose has been used most extensively in experimental studies. In man treatment with galactoflavin results in the usual effects on the mouth and skin (see Table 3.1). In addition a normochromic and normocytic anemia has been described (Lane and Alfrey, 1970). The anemia is accompanied by decreased incorporation of radioactive iron (^{59}Fe) into erythrocytes and bone marrow red cell hypoplasia. (See Chapter 16.) This condition is cured by riboflavin and is assumed to be a manifestation of riboflavin deficiency in humans. A similar syndrome has been observed in baboons fed a riboflavin-deficient diet (Foy and Kondi, 1968).

Diethylriboflavin, another riboflavin antagonist, was shown to possess a potent antivitamin effect in rats. (See Lambooy, 1955.) This compound was found to be useful in studies designed to elucidate the mechanism of action of the flavoprotein enzymes. Other riboflavin antagonists also have been described (Lambooy, ibid). Some of these compounds have been shown to retard malignant tumor growth in experimental animals. (See Rivlin, 1970a.)

A substance antagonistic to riboflavin was found to occur naturally in a limited number of foods, as for example the ackee fruit that is consumed in Jamaica (Fox and Miller, 1960).

Niacin (Nicotinic Acid and Nicotinamide)

Pellagra apparently has been known for several centuries and has long been associated with dietaries in which corn is a major staple food. The disease was endemic in the southern United States during the early part of the twentieth century and reached such proportions in institutions in the south that in 1914 a U.S. Public Health team headed by Dr. Joseph Goldberger was sent to the area to determine the cause and possible treatment of the disease. At that time it was generally believed that pellagra was caused either by an infectious agent or a toxic substance present in corn.

Goldberger's work on pellagra represents one of the most fascinating chapters in the history of nutrition. He observed that the disease occurred among institution inmates but not among staff who lived in the same environment but who invariably had a better diet including more animal protein food. Through carefully conducted studies he was able to produce pellagra in a group of prisoner volunteers by feeding them a diet similar to that consumed by persons who developed the disease (Goldberger and Wheeler, 1915). He was able to show also that the disease was not infectious since it could not be induced by exposure of healthy, well-fed volunteers to secretions or excreta from pellagrous patients (Goldberger, 1916). Finally, Goldberger and Wheeler (1928) produced black tongue in dogs, a disease comparable to human pellagra, by feeding a diet then known to produce pellagra in humans.

It was not until the middle 1930s that the pellagra-preventive factor in food was identified. Interestingly enough, nicotinic acid had been known for some time. It had even been isolated by Funk in the early part of this century when he was searching for an antiberiberi factor but was discarded when it was ineffective against beriberi! However, the discovery of nicotinamide as a component of coenzyme II (now NADP) by Warburg and Christian (1935) suggested that the substance was of metabolic importance. When Elvehjem et al. (1938) were able to cure black tongue in dogs with nicotinamide isolated from liver, the vitamin was firmly established as the pellagra-preventive factor. Subsequent treatment of pellagrous humans with the compound added final confirmatory evidence (Spies et al., 1938).

The history of pellagra and the discovery of niacin as the protective dietary component in the prevention of the disease were reviewed by Sydenstricker (1958).

CHEMISTRY

Niacin is the official name for the vitamin and includes both nicotinic acid and nicotinamide. Nicotinic acid is pyridine-3-carboxylic acid, a white crystalline solid that is easily converted to the physiologically active compound, nicotinamide. Both are soluble in water and in alcohol, but nicotinamide has a much higher solubility than nicotinic acid. Both are stable in the dry state and in solution at temperatures not exceeding 120°C.

Nicotinic Acid   Nicotinamide

Chemical determination of the vitamin depends on the reaction of the pyridine ring with cyanogen bromide to form a yellow color. (See György, 1950.) This method detects both nicotinic acid and nicotinamide, but it is less sensitive than some other procedures. Microbiological methods, for example, appear to be more accurate (Snell and Wright, 1941; Baker and Frank, 1968). Modern methods involving fluorometry (see McCormick and Wright, 1980a) and high performance liquid chromatography (Shaik et al., 1977; Hengen et al., 1978; DeVries et al.,

1980) have emerged as promising tools for determination of nicotinic acid and nicotinamide.

BIOCHEMICAL FUNCTION

Niacin functions metabolically as a component of the coenzymes nicotinamide adenine dinucleotide (NAD) and nicotinamide adenine dinucleotide phosphate (NADP). The coenzymes were previously known as coenzymes I and II and then DPN and TPN. Like the flavin coenzymes the nicotinamide nucleotides function in redox reactions (transfer of electrons and hydrogens). In the reduced state they are designated NADH and NADPH. Hydrogens are attached at the number 4 carbon of the pyridine ring, indicated by asterisks in the formulas for the coenzymes.

The influence of these coenzymes is so widespread in cellular metabolic processes that a lack of the vitamin results in major damage to cellular respiration. Enzyme systems in which NAD participates include alcohol dehydrogenase, glycerolphosphate dehydrogenase, lactic dehydrogenase, and glyceraldehyde-3-phosphate dehydrogenase to name only a few. Either NAD or NADP participates in reactions involving isocitric dehydrogenase and glutamic dehydrogenase; NADP is specifically involved with malic enzyme, glucose-6-phosphate dehydrogenase, and as cosubstrate for the mixed-function oxidase system, when in the NADPH form.

$$\frac{+H^+ + 2e}{-H^- - 2e}$$

NAD

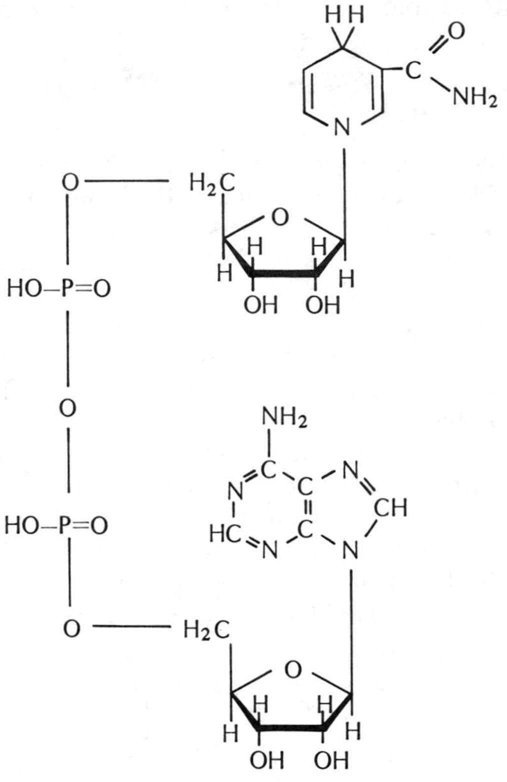

HH

C≡O
-C
NH₂

N

O —— H₂C
O
H   H
H   H
HO—P=O
OH   OH

O

NH₂

N≡C–C–N≡
HO—P=O   CH
HC≡N–C–N

O —— H₂C
O
H   H
H   H
OH   OH

NADH

Reduced NAD (NADH) usually donates its hydrogens to FAD and thus to the cell respiratory chain responsible for energy release. (See Chapter 13.) NADPH gives up its hydrogens most often to cellular biosynthetic processes. For example, the synthesis of fatty acids specifically requires NADPH. For detailed discussion of reactions involving niacin coenzymes, see Chaykin (1967); Sund (1968); and Slater et al. (1970).

Niacin is synthesized by mammalian cells from the amino acid tryptophan (Krehl et al., 1945a; 1945b) and, therefore, is not a vitamin in the strictest sense of the word. Numerous studies with microorganisms and animal tissues helped to elucidate the pathway by which tryptophan is converted to the vitamin. The final step in the synthesis of niacin eluded investigators for many years but eventually was shown to involve the conversion of the key intermediate quinolinic acid to nicotinic acid mononucleotide (Nishizuka and Hayaishi, 1963) and thus to NAD (Fig. 3.2). Nicotinic acid mononucleotide also is an intermediate in the conversion of nicotinic acid to NAD.

Confirmation of nicotinic acid synthesis from tryptophan supported early observations on the efficacy of animal protein in the prevention and cure of pellagra. Experiments with humans indicate that approximately 60 mg of tryptophan are

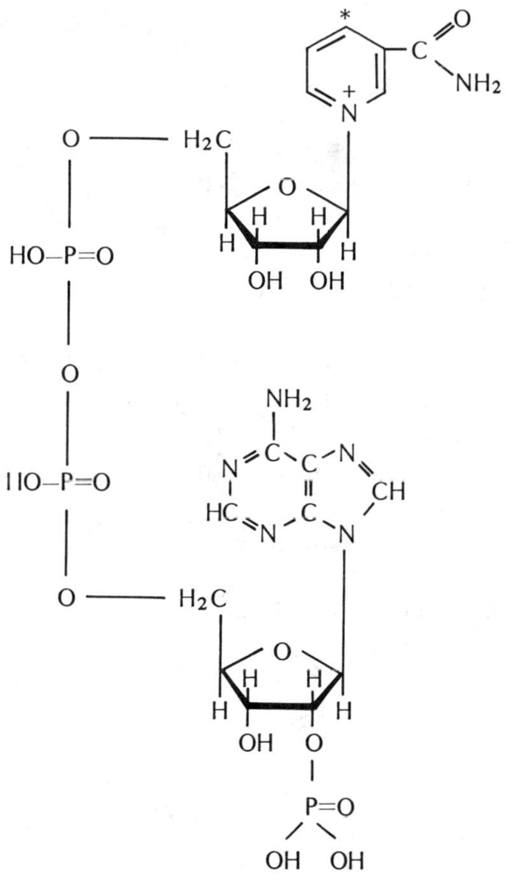

$$O = C - NH_2$$

$$O — H_2C$$

$$HO—P=O$$

$$O$$

$$HO—P=O$$

OH   OH

$$NH_2$$

$$O — H_2C$$

OH   O

$$P=O$$

OH   OH

NADP+

equivalent to 1 mg of nicotinic acid (Horwitt et al., 1956a; Goldsmith et al., 1961). The total amount of available niacin in the diet thus may be expressed in terms of niacin equivalents (mg equiv), which includes both preformed niacin and niacin synthesized from tryptophan. (See Chapter 25.) Since food tables list niacin values in milligrams a rough calculation of available niacin may be made on the assumption that tryptophan comprises approximately 1 percent of dietary protein. The resulting figure added to preformed niacin yields total niacin in foods. More precise figures for tryptophan content of various foods have been derived: corn products 0.6 percent; other grains, fruits, and vegetables 1.0 percent; meats 1.1 percent; and eggs 1.5 percent (Horwitt et al., 1981). For most practical purposes, the use of 1 percent of dietary protein as tryptophan and the 60:1 ratio of tryptophan to niacin appear to be adequate (ibid.).

The turnover of nicotinamide nucleotides in the mammalian body is very high. (See Dietrich, 1971.) However, under normal conditions the vitamin appears to be utilized efficiently. Metabolism of the nicotinamide nucleotides appears to be

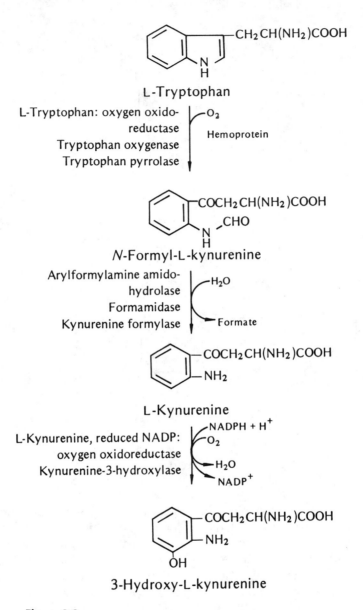

L-Tryptophan

L-Tryptophan: oxygen oxido-
reductase
Tryptophan oxygenase
Tryptophan pyrrolase

O_2

Hemoprotein

N-Formyl-L-kynurenine

Arylformylamine amido-
hydrolase
Formamidase
Kynurenine formylase

H_2O

Formate

L-Kynurenine

L-Kynurenine, reduced NADP:
oxygen oxidoreductase
Kynurenine-3-hydroxylase

NADPH + H^+
O_2

H_2O
$NADP^+$

3-Hydroxy-L-kynurenine

Figure 3.2
Conversion of tryptophan to NAD. (From S. Dagley and D. E.
Nicholson, *An Introduction to Metabolic Pathways,* John Wiley,
New York, 1970, pp. 238–239.)

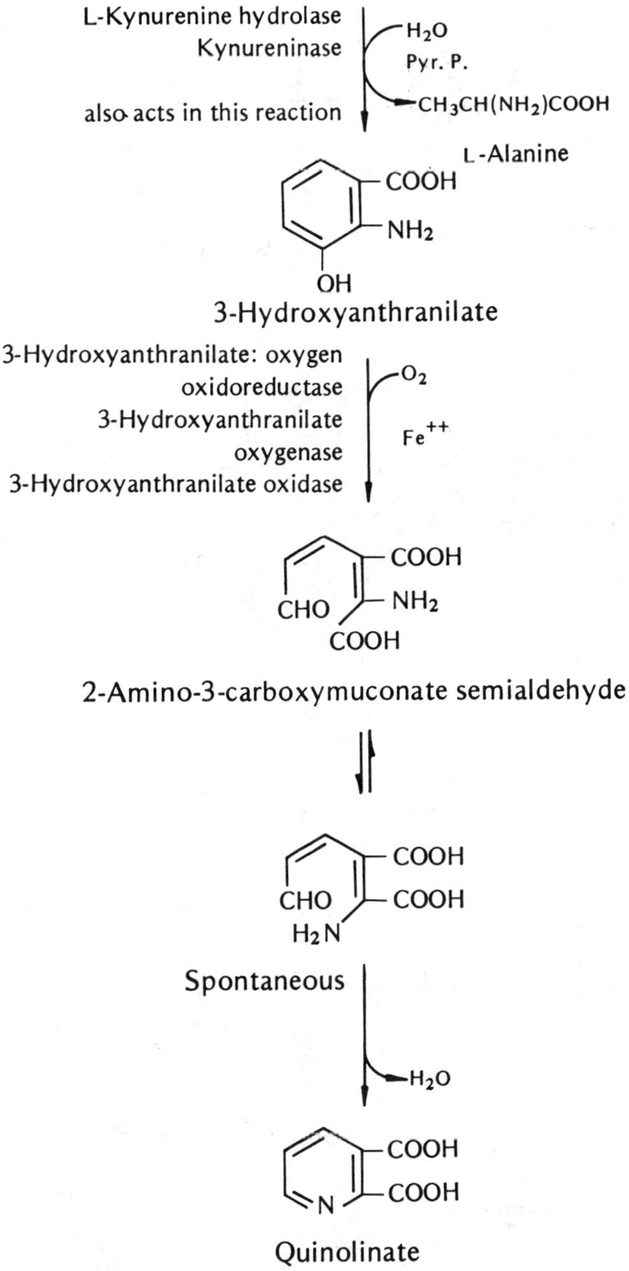

L-Kynurenine hydrolase
Kynureninase

also acts in this reaction

H_2O
Pyr. P.

$CH_3CH(NH_2)COOH$

L-Alanine

COOH

NH_2

OH

3-Hydroxyanthranilate

3-Hydroxyanthranilate: oxygen
oxidoreductase
3-Hydroxyanthranilate
oxygenase
3-Hydroxyanthranilate oxidase

O_2

Fe^{++}

COOH

NH_2

CHO

COOH

2-Amino-3-carboxymuconate semialdehyde

COOH

COOH

CHO

H_2N

Spontaneous

H_2O

COOH

COOH

N

Quinolinate

Figure 3.2 (continued)

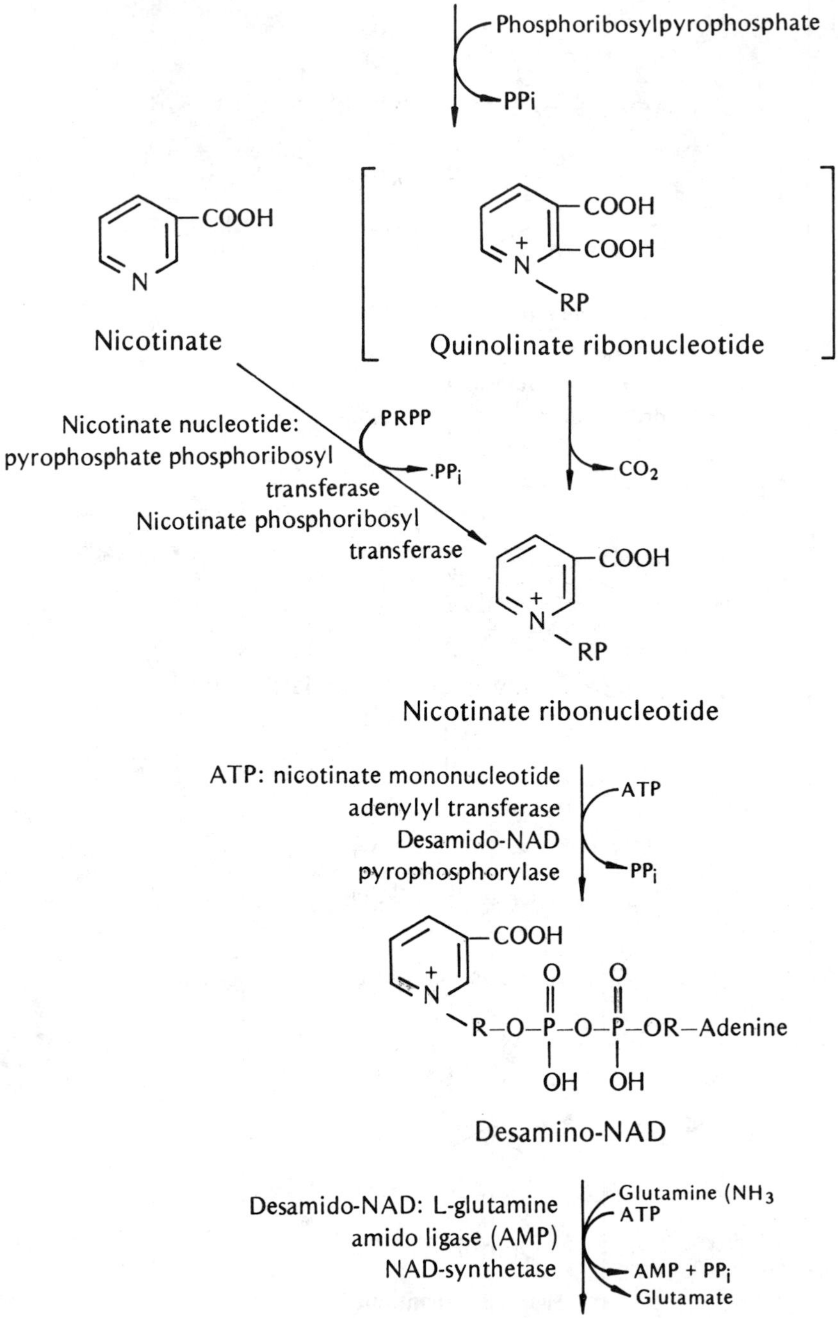

Figure 3.2 (continued)

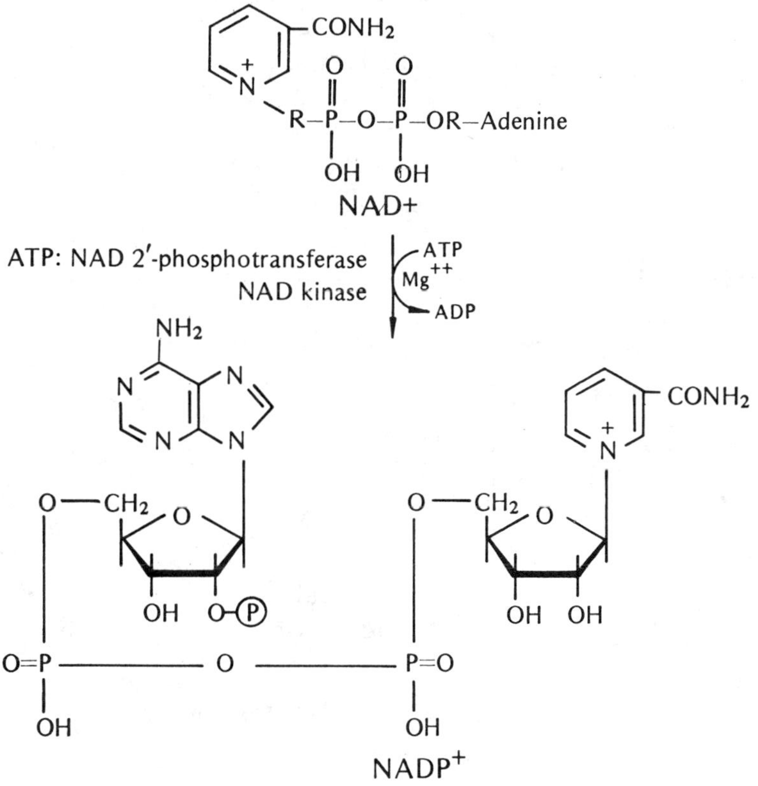

R represents the ribosyl group and RP ribosyl phosphate

Figure 3.2 (continued)

regulated both at the cellular (Gholson, 1966) and systemic levels (Dietrich et al., 1968) by an intricate series of enzyme activations and inhibitions involving the synthesis and degradation of the niacin coenzymes.

In the liver, tryptophan and nicotinic acid are converted to NAD as shown in Fig. 3.3. Catabolism of NAD releases nicotinamide that, along with absorbed vitamin, is converted to NAD in other tissues where the cycle is repeated. Some nicotinamide is believed to be excreted into the gastrointestinal tract where it may be converted by intestinal bacteria to nicotinic acid. At least some of the nicotinic acid so formed may be absorbed and returned to the general circulation. Nicotinamide also is converted in the liver to N^1-methyl nicotinamide, a major niacin metabolite that is excreted in the urine. For a review of niacin metabolism, see Henderson (1983).

Marginal deficiency of niacin produces a glossitis similar to that which occurs in riboflavin deficiency. Severe niacin deficiency leads to pellagra, which is characterized by the three "D's": dermatitis, diarrhea, and dementia. The der-

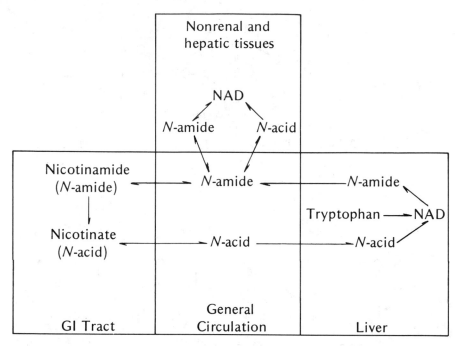

Figure 3.3
Systemic pyridine nucleotide cycle. (From L. S. Dietrich, *Am. J. Clin. Nutr.* 24:802, 1971.)

matitis of pellagra most commonly occurs in a broad band around the neck, the upper chest and back and is called Casal's Necklace. The dermatitis may occur elsewhere on the body but most particularly in areas exposed to sunlight. How these symptoms relate to the biochemical reactions that require niacin is not known. Moreover, because of the pervasive involvement of niacin coenzymes in cellular metabolism it is difficult to identify any specific enzymatic reaction requiring these coenzymes for use in determining niacin status.

NIACIN METABOLITES

As mentioned above, in humans and other monogastric animals nicotinamide is methylated before it is excreted. N^1-methylnicotinamide and the 2- and 6-pyridones of N^1-methylnicotinamide are excreted in the urine. Determination of N^1-methylnicotinamide excretion in urine is commonly used as an indicator of niacin nutritional status. (See Chapter 26.) Other known metabolites of niacin are nicotinuric acid, nicotinamide-N-oxide, N^1-methyl-2-pyridone-5-carboxamide, and N^1-methyl-4-pyridone-3-carboxamide, 6-hydroxynicotinamide, and 6-hydroxynicotinic acid (Lee et al., 1969). Many of these compounds were identified in urine following injection of ^{14}C-labeled nicotinamide or nicotinic acid. The compounds that were excreted have been shown to vary both with the form of the vitamin administered and the size of the injected dose. Recently high performance liquid chromatography has been used as a means of quantifying niacin metabolites in urine (Hengen et al., 1978; Sandhu and Fraser, 1981; Carter, 1982).

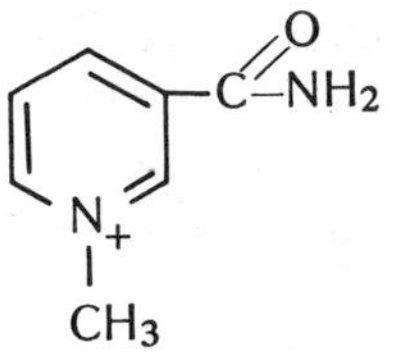

**N'-Methyl
Nicotinamide**

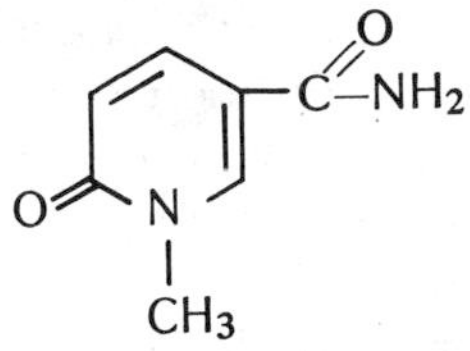

**6-Pyridone of
N'-Methyl Nicotinamide**

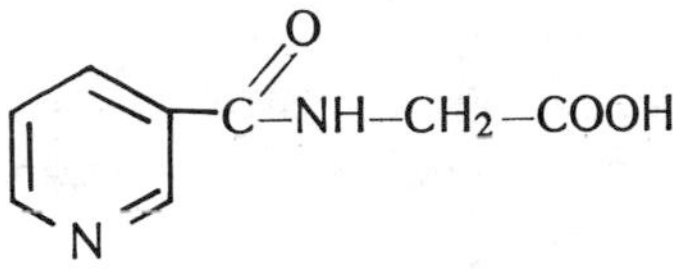

Nicotinuric Acid

NIACIN ANTAGONISTS

One of the first niacin antagonists to be discovered was 3-acetyl pyridine (Woolley, 1945), and this compound and 6-aminonicotinamide have received the most attention (Kodicek, 1966). Other niacin antagonists include pyridine-3-sulphonamide, 7-aminonicotinamide, and 4-acetyl pyridine.

The development of pellagra on predominantly maize diets has been attributed to binding of niacin with a complex substance such that niacin is not absorbed or is otherwise made unavailable. The low incidence of pellagra in Mexico where maize is treated with lime and baked into tortillas led to the belief that lime treatment freed niacin and thus made it available for metabolism. (See Carpenter, 1981.) Other cereals such as wheat bran also contain niacin bound to large macromolecules (Mason et al., 1973), and the availability of bound niacin appears to be affected by the method of processing. Carter and Carpenter (1982), for example, found alkali-treated wheat bran to be about 62 percent available to human subjects when urinary N^1-methylnicotinamide and N^1-methyl-2-pyridone-5-carboxamide levels were used as indicators of niacin status. In contrast, niacin from untreated wheat bran was largely unavailable. These findings are of practical importance in areas of the world where cereal grains comprise the bulk of the diet.

Vitamin B₆ (pyridoxine, pyridoxal and pyridoxamine)

The term vitamin B_6 is the official name for the 2-methyl pyridine derivatives having the biological activity of pyridoxine and includes the aldehyde, pyridoxal, and the amine, pyridoxamine.

Vitamin B_6 was first defined by György (1934) as "that part of the vitamin B complex responsible for the cure of a specific dermatitis developed by rats on a vitamin-free diet supplemented with vitamin B_1 and lactoflavin (riboflavin)." The dermatitis of vitamin B_6 deficiency in rats is a characteristic scaliness about the paws and mouth; these areas eventually become denuded as the scales slough off. Hence the vitamin was first identified as the rat antidermatitis factor. Alopecia (loss of hair) also is a commonly observed symptom of vitamin B_6 deficiency in rats.

The vitamin B_6 alcohol, pyridoxine, was isolated first by Kerestezy and Stevens (1938) and later in the same year by four independent groups including György (1938) and Lepkovsky (1938). Synthesis of the vitamin was accomplished in the following year by Harris and Folkers (1939). It was not until 1945, however, that the multiple nature of the vitamin was recognized and the other compounds of the complex identified as pyridoxal and pyridoxamine (Snell, 1945). Pyridoxine predominates in plant products, but pyridoxamine and pyridoxal are the principal forms of the vitamin in animal tissues (Rabinowitz and Snell, 1948).

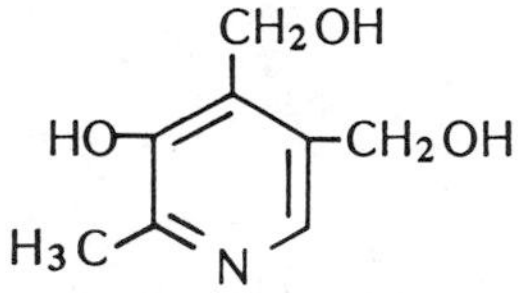

Pyridoxine

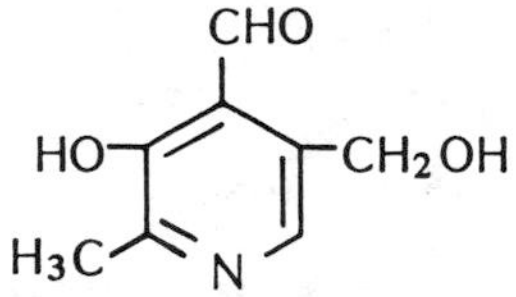

Pyridoxal

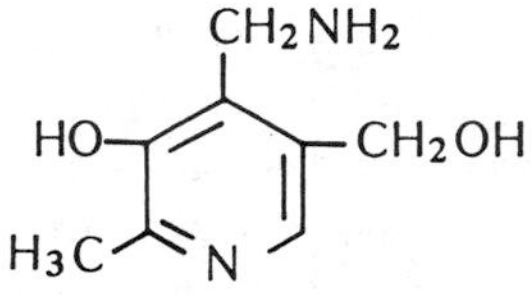

Pyridoxamine

CHEMISTRY

Pyridoxine is readily soluble in water and slightly soluble in alcohol and acetone. It is stable to heat in acid solution and somewhat less stable in alkaline medium. It is quite unstable to visible and ultraviolet light in neutral and alkaline solution and therefore must be protected during laboratory analysis. In acid solution very little of the vitamin is destroyed by light.

The microbiological method has long been a preferred method for the determination of the vitamin. (See Haskell and Snell, 1970.) For many assays, *Sacchromyces uvarum* (formerly *Sacchromyces carlsbergensis*) has been the organism of choice (Polansky, 1980; Miller and Edwards, 1980). Under some conditions, the method is complicated by different growth responses to the three forms of the vitamin. A satisfactory modification has been the separation of the three compounds on a chromatographic column and assay of each by microbiological assay

(Toepfer and Lehmann, 1961; Polansky, 1980). However, Guilarte et al. (1980) report that *Kloeckera brevis* (renamed *Kloeckera apiculata*) shows an equal growth response to the three forms of the vitamin.

Recently, HPLC has been found to be a promising method for analysis of the B_6 vitamins in plasma and other animal tissues (Vanderslice et al., 1979; Vanderslice and Maire, 1980; Gregory, 1981; Vanderslice et al., 1981).

BIOCHEMICAL FUNCTION

The active form of vitamin B_6 is the coenzyme pyridoxal phosphate (PLP) identified by Umbreit and Gunsalus (1945). All three forms of the vitamin are converted to the active coenzyme or to their respective phosphates. Phosphorylation requires ATP.

Pyridoxal Phosphate

All reactions catalyzed by enzymes requiring PLP as coenzyme are characterized according to the chemical group removed from the compound being metabolized. (See Gershoff, 1976.)

1. Type I reactions: e^- withdrawal from bond ⓐ resulting in H^+ liberation followed by addition of another group.

2. Type II reactions: e^- withdrawal from bond ⓑ resulting in liberation of $(COOH)^+$, which is $CO_2 + H^+$, followed by addition of another group, often H^+, in place of the carboxyl group.
3. Type III reactions: e^- withdrawal from bond ⓒ resulting in liberation of R^+, followed by addition of another group.

Some of the most common examples of these types of reactions are as follows.

Type I: Transaminations

For example, alanine + α-ketoglutarate $\rightleftharpoons$ pyruvate + glutamate

Racemase Reactions

For example, L-alanine $\rightleftharpoons$ D-alanine
        also for D- and L-methionine and D- and L-glutamate

α,β-Addition or Elimination Reactions

For example, L-serine $\rightarrow$ pyruvate + H_2O

α,γ-Addition or Elimination Reactions

For example, homocysteine + serine $\rightarrow$ cystathionine + H_2O
        cystathionine + H_2O $\rightarrow$ cysteine + homoserine

Type II: Amino Acid Decarboxylations

For example, dopa $\rightarrow$ dopamine + CO_2
        tyrosine $\rightarrow$ tyramine + CO_2
        5-hydroxytryptophan $\rightarrow$ serotonin + CO_2
        histidine $\rightarrow$ histamine + CO_2

Type III: Aldol Reactions

For example, serine + THFA $\rightarrow$ $N_{5,10}$-methylene THFA + glycine

Anhydride Condensations

For example, glycine + succinyl CoA $\rightarrow$ ALA (δ-aminolevulinic acid)
        2 ALA $\rightarrow$ porphobilinogen

These examples are only a few of the best known and most important reactions catalyzed by PLP-requiring enzymes. In each of these, PLP is a crucial part of the active center of the enzymes. PLP is required for many specific reactions of individual amino acids, and is a coenzyme for phosphorylase (Cori and Illingworth, 1957) in which it is covalently linked to a lysine residue and stabilizes the enzyme without taking a direct part in the catalysis.

Whereas the formyl group of PLP appears to be the major site for coenzyme binding, the phosphate group, 2-methyl group, 3-hydroxy group, and the heterocyclic N atom all are involved in coenzyme-apoenzyme interaction (Hayaishi and Shizuta, 1970). In fact, every side chain of the PLP molecule likely plays a role in apoenzyme binding, but the importance of the group involved varies from one enzyme system to another. (See Fasella, 1967.)

Not unexpectedly vitamin B_6 deficiency results in profound effects upon protein and amino acid metabolism. Since PLP is required for the action of the kynureninase enzyme involved in the metabolism of tryptophan (see Fig. 3.2), nicotinic

TABLE 3.2
Vitamin B₆ Genetic Diseases

Abnormal Condition	Biochemical Defect
Infant convulsive seizures	Decreased synthesis of γ-aminobutyric acid due to reduced activity of glutamic decarboxylase.
Vitamin B₆-responsive anemia (microcytic, hypochromic)	Decreased formation of δ-aminolevulinic acid from glycine and succinyl CoA in heme synthesis.
Cystathionuria	Decreased interconversion of homoserine and cystathionine due to reduced activity of cystathionase.
Xanthurenic aciduria	Decreased conversion of kynurenine to anthranilic acid due to reduced activity of kynureninase.
Homocystinuria	Decreased conversion of homocysteine to cystathionine due to reduced activity of cystathionine β-synthase.

acid formation may be reduced as a consequence of the deficiency. In addition, tryptophan metabolism is diverted from its normal course which results in the formation of xanthurenic acid, an abnormal metabolite of the amino acid. The excretion of xanthurenic acid following a test dose of tryptophan thus can be used as a means of detecting vitamin B₆ deficiency. (See Chapter 24.)

Some other symptoms associated with vitamin B₆ deficiency can be associated with a specific biochemical defect. The role of PLP in glycogen phosphorylase activity may account for decreased glucose tolerance observed in vitamin B₆ deficiency. The involvement of PLP in the synthesis of the neurotransmitters, serotonin and norepinephrine (from dopamine), may explain the symptoms of nervousness and irritability. (See Rose, 1978a; Chapter 19.)

A number of genetic diseases involving vitamin B₆-dependent enzyme systems have been reported. (See Mudd, 1971; György, 1971; Brown, 1972; Mudd and Levy, 1978.) Some of the reported diseases and reactions affected are shown in Table 3.2. The basic defect in many of these diseases appears to be a decrease in binding of PLP to the apoenzyme; in some cases, the amount of the apoenzyme is low. Many of these defects respond to massive doses of the vitamin in the order of 100 to 1000 mg per day (Valle et al., 1980).

VITAMIN B₆ METABOLITES

A major metabolite of vitamin B₆ is 4-pyridoxic acid. Following injection of pyridoxine about 50 percent of the dose is excreted in the urine as pyridoxic acid. This compound can be measured fluorometrically (Reddy et al., 1958). Following oral dosage with the vitamin approximately 20 to 40 percent has been recovered in the urine as pyridoxic acid (Johansson et al., 1966; Tillotson et al., 1968).

Pyridoxic acid is similar in structure to the vitamin but is inactive metabolically.

Pyridoxic Acid

An intermediary metabolite in the formation of pyridoxic acid has been identified in rat tissues as 4-pyridoxic acid-5'-phosphate (Contractor and Shane, 1970). Apparently pyridoxal phosphate is oxidized to pyridoxic acid phosphate, which is hydrolyzed to pyridoxic acid and excreted. Determination of urinary 4-pyridoxic acid can be used as an indicator of vitamin B_6 nutritional status. (See Chapter 24.)

Other metabolites of vitamin B_6 have been found in urine. Those that have been identified include pyridoxal, pyridoxamine, PLP, pyridoxamine phosphate, and traces of pyridoxine. At least nine other unidentified compounds are excreted following a radioactive dose of vitamin B_6 (Tillotson et al., 1968).

VITAMIN B_6 ANTAGONISTS

Many compounds are effective antagonists of pyridoxine. (See Umbreit, 1955; Sauberlich, 1968; Hullar, 1969.) Some of the structural requirements for antagonism are suggested by the formulas for three of the most common and effective: 4-deoxypyridoxine, isoniazid (an antituberculosis drug), and toxopyrimidine.

4-Deoxypyridoxine   **Isoniazid**   **Toxopyrimidine**

Of these compounds 4-deoxypyridoxine has been utilized most frequently in experimental studies. The first studies of vitamin B_6 deficiency in humans were made with the use of deoxypyridoxine (Mueller and Vilter, 1950). Deoxypyridoxine apparently can be phosphorylated and thus competes with PLP for binding to the apoenzyme.

Isoniazid, a drug used in the treatment of tuberculosis, also is a potent antimetabolite of the vitamin B_6 group (Biehl and Vilter, 1954). This compound as well as other hydrazines form hydrazones with pyridoxal that inhibit pyridoxal kinase activity thus preventing formation of the coenzyme. Cycloserine, another antituberculosis drug, leads to an increased excretion of pyridoxine in the urine and, like isoniazid, produces neurological symptoms similar to those seen in vitamin B_6 deficiency (Cohen, 1969). Deoxypyridoxine does not produce the neurological symptoms.

Certain drugs such as amphetamine, chlorpromazine, reserpine, and birth control pills affect either the concentration of the vitamin in various tissues or enzymes involved in vitamin B_6 metabolism. The effect of birth control pills on vitamin B_6 requirement has received considerable attention. Much of the work has been reviewed by Mason et al. (1969), Brown et al. (1969), György (1971), Brown (1972) and Rose (1978b). Tryptophan metabolism is markedly affected in women taking the pill Leklem et al., (1975a; 1975b). This results in increased excretion of tryptophan metabolites and other biochemical manifestations of abnormal vitamin B_6 metabolism. Biochemical evidence of vitamin B_6 deficiency also has been observed in normal pregnancy (Wachstein, 1964; Hamfelt and Tuvemo, 1972).

Pantothenic Acid

Pantothenic acid was isolated and synthesized long before its metabolic role was identified. The vitamin was purified from liver and yeast along with pyridoxine, and the two vitamins were separated by adsorption chromatography. Pyridoxine was adsorbed on a column of Fuller's earth and subsequently eluted; pantothenic acid was not adsorbed and was recovered in the filtrate leaving the column. For this reason, pantothenic acid was designated the *filtrate factor* and pyridoxine, the *eluate factor*.

At about the same time several groups of investigators were searching for the identification of the vitamin known to be necessary for growth of lactic acid bacteria, prevention of dermatitis in chicks, and prevention of graying in black rats. Pantothenic acid was isolated by R. J. Williams and his associates (1938) and was synthesized by Stiller et al. (1940). Later tests with the purified vitamin proved it to be the factor required by bacteria, chicks, and rats for preventing the dissimilar deficiency symptoms.

Pantothenic acid attracted only mild interest for more than 10 years after it was recognized as a vitamin. The first breakthrough came with the identification of coenzyme A (CoA) as the active factor required for metabolic acetylation processes (Lipmann and Kaplan, 1946); this discovery earned a Nobel Prize for Dr. Lipmann. The identification of pantothenic acid as a constituent of CoA was accomplished by a group in the same laboratory (DeVries et al., 1950). With this discovery the metabolic importance of pantothenic acid was clearly recognized.

Pantoic Acid   **β-Alanine**

Pantothenic Acid

CHEMISTRY

The pantothenic acid molecule is a condensation product of β-alanine and a hydroxyl- and methyl-substituted butyric acid, pantoic acid. It is an unstable pale yellow oil. Commercially it is available as the stable white crystalline calcium or sodium salt. The salt is soluble in water and glacial acetic acid. In neutral to slightly acid medium, pH 5-7, it is relatively stable at high temperatures.

Microbiological methods are generally reliable methods for determination of the vitamin in biological materials. *Lactobacillus casei* (Pennington et al., 1940), *Lactobacillus arabinosus* (Skeggs and Wright, 1944), and *Tetrahymena pyriformis* (Baker and Frank, 1968), and *Lactobacillus plantarum* (ibid.; Association of Official Analytical Chemists, 1980) are among the organisms that have been used. A major problem in the analysis is to free the vitamin from the coenzyme molecule and other bound forms; these compounds must be hydrolyzed to free pantothenic acid or analyzed separately.

More recently a radioimmunoassay for pantothenic acid in blood and other tissues was described (Wyse et al., 1979). High performance liquid chromatography also has been suggested as a means of separating coenzyme A and its precursors (Halvorsen and Skrede, 1980).

BIOCHEMICAL FUNCTION

Pantothenic acid is a component of CoA and is the prosthetic group on acyl carrier protein (ACP). It is required in the metabolism of fat, protein, and carbohydrate through the citric acid cycle. (See Chapter 13.) More than 70 enzymes are known to use CoA or ACP.

The CoA molecule contains β-mercaptoethylamine, adenine, ribose, and phosphoric acid in addition to the vitamin. Pantotheine, the β-mercaptoethylamine derivative of pantothenic acid, is the functional unit of CoASH. The sulfhydryl group of β-mercaptoethylamine is the site at which acyl groups are linked for transport by the coenzyme. The discovery of the thioester linkage was reported

Coenzyme A

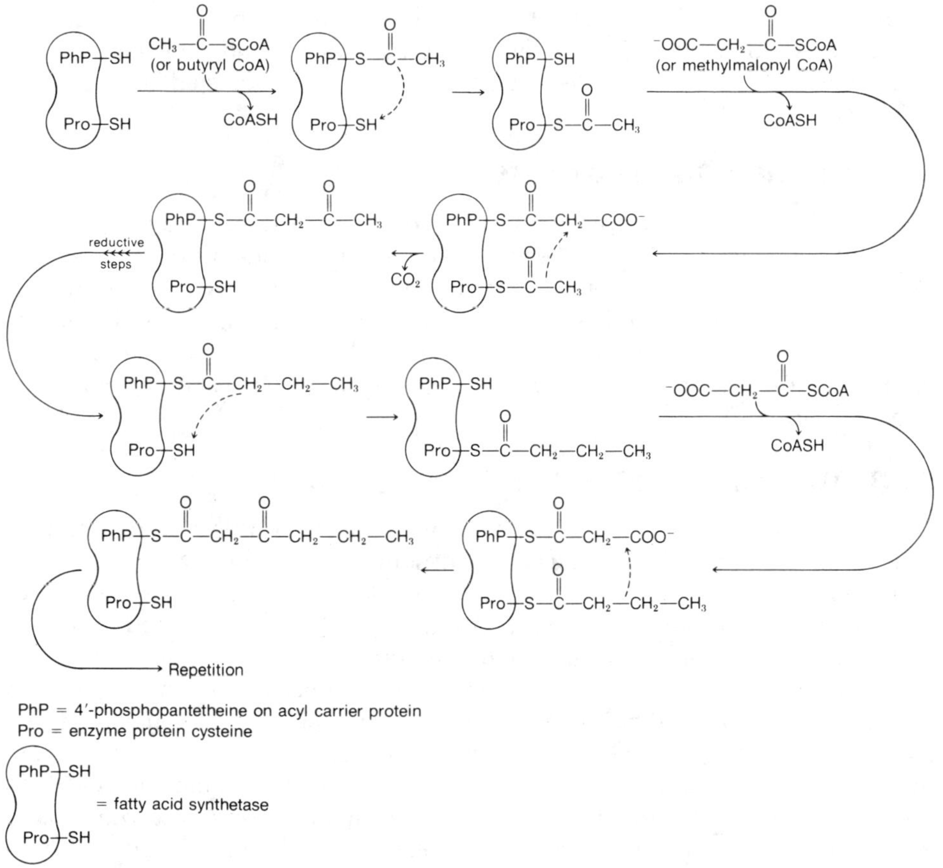

PhP = 4'-phosphopantetheine on acyl carrier protein
Pro = enzyme protein cysteine

= fatty acid synthetase

Figure 3.4
Mechanism of pantothenic acid in ACP function. (From Devlin, *Textbook of Biochemistry*, John Wiley, New York, 1982, p. 451.)

by Lynen and Reichert in 1952. Since then CoASH has been demonstrated to be by far the most important acyl transfer coenzyme in biological systems.

The ability of CoA to form thioesters with carboxylic acids is responsible for the vital role of the coenzyme in numerous metabolic processes. A key reaction is the formation of acetyl CoA, *active acetate*, which condenses with oxaloacetate to form citrate and thus introduces two-carbon fragments into the tricarboxylic acid cycle, the common pathway of nutrient oxidation in the cell.

An essential reaction in fatty acid synthesis is the binding and transfer of acyl groups by ACP. The structure of ACP involves a 4-phosphopantotheine cofactor which is identical to part of the structure of CoA. The sulfhydryl groups in the pantotheine and in the protein are in close proximity allowing the growing acyl chain to be shuttled between the two (Fig. 3.4).

Because of the importance of CoA and ACP in many diverse aspects of metabolism, one might expect pantothenic acid deficiency to be a major problem. However, pantothenic acid is widely distributed in foods, and clinical symptoms of deficiency are not easily distinguished from those associated with other B vitamins.

PANTOTHENIC ACID METABOLITES

Metabolic products of pantothenic acid have not been studied extensively. Although degradation products of the vitamin have not been identified it was shown that pantolactone probably is not a metabolite of pantothenic acid in humans (Sarett, 1945) as in some other species. Pantothenic acid administered orally or by injection is rapidly excreted in the urine (Silber and Unna, 1942). Larger amounts of the vitamin are excreted following oral dosage than after subcutaneous injection.

PANTOTHENIC ACID ANTAGONISTS

A large number of pantothenic acid antagonists have been described. (See Bird et al., 1955; Copping, 1966.) The activity of some of these compounds, however, varies among species. For example, pantothenol, a simple alcohol derivative of the vitamin, is a powerful antagonist for many bacteria but is utilized as readily as the vitamin by higher animals, including humans.

The most important of the pantothenic acid antimetabolites in studies with experimental animals and man is ω-methyl pantothenic acid, a compound produced by substitution of a methyl group for the hydrogen in the pantoyl part of the molecule. This antagonist was used in the first studies of pantothenic acid deficiency in humans (Bean and Hodges, 1954). Symptoms were observed in little more than a month in subjects given the antagonist and a diet deficient in pantothenic acid.

Other reported pantothenic acid antagonists include homopantothenic acid (Nishizawa and Matsuzaki, 1969) and N'-substituted pantothenamides (Clifton et al., 1970).

Folacin (Folic Acid)

Many different species played significant roles in the identification of folacin as a vitamin. In the early 1930s Dr. Lucy Wills in India observed a megaloblastic anemia in pregnant women whose diets consisted primarily of white rice and bread. Since the anemia could be produced in monkeys maintained on a similar monotonous diet and responded to supplements of yeast, it was apparent that the anemia was of nutritional origin (Wills, 1933). The unidentified factor was known as the Wills factor. Various other nutritional factors protective in other species were later shown to be identical with the original Wills factor: vitamin M, a factor protective against cytopenia in monkeys; factor U, a growth factor for chicks; vitamin B_c, protective against anemia in chicks; *L. casei* factor, necessary for growth of *Lactobacillus casei;* citrovorum factor, necessary for growth of *Leuconostoc citrovorum* (now *Pediococcus cervisiae*).

The name folic acid was proposed by Mitchell et al. (1941) for a compound isolated from spinach and shown to be necessary for growth of *Streptococcus faecalis R.* Eventually the structure and synthesis of pteroylglutamic acid were determined by Angier et al. (1946) and Pfiffner et al. (1946). A few years later it was clear that all the factors were forms of the vitamin now known as folacin, a collective term that comprises folic acid (pteroylmonoglutamic acid) and its derivatives.

| Pteridine nucleus | *p*-Aminobenzoic acid | Glutamic acid |

Pteroic acid

Folic Acid (pteroylmonoglutamic acid)

CHEMISTRY

Folic acid consists of a pteridine nucleus, *p*-aminobenzoic acid, and glutamic acid, hence the name pteroylmonoglutamic acid. The portion of the molecule containing pteridine and *p*-aminobenzoic acid is designated pteroic acid. At one time both *p*-aminobenzoic acid and pteroylglutamic acid were considered to be vitamins, but it is now apparent that the species requirement is for one or the other of the two. Pteroylglutamic acid is the vitamin for most mammals, whereas *p*-aminobenzoic acid is essential to certain bacteria that are able to synthesize the larger molecule.

The compound is a dull yellow substance very slightly soluble in water. Its sodium salt is considerably more soluble. When in dilute acid solution pteroylglutamic acid is stable at temperatures below 100°C; stability to heat increases as pH increases. Solutions of both the acid and its salts are unstable to light.

Other biologically active forms of folic acid have been isolated from liver and yeast. These compounds contain three or more glutamic acid molecules. The tri- and heptaglutamyl peptides are most prevalent.

The microbiological procedure is preferred for the determination of folacin in biological materials (Hoppner et al., 1977). Because of the many different forms of the vitamin, major problems are encountered due to variance in response and to the small amounts and instability of many naturally occurring folates. (See Baugh and Krumdieck, 1971.) *Streptococcus faecalis, Lactobacillus casei* and *Pediococcus cervisiae* have been used for assay. Of these, *Lactobacillus casei* appears to be most satisfactory for detection of folate nutritional status in humans and animals (Baker et al., 1958; Cooperman, 1971). However, there is no one method at present that will measure *all* folic acid active compounds.

Enzymatic methods, radioisotope assay, and column chromatography have been used for the determination of folic acid activity. (See McCormick and Wright, 1971a; Waxman and Schrieber, 1977.)

BIOCHEMICAL FUNCTION

The active form of the vitamin is tetrahydrofolic acid (THFA). Folic acid is reduced to dihydrofolic acid by an enzyme, folic acid reductase. Dihydrofolic acid, in turn, is reduced to the active THFA. Both reductions require NADPH.

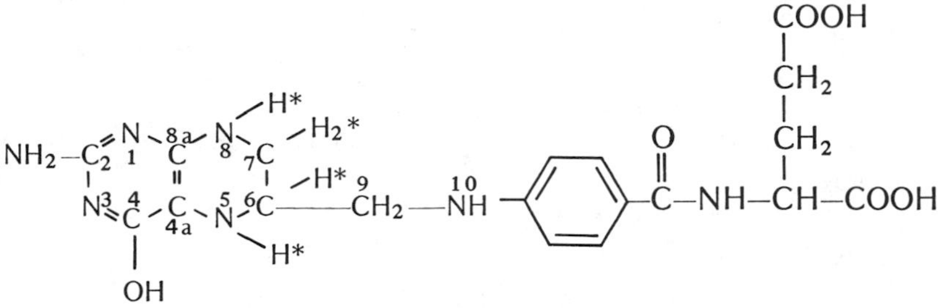

Tetrahydrofolic Acid (THFA)

Just as COA is a carrier for acyl groups, THFA is carrier for single carbon groups: formyl, formaldehyde, and methanol. One-carbon donors include formylglutamate, purines, serine, glycine, and histidine. Several coenzyme forms are involved in folate metabolism: N^{10}-formyl THFA, N^5-formyl THFA, $N^{5,10}$-methenyl THFA, $N^{5,10}$-methylene THFA, and N^5-formimino THFA. The interconversions of these compounds and some of the reactions in which they participate are shown in Fig. 3.4. Folic acid in plasma occurs primarily in the N^5-methyl THFA form and is produced by the reaction of serine with THFA giving $N^{5,10}$-methylene THFA which is then reduced to N^5-methyl THFA (Fig. 3.5). As shown in the figure, the only major pathway by which N^5-methyl THFA can be returned to the primary folate pool is via the vitamin B_{12}-dependent conversion of homocysteine to methionine. In vitamin B_{12} deficiency, folacin enters this "methyl trap" and accumulates in the form of N^5-methyl THFA, because vitamin B_{12} is not available to catalyze its conversion back to THFA. Either vitamin B_{12} or methionine is capable of releasing folacin from the "methyl trap" (Jagerstad et al., 1980).

THFA is a carrier for single carbon groups, that is, it is the primary nutrient involved in "one-carbon" metabolism. THFA, $N^{5,10}$-methenyl THFA, N^{10}-formyl-THFA, and N^5-methyl THFA all are involved in reactions that are important in the metabolism of other substances, notably amino acids and nucleic acid bases. Although not shown in Fig. 3.4, N^{10}-formyl THFA can be produced from THFA

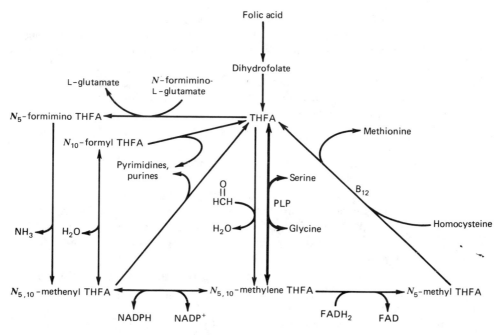

Figure 3.5
The roles of tetrahydrofolic acid in one-carbon metabolism.

by reaction with formic acid; this reaction requires ATP. Also, the formic acid must be produced from formaldehyde which usually is in limited supply in mammalian systems. The major pathway for production of N^{10}-formyl THFA is through the reaction of serine with THFA to produce $N^{5,10}$-methylene THFA, its oxidation to $N^{5,10}$-methenyl THFA, and subsequent conversion to the formyl derivative.

N^{10}**-Formyl THFA** $N^{5,10}$**-Methenyl THFA**

The single-carbon units transferred by THFA and its derivatives are important in the biosynthesis of purines and pyrimidines, in amino acid interconversions, and in certain methylation reactions. Some specific reactions in which THFA participates are conversion of glycine to serine, methylation of ethanolamine to choline, methylation of homocysteine to methionine, methylation of nicotinamide to N^1-methylnicotinamide, methylation of a pyrimidine intermediate to thymine, and introduction of carbons 2 and 8 in the purine ring structures. Vitamin B_{12} is intimately involved in some of these reactions. There is evidence that, in these instances, a methyl group is transferred from N^5-methyl THFA to form methyl-B_{12}.

The involvement of folacin in purine and pyrimidine syntheses appears to be the most significant of its metabolic functions. Folacin, however, makes a significant contribution to the available methionine pool by remethylation of homocysteine. Betaine, an oxidized form of choline, contributes to the remethylation of homocysteine. The most dramatic effect of folacin deficiency is the inhibition of DNA synthesis because of decreased availability of purines and thymidine. This inhibition leads to an arrest of cell division and the characteristic "megaloblastic" appearance of erythrocyte precursor cells in folacin-deficiency anemia. (See Chapter 16.)

One-carbon metabolism appears to be influenced only by the THFA form of folacin; the specific THFA compounds involved include the penta-, hexa-, and heptaglutamates (Brody et al., 1982). At the pentaglutamate level, 5-methyl THFA is the major form; at the hexaglutamate level, THFA and 5-methyl THFA are major forms; and at the heptaglutamate level, THFA predominates but a small amount of 5-methyl THFA also is present. All three folates of 5-methylTHFA(glu^{5-7}) are metabolically active in liver.

A folate-binding protein is present in human placenta. This protein also binds glutamates, but the number of glutamates attached apparently does not affect binding for folacin (Antony et al., 1981).

Formyl THFA, but not vitamin B_{12}, is effective in correcting thymidine (and therefore DNA) biosynthesis in folacin deficiency, but either THFA or vitamin B_{12} corrects thymidine biosynthesis in vitamin B_{12} deficiency (Taheri et al., 1982). Folacin alone will correct the megaloblastic anemia without preventing the longer-term and more harmful central nervous system effects of vitamin B_{12} deficiency.

The clinical pathology of folic acid deficiency includes glossitis, gastrointestinal disturbances, diarrhea, megaloblastic anemia, and neurological damage (Herbert, 1967; 1968). The time sequence of developing symptoms in experimental folacin deficiency in humans was described by Herbert (1967). Within one month serum folacin activity as measured by *Lactobacillus casei* assay is depressed. By three months, erythrocyte and liver stores are depleted and urinary excretion of formiminoglutamate (FIGLU), urocanate, formate, and aminoimidazole carboxamide (AIC) increases. Excretion of these compounds with or without a test dose of histidine can be used as a measure of folacin nutritional status (Herbert et al., 1964; Herbert, 1968). Excretion of AIC, however, also is increased in vitamin B_{12} deficiency (Herbert et al., 1964; Marston and Allen, 1970).

A high incidence of megaloblastic anemia in pregnancy has been reported (Halstead, 1978). The incidence is highest in the underdeveloped countries where diets are likely to be poor in quality. The incidence of megaloblastic anemia also is somewhat higher during the last trimester of pregnancy, which suggests an increased maternal need for the vitamin in response to increased demands by the fetus in late pregnancy. The finding that levels of folacin are significantly higher in fetal than in maternal blood at term (Baker et al., 1958) adds support to this argument. Aside from the needs of the developing fetus, however, hormonal changes during pregnancy conceivably could play a role in the apparent increased requirement for folacin. A relative deficiency of folacin has been demonstrated in women taking birth control pills (Streiff, 1970; Necheles and Synder, 1970; Kahn et al., 1970; see Rose, 1978a). The significance of this finding is not well understood. Since oral contraceptive therapy apparently simulates the state of pregnancy, it seems possible that either estrogen or progesterone, or both hormones, could be involved in producing the effect on folacin metabolism.

FOLACIN METABOLITES

Metabolites of folacin have been as difficult to identify as have been the many forms of the vitamin itself. N^5-formyl THFA is excreted in the urine in extremely small amounts. Since only 0.1 percent of a 50 mg oral dose of pteroylglutamic acid could be recovered in this form (Broquist et al., 1951), it would seem that the compound is metabolized further in tissue cells. A heat-labile metabolite that stimulated the growth of *Lactobacillus citrovorum* also has been identified in urine (Silverman et al., 1956). Presumably this factor is N^{10}-formyl THFA. Other compounds isolated from human urine include xanthopterin (Koschara, 1936), isoxanthopterin (Blair, 1958), and biopterin (Patterson et al., 1956). It seems likely that they are true end products of folacin metabolism (Scott, 1980).

FOLACIN ANTAGONISTS

A large array of folacin antagonists have been identified (Burchenal, 1955; Robinson, 1966). Of these, the 4-amino derivatives of pteroylglutamic acid have been studied most extensively both in the induction of experimental folacin deficiency and as cancer chemotherapeutic agents. Aminopterin is the preferred antimetabolite for nutritional studies. It is partly competitive in action but certain cells, such as chick embryo osteoblasts and fibroblasts, and mouse liver can inactivate the antimetabolite; normal bone marrow or normal lymphoblasts and lymphocytes cannot (Jacobson and Cathie, 1960).

Beginning with the discovery by Farber et al. (1948) that aminopterin produced temporary remission in leukemia in children, several related compounds have been developed as cancer chemotherapeutic agents. Of these compounds, 4-amino-N_{10}-methylfolic acid (methotrexate, MTX) has shown most promise against tumor growth. The selectivity of the antimetabolite in inhibiting tumor growth seems to depend on the vulnerability of rapidly proliferating tumor cells to folacin antagonists. (See Hryniuk and Bertino, 1971.) Methotrexate blocks the synthesis of thymidine through inhibition of one-carbon transfers (Waxman et al., 1970). Because cell division is dependent upon thymidine, cell division, including that of cancer cells, stops. The more rapidly growing cancer cells are most affected; thus, the net result is beneficial. However, other rapidly dividing cells such as those in bone marrow also are sensitive to the drug and prolonged use may cause anemia. In addition, tumor cells may become resistant by producing large amounts of the dihydrofolate reductase or by a compensatory increase in thymidine kinase activity, which permits tumor cell growth to continue. For these reasons, control and timing of dosage of the antagonist are critical determinants in the effectiveness of treatment.

Although a large amount of administered antagonist is recovered in the urine, contrary to earlier supposition, folate antagonists are metabolized to some degree by the animal body (Johns and Valerino, 1971). Tissue distribution of folate antagonists also has been extensively studied (Oliverio and Zaharko, 1971); these data provide valuable insight into the relative efficiency of antagonists in limiting tumor growth in various tissues.

Vitamin B₁₂ (Cyanocobalamin)

The search for vitamin B_{12} began with the discovery by Minot and Murphy (1926) of the efficacy of liver in the treatment of pernicious anemia, a disease characterized by a severe megaloblastic anemia and, if untreated, eventual extensive neurological damage. Much of the work leading to the isolation of the active principle in liver was reviewed by SubbaRow et al. (1948). Crystalline B_{12} was isolated independently by two groups, Rickes et al. (1948) in the United States and Smith and Parker (1948) in England and was shown to be active in the treatment of pernicious anemia (West, 1948). The substance was also shown to be identical with the *animal protein factor,* a growth factor present only in animal products, which had been known for some time and rightly believed to be an unidentified vitamin.

CHEMISTRY

The vitamin B_{12} molecule is the most complex of the vitamins. Elucidation of the structure of the vitamin was accomplished seven years after its isolation and resulted from a brilliant series of x-ray crystallographic analyses by Hodgkin and associates (1955; 1957). The vitamin is distinguished by the presence of cobalt in the molecule, which is responsible for its dark red color.

The cobalt is bordered by a corrin ring that consists of four nitrogen-containing five-membered rings joined through three methylene bridges. The corrin ring is similar to the porphyrin ring of chlorophyll. (The term *corrinoids* applies to all compounds containing the corrin nucleus and though chemically related to the vitamin they are not synonymous with vitamin B_{12}.)

Cyanocobalamin, the usual commercial form of the vitamin, contains a cyanide group attached to the central cobalt (see formula). Apparently cyanide is present due to contamination from reagents used in isolation of the vitamin and little, if any, of the cyanide form occurs naturally. (See Stadtman, 1971.) However, other forms of the vitamin in which cyanide is replaced by another group occur in nature. For example, *hydroxycobalamin* contains a hydroxyl group in place of cyanide; this compound has been isolated from liver extracts. Certain bacteria have been found to contain a *nitritocobalamin*. In foods, vitamin B_{12} usually

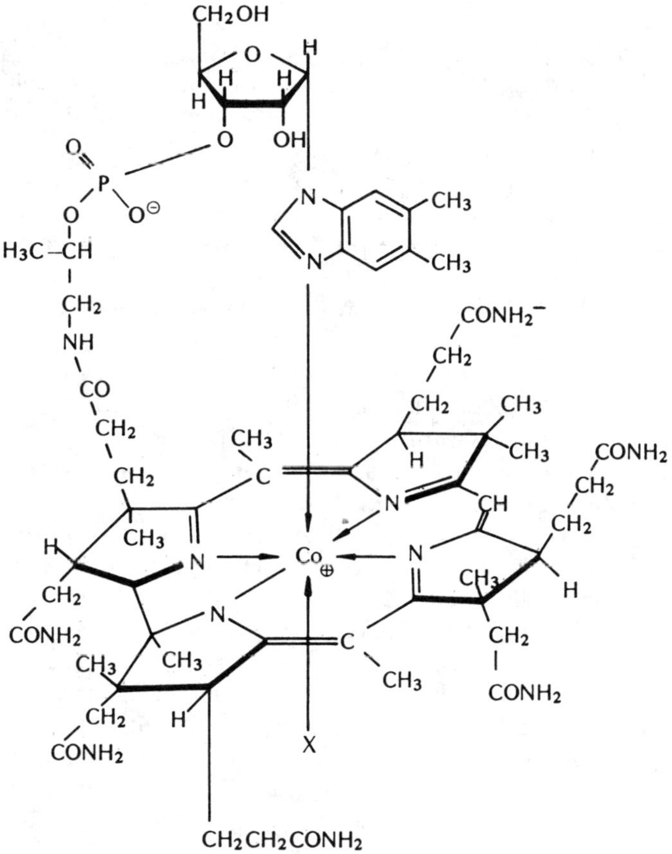
CH2OH
O
H
H
H
H
O
OH
O
P
O
O⊖
H3C–CH
CH2
NH
CO
CH2
CH2
N
N
CH3
CH3
CONH2⁻
CH2
CH2
CH3
CH3
H
CH3
C
CONH2
CH2
CH2
N
CH
CH3
H
N
Co⊕
N
CH3
H
CH2
CONH2
N
C
CH3
CH3
CH3
CH2
H
CH2
CONH2
CH3
CONH2
X
CH2CH2CONH2

Vitamin B_{12}

X = $-CN$ in cyanocobalamin
= $-OH$ in hydroxycobalamin
= $-CH_3$ in methylcobalamin
=

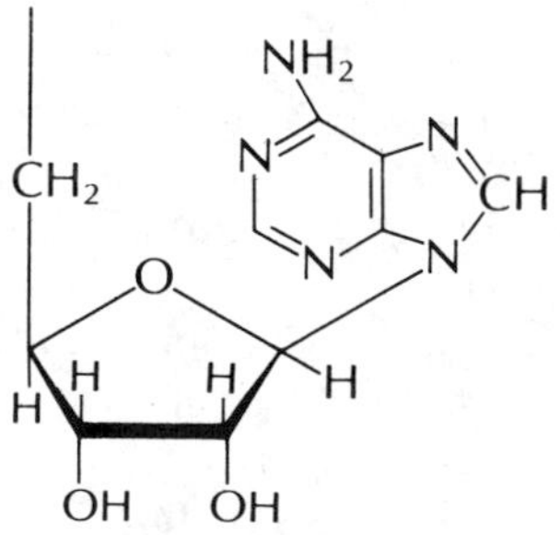
NH2
N
N
CH
N
N
CH2
O
H
H
H
H
OH
OH

in 5′-deoxyadenosylcobalamin

occurs bound to protein in the methyl or 5'-deoxyadenosyl forms, both of which are coenzymes.

A major breakthrough in the chemistry of vitamin B_{12} came with the synthesis of the vitamin 25 years after its isolation. (See Maugh, 1973.) This work represented a joint effort directed by R. B. Woodward of Harvard University in the United States (who won the Nobel Prize in 1965 for the synthesis of chlorophyll) and A. Eschenmoser of the Eidgenössische Technische Hochschule, Zurich, Switzerland. The enormity of the task can be appreciated when one considers that the project involved 99 scientists from 19 countries working over a period of 11 years! The final stages of the synthesis began with a compound aptly designated B-corrnorsterone by Woodward because it is the "cornerstone" of the plan for completion of the cyanocobalamin molecule (Woodward, 1971).

Both spectrophotometric and chemical methods of assay are suitable for determination of vitamin B_{12} in pharmaceutical preparations or in substances relatively free of interfering substances. (See Rosenthal, 1968.) However, for complex biological materials the microbiological assay is the preferred method of analysis. *Lactobacillus lactis* Dorner (LLD) has been used as a test organism for determining antipernicious anemia activity of liver extracts. Bioassays run with this organism aided in identifying the crystallized vitamin as the antipernicious anemia factor (Shorb, 1948). This organism is more erratic in response, however, than *Lactobacillus leichmanii*. (See Association of Official Analytical Chemists, 1980.) Methods using *Ochromonas malhamensis* and *Euglena gracilis,* z strain, are described in detail by Baker and Frank (1968) and are equally suitable for urine, blood, and animal tissues. Vitamin B_{12} can be measured in serum using radio dilution assay using $^{57}CoB_{12}$ and intrinsic factor (Rothenberg, 1961). However, these assays are not always specific and may measure analogs of the vitamin as well (Kolhouse et al., 1978).

BIOCHEMICAL FUNCTION

The first coenzyme form of vitamin B_{12} was discovered by Barker and his coworkers (1958) in the course of studying the conversion of glutamic acid to β-methylaspartate in an obscure anaerobic bacterium, *Clostridium Tetanomorphum*. They found that a derivative of pseudovitamin B_{12} was involved in the reaction. The same group later isolated a similar derivative containing 5,6-dimethylbenzimidazole from *Clostridium tetanomorphum,* animal liver, and propionic acid bacteria (Weissbach et al., 1959). The structure of the coenzyme which contained a 5-deoxyadenine nucleoside was determined by Lenhert and Hodgkin (1961) using the x-ray crystallography technique, which had been instrumental in determining the structure of the vitamin.

In addition to the 5'-deoxyadenosyl derivative, vitamin B_{12} also exists as a methyl coenzyme. The 5'-deoxyadenosyl derivative is required for the conversion of methylmalonylCoA to succinyl CoA; the methyl derivative is a coenzyme for the conversion of homocysteine to methionine. The structures of the coenzyme forms may be visualized by substituting the methyl or 5'-deoxyadenosyl group for the X in the structure of vitamin B_{12} shown on page 123. All bonds to the cobalt atom in vitamin B_{12} are coordinate bonds. The electronegativities of the different species of X in the structure will influence the relative proportions of the covalent and the ionic character of the bond to the cobalt atom. Also, the valence of the X group will influence the net charge of the cobalt ion in the structure. In the coenzyme forms, the X group is electrically neutral and therefore the net charge on the molecule is more positive than it is when X is either CN^- or OH^-.

Vitamin B_{12} is known to participate in a number of enzymatic reactions in bacteria, but only two vitamin B_{12}-dependent enzyme systems of significance— methylmalonylCoA mutase and 5-methyl THFA:homocysteine methyltransferase—have been demonstrated in mammalian tissues. (See Stadtman, 1971.) A vitamin B_{12}-dependent enzyme that catalyzes the formation of leucine from β-leucine, was demonstrated originally in plants and has been shown to occur in rat and human tissues (Poston, 1980). The metabolic significance of this reaction is uncertain.

Methylmalonyl CoA is the intermediary compound in the metabolism of propionate in mammalian tissues; the enzyme converts methylmalonyl CoA to succinyl CoA. The reaction is essentially a carbon-carbon bond cleavage (see below). In vitamin B_{12} deficiency excretion of methylmalonate in the urine is increased (Cox and White, 1962).

$$
\begin{array}{ll}
& O \\
& \| \\
① & C-S-CoA \\
& | \\
② & CH-CH_3 \\
& |\ \ ③ \\
④ & COOH
\end{array}
\qquad \rightleftharpoons \qquad
\begin{array}{ll}
& O \\
& \| \\
① & C-S-CoA \\
& | \\
② & CH_2 \\
& | \\
③ & CH_2 \\
& | \\
④ & COOH
\end{array}
$$

Methylmalonyl CoA **Succinyl CoA**

The mutase reaction is a key step in the metabolism of some branched-chain amino acids and branched-chain fatty acids and may be involved in the neurological disorders that occur in pernicious anemia. These disorders reflect a progressive demyelination of nerve tissue. When the mutase reaction is blocked, the methylmalonylCoA that accumulates may inhibit myelin sheath formation by competitive inhibition of malonylCoA in fatty acid synthesis or by substitution of branched-chain fatty acids for malonylCoA in the myelin sheath. (See Chapter 20.)

The vitamin B_{12}-methyltransferase is responsible for the methylation of homocysteine to form methionine. This reaction involves N^5-methyl THFA; the methyl group is transferred to homocysteine to form methionine and as a result, THFA is regenerated. (See Fig. 3.5.)

The megaloblastic anemia and the changes in bone marrow associated with the pernicious anemia syndrome suggest that, like folacin, vitamin B_{12} is essential for DNA synthesis which, in turn, is necessary for normal development of mature

red blood cells. (See Beck, 1968.) However, neither the methylmalonyl CoA reaction nor methionine synthesis per se provided clear evidence of precisely how
vitamin B_{12} is related either to folacin metabolism and one-carbon transfers or to
DNA synthesis. In an attempt to clarify this, Herbert and Zalusky (1962) proposed
that the function of vitamin B_{12} in DNA synthesis may be through its involvement
in methionine synthesis and subsequent regeneration of THFA. If methionine
synthesis is inhibited by vitamin B_{12} deficiency, then the ability to regenerate
THFA from N^5-methyl THFA also would be inhibited. (See Fig. 3.5.) Further, if
the synthesis of methionine from homocysteine is the major pathway for regeneration of THFA, then a deficiency of vitamin B_{12} could result in an excess of
N^5-methyl THFA and subsequent accumulation of folacin in the "methyl trap."

Dietary supplementation with high levels of folacin can prevent or cure the
megaloblastic anemia of pernicious anemia but has no effect in preventing the
neurological damage resulting from the disease. Thus, it appears that these two
symptoms may stem from different biological mechanisms, anemia from folacin
accumulation as 5-methyl THFA and neurological damage from inadequate
methylmalonylCoA mutase activity.

Pernicious anemia (or vitamin B_{12} deficiency) is most often due to malabsorption
of the vitamin that results from a hereditary lack of the factor required for vitamin
B_{12} absorption. (See Thedering, 1968; also see Chapter 6.) However, since vitamin
B_{12} occurs only in animal products, a dietary deficiency of the vitamin has been
known to occur in complete vegetarians, that is, those persons who include no
animal products in their diet.

Vitamin B_{12}, thus, is a vitamin in which cellular deficiency is the result, most
often, not of a dietary lack but, instead, of the inability of the individual's absorptive mechanism to make the vitamin available for cellular metabolism.

VITAMIN B_{12} METABOLITES

Very little is known of the end products of vitamin B_{12} metabolism. Absorbed
vitamin B_{12} that is not required immediately is stored in body tissues, particularly
in the liver. Total body stores in the human have been estimated as 2–4 mg of
which 30–60 percent is in the liver, 30 percent in muscle, skin, and bone, and
smaller amounts in the lungs, kidneys, and spleen (Reisner, 1968). Surprisingly
little vitamin B_{12} is stored in bone marrow. The vitamin is excreted in the urine,
but when given in physiological amounts, a large amount is excreted in the bile
(Reizenstein, 1959). In fact, more vitamin B_{12} is excreted daily in the bile than
is contained in the entire blood volume. It is assumed that most of the vitamin
B_{12} in bile is from hepatic stores. Fecal excretion, although higher than urinary
excretion, is less than biliary loss. Thus some reabsorption of biliary vitamin B_{12}
probably occurs.

VITAMIN B_{12} ANTAGONISTS

Vitamin B_{12} analogs and antagonists were reviewed by Friedrich (1966) and Moore
and Folkers (1968). Although many derivatives of vitamin B_{12} possess vitamin

activity, and many are antagonistic to bacterial growth and survival, relatively few compounds inhibit vitamin B_{12} activity in higher animals. The antagonists active in animals include a lactam of vitamin B_{12} prepared by Beiler et al. (1951) and several competitive inhibitors involving modification of one or more of the propionamide side chains of vitamin B_{12}. (See Cuthbertson et al., 1956.)

Biotin

Biotin was first described as the factor protective against egg-white injury. Rats fed large amounts of raw egg white developed an eczemalike dermatitis, paralysis of the hind legs, and a characteristic alopecia around the eyes, aptly termed *spectacle eye*. However, cooked egg white fed to rats was not toxic. A protective factor present in liver and yeast was designated vitamin H by György (1939), and the "factor protective against egg white injury" by Parsons et al. (1937). This factor was later designated biotin and was shown to be identical to *bios* or *Coenzyme R,* a growth factor for certain microorganisms that previously had been isolated from egg yolk as the crystalline methyl ester (Kögl and Tönnis, 1936). The synthesis of biotin was accomplished several years later by Harris et al. (1945).

The heat-labile biotin antagonist in raw egg white is avidin, a glycoprotein that binds with biotin in the intestinal tract and thus inhibits biotin absorption.

CHEMISTRY

Biotin is a relatively simple monocarboxylic acid. It is soluble in methanol, ethanol, acetone, and chloroform but is almost insoluble in water. Salts of the acid, however, are quite soluble. Biotin is destroyed by severe treatment with acids and alkalies but, in general, it tends to be more stable than most other vitamins to acid and alkali treatment.

Biotin

A number of microorganisms have been tested for use in a biotin assay (see Baker and Frank, 1968), but because of a lack of specificity for the vitamin, few are suitable for determination of the vitamin in biological materials. Baker et al. (1962) found the flagellate, *Ochromonas danica,* to be both specific and sensitive as an assay organism for biotin. This organism has been used for biotin assay in blood, urine, and animal tissues. More recently a colorimetric reaction has been described that allows for separation of biotin and its analogs by paper or thin-layer chromatography (McCormick and Roth, 1970). Spectrophotometric techniques for determination of both biotin and avidin also have been developed (Green, 1970); these methods are somewhat less sensitive than the microbiological assay but are described as more convenient, more precise, and applicable over a wide range of pH and salt concentrations. More recently a radioisotope dilution method was described that compares favorably with results obtained using the microbiological assay with *Ochromonas danica* as the assay organism (Sangvi et al., 1982).

BIOCHEMICAL FUNCTION

Biotin is known to function in two general types of carboxylation reactions. The first type is energy dependent and involves the cleavage of ATP to ADP and inorganic phosphate (see below). Most biotin-requiring reactions in mammalian tissues appear to be of this type.

$$ATP + HCO_3^- \qquad ADP + Pi$$

Biotin-protein $\qquad {}^-O_3C-biotin-protein$

$$RCO_2^- \qquad RH$$

The second type involves only an exchange of carboxyl groups; free CO_2 does not participate nor is ATP or any other energy source needed for the reaction.

The biotin-catalyzed carboxylase systems have been shown to consist of three types of subunits: biotin carboxylase (BC), carboxyl transferase (CT), and carboxyl carrier protein (CCP). (See McCormick, 1975.) Biotin is covalently linked to CCP through a peptide bond to the ϵ-amino group of lysine. This biotin-lysine structure is known as biocytin and was identified first by Lane and Lynen (1963) for propionyl carboxylase, a biotin-dependent enzyme. In the process of carboxylation, bicarbonate becomes attached to the 1'-N atom of the ureido moiety of biotin.

$$HN \overset{\displaystyle \overset{O}{\|}}{\quad} NH$$

$$S-(CH_2)_4-\overset{O}{\overset{\|}{C}}-\overset{H}{\overset{|}{N}}-(CH_2)_4-\overset{NH^-}{\underset{H}{\overset{|}{C}}}-CO^-$$

Biocytin

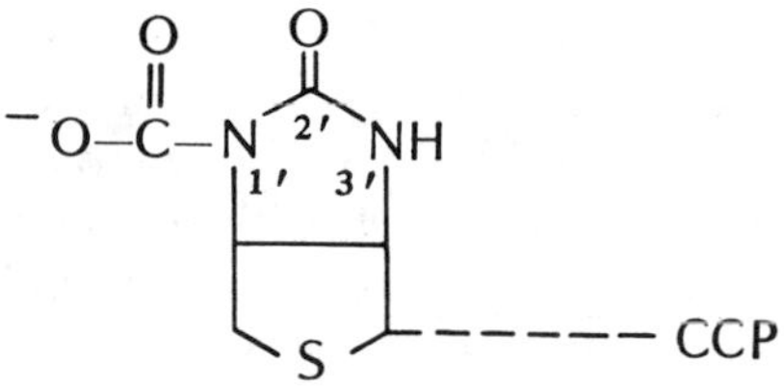

$$
\begin{array}{cc}
O & O \\
\parallel & \parallel \\
^-O-C-N & \overset{2'}{} NH \\
\end{array}
$$

During catalysis, the attached carboxyl group becomes tautomerized with the 2'-CO with a resulting interchange of these two carbon atoms (see above).

The most important of the biotin-dependent carboxylation enzymes are (1) pyruvate carboxylase and (2) acetyl CoA carboxylase. A third biotin-dependent carboxylation enzyme, propionyl CoA carboxylase, is of lesser metabolic importance. The reactions catalyzed by these enzymes are shown as follows.

1. $CH_3COCOOH + HCO_3^- + ATP \xrightarrow[\text{Pyruvate carboxylase}]{CH_3COSCoA + Mg^{++}}$
Pyruvate

$HOOCCH_2COCOOH + ADP + P_i$
Oxaloacetate

Pyruvate carboxylase appears to be dependent on the presence of acetyl CoA or propionyl CoA; acetyl CoA is not incorporated into the oxaloacetate molecule.

2. $CH_3COSCoA + HCO_3^- + ATP \xrightarrow[\text{Acetyl CoA carboxylase}]{Mg^{++}}$
Acetyl CoA

$$
\begin{array}{c}
COO^- \\
| \\
CH_2COSCoA + ADP + P_i
\end{array}
$$
Malonyl CoA

Acetyl CoA carboxylase enzyme plays an essential role in the initial stage of the biosynthesis of fatty acids.

3. $CH_3CH_2COSCoA + HCO_3^- + ATP \xrightarrow[\text{Propionyl CoA carboxylase}]{Mg^{++}}$
Propionyl CoA

$$
\begin{array}{c}
COO^- \\
| \\
CH_3CHCOSCoA + ADP + P_i
\end{array}
$$
Methylmalonyl CoA

Propionyl CoA arises from various pathways including degradation of isoleucine and the oxidation of odd-numbered fatty acids. Travis et al. (1972) found that linoleate is catabolized by way of propionyl CoA. Thus, the reaction is both biotin- and vitamin B_{12}-dependent (Dupont and Mathias, 1969). (Note that methylmalonyl CoA is an intermediary in the conversion of propionyl CoA to succinyl CoA.)

Biotin also is involved in the action of β-methyl crotonyl CoA carboxylase, which catalyzes the conversion of β-methyl crotonyl CoA to β-methyl glutaconyl CoA. This reaction is an intermediary step in the oxidative degradation of leucine to acetoacetate and acetyl CoA. A transcarboxylation of methylmalonyl CoA with pyruvate to form propionyl CoA and oxaloacetate requires biotin in microorganisms (Dimroth, 1982); this reaction is not known to be of significance in mammalian tissues.

In biotin-deficient rats, brain biotin levels and carboxylase activity are in the normal range when liver stores are almost totally depleted (Sander et al., 1982). This finding is in contrast to observed low carboxylase activity in brain and other tissues in genetically determined biotin-responsive diseases in humans. Large amounts of oral biotin (10 mg/day) corrects an apparent genetic multiple carboxylase deficiency in some persons so afflicted (Thoene et al., 1981). This condition involves deficiencies of propionyl-CoA carboxylase, 3-methylcrotonyl-CoA carboxylase, and pyruvate carboxylase.

Biotin deficiency is rarely encountered in humans although low levels in blood and urine have been reported in pregnant women, infants with seborrheic dermatitis, alcoholics, and in persons with achlorhydria. (See Bonjour, 1977.) The vitamin is widely distributed in foods. It also is synthesized in the gastrointestinal tract and some of this appears to be absorbed. A few cases of biotin deficiency due to excessive intake of raw eggs, however, have been reported (Scott, 1958; Baugh et al., 1968). Paradoxically, although egg white is the best known source of avidin, the biotin antagonist, egg yolk is a very rich source of the vitamin.

For additional information on biotin metabolism and nutrition, see Knappe (1970), Balnave (1977), Bonjour (1977), and Murphy and Mistry (1977).

BIOTIN METABOLITES

Very little breakdown of biotin apparently occurs in either rats or man (Fraenkel-Conrat and Fraenkel-Conrat, 1952; Wright et al., 1956). A high proportion of administered biotin is recovered intact in the urine. The rapid clearance of injected radioactive biotin in experiments with rats further suggests that the rat possesses a very low renal threshold for reabsorption of biotin (Lee et al., 1972). The same situation probably holds for the human as well. Biotin excretion in the human, like that of most water-soluble vitamins, is closely related to intake (Sydenstricker et al., 1942).

The degradation that does take place involves only the side chain of the vitamin. When ring-labeled ^{14}C-biotin is administered, little or no radioactive CO_2 is recovered in expired air (Dakshinamurti and Mistry, 1963; Lee et al., 1972). These data strongly suggest that the biotin ring remains intact.

In addition to the high amounts of intact biotin, however, small amounts of biotin metabolites have been recovered in the urine following administration of the radioactive vitamin. These include the d- and l-sulfoxides, bisnorbiotin (a compound with two carbons less in the side chain), and a neutral unidentified ketone (Lee et al., 1972). All of these compounds involve changes in the side chain of the vitamin.

In later studies (Lee et al., 1973), small amounts of biotin sulfone and tetra-norbiotin (four carbons less in the side chain) also were recovered in urine. The excretion rate of the metabolites is exceedingly rapid, thus following the excretion pattern of the vitamin. Kidney clearance appears to be related to the degree of water solubility of the compounds excreted.

BIOTIN ANTAGONISTS

Avidin is the most important of the biotin antagonists in mammalian metabolism. As mentioned earlier, the antibiotin effect of this compound was responsible for the discovery of the vitamin. Avidin has been shown to be an oligomer with molecular weight of about 70,000 comprising four polypeptide chains and four binding sites for biotin (Green, 1968).

A number of other antagonists including desthiobiotin, desthioisobiotin, 4-imidazolidone-2-caproic acid, biotin sulfone, and ureylenecyclohexylvaleric acid are active against various bacteria and insects (Kodicek, 1966; Langer and György, 1968).

Ascorbic Acid

Historically the disease scurvy became widely recognized when man learned to build ships capable of long sea voyages, and it is probably true that on long-term explorations more deaths were caused by scurvy than any other single factor. The dietary prevention of scurvy was well documented by Lind in 1750. It is typical of the time span between discovery and application of knowledge that Lind's recommendation of providing fresh foods for sailors on long sea voyages was not introduced until some 30 years later when Captain Cook sailed to the Pacific and subsequently discovered the Hawaiian Islands.

The identification of ascorbic acid was aided by Holst and Frölich (1907) who accidentally produced scurvy in guinea pigs and thus provided a test animal for later studies. Of the mammals, only humans, monkeys, and guinea pigs require the vitamin; other mammalian species possess the necessary enzyme to synthesize ascorbic acid.[1] The fruit bat, the pipistrelle and some birds of the Passeriformes order (Chaudhuri and Chatterjee, 1969; Chatterjee, 1970; Chatterjee et al., 1975) as well as the channel and blue catfish (Lovell, 1973) and trout (Halver et al., 1975) have been shown to require the vitamin.

Ascorbic acid was isolated first by Szent-Györgi (1928) from orange juice, cabbage juice, and adrenal cortex; he named the compound hexuronic acid in recognition of the six carbon atoms in the molecule and, at the time, was concerned chiefly with the reducing property of the acid. Four years later ascorbic acid was isolated again by Waugh and King (1932), who demonstrated its anti-

---

[1]Synthesis of ascorbic acid is by way of D-glucuronic acid→L-gluconic acid→L-gulonolactone→3-keto-L-gulonolactone→L-ascorbic acid. Species that require a dietary source of the vitamin lack the enzyme, L-gulonoxidase, which converts L-gulonolactone to 3-keto-L-gulonolactone.

scorbutic activity in guinea pigs. The compound was subsequently shown to be identical with hexuronic acid by Svirbely and Szent-Györgyi (1932).

CHEMISTRY

Ascorbic acid is a hexose derivative and is properly classified as a carbohydrate. It is a white crystalline substance, highly soluble in water, and also soluble in ethyl alcohol and glycerol. The vitamin is quite stable in the dry state but is easily oxidized when in solution. It is stable in acid solutions below pH 4.0 but the instability of ascorbic acid in solution increases markedly as the alkalinity of the solution increases. Ascorbic acid also is unstable in the presence of oxygen and catalysts such as the ions of iron and copper.

Ascorbic Acid   **Dehydroascorbic Acid**   **Diketogulonic Acid**

Ascorbic acid (reduced ascorbic acid) is easily oxidized to form dehydroascorbic acid that is just as easily reduced back to the original form. The ease with which the two active forms of the vitamin are interconverted is probably related to at least some of the physiological properties of the vitamin. Further oxidation of dehydroascorbic acid results in irreversible formation of diketogulonic acid and loss of vitamin activity.

In mammalian tissues reduction of dehydroascorbic acid to reduced ascorbic acid is aided by the sulfhydryl tripeptide glutathione. The formation of reduced glutathione involves coenzymes of both niacin and riboflavin. In analytical procedures that measure only the reduced form of ascorbic acid, hydrogen sulfide may be passed through the solution for the same purpose.

The strong reducing property of ascorbic acid is the basis for an analytical procedure in which the dye 2,6-dichlorophenolindophenol is reduced by the vitamin; only the reduced form of the vitamin is measured by this method. Total ascorbic acid may be measured by reaction with 2,4-dinitrophenylhydrazine (Roe et al., 1948; Roe and Kuether, 1943). The latter method is probably the most widely used method. A liquid chromatographic assay for determination of ascorbic acid in lymphocytes was described recently (Lee et al., 1982). Other methods for the determination of ascorbic acid have been reviewed by Omaye et al. (1979), Sauberlich (1981), and Sauberlich et al. (1981).

BIOCHEMICAL FUNCTION

The mechanism by which ascorbic acid acts in biological systems remains obscure; if a coenzyme form exists for the vitamin, it likely is a highly unstable molecule since it has eluded investigators for so long. Ascorbic acid is known to function as a reducing agent, but since in some cases other reducing agents perform equally well, the effect may be largely nonspecific for the vitamin.

Abnormalities of connective tissue observed in scurvy have long suggested that ascorbic acid is involved in the synthesis of collagen or mucopolysaccharides. There is now ample evidence to support a role of the vitamin in collagen biosynthesis as first suggested by the studies of Robertson and Hewett (1961). Stone and Meister (1962) and Peterkafsky and Udenfriend (1965) demonstrated that the vitamin is necessary for the hydroxylation of proline to form hydroxyproline, an unusual amino acid that occurs almost exclusively in collagen. In in vitro studies, Gottlieb et al. (1966) presented evidence of a collagenlike protein containing little hydroxyproline. This protein is formed in response to ascorbic acid deficiency or when hydroxylation is impaired by lack of oxygen and was believed to be responsible for the structural changes observed in scorbutic tissues. In in vivo experiments, however, Barnes (1969) reported that collagen synthesis is impaired in scorbutic animals but that there is not an accumulation of an unhydroxylated collagen precursor as was observed in vitro. These data suggested that proline (and lysine) are hydroxylated after incorporation into the polypeptide chain.

Without hydroxyproline and hydroxylysine protocollagen does not properly cross-link to form fibrous collagen. (See Chapter 17.) Since collagen is a crucial part of the structure of normal connective tissue, connective tissue involved in wound healing, and of the organic matrix of bone, ascorbic acid deficiency involves abnormalities in all these structures. Collagen is a component of the ground substance surrounding capillary wall cells; scurvy always involves bleeding into joints and periosteal spaces because of this inadequacy in capillary structure (Barnes, 1975; Chaney, 1982).

Other hydroxylation reactions also have been reported to require the vitamin including the oxidation of tryptophan to 5-hydroxy-tryptophan (Cooper, 1961), the conversion of 3,4-dihydroxyphenylethylamine to norepinephrine (Levin et al., 1960), and hydroxylation of p-hydroxyphenylpyruvate to homogentisic acid in tyrosine metabolism (Sealock and Silberstein, 1939). All the hydroxylations carried out by the cytochrome P_{450}-dependent mixed-function oxidase system in mitochondria and smooth endoplasmic reticulum require ascorbic acid (Zannoni et al., 1978; Chaney, 1982). Substrates for the mixed-function oxidase system include many drugs, pesticides, carcinogens, environmental chemicals, and both endogenous and exogenous steroids. Because ascorbic acid is concentrated in the adrenal gland, it has been postulated to be important in the biochemical functions of this organ, especially in the production of the adrenal steroids and the epinephrines.

Ascorbic acid functions, along with vitamin E to a certain extent, as a nonenzymatic reducing agent; it enhances the absorption of nonheme iron in the intestine by reducing it to the ferrous state in the stomach and, perhaps, by chelation and acidification effects. (See Chapter 6.) This vitamin also is involved in the transfer of plasma iron to the liver and its incorporation in ferritin, the primary iron storage form in liver (Mazur, 1961), and in the distribution of iron among the different iron-binding proteins (Lipschitz et al., 1971). In ascorbic acid-deficient guinea pigs, ferritin was reported to be decreased and hemosiderin increased in liver and spleen. When ascorbic acid was fed, the distribution of iron between these compounds returned to normal.

Ascorbic acid enhances the conversion of folate to tetrahydrofolate, but the possible involvement of enzymes in this function is not clear. The reducing capacity of ascorbic acid helps protect vitamin A, vitamin E, and some of the B vitamins from oxidation.

Ascorbic acid needs are increased by exposure to certain chemicals such as ozone and the aldehydes in cigarette smoke. These increases may be mediated through its nonenzymatic antioxidant effects. Ascorbic acid reacts with nitrite (a food component and a food additive) and thereby prevents the reaction with secondary amines to produce carcinogenic nitrosamines. In this reaction, it is converted to dehydroascorbic acid in a nonenzymatic reaction (Archer, 1982).

Thus, the participation of ascorbic acid in a number of metabolic reactions has been demonstrated and, for the most part, these reactions tend to relate to clinical symptoms of ascorbic acid deficiency. A role for the vitamin in the prevention of the common cold has been suggested when the vitamin is taken in massive doses (Pauling, 1970; 1971). Although there is some evidence that symptoms of a cold are somewhat lessened among persons taking large quantities of ascorbic acid (Anderson et al., 1972; Coulehan et al., 1974) any such effect likely should be classed as pharmacologic rather than physiologic. *In vitro* studies indicate that ascorbic acid is effective in the detoxication of histamine (Subramanian et al., 1973). Since histamine formation is known to be increased under many conditions of body stress (including the common cold) these workers suggest that any beneficial effect of ascorbic acid is due to its detoxication of excess histamine.

ASCORBIC ACID METABOLITES

Very little is known of the end products of ascorbic acid metabolism. Apparently much of ingested ascorbic acid is excreted intact (Baker et al., 1971b). Various unidentified 6-carbon compounds are excreted following administration of labeled ascorbic acid but because of the labile nature of the vitamin, the identification of these compounds as true metabolites or as breakdown products in urine is difficult. Oxalate has been shown to be derived from ascorbic acid (Hellman

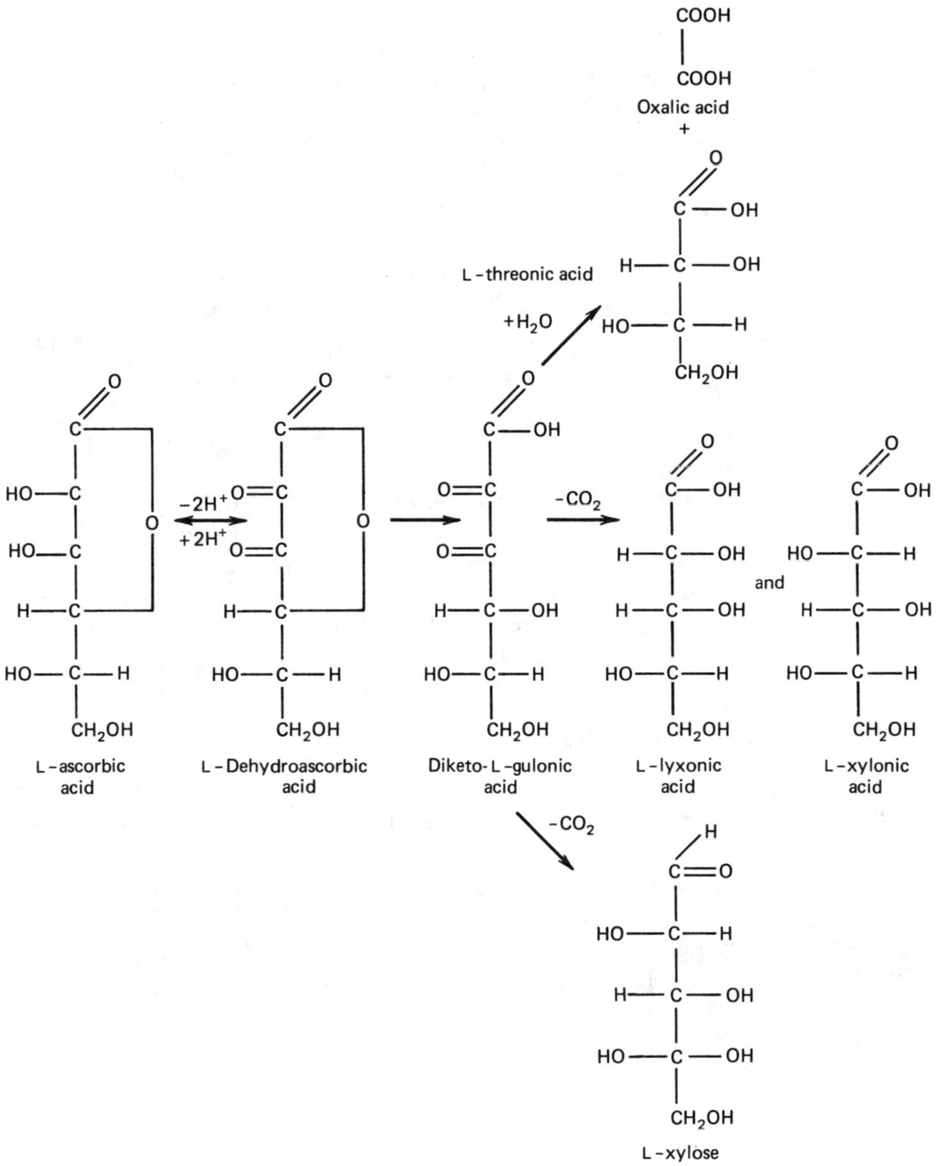

Figure 3.6
Metabolism of ascorbic acid.

and Burns, 1958; Baker et al., 1966). Ascorbate-3-sulfate also has been identified as a metabolite of the vitamin (Baker et al., 1971a).

Mammalian cells contain two enzymatically produced ascorbic acid derivatives, ascorbate-2-sulfate and ascorbate-2-phosphate (Baker et al., 1971a). The involvement of these metabolites in any of the essential functions of ascorbic acid is not clear. However, ascorbate-2-sulfate has ascorbic acid activity for the channel catfish (Murai et al., 1978) but not for the guinea pig nor the rhesus monkey (Machlin et al., 1976).

A small amount of ascorbic acid is excreted in expired air as CO_2, but only 2 percent of a radioactive dose of the vitamin has been accounted for in that form (Baker et al., 1971b). At least one source of CO_2 appears to be 2,3-diketo-L-gulonic acid that is formed by hydrolysis of dehydro-L-ascorbic acid. The enzyme involved is known to be aldonolactonase. (See Kagawa and Shimazono, 1970.) In turn, 2,3-diketo-L-gulonic acid is hydrolyzed to L-xylonic acid (or L-lyxonic acid) and CO_2. (See Fig. 3.6.)

In humans, catabolism of ascorbic acid appears to represent about 3 percent of the body pool per day. When subjects were depleted of the vitamin, a body pool of approximately 300 mg appeared to be associated with appearance of clinical symptoms of scurvy. The average pool of healthy male subjects was calculated to be 1500 mg. Once this level is reached, excretion of ascorbic acid in the urine markedly increases (Baker et al., 1971b).

ASCORBIC ACID ANTAGONISTS

Only one antagonist of ascorbic acid, glucoascorbic acid, is known and it appears that this compound may have toxic as well as antimetabolite properties (Woolley and Krampitz, 1943). When fed to rats, mice, and guinea pigs, glucoascorbic acid induced growth failure and lesions similar but not identical to scurvy. Effects of the compound were alleviated by adding ascorbic acid to the diet of the guinea pig, which requires the vitamin, but not to rats or mice, which synthesize ascorbic acid (Woolley, 1944b). This compound is of little current interest.

chapter 4

fat-soluble and other vitamins

Fat-Soluble Vitamins

The fat-soluble vitamins appear to be more unlike the water-soluble vitamins in biological function than can be attributed to their solubility properties alone. Solubility, of course, affects the transport, distribution, storage, and excretion of the vitamins, but the concept of very fundamental differences in mode of action of some of these vitamins has emerged. The search for a coenzyme function comparable to those of the B-vitamins has given way to investigation of other mechanisms by which the fat-soluble vitamins exert their influence in biochemical systems.

Recent evidence suggests, for example, that vitamin D fulfills the functional requisites for classification as a hormone, that is, the active "vitamin" is elaborated by one organ but acts on other target organs. Although no such clearly defined mode of action has yet been attributed to the other fat-soluble vitamins, the separation of these substances from the water-soluble vitamins is far more than a question of solubility. They are, indeed, a class unto themselves.

VITAMIN A (RETINOL, RETINAL, RETINOIC ACID)

Vitamin A was the first of the accessory food factors to be identified as a component of specific foods. In 1913 McCollum and Davis reported that rats failed to grow on diets containing carbohydrate, protein, lard, and salts. Addition of an ether extract of butter or eggs promoted growth and established that the missing factor was a fat-soluble substance. A lack of the *fat-soluble growth factor* later was shown to result in necrosis of the cornea in rats. This condition was similar to an eye disease (xerophthalmia) seen in humans, then believed to be due to a lack of dietary fat. Mori (1922) clearly established that the disease was due to lack of a fat-soluble factor (vitamin A) but not to a lack of dietary fat per se.

By the middle 1920s the relationship between dark adaptation and vitamin A was established, but it was nearly 10 years later that Wald discovered that the pigment rhodopsin (visual purple), responsible for sight in dim light, contained vitamin A in combination with protein (Wald, 1933). Wald's subsequent elucidation of the reactions involved in bleaching and regeneration of rhodopsin still provides the only well-defined role of the vitamin in mammalian systems. For this contribution Wald was awarded the Nobel Prize for Medicine in 1967.

Early feeding experiments with rats indicated that vitamin A was associated with plants containing the yellow-, orange-, or red-colored carotenoid pigments. Moore (1930) demonstrated that the most common of these, the carotenes, were related structurally to vitamin A and some of them were converted in vivo to the vitamin.

Vitamin A was isolated in large amounts from fish liver oils by Karrer et al. (1931) and subsequently by several groups. It was not until the late 1940s, however, that synthetic vitamin A became available on the commercial market.

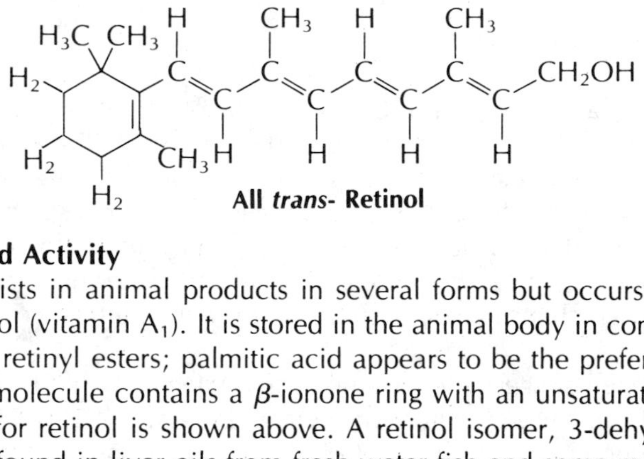

All trans- Retinol

Chemistry and Activity

Vitamin A exists in animal products in several forms but occurs largely as the alcohol, retinol (vitamin A_1). It is stored in the animal body in combination with fatty acids as retinyl esters; palmitic acid appears to be the preferred fatty acid. The vitamin molecule contains a β-ionone ring with an unsaturated side chain. The formula for retinol is shown above. A retinol isomer, 3-dehydroretinol (vitamin A_2), is found in liver oils from fresh water fish and some marine fish. This compound has an additional double bond between carbon atoms 3 and 4 in the ring and is about 40 percent as active as retinol (Shantz, 1948).

Recent studies have shown that vitamin A_2 can be converted to retinol (A_1) in rats (Border and Pitt, 1981). Overall, 3-dehydroretinol has about 40 percent of the biological activity of retinol (Shantz, 1948). It has been proposed that the term "retinoids" be used to designate all compounds derived from retinol by modification of the ring or side chain (Sporn et al., 1976). The term "vitamin A" includes only those β-ionone derivatives, other than provitamin A carotenoids, which exhibit activity resembling that of all trans retinol.

Retinol is converted in vivo to an aldehyde, retinal, which has been isolated from the retina of the eye and is the form in which the vitamin functions in dark adaptation. Retinoic acid (vitamin A acid) is formed from retinol via retinal in the animal body, but a reverse reaction does not occur. Synthetic retinoic acid, for example, will promote growth in animals, but it is not active in the visual process (Dowling and Wald, 1960) nor in the support of normal reproduction (Thompson et al., 1964).

Retinol is a light yellow crystalline substance and is soluble in all fat solvents. It readily undergoes oxidation in air and isomerizes when exposed to light. Esters of retinol are more stable. The basis for the earliest chemical determinations for vitamin A is the Carr-Price reaction, in which the vitamin forms a blue color with antimony trichloride in chloroform (Carr and Price, 1926). An improved modification of this reaction uses trifluoroacetic acid in place of antimony trichloride (Neeld and Pearson, 1963). The vitamin can also be determined from its ultraviolet absorption or its fluorescence. The method of choice for blood is high performance liquid chromatography (Bieri et al., 1979).

Vitamin A activity in plants resides in the carotenoid pigments that are precursors to the vitamin in the animal body and, therefore, are designated the provitamins A. Conversion of the provitamins to the vitamin occurs in cells of the intestinal mucosa and, to some extent, in the liver and possibly in the kidney. Beta-carotene is the most widely distributed of the carotenoid pigments and is the most active in terms of vitamin A activity.

The β-ionone ring is essential for vitamin A activity. The β-carotene molecule is a double retinol structure (see formula) and theoretically should give rise to two molecules of retinol. Biologically, however, the activity of pure β-carotene in rat bioassays is only about half that of retinol. Due to inefficiency in intestinal absorption from vegetables and fruits, food sources of β-carotene are only about one-sixth as active as retinol (National Research Council, 1980). The enzyme responsible for carotene cleavage to retinal has been referred to as β-15,15' dioxygenase (Olson and Hayaishi, 1965) and is known to split the two central carbon atoms of β-carotene in the presence of molecular oxygen to yield two molecules of retinal. Retinal so produced is converted to retinol by a nonspecific aldehyde reductase for which either nicotinamide adenine dinucleotide, reduced form, (NADH) or nicotinamide adenine dinucleotide phosphate, reduced form, (NADPH) can serve as cofactor. (See Goodman, 1969a, Olson and Lakshmanan, 1970.) Some carotenoids may enter the lymphatic system intact and are partially converted to the vitamin in the liver or possibly in the kidney. (See Chapter 6.)

The disparity between the chemical structure and biological activity of carotene compounds is primarily the result of inefficiency of carotene absorption but also, in part, of the oxidation of some of the retinal formed from carotene cleavage to retinoic acid. The retinoic acid, in turn, is rapidly oxidized and excreted. (See below.)

Many different carotenoids occur in nature. In addition to β-carotene, likely only α-carotene and cryptoxanthin are significant in human nutrition. The latter two carotenoids are about half as efficient as β-carotene in the ultimate yield of retinol. Naturally occurring carotenoids are believed to have only the all-*trans* configuration of double bonds in their chains, but on heating, some of these bonds readily change to the cis-configuration. Analyses of foods as consumed usually show significant amounts of these isomers. The analyses of carotenoids is best done by column or thin layer chromatography although high-performance liquid chromatography has been used for some plants. The biopotencies of some active carotenoids are shown in Table 4.1.

Beta-carotene

Biochemical Function

The physiological functions of vitamin A have been well defined for many years. The vitamin is necessary for growth, reproduction, the maintenance of epithelial tissues, and for normal vision. Of these functions, only the latter—the visual function—has been delineated in terms of biochemical action. The role of the vitamin in growth is less well understood. Its role in reproduction and epithelial tissues, although still an enigma, at least can be characterized by a series of events that are associated directly or indirectly with vitamin A.

In the visual function vitamin A is combined with a hexose and hexosamine-containing protein, opsin, to form the visual pigment rhodopsin. This pigment is present in the rod cells of retina of most, but not all, vertebrates. Functionally, 11-cis-retinal is the active form of the vitamin moiety of rhodopsin and combines with opsin through an ϵ-amino group of a specific lysine residue of the protein and possibly through the sulfhydryl group of a cysteine residue (Heller, 1968). Other light-sensitive pigments also contain a form of vitamin A. Iodopsin, a pigment of the cone cells, contains retinal, but the opsin is different from that of rod cells; porphyropsin, found in rod cells of fresh-water fish, contains 3-dehydroretinal.

The reactions involved in the visual cycle were identified principally by Wald and his associates. (See Wald, 1953.) The pigment rhodopsin (visual purple) is bleached by light, resulting in liberation of protein and retinal in all trans form via a series of intermediary compounds (Matthews et al., 1964). In the dark, the pigment is regenerated; this process requires that retinal be isomerized back to the cis form. The series of reactions is shown in Fig. 4.1. Some of the vitamin is degraded in the overall process, and night blindness results when there is not sufficient vitamin present for regeneration of the rhodopsin molecule. The effect of light on degeneration of rhodopsin and the maintenance of rhodopsin content of the eye have been shown in rats to be highly dependent on the level of illumination to which the animals are exposed. Animals that were depleted of

TABLE 4.1
All-*Trans* Carotenoids with Vitamin A Activity

Compound	Moiety Structure[a]	Relative Biological Activity[b]
Retinol	—	200
3-Dehydroretinol	—	80
Hydrocarbons		
β-Carotene	(Retinyl:)$_2$	100
3-Dehydro-β-carotene	Retinyl:3-dehydroretinyl	75
α-Carotene	Retinyl:α-retinyl	53
γ-Carotene	Retinyl:geranyl-geranyl-4,8-diene	43
β-Zeacarotene	Retinyl:geranyl-geranyl-4-ene	40
Homo-β-carotene	Retinyl:retinylvinyl	20
Bis-3,3'-dehydro-β-carotene	(3-dehydroretinyl:)$_2$	38
Oxygenated derivatives		
Cryptoxanthin	Retinyl:3-hydroxyretinyl	57
Echinenone	Retinyl:4-ketoretinyl	44
5,6-Epoxy-β-carotene	Retinyl:5,6-epoxyretinyl	21
Torularhodin	Retinyl:geranyl-geranyl-4,8,12-tetraen-16-oic acid	<50
Apocarotenol derivatives		
β-Apo-14'-carotenol	Retinyl:ethanol	(7)
β-Apo-12'-carotenal	Retinyl:α-methylbutenal	(125)
Methyl β-apo-12'-carotenoate	Retinyl:methyl α-methylbutenoate	(200)
β-Apo-10'-carotenal	Retinyl:γ-methylhexadienal	(>100)
β-Apo-8'-carotenal	Retinyl:α,ε-dimethyloctatrienal	(40), 72

Source: Adapted from J. A. Olson and M. R. Lakshmanan, in *The Fat-Soluble Vitamins*, H. F. DeLuca and J. W. Suttie, eds., The University of Wisconsin Press, Madison, 1969, p. 216.

[a]Colon(:) indicates a double bond joining two moieties head to head.

[b]In reference to activity of β-carotene (= 100).

vitamin A and kept in the dark maintained rhodopsin content of the retina for 5 to 6 months whereas those kept in weak cyclic light lost rhodopsin continuously (Noell and Albrecht, 1971).

Both retinol and retinal will prevent night blindness, but retinoic acid is not effective in the visual process. As shown in Fig. 4.2, the alcohol and aldehyde forms of the vitamin are interconvertible. Retinoic acid is a normal metabolite of retinol and retinal, but it cannot be converted *in vivo* to either of these compounds. The acid, however, is fully active in promoting growth in experimental animals.

The role of the vitamin in the growth process is poorly understood. Vitamin A-deficient animals lack appetite and fail to grow. Loss of appetite has been attributed in part to loss of the sense of taste due to keratinization of taste buds and atrophy of accessory glandular tissue (Bernard and Halpern, 1968). Death appears to be

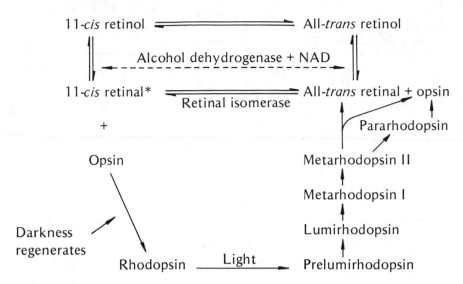

Figure 4.1
Role of vitamin A in the visual cycle. The asterisk (*) indicates the active form.

due to infection. Bieri et al. (1969) found that conventional animals reared under standard laboratory conditions died within 54 days when fed a vitamin A-deficient diet whereas germ-free animals lived up to 272 days. Marginal vitamin A deficiency in young rats has been shown to reduce the number of cells (DNA) in most organs (Zile et al., 1979). Thus, a direct role of vitamin A in cell division has been postulated.

An explosion in vitamin A research occurred during the decade 1970 to 1980 with the demonstration by Saffiotti et al. (1967) that retinol and other derived retinoids could delay or prevent the development of certain epithelial carcinomas. Most interest centered initially on retinoic acid, but because of the general toxicity of this compound in the high concentrations required to inhibit tumor induction, hundreds of derivatives were synthesized in an attempt to find a suitable compound. This action of retinoids in inhibiting epithelial carcinomas and also chem-

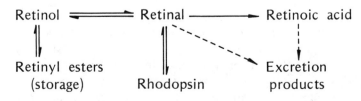

Figure 4.2
Interrelationship between retinol, retinal, and retinoic acid.

ical transformation of cells is considered to be related to the normal action of vitamin A on epithelial tissues. For a recent symposium on this topic, see DeLuca and Shapiro (1981).

Attempts to relate the activity of specific enzymes to vitamin A status of tissues have not produced clear-cut relationships. Because the vitamin A-deficient state in animals is accompanied by varying degrees of inanition, infection, stress, and morphological changes in many tissues, alteration in enzyme activity compared with normal controls cannot be assigned unequivocally to vitamin A. Claims that the vitamin is directly involved in steroidogenesis have not been verified (Rogers, 1969).

A role for vitamin A in the maintenance of epithelial tissue integrity was offered by DeLuca et al. (1972) who studied the effect of vitamin A deficiency on intestinal tissue. In most epithelial tissues, vitamin A deficiency is characterized by replacement of normal mucus-secreting cells by keratinized epithelia. Intestinal mucosa does not become hyperkeratinized but instead there is a significant reduction in the number of goblet cells. In addition, goblet cells were shown to contain a specific fucose-containing glycopeptide and the synthesis of this compound also is decreased in vitamin A deficiency. DeLuca and coworkers (1972) hypothesized that vitamin A, a short-chain polyprenol derivative, may function in mammals by forming retinyl-phosphate-sugar intermediates that act as donors of sugar to acceptor proteins in membrane structures. This hypothesis is based on an analogy between vitamin A function in higher animals and the known function of polyisoprenols in bacteria in the transfer of mono- or oligosaccharides into acceptor proteins to synthesize glycoproteins.

Recent interest has centered on glycosylation of glycoproteins, specifically the incorporation of mannose. Quill and Wolf (1981) and Shidoji et al. (1981) hypothesize that retinyl phosphate functions as a carrier of mannosyl residues in membranes. The active compound, mannosylretinyl phosphate (MRP), has been demonstrated in mammalian cells and is highly specific for mannose. Attractive as this hypothesis is, it does not explain how retinoic acid, which cannot give rise to retinylphosphate, maintains normal glycosylation of proteins.

Vitamin A Metabolites

Several lines of reasoning have led biochemists to infer that there must be a metabolite of retinol that is the ultimate "active" form of vitamin A at the molecular level. Two metabolites, retinal and retinoic acid, have been well characterized as functioning in specific tissues. Retinoic acid, although capable of sustaining the growth and epithelial tissue functions of retinol, is not able to support normal testicular function, gestation, or the visual process (Chole and Quick, 1978). It cannot be ruled out that retinol is the active form of the vitamin, but the discovery of several active metabolites of vitamin D (see below) has sustained hopes that functional metabolites may exist for vitamin A.

Numerous end products of retinol metabolism are known to be present in tissues or excreted in urine and bile but only a few have been identified. All identified metabolites are derived from retinoic acid (Roberts and DeLuca, 1967). An isomer, 13-*cis*-retinoic acid, has been found in rat tissues (Zile et al., 1967). Several oxidation products of retinoic acid have also been identified. From intestinal mucosa, McCormick et al. (1978) isolated 5,6-epoxyretinoic acid. From hamster trachea and liver, Roberts and Frolik (1979) found at least five radioactive peaks by high performance liquid chromatography after administering H^3-retinoic acid. Two of these were identified as 4-hydroxyretinoic acid and 4-ketoretinoic acid; the latter is presumably a further oxidation product of the former. All of these identified metabolites have biological activity in various test systems, but most are no more active than retinoic acid.

Retinoic acid and its metabolites are excreted in the urine and also in bile, primarily in bile as their glucuronides. Compounds identified from these excretory pathways are 4-ketoretinoic acid, 5'-hydroxyretinoic acid, and two further products, one of which has been decarboxylated (Hanni et al., 1976; Hanni and Bigler, 1977). At the present time, there is no evidence that any metabolite of retinoic acid has a function different from that of retinoic acid itself. Also, it is not certain that retinol is not the "active" form of vitamin A for maintaining growth and normal epithelial tissues. However, the greater *in vitro* activity of retinoic acid, compared with retinol, in affecting membrane properties suggests that this form of the vitamin is the functional metabolite in epithelial cells. For further discussion on vitamin A metabolism, see Goodman (1980) and Zile and Cullum (1983).

Vitamin A Toxicity

It seems paradoxical that vitamin A deficiency is a major nutritional problem in many areas of the world and at the same time, vitamin A toxicity resulting from excessively high intakes is also a problem, albeit to a lesser degree. Both acute and chronic toxicities are reported in the literature.

Acute toxicity has been known to occur in Arctic explorers who consumed large quantities of polar bear liver. Polar bear liver contains nearly 600 mg retinol/100 gm (2 million I.U./100 gm). Acute toxicity also has been observed in infants and children given a single massive dose of the vitamin. The chief symptoms are transient hydrocephalus and vomiting. In very young children bulging of the fontanelle is a typical symptom. (See Canadian Pediatric Society, 1971.)

Chronic toxicity has been reported in cases where 40,000 to several hundred thousand I.U. were ingested over a period of years or months. When aqueous preparations of vitamin A are taken, as little as 18,500 to 60,000 I.U. for periods as short as 1 to 3 months may be toxic to children (Persson et al., 1965). Anorexia, loss of weight, nausea, vomiting, vague abdominal pain, and irritability are common symptoms. Drying and scaling of the lips and various types of skin rashes may occur without any other sign of toxicity. Loss of hair is not uncommon (Morrice et al., 1960). A characteristic symptom is pain and tenderness over the long bones, possibly with swelling of the joints. Other symptoms reported to occur include headache, pseudotumor cerebri, enlargement of the liver, spleen, and lymph glands, polydipsia, polyuria, and hypercalcemia (Dalderup, 1967; Lippe et al., 1981).

The clinical picture of vitamin A toxicity is variable, and one or two or many of the symptoms may be seen in any one case. It seems that many cases of minor chronic toxicity would not easily be detected. In clinically diagnosed cases, blood levels of vitamin A range from 85 to 2,200 μg/dl as compared with a normal range of 20 to 70 μg/dl (Roe, 1966). Chronic toxicity is a function of dose and duration of intake. Thus, both factors must be considered when evaluating potentially toxic doses (Korner and Vollm, 1975).

In experimental animals, excess vitamin A given during pregnancy resulted in congenital malformations in the young (Cohlan, 1953; Murakami and Kameyama, 1965). For further discussion of molecular effects of vitamin A excess, see Chapter 14.

Vitamin A Antagonists
Several chemically unrelated compounds have been shown to be antagonistic to vitamin A. The nature of the antagonistic action is not known since the metabolic function of the vitamin itself is not understood. However, it appears that the antagonisms are quite different from those of the water-soluble vitamins which usually are associated with the coenzyme function of the vitamin.

A number of compounds at toxic levels in the diet produce symptoms similar to those seen in vitamin A deficiency (Meunier et al., 1949). Some of these toxicities are reversed by additional vitamin A, which suggests that the compounds may be destroying the vitamin. This is probably the mechanism by which numerous organic halogen compounds antagonize vitamin A (Haley and Samuelsen, 1943; Copenhaver and Bell, 1954). These compounds are sources of free radicals that initiate oxidative reactions leading to tissue damage. (See Vitamin E, below.) It has been known for 40 years that vitamin E protects liver reserves of vitamin A. For further discussion of vitamin A antagonists, see Green (1966a).

VITAMIN D (ERGOCALCIFEROL, CHOLECALCIFEROL)

It has been said facetiously that civilization changed vitamin D from a hormone into a vitamin. Certainly the ambiguous nature of this vitamin has been evident since Mellanby (1919) demonstrated the beneficial effect of cod liver oil and other foods in the prevention and cure of rickets, and in the same year Huldschinsky (1919) reported healing rickets in young children by exposure to sunlight or artificial ultraviolet light. In the middle 1920s Steenbock (1924) demonstrated that irradiation of foods also produced antirachitic activity. Later the phenomenon was shown to be due to activation of a sterol in foods. The Steenbock irradiation process was patented and royalties obtained helped to begin the Wisconsin Alumni Research Foundation at the University of Wisconsin.

The factor responsible for prevention of rickets was named vitamin D and was clearly distinguished from the vitamin A also present in oils when it was discovered that antirachitic activity remained even after vitamin A activity had been destroyed by oxidation (McCollum et al., 1922). It was not until 1934, however, that it was demonstrated that the vitamin D synthesized in the animal body was chemically different from that derived from plant sources (Waddell, 1934).

Chemistry

Several forms of vitamin D exist; nearly all arise from the irradiation of sterols that are provitamins or precursors of the vitamin. The two most important forms of vitamin D in human nutrition are ergocalciferol and cholecalciferol. Ergosterol, which occurs in plants, is activated by sunlight to form ergocalciferol (vitamin D_2, calciferol). The form synthesized in animal epidermal cells is cholecalciferol (vitamin D_3) which is derived from 7-dehydrocholesterol. The formulas for these two forms of vitamin D are shown below.

Ergocalciferol differs from cholecalciferol only by a double bond at the 22,23 position and a methyl group at the 24 position. Both forms possess equal activity for humans, rats, and most mammalian species (Hess et al., 1925) with the exception of the new world monkey (Hunt et al., 1967). However, ergocalciferol is only one-tenth as potent in curing rickets in chicks (Chen and Bosmann, 1964).

Although ultraviolet irradiation produces the vitamins from their sterol precursors, the active forms, ergocalciferol and cholecalciferol, are unstable to irradiation. Excessive irradiation will produce some toxic products. The vitamins D are

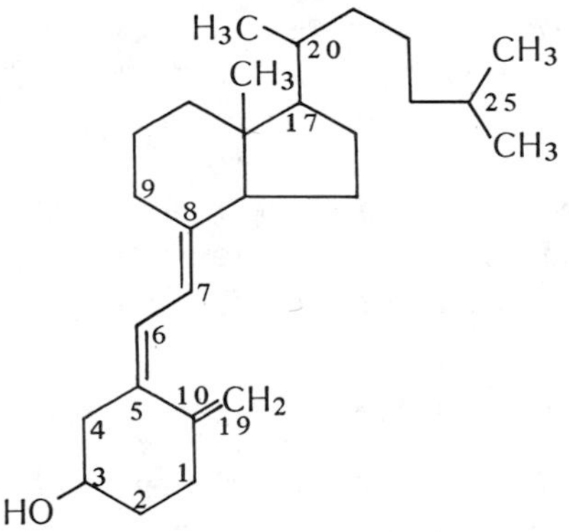

Vitamin D_3
Cholecalciferol

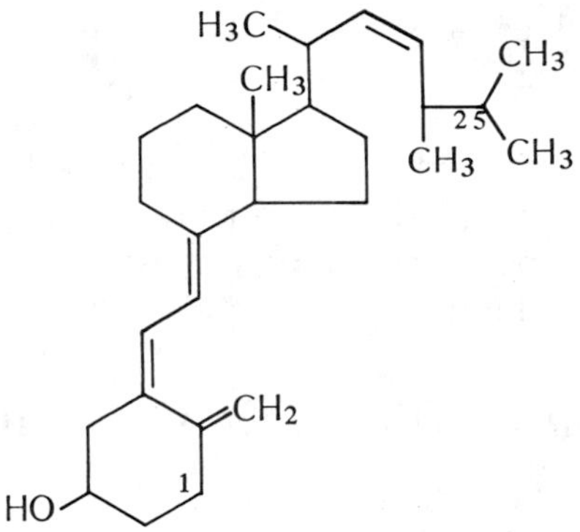

Vitamin D_2
Ergocalciferol

not affected by oxidation or by temperatures below 140°C. In acid media the vitamins are relatively unstable, the instability increasing with increase in temperature. In alkaline solution vitamin D compounds are stable even at elevated temperatures.

Assay of total vitamin D activity in natural materials was originally made by biological testing in rats made rachitic. The healing of bone, as shown by staining the tibia with silver nitrate, was examined histologically and scored. (See DeLuca and Blunt, 1971.) Pure vitamin D can be measured by its ultraviolet absorption or by its color reaction with antimony trichloride-acetyl chloride (U.S. Pharmacopeia, 1960). Gas chromatography has also been used (Sheppard and Hubbard, 1971) but recently high performance liquid chromatography (HPLC) has become the method of choice because of its high sensitivity and resolving power (Horst et al., 1979). This highly versatile technique is particularly useful for analyzing the various metabolites of calciferol. Because of the very low concentrations of vitamin D metabolites in plasma and tissues, purification steps are usually required prior to HPLC analysis. Some metabolites have also been estimated by using radioimmunoassay. For a comprehensive review of methodology, see Seamarks et al. (1981).

Biochemical Function
The biochemical function of vitamin D has been succinctly summarized by Omdahl and DeLuca (1973).

1. *Vitamin D must first be metabolically altered before it functions.*
2. *Functional metabolites of vitamin D are generated in organs other than their sites of action.*
3. *The rates of synthesis and secretion of these functional forms are feedback regulated.*
4. *This regulation is effected through humoral agents that probably involve the parathyroid hormone and possibly calcitonin.*
5. *The final functional form of vitamin D that controls calcium movement from both intestine and bone is a major humoral substance responsible for regulating plasma calcium concentration.*

On the basis of these functions, vitamin D may be considered a *prohormone* and its active metabolites as *hormones*. This distinction is based largely on two points. First, the active metabolite is elaborated by one organ but acts on other target organs. Second, a feedback mechanism exists for controlling the rate of synthesis and secretion of the active metabolite. Both of these functions comply with the classic definition of a hormone, but not a vitamin, at least not in the same sense that we have come to think of the action of the water-soluble vitamins.

The overall effect of vitamin D is to bring about the mineralization of bone. (See Chapter 17.) In absence of the vitamin, rickets (or demineralization of bone) results. The mechanism by which vitamin D accomplishes mineralization lies in stimulating the absorption of calcium and phosphate from the intestinal lumen to the blood (Nicolaysen, 1937). Thus, plasma calcium and phosphorus levels are elevated so that these ions are present in good supply in the extracellular fluid surrounding the sites of calcification. The possibility that vitamin D functions in a more direct fashion in calcification of bone remains speculative. However, the vitamin is known to stimulate the mobilization of calcium from bone to blood.

A lag period of from 10 to 12 hours occurs after administration of vitamin D to rachitic animals before functioning of the calcium transport system or mobilization of calcium from bone. This observation led to the belief that some transformation of the vitamin was required before it became active *in vivo*. Following the preparation of a tritiated vitamin D, extensive work from several laboratories has shown that Vitamin D_3 is first acted upon by an enzyme in the liver, calciferol-25-hydroxylase, which introduces one hydroxyl group to give 25-hydroxycholecalciferol, $25(OH)D_3$ (Blunt et al., 1969). This enzyme was shown to be regulated by a feedback mechanism. Rats pretreated with labeled or unlabeled vitamin D_3 showed decreased levels of liver calciferol-25-hydroxylase activity and the degree and length of low activity depended on the amount of vitamin administered (Bhattacharyya and DeLuca, 1973). The regulation of enzyme activity may be important both in protecting against vitamin D toxicity and in conserving vitamin D during periods when dietary intake and/or formation of vitamin D in skin are low.

Studies of the ability of $25(OH)D_3$ to stimulate intestinal calcium absorption revealed a time lag of 2 hours, suggesting that further metabolism of the vitamin may occur. This anticipated next step was demonstrated almost simultaneously at the Cambridge laboratory (Lawson et al., 1971) and DeLuca's laboratory at Wisconsin (Holick et al., 1971) in rats, and shortly thereafter confirmed in human subjects (Mawer et al, 1971). A second metabolite of vitamin D was isolated and identified as $1,25(OH)_2D_3$ (Holick et al., 1972a). The kidney was shown to be the site where $1,25(OH)_2D_3$ is synthesized (Fraser and Kodicek, 1970). This metabolite was shown to act much more rapidly than $25(OH)D_3$ in both the calcium transport system and the bone calcium mobilization system. Further, $1,25(OH)_2D_3$ is about 10 times more potent than the $25(OH)D_3$ compound in the prevention and cure of rickets (Tanaka et al., 1973).

The synthesis of $1,25(OH)_2D_3$ is under feedback regulation by calcium availability. This finding helps to explain the well-known ability of man and experimental animals to adapt to low levels of dietary calcium by increasing calcium absorption. Indeed, Boyle et al. (1971) demonstrated that rats fed low-calcium diets synthesize large amounts of $1,25(OH)_2D_3$, but when calcium intake is increased the synthesis of $1,25(OH)_2D_3$ is reduced. These data are in accord with the more recent finding of a feedback mechanism regulating the activity of calciferol-25-hydroxylase activity as mentioned previously. Furthermore, when $1,25(OH)_2D_3$ synthesis is depressed, another metabolite identified as $24,25-(OH)_2D_3$ is formed (Holick et al., 1972b). This compound is very active in intestinal calcium transport but has only slight activity in mobilization of calcium from bone.

A fourth metabolite of vitamin D_3 was identified as $1,24,25(OH)_3D_3$, which is generated from $25(OH)D_3$ (Holick et al., 1973). This compound is preferentially more active in inducing calcium transport in the intestine than in mobilizing calcium from bone. It is about 60 percent as effective as vitamin D_3 in curing rickets. A fifth metabolite, $25,26(OH)_2D_3$, also was identified (Suda et al., 1970). This compound is active in calcium intestinal transport but has little activity in the laying down or mobilization of calcium from bone. Still other unidentified metabolites of vitamin D_3 have been detected (Schnoes and DeLuca, 1980).

Evidence suggests that parathyroid hormone stimulates synthesis of $1,25(OH)_2D_3$ (Garabedian et al., 1972; Fraser and Kodicek, 1973). The feedback mechanism is shown in Fig. 4.3. When serum calcium falls below the norm of 10 mg/dl the parathyroid glands are stimulated to secrete parathyroid hormone, which stimulates synthesis of $1,25(OH)_2D_3$ in kidney. This compound then stimulates calcium intestinal absorption and mobilization from bone. When serum calcium returns to normal, the parathyroid secretion is cut off, and the feedback loop is completed. (See Omdahl and DeLuca, 1973.) The role of the parathyroid hormone in calcium metabolism in bone will be discussed in Chapter 17.

The mechanism by which $1,25(OH)_2D_3$ facilitates calcium transport across the intestinal mucosal cell has been an area of intense study and controversy. It is

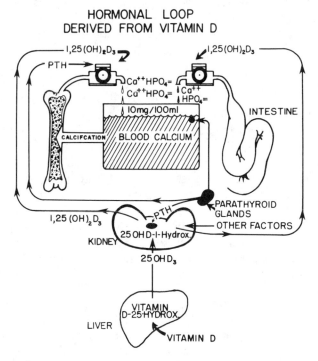

Figure 4.3

Diagrammatic representation of the regulation of plasma calcium (ECF) concentration by the vitamin D endocrine system and the parathyroid glands. Low plasma calcium is detected by parathyroid glands. Parathyroid hormone stimulates production of $1,25(OH)_2D_3$. The two hormones act either independently or in concert to mobilize calcium from bone, kidney tubules, and small intestine, bringing about an elevation of plasma calcium concentration that in turn suppresses parathyroid hormone secretion. (Courtesy of H.F. DeLuca.)

known that mucosal cells contain a low molecular weight protein that binds calcium (calcium binding protein, CaBP; Wasserman, 1970), and the synthesis of this protein appears to be controlled by $1,25(OH)_2D_3$ (Bronner et al., 1982). A higher molecular weight protein isolated from microvillus membranes, termed intestinal membrane calcium-binding protein or IMCal, is also postulated to be under the control of $1,25(OH)_2D_3$ (Schachter and Kowarski, 1982). Another complicating factor in our understanding of how vitamin D regulates calcium absorption is the observation that $1,25(OH)_2D_3$ affects the synthesis of phosphatidylcholine in microvillus membranes, thus affecting membrane fluidity and calcium transport (Rasmussen et al., 1982). A receptor molecule that transports $1,25(OH)_2D_3$ from the cytosol of the mucosal cell to the nucleus has been postulated (DeLuca et al., 1982). It is apparent that $1,25(OH)_2D_3$ may be acting at several sites in the cell and future work is needed to clarify this complex picture. (See Chapter 6 for details about calcium absorption.)

For a review of vitamin D, see DeLuca and Schnoes (1983).

Vitamin D Toxicity

Vitamin D toxicity in humans is more likely to occur in infants and young children, but toxic symptoms have been reported in adults as well. In mild toxicity, hypercalcemia is the chief symptom. In severe toxicity, typical facies, supravalvular aortic stenosis, and mental retardation have been reported (Anning et al., 1948; American Academy of Pediatrics Committee on Nutrition, 1963). Intakes in the range of 2,000 to 3,000 I.U. per day have been associated with hypercalcemia. However, lower intakes also have been implicated (Taussig, 1966) and individual hypersensitivity to the vitamin may be a causal factor in such cases (Fraser et al., 1966).

Although the population at risk is believed to be relatively small, the dangers associated with vitamin D toxicity and the rather low levels of intake that have been reported to be toxic prompted the American Academy of Pediatrics Committee on Nutrition (1965) to recommend extreme caution in supplementation of foods other than milk with vitamin D.

Excessive levels of vitamin D_2 (150,000 I.U. daily for 10 to 14 days) were found to stimulate oxidation of tissue lipids (Spirchev and Blazheievich, 1969). Antioxidants and especially tocopherols reduced peroxidation and deposition of calcium in aorta and kidney. The effect of vitamin D and the opposing effect of tocopherols and antioxidants was believed to be due to corresponding effects on mitochondrial and lysosomal membranes. (See Chapter 9.) This finding may prove to be significant in explaining the mechanism of vitamin D toxicity.

Vitamin D Antagonists

No antagonists of vitamin D are known at present.

VITAMIN E

Vitamin E has been known as the antisterility vitamin since its discovery in 1922 by Evans and Bishop as the fat-soluble factor that prevented resorption of fetuses in female rats and testicular degeneration in males. The early history of the vitamin has been reviewed by Evans (1963) including the work of Karrer, Fernholz, the Emersons, and others in the isolation and synthesis of the tocopherol compounds. The name tocopherol was derived from the Greek *tokos* (childbirth) and *phero* (to bear), but the influence of the tocopherols is vastly greater than the original designation implies.

Chemistry and Occurrence

Two distinct classes of compounds comprise the vitamin E group. They are all derivatives of chroman-6-ol. The first series—the tocopherols—derive from tocol, which contains a 16-carbon saturated isoprenoid side chain. The second series, the tocotrienols, contain a triply unsaturated side chain. Within each series the compounds differ only in the number and position of methyl groups in the ring structure. The ring structure of the corresponding tocotrienol is similar to the tocopherols designated α, β, γ, δ. (See Table 4.2.) Alpha tocopherol is the most widely distributed in nature and is the most active biologically of the compounds. The formula is as follows.

α-Tocopherol
(5,7,8-trimethyltocol)

Vitamin E is found mostly in plants and is present in highest concentration in many of the seed oils such as soybean, cottonseed, corn, sunflower, and wheat germ oil. Olive, coconut, and peanut oils are low in the vitamin. Animal tissues contain small amounts of the vitamin, as do vegetables and fruits. The dietary content of vitamin E is expressed as "mg α-tocopherol equivalents," an expression that takes into consideration the biological activity of the significant amounts in foods of β- and γ-tocopherols and also α-tocotrienol, as well as that of α-tocopherol (Bieri and McKenna, 1981).

The hydroxyl group on the chroman ring is readily oxidized by air at elevated temperatures or in the presence of alkali. Iron salts are especially effective oxidants, and this property is the basis for the most common assay method, the Emmerie-Engel reaction. In this reaction between ferric iron and tocopherol, the resulting ferrous iron complexes with dipyridyl to give an intense pink color. (See Quaiffe and Harris, 1948.) A more recent modification uses bathophenanthroline instead of bipyridyl, resulting in greater sensitivity. Usually, partial purification of α-tocopherol from plant or animal tissues by thin layer chromatography is required prior to the colorimetric reaction (Bieri, 1969). Other analytical procedures include spectrophotometry, fluorimetry, and gas chromatography, but interfering materials cause some difficulties. Recently, high performance liquid

TABLE 4.2
Naturally Occurring Forms of Vitamin E

Tocols	Basic Structure	CH₃ Substitution

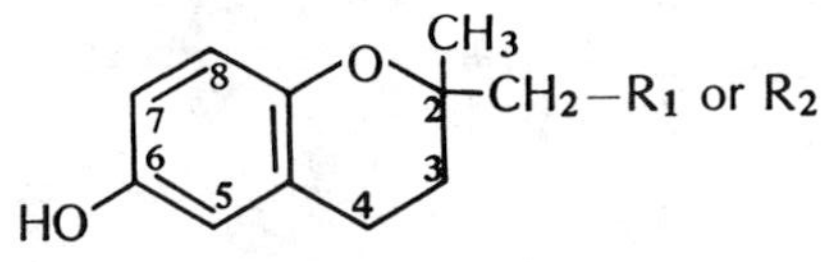

Basic Structure

R_1 = (CH₂—CH₂—CH—CH₂)₃H with CH₃

Tocols

R_2 = (CH₂—CH=C—CH₂)₃H with CH₃

Tocotrienols

Tocols		CH₃ Substitution
α-T	α-T-3	5,7,8-Trimethyl
β-T	β-T-3	5,8-Dimethyl
γ-T	γ-T-3	7,8-Dimethyl
δ-T	δ-T-3	8-Methyl

chromatography has been used for plasma (Bieri et al., 1979) and for foods and tissues (Thompson and Hatina, 1979).

Biological assays include the original fetal resorption test in rats and also the *in vitro* hemolysis of red cells in the presence of an oxidizing agent. The prevention of an increase in the enzyme, pyruvate kinase, in rat serum has recently been described (Machlin et al., 1982).

Biochemical Function

The early observation that the tocopherols were effective antioxidants *in vitro* led to the postulation that this action also occurred *in vivo*. Many experiments in animals indirectly supported this theory, but certain anomalies led some investigators to question it. However, it is now widely believed that the ability of α-tocopherol to protect against lipid peroxidation is the basis for its manifold effects observed at the cellular level. (See Tappel and Dillard, 1981.) It has become increasingly apparent to biochemists that cells produce a variety of potentially damaging oxidative products, and that the body has numerous protective defense mechanisms to deal with them. Vitamin E is only one part of this defense system, but probably it is the first line of defense and one that is readily affected by nutritional factors (Chow, 1979).

In its protective role, the vitamin prevents oxidative damage primarily of poly-unsaturated fatty acids (PUFA) in membranes. Such damage results in membrane changes with subsequent cascading effects that lead ultimately to the biochemical changes and overt symptoms seen in deficient animals (Molenaar et al., 1980). The tissue requirement for vitamin E is related to its content of PUFA, and since the latter can be altered by dietary means, it is easy to understand why discrepancies in research findings have characterized the work on vitamin E (Bieri and Farrell, 1976). In addition to the antioxidant action, other theories of function have been proposed. Although there is not sufficient evidence so far to give them credence, it is not yet known if vitamin E is involved in more than one type of function (McCay et al., 1982). Other defense systems, the glutathione peroxidases, can affect the vitamin E requirement since one of these enzymes is dependent on selenium status. (See Chapter 5.) Thus, some tissues can be protected solely by glutathione peroxidase activity, but most require vitamin E.

The relationship between dietary PUFA and vitamin E is well documented in experimental animals (Dam, 1962) and humans (Horwitt, 1962). The requirement for vitamin E is increased as the PUFA content of the diet is increased and, consequently, the severity of symptoms due to a lack of vitamin E in the diet is increased by the level of dietary PUFA.

Most (but not all) of the symptoms of vitamin E deficiency can be prevented by a nonspecific antioxidant (Table 4.3). Encephalomalacia and exudative diathesis in chicks are typical examples of this phenomenon. The clinical signs of encephalomalacia are ataxia, spasms, or paralysis. Exudative diathesis is characterized by accumulation of fluid in subcutaneous tissues, muscles, or connective tissues and is caused by exuding of plasma from the capillaries. These symptoms

TABLE 4.3
The Vitamin E Deficiency Diseases

Disease	Experimental Animal	Tissue Affected	Severity Dependent Upon Dietary PUFA	Prevented by			
				Vitamin E	Selenium	Synthetic Antioxidants	Sulfur Amino Acids
REPRODUCTIVE FAILURE							
Embryonic degeneration							
Type A	Rat, hen, turkey	Vascular system of embryo	Yes	Yes	No	Yes	No
Type B	Cow, ewe	Vascular system of embryo	No	No[a]	Yes[b]	No	No
Sterility	Male rat, guinea pig, hamster, dog, cock	Male gonads	No	Yes	No	No	No
LIVER, BLOOD, BRAIN, CAPILLARIES, ETC.							
Liver necrosis	Rat, pig	Liver	No	Yes	Yes	No	No
Erythrocyte hemolysis	Rat, chick, human (premature infant)	Erythrocytes	Yes	Yes	No	Yes	No
Plasma protein loss	Chick, turkey	Serum albumin	No	Yes	Yes	No	No

Condition	Species	Tissue					
Anemia	Monkey	Bone marrow	No	Yes	No	Yes	No
Encephalomalacia	Chick	Cerebellum	Yes	Yes	No	Yes	No
Exudative diathesis	Chick, turkey	Vascular system	No	Yes	Yes	No	No
Kidney degeneration	Rat, monkey, mink	Kidney tubular epithelium	Yes	Yes	Yes	No	No
Depigmentation	Rat	Incisors	Yes	Yes	No	Yes	No
Steatitis (yellow fat disease)	Mink, pig, chick	Adipose tissue	Yes	Yes	No	Yes	No

NUTRITIONAL MYOPATHIES

Condition	Species	Tissue					
Nutritional muscular dystrophy							
Type A	Rabbit, guinea pig, monkey, duck, mouse, mink	Skeletal muscle	No	Yes	No	No?	No
Type B	White muscle disease of lamb, calf, kid	Skeletal and heart muscles	No	No[a]	Yes[b]	No	No
Type C	Turkey	Gizzard, heart	No	No[a]	Yes	No	No
Type D	Chicken	Skeletal muscle	No[c]	Yes	No	No	Yes

Source: From M. L. Scott, *The Fat Soluble Vitamins*, H. F. DeLuca and J. W. Suttie, eds., The Univ. of Wisconsin Press, Madison, 1969, p. 357.

[a]Not effective in diets severely deficient in selenium.

[b]When added to diets containing low levels of vitamin E.

[c]A low level (0.5%) of linoleic acid is necessary to produce dystrophy; higher levels did not increase vitamin E required for prevention.

were first described by Pappenheimer and Goettsch (1931) and do not occur in chicks given a fat-free vitamin E-deficient diet. Furthermore, lipofuscin or ceroid pigmentation, a yellow-brown coloration of adipose tissue, liver, and other tissues, which is highly characteristic of vitamin E deficiency, is known to be dependent on the *in vivo* autoxidation of polyunsaturated acids (Dam and Granados, 1945).

The wide range of deficiency symptoms that occur in various species of animals (Table 4.3), and their reversal by several modifications of diet other than vitamin E (e.g., selenium, PUFA content, sulfur amino acids), has been partly responsible for the lack of agreement about the biochemical function of tocopherol.

Wasserman and Taylor (1972) classified vitamin E deficiency diseases into two categories: those that respond to an antioxidant as well as to the vitamin and those that respond to the vitamin but are not affected by antioxidants. The antioxidant-responsive symptoms include encephalomalacia, *in vitro* erythrocyte hemolysis, formation of ceroid pigments, and reproductive failure in some species (Table 4.3). The symptoms that respond to vitamin E but do not respond to antioxidants include muscular dystrophy in most species, testicular degeneration in the rat, and anemia in monkeys.

Vitamin E deficiency in the human was not documented until 1966 when several premature infants were given a formula with insufficient vitamin E. Earlier, it had been known that low blood vitamin E levels occurred in newborn infants and in individuals who for a variety of reasons did not absorb fat normally. (See Bieri and Farrell, 1976.) In newborn infants, the low plasma levels are a result of low β-lipoproteins in blood, the primary transport protein, and possibly are due also to impaired placental transfer (Hågå and Kran, 1981). Few, if any, clinical signs of deficiency are apparent but in long-standing deficiency (many years), damage to some neurological centers leads to neuromuscular problems (Sung et al., 1980).

The role of vitamin E in hematopoiesis is unclear at the present time, but the anemia seen in several animal species, and also in the human infant, indicate a key function of the vitamin in this system. Other systems in which tocopherol has been implicated are that of immune response (Tengerdy, 1980) and platelet function as related to clotting (Whiton et al., 1982). Both of these areas are under active investigation. For further discussion on vitamin E function see Scott (1980) and Lubin and Machlin (1982).

Vitamin E Metabolites

Very little is known of the metabolic fate of vitamin E. The formation of a dimer and a trimer in rat and pig liver has been reported as the result of α-tocopherol oxidation (Csallany and Draper, 1963; Draper et al., 1967). Neither compound has vitamin E activity, but they are believed to be formed in animal tissues since oral administration of the synthetic dimer indicated extremely poor absorption from the intestinal lumen. It does not seem likely, therefore, that these compounds are formed in the gut.

A large number of oxidation products of α-tocopherol have been produced in the laboratory, including dimers and trimers. There has been considerable controversy about the initial oxidative attack on α-tocopherol, but most evidence supports the formation of a 9-hydroxytocopherone, which readily oxidizes further to the stable α-tocopherolquinone (Kasparek, 1980).

Vitamin E Antagonists

No true metabolic antagonists of vitamin E are as yet known.

Vitamin E Toxicity

Available evidence suggests that vitamin E has a low level of toxicity in the human (Hillman, 1957) and, in general, there has been little concern over the likelihood of overdosing. Hypervitaminosis E, however, has been demonstrated in chicks given 2,200 I.U. vitamin E/kg of diet (March et al., 1973). Depression in growth, bone calcification, hematocrit levels, and in respiration of skeletal muscle mitochondria was observed as well as increased prothrombin times. The effects on bone calcification and prothrombin time suggested that requirements for vitamin D and vitamin K were increased by hypervitaminosis E. Interference with blood clotting in a man on anticoagulant therapy and self-dosed with 800 I.U. of vitamin E daily has been described (Corrigan and Marcus, 1974).

Large doses of vitamin E have been proposed by various individuals and groups for the treatment of heart disease, infertility, muscular dystrophy, as well as numerous other ailments. There is no convincing evidence, however, in favor of giving vitamin E supplements for any of these disorders (Committee on Nutritional Misinformation, 1973; Olson, 1973). In view of the recent evidence of hypervitaminosis E in chicks, the possibility of adverse effects occurring in man as a result of overzealous supplementation with vitamin E should not be discounted.

VITAMIN K

Vitamin K was identified in 1935 by Dam as a factor present in green leaves which prevented a hemorrhagic syndrome observed in chicks maintained on a low fat diet. The new fat-soluble vitamin was designated vitamin K for the Danish word, *koagulation*. The purified compound was isolated from alfalfa by Dam and associates in 1939. (See Dam, 1948.)

Chemistry

Vitamin K exists in nature in two series of compounds: the phylloquinone (K_1) series and the menaquinone (K_2) series. A third series is related to the synthetic compound, menadione (2-methyl-1,4-naphthoquinone or vitamin K_3), a ring compound which is the basic structure of the naturally occurring vitamins and is about one-third as active biologically, on a molar basis, as vitamins K_1 and K_2.

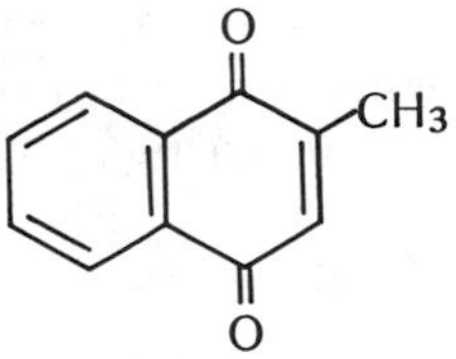

Menadione

The naturally occurring vitamins are 2-methyl-1,4-naphthoquinones substituted in the 3-position by isoprenoid chains. Vitamin K_1 contains a monounsaturated side chain with 20 C atoms (2-methyl-3-phytyl-) and occurs in green plants. The K_2 compounds contain a polyunsaturated side chain with 30 to 45 C atoms comprised of 6 to 9 isoprenoid units (2-methyl-3-difarnesyl-). These compounds are synthesized in many microorganisms including bacteria of the intestinal tract of a large number of species. Phthiocol (2-methyl-3-hydroxy-1,4-naphthoquinone), a pigment first isolated from bacteria, also has vitamin K activity.

Total vitamin K activity in natural materials is determined by a bioassay with chicks in which blood clotting time or whole blood prothrombin level is the criterion. The relative potency of the various forms of vitamin K in this test has been reviewed (Griminger, 1966). The pure vitamin can be determined by a

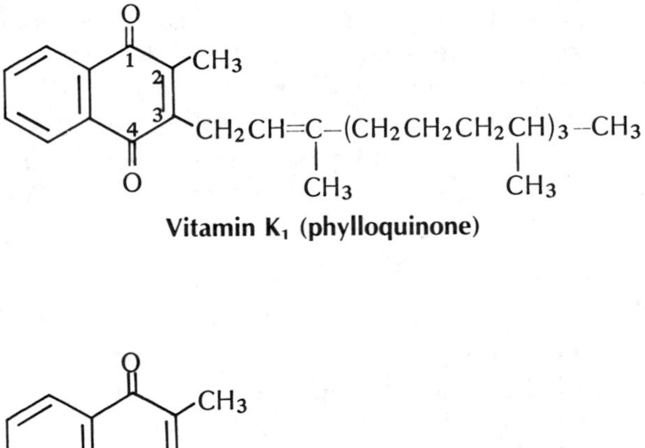

Vitamin K₁ (phylloquinone)

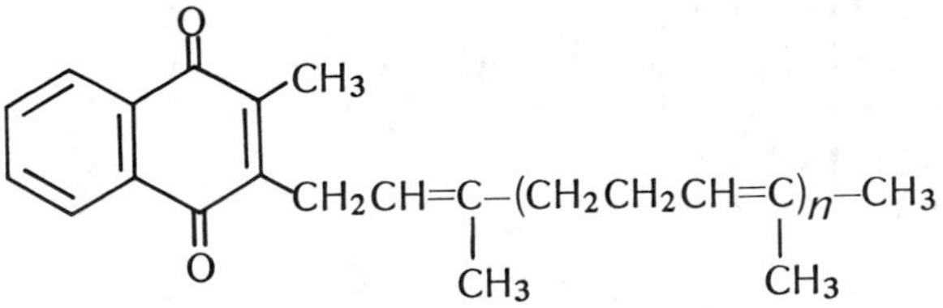

Vitamin K₂ (menaquinone)

variety of physical methods such as ultraviolet absorption, polarography, and thin layer or gas chromatography (Sommer and Kofler, 1966). Because the vitamin and its metabolites are present in blood and tissues in very low amounts, their measurement was handicapped until the advent of high performance liquid chromatography (Lefevere et al., 1979). This method is now the primary tool for studies of vitamin K.

Biochemical Function

The active form of vitamin K and its specific role in mammals are not known. The vitamin is known, however, to be essential for the synthesis of prothrombin and of other factors involved in blood clotting.

Early work by Dam et al. (1936) and Quick (1957) indicated that prothrombin was lacking in hemorrhagic disease of chicks and that the disease was of dietary origin. The deficiency was later shown to be due to a lack of vitamin K (Brinkhous, 1940). For many years it was thought that vitamin K exerted its influence on blood clotting only through its effect on prothrombin synthesis in liver. However, during the 1950s, three other factors involved in the complex series of events leading to blood coagulation were shown to be vitamin K-dependent: Factor IX, Factor VII, and Factor X. (See Table 4.4.)

It had been known for a number of years that there was a precursor of prothrombin in liver and blood of vitamin K-deficient animals. This "abnormal prothrombin" was purified and shown to have different calcium-binding properties than did prothrombin (Nelsestuen and Suttie, 1972). Other properties of the two proteins were similar but a breakdown of their structures to peptides revealed that the glutamic acid residues in prothrombin were present as a new amino acid, α-carboxyglutamic acid (Stenflo et al., 1974). For a review, see Suttie (1978).

This vitamin K-dependent carboxylation is effected by a liver microsomal enzyme and requires reduced vitamin K (or its epoxide) and CO_2. The exact mechanism by which vitamin K participates in this carboxylation is not understood. Several theories as to how the vitamin K antagonists, coumarins, function in relation to prothrombin synthesis have been reviewed (Suttie, 1978; 1980a; 1980b).

In addition to the vitamin K-dependent proteins in plasma, all of which are involved in blood clotting, there is a Gla-containing protein in bone and also in

$$
\begin{array}{c}
COOH \\
| \\
HC\!-\!NH_2 \\
| \\
CH_2 \\
| \\
HC\!-\!COOH \\
| \\
COOH
\end{array}
$$

γ-Carboxyglutamic Acid (Gla)

kidney (Hauschka et al., 1975; 1976). The physiological role of these nonclotting factor vitamin K-dependent proteins is not known, but their presence suggests a wider role for this vitamin than previously suspected.

In bacteria, quinone reductases can effect a reversible oxidation reduction of vitamin K. Some organisms use this system as part of their respiratory chain in a manner similar to that of ubiquinone, (coenzyme Q, see below). Participation of vitamin K in oxidative phosphorylation is not clearly established (Suttie, 1978).

TABLE 4.4
Scheme of Blood Coagulation

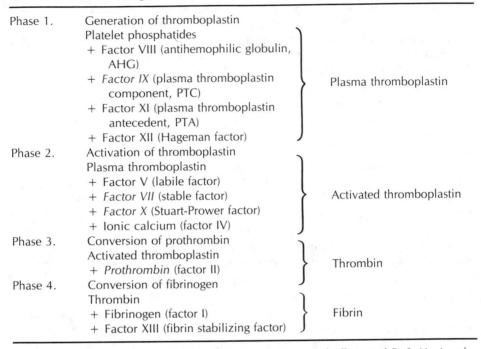

Phase 1.	Generation of thromboplastin	
	Platelet phosphatides	
	+ Factor VIII (antihemophilic globulin, AHG)	
	+ *Factor IX* (plasma thromboplastin component, PTC)	Plasma thromboplastin
	+ Factor XI (plasma thromboplastin antecedent, PTA)	
	+ Factor XII (Hageman factor)	
Phase 2.	Activation of thromboplastin	
	Plasma thromboplastin	
	+ Factor V (labile factor)	
	+ *Factor VII* (stable factor)	Activated thromboplastin
	+ *Factor X* (Stuart-Prower factor)	
	+ Ionic calcium (factor IV)	
Phase 3.	Conversion of prothrombin	
	Activated thromboplastin	Thrombin
	+ *Prothrombin* (factor II)	
Phase 4.	Conversion of fibrinogen	
	Thrombin	
	+ Fibrinogen (factor I)	Fibrin
	+ Factor XIII (fibrin stabilizing factor)	

Source: From C. A. Owen, Jr., *The Vitamins*, Vol. III, W. H. Sebrell, Jr. and R. S. Harris, eds., Academic Press, N. Y., 1971, p. 472.

Vitamin K Metabolites

Menadione, phylloquinone, and the menaquinones are rapidly metabolized and a variety of products are excreted in the urine and bile, primarily as glucuronides. For vitamins K_1 and K_2, the primary attack appears to be on the side chain resulting in the formation of numerous carboxy acids with shorter side chains. The most significant metabolite is the 2,3-epoxide, called "vitamin K oxide" (Matschiner, 1970). The amount of this metabolite in liver and plasma greatly increases after treatment with coumarins such as warfarin. An enzyme in liver, epoxide reductase, can convert the metabolite back to vitamin K. The exact role of the epoxide in vitamin K function is uncertain.

Vitamin K Antagonists

A number of vitamin K antagonists are known. The hemorrhagic effect of a substance present in spoiled sweet clover was isolated and identified by Campbell and Link (1941) as dicoumarol. This compound is one of a large number of 3-substituted 4-hydroxy coumarin compounds with anti-vitamin K activity. It is assumed that coumarin antagonists compete directly with vitamin K at the site where vitamin K exerts its biological activity. Warfarin, the rodenticide, and

Tromexan, which is used clinically in the treatment of thromboembolisms, are dicoumarol derivatives. The anticoagulant effect of these compounds is reversed by phylloquinone or menaquinones but not by menadione.

A number of 1,3-indanedione derivatives also possess anti-vitamin K activity (see Arora and Mathur, 1963), and 2-chloro-3-phytyl-1,4-naphthoquinone was shown to be a competitive antagonist of vitamin K (Lowenthal and MacFarlane, 1967). For a detailed discussion of vitamin K antagonists, see Green (1966b).

Other Vitamins and Vitaminlike Compounds

CHOLINE

$$\begin{array}{c} CH_2\,CH_2\,OH \\ | \\ +N\!-\!CH_3 \\ | \diagdown CH_3 \\ CH_3 \end{array}$$

Choline

Choline is a trimethylated hydroxide compound and occurs in biological tissues in the free form and as a component of lecithin, acetylcholine, and certain of the plasmalogens and sphingomyelins. Choline is important as a source of labile methyl groups and is also synthesized by methylation of dimethylaminoethanol, the needed methyl group being supplied by methionine (Fig. 4.4).

A choline deficiency has never been demonstrated in humans, and it is not known if a dietary supply is required in addition to that formed by biosynthesis. Because choline is widely distributed in plant and animal tissues, however, it seems unlikely that a deficiency would occur except under the most severe circumstances. Choline is known to be required by a number of animal species including the rat, the chick, the pig, and the dog. For this reason it is classified as a vitamin.

The two most significant results of choline deficiency in rats are fatty liver (Best and Huntsman, 1932) and hemorrhagic degeneration of kidneys (Griffith and Wade, 1939). In rats fed a choline-deficient diet, these conditions can be prevented by other methyl donors, betaine and methionine, or by folic acid and vitamin B_{12}. The coenzymes of the latter two nutrients catalyze reactions leading to *de novo* synthesis of methyl groups that can be transferred to homocysteine to form methionine (Fig. 4.4). Perosis or slipped tendon disease is the chief sign of choline deficiency in poultry. This disease responds to treatment with choline, but not to betaine, methionine, folic acid, or vitamin B_{12} (Table 4.5).

There are three important pathways for choline metabolism in the animal body: (1) formation of phospholipids via phosphorylcholine; (2) oxidation to betaine, a source of labile methyl groups; and (3) formation of acetylcholine, a neurotransmitter.

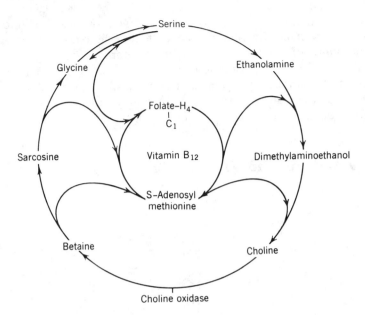

Figure 4.4
Labile methyl metabolism.

One of the earliest effects of choline deficiency in the rat is an interference with the secretion of triglycerides in the form of low-density lipoproteins from liver into the plasma. This defect seems to be the major cause for development of fatty liver in choline deficiency (Mookerjea, 1971). The exact mechanism of this defect in fat mobilization is not known, but it may be due to a deficient biosynthesis of one or more specific phosphatidylcholines. (See Kuksis and Mookerjea, 1978a.) Changes in the fatty acid components of phosphatidylcholines are known to occur in choline deficiency. Beare-Rogers (1971) proposed the involvement of the fatty acid chain elongation and desaturase systems in these transformations.

The hemorrhagic kidney disease in choline-deficient weanling rats has been hypothesized to be due to two factors. First, decreased acetylcholine concentration in the kidney results in increased production of renal vasopressin and necrosis of the proximal convoluted tubules. Second, choline deficiency has been shown to result in a deficiency of the Factor V involved in blood clotting. The latter could account for massive hemorrhages observed in kidneys of depleted animals. Working alone, neither factor likely could account for the hemorrhagic disease, but concomitantly, these two factors could cause the hemorrhagic degeneration observed in choline-deficient weanling rats (Wells, 1971).

Perosis in poultry appears to be independent of the labile methyl function of choline in that it is not alleviated by the usual methyl donors. It is possibly due to a defect in phospholipid synthesis and thus to effects on cell membrane function (Griffith and Nyc, 1971).

TABLE 4.5
Effect of Choline and Other Dietary Factors on Symptoms Produced by Choline Deficiency

Symptom	Choline	Methionine	Betaine	Folic acid + Vit. B_{12}
Fatty liver (rats)	+	+	+	+
Hemorrhagic kidneys (rats)	+	+	+	±
Prevention of perosis (chicks and turkeys)	+	−	−	−

Source: Adapted from T. H. Jukes, *Fed. Proc., 30:*156 (1971).

Dietary choline has been shown to affect the acetylcholine levels in brain. Since acetylcholine is one of the key neurotransmitters, there has been considerable interest recently in using high intakes of choline as a dietary means of modifying certain neuropsychiatric diseases (Growdon and Wurtman, 1979). Results to date have been equivocal. For a recent review of choline metabolism, see Zeisel (1981).

myo-Inositols

Inositols are cyclic alcohols (cyclohexanehexols) that, because of the presence of several hydroxyl groups and the configuration of the molecule, are related chemically to the sugars. Like the sugars, *myo*-inositol is a white chrystalline sub-

myo-**Inositol**

stance and has a sweet taste. Several isomers of inositol exist in nature. *Myo*-Inositol occurs in animal tissues as a constituent of phospholipids. In plants it is usually found as phytic acid, the hexaphosphate ester of inositol. It is present mostly in seeds and whole grains. Large amounts of phytic acid in the diet may interfere with the absorption of calcium and iron. (See Chapter 5.) Paradoxically, a beneficial effect of phosphates primarily in the form of phytates of whole grain cereals has been demonstrated in the prevention of dental caries (McClure, 1964).

Symptoms of inositol deficiency vary widely among different species of animals, due to differences in rates of endogenous synthesis in various tissues. In the rat, fatty liver occurs; in the gerbil, fat accumulates in the intestinal mucosa. The exact mechanism of lipid accumulation in tissues is unknown, but an inhibition of proper lipoprotein formation or secretion seems to be the major cause. (See Kuksis and Mookerjea, 1978b.) Changes in cell membrane properties in inositol-deficient cells are thought to be a result of abnormal phospholipid composition.

There is no evidence that *myo*-inositol is required in the human diet. However, it is widely distributed in the body of humans and has been demonstrated to exert a lipotropic action in patients with fatty infiltration of the liver (Milhorat, 1971).

Myo-inositol is thought to have three metabolic pathways in the animal body: (1) oxidation to CO_2, (2) synthesis of phospholipids, and (3) use in gluconeogenesis (Alam, 1971). *Myo*-inositol gives rise to glucose through glucuronic acid in the following sequence:

D-Glucuronic acid ⟶ L-Gulonic acid

⟱

D-Xylulose ⟵ Xylitol ⟵ 3-Oxogulonic acid

⟱ Pentose phosphate shunt

Glucose

It is through this reaction that myoinositol may be used in gluconeogenesis or oxidized to CO_2. The role of *myo*-inositol as a component of phospholipids appears to account both for its wide distribution in the animal body and for its apparent lipotropic action.

LIPOIC ACID

Lipoic acid was discovered as a growth factor for certain microorganisms. (See Gunsalus, 1953.) It is not likely a vitamin for mammals since it appears to be synthesized in adequate amounts in the mammalian cell. It is a coenzyme for a number of enzyme systems, the most significant of which are the pyruvate dehydrogenase complex and the α-ketoglutarate dehydrogenase complex. (See Schmidt et al., 1969.)

$$
\begin{array}{cc}
\underset{\text{Oxidized lipoic acid}}{\overset{\displaystyle CH_2}{\underset{\displaystyle S\text{---}S}{CH_2 \qquad CH-(CH_2)_4COOH}}} &
\underset{\text{Reduced lipoic acid}}{\overset{\displaystyle CH_2}{\underset{\displaystyle SH \qquad SH}{CH_2 \qquad CH-(CH_2)_4COOH}}}
\end{array}
$$

Oxidized lipoic acid   **Reduced lipoic acid**

Lipoic acid exists in the oxidized (disulfide) or the reduced (sulfhydryl) form. In the pyruvate and α-ketoglutarate dehydrogenase systems, lipoic acid works along with thiamin in the transfer of acyl groups that, in effect, are generated by lipoic acid. The latter compound reacts with an acylol-thiamin complex to form a larger complex that rearranges to yield a free thiamin residue and an acyl-lipoic acid complex. (In the course of the reaction the acylol moiety is oxidized to an acyl group and the oxidized lipoic acid is reduced.) Finally, the acyl group is transferred to coenzyme A and the reduced lipoic acid is oxidized by an FAD-enzyme to yield the oxidized lipoic acid. (See Chapter 13.)

In enzyme binding, lipoic acid seems to be bound to the lysine residues of the enzyme protein. Hydrolysis of lipoic acid-protein complexes yields ϵ-N-lipoyl-L-lysine, a compound that is similar to biocytin (ϵ-N-biotinyl-L-lysine).

Lipoic acid, thus, is of vital importance in cellular oxidative processes. It is, however, of little significance as a dietary component in mammals.

UBIQUINONE

Ubiquinone (coenzyme Q) is a collective name for a group of lipidlike compounds consisting of a substituted benzoquinone ring with a long isoprenoid side chain.

Ubiquinone$_{10}$

Several forms of the compound exist in nature varying only in the number of isoprenoid units in the chain. Ubiquinone$_{10}$ is the form that is commonly found in mammalian respiratory systems. Ubiquinones with six to nine isoprenoid units are found in lower organisms. A chemically similar compound, plastoquinone, is found in plant tissues and apparently is functionally analogous to the ubiquinones in animal tissues.

Ubiquinone is synthesized in animal tissues and for this reason it is not a true vitamin. It functions in cellular electron transport, acting between the flavin coenzymes and the cytochromes. (See Chapter 13.) Like all quinones, ubiquinone is easily reduced to the hydroquinone.

Synthetic derivatives of reduced ubiquinone with a much shortened side chain (hexahydrocoenzyme Q_4) have been shown to have some biological effects resembling those of vitamin E.

Ubiquinone has been reported to improve reproductive performance of rats on a vitamin E-deficient diet (Scholler et al., 1968; Jones et al., 1971). The physical performance of genetically dystrophic mice also has been reported to be improved by administration of hexahydrocoenzyme Q_4, which can substitute for ubiquinone$_{10}$

(Scholler et al., 1968). Ubiquinone has also been shown to be of value in treatment of anemia of severe human malnutrition (Majaj and Folkers, 1968). These are most probably nonspecific actions shown by a number of antioxidants. A specific role for, or effect of, ubiquinone in any deficiency or metabolic disease has not been unequivocally demonstrated. An impaired synthesis of ubiquinone in some diseases may eventually reveal a medical use for this ubiquitous family of compounds.

chapter 5

minerals and water

". . . Fish, amphibian, and reptile, warm-blooded bird and mammal—each of us carries in our veins a salty stream in which the elements sodium, potassium and calcium are combined in almost the same proportions as in sea water. This is our inheritance from the day, untold millions of years ago, when a remote ancestor, having progressed from the one-celled to the many-celled stage, first developed a circulatory system in which the fluid was merely the water of the sea. In the same way, our lime-hardened skeletons are a heritage from the calcium-rich ocean of Cambrian time. Even the protoplasm that streams within each cell of our bodies has the chemical structure impressed upon living matter when the first simple creatures were brought forth in the ancient sea. . . ."

Rachel Carson, *The Sea Around Us*

The bulk of the total mineral content of the animal body is represented by the skeletal minerals. Lesser amounts of minerals are constituents of essential molecules such as thyroxine and hemoglobin, are an integral part of various metalloenzymes such as alkaline phosphatase and carbonic anhydrase, exist as free ions, or more frequently are loosely bound to proteins and other substances in the body tissues. Activation of cellular enzyme systems, the critical pH of body fluids necessary for the control of metabolic reactions, and the osmotic balance between the cell and its environment all largely depend on mineral elements.

The minerals that are known to be essential and that are present in fairly large quantities are calcium, phosphorus, potassium, sodium, chloride, magnesium, and sulfur. The principal minerals present in lesser quantities and for which essential roles in humans have been identified include iron, copper, cobalt, manganese, zinc, iodine, molybdenum, selenium, chromium, and fluoride. Accumulating evidence indicates that nickel, silicon, tin, and vanadium are essential for some animals and likely also for humans.

Essential elements characteristically tend to concentrate in body tissues in a fairly consistent fashion; absorption from the gut and excretion through the kidney, bile, or other intestinal secretions are precisely regulated by body homeostatic mechanisms. However, the homeostatic mechanism can be overloaded when excessive amounts gain entrance to the body through food, water, or air. A number of minerals that are essential in minute amounts to body functioning are toxic when accumulated in large amounts. Iron and manganese as well as some of the newly detected essential trace minerals are in this category.

In order to analyze minerals that are present in biological materials the elements must be freed from the organic complexes to which they are bound. Removal of organic substances is accomplished by ashing. Dry ashing involves heating the dried material to high temperatures in a muffle furnace; wet ashing is accomplished by digesting with strong acids. When minerals are present in fairly large amounts, methods of assay are usually quite precise. A number of reasonably simple colorimetric methods have been used for years. (See Sandell, 1959; Association of Official Agricultural Chemists, 1960.) More precise analysis of the resultant material for the element(s) in question can be performed by a variety of techniques including atomic absorption spectrophotometry, emission spectroscopy, neutron activation, and atomic fluorescence spectroscopy, to name a few. (See Brätter and Schramel, 1980.) The development of newer methods has permitted the analysis of many elements present at very low concentrations (less than 1 ng/gm) to be accomplished with great precision.

Calcium

The human body contains about 22 gm Ca/kg fat-free body weight, about 99 percent of which is concentrated in the hard structures of bones and teeth. The precise composition and structure of bone salt are not known; it is generally assumed to resemble a hydroxyapatite similar to $Ca_{10}(PO_4)_6(OH)_2$. (See Bronner, 1964.) Other minerals such as magnesium, sodium, and strontium in combination with phosphates and carbonates or citrates are adsorbed on the surface of bone crystals or trapped in the latticelike network characteristic of bone. (See Chapter 17.) Some minerals such as strontium probably are not essential to bone structure but are incidental though harmless contaminants. Other minerals that are harmful, such as lead, are also sequestered by bone, perhaps thereby lessening their toxicity (Waldron and Stofen, 1974). Bone provides an enormous depot of calcium on which the body can draw by various hormonal stimulations.

The calcium in blood, extracellular fluid, and extraosseus compartments account for the remaining 1 percent of total body calcium. The level of calcium circulating in blood is independent of dietary intake. It remains remarkably constant, ranging between 2.25 and 2.75 mM, with an average value of 2.5 mM (10mg/dl). Calcium exists in three forms in blood and body fluids: protein-bound calcium (46 percent), diffusible calcium complexed with citrate, sulfate, or phosphate (6.5 percent), and ionized calcium (47.5 percent). The physiological functions of calcium are associated with this last (ionized) fraction. Plasma ionized calcium concentrations normally range between 0.94 and 1.33 mM. The maintenance of plasma ionized calcium levels within this narrow range is essential; hypercalcemia may lead to respiratory failure, and hypocalcemia results in tetany.

The role of ionized calcium in a wide variety of intra- and extracellular processes, such as neuromuscular excitability, blood coagulation, cellular adhesiveness, and maintenance and function of cell membranes, have been well documented. (See Carafoli, 1982.) A role of calcium in muscle contraction was suggested as early as 1882 by Ringer, who showed that the contraction of excised heart muscle depended on the concentration of calcium in solutions bathing the muscle. (Muscle contraction and the effect of calcium will be discussed in detail in Chapter 18.)

The role of calcium in blood clotting has been mentioned in connection with vitamin K. Apparently extremely minute quantities of calcium are required for prothrombin activation since blood clotting proceeds normally even in the presence of hypocalcemic tetany. Calcium also is involved in maintaining the integrity of the intercellular cement substance. Calcium is necessary for the activation of certain enzymes including pancreatic lipase, plasma lipoprotein lipase, phospholipase A, and phosphorylase kinase, and the release of neurotransmitters such as acetylcholine, serotonin, and norepinephrine. (See Chapter 19.)

Extracellular calcium influences DNA synthesis in normal cells. Calcium also participates in stimulus secretion coupling as in the release of neurohormones from nerve endings after depolarization (West, 1982) and subsequent transmission of nerve signals (Llinás, 1982). Many of these events involve the interaction of calcium with calmodulin, a heat stabile, acidic polypeptide that contains four calcium-binding sites (Cheung, 1982a). Calmodulin has been shown to participate in the calcium-dependent activation of several enzymes including adenylate cyclase, myosin light chain kinase, phosphorylase b kinase, glycogen synthase, actomyosin ATPase, and erythrocyte Mg^{++},Ca^{++}ATPase (Cheung, 1980; 1982b). It also functions in the calcium-dependent release or synthesis of certain hormones and neurohormones, and the calcium-dependent inhibitory effects of microtubule polymerization (Cheung, 1982a).

The maintenance of normal levels of calcium in the body is accomplished by hormonal controls of resorption or synthesis of bone, intestinal absorption, and renal reabsorption, as well as renal and intestinal excretion. Absorption of calcium is dependent on body needs, vitamin D status, the form of calcium ingested, the effects of other dietary components such as fiber, oxalates, and phytates, as well as various disease states. (See Allen, 1982 and Chapter 6.) The excretion of calcium is through the intestine and the kidney. Secretion of calcium into the gut is largely independent of dietary calcium intake or calcium status; however, much of this calcium may be reabsorbed if calcium needs are increased. Renal excretion is sensitive to several hormones, particularly parathyroid hormone (PTH) and vitamin D metabolites. In a hypocalcemic state, increased PTH and $1,25\text{-}(OH)_2$ D_3 will increase the reabsorption in the proximal convoluted tubule and in the ascending limb of Henle's loop.

The metabolism of calcium in relation to vitamin D has been discussed in Chapter 4 and will be discussed further in Chapter 17.

Phosphorus

The human body contains roughly 12–14 gm P/kg fat-free tissue; of this amount, about 85 percent is contained in the inorganic phase of skeletal structures. The phosphorus content of plasma is about 3.5 mg/dl; when red cell phosphorus is also included the total phosphorus content of blood ranges between 30 to 45 mg/dl.

Organic phosphates are a part of the structure of all body cells and are intimately involved in cellular functions. Phosphorus is a constituent of the high energy compound ATP and thus is necessary for energy transductions essential for all cellular activity. The oxidation of carbohydrate leading to the formation of ATP also requires phosphorus since phosphorylation is an obligatory step in the metabolism of the monosaccharides. The active coenzyme form of certain of the B vitamins also functions as the phosphorylated derivatives. Phospholipids are constituents of all cellular membranes and are active determinants of cellular permeability. Deoxyribonucleic acid (DNA) and RNA, the genetically significant compounds responsible for cell reproduction and therefore for growth and all protein syntheses, are phosphorylated compounds. Indeed, all nucleotides contain phosphorus.

Phosphorus is more completely absorbed than is calcium; 60 to 70 percent is absorbed on a normal intake and maximal absorption (up to 90 percent) is achieved on very low intakes. Phosphorus occurs in foods in both inorganic and organic forms; the latter are hydrolyzed in the lumen of the small intestine by phosphatases prior to absorption as inorganic phosphate. Some forms of dietary phosphates, for example phytic acid of cereals and seeds, appear to be generally unavailable for absorption, and other dietary components such as unsaturated fatty acids, iron, and aluminum may interfere with absorption. (See Avioli, 1980.) Fecal phosphorus represents both unabsorbed phosphate and that secreted into the gastrointestinal tract. Urinary phosphorus is largely inorganic phosphate. In humans, the tubular reabsorption of phosphate is normally 85 to 95 percent but may be decreased by elevated levels of PTH or increased by hypophosphatemia (Lee et al., 1981).

Because of the widespread presence of phosphorus in most foodstuffs, a dietary deficiency is not likely to occur in the human. However, phosphorus depletion in humans can occur as a result of prolonged treatment with nonabsorbable antacids such as magnesium hydroxide and aluminum hydroxide. This depletion is characterized by weakness, anorexia, malaise, stiff joints, and fragile bones. (See Knochel, 1977.) A phosphorus depletion syndrome also has been observed in grazing animals subsisting on grasses and hay that are high in calcium but low in phosphorus.

The ratio of dietary calcium to phosphorus is critical in rats. Diets with a low Ca:P ratio have led to progressive bone loss secondary to hyperparathyroidism (Krishnarao and Draper, 1972; Draper and Scythes, 1981). However, similar effects have not been observed in human adults (Malm, 1953; Spencer, 1965; see Allen, 1982). Provision of a cow's milk-based formula containing more phosphorus than calcium (in contrast to a Ca:P ratio of approximately 2:1 in human breast milk) may contribute to the syndrome of "idiopathic hypocalcemia" and tetany in infants (Mizrahi et al., 1968).

Magnesium

Of the total body magnesium, about 0.5 gm/kg fat-free body weight, approximately 60 percent is located in bone. The function of magnesium in bone is not known, although it may serve as a magnesium reserve for the body. One-third of the magnesium is in combination with phosphate, and the remainder appears to be adsorbed loosely on the surface of the mineral structure. Approximately 1 percent of the total body content of magnesium is extracellular. The levels of magnesium in serum of healthy people are remarkably constant at about 2 mg/dl and vary less than 15 percent from this mean value. Approximately 35 percent of the extracellular magnesium is bound nonspecifically to plasma proteins; the remaining 65 percent, which is diffusible or ionized, appears to be the biologically active component.

Magnesium is absorbed mainly from the small intestine. When fed a diet containing a normal amount of magnesium, subjects absorb about 44 percent of it; with severe dietary restriction, the percent absorption rises to 76 percent (Graham et al., 1960). A substantial amount of magnesium is secreted into the intestinal tract from bile and from pancreatic and intestinal juices; however, in normal people, most of the secreted magnesium is reabsorbed. Magnesium is excreted by the kidney; some is excreted also in sweat. Under extreme conditions, however, sweat can account for 25 percent of the magnesium lost daily.

All organisms require magnesium to function normally. The metal has many biochemical roles in cells: it activates enzymes, it maintains the conformation of nucleic acids, and it regulates a number of important biochemical processes. Magnesium is required for most reactions in protein synthesis, from the formation of the aminoacyladenylate to the stabilization of the structure of the aminoacyl-tRNA complex to the maintenance of the structure of ribosomal particles. (See

Wacker, 1980.) Many enzymes require magnesium for activation. Phosphatases, kinases, enolases, and nucleic acid polymerases all are involved in phosphate metabolism and all require magnesium probably because phosphate ligands form more stable complexes with magnesium than with any other cation. This property is useful for the formation of enzyme substrate complexes through magnesium, for the maintenance of substrate conformation, for the reduction of charged phosphate substrates and phosphorylated enzymes, and for the enhancement of the positive dipolarity of phosphorus in phosphate groups (ibid).

Acute magnesium deficiency in the rat was first described by Kruse et al. (1932) and is characterized by progressive hyperkinetic behavior when the animal is disturbed. This condition later develops into tonic-clonic convulsions that are often fatal. Chronic deficiency produces reduced growth, alopecia, skin lesions, edema, and swollen gums. Calcification and degenerative changes in various organs, especially kidneys, have also been reported. (See Aikawa, 1981.)

Magnesium deficiency has been induced experimentally in human subjects (Shils, 1964). With magnesium depletion (plasma levels 10 to 30 percent of those from control periods), hypocalcemia occurred despite adequate calcium intake and absorption, and hypocalciuria and hypokalemia were also reported. Anorexia, nausea, and apathy occurred frequently and heralded exacerbation of neurological changes including personality change, spontaneous generalized muscle spasm, tremor, twitching, and Trousseau and Chvostek's signs. (See Shils, 1980.)

Magnesium deficiency does not appear to be a problem in most human dietaries since the mineral element is widely distributed in foodstuffs. In a normal adequate diet about 30 percent of the total magnesium intake may come from green vegetables that contain the magnesium porphyrin, chlorophyll.

Magnesium deficiency, however, can occur in man as a result of prolonged episodes of vomiting or malabsorption as in severe diarrhea. Gastric juice contains a fair amount of magnesium and excessive vomiting could result in substantial losses of the mineral in addition to the loss resulting from the failure to retain ingested food. Certain drugs—ammonium chloride and mercurial diuretics—result in loss of magnesium through the urine (Martin et al., 1952). Magnesium deficiency has been reported in children with protein-calorie malnutrition due primarily to diarrhea which increases fecal loss of the mineral (Caddell, 1969). Recovery was more prompt when diets were supplemented with magnesium (ibid.). Magnesium deficiency can occur also as a result of prolonged fasting, increase in intestinal transit time, distal small intestine resection, acute alcoholism, burns, and renal disease. (See Aikawa, 1981.) For a review of magnesium deficiency and excess, see Rude and Singer (1981).

Sodium

The value of salt has been recognized for centuries. The common expressions "salt of the earth" and "worth his salt" and even the word "salary" all derive from the high value placed on salt throughout history. The requirement for sodium is not well defined, but human dietaries generally contain more sodium than necessary. A human adult can maintain sodium balance with intakes of less than 200 mg/day under conditions of moderate ambient temperature and humidity, and excluding any substantial increase in sodium loss due to excessive sweating. Intakes vary widely; about 10 gm NaCl/day appears to be usual for most Americans, whereas intakes of 30 to 40 gm/day are not uncommon in some Oriental countries where soy sauces and monosodium glutamate are favored as flavoring agents.

The content of sodium in the normal human adult is 1.1 to 1.4 gm/kg body weight. From 35 to 40 percent of total body sodium is in the skeleton, bound for the most part on the surface of bone crystals. Only 25 to 35 percent of skeletal sodium is exchangeable and hence part of the active labile sodium pool of the body. (See Chapter 17.)

The content of sodium in serum normally ranges between 136 and 145 mEq/liter (313 to 334 mg Na/dl). Since sodium is the chief cation of the extracellular fluid, the control of body fluid osmolarity and therefore body fluid volume is largely dependent on sodium ions and the ratio of sodium to other ions.

Sodium is capable of permeating the cell membrane, and muscle contraction and nerve transmission involve a temporary exchange of extracellular sodium and intracellular potassium. (See Chapters 18 and 19.) The subsequent transfer of sodium out of the cell is by means of an active mechanism or *pump*. (See Chapter 9.) A very small amount of sodium occurs intracellularly.

Sodium metabolism is regulated primarily by aldosterone, a hormone of the adrenal cortex that promotes the reabsorption of sodium from the kidney tubules. In the absence of this hormone, sodium excretion is increased and symptoms of deficiency ensue. Other adrenal mineralocorticoids, deoxycorticosterone and hydrocortisone, are involved in regulation of sodium excretion but are less potent in action.

Dietary deficiency of sodium probably never occurs in the human. The element is widely distributed in foodstuffs. Plant sources contain less than animal products and are therefore prominent on low sodium diets. Processed foods of all kinds tend to have a high sodium content since many sodium compounds are used in preserving, tenderizing, and flavoring.

Excessive losses of sodium leading to hyponatremia have been observed in a variety of clinical and environmental circumstances. Abnormal loss of sodium without adequate replacement accompanying diarrhea, vomiting, and excessive sweating can lead to a hyponatremic state. Depletion is usually, although not always, associated with concurrent water loss. If the balance is maintained between water and sodium loss, plasma sodium values might remain within the normal range even though the individual is undergoing sodium depletion and reduction of total body fluids. Thus the determination of plasma sodium may not accurately reflect total body sodium.

The results of sodium depletion are closely related to the state of water balance. If only sodium is lost and water is retained, serum sodium concentration eventually will decrease, as when water only is replaced following excessive sweating. As a result, water will migrate into the cells and symptoms of water intoxication develop: loss of appetite, weakness, mental apathy, and muscle twitching. If sodium loss is accompanied by water loss, symptoms of extracellular fluid depletion develop: low blood volume, high hematocrit, collapse of veins, low blood pressure, and muscle cramps.

Sodium balance is so well controlled by homeostatic mechanisms in normal individuals that little attention usually was given to sodium intake. Recently, however, interest has focused on the potential role of excessive sodium intake in the development of hypertension. Epidemiological studies relating salt consumption with the prevalence of hypertension between and within populations, the development of hypertension in experimental animals (especially those genetically susceptible to hypertension) fed diets high in salt, and the responsiveness of hypertensive patients to a drastically curtailed intake of sodium have all been used to implicate high salt intake as a causative factor in the development of hypertension (Weinsier, 1976). Such information does not constitute proof of a causative role, but there may be a fraction of the population who are sensitive to high salt intake and for whom the "normal" salt consumption may present a hazard.

In response to pregnancy, the glomerular filtration rate increases and the level of progesterone increases, reducing sodium reabsorption at the tubular level. (See Vander, 1980.) These changes, accompanied by the increase in body mass and body water, increase sodium requirements during pregnancy (Pike and Smiciklas, 1972). When this additional requirement is not met, the sodium-conserving mechanisms operate to increase sodium reabsorption. The resulting stress during pregnancy in rats has been documented through electron microscopic and histochemical evidence as severe pathology in the adrenal gland (Smiciklas et al., 1971a; 1971b) and by changes in the secretory capacity of the adrenal (Khokhar and Pike, 1973). These findings further support the suggestion that the once common practice of restricting salt intake in pregnancy be critically evaluated (Committee on Maternal Nutrition, 1970; National Research Council, 1980).

Chloride

Total body chloride averages about 33 mEq/kg body weight (1.2 gm/kg) in a normal adult male. Chloride ion is the major anion of the extracellular fluid and occurs for the most part in combination with sodium, although small amounts may be bound loosely to protein and other substances. Although predominantly extracellular, chloride is found in low concentration in bone and is probably loosely bound in connective tissue. Less than 15 percent of total body chloride is located intracellularly; erythrocytes have the highest cellular concentration with gastric mucosa, gonads, and skin containing lesser amounts. Chloride in blood easily transfers between plasma and erythrocytes in what is commonly known as the chloride shift, a primary homeostatic mechanism for the control of blood pH. Chloride is also essential for the formation of gastric hydrochloric acid.

In many physiologic and clinical conditions, chloride plays an important role in the control of electrolyte and acid base equilibria. The role of chloride in the genesis, maintenance, and correction of metabolic alkalosis and potassium deficiency is well recognized. (See Simopoulos and Bartter, 1980.) Hypochloremia may occur in response to sodium chloride deprivation if there is fluid retention, as a result of excess loss of sodium chloride in sweat as in cystic fibrosis patients, as a consequence of loss of hydrochloric acid due to repeated vomiting, and with the use and abuse of diuretics. Dietary chloride deprivation has not been a cause for concern, but the recent report of hypochloremic metabolic alkalosis resulting from consumption of a chloride-deficient infant formula has demonstrated the importance of adequate chloride consumption (Roy and Arant, 1979). Long-term consequences to the infants appear to include polydipsia, perhaps an excessive salt appetite, growth retardation (especially head growth), and delayed development of speech. (See Simopoulos and Bartter, 1980.)

Potassium

Potassium is the principal cation of intracellular fluid. Within the cell, it functions, as does sodium, by influencing acid base balance and osmolarity. The human body contains about 2.6 gm K/kg fat-free body weight; values are found to be higher in trained athletes with larger than normal muscle mass. Nerve and muscle cells are especially rich in potassium but all cells, both plant and animal, tend to concentrate the mineral. High intracellular potassium concentrations are essential for several important biochemical functions including protein biosynthesis by ribosomes and glycogen synthesis. A number of enzymes, including pyruvate kinase, require potassium for maximal activity.

Potassium ion is found in small amounts in the extracellular fluid. Serum levels in a normal individual range from 3.5 to 5.0 mEq/liter (14 to 20 mg/dl). Serum potassium concentration is not a reliable index of total body potassium and only the extremes of high and low concentration are clinically diagnostic. Serum values of less than 3.5 mEq/liter are often accompanied by disordered smooth muscle function; paralysis of skeletal muscle and abnormalities in conduction and activity of cardiac muscles can occur. (See Randall, 1980.) Serum values greater than 6 mEq/liter can lead to cardiac and central nervous system depression and ultimately to cardiac arrest.

A deficiency of potassium is unlikely to occur as a result of insufficient dietary intake. However, body potassium can be depleted leading to a hypokalemic state in the following ways: by loss of chloride and potassium due to vomiting and thus leading to hypokalemic alkalosis, the administration of diuretics, chronic renal disease where there is wastage of potassium, hyperfunction of the adrenal cortex (or administration of adrenal steroids), and diabetic acidosis. Hyperkalemia can occur with acute or chronic renal failure, with acute dehydration, adrenal insufficiency, severe metabolic or respiratory acidosis, or shock. (See Rose, 1977).

Sulfur

The bulk of the sulfur present in the animal body is derived from the three sulfur-containing amino acids—methionine, cystine, and cysteine—which provide the sulfur needed for synthesis of other sulfur-containing compounds. Inorganic sulfates and sulfides are a small fraction of the total sulfur. Thiamin and biotin also contribute small amounts of sulfur to the total body supply.

The metabolic importance of some sulfur-containing compounds resides in the easy interconvertibility of disulfide and sulfhydryl groups in oxidation-reduction reactions. The reduction of cystine (disulfide) to cysteine (sulfhydryl) demonstrates the kind of reaction involved.[1]

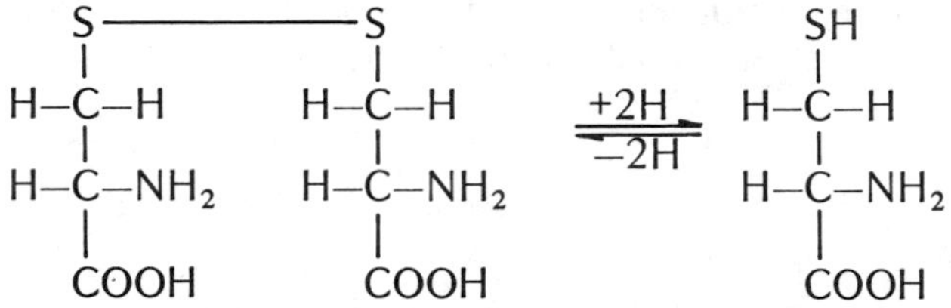

$$
\begin{array}{ccc}
\text{S} \!-\!\!-\!\!-\!\!-\!\!-\!\!-\!\!-\! \text{S} & & \text{SH} \\
| \qquad\qquad\quad | & & | \\
\text{H--C--H} \qquad \text{H--C--H} & \xrightarrow[-2H]{+2H} & \text{H--C--H} \\
| \qquad\qquad\quad | & & | \\
\text{H--C--NH}_2 \quad \text{H--C--NH}_2 & & \text{H--C--NH}_2 \\
| \qquad\qquad\quad | & & | \\
\text{COOH} \qquad \text{COOH} & & \text{COOH} \\
\textbf{Cystine} & & \textbf{Cysteine}
\end{array}
$$

Other reactions utilizing the reversible formation of disulfide bonding include those that require glutathione (γ-glutamylcysteinylglycine) as a reducing agent. For example, in the erythrocyte, hydrogen peroxide is destroyed by the following reaction: two molecules of reduced glutathione react with hydrogen peroxide

$$2\ \text{G-SH} + \text{H}_2\text{O}_2 \xrightarrow{\text{glutathione peroxidase}} \text{G-S-S-G} + 2\text{H}_2\text{O}$$

The oxidized glutathione is then reduced by reaction with NADPH which is formed in the erythrocyte via the pentose phosphate pathway

$$\text{G-S-S-G} + \text{NADPH} + \text{H}^+ \xrightarrow{\text{glutathione reductase}} 2\ \text{G-SH} + \text{NADP}^+$$

Other reactions involving a sulfhydryl group include those used in the formation of high energy-thioester linkages as in the formation of acyl-coenzyme A derivatives during fatty acid activation:

$$\text{fatty acid} + \text{CoA-SH} + \text{ATP} \xrightarrow{\text{thiokinase}} \text{acyl-S-CoA} + \text{AMP} + \text{PP}_i$$

---

[1]The cystine content of hair and animal fur is roughly 15 percent; human hair contains somewhat more cystine than that of other species. The presence of disulfide or sulfhydryl bonds in the protein molecule forms the molecular basis for the permanent wave. Disulfide bonds are opened and reformed in a second position; hence the proper curl is held in place.

In addition to its role in oxidation-reduction reactions, sulfur is a component of other essential compounds and active metabolites. Taurine, the precursor to the bile acid taurocholic acid, is formed from cysteine. The mucopolysaccharides, specifically, the chondroitin sulfates and heparins, contain sulfated sugar derivatives. Sulfates are also metabolically important in detoxication reactions and form esters with potentially toxic compounds. Prior to ester formation, sulfates are activated by ATP which gives rise to 3-phosphoadenosine 5'-phosphosulfate (PAPS); the reaction requires magnesium. This compound was originally designated active sulfate by Hilz and Lipmann (1955). Such sulfation steps are essential for the formation of various proteoglycans, glycolipids, and glycoproteins. In addition, potentially important roles have been suggested for the sulfated steroid hormones in the control of various aspects of metabolism. (See Singer, 1982.)

Iron

The iron content of the adult human male is about 49 mg/kg body weight and the adult female about 38 mg/kg; some of the difference reflects variation in body composition between the sexes. Essential body iron in humans (about 35 mg/kg) is generally proportional to lean body mass. In addition, there is a variable amount of storage iron.

Essential tissue iron is composed of two general types of compounds, heme and nonheme. The heme molecule is comprised of ferrous or ferric iron in the center of a porphyrin ring. Hemoglobin contains four porphyrin units bound to the protein globin. (See Chapter 16.) Myoglobin, a similar type of compound present in skeletal and heart muscle, contains only one ferrous porphyrin group per molecule. Both hemoglobin and myoglobin enter into a reversible combination with oxygen; myoglobin has the greater affinity and this property enables it to serve as a cell reservoir of oxygen. About three-fourths of the total body iron is contained in these two compounds.

Less than 0.3 percent of total body iron is present in the form of intracellular heme enzymes. These enzymes include cytochromes a, a_3, b, c_1, c, b_5, and P450 as well as catalases and tryptophan pyrrolase.

The group of nonheme compounds is composed of iron-containing enzymes. These include various "iron-sulfur" proteins which take part in electron transfer reactions and which include iron in an active site covalently associated with either acid labile sulfide or cysteinyl sulfur (Hall et al., 1974). In addition, various other enzymes such as xanthine oxidase, aconitase, and phenylalanine hydroxylase also contain iron.

A large amount of iron, about 26 percent of total body content, is stored in cells of liver, spleen, and bone in the form of two compounds, ferritin and hemosiderin; lesser amounts are stored in other tissues. These compounds are iron-protein complexes containing ferric hydroxide and are closely related in structure. Ferritin is a polyhydroxy iron polymer with a molecular weight of about

150,000 surrounded by a protein coat of molecular weight 465,000. The specific protein to which iron is attached is known as apoferritin. The hemosiderin molecule apparently is more complex. When normal amounts of iron are stored, ferritin appears to predominate; when large stores accumulate, the storage form is chiefly hemosiderin. Apparently ferritin is a constituent of the hemosiderin structure, and grouping of ferritin molecules occurs as the compound accumulates. Ferritin has a high capacity for iron storage incorporating as much as 4,500 atoms as the ferric oxide hydrate (Macara et al., 1972; see Harrison et al., 1974).

Hemosiderin is the insoluble form of storage iron in the cell and appears as golden brown granules by light microscopy. Electron microscopy shows that hemosiderin granules include a range of materials from crystalline arrays of intact ferritin molecules to amorphous aggregates of iron. Because a variety of organic constituents are also included in the aggregate, these are believed to be disintegrated, ferritin loaded, cellular organelles. (See National Research Council, 1979.)

In addition to the large amount of iron in the erythrocytes, iron is also present in serum bound to transferrin, a β-globulin sometimes called siderophilin. This glycoprotein is synthesized as an apoprotein by the liver and is used to transport iron between tissues through the extravascular fluids and plasma. Transferrin has a single polypeptide chain of molecular weight 80,000, contains about 6 percent carbohydrate, and has two specific sites on the protein at which iron (Fe^{+++}) is bound (Morgan, 1974). The concentration of transferrin is influenced by the availability of body stores of iron and by the rate of erythropoiesis. (See Chapter 7.) Serum iron ranges from 70 to 140 μg/dl, although approximately 360 μg or more could be bound to the protein present. The quantitative ability of transferrin to bind iron is designated *iron-binding capacity* of serum. Practically no ionic iron exists in the animal body. Regardless of iron status (other than in acute iron toxicity), the largest fraction of transferrin does not have iron bound to it. Among individuals with adequate iron status, serum transferrin is only 20 to 40 percent saturated with iron; depletion of iron stores results in saturation falling to less than 15 percent. (See Chapter 16.)

Virtually all metabolic processes involving iron are dependent on the interconversion of ferrous and ferric iron (Frieden, 1973). Iron must be in a ferrous state (Fe^{++}) to be absorbed into the intestinal mucosal cell, but it must be oxidized to the ferric state (Fe^{+++}) before binding to apotransferrin and transported in the plasma. The oxidation of Fe^{++} to Fe^{+++} is accomplished by the copper-containing enzyme ceruloplasmin. (See Frieden, 1981; also see Chapter 6.) Iron is present in the Fe^{++} state in hemoglobin and in the Fe^{+++} state in methemoglobin, transferrin, and ferritin. The relationship of iron transport, storage, mobilization, and function to ceruloplasmin action is shown in Fig. 5.1.

The degradation of hemoglobin is discussed in detail in Chapter 16. It is enough to mention here that the pathway is through oxidation to methemoglobin, which contains ferric iron and is degraded to yield iron, globin, and protoporphyrin. Iron so released is reused for synthesis of hemoglobin or other iron-containing compounds. The globin portion gives rise to its component amino acids, and the protoporphyrin is degraded to form the bile pigments.

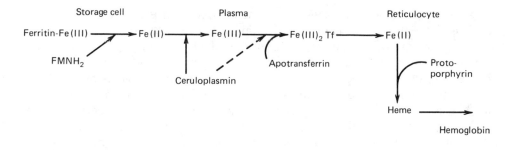

Figure 5.1
(a) Steps in the release of iron from liver storage cells to transferrin in the plasma
and then to reticulocytes for hemoglobin synthesis. (b) The central role of ceruloplasmin (ferroxidase) in iron mobilization and transport. The Fe(II) to Fe(III) cycles
of iron are shown in relation to the metabolism of the major iron compound of the
vertebrates, hemoglobin. aFt = apoferritin; aTf = apotransferrin. From E. Frieden,
Ciba Foundation 79 (new series), 1980, p. 107.

In simplest terms, iron serves a primary role in the animal body as a mediator
of oxidative processes. Heme compounds are the carriers of oxygen to cells and
the transporters of hydrogen to molecular oxygen as a part of the cellular electron
transport system. In iron deficiency, the lowered capacity to provide oxygen is
largely responsible for the fatigue and apathy characteristic of iron-deficiency
anemia, and, for that matter, of all anemias.

Iron-deficiency anemia occurs almost exclusively in young children and women
of child-bearing age. Because iron is conserved by the body, adult males rarely
develop the anemia of iron-deficiency except following excessive blood loss. (See

Chapter 23.) In the early stages of iron deficiency, iron is released from stores and used for the synthesis of hemoglobin and other iron-containing proteins. Once the stores are depleted, if further iron depletion continues, a fall in plasma iron occurs. With continuation of insufficient iron intake, a severe iron deficiency can ensue, characterized by a variety of morphological and biochemical manifestations. Lesions of the gastrointestinal tract, particularly mucosal cell atrophy as well as changes in the integument (progressive changes in fingernails from brittleness to thinning, flattening, and eventual concaving) have been related to the deficiency. When iron deficiency is extensive, hemoglobin synthesis is impaired and a hypochromic, microcytic anemia develops. A variety of iron-enzyme defects have been described in iron-deficient tissues (see Dallman, 1974) but there is considerable variation in the response of individual tissues. Thus myoglobin can be reduced dramatically in skeletal muscle but may be unaffected in heart muscle. Depletion of cytochromes and impaired activity throughout the electron transport pathway in heart mitochrondria have been reported (Blayney et al., 1976). Mitochondria become enlarged, radiolucent, and abnormally fragile in response to iron deficiency. (See Dallman, 1974.) There also appears to be functional consequences of iron deficiency, as Gardner et al. (1977) have noted a considerable impairment of work performance in subjects with hemoglobin concentrations below 12 gm/dl.

Other Trace Elements

For many years the importance of trace elements in human dietaries was given little attention. The following statement from the first edition of this book was typical of the prevailing opinion.

> Trace elements are required in extremely small amounts in the diet and are so widely distributed in foodstuffs that even diets inadequate in other respects usually contain sufficient quantities of these nutrients.

With the development of improved methods for the detection of trace elements and the resulting intensified research in this area, it is now clear that some human dietaries *are* marginally deficient in some trace elements and that functional impairments due to these deficiencies may be more prevalent than had been suspected.

Many of the difficulties of trace element research were the result of the relative insensitivity of methods for detecting the minute amounts present in biological materials and the inability to prevent contamination during feeding experiments. The development of an "ultraclean environment" (Smith and Schwartz, 1967) made possible the study of trace element deficiencies in small animals in a controlled environmental system similar to germfree isolators.

Because of the small amounts of trace minerals present in the body, it is clear that they play primarily catalytic roles in cellular metabolism and therefore function in much the same way as vitamins. Some, such as cobalt and iodine, appear to function entirely as components of larger molecules whose metabolic role, however, also is fundamentally catalytic. The functions and deficiency symptoms (where known) of some of the more significant trace minerals are shown in Table 5.1.

Deficiencies of several of the trace elements have been known to occur naturally in cattle and sheep allowed to graze on pastures in which the soil was grossly deficient in an essential mineral. Some pathological conditions observed in grazing animals, however, also may result from toxic effects of excessive amounts of certain elements in the soil. Experimental studies have for the most part been performed on animals, and these studies have provided useful clues to mineral function in humans. A few rare disease conditions that occur in humans appear to result in or from abnormalities in trace mineral metabolism. Some of these diseases will be mentioned briefly in the section that follows.

For a review of the bioavailability of trace elements, see Forbes and Erdman (1983).

COPPER

Although copper had been recognized as a constituent of plant and animal tissues for more than 150 years, it was not until 1928 that conclusive evidence for the essentiality of this trace element emerged from studies of milk anemia in rats. Hart et al. (1928) reported that copper, in addition to iron, was necessary for hemoglobin formation. (See Chapter 16.) Subsequently, this and other effects of copper deficiency were recognized in domestic animals grazing on pasture lands with low copper content or fed copper-deficient diets.

Dietary copper is absorbed in the stomach or proximal small intestine, although the mechanisms are not yet understood. Copper, on entering the blood, becomes immediately attached to albumin or to plasma amino acids. This exchangeable copper is rapidly transferred to the liver. It appears that the amount of copper absorbed is far in excess of metabolic needs and most copper is returned to the intestine in the bile. The copper retained by the liver may be stored, presumably bound to metallothionein (Bremner et al., 1978), or used for the synthesis of various copper-containing proteins. One of these, ceruloplasmin, is a glycoprotein of the α_2-globulin fraction of human plasma. It is synthesized as an apoceruloplasmin, but for enzymatic activity requires the addition of six copper atoms prior to release from the liver. In severe copper deficiency, apoceruloplasmin is secreted by the liver. More than 90 percent of the copper in plasma is in the form of ceruloplasmin. Roles for this multifunctional copper-containing protein likely include the oxidation of ferrous iron for binding to transferrin, the transport of copper, and the regulation of biogenic amines. (See Frieden, 1981.) Other copper proteins synthesized in the liver and in extrahepatic tissues of the body include superoxide dismutase, cytochrome c oxidase, lysyl oxidase, tyrosinase, and dopamine β-hydroxylase.

Copper excreted in the bile is largely eliminated in the feces with only a small amount being reabsorbed. This biliary copper is comprised of both the copper

TABLE 5.1
Classification of the Essential Trace Elements

Element	Function	Deficiency Signs		Occurrence of Imbalances in Humans
		Animals	Humans	
Fluorine	Structure of teeth, possibly of bones; possibly growth effect	Caries; possibly growth depression	Increased incidence of caries; possibly risk factor for osteoporosis	Deficiency and excess known
Silicon	Calcification; possibly function in connective tissue	Growth depression; bone deformities	Not known	Not known
Vanadium	Not known	Growth depression, change of lipid metabolism, impairment of reproduction	Not known	Not known
Chromium	Potentiation of insulin	Relative insulin resistance	Relative insulin resistance, impaired glucose tolerance, elevated serum lipids	Deficiency known in malnutrition, aging, total parenteral alimentation
Manganese	Mucopolysaccharide metabolism, superoxide dismutase	Growth depression, bone deformities, β-cell degeneration	Not known	Deficiency not known; toxicity by inhalation
Iron	Oxygen, electron transport	Anemia, growth retardation	Anemia	Deficiencies widespread; excesses dangerous in hemochromatosis; acute poisoning
Cobalt	As part of vitamin B_{12}	Anemia; growth retardation in ruminant species	Only as vitamin B_{12} deficiency	Inability to absorb vitamin B_{12}; low B_{12} intake from vegetarian diets

Element	Biochemical function	Signs of deficiency (animals)	Signs in humans	Occurrence in humans
Nickel	Interaction with iron absorption	Growth depression, anemia, ultrastructural changes in liver; impaired reproduction	Not known	Not known
Copper	Oxidative enzymes; interaction with iron; cross-linking of elastin	Anemia, rupture of large vessels, disturbances of ossification	Anemia, changes of ossification; possibly elevated serum cholesterol	Deficiencies in malnutrition, total parenteral alimentation
Zinc	Numerous enzymes involved in energy metabolism and in transcription and translation	Failure to eat, severe growth depression, skin lesions, sexual immaturity	Growth depression, sexual immaturity, skin lesions, depression of immuno-competence, change of taste acuity	Deficiencies in Iran, Egypt, in total parenteral nutrition, genetic diseases, traumatic stress
Arsenic	Not known	Impairment of growth, reproduction; sudden heart death in third generation lactating goats	Not known	Not known
Selenium	Glutathione peroxidase; interaction with heavy metals	Different, depending on species; muscle degeneration (ruminants), pancreas atrophy (chicken)	Endemic cardiomyopathy (Keshan disease) conditioned by selenium deficiency	Deficiency and excess in areas of China; one case resulting from total parenteral alimentation
Molybdenum	Xanthine, aldehyde, sulfide oxidases	Difficult to produce; growth depression	Not known	Excessive exposure in parts of Soviet Union associated with goutlike syndrome
Iodine	Constituent of thyroid hormones	Goiter, depression of thyroid function	Goiter, depression of thyroid function, cretinism	Deficiencies widespread; excessive intakes may lead to thyrotoxicosis

Source: From W. Mertz, *Science 213*:1336 (1981).

absorbed in excess of body needs and copper from the catabolism of copper-containing proteins in extrahepatic tissues. Urinary excretion of copper is very small as there is virtually no ionic plasma copper, and likely only the small fraction bound to amino acids (less than 1 percent of nonceruloplasmin copper) could filter through the glomeruli and be lost in urine.

Copper deficiency has been observed in a number of animal species both among domesticated animals consuming a diet insufficient in copper and in experimental animals fed a copper-deficient semipurified diet. The expression of deficiency symptomology is somewhat dependent on the species and its age and sex, but may include anemia, bone abnormalities, demyelination and degeneration of the nervous system leading to neonatal ataxia, impaired reproductive performance, lesions in the cardiovascular system and depigmentation of hair, wool, or skin. (See Underwood, 1977.) It has been possible to relate many of these symptoms to decreases in the activities of individual key enzymes that require copper for activity. Thus the anemia seems to be caused by impaired ceruloplasmin synthesis, since this enzyme apparently is required for iron absorption from the gastrointestinal tract and for mobilization from iron stores. (See Frieden, 1981.) Skeletal and cardiovascular defects apparently are due to impaired collagen and elastin cross-linking. An initial step in cross-linking is the conversion of lysyl or hydroxylysyl residues to the corresponding α-aminoadipic-δ-semialdehyde or α-amino-γ-hydroxyadipic-δ-semialdehyde derivatives which are then subjected to a variety of condensation reactions; the initial modification of lysyl or hydroxylysyl residues is catalyzed by lysyl oxidase, a copper metalloenzyme (Rucker and Murray, 1978). Achromotricia has been related to impaired conversion of tyrosine to melanin due to decreased tyrosinase activity (Mason, 1979). Demyelination and degeneration of nerves may be related to impaired cytochrome c oxidase activity in the nerve cell body leading to decreased oxidative phosphorylation in nerve cell mitochondria (Howell and Davison, 1959).

Severe copper deficiency is rare in humans, but has been reported in children with protein-energy malnutrition and in some individuals maintained on total parenteral alimentation. (See Mason, 1979.) The milk-fed, premature infant is at greatest risk of developing copper deficiency. As the majority of the very high intrahepatic stores of copper are laid down late in gestation, the premature infant is born without such large stores, and on a human milk diet (which is low in copper) may develop a copper deficiency (Dauncey et al., 1977). The deficiency is most frequently characterized by severe anemia, leukopenia, neutropenia, and occasionally by demineralization of bone, decreased pigmentation of skin, and neurological abnormalities. (See Mason, 1979.)

Two inherited diseases that are directly related to copper metabolism are known. Menkes steely hair disease is an X-linked, invariably fatal, disorder characterized by progressive psychomotor retardation, short, broken, spirally twisted scalp hair with loss of pigment, poor weight gain, hypothermia, scurvylike changes in long bones, and widespread tortuosity of arteries. (See Mason, 1979.) Most of these symptoms are similar to those seen in severe copper deficiency and, in fact, appear to be due to insufficient amounts of the appropriate copper-containing enzymes, but there are some differences. The anemia and neutropenia found in dietary copper deficiency are not observed in children with Menkes' disease. This disease is characterized by profound derangement of copper metabolism, with some tissues having markedly elevated copper levels (intestine, skin fibroblasts, and renal cells), but other tissues, liver and brain, having much reduced levels. The nature of the defect that results in diminished absorption of copper from the intestinal tract and in alterations in retention of copper by the liver are not completely understood (Dekeban et al., 1975).

The other disease of an inborn error of copper metabolism is Wilson's disease or hepatolenticular degeneration. This autosomal recessive disease is characterized by low levels of serum copper (and ceruloplasmin), abnormally high liver copper with chronic liver disease, progressive accumulation of copper in brain leading to a wide variety of neurological disorders, accumulation of copper in kidneys with renal damage, deposition of copper in cornea leading to formation of Kayser-Fleischer rings, and episodes of hemolysis. Copper absorption appears normal in Wilson's disease patients, but there is a striking reduction in biliary excretion. Consequently, the liver becomes saturated with copper. Ceruloplasmin synthesis is inhibited and thus this mechanism for copper transport out of the liver is reduced also. Some of the stored copper may be released unbound to ceruloplasmin and accumulates in other tissues of the body such as brain, kidney, and cornea (Aspin and Sass-Kortsak, 1981). Wilson's disease is invariably fatal if untreated, but with the advent of chelation therapy, particularly using penicillamine, patients can be treated with some success.

Iodine

As far as is known, the role of iodine in the animal body is related solely to its function as a constituent of the thyroid hormones (triiodothyronine, T_3, and tetraiodothyronine, thyroxine, T_4). The adult body contains 10 to 20 mg iodine, of which 70 to 80 percent is concentrated in the thyroid gland. Although certain tissues (salivary glands, gastric mucosa, and lactating mammary glands) have the ability to concentrate iodine, only the thyroid is capable of synthesizing the thyroid hormones.

Dietary iodine is converted largely to iodide in the gastrointestinal tract and it is in this form that it is absorbed. Absorption is rapid and the iodide ion is distributed throughout the extracellular fluid. The iodide ion is selectively accumulated by thyroid follicular cells, apparently by an energy-dependent, active transport mechanism in the follicular cell basal membrane. Once within the thyroid gland, iodide is rapidly oxidized by iodine peroxidase to a higher oxidation state forming "active iodide," a form of inorganic iodide that readily binds to the phenolic ring of tyrosine. The tyrosine residues that are iodinated are constituents of thyroglobulin, a large (molecular weight 670,000) glycoprotein synthesized on the rough endoplasmic reticulum of the follicular cells and packaged into membrane-bound secretion granules in the Golgi apparatus. (See Chapter 14.) Iodination of tyrosine residues in the completed thyroglobulin molecule occurs at the cell-colloid interface. The products of this iodination reaction include 3-monoiodotyrosine and 3,5-diiodotyrosine, with the quantities of each determined by the amount of "active iodine" available.

The exact way in which thyroid hormones are formed from iodinated tyrosines is not known, although it presumably occurs between adjacent residues in the folded, globular thyroglobulin molecule. Coupling involves two iodinated tyrosine molecules, either monoiodotyrosine or diiodotryosine. The alanine side chain of one of the iodinated tyrosines is cleaved off and the remaining iodinated phenolic ring is joined to the other iodinated tyrosine through formation of an ether linkage (Fig. 5.2). The resultant structure is known as an iodinated thyronine, forming either 3,5,3'-triiodothyronine (T_3) or 3,5,3',5'-tetraiodothyronine (T_4, thyroxine) depending on the iodinated tyrosines used in the coupling. Only about 30 percent of the iodinated tyrosines are used to synthesize the iodinated thyronines; the

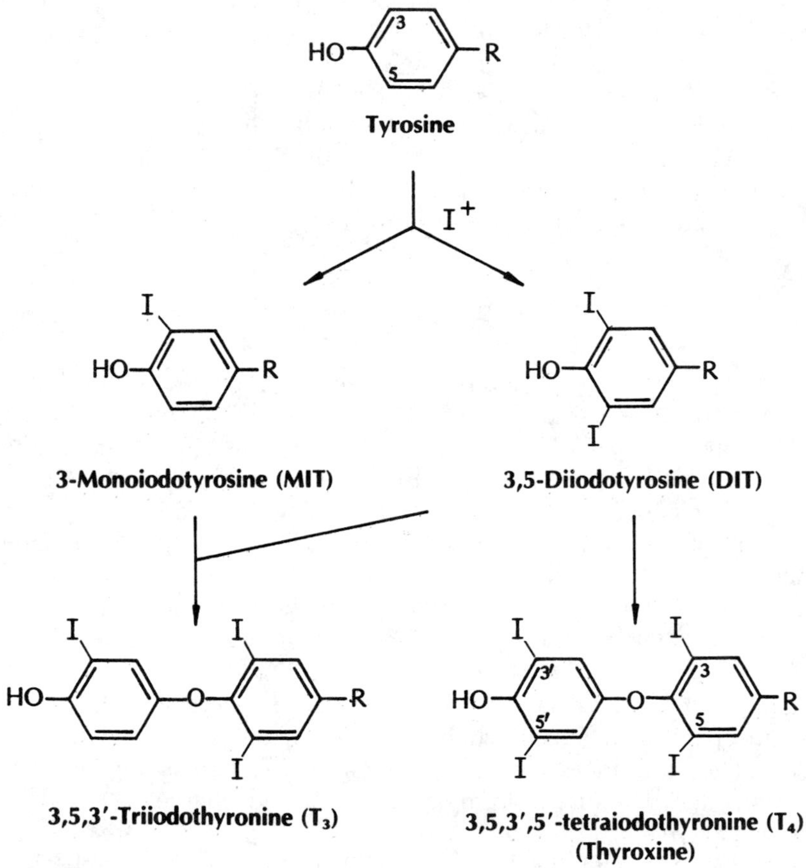

Figure 5.2
Iodinated compounds.

balance is in the form of mono- and diiodotyrosine residues in the thyroglobulin molecule. Such modified thyroglobulin molecules are stored in the lumen of the follicle in a proteinaceous fluid called the colloid.

Release of the thyroid hormones requires the proteolysis of the iodinated thyronine containing thyroglobulin. On stimulation with thyrotropin, a portion of the colloid is engulfed by endocytosis. Within the follicular cell, the colloid droplets become associated with lysosomes forming phagolysosomes. (See Chapter 14.) Hydrolysis of the thyroglobulin within the phagolysosomes releases monoiodotyrosine, diiodotyrosine, T_3, and T_4, which diffuse into the cytosol. T_3 and T_4 diffuse from the cells into the blood; mono- and diiodotyrosine are hydrolyzed to tyrosine and iodide ions by the enzyme deiodinase, found in the cytoplasm of the follicular cells. The released iodide ion can then be reoxidized and used for subsequent iodinations, thereby conserving the available iodine.

T_3 and T_4, which diffuse from the thyroid gland, are bound reversibly to three major transport proteins in human plasma. About 75 percent of thyroxine is bound to thyroxine binding α-globulin, 15 percent to prealbumin (or transthyretin according to more recent nomenclature), and 10 percent to albumin. Only a very small fraction (less than 1 percent) of the thyroxine is not protein bound, although the unbound moiety is in equilibrium with the bound fraction of each protein and likely represents that fraction able to penetrate cells. Although under normal conditions the concentration of T_4 is more than 30 times as great as that of T_3, the latter is much less firmly bound to all three protein carriers and hence has a relatively greater proportion in the unbound diffusible state. T_3 is now believed to have a major role in normal physiology. Of the circulating T_3, less than one-third is of thyroidal origin, the rest arising from peripheral deiodination principally in the liver and kidney. (See Sterling and Lazarus, 1977.) It is thought that 33 to 40 percent of the circulating T_4 is monodeiodinated to T_3; about 15 to 20 percent is changed to tetraiodothyroacetic acid and lost in urine or bile; and the remainder converted to "reverse T_3" (3',5',3-triiodothyronine), which has no biological activity and is rapidly excreted.

Although the exact mechanism by which T_3 and T_4 exert their biological effects is not known, several functions based on experimental findings have been proposed. (See Chopra, 1981.) On entering the target cells, the thyroid hormones bind to nuclear receptors and increase transcriptional and translational activity leading to increased synthesis of proteins and enzymes. It has been demonstrated also that there exists a high affinity binding site for the thyroid hormones on the inner membrane layer of the mitochondria which modulates the stimulation of oxygen consumption due to the thyroid hormones. These hormones also have been shown to influence the permeability of cell membranes in some fashion not requiring protein synthesis. It has been suggested that the thyroid hormones may stimulate the synthesis of the enzyme adenyl cyclase which may then be activated by other hormones to increase cAMP. (See Chopra, 1981.)

The hypothalamus exerts regulatory control, through release of thyrotropin-releasing hormone (TRH), over the secretion of thyrotropin from the adenohypophysis. Thyrotropin enhances uptake of iodine by the thyroid gland, synthesis of thyroglobulin, and induces the engulfment and hydrolysis of thyroglobulin in the colloid, thereby increasing the release of thyroid hormones to the blood. (See Ingbar and Woeber, 1981.) The release of thyrotropin is regulated by negative feedback inhibition by the thyroid hormones. Continued stimulation by thyrotropin causes structural changes in the follicular cells resulting in hypertrophy. Chronic stimulation may also result in hyperplasia. Enlargement of the thyroid gland due to hypertrophy or hyperplasia leads to formation of a goiter.

Simple goiter is endemic in many areas of the world and is associated most often with a deficiency of iodine. Iodine content of foods varies widely depending on the geographic origin of the food supply. Foods grown in iodine-poor soil contain little or none of the element. Very low intake of iodine reduces the synthesis of the thyroid hormones, particularly T_4, leading to a hypothyroid state. Factors other than iodine deficiency, however, can contribute to the development of simple nontoxic goiter. Certain ions (especially thiocyanate, SCN^-, and perchlorate, $HClO_3^-$) inhibit the uptake of iodide ions by the thyroid, and other compounds (termed goitrogens) inhibit iodination of tyrosines. (See Yamada et al., 1974.) These latter compounds include various drugs such as thiourea and propylthiouracil, and progoitrin, a constituent of many of the plants of the Brassicae (cabbage, Brussel sprouts, rutabaga, and turnips) which is converted enzymatically to the goitrogenic compound goitrin (5-vinyl-2-thiooxazolidone). It is doubtful that humans consume enough of any potentially goitrogenic food to seriously affect thyroid activity, but high intakes of progoitrins may accentuate the effects of low iodine intake. Goiter can also occur as a result of various biochemical defects in thyroid iodine metabolism. (See Stanbury, 1978.)

The enlargement of the thyroid gland seen in simple goiter does not seem to have adverse effects on a person other than in physical appearance. However, more severe iodine deprivation can lead to severe consequences. Children born to iodine-deficient women can develop cretinism. Such afflicted children demonstrate growth retardation, thickened coarse skin, thick lips, an enlarged tongue, and enlarged, protruding abdomen, and severe mental retardation as well as hypothermia. Hypothyroid function in an adult can lead to myxedema which is characterized by lethargy, coarse dry hair, yellowish skin, low pulse rate, and low body temperature.

MANGANESE

The adult human body contains about 20 mg manganese. The highest concentration is in bone where it is found in both inorganic salts and in the cells of the organic matrix. Pituitary, liver, kidney, pancreas, pineal gland, and lactating mammary gland also contain relatively high concentrations (about 2 to 3 $\mu g/gm$). Within the cells, manganese concentrations tend to be highest in the mitochondria.

Only a small percentage of ingested manganese is absorbed. Manganese absorption can be altered by the presence of other nutrients in the digestive tract such as high dietary concentrations of calcium, phosphorus, or iron which tend to decrease manganese absorption; alcohol may enhance uptake. (See Leach and

Lilburn, 1978.) Although the mechanism of absorption is not completely understood, it is probably absorbed as Mn^{++} and generally is proportional to dietary manganese concentration. In the portal blood, it is likely that most of the manganese binds to an α_2-macroglobulin for transport to the liver (ibid). A small proportion of the manganese is oxidized to Mn^{+++} before binding to transferrin for transport to the extrahepatic tissues. Manganese is excreted largely through the intestinal tract, primarily through the bile (Papavasiliou et al., 1966).

Manganese deficiency has been induced in a variety of animal species. Although the symptoms are somewhat specific and dependent on the severity of the deficiency, they generally include reduced growth, reproductive dysfunction, bone abnormalities, congenital ataxia, and structural defects in a number of cellular organelles. (See Underwood, 1977.) Manganese deficiency affecting a human has been reported for only one individual and was manifested by impaired blood clotting, hypocholesterolemia, slowed hair and nail growth, weight loss, and reddening of hair and beard (Doisy, 1972).

Specific biochemical roles for manganese were for many years difficult to define. There are relatively few manganese-containing metalloenzymes, although there are a considerable number of enzymes that are activated by manganese (Vallee and Coleman, 1964). Such activation of the enzymes may be relatively nonspecific for manganese, however. Two manganese-containing metalloenzymes, pyruvate carboxylase and superoxide dismutase, are found in the mitochondria. In a manganese deficiency, the activity of pyruvate carboxylase is maintained by substitution of magnesium for manganese with little change in activity; superoxide dismutase activity does decline, however. (See Leach and Lilburn, 1978.) It is likely that many of the symptoms of manganese deficiency can be related to its role in glycosaminoglycan metabolism. The ability of manganese to activate one general class of enzymes, the glycosyltransferases, appears to explain the aberrations in glycosaminoglycan metabolism that are associated with manganese deficiency (Leach, 1971).

Manganese toxicity has been reported to occur via inhalation among manganese miners and through oral ingestion of manganese contaminated drinking water. Symptoms include hypokinesia, akinesia, rigidity, tremor, and a peculiar masklike facial expression. These symptoms appear to be due to damage to the extrapyramidal system in the brain with depletion of dopamine and serotonin in the caudate nucleus. Increased susceptibility to manganese poisoning has been reported in anemic adults and in newborn and premature children, apparently due to increased intestinal absorption of manganese. (See Mena, 1981.)

MOLYBDENUM

Molybdenum is an essential trace element required for both plants and animals, although its essentiality for humans has not yet been demonstrated conclusively. As a transition element, molybdenum readily changes its oxidation state and can thus act as an electron transfer agent in oxidation-reduction reactions. Molybdenum has been identified as a constituent of several enzymes and it is likely that through these enzymes it plays its biochemical roles.

The metabolism of molybdenum is incompletely described, but it is clear that molybdate is rapidly and extensively absorbed and very rapidly excreted in the urine. The rapid elimination of excess molybdate reduces accumulation (and thus its toxicity) and appears to be the primary mechanism for maintaining homeostasis. The molybdenum retained in the body is incorporated into various metalloproteins or is stored in the form of a small, nonprotein, pterin molecule. This compound, known as the molybdenum cofactor, contains molybdenum, iron, and sulfur in the ratio of 1:8:6 and a novel, reduced, complex pterin (Rajagopalan et al., 1982). Molybdenum cofactor is bound to the mitochondrial outer membrane and can be transferred to an apoenzyme to form an active, holoenzyme (Johnson et al., 1980a). Enzymes from mammalian tissues shown to be molybdenum-dependent include xanthine oxidase, aldehyde oxidase, sulfite oxidase, and xanthine dehydrogenase. The essentiality of sulfite oxidase and xanthine oxidase activities has been demonstrated in a young child unable to synthesize the molybdenum cofactor; symptomology included displaced occular lenses and neurological abnormalities leading to early death (Johnson et al., 1980b). Human molybdenum deficiency due to insufficient dietary intake has not been demonstrated.

FLUORIDE

Fluoride is present in humans and other animals in highly variable amounts depending on the diet and water supply. It is not known if fluoride is essential to life. Studies reporting impaired growth and reproduction and lowered hematocrit (see Messer et al., 1974), could not be confirmed by Tao and Suttie (1976). The earlier work may have utilized diets that were marginal in certain nutrients, particularly iron. The beneficial effects of fluoride on dental health, however, are well documented (Ast et al., 1956).

Fluoride intake from food is variable and contents range from traces to nearly 2 mg/kg. An exception of interest to nutritionists is fish protein concentrate (FPC), which has been proposed as an inexpensive source of high quality protein. It may contain 150 to 300 mg F/kg (Zipkin et al., 1970); the addition of 10 to 15 gm of FPC in the daily diet could add 1.5 to 4.5 mg F, an amount sufficient to damage the appearance of teeth in children less than 8 years of age. Fluoride levels in drinking water can vary appreciably depending on the fluoride naturally present in water and that added through fluoridation. Fluoride can also be absorbed from the pulmonary tract when atmospheric exposure occurs (Hodge and Smith, 1977).

Fluoride is very readily absorbed (88 to 95 percent) from the gastrointestinal tract, apparently by purely physiochemical means. Ingested fluoride rapidly enters the circulating blood and is distributed through the extracellular fluid of all organs and tissues. A major site for tissue deposition of fluoride is the skeleton. The accretion of fluoride by bone seems to involve surface exchanges in which fluoride ions from the extracellular fluid exchange with hydroxyl ions in the surface layer of the hydroxyapatite crystals. Fluoride is incorporated into the inner layers of the crystal lattice as well as onto the surface of the newly formed crystals. (See Chapter 17.) Fluoride is deposited in the dental tissues during tooth mineralization as it is in bone. A large fraction of absorbed fluoride is rapidly excreted in the urine, the major pathway for excretion. Fecal and sweat excretory routes appear to be quantitatively much less important.

The beneficial effects of adequate fluoride on dental health are well documented, but incompletely understood. (See Shaw and Sweeney, 1980.) In addition, supplementation with fluoride has been shown to be helpful in increasing bone mass and reversing the osteoporotic process in some individuals with osteoporosis. Otosclerosis also has been treated with fluoride with some success (Shambaugh and Causse, 1974).

It is important also to recognize the toxic effects of fluoride. With low levels of excess fluoride intake, children may develop mottling of tooth enamel (Aasenden and Peebles, 1974). When higher concentrations are ingested, some will develop cosmetically damaging fluorosis (chalky or brown-stained enamel with intact surface or pitted, grooved, stained surface). With the chronic ingestion of large amounts of fluoride (as with industrial exposure and among individuals in parts of India and China with high natural fluoride levels in water), osteofluorosis can develop (Johnson, 1965). This condition may involve hypermineralization of the pelvic vertebrae, osteoporosis of the cortex of bone, osteomalacia with wide uncalcified osteoid seams, and the presence of new bone tissue, including streamers of woven bone and tendon bone. In extremely high dosages (5 to 10 gm NaF), fluoride can be lethal. (See National Research Council, 1971.)

SELENIUM

Selenium, the element once considered to be of biological importance solely because of its toxic properties, is now recognized as one of the essential trace elements for mammals (including humans), birds, and several bacteria. Evidence for the essentiality of selenium was provided initially by Schwarz and Foltz (1957) who demonstrated that liver necrosis in vitamin E-deficient rats could be prevented by selenium. Several diseases among livestock were subsequently reported to be responsive to selenium and vitamin E; these included exudative diathesis in poultry, mulberry heart in swine, and white muscle disease in lambs and calves. (See Underwood, 1977.) The essentiality of selenium apart from its role in vitamin E metabolism was demonstrated by Thompson and Scott (1969) who found that selenium prevented pancreatic degeneration in chicks fed vitamin E-adequate diets. (See Chapter 4.) McCoy and Weswig (1969) reported that offspring of selenium-deficient animals fed adequate vitamin E grew slowly, and failed to reproduce.

Evidence for the essentiality of selenium for humans has been less readily obtained, perhaps because selenium deficiency does not appear to occur with any great frequency in most populations. Even among those populations exposed to extremely low levels of selenium in the environment, such as New Zealanders, the consequences of low selenium status on health are not readily apparent

(Thomson and Robinson, 1980). If individuals are severely depleted of selenium, however, manifestations of the deficiency syndrome may occur. A selenium-responsive syndrome involving pain in the thigh muscles was reported in a patient on total parenteral nutrition; 100 μg Se as selenomethionine for 1 week as the sole treatment corrected the symptoms (Van Rij et al., 1979). Keshan disease, a cardiomyopathy that affects children who live in a region of China where selenium levels are low, was virtually eliminated after selenium supplementation (Keshan Disease Research Group, 1979). A cardiomyopathy syndrome linked to selenium deficiency also was reported in a patient undergoing long-term total parenteral alimentation (Johnson et al., 1981). Although selenium-responsive symptoms appear to be manifest only in the severely depleted individual, considerable interest in selenium has been generated by reports of an interaction between suboptimal selenium status and cancer (Schrauzer, 1976) and cardiovascular disease (Frost and Lish, 1975). It will require a considerable amount of research to establish these relationships, if they do exist.

Animals have mechanisms to maintain selenium homeostasis, if intakes are not excessive. The level of control does not appear to be at the absorptive step as there is no evidence of altered rates of absorption in response to deficient or toxic states. True intestinal absorption of selenium in food was estimated at approximately 80 percent in young women given tracer doses of radioactive selenium or selenomethionine (Stewart et al., 1978). The level of selenium absorbed from the diet can be influenced by other dietary factors such as the solubility of the selenium compound and the level of sulfur in the diet. Selenium homeostasis appears to be accomplished by production of excretory metabolites. Urinary selenium excretion is markedly higher than fecal excretion (Levander et al., 1981); the major urinary metabolite is trimethylselenonium ion. Very high intakes of selenium may be associated with the production of dimethylselenide which is excreted from the lung as a volatile compound.

A clear role for selenium in mammalian and avian tissues has been shown by the demonstration that glutathione peroxidase is a selenometalloenzyme. Glutathione peroxidase, an enzyme with a molecular weight of 80,000, is composed of four identical subunits with a molecule of selenocysteine incorporated into the peptide chain of each subunit (Sunde and Hoekstra, 1980). This enzyme appears to function by reducing organic and inorganic hydroperoxides. Various prooxidant compounds including hydrogen peroxide, hydroperoxides, superoxide, and hydroxy radicals can occur in cells as a result of normal cellular functions or from the metabolism of toxic substances. Depending on the origin and target of these prooxidants, various antioxidants are needed to protect the cells. Thus, lipid-soluble vitamin E scavenges free radicals in membranes, glutathione peroxidase reacts with peroxides in the cytosol and superoxide dismutase with superoxide in the mitochondrial matrix space, and catalase destroys hydrogen peroxide in the peroxisomes (ibid.). Some of the interrelationships between selenium and vitamin E may be based on such an interactive system of protection against peroxidative damage.

Other selenium-containing proteins have been reported in addition to gluta-thione peroxidase. Selenium-deficient lambs suffering from nutritional muscular dystrophy apparently fail to synthesize a selenium-containing protein found in the muscle of selenium-adequate lambs (Black et al, 1978). The function of this protein has not yet been elucidated. There are reports also of an uncharacterized 15,000 to 20,000 molecular weight selenoprotein in spermatozoa, but again, no function has yet been ascribed to it (McConnell et al., 1979).

For a review of the biological activity of selenium, see Burks (1983).

In greater than trace amounts, selenium is toxic to animals. Selenium poisoning in animals has been known since the middle of the nineteenth century, but it was not until the 1930s that the disease was recognized as the result of high concen-tration of selenium in soils. "Blind staggers" disease, seen in animals consuming limited amounts of plants that accumulate selenium, may be due in part to the alkaloids derived from the plant. Afflicted animals wander aimlessly, stumble, have impaired vision, and some signs of respiratory failure. "Alkali disease" is due to ingestion of feeds containing 5 to 40 ppm Se for weeks or months. Man-ifestations include lameness, hoof malformations in cattle and horses, loss of body hair, and emaciation. Acute intoxication occurs when grazing animals eat enough selenium accumulator plants or when accidental poisoning occurs with admin-istration of selenium supplements. This toxicosis appears as labored breathing, ataxia, abnormal posture, prostration, diarrhea, coma, and death. Recommen-dations of selenium intakes range from 0.1 to 0.3 μg/gm of dry matter and toxic dietary levels are about 10 to 50 times greater. (See National Research Council, 1980.)

ZINC

The total amount of zinc in the human body has been estimated to be between 2 and 3 gm. Zinc is found in all human tissues, varying from 1 to 60 μg/gm wet weight. Levels are remarkably higher than this for tissues of the male reproductive tract (90 μg/gm for normal human prostate).

Parakeratosis, a naturally occurring disease of pigs and cattle, has been shown to be due to zinc deficiency. High levels of calcium accentuate the development and the severity of the disease. This antagonistic action of calcium appears to be mediated primarily through a reduction in zinc absorption (Forbes, 1960).

In rats, zinc deficiency is characterized by growth failure, testicular atrophy, decreased size of the accessory sex glands, and dermatitis and keratinization of epithelial tissues. Delayed healing of experimental wounds has been observed in the zinc-deficient rat (Sandstead et al., 1970).

Growth retardation associated with reduction of voluntary food intake, the appearance of parakeratotic skin and esophageal lesions, and hair loss are symp-toms of zinc deficiency that are common to most species. Reproductive perfor-mance also has been shown to be seriously impaired as a result of zinc deficiency. (See Underwood, 1977.) In the young, there is a lack of sexual development and in the adult, there is aspermatogenesis and loss of libido in the male and loss of estrus cycle in the female. Zinc deficiency during gestation results in difficulties in parturition and the presence of various birth defects in the offspring. Other symptoms include hypogeusia, impaired wound healing, and disorders of bone development (ibid.).

Zinc deficiency in humans was first described by Prasad et al. (1963) in areas of the Middle East where the diet consisted chiefly of cereals with little or no animal protein. The syndrome is similar to that seen in experimental animals: severe growth retardation resulting in dwarfism, hypogonadism, and low levels of zinc in plasma and red blood cells. Treatment with zinc resulted in improved growth and sexual development and a return of zinc blood levels to normal. More recently, hypogeusia (decreased taste acuity) has been shown to be a consequence of zinc deficiency (Henkin et al., 1971). Marginal zinc deficiency in a group of children in the United States has been reported (Hambridge et al., 1972). The symptoms were poor appetite, poor growth, hypogeusia, and low levels of zinc in the hair; all symptoms were improved by zinc therapy. The observation that wound healing in man can be accelerated by treatment with zinc sulfate (Pories et al., 1967) further suggests that marginal zinc deficiencies may not be uncommon.

Some studies have revealed evidence of zinc deficiency among infants, children, adolescents, pregnant women, and the elderly in the United States and elsewhere. (See Sandstead, 1981.) In addition, a heightened incidence of the deficient state has been observed among individuals with a variety of clinical problems including alcoholism with Laennec's cirrhosis, inflammatory bowel disease and malabsorption, renal disease, and hemolytic anemia (Sandstead et al., 1976).

The mechanism for zinc absorption across the gastrointestinal mucosa is incompletely characterized. (See Chapter 6.) Absorption appears to be responsive to zinc status and is in excess of 90 percent in deficient animals; in animals with adequate zinc status, absorption typically ranges about 25 percent. With exposure to zinc in the atmosphere, absorption can occur through the alveolocapillary membrane or across the epithelial membrane of the skin. (See National Research Council, 1980.)

Once zinc enters the body, it is bound to albumin or to amino acids (a much smaller fraction) for transport to the liver. About two-thirds of the zinc found in the peripheral circulation is bound loosely to albumin, approximately another third is firmly complexed with α_2-macroglobulin, and a small portion is bound to amino acids. Zinc that is bound to albumin and amino acids is readily taken up by tissues.

The primary route for zinc excretion is the gastrointestinal tract. Endogenous zinc enters the intestinal lumen as a constituent of metalloproteins secreted by the intestinal mucosa and the pancreas, by the catabolism of desquamated intestinal mucosal cells, and by direct passage across the mucosa involving an unidentified mechanism. Lesser amounts are excreted in the urine and sweat.

The various roles for zinc within the body have not been completely identified but much of the zinc is incorporated into a large number of zinc-requiring enzymes. The zinc enzymes have been divided into two groups based on their affinity for zinc; zinc-enzyme complexes and zinc metalloenzymes. Within the enzyme, zinc may be involved in the catalytic process, may function to stabilize the structure of the protein, or both. Other functions that have been proposed for zinc include roles in cell replication, in the expression of genetic information, and in the stabilization of biological molecules other than enzymes. (See Chesters, 1978.) It is not possible to ascribe all the biological functions of zinc to any single role or to relate all the deficiency symptoms to the decrease in activity of one or several enzymes.

A genetic disorder in humans, acrodermatitis enteropathica, resulting in alterations in zinc metabolism has been reported. (See Walravens et al., 1978.) The disease is transmitted by an autosomal recessive gene and is characterized by severe dermatitis, loss of body hair, diarrhea, irritability, failure to thrive, infections, and death. Symptoms usually appear after weaning from breast milk and are likely due to a severe zinc deficiency as a consequence of impaired ability to absorb dietary zinc. As the symptoms do not appear while the child is receiving human milk, there appears to be a factor in the milk which facilitates zinc absorption. The nature of this factor continues to be a source of controversy. Evans and Johnson (1976) believe that the factor is picolinic acid, but Hurley and associates (Eckhert et al., 1977) believe that citrate is the factor. It is possible, however, to supply sufficient zinc for the child by supplementation; the levels required, however, are much greater than normal requirements for zinc. (See Walravens et al., 1978.)

CHROMIUM

Studies by Schwarz and Mertz (1959), investigating glucose intolerance in rats fed a Torula yeast diet, led to the identification of chromium (Cr^{+++}) as a factor essential for normal glucose tolerance. The essentiality of chromium was subsequently demonstrated by Schroeder (1966) who induced a severe deficiency in rats and noted fasting hyperglycemia, glycosuria, and impaired growth.

Most inorganic, trivalent chromium compounds are absorbed with an efficiency of less than 1 percent. In contrast, 10 to 25 percent of chromium from organic chromium complexes extracted from Brewer's yeast may be absorbed (Mertz and Roginski, 1971). Once absorbed, some of the inorganic chromium may pass to the liver and be incorporated into an organic chromium complex known as *glucose tolerance factor*. The exact structure of glucose tolerance factor is not known, although it appears to be a tetraaquodinicotinatochromium (III) complex which contains nicotinic acid and is stabilized by the binding of several amino acids (Mertz et al., 1974). It is likely, although not yet proven, that this factor forms a ternary complex with insulin and insulin receptor sites thus potentiating the action of insulin *in vivo*. Chromium is present in relatively high concentrations in the fetus and newborn, but it appears that chromium can only cross the placenta in the form of glucose tolerance factor.

Excretion of chromium from the body is primarily in the urine (90 to 95 percent of endogenous loss); fecal losses contain predominantly nonabsorbed chromium. Urinary chromium excretion in adults is now thought to be less than 1 μg/day (Guthrie et al., 1978) and it thus appears that the requirement for intestinal absorption of chromium is approximately 1 μg/day to achieve chromium balance.

The earliest known effect of a chromium deficiency is an impairment of glucose tolerance. A more severe degree of deficiency in animals results in hyperglycemia, glycosuria, impaired growth rates, corneal lesions, increased mortality, and decreased longevity. There is one well-documented report of severe chromium deficiency in a woman maintained on total parenteral nutrition for 3½ years (Jeejeebhoy et al., 1977). This deficiency was characterized by glucose intolerance, an inability to utilize glucose for energy, and neuropathy in the presence of normal insulin levels. Another study suggests that chromium deficiency is associated with increased plasma cholesterol and total lipids accompanied by hyperinsulinemia (Offenbacher and Pi-Sunyer, 1980). The consequences of marginal or moderate chromium deficiency on human health are not well understood. Chromium status may play a role in the development of maturity-onset diabetes and may also influence the development of ischemic heart disease by way of its role in the normalization of insulin levels. (See Mertz, 1979.)

NICKEL, SILICON, TIN, AND VANADIUM

Evidence for the essentiality of many of the trace elements for humans is often difficult to obtain directly. Essentiality can be predicted from evidence obtained from other mammalian species and from identification of given elements as part of normal human enzyme systems. Nickel and silicon are trace elements whose essentiality for a mammalian species has been demonstrated; a requirement has not yet been demonstrated in humans. The essentiality of tin and vanadium as well as arsenic has not been conclusively proven, although there is some evidence for essential roles. (See Nielsen, 1980.) Deficiencies of these trace elements have only been produced in experimental animals under carefully controlled conditions.

Nickel appears to have a role in maintaining the structure of nucleic acids and membranes and in lipid metabolism. Nielsen and Sandstead (1974) suggested, by extrapolation from animal data, that the dietary requirement for adults is about 0.05 to 0.08 μg/gm diet (about 30 μg/day); daily intakes are generally 100 to 200 μg with highest concentrations of nickel being in foods of plant origin (Myron et al., 1978).

A number of investigators have reported adverse effects of feeding vanadium-deficient diets; unfortunately there has been considerable inconsistency in the reported symptomology. Vanadium appears to have a role in lipid metabolism, but again the lack of consistency in experimental findings does not allow a clear understanding of that role. (See Nielsen, 1980.)

Silicon is essential for the normal growth of the chick. It is involved in the formation of cartilage, bone, and other connective tissues and is localized in the mucopolysaccharide fraction (Carlisle, 1974; 1982). Silicon is plentiful and ubiquitous in the environment and it is unlikely that a human deficiency would arise under normal conditions.

WATER

Water is by far the most critical of all nutrients. Animals will succumb to water deprivation sooner than to starvation. Water is an essential component of all cell structures and is the medium in which all the chemical reactions of cellular metabolism take place. Just as the life of the one-celled organism depends on contact with its watery environment for sustenance, the cells of higher organisms are dependent on the aqueous medium within and surrounding cell structures.

The water available to the animal body includes that present in liquids and solid food consumed, and water formed in the cells as a result of the oxidation of foodstuffs. This endogenous water is designated *metabolic water* or *water of oxidation*. Metabolic water amounts to roughly 15 percent of the daily total water available from an ordinary intake of food and drink. The water of oxidation has been computed for the major foodstuffs by Newburgh et al. (1930) and Peters et al. (1933). The figures vary slightly for carbohydrate and protein, as shown below.

Foodstuff (100 gm)	Water of Oxidation (gm)	
	Newburgh	Peters
Protein	41	40
Carbohydrate	60	56
Fat	107	107

The total amount of water available to the body thus may be calculated when the composition of the diet as well as the consumption of water and other beverages are known. Accurate determination of water balance, for example, must include the metabolic water. The data shown in Table 5.2 illustrate a typical water balance.

The animal body contains more water than any other compound. Approximately 70 percent of the fat-free body is water. Water is compatible with more substances

TABLE 5.2
Typical Daily Water Balance—Average-sized, Normal Adult Male

Water Intake	Grams	Water Output	Grams	
Drinking water	400	Skin	500	
Water in other beverages	580	Expired air	350	
Preformed water in solid foods	720	Urine	1100	
Metabolic water	320	Feces	150	
Total	2020	Total	2100	Balance = −80 gm

Source: J. M. Orten and O. W. Neuhaus *Human Biochemistry*, 10th ed., C. V. Mosby Co., St. Louis, 1982, p. 526.

than any other known solvent, and therefore it is an ideal medium for transporting nutrients to the cells and for the chemical reactions of cellular metabolism to take place. Its role, however, is more than that of a passive reaction medium; in hydrolytic and hydration reactions, water is an active participant in body metabolism.

The regulation of body temperature is dependent partially on the high conductivity property of water to distribute heat evenly within the body and eventually to remove by vaporization the excess heat released by metabolic reactions within the cells. (As environmental temperature decreases, radiation and conduction are more important means of disposing of body heat.) Drastic changes in body temperature, moreover, are prevented by other properties of water: high specific heat and high latent heat of vaporization. In other words, more heat is required to change water from liquid to vapor or liquid to solid than almost any other substance. These properties alone establish water as a superior medium for metabolic activity. Sudden and violent changes in temperature obviously would disrupt the enzymatic machinery of the animal cell.

Excessive water loss from the body, as in profuse sweating, diarrhea, or prolonged episodes of vomiting, results in dehydration and in loss of electrolytes. The danger of replenishing the body water without concurrent repletion of electrolytes leads to water intoxication and has been discussed in the section on sodium. Body water distribution and compartments are discussed in Chapters 7 and 22.

part two

physiological aspects of nutrition

The integration of biological mechanisms and the arbitrary divisions between branches of the biological sciences are well illustrated by the chapter title. Nutritionists refer to the physiological aspects of nutrition; physiologists to the nutritional aspects of physiology, and biochemists to the nutritional or physiological aspects of biochemistry. Each, however, is concerned with the biochemical activity in the physiological process of digestion through which nutrients are released and converted to forms capable of passing through a membrane. Understanding the details of the actual process of membrane transport calls for the talents of the biophysicist. The simpler the organism, the fewer the membranes or barriers to be crossed before entering cellular metabolism. In the complex organism, the first barrier is the intestinal mucosal membrane that is, in reality, the lumenal surface of each cell in the convoluted sheet of epithelium lining the tract. The accepted nutrients must then leave the cell, enter the extracellular fluid, the transport system and, eventually, leave the capillaries to enter the external environment, or the fluid, surrounding each of the individual cells throughout the body. It is at this point that the nutrients function and, depending on perspective, come within the purview and, hence, the domain of the cell physiologist, geneticist, molecular biologist, biophysicist, biochemist, and nutritionist. Such convergence of interest has led to the enormous acceleration of activity in this area of investigation in recent years. It is inevitable that progress toward an understanding of the common denominator should be the cooperative achievement of such a spectrum of scientific disciplines. The divisions of science, like the joinings and juxtapositions of a mosaic, are a means to an end and should not be permitted to detract from the unity of the image. If it is recognized that there is a broad spectrum of knowledge that sometimes can be examined only in segments, then we can proceed with what might otherwise have been considered a parochial view: the physiological aspects of nutrition.

In order to discuss the activities of the gastrointestinal tract in the preparation of food for absorption into the body, one must assume that it is taken into the mouth, however eagerly or reluctantly. However, admission of food to the gastrointestinal tract, the obvious first step, does not assure admission to the body. Despite the activities of the tract in the breakdown of the complex foodstuffs, they are still "outside." Only after each of the individual nutrients breaches the barrier of the intestinal mucosa are they "in." Absorption, then, is the final and crucial hurdle. After that hurdle is passed, what were the foods become the nutrients en route to their site of action: the cells.

All cells depend on their external environment for their supply of nutrients. In a complex organism only those cells forming the mucosa of the gastrointestinal tract are in direct contact with the essential nutrients available in the external environment. It becomes obligatory, therefore, for these mucosal cells to take in all the nutrients essential not only for their own metabolism, but also for that of the whole organism. The mucosal cells are uniquely adapted to perform this primary function: transporting from the external environment (lumen of the tract) to the internal environment (extracellular fluid) the nutrients essential for all of the cells that comprise the total organism. As a corollary to this function, the cells also can exert control over the quantities of certain nutrients absorbed, such as iron, an excess of which leads to physiological embarrassment. Unfortunately, this capacity for exclusion does not extend to surplus energy-yielding nutrients that may also lead to embarrassment.

Disorders of nutrition may be due to failure at any step: inadequate intake, impaired digestion, or inefficient absorption. Despite seemingly adequate intake, psychomotor effects on motility of the gastrointestinal tract may so rush the passage of foods that breakdown and absorption cannot take place; genetic error may interfere with synthesis of enzymes or accessory factors essential to digestion or absorption; parasitic infestation, a fortuitous nutritional arrangement for the parasite, may prove rather less fortunate for the deprived host.

chapter 6

digestion and absorption

Gastrointestinal Hormones

Early studies on the motility and secretory activity of the gastrointestinal tract indicated that control was not only by the autonomic nervous system but also by a series of gastrointestinal hormones whose release is stimulated when specific hormones reach particular loci in the tract. Hormones were originally identified by four primary actions (Table 6.1). When it became apparent that the activities ascribed to cholecystokinin (CCK) and to pancreozymin could not be separated and were performed by a single substance, Grossman (1970) proposed that the

TABLE 6.1
Identifying Actions of Gastrointestinal Hormones

Hormone	Action	Reference
Secretin	Stimulates secretion of HCO_3 and H_2O	Bayless and Starling, 1902
Gastrin	Stimulates gastric secretion of acid	Edkins, 1906
Cholecystokinin (CCK)	Contracts gallbladder	Ivy and Oldberg, 1928
Pancreozymin (PZ)	Stimulates pancreatic secretion of enzymes	Harper and Raper, 1943

hormone performing both functions be called cholecystokinin since it was discovered first. The identifying and the additional physiological actions of the three originally purified hormones, secretin, gastrin, and cholecystokinin, are shown in Table 6.2 (Grossman, 1977). Gastric inhibitory peptide (GIP) which also meets the criteria set for a hormone exerting physiological rather than pharmacological events is also shown.

Rapid advances in identifying and localizing other peptides that regulate gastrointestinal function soon showed that the term "gastrointestinal hormone" was too restrictive since the regulatory substances were not solely gastrointestinal in origin nor were they all hormones. In fact, it became increasingly clear that the so-called gastrointestinal hormones were part of a much broader group of regulatory secretions and, further, that the same or similar peptides were produced by cells in the brain as well as in the gut (Grossman, 1979). These peptide secretions function as *endocrine* (circulated by the blood to reach and affect a distant target cell), *paracrine* (diffused through extracellular fluid to influence neighboring cells), and/or *neurocrine* agents (delivered by a neuron across a short synaptic gap to a target cell). Grossman (1970) suggested that the term "regulator cells" be used to designate the neural, endocrine, and paracrine cells as a group and that the chemical messengers they produce be called "regulins."

Table 6.3 presents a list of 20 identified peptides of the alimentary tract and pancreas. More than half of the listed peptides have been sequenced, and the others either partially sequenced or identified by immunoreactivity. Though the list of peptide hormones grows, progress in identifying physiological function is difficult because the source of a secretion is not confined to a single discrete locus but rather to specific cell types scattered throughout the tract. As a result, the physiological roles of many of the identified peptides have yet to be found.

The classic studies by Pavlov (1910) demonstrated nervous control of gut function; those of Bayless and Starling (1902) demonstrated control by chemical messengers or hormones. Both have led to lines of research revealing a complex pattern of gastrointestinal responses to normal physiological stimuli. However, the pattern has become extremely intricate and still is largely obscure.

The list of peptides common to the gastrointestinal tract and the brain continues to grow. Physiological function for some of these peptides has been established

TABLE 6.2
Major Gastrointestinal Hormones

Hormone	Number of Amino Acid Residues	Hormone Family	Region Where Found	Action
Gastrin	17 or 34	Gastrin	Antral and duodenal mucosa	Stimulates HCl release by stomach, and pancreatic enzyme secretion. Increases motor activity in intestine.
Secretin	27	Secretin	Duodenal and jejunal mucosa	Stimulates pancreatic bicarbonate and water secretion, and gastric pepsin secretion. Augments action of CCK on pancreatic enzymes. Inhibits gastric acid secretion and smooth muscle contraction in GI tract.
Cholecystokinin[a] (CCK)	33 or 39	Gastrin	Jejunal, duodenal, and ileal mucosa	Stimulates pepsin secretion, gall-bladder contraction, and pancreatic enzyme secretion. Some inhibition of stomach emptying.
Gastric inhibitory peptide (GIP)	43	Secretin	Endocrine cells of duodenum and jejunum	Inhibits stomach acid secretion. Stimulates insulin release from pancreas, and intestinal mucosa secretion.

Source: Tabulated from material presented by McGuigan (1978) and Williams (1981).

[a]Also known as cholecystokinin–pancreozymin (CCK–PZ)

TABLE 6.3
Peptides of the Alimentary Tract and Pancreas

Sequenced peptides	Partially sequenced peptides
Cholecystokinin	Chymodenin
Gastrin	Glicentin
Gastric inhibitory peptide (GIP)	Gastrozymin
Glucagon	PI-HIA-27
Insulin	
Motilin	**Immunoreactivities**
Neurotensin	
Pancreatic polypeptide	Bombesin-like
Secretin	Enkephalin-like
Substance P	Somatostatin-like
Urogastrone	Thyrotropin-releasing-hormone-like
Vasoactive intestinal peptide (VIP)	

in the gut but their roles in the brain are, for the most part, just beginning to be revealed. CCK appears to affect the regulation of feeding behavior. Strauss and Yalow (1979) found a strikingly lower content of CCK in cerebral cortex of genetically obese hyperphagic mice compared with their lean littermates and other normal mice. Similarly, when CCK activity was blocked by injection of antibody to CCK in sheep, food intake was increased by 100 percent. However, when CCK was administered directly into the cerebral ventricles of sheep, there was a sharp decrease in food intake (Della-Fera and Baile, 1979; 1981). It appears, therefore, that an inverse relationship exists between the amount of CCK in the cerebral cortex and the amount of food consumed. The possibilities for the exploitation of such findings are frightening.

Intracranial injections of gastrin increase gastric acid secretion in rats by acting on the hypothalamus as well as on the stomach (Tepperman and Evered, 1980). Since this action does not occur following intravenous injection, it appears that gastrin endogenous to the hypothalamus may act as a neurohormone or neurotransmitter in the neural control of gastrointestinal function. Gastrin also has been shown to stimulate RNA, DNA, and protein synthesis along almost the entire length of the gut, excluding only the esophagus and antrum, thereby participating in the rapid proliferation of intestinal mucosa (Enochs and Johnson, 1977). Each tissue subject to the trophic effect of gastrin also has been shown to secrete a hormone or peptide that inhibits gastrin release, indicating tight control of gastrin secretion.

Somatostatin, initially extracted from the hypothalamus and found to inhibit growth hormone release, also has wide distribution in the gut. Pimstone et al. (1979) reported that the circulating levels of somatostatin vary widely with ingestion of food. They concluded that somatostatin might participate in the regulation of food intake and also play a hormonal role in nutrient homeostasis within the gastrointestinal portal system. Feeding behavior and the factors that affect it have been the subject of intense study for many years. Only now are there some specifics emerging concerning biochemical mechanisms.

For detailed discussion of gastrointestinal hormones, see Grossman et al. (1977); Bloom (1978); Glass (1980); Walsh (1981). For an interesting and humbling theory that relates hormones and neurotransmitters of vertebrates to each other and to their origin in unicellular organisms, see Roth et al. (1982).

Digestion

CARBOHYDRATES

Some polysaccharides such as the celluloses, hemicelluloses, and pectins are completely indigestible and are the major components of dietary fiber. Inulin, galactogens, mannosans, and raffinose that occur in certain fruits and vegetables are partially digested to monosaccharides.

The only polysaccharides in food that are digested to any degree by humans are the starches that are glucose polymers. They must be broken down into monosaccharides, the molecules suitable for passage through the intestinal mucosal cells. This process of digestion could start in the mouth since a salivary amylase is secreted that can hydrolyze cooked starch to maltose *in vitro;* its efficacy *in vivo*, however, depends on the degree of mixing with saliva and on the amount of time that the enzyme remains in contact with the substrate. Generally, eating habits permit too short a time for enzyme-substrate interaction and activity is, therefore, insignificant. After the food reaches the stomach further amylase activity depends on the time it takes for the pH to be brought below the 6.6–6.8 range, which is optimum for amylase. Davenport (1971) suggests that up to 50 percent of the starch may be broken down depending on the rate of gastric mixing and emptying time.

No carbohydrate-digesting enzymes are secreted into the gastric juice. Theoretically there is a possibility of some acid hydrolysis of sucrose taking place in the stomach but it is probably negligible (Dahlqvist and Borgström, 1961). Therefore, no further digestion of carbohydrate takes place until the stomach contents, or *chyme,* enter the duodenum.

The major carbohydrate-digesting enzyme, α-amylase, is secreted with the pancreatic juice and is effective on raw as well as cooked starch. It hydrolyzes the α-1,4 glycosidic bonds. If the starches are unbranched, the end products are maltose and maltotriose; but if the starches are branched, there will be, in addition, a mixture of dextrins averaging six glucose residues per molecule containing the 1,6 linkages. Through the complimentary action of α-dextrinase (isomaltase) and sucrase, single glucose units are removed sequentially from the α-dextrins (Gray et al., 1979). A striking adaptation in pancreatic enzyme activity has been shown to occur with long-term alterations in the diet. In Desnuelle's laboratory (Marchis-Mouren et al., 1963) an eight-to tenfold increase in rate of amylase synthesis has been shown to occur in rats with a diet high in carbohydrate compared with a diet high in protein. At the same time, there was a two- to threefold decrease in the rate of synthesis of chymotrypsinogen, a protease precursor.

No further hydrolysis of carbohydrate takes place in the intestinal lumen since the disaccharidases (see Table 6.4) responsible for the final hydrolysis are located in the outer protein coat of the membrane of the intestinal mucosal cells (Miller and Crane, 1961a; 1961b; Eichholz and Crane, 1965; Overton et al., 1965). The development of disaccharidase activity within the villus cells as they migrate up toward the tip was demonstrated by Dahlqvist (1967) and the higher enzyme activity was observed in the region of the villi where the most active absorption of monosaccharides occurred.

Although the detection in the intestinal lumen of monosaccharides or the various enzymes responsible for the final stages of hydrolysis has been cited as evidence of lumenal digestion, the presence of these enzymes can be explained. Either the membrane-bound enzyme may be at the outermost edge of the intestinal coat permitting hydrolysis while the disaccharides are still in the lumen, or desquamation of mucosal cells from the tip of the villi contributes the membrane-bound enzymes to the lumenal contents. According to Ugolev (1965), hydrolysis on the external surface of the cell, or membrane digestion, is midway between digestion and absorption and ensures absorption at the final stages of hydrolysis. This is brought about by the intestinal enzymes present in or on the brush borders of the cells themselves. Thus, the digestion taking place in the lumen and in the membrane are interacting mechanisms that provide optimum conditions for absorption. Ugolev (1974) suggests a three-link system: hydrolysis in the lumen—membrane digestion—absorption. This relationship is depicted in Fig. 6.1. A schematic representation of a section of brush border, according to Gray (1981), is shown in Fig. 6.2. A disaccharidase, though an integral part of the membrane, has its glycoprotein active site readily available to substrate in the lumen. Also in the membrane and close by is the transport protein that accepts the released monosaccharides for transit into the cell (see below). Membrane digestion takes place not only for the final hydrolysis of carbohydrates but also for the lipids and proteins to be discussed subsequently.

A disaccharidase deficiency prevents the final hydrolysis of carbohydrate prior to its absorption and produces a condition of disaccharide intolerance (Dahlqvist, 1962). Accumulation of disaccharides in the lumen is associated with diarrhea, flatulence, nausea, and a sense of fullness—partly due to the osmotic activity of the disaccharides and partly due to bacterial fermentation. Any condition that produces damage to the mucosa by preventing the rapid proliferation of cells, such as occurs in protein-energy malnutrition or celiac disease (Plotkin and Isselbacher, 1964), is associated with enzyme deficiency.

The most widespread disaccharidase deficiency was attributed to a defect in the synthesis of lactase (Holzel et al., 1959). The consequent lactose intolerance was observed in 30 percent of apparently healthy white adults (Friedland, 1965; Newcomer and McGill, 1966) and 80 percent of nonwhite subjects (Bayless and Rosensweig, 1966). On the assumption that continuance of lactase synthesis was

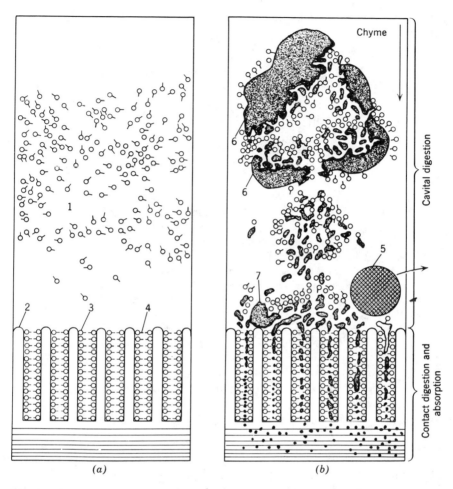

Figure 6.1
Detailed diagram of relation between cavital and membrane digestion in the intestinal cavity in the presence (a) and absence (b) of foodstuff. (1) Enzymes in intestinal cavity (distributed chaotically); (2) microvilli; (3) enzymes on surface of microvilli (strictly orientated); (4) pores of brush border; (5) microbes not penetrating brush border; (6,7) food substances at various stages of hydrolysis. (From A.M. Ugolev, *Physiol. Rev.* 45:557, 1965.)

normal for the human adult, lactase deficiency was attributed either to a genetic defect (Huang and Bayless, 1968) or to a regression of enzyme activity in a postweaning diet low in lactose (Bolin et al., 1969). Since, worldwide, more people are lactose intolerant than tolerant, and since a rapid rise in lactase activity just prior to birth and its regression as part of the normal growth pattern is observed in all mammals studied (Deren, 1968), it is evident that tolerance is the more unusual situation. It was then suggested that lactase is an adaptive enzyme and

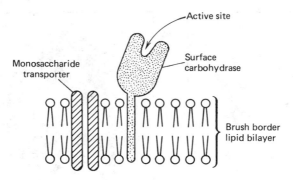

Figure 6.2
Schematic representation of association of integral carbohydrases and monosaccharide carriers with the brush border surface membrane. The hydrolases are anchored by means of a hydrophobic segment but the bulk of the glycoprotein is exterior to the bilayer so that its active site is readily available to oligosaccharide substrates in the intestinal lumen. In contrast, the monosaccharide transporters are probably highly hydrophobic and completely imbedded in the membrane. A hydrophylic interior may serve as the route of transfer for the polar monosaccharide. (From G. M. Gray, *Physiology of the Gastrointestinal Tract,* Vol. 2, L. R. Johnson, ed., Raven Press, New York, 1981, p. 1064.)

that tolerance is the result of the continued presence of milk in the adult diet (Cuatrecasas et al., 1965). No apparent correlation, however, could be demonstrated between milk consumption and lactose intolerance (Nandi and Parham, 1972; Gilat et al., 1972). It now appears likely that the development of lactose-tolerant population groups resulted from a genetic mutation inherited as a dominant characteristic. The dominance of the trait explains the increased lactose tolerance in mixed population groups (Ransome-Kuti et al., 1975). For an interesting presentation of the historical and geographical selection involved in the development of lactose-tolerant population groups, see Simoons (1981).

The prevalence of lactose malabsorption in older children and adults in the majority of the human species brought into question the use in many countries of large-scale supplementary feeding of whole or skim milk powder. This prompted the publication of a United Nations report (Protein Advisory Group, 1972) alerting authorities to the problem and suggesting that milk, when used, be introduced gradually.

The tests first used to detect lactose intolerance involved the administration of

50 gm of lactose, an amount approximating the lactose content of one liter of milk. It was shown by Bell et al. (1973) that Eskimo adults and children with a high incidence of lactose intolerance to the test dose could consume one cup of milk without adverse effects. Other studies confirmed that individuals with positive tests for lactose intolerance can consume nutritionally useful quantities of milk without developing symptoms (Stephenson and Latham, 1974; Woteki et al., 1976). The Committee on Nutrition of the American Academy of Pediatrics (1978) recommended that it would be inappropriate to discourage milk-feeding programs targeted at children on the basis of lactose intolerance, and that milk consumption should not be discouraged unless it caused severe diarrhea. Paige et al. (1975) found a significant improvement in absorption when lactose-hydrolyzed milk was fed to lactose-intolerant individuals and recommended prehydrolyzed milk for high-risk populations.

A variety of tests other than the lactose tolerance test have been devised for investigation of lactase deficiency. The test showing the greatest promise, especially for field screening, is the hydrogen breath test first introduced by Calloway et al. (1969). This test is based on the stoichiometric relationship between hydrogen evolved and the amount of unabsorbed carbohydrate fermented by bacteria in the human colon.

For a comprehensive review of both the clinical and nutritional implications of lactose intolerance, see Paige and Bayless (1981).

Sucrase deficiency as well as deficiencies in maltase and isomaltase have been detected in children (Semenza et al., 1965). However, when there is a change from a sucrose-free diet to one high in sucrose, sucrase and maltase activity is doubled (Rosensweig and Herman, 1968). Recently, sucrase deficiency has been established as the cause of a nonspecific chronic diarrhea, and was traced to an inherited recessive defect in the ability to synthesize sucrase (Gray et al., 1976).

LIPIDS

The initial event in the digestion of dietary lipids begins in the mouth. Although no hydrolysis of triacylglycerol occurs in the mouth, lipids stimulate the secretion of "lingual lipase" from the serous glands (glands of Ebner) at the base of the tongue. Lingual lipase, which exhibits optimum activity between pH 4.5 and 5.4 (Hamosh and Scow, 1973), becomes active in the stomach. This enzyme accounts for 20 to 30 percent of the lipid digestion that occurs in the stomach. Lingual lipase prepared from bovine tongue also has a commercial use in the manufacture of mozzarella cheese.

Although a gastric lipase is secreted, it is not of major physiological importance. It is a tributyrase and responsible mainly for the hydrolysis of tributyrin to free fatty acids. The activity of this lipase decreases with increasing chain length of the fatty acids in the triacylglycerols. This enzyme is virtually ineffective for releasing fatty acids with ten carbons or more.

The presence of fat in the duodenum elicits the release of the postulated hormone, enterogastrone, which is purported to decrease gastric secretion and motility thereby slowing gastric emptying time. Whether the inhibitory mechanism is due to a distinct and separate hormone or a combination of other effects is still a moot question (Andersson, 1967). Nevertheless, the rate at which fat enters the duodenum is regulated and appears to be correlated with the capacity of the lipolytic enzymes from the pancreas to handle entering fat.

In the duodenum, the major source of lipolytic enzymes is the pancreatic juice. Several pancreatic hydrolases have been identified. A glycerol ester hydrolase, which hydrolyzes insoluble esters of glycerol, and a cholesterol esterase, which hydrolyzes esters of cholesterol, are both dependent on bile salts for their action. The bile salts along with fatty acids and glycerol have a detergent action on fat and aid in the emulsification of triacylglycerols. Since pancreatic lipase acts on the interface of triacylglycerol emulsions, it follows that there is increased activity with increased surface area. Bile salts also promote the downward shift in lumen contents to a pH of 6.0, which is the optimum for pancreatic lipase activity. The pancreatic lipases have a specificity for the 1 and 3 positions of the triacylglycerol molecule. If short chain fatty acids are in the 2 position, these may be hydrolyzed to a considerable degree. However, since short- and medium-chain fatty acids isomerize at a high rate, it is possible that isomerization to the 1 position might account for the hydrolysis (Benzonana et al., 1964). The major end products following triacylglycerol lipolysis by pancreatic lipase, therefore, are the 1-, 3-fatty acids and the remaining 2-monoacylglycerols. Furthermore, bile salts along with monoacylglycerol and fatty acids play a fundamental role in the formation of aggregates called *micelles* (Johnston, 1968). Under normal conditions, conjugated bile salts in the intestinal lumen are above the concentration critical for micellar formation. As a result, monoacyglycerols liberated from triacylglycerols are immediately trapped by the bile salts to form micelles which then dissolve free fatty acids. Cholesterol and fat-soluble vitamins are also dissolved in the micelles. (See Davenport, 1971.) According to Hofmann and Borgström (1962), mixed micelles of fatty acids, cholesterol, and monoacylglycerols with bile salts acting as detergents are brought into contact with the microvilli of the intestinal mucosa. The role of the micelle in lipid and in fat-soluble vitamin absorption will be discussed in a later section.

The enzymes located in the intestinal mucosal cells and concerned with lipid digestion are a lipase (Holt and Miller, 1962) and lecithinase (Winkler et al., 1967). The appearance of these enzymes in the lumen is due to the sloughing off of cells.

Abnormalities of lipid digestion can occur as the result of interference with enzyme synthesis, which may be due to a genetic defect, or to interference with enzyme secretion associated with pancreatic disease. In either case, undigested lipid remaining in the lumen will result in a condition known as *steatorrhea* in which the stools are fatty, bulky, and very light in color. Lipid in the stools would, of course, carry with it lipid-soluble substances. As a result, the disorder that develops is due not only to deficiency of lipid as an energy source but also to the deficit of essential linoleic acid and fat-soluble vitamins. Cases of congenital pancreatic lipase deficiency have been described (Sheldon, 1964).

The detergent action of bile salts may not always be to an individual's advantage. Many patients with gastric ulcers have been found to have bile salts in the stomach that apparently were carried there by regurgitation of intestinal contents during digestion. The detergent action of the bile is believed to break the gastric mucosal barrier making it vulnerable to self-digestion, or ulceration (Davenport, 1972).

For a review of lipid digestion, see Patton (1981); Carey et al. (1983).

PROTEINS

The distention of the stomach as well as the chemical stimulation produced by the presence of food liberates the hormone gastrin (see Table 6.2) from the gastric mucosa. Gastrin then stimulates the parietal cells of the mucosa to secrete hydrochloric acid. The hydrochloric acid plays a dual role in protein digestion: it promotes the swelling of protein and it activates pepsinogens (protease precursors) secreted by the zymogenic cells of the mucosa. The activation process is auto-catalytic, that is, after the initial conversion of pepsinogen to pepsin, the pepsin itself can activate additional pepsinogen.

The mechanisms by which the stomach protects itself from both the strong acid and the proteolytic enzymes has been the subject of both speculation and sound research. The known physical and chemical mechanisms by which the stomach maintains its mucosal barrier are interestingly discussed by Davenport (1972).

Seven distinct pepsinogens have been identified and each is thought to produce a distinctive pepsin (Rudick and Janowitz, 1974). The physiological significance of the various pepsinogens and pepsins is not clear. Pepsins hydrolyze the peptide bonds that link aromatic amino acids to other amino acids to give polypeptides of varying lengths with N-terminal amino acids. In addition, small quantitites of oligopeptides and amino acids are released (Meyer and Kelly, 1976).

The efficiency of peptic digestion of protein can vary enormously from person to person, and the protein entering the duodenum from the stomach is a mixture of intact protein, large polypeptides, and not more than 15 percent as amino acids. However, gastric hydrolysis does not appear to be an essential phase of protein digestion since individuals with achlorhydria have no difficulty in digesting protein nor do those who have undergone total gastrectomies.

The action of the gastric proteolytic enzymes is halted when the acid content of the stomach reaches the duodenum and the pH is increased from approximately 2.0 to about 6.5. However, acid chyme entering the duodenum elicits the secretion of the hormone secretin which stimulates the secretion of an aqueous, enzyme-poor pancreatic juice. The products of protein digestion entering the duodenum stimulate the secretion of another hormone, cholecystokinin (CCK), which affects the enzyme content but not the volume of pancreatic juice.

The zymogens, or inactive proteolytic enzymes, in the pancreatic juice are trypsinogen, chymotrypsinogen, and procarboxypeptidase. Activation is triggered

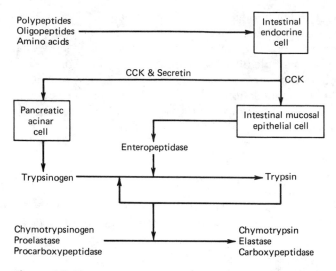

Figure 6.3
Secretion and activation of pancreatic enzymes. (From H. J. Freeman and Y. S. Kim, *Ann. Rev. Med.* 29:99, 1978.)

by the conversion of the trypsinogen to trypsin by the enzyme enteropeptidase secreted by the intestinal mucosa. This activation results from the removal of a hexapeptide from the amino terminus. After the initial activation, trypsin acts autocatalytically activating more trypsinogen. Trypsin also activates the rest of the pancreatic enzymes: chymotrypsinogen, proelastase, and procarboxypeptidase to chymotrypsin, elastase, and carboxypeptidase respectively. Activation, in each case, is cleavage of a peptide bond adjacent to an arginine or a lysine residue near the beginning of the chain of the zymogen (Neurath, 1964). It appears that a further change is required in the activation of procarboxypeptidase. A summary of the secretion and activation of pancreatic proteases is shown in Fig. 6.3.

The pancreatic proteolytic enzymes are classified as *endopeptidases* and *exopeptidases*. These enzymes can perform their proteolytic functions whether or not peptic digestion has taken place. The *endopeptidases,* trypsin, chymotrypsin, and elastase, cleave specific peptide bonds in the inner portion of the protein molecule. Trypsin acts at a bond where a dibasic amino acid contributes the carboxyl group; chymotrypsin at a bond where an aromatic amino acid contributes the carboxyl group. The *exopeptidases,* mainly carboxypeptidase A and carboxypeptidase B, hydrolyze in sequence the terminal peptide bonds at the carboxyl end of the peptide. Carboxypeptidase A attacks neutral or aromatic residues, and carboxypeptidase B hydrolyzes basic residues. The endo- and exopeptidases work in conjunction with each other and operate more efficiently as digestion proceeds, the endopeptidases increasing the substrate concentration for the two carboxy-

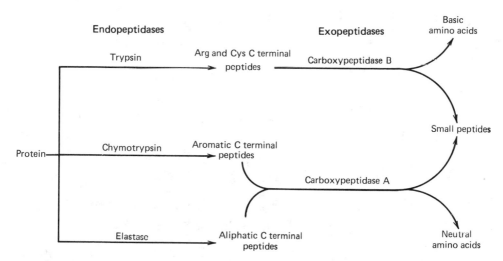

Figure 6.4

Intraduodenal sequential action of pancreatic endopeptidases and exopeptidases on dietary protein. Final products at right are substrates that enter the mucosal cell. Arginine (Arg), Cysteine (Cys). (From G. M. Gray and H. L. Cooper, *Gastroenterology* 61:535, 1971.)

peptidases. The combined action of these groups of enzymes results in a mixture of amino acids and short peptides (Fig. 6.4). Thus, oligopeptides are the major products of protein digestion in the intestinal lumen. In fact, after a meal, the lumen content of amino acids in peptide form is four times the amount of free amino acids (Adibi and Mercer, 1973). The reported appearance of intestinal proteolytic enzymes in the lumen contents of the small intestine is acknowledged to be due to the sloughed off mucosal cells since carefully prepared cell-free juice is free of intestinal digestive enzymes. (See Davenport, 1971.)

The final hydrolyses of oligopeptides of from four to eight amino acids in length occurs in the membranes of the microvilli. The di- and tripeptides released along with some amino acids are considered the end products of protein digestion. Thus, the last stage of protein digestion, like the last stage of carbohydrate digestion, is a membrane function and is the link between digestion and absorption.

For detailed discussion of protein digestion, see Freeman and Kim (1978) and Adibi and Kim (1981).

The coordinated timing and action of hormonal secretions and neuromuscular and secretory activity in the presence of substrate results in an orderly and sequential digestive process summarized in Table 6.4. The nutrients released from the carbohydrate, lipid, and protein can now make the final transition from being constituents in food to being nutrients and metabolties in the body. They are now ready for the final hurdle through the mucosal cell, the intricate process of absorption.

Table 6.4
Source and Action of Digestive Enzymes

Source of Secretion	Stimulus	Enzyme or Secretory Product	Action
Mouth Salivary glands (3 pair)	Psychic Mechanical Chemical	Salivary amylase	Glycogen, Starch, Dextrin → branched oligosaccharides, some maltose Action of minor importance
Stomach Gastric glands (35,000,000)	Acetylcholine Gastrin Histamine	HCl	Pepsinogen → pepsin $Fe^{+++} \rightarrow Fe^{++}$ Swelling of proteins Antibacterial effect Acid-combining power
	↓ Gastric pH Gastric irritants	Mucus	Protective to mucosa
	Vagal stim. Histamine	Pepsinogen (pepsin)	Hydrolyze peptide bonds → large polypeptides between aromatic and amino acids dicarboxylic acids
	Gastrin continuous secretion, inc. with stim. to gastric secretion	Intrinsic factor	Essential for absorption of vitamin B_{12}
Pancreas Exocrine secretion	Secretin Cholecystokinin Acetylcholine Gastrin	Trypsinogen Chymotrypsinogen Procarboxypeptidase	Activated by enterokinase and by trypsin Activated by trypsin Activated by trypsin

Enzyme	Action
Endopeptidases	
Trypsin	Protein and polypeptides → small polypeptides
Chymotrypsin	Protein and polypeptides → small polypeptides
Exopeptidases	
Carboxypeptidase A	Polypeptides with free carboxyl group → lower peptides and aromatic amino acids
Carboxypeptidase B	Polypeptides with free carboxyl group → lower peptides and dibasic amino acids
Elastase	Hydrolyzes fibrous proteins
Collagenase	Hydrolyzes collagen
Ribonuclease	Ribonucleic acid → nucleotides
Deoxyribonuclease	Deoxyribonucleic acid → nucleotides
α-Amylase	Starch → dextrins and maltose
Lipase (requires bile salts)	Fats → monoacylglycerols, fatty acids, glycerol
Phospholipase A	Lecithin → lysolecithin (= removal of one fatty acid)
Retinyl ester hydrolase	Hydrolyzes retinyl esters
Cholesterol esterase (requires bile salts)	Free cholesterol → esters of cholesterol with fatty acids

Table 6.4 (continued)

Source of Secretion	Stimulus	Enzyme or Secretory Product	Action
Small intestine Most enzymes located in microvilli of mucosal cells	Gastrin Secretin Cholecystokinin Vasoactive inhibitory peptide	Aminopeptidases	Polypeptides with → lower peptides and free amino group free amino acids
		Dipeptidases	Dipeptides → amino acids
		Nucleotidase	Nucleotides → nucleosides and H_3PO_4
		Nucleosidase	Nucleosides → purines, pyrimidines, and pentose
	Gastric inhibitory peptide Calcitonin Glucagon	Alkaline phosphatase	Organic phosphates → free phosphates
		Monoglyceride lipase	Monoglycerides → fatty acids and glycerol
		Lecithinase	Lecithin → fatty acids, glycerol, phosphoric acid, and choline
		Disaccharidases	
		Sucrase	Sucrose → glucose and fructose
		Maltase	Maltose → glucose
		Lactase	Lactose → glucose and galactose
Gallbladder Liver	Secretin Cholecystokinin Hepatocrinin	Bile	Emulsifies fat Stabilizes emulsions Neutralizes acid chyme Accelerates action of pancreatic lipase Path for pigment and cholesterol excretion

Absorption

MUCOSAL STRUCTURE

The small intestine is approximately 380 cm long but with an epithelial lining that presents a surface area many times this linear measurement. The entire lining has its surface extended by villi, fingerlike protuberances extending into the lumen, each of which is 0.5–1.5 mm long. There are 20–40 villi per mm^2, giving a total estimated surface of approximately 300 m^2 (Blankenhorn et al., 1955) or about 3,000 square feet! This enormous surface area is further increased by the brush borders, revealed by the electron microscope to be microvilli, which extend as slender, closely packed projections from the entire free surface of the villi epithelial cells (Fig. 6.5).

In man and other mammals, the microvilli of the absorptive cells average 1 μ in length and 0.1 μ in width (Palay and Karlin, 1959a) becoming increasingly longer along the villi, attaining greatest length and number toward the tip. There may be 2,000–4,000 microvilli on the free surface of each intestinal cell and in one mm^2 of intestine, the estimates range from 50,000–200,000 (Ugolev, 1965) to 200,000,000 (DeRobertis et al., 1970), increasing the effective absorptive surface of the intestine approximately thirtyfold. A surface coat or glycocalyx (see Chapter 9) covers the microvillus surface. It is in this glycocalyx-microvillus membrane complex that the enzymes involved in the terminal digestion of carbohydrates and proteins and the specific receptors and carriers for absorption of these and other nutrients are located.

At the base of the villi, and with epithelium continuous with the villus epithelium, are the crypts of Lieberkühn. These are simple tubes 0.3–0.5 mm deep. Each villus has three of them, and they comprise the proliferative area, the area of mitotic activity, where the epithelial cells of the intestinal mucosa are formed. Cells formed in the crypts migrate up the length of the villus and are extruded from the tip into the intestinal lumen when their short (1 to 3 day) life-span is completed (Leblond and Messier, 1958). The average height of a column of cells in the crypt is 30 cells and each of these columns produces one new cell every three hours. However, each villus loses one cell per hour from its tip; consequently cellular production from three crypts is needed to maintain each villus. The extrusion of these cells into the intestine of man is estimated to be at a rate of 20–50 million cells per minute and amounts to 250 gm of cells each day. (See Lipkin, 1981.) With increasing age, as cells approach the tip of the villus, comes increased efficiency, the absorptive capacity being greater in the oldest cells (Padykula, 1962). The villus cell clearly exemplifies the manner in which morphological differentiation and development are correlated with the development of specific functional capabilities (Rubin, 1971). The undifferentiated crypt cell acquires numerous enzymes, receptors, and carriers to become the highly selective and biochemically sophisticated mature cell. It functions impressively but reaches its nadir and oblivion in short order.

The extremely rapid rate of renewal of mucosal cells has been demonstrated by following the incorporation of tritiated thymidine into newly synthesized DNA

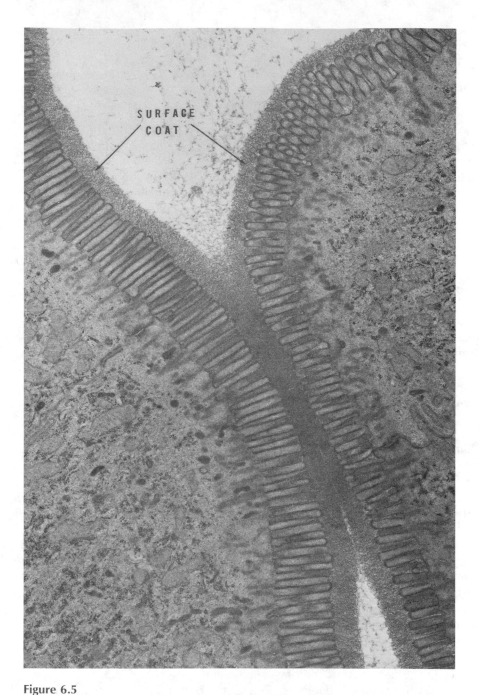

Figure 6.5
The brush border or microvilli of two adjacent intestinal villi showing the surface coat which is a product of the cells whose surface it covers. Among the probable functions of this coating is the role as barrier to large particles while permitting substances in solution, emulsified lipid, and colloidal particles to pass freely. It is resistant to a wide variety of proteolytic and mucolytic agents. Intestinal epithelium of cat. Magnification 51,000. (Courtesy of Dr. Susumu Ito.)

by autoradiography techniques. Lipkin (1965) has shown that most of the epithelial lining of the human tract is replaced in 3 to 6 days. The mean rate of cell proliferation was calculated as 1 to 2 cells/100 cells/hour. A similar technique used earlier in rats and mice indicated that replacement of the epithelial lining occurred within 2 to 3 days (Hooper, 1956). The very brief life-span of the intestinal epithelial cell (compared with 120 days for the erythrocyte and far slower rates for connective tissue and muscle cells) makes it very clear why the intestinal mucosa is an early target when there is interference with cell division, as in vitamin B_{12} deficiency.

A reduction in the number of microvilli has been observed in various malabsorption syndromes (Ugolev, 1965). Stanfield et al. (1965) reported that in infants with protein-energy malnutrition there are gross changes in the appearance of the villi: flattening, broadening, and atrophy, drastically decreasing the membrane surface. They also observed associated disaccharidase deficiency. It appears reasonable to suggest that severe protein deficiency of protein-energy malnutrition prevents the rapid cellular proliferation of the mucosa, which normally offsets the desquamation of cells from the villus tip, and that this in time leads to the atrophy observed.

The core of each villus contains a capillary network and a lacteal. The capillaries drain into venules and eventually to the portal vein, which carries the blood and all that it contains to the liver before entering the systemic circulation. The lacteal or lymphatic capillary empties into the lymphatic channels and, via the left thoracic duct, into the systemic circulation. By means of these two entries into the transport system, the absorbed products of digestion reach the distant cells of the organism.

The distance traveled by each nutrient before absorption is related to the rate and mechanism of absorption. Absorption of most nutrients takes place in the duodenum and the first part of the jejunum; those absorbed by passive diffusion usually leave from the duodenum although some absorption also occurs further along the tract. Vitamin B_{12} and bile salts are unique in that they are not absorbed until they reach the ileum where their specific active transport mechanisms are located (Booth, 1968). The known sites for absorption are shown in Fig. 6.6.

For an in-depth review of the morphology of the mucosa of the small intestine, see Trier and Madara (1981).

MUCOSAL FUNCTION

Often it is glibly stated that the end products of digestion leave the intestinal lumen and enter the blood. This statement discloses the end and ignores the means. The end result is fact and accepted, but the means are illusive, intriguing, and in many ways, mystifying. It is the passage between the lumens, intestinal and vascular, that is the big step from outside to inside. This step, absorption, is the primary assignment and main function of the mucosal cells.

The mucosal membrane is the first in the series of membranes interposed between the incoming nutrients and the cells to which they must be transported for

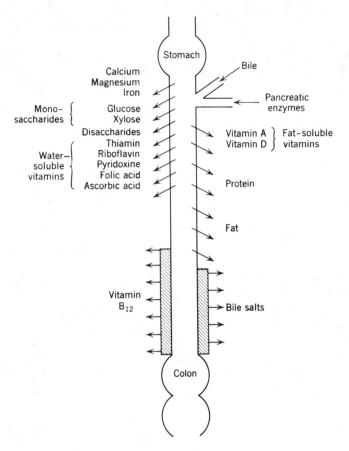

Figure 6.6
Known sites of absorption in the small intestine. (From C. C.
Booth, *Handbook of Physiology*, Section 6, Vol. 3, C. F. Code,
ed., American Physiological Society, Washington, D.C., 1968,
p. 1524.)

metabolism. Once inside the mucosal cell, the nutrients must traverse the cell,
leave through the serosal membrane, and ultimately enter the interstitial fluid.
From this compartment the nutrients finally can pass through the wall of the
vascular or lymphatic capillary and be transported to other loci for metabolism.
The mucosal cell, therefore, must participate actively or passively in the transport
of any substance from the lumen of the small intestine into the body. If this
specialized membrane either fails to accept or rejects specific molecules, the
effects will eventually become apparent in the metabolism of the total organism.
For discussion of hereditary disorders of intestinal transport, see Milne (1974).

The mechanisms of membrane transport will be discussed in Chapter 9.

Carbohydrate Absorption

It has been known for over 60 years that the small intestine absorbs certain hexoses faster than others (Csaky, 1963). The first suggestion of selectivity of the intestinal membrane for simple sugars was made by Cori (1925). He found that sugars administered to rats by stomach tube disappeared from the intestine at strikingly different rates: Galactose > glucose > fructose > mannose > xylose > arabinose. It was established that galactose and glucose were actively absorbed against a concentration gradient and that fructose, mannose, xylose, and arabinose did not enjoy active transport. The minimal structural requirements for active transport of sugar by the intestine suggested by Wilson and Landau (1960) and by Crane (1960) provided an explanation for the differences in rate. For active transport, the sugar must contain six carbons in the form of a D-pyranose ring with an intact —OH at the carbon-2 position (Fig. 6.7). It therefore became understandable, on the basis of the minimal structural requirements, why certain of the sugars were transported against a concentration gradient and others were not (Table 6.5).

Despite the inability of fructose to qualify structurally for active transport and its consequent slower rate of absorption than galactose and glucose, it traverses the membrane by means of facilitated diffusion (see Chapter 9) and at a rate faster than mannose, xylose, and arabinose.

The story of the attempts to unravel the intricacies of sugar transport across the intestinal mucosa illustrates another instance where a forgotten discovery was rediscovered after a lapse of almost 60 years. Schultz and Curran (1968) point to the report of Reid (1902) as the first indication that the presence of Na^+ in the intestinal lumen enhanced the absorption of glucose. The importance of Na^+ in the small intestine for the active transport not only of sugars but also amino acids and other nonelectrolytes was then rediscovered and extensively studied (Riklis and Quastel, 1958; Csaky, 1961; Bihler and Crane, 1962; Schultz et al., 1966).

Crane (1960; 1965) studied sugar transport using the everted gut sac technique first described by Wilson and Wiseman (1954) which permitted monitoring of net transport of sugar. The model they proposed to explain the dependence on Na^+ for sugar transport came to be known as the Na^+-gradient hypothesis for energy

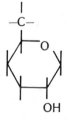

Six carbons
Intact —OH at carbon 2
D-pyranose ring

Figure 6.7
Minimal structural requirements for active transport of sugar by intestine. (From R. K. Crane, *Physiol. Rev.* 40:789, 1960; Wilson et al., *Fed. Proc.* 19:870, 1960.)

TABLE 6.5
Partial Specificity of Sugar Active Transport in Hamster Small Intestine *in Vitro*

Actively Transported	Not Actively Transported
Glucose	Fructose
Galactose	Mannose
3-O-Methylglucose	Xylose
1-Deoxyglucose	2-Deoxyglucose
6-Deoxyglucose	Sorbitol
6-Deoxy-D-galactose	6-Deoxy-L-galactose

Source: From R. K. Crane, *Fed. Proc.* 21:891 (1962).

coupling. The model suggested that glucose associated with a carrier and with Na^+ in the microvilli and the complex traveled to the inner side of the membrane where it dissociated, releasing glucose and Na^+ into the cytoplasm. The Na^+ was then actively transported out of the cell. The stored energy in ATP in the cell, trapped through the metabolism of glucose molecules previously brought in or by fatty acids (Crane and Mandelstam, 1960) indicated a reciprocity; Na^+ helped to move glucose into the cell and the metabolic energy in ATP moved Na^+ out. A model proposed by Crane (1968) of the functional activities of the disaccharidases in the membrane and Na^+ involvement in the mechanism of active sugar transport is shown in Fig. 6.8.

In the transport model proposed by Crane (1968) one Na^+ attached to the carrier along with the glucose molecule. During the 1970s, when it became possible to study transport in isolated intact intestinal cells, the same characteristics of Na^+ described earlier using everted gut sacs were evident. Later, however, Kimmich and Randles (1980) demonstrated that the stoichiometric ratio of Na^+ to glucose was 2:1. The transport protein with high affinity for glucose attaches to it along with two Na^+. When the glucose and Na^+ reach the inner aspect of the membrane, both Na^+ and glucose are released into the cell. Part of the energy for the uphill movement of glucose is provided by a sodium pump at the lateral membrane which sends Na^+ into the intercellular space. Further refinement in laboratory techniques made possible the study of isolated membranes and membrane vesicles from both the mucosal and serosal boundaries of the intestinal epithelial cell. From studies on the isolated membranes it became apparent that the energy coupling involved in sugar transport could not be explained solely on the basis of a chemical potential difference for Na^+. The use of microelectrodes demonstrated that actively transported sugars produce a dramatic change in membrane potential across the brush border indicating that both chemical and electrical potential differences are involved in the function of the Na^+-dependent sugar carrier in the mucosal cell (Okada et al., 1977a; 1977b).

The study of net transport through the cell involves not only the activities of the brush border on the mucosal side but also those of the organelles within the

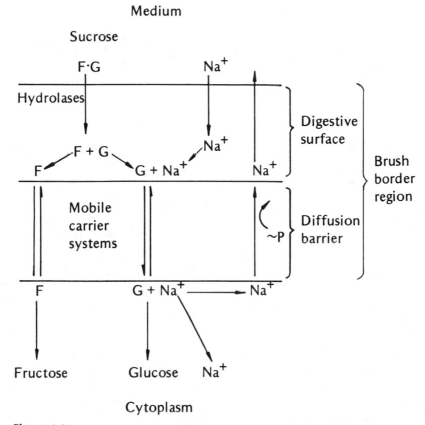

Figure 6.8
Model of functional activities of the brush border membrane of intestinal epithelial cell indicating the diffusion of fructose (F) and the transport of the combined glucose (G) and Na^+ through the membrane. (From R. K. Crane, *Handbook of Physiology*, Section 6, Vol. 3, American Physiological Society, Washington, D.C., 1968, p. 1338.)

cell and the mechanisms involved in the exit through the lateral or serosal membranes. The glucose in the mucosal cell appears to leave by three different routes (Gray, 1981). An estimated 15 percent leaks back through the brush border into the intestinal lumen and about 25 percent diffuses out through the basolateral membrane. The major portion of glucose, approximately 60 percent, leaves the cell by means of a yet-to-be isolated carrier in the serosal membrane. This carrier is independent of Na^+ and its capacity for glucose transport is greater than that of the Na^+-dependent carrier on the mucosal side. Because the capacity to carry glucose out is greater than the capacity to bring it in, glucose does not accumulate in the mucosal cell. In addition, the glucose absorption mechanism is so efficient that practically all of the digested carbohydrate has been transported through the

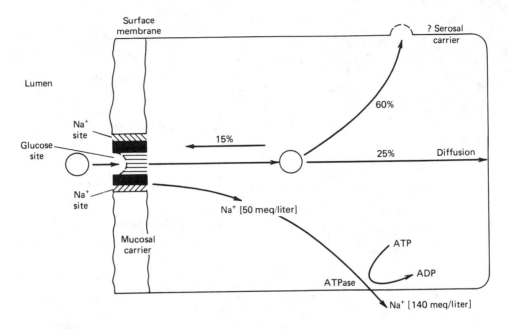

Figure 6.9
Model of the active transport of glucose or galactose. The membrane carrier has high affinity at the luminal surface for both monosaccharide and Na$^+$. There are probably two Na$^+$ binding sites on the carrier. The polar glucose passes through a hydrophylic core of the carrier to be discharged in the cell interior. The energy for monosaccharide transport is provided by the Na$^+$-K$^+$ ATPase pump at the basolateral membrane and exit of glucose appears to be facilitated by a serosal carrier. Carrier proteins have not been isolated but their functional role has been studied in intact cells and isolated membrane vesicles. (From G. M. Gray, *Physiology of the Gastrointestinal Tract*, Vol. 2, L. R. Johnson, ed., Raven Press, New York, 1981, p. 1069.)

intestinal wall by the time the contents reach the lower portion of the jejunum. A modification of Crane's original model of glucose transport through the intestinal cell is shown in Fig. 6.9.

For extensive review of the intestinal absorption of sugar, see Kimmich (1981); Gray (1981).

Lipid Absorption
Lipid absorption has been a subject of controversy since 1856 when Claude Bernard observed that the lymphatics distal to the pancreatic duct became cloudy after a fat-containing meal. He suggested that pancreatic juices were involved and that absorption was by way of the lymphatic system. A brief history of some of the early investigations and speculations concerning fat absorption are well told by Johnston (1963; 1968) and are, therefore, only briefly reviewed here.

The mechanism by which fat reaches the lymphatics was debated with great fervor by two opposing schools. The adherents of the *particulate theory* held that fat was absorbed as a fine emulsion and crossed the intestinal epithelial cells to enter the lymphatic ducts in the villi. The opposing school, adherents of the *lipolytic theory,* held that triacylglycerols had to be completely hydrolyzed to fatty acids before they could be absorbed. The lipolytic theory gained more adherents, and it was generally accepted that hydrolysis was complete in the lumen. It was accepted that emulsification was advantageous but not obligatory prior to hydrolysis. Following hydrolysis, it was hypothesized that the fatty acids and glycerol were taken into the mucosal cells and reconverted into triacylglycerols which appeared as small globules. This theory remained popular well into the 1930s. At that time Verzar (see Verzar and McDougall, 1936), a strong proponent of the lipolytic theory, emphasized the importance of bile acids in the solubilization of the fatty acids and suggested that α-glycerophosphate might be involved in the resynthesis of the triacylglycerols.

The suggestion that some fat was partitioned into the portal circulation and other fat into the lymph and that bile salts, monoacylglycerols, and fatty acids were involved in the emulsification of triacylglycerols (Frazer, 1938) remained dormant for 25 years and then emerged in the 1960s with the work of Borgström (1962; 1963) and Hofman and Borgström (1962; 1963) establishing the importance of micelles in lipid absorption. Bile salts aggregate above a certain concentration, known as the critical micellar concentration (CMC), dependent on species of bile salt, pH, and temperature, to form pure micelles (Chapman, 1968). Monoacylglycerols, phospholipids, cholesterol, and fatty acids become solubilized by the pure micelles to form mixed micelles. In this way fat-soluble compounds are incorporated into a more water-soluble phase.

From the mixed micelles the monoacylglycerols and fatty acids as well as cholesterol must cross the unstirred water layer lining and intestinal cells and then permeate the plasma membrane (Thomson and Dietschy, 1981). The unstirred water layer is thought to be physiologically important in determining the rate of absorption (Lukie et al., 1974; Thomson and Dietschy, 1980).

How the material in the mixed micelle is taken up by the mucosal cell is not understood completely. Three mechanisms have been suggested (Thomson and Dietschy, 1981):

1. The micelle is taken up intact. This mechanism is unlikely since the individual constituents of the mixed micelle are taken up at different rates (Hoffman, 1970; Simmonds, 1972).
2. The micelle binds or interacts with the plasma membrane of the cell resulting in the transfer of material into the cell. Experimental data to support this theory is lacking (Westergaard and Dietschy, 1976).
3. Absorption of substances in the micelle occurs through partitioning from the micelle into the aqueous phase followed by uptake by the plasma membrane. This is the mechanism that appears to be physiologically important (Thomson and Dietschy, 1981).

The process of uptake of fatty acids and monoacylglycerols is a passive process (Johnston and Borgström, 1964; Johnston, 1968). Both biochemical and autoradiographic data support the hypothesis that the intestinal uptake of lipids in micellar form occurs by simple diffusion (Strauss, 1964; 1966; 1968), and that chemical synthesis of higher acylglycerols within the cell was subsequent to diffusion of lipid into the cells, and independent of uptake (Strauss and Ito, 1965). Most of the monoacylglycerol and fatty acid absorption takes place in the first half of the intestine.

Ockner et al. (1972) reported the presence of a binding protein for long chain fatty acids in jejunal mucosa and other mammalian tissues. The fatty acid binding protein (FABP) was offered as an explanation for the differences in intestinal absorption among fatty acids since FABP appears to have greater affinity for unsaturated than saturated fatty acids (Ockner and Manning, 1974). This property may play a role in regulation of esterification of fatty acids by the endoplasmic reticulum. Within the endoplasmic reticulum free fatty acids must be activated to form the acyl-coenzyme A derivative (Ockner and Isselbacher, 1974). This is an energy-requiring step utilizing ATP that is catalyzed by fatty acid-coenzyme A ligase (Brindley and Hubscher, 1966). The fatty acyl-CoA can then be incorporated onto α-glycerophosphate, monoacylglycerols, or diacylglycerols to ultimately yield triacylglycerols (Fig. 6.10). α-Glycerophosphate is provided by either glycerol or glucose.

The source of α-glycerophosphate that forms the glycerol backbone of the triacyglycerol has been a subject of controversy. It had been generally believed that the glycerol liberated in the lumen by the complete hydrolysis of triacylglycerol could not be reused for triacylglycerol synthesis. The investigators supporting this hypothesis suggested that the acylglycerol glycerol came from glycolysis in the mucosal cell. These conclusions were based on labeling experiments and on the assumption that the intestine did not contain a glycerokinase (Buell and Reiser, 1959). However, Haessler and Isselbacher (1963) demonstrated that glycerol is metabolized by intestinal mucosa and that it can serve as a precursor of glycerophosphate. In addition, it was shown by these workers and by Clark and Hubscher (1962) that a glycerokinase was present in the cytoplasm of the intestinal mucosal cells and acted in the formation of glycerophosphate from glycerol and ATP. The monoacylglycerol pathway is believed to be of more importance in intestinal triacylglycerol resynthesis than the α-glycerophosphate pathway (Ockner and Isselbacher, 1974).

Triacylglycerol resynthesized in the smooth endoplasmic reticulum is packaged into a lipoprotein by the addition of phospholipids, cholesterol, cholesterol esters, and a specific protein, apoprotein B (Hamilton, 1972). The chylomicrons migrate to the Golgi apparatus where glycoproteins may be added to the particle (Lo and Marsh, 1970). From data reported by Ockner et al. (1969), it appears that specific micellar fatty acids can regulate the synthesis of lipoproteins by the intestinal mucosa and, in this way, affect the circulating lipids. The amounts of specific monoacylglycerols or of the fatty acids that have been split off may determine whether triacylglycerol or phospholipid synthesis takes place, as well as the char-

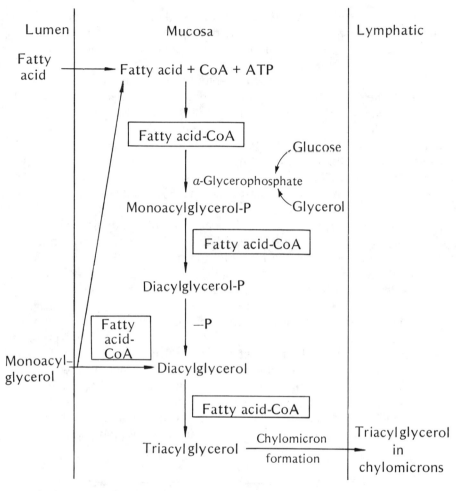

| Lumen | Mucosa | Lymphatic |

Fatty acid ──→ Fatty acid + CoA + ATP

Fatty acid-CoA

Glucose

a-Glycerophosphate

Monoacylglycerol-P   Glycerol

Fatty acid-CoA

Diacylglycerol-P

Fatty acid-CoA   −P

Monoacyl-glycerol   Diacylglycerol

Fatty acid-CoA

Triacylglycerol ── Chylomicron formation ──→ Triacylglycerol in chylomicrons

Figure 6.10
Major biochemical reactions in transport of long chain fatty acids and monoacylglycerols by intestinal mucosa. (From K. J. Isselbacher, *Fed. Proc.* 24:16, 1965.)

acter of the lipoprotein coat. The triacylglycerol in food finally emerges from the intestinal cell with a coat of protein. Water-insoluble triacylglycerol can now be transported as lipoprotein in an aqueous medium. Lipoprotein characteristics depend on the relative proportions of protein in the molecule and the kind and amount of lipid. (See Chapter 2.) The pattern of the circulating lipoproteins and the possibility of a relationship to dietary fat is being avidly pursued by investigators in the area of cardiovascular disease. (See Chapter 25.)

Karmen and colleagues (1962; 1963) showed that the fatty acids in the chylomicrons of the lymph are not exclusively from fed fat but include fatty acids from endogenous sources. Baxter (1966) suggested that 50 percent of the endogenous fatty acids are derived from the fatty acids present in bile.

Chylomicrons must leave the mucosal cell, and it was suggested (Palay and Karlin, 1959a; 1959b) that they are discharged through the side of the cell and into the extracellular space. They then enter the lymph through the wall of the lacteal en route to the thoracic duct. Lipid that has been hydrolyzed, resynthesized, and protein-coated enters the circulation as chylomicrons.

Obligatory triacylglycerol synthesis in the mucosal cell and subsequent entry into the lymph occurs only for the long chain fatty acids and monoacylglycerols. Those fatty acids with a chain length of 10–12 carbons or less are transported unesterified and leave the mucosa via the portal vein and are transported directly to the liver. Triacylglycerols containing fatty acids of medium chain length have been shown to enter the mucosal cell without prior hydrolysis and to be subjected to hydrolysis after entry by a lipase or esterase present in the microsomal fraction (Playoust and Isselbacher, 1964). These medium chain fatty acids then leave the cell and enter the blood for transport (Fig. 6.11).

The major portion of ingested phospholipid undergoes complete hydrolysis in the lumen to fatty acids, glycerol, phosphate, and other compounds. Absorption presumably parallels that of the breakdown products from ingested triacylglycerols.

Bile acids are reabsorbed by an energy-dependent process in the ileum (Baker and Searle, 1960). The reabsorbed bile acids are taken up by the liver for reuse in the digestive process (Glasinovic et al., 1975). This is known as enterohepatic circulation. Each bile salt molecule is reused 15 to 20 times (Tyor et al., 1971).

Most of the dietary fat ingested is digested and absorbed. Approximately 95 percent is absorbed and the remaining 5 percent is excreted in the feces (Kasper, 1970). Conditions that interfere with bile salt synthesis or reabsorption or pancreatic lipase function can lead to decreases in fat absorption and steatorrhea.

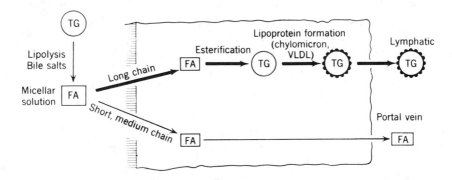

Figure 6.11
A scheme showing the major steps in lipid uptake by the mucosal cell, its metabolism, and its exit into the lymph as chylomicra or short-chain fatty acids. (Adapted from K. J. Isselbacher and R. M. Glickman, *Transport Across the Intestine*, W. L. Burland and P. D. Samuel, eds., Churchill Livingstone, Edinburgh, 1972, p. 245.)

The fate of circulating lipid may range from the evanescent provider of energy, to the invisible component of cell substance, to the far-too-visible package of adipose tissue stored for future contingencies that all too often fail to materialize.

Cholesterol Absorption

Cholesterol in the lumen of the intestine is derived from both endogenous and exogenous sources. Most of the endogenous cholesterol, which comprises about one-half of the total, is derived from bile. Cholesterol esters comprise about 15 percent of the cholesterol in the lumen. They cannot be absorbed intact but must be hydrolyzed before the cholesterol moiety can be transferred through the mucosa (Hyun et al., 1964). The esters, therefore, will remain in the lumen for either eventual hydrolysis and absorption, or will continue on to the large intestine and be excreted.

Bile acids are necessary for the absorption of cholesterol (Siperstein and Guest, 1960). Bile acids appear to increase the solubility of cholesterol and may in some way change the permeability of the brush border. The presence of fatty acids, particularly oleic acid, also stimulates the absorption of cholesterol (Treadwell et al., 1962). These authors also showed that absorption is stimulated by pancreatic juice which increases the level of cholesterol esterase in the mucosa, thereby promoting micellar formation and entrance into the cell, and by bile which influences the level of esterifying activity and chylomicron formation in the cell.

Cholesterol absorption is particularly difficult to study because at the same time that it is being absorbed it is being returned to the intestinal lumen as bile acids, the end products of its metabolism, or in the form of cholesterol esters from desquamated intestinal cells (Thomson and Dietschy, 1981). However, Goodman and Noble (1968) calculated that 34 to 63 percent of dietary cholesterol was absorbed by the subjects they studied.

How cholesterol enters the mucosal cell is not clear. It appears likely that the involvement of cholesterol in a bile salt micelle is required for the initial transfer of free cholesterol into the mucosal cell (Treadwell and Vahouny, 1968). It has been postulated that entry is through solution in the lipid portion of the membrane. It also has been suggested that the cholesterol in micellar form in the lumen is transferred to a mucoprotein carrier on the cell surface (Green, 1963).

Cholesterol absorption occurs primarily in the jejunum (Arnesjo et al., 1969). Cholesterol is absorbed much more readily than plant sterols. It had been believed that plant sterols were not absorbed and that they, in fact, blocked the absorption of cholesterol (Blomstrand and Ahrens, 1958). This block in absorption was attributed to competition for a carrier and the ingestion of plant sterols was recommended in order to reduce the quantity of cholesterol absorbed. However, it has been shown that the phytosterols that occur in plants can be absorbed by the same mechanism and influenced by the same factors as cholesterol but that the quantity absorbed is considerably less (Swell et al., 1959a; 1959b). From a study on humans, Grundy et al. (1969) concluded that with large doses of plant sterols absorption of both endogenous and exogenous cholesterol was impaired, and this was reflected in increased fecal excretion. Whether the decreased absorption was due to competitive inhibition of absorption, esterification, or micelle formation was not clear. However, when reabsorption was diminished by feeding plant sterols, cholesterol synthesis increased.

Within the intestinal cell cholesterol enters a pool of free cholesterol. Cholesterol from this pool is withdrawn and reesterification of cholesterol occurs. This reaction can be catalyzed by either acyl-CoA-cholesterol acyltransferase (ACAT) (Haugen and Norum, 1976) or mucosal cholesterol esterase (Hernandez et al., 1955). Movement through the cell is slow. It has been suggested that cholesterol may enter the triacylglycerol droplets in the cell and leave with the triacylglycerols to enter the lymph (Wilson, 1962). The major portion of cholesterol in the lymph is esterified with fatty acids that are apparently drawn from pools of fatty acids derived from both exogenous and endogenous sources. The absorption of cholesterol is, therefore, intimately related to and possibly dependent on the concurrent absorption of fats. Fig. 6.12 illustrates the degree of synchronization required to bring lipids, including cholesterol and cholesterol esters, from the lumen of the intestinal tract to the point of incorporation into chylomicrons which leave the cell for transit to the lymph.

For comprehensive accounts of lipid absorption, see Brindley (1974), Borgström (1974), Thomson and Dietschy (1981), Carey et al. (1983).

Protein Absorption

Of the total protein in the intestinal lumen, a relatively small part is derived from the ingested food; the major portion is derived from endogenous sources: digestive secretions and desquamated cells. The digestive secretions in humans can contribute from 60 to 260 gm protein/24 hr as calculated by Nasset (1965). In addition, Nasset estimates that 90 gm protein/day are released into the lumen by desquamated cells. In a feeding experiment using labeled protein it was found that the endogenous protein diluted that obtained from food by approximately sevenfold (Nasset and Ju, 1961), but more recent estimates tend to be smaller (Nixon and Mawer, 1970a; 1970b; Johansson, 1975). However, since only 1 to 2 gm of fecal nitrogen (6 to 12 gm protein) are excreted per day, it is apparent that digestion and absorption of both exogenous and endogenous protein is extremely efficient. (See Freeman and Kim, 1978.)

The passage of intact protein molecules across the intestinal mucosa of adult animals is insignificant, but it does occur. In humans, intact protein absorption may produce allergic reactions in sensitive individuals. However, in newborn mammals, the transfer of protein by pinocytosis (Clark, 1959) during the first hours or days of life performs an extremely important function. Since the fetal mammal does not synthesize its own antibodies and is, therefore, born practically devoid of gamma globulins, the absorption of these intact proteins carried by the colostrum allows the newborn in some species—but probably not in humans—to obtain passive immunity from the mother. For reasons not understood, the intestinal mucosa loses this capacity to absorb protein by the time milk proteins are ingested, at which time the gamma globulin concentration equals the adult level. Payne

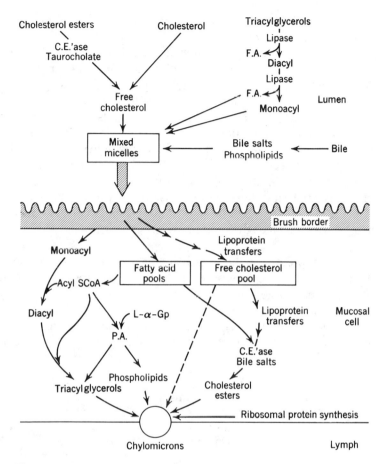

Figure 6.12
Mechanism of cholesterol absorption. C.E.'ase, cholesterol esterase; F.A., fatty acids; Diacyl, diacylglycerols, Monoacyl, monoacylgly-cerols; L-α-GP, L-α-glycerophosphate; P.A., phosphatidic acid. (From C. R. Treadwell and G. V. Vahouny, *Handbook of Physiology*, Section 6, Vol. 3, American Physiological Society, Washington, D.C., 1968, p. 1432.)

and Marsh (1962), administering fluorescein-labeled gamma globulins to the newborn pig, showed that the intestinal cells absorbed the gamma globulin until they became so packed that the nuclei were pushed aside. When the cells apparently could take in no more, the gamma globulin passed into the lymphatics. This ability to absorb intact protein ceased when the microvilli of the epithelial cells were exposed to a yet-to-be identified protein contained in milk. In humans and other primates, passive immunity at birth is the result of placental transfer of maternal antibodies, and the transfer of passive immunity by absorption of intact gamma globulin from colostrum is probably negligible. (See Morris, 1968.)

Amino Acids.   Amino acid absorption is rapid and active. It has been established by a long series of studies, reviewed by Wilson (1962) and Schultz and Frizzell (1975), that the interaction of an amino acid with its carrier depends on the following criteria: optical specificity (the D-stereoisomer does not appear to be transported actively); an intact α-carboxyl group; an α-amino group; an α-hydrogen; pyridoxal phosphate; and solubility of the side chain in the lipid-rich membrane of the mucosal cells. Wilson (1962) suggests that the solubility of the side chain in the lipid-rich membrane is decisive in permitting the carboxyl group, amino group, and α-hydrogen to gain access to the active site of the carrier. In a study of neutral amino acids that inhibit valine absorption by rat intestine, those with very lipophilic side chains had a greater effect than did those amino acids that were poorly lipophilic (Reiser and Christensen, 1965). This may be related to the findings of Imami et al. (1970) that vitamin E is specifically concerned with the transport of valine across the membrane of the intestinal mucosal cells in the rat.

Separate carriers present in the microvillus membrane are responsible for the active transport of four specific groups of amino acids across the membrane and into the mucosa cell (Table 6.6).

Competition among the groups of amino acids for the shared transporting mechanism is on a "first come, first served" basis. The relative absorption rates of the eight essential amino acids have been studied in humans using a perfusion tech-

TABLE 6.6
Intestinal Amino Acid Transport Mechanisms

Type	Amino Acids Transported	Type of Transport	Relative Rate
Neutral (monoamino-monocarboxylic)	Aromatic (tyrosine, tryptophan, phenylalanine Aliphatic (glycine[a], alanine, serine, threonine, valine, leucine, isoleucine) Methionine, histidine, glutamine, asparagine, cysteine	Active, Na^+-dependent	Very rapid
Dibasic (diamino)	Lysine, arginine, ornithine, cystine	Active, partially Na^+-dependent	Rapid (10% of neutral)
Dicarboxylic (acidic)	Glutamic acid, aspartic acid	Carrier-mediated, active, partially Na^+-dependent	Rapid
Imino acids and glycine	Proline, hydroxyproline, glycine[a]	Active, ?Na^+-dependent	Slow

Source: From G. M. Gray and H. L. Cooper, *Gastroenterology* 61:540 (1971).
[a]Shares both the neutral and imino mechanism with low affinity for the neutral.

nique (Adibi and Gray, 1967). A consistent sequence was observed in the way the amino acids were absorbed from the mixture indicating a specific affinity of each amino acid for the transport mechanism as well as competition among them for the carrier. Supportive data based on *in vitro* work with rat intestine indicate that methionine, isoleucine, leucine, and valine have the greatest affinity for their carrier and were most rapidly bound; threonine had the lowest affinity and was the slowest to be absorbed. From these data it is assumed that methionine and branched-chain amino acids, having highest affinity for carriers, would therefore have the greatest rates of absorption and would inhibit transport of the amino acids having lower affinities.

The basic amino acids lysine, arginine, and ornithine share a carrier system with cystine and are transported at a rate that is one-tenth to one-twentieth the rate for glycine and alanine (Wiseman, 1956). This difference may be explained, in part, by their charge which causes basic amino acids to be transported against the electrical gradient.

Information concerning the common carrier for basic amino acids was revealed when it was shown that the genetic defect that led to cystinuria prevented the absorption from the intestine of lysine and ornithine as well as cystine (Milne et al., 1961). It was later shown that arginine absorption was also reduced in cystinurics (Asatoor et al., 1962). Apparently a similar carrier is present in both the kidneys and the intestines for these amino acids. The defect in the intestinal carrier is of doubtful clinical importance since absorption abnormalities become apparent only when the affected amino acids are presented for absorption in the free form. However, the defect in renal absorption in cystinurics involving the same carrier protein is clinically important (Milne, 1968).

The mechanism of glutamic and aspartic acid absorption is still not entirely clear. It had been suggested that these were not actively transported since relatively small amounts were recoverable in the portal blood after feeding. However, Neame and Wiseman (1957) have shown in dogs that introduction of glutamic acid into the lumen resulted in an increase in alanine in the blood rather than glutamic acid. Transamination during glutamic acid absorption also has been demonstrated for the cat and rabbit (Neame and Wiseman, 1958) and the rat (Peraino and Harper, 1962).

The transport system for imino acids originally described as specific for proline, hydroxyproline, and N-methylated glycines now includes β-alanine, D-alanine, betaine, γ-aminobutyric acid, and taurine. Proline and hydroxyproline can be absorbed by the neutral amino acid pathway, but Wilson (1962) suggests that competition for the neutral amino acid carrier might lead to their exclusion and that the imino acid transport system is the one normally used by these two amino acids.

The absorption of amino acids is coupled with Na^+ absorption and is energy-dependent. The dependence of amino acid transport on Na^+, shown for the entry of glycine into the ascites tumor cell (Kromphardt et al., 1963), suggests a direct interaction of Na^+ with the substrate carrier. This effect of Na^+ on glycine uptake was further demonstrated by Vidaver (1964a; 1964b; 1964c), who showed that the interaction was similar to that observed for sugar in the intestine. The absorption of L-alanine *in vivo* in the dog reported by Fleshler and Nelson (1970) depended on the associated movement of Na^+ from the blood to the gut lumen. The dependency of L-alanine absorption on Na^+ transport operated over a wide range and was observed even when the concentrations of L-alanine were higher than blood levels. Curran et al. (1970) demonstrated that the unidirectional Na^+ flux from mucosal solution into the cell was increased in the presence of L-alanine and was related to the unidirectional influx of the L-alanine into the cell. These workers suggested that the effect of L-alanine in stimulating Na^+ transport was the result of an interaction at the mucosal border of the cell leading to an increased rate of Na^+ entrance into the intestinal cell.

Pyridoxal appears to play a part in the uptake of amino acids by intestinal cells but the way in which it augments amino acid absorption is not known. Christensen (1962) suggests that perhaps pyridoxal decreases loss of amino acids from cells by altering membrane permeability, but Asatoor et al. (1972) suggest that pyridoxal is more likely to affect the exit of amino acids from the mucosal cells rather than their entrance.

For further details on amino acid absorption, see Wiseman (1974) and Munck (1981).

Peptides.   Until the 1960s it was generally accepted that complete hydrolysis of protein to its constituent amino acids occurred in the intestinal lumen and that only free amino acids were taken up by the mucosal cell. Toward the end of that decade mucosal uptake of dipeptides followed by intracellular hydrolysis was reported for rats (Matthews et al., 1968) and for humans (Adibi and Phillips, 1968). These reports soon were followed by observations on the uptake of tri-peptides (Adibi et al., 1975) and the probable inability to absorb tetrapeptides (Adibi and Morse, 1977). Early observations that amino acid absorption from peptides was more rapid than from equivalent mixtures of free amino acids have been confirmed for most di- and tripeptides that have been studied (Adibi and Mercer, 1973; Chung et al., 1979). It now seems evident that protein hydrolyzed to the di- and tripeptide stages are the major candidates for absorption by the intestinal mucosal cells. The isolation of a dipeptidase with broad specificity (Das and Radhakrishnan, 1973; Noren et al., 1973) and an aminotripeptidase (Dou-meng and Maroux, 1979) from the cytoplasmic fraction of intestinal mucosal cells indicates that the final steps in peptide hydrolysis occur inside the cell because protein digestion products leave the mucosal cell for entry into the portal blood almost entirely as free amino acids. However, there is some evidence of absorption of unhydrolyzed dipeptides in portal blood in animals (Sleisenger et al., 1977) and in humans (Adibi, 1971), and peptide hydrolase has been found in the cytoplasm of various tissues of rats (Krzysik and Adibi, 1977).

Two genetic diseases, Hartnup disease and cystinuria have contributed signif-icantly to the understanding of peptide and amino acid absorption. In individuals with Hartnup disease there is a defect in the ability to transport free neutral amino acids; cystinurics, as noted above, have reduced capacity to absorb dibasic amino acids and cystine. Despite these defects in transporting even essential amino acids such individuals show no evidence of protein malnutrition (Milne, 1964). Studies on patients with these genetic defects showed clearly that despite the inability to absorb specific free amino acids, there was no interference with their absorption when they were presented in the form of dipeptides (Asatoor et al., 1970; 1971; Leonard et al., 1976). These studies show clearly that the absorption of peptides and amino acids occurs independently of each other in humans. Additional evidence that the two mechanisms are separate comes from the location of sites of maximal absorption which for peptides is more likely to be the jejunum and for free amino acids, the ileum. This difference appears to be true for both humans (Silk et al., 1974) and experimental animals (Crampton et al., 1973; Heading et al., 1977).

As in all carrier-mediated transport, factors related to the molecular structure of the peptide are crucial. The factors affecting the interaction of peptides with

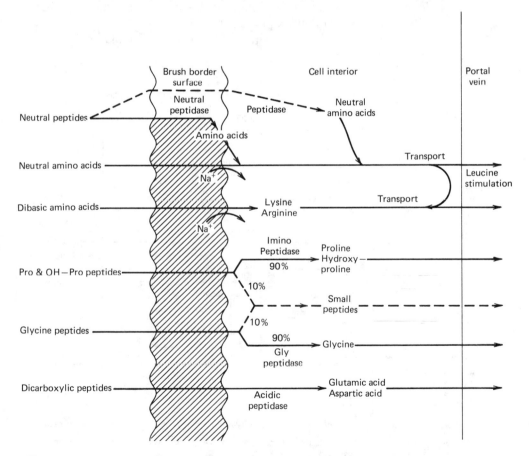

Figure 6.13
Outline of the major routes of oligopeptide and amino acid entry into the intestinal cell. The peptides probably average three to four amino acid residues. Proline (Pro), Glycine (Gly). (From G. M. Gray and M. L. Cooper, *Gastroenterology* 61:540, 1971.)

their carriers are (1) stereoisomerism, (2) length of the side chain, (3) substitutions on N- and C- terminals, and (4) the number of amino acid residues. (See Adibi and Kim, 1981.)

The evidence appears quite clear that there is a single carrier system for dipeptides in both human and monkey intestine (Das and Radhakrishnan, 1973) and that, in contrast to amino acids, neutral, basic, and acidic dipeptides share the carrier system (Fig. 6.13). The carrier system appears to be Na^+-dependent (Addison et al., 1972) although there is also evidence that an appreciable amount of dipeptide uptake may be independent of Na^+ (Matthews et al., 1974). In studies with human subjects, dipeptides added to the perfusion solution greatly enhanced the absorption of Na^+ from the jejunum (Silk et al., 1975). Whether or not there is a direct link between Na^+ and peptide absorption requires further study, especially since results of *in vivo* and *in vitro* experiments vary.

For detailed reviews of intestinal absorption of peptides, see Matthews (1975a; 1975b), Silk (1980), and Adibi and Kim (1981).

Figure 6.14 presents a summary of the role of the gastrointestinal tract in amino acid metabolism.

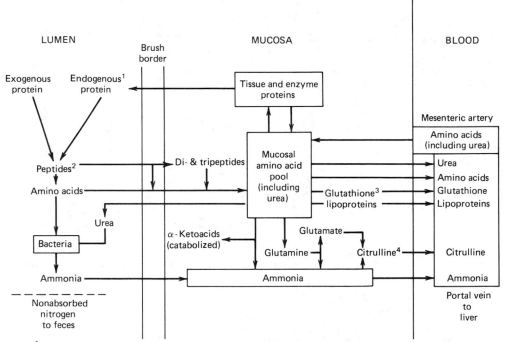

[1] Includes gastric and pancreatic enzymes. Not necessarily absorbed in same region as exogenous protein.

[2] Only di- and tripeptides are absorbed. Brush border peptidases and cytoplasmic peptidases are both involved in the hydrolysis of peptides to amino acids.

[3] Major role of glutathione in mucosa may be in amino acid transport.

[4] Several steps involved in synthesis.

Figure 6.14
Role of the gastrointestinal tract in amino acid metabolism. (Courtesy of Dr. Peter Pellett.)

Nucleic Acid Absorption

Nucleic acids are almost completely absorbed from the small intestine after being split to the free base or only partially fragmented to nucleotides or nucleosides. According to Wilson and Wilson (1958) nucleotides can be split in the intestinal mucosal cell to nucleosides, which then pass through the serosal side of the cell by diffusion.

Water-Soluble Vitamin Absorption

Although chemically diverse, most water-soluble vitamins are of relatively low molecular weight and, except for vitamin B_{12}, all are readily absorbed. Until recently the mechanism involved was assumed, in most instances, to be simple diffusion. However, evidence has been appearing in the literature that suggests that probably more of the water-soluble vitamins attain passage through the intestinal mucosal cell via energy-dependent and carrier-mediated transport systems than by passive diffusion.

Ascorbic Acid.   Spencer et al. (1963) studied ascorbic acid absorption in the rat and hamster and reported that absorption occurred by passive diffusion. This was generally accepted as a model for other species. However, Stevenson and Brush (1969) pointed out that the rat and hamster do not have an ascorbic acid requirement whereas guinea pigs, humans, and other primates do. They hypotheiszed that the mode of intestinal absorption of ascorbic acid in a given species would reflect the presence or absence of a dietary requirement. Therefore, they chose the guinea pig for study and did indeed find that ascorbic acid transport had the characteristics of a Na^+-dependent, gradient-coupled carrier mechanism that was located in the distal region of the small intestine. They noted further that it was ascorbic acid that was involved in the active transport system and that if dehydroascorbic acid entered the epithelial cell its absorption rate was very low. Since they were unable to demonstrate a similar active transport system in the rat, they suggested that a species-specific transport mechanism for ascorbic acid is related to a species-specific nutrient requirement.

Absorption of ascorbic acid occurs also by simple diffusion but the rate is low and may be of significance only when the concentration of ascorbic acid in the lumen is very high (Mellors et al., 1977). Since the maximal absorption of ascorbic acid is dependent on the availability of the carrier and since the rate of absorption through simple diffusion is relatively low, the absorption of extremely high intakes is probably inefficient. (See Rose, 1980; 1981.)

Thiamin.   The absorption of thiamin is rapid and largely from the proximal small intestine. Since the absorptive capacity for thiamin in humans is very restricted, amounting to only a few milligrams per dose, it was attributed to a special mechanism (Morrison and Campbell, 1960). *In vivo* data from chicks, in which intestinal loops and a thiamin antagonist were used, suggested that thiamin uptake was an active process superimposed on some passive absorption (Polin et al., 1963). Studies on everted sacs in rats demonstrated a net transport of thiamin against a concentration gradient with the serosal concentration increasing up to

2.1 times the initial concentration (Ventura and Rindi, 1965). Both metabolic inhibitors and reductions in incubation temperatures depressed serosal accumulation of thiamin, supporting the conclusion that an active transport mechanism was operating. Pyrithiamin was shown to inhibit uphill transport of thiamin whereas oxythiamin did not. Since pyrithiamin but not oxythiamin is a potent inhibitor of thiamin phosphorylase from rat intestine, it was concluded that phosphorylation is the basic mechanism of intestinal uphill transport of thiamin (Ventura and Rindi, 1965). Although the exact relationship between phosphorylation of thiamin and its intestinal transport was not established, it was assumed to be the primary mechanism for absorption (Rindi et al., 1966).

When an increase in thiamin intake above 10 mg did not significantly increase its level in the blood or urine, Thomson et al. (1971) concluded that intestinal transport of thiamin involved a rate-limiting process. The maximum absorption of thiamin in a normal man after a single 20 mg dose was found to be approximately 8 mg (Thomson and Leevy, 1972). However, it was not the phosphorylation step that was the rate-limiting one (Thomson et al., 1971). Evidence obtained from *in vivo* and *in vitro* studies in rats showed that thiamin absorption is a saturable process inhibited by inhibitors of $Na^+,K^+ATPase$ and by a lack of sodium (Hoyumpa et al., 1975a). It appears, therefore, that thiamin absorption, like that of glucose, amino acids, and other nutrients, is by a carrier linked to sodium transport, and this is the mechanism of absorption when concentrations in the lumen are low. However, as with ascorbic acid, passive absorption takes place when concentrations in the lumen are high.

Alcoholics frequently exhibit a marked reduction in thiamin absorption (Leevy and Baker, 1968). Thomson et al. (1970) found that thiamin absorption in malnourished alcoholics was one-third that of normal volunteers after a 20 mg dose but returned to normal following nutritional improvement or abstention from alcohol. These investigators (Thomson and Leevy, 1972) suggested that the decrease in thiamin absorption in alcoholic patients could be due to a decrease in the number of available receptor sites. However, *in vitro* studies using everted jejunal sacs from rat intestine showed that it was not the mucosal uptake of thiamin that was depressed by alcohol but the transfer through the serosal membrane, and that this inhibition occurred when the concentrations of thiamin were low (Hoyumpa et al., 1975b). Since similar results were obtained with inhibitors of both $Na^+,K^+ATPase$ and sodium transport, it appears that alcohol interferes with the $Na^+,K^+ATPase$ pump which is involved in the transport of thiamin through the basolateral membrane of the mucosal cell.

Riboflavin. According to Spencer and Zamchek (1961) riboflavin absorption occurs through passive diffusion in the proximal part of the small intestine. This study was carried out using the everted sac technique in the rat and hamster. In studies of riboflavin and riboflavin-5'-phosphate (flavin monophosphate, FMN) absorption, it was found that absorption took place only in the proximal small intestine and that the site could be saturated (Levy and Jusko, 1966; Jusko and Levy, 1970). Extensive evidence has been presented that FMN is rapidly and almost completely dephosphorylated to free riboflavin in the small intestine (Jusko and Levy, 1967). A specialized transport process involves subsequent rephos- phorylation of riboflavin to FMN in the intestinal wall (Jusko and Levy, 1967). An apparent conflict exists when it is suggested that riboflavin absorption is carried out by simple diffusion (Spencer and Zamchek, 1961) and requires phosphory- lation (Jusko and Levy, 1967), since phosphorylation of riboflavin to FMN requires ATP. One wonders whether the specialized transport process may indeed be energy-requiring. In addition, riboflavin absorption is decreased when sodium is lacking which suggests the involvement of a sodium-mediated, energy-requiring transport system.

In a study on humans ranging in age from 0.25 to 40 years, Jusko et al. (1970) observed increased absorption with increased age when FMN was administered orally. The authors suggested that retention of the vitamin at intestinal absorption sites was responsible but indicated that secretions, motility, and length of the intestine might also be involved in the increase in riboflavin absorption with age. Although the dephosphorylation rate was ruled out since phosphatase decreases rather than increases with age, no mention was made of the possibility that retention of the vitamin might be due to the increased number of absorption sites or, perhaps, to an increased rephosphorylation rate with age. Further work is needed to clarify the mechanism.

Niacin.   Absorption of niacin is diminished under sodium-free conditions which suggests an energy-requiring mechanism. This limited evidence is in contrast to the general assumption that niacin is absorbed by passive diffusion. However, active transport at low concentrations may be obscured by passive transport which occurs at higher and the more usual concentrations.

Pyridoxine.   The absorption of pyridoxine was investigated by Booth and Brain (1962) using tritium-labeled pyridoxine hydrochloride. Absorption was remark- ably rapid in the rat and occurred primarily in the jejunum although some ab- sorption also took place in the ileum. The criteria for passive diffusion were that absorption of the oral dose was in the proximal part of the intestine and that the site of absorption was independent of the dose given. It was concluded, therefore, that pyridoxine absorption occurred by passive diffusion. In a study on humans using tritiated pyridoxine (Brain and Booth, 1964), absorption was maximal be- tween 60 and 90 minutes. There was no effect on the amount of pyridoxine absorbed in conditions that contributed to malabsorption, such as steatorrhea or resection of major sections of the small intestine. Again, it was concluded that passive diffusion accounted for pyridoxine absorption.

Pyridoxine appears to be bound in blood or tissues after transport through the mucosa thereby reducing the free concentration of the vitamin in the lumen. As a result, the concentration gradient favors an increased rate of passive diffusion (Hamm et al., 1979; Mehansho et al., 1979). The binding and chemical tran- formations associated with pyridoxine absorption have complicated study of the mechanisms involved. However, in contrast to most other water-soluble vitamins for which recent evidence indicates active transport, the evidence that pyridoxine is transported from the intestinal lumen to the blood by passive diffusion remains strong.

Folacin. The primary site for the absorption of folacin is the proximal portion of the small intestine (Hepner et al., 1968) and at a location more distal than pyridoxine (Booth, 1968). Most naturally occurring folates found in food are in the form of polyglutamates but only monoglutamates are detected in the serum. It was concluded, therefore, that the polyglutamates must be deconjugated before absorption takes place (Rosenberg et al., 1969; Bernstein et al., 1970). In a series of studies on dogs, in which folic acid conjugates with side chains of varying lengths were used, it was shown that the intestinal mucosa was capable of absorbing the diglutamate as well as the monoglutamate (Baugh et al., 1971), and that the rate of absorption was inversely proportional to the length of the γ-glutamyl side chain. However, Butterworth et al. (1969) administered labeled synthetic folates orally to human subjects and found that only the monoglutamate was absorbed.

Whether the enzymatic deconjugation of the polyglutamates takes place in the mucosal membrane or within the cell remains controversial. Guinea pig mucosa contains a high concentration of a pteroylpolyglutamate hydrolase (folate conjugase) (Hoffbrand and Peters, 1969) and *in vitro* studies by Halstead et al. (1976) indicate the enzyme is located within the mucosal cell. According to Reisenauer et al. (1977), a folate conjugase is present in the brush border as well as within the cell, and the two enzymes have different characteristics.

Some reports on folacin absorption suggested passive diffusion (Turner and Hughes, 1962) and others suggested active transport (Herbert and Shapiro, 1962; Cohen et al., 1964). A more recent report (Rose et al., 1978) provides evidence that folacin is absorbed through the brush border by a sodium-dependent saturable carrier mechanism (Fig. 6.15), similar to that for ascorbic acid.

Another point of controversy is whether folic acid is absorbed unchanged as suggested by some (Baugh et al., 1971; Melikian et al., 1971) or whether it is methylated in the intestinal mucosa (Chanarin and Perry, 1969). As so often happens, the conditions of the experiments produced the contradictory results. Oral doses ranging from 0.5 to 3 mg of folic acid appeared in human portal blood unchanged (Melikian et al., 1971), but with lower concentrations used in *in vitro* preparations folic acid was reduced and methylated during absorption (Olinger et al., 1973). These controversial findings emphasize that divergent results can be obtained when testing under physiologic and unphysiologic conditions.

Folate deficiency has been observed in women taking oral contraceptives (Shojania et al., 1968). In a clinical study, Strieff (1970) found that absorption of polyglutamates was decreased by 50 percent when oral contraceptives were used. Similar findings were reported by Necheles and Snyder (1970). Strieff (1970) concluded that interference by oral contraceptives probably occurred at the step of enzymatic deconjugation through inhibition of folate conjugase. The chance of folate deficiency developing when the folate intake is low should not be over-

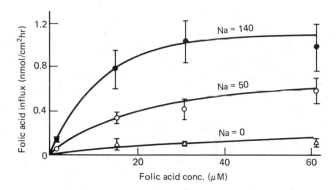

Figure 6.15
Folic acid influx into mammalian small intestine at three
Na concentrations. Each bracket is mean ± SE of at least
four influx determinations. (From R. Rose et al., *Am. J.
Physiol.* 235:E678, 1978.)

looked and could be of particular concern in malnourished populations in developing countries.

Reports on the effects of oral contraceptives on folate absorption are controversial and it appears that much work remains to be done before a clearer understanding of the mechanisms is obtained. For a review of the effects of oral contraceptives on nutrient absorption, see Rose (1978). For comprehensive reviews of folate absorption in man, see Rosenberg (1981).

Vitamin B_{12}. The absorption of vitamin B_{12} is unique and, despite extensive study, some of its aspects remain obscure. Vitamin B_{12} is the largest and most complex of the B vitamins and for the absorption of microgram quantities of this large molecule the presence of a still larger molecule, gastric intrinsic factor (IF), is required.

The chemistry of IF has been studied intensively and a highly purified form has been prepared that is active at a dose as small as 50 μg, one-millionth the dose of 40 years ago. IF is a glycoprotein with a ratio of protein to carbohydrate of 3:2 (Highly et al., 1967), and with a molecular weight of approximately 50,000 (Gräsbeck et al., 1966). The polysaccharide moiety contains up to 5 percent fucose and 10 percent hexosamine and hexoses. Neuraminic acid is also present. The chemical characteristics of IF are closely related to those of the mucopolysaccharides forming the cell coat (see Chapter 9), and this is interesting in light of the function of IF in absorption. The specific affinity of IF-B_{12} for the absorption site suggests that the binding forces are similar to those concerned in antigen-antibody reactions. Many excellent review articles on both the historical and current aspects of IF are available (Herbert and Castle, 1964; Castle, 1968; Glass, 1974; Jacob et al., 1980).

It is generally acknowledged that IF is secreted by the cells in the fundic region of the stomach. In the rat and mouse the chief or pepsinogen-secreting cells appear to be responsible for the secretion of IF, whereas in human preparations the parietal or acid-secreting cells are responsible (Hoedemaker et al., 1964). The IF secreted into the stomach binds with vitamin B_{12}, part of which is released from food by cooking and part of which enters the stomach bound to animal protein and then is released in the acid medium of the stomach by gastric protease (Abels and Schilling, 1964).

The binding capacity of IF for vitamin B_{12} is its unique biological property and is related to the absorption of the vitamin. The nature of the bond or bonds between the two molecules, or the bonding sites, remains unclear. Once binding has taken place, however, advantages accrue to each molecule: the thermolability of IF and its sensitivity to proteolytic enzymes is abolished; and vitamin B_{12} is protected from intestinal microflora in its passage to receptor sites in the ileum.

The pancreas has been implicated in the protection and maintenance of the IF-B_{12} complex in a form available for absorption. Toskes et al. (1971) found that vitamin B_{12} malabsorption which accompanied pancreatic insufficiency was corrected by administration of pancreatic extract. In a subsequent study employing partially depancreatized rats as an animal model (Toskes and Deren, 1972), vitamin B_{12} absorption was found to be defective but could be corrected by the administration of pancreatic extract. The authors postulated that the pancreatic extract either protected the complex or blocked an inhibitor of complex formation.

The site for passage through the mucosa has been determined in the human, monkey, rat, dog, and other animals. The absorption of vitamin B_{12} by the ileal cells was established (Booth and Mollin, 1959), and transplant experiments demonstrated that the absorptive capacity is due to specific characteristics of these cells rather than to their distal location in the tract (Drapenas et al., 1963). Histochemical staining of the ileal cells has shown high concentrations of certain enzymes on the mucosal surface (Wilson, 1962). The specific receptor sites postulated by Abels et al. (1959) and Herbert (1958) were shown to be on the microvilli or brush border of the ileal mucosal cells (Donaldson et al., 1967; Rothenberg, 1968; MacKenzie et al., 1968).

The attachment of IF-B_{12} complex to the ileal cell surface does not appear to be an energy-requiring process since it occurs almost immediately and is not affected by oxygen or temperature (Donaldson et al., 1967). It seems, therefore, that the process is one of physical adsorption. The receptor site for the complex, like IF itself, probably is a glycoprotein or a mucopolysaccharide. This is consistent with both the location of the site on the microvillus surface and with the character of the attachment that probably takes place (MacKenzie and Donaldson, 1969). Studies on both everted sacs and ileal homogenates (Herbert, 1959; Herbert et al., 1964) demonstrated that, in the presence of Ca^{++} and a pH in the neutral to slightly alkaline range, the IF-B_{12} complex attaches to the receptor sites on the surface of the ileal mucosal membrane (Fig. 6.16). It appears that the IF molecule has different binding sites for vitamin B_{12} and Ca^{++} since the initial complexing of IF and B_{12} does not require Ca^{++} but the attachment of the complex to the receptor does (Castle, 1968). A proper fit into the receptor site appears to require

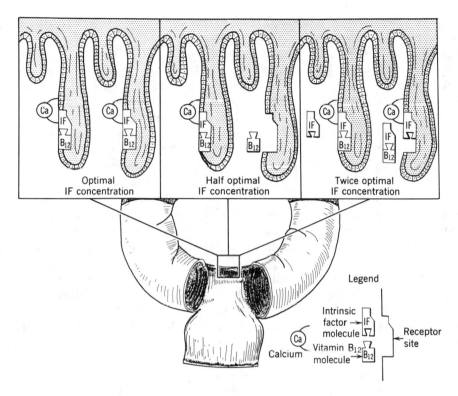

Figure 6.16
Mechanism of vitamin B_{12} absorption and intrinsic factor action. (From V. Hebert et al., *Medicine* 43:679, 1964.)

the prior complexing of IF with vitamin B_{12}. The receptor sites have little or no affinity for the free vitamin and insufficient quantity of IF leads to inadequate B_{12} absorption. However, if excessive quantities of IF are present in the lumen, some IF molecules may attach to receptor sites without the vitamin, thereby blocking receptor sites for the IF-B_{12} complex.

How the vitamin B_{12} molecule progresses from the receptor site through the cell and into the circulation is not known. The location of receptor sites on the microvilli suggested to some that the mode of entrance of vitamin B_{12} into the cell is by pinocytosis, especially if entry occurs as the large IF-B_{12} complex (Abels et al., 1959; Wison, 1963). This, however, is purely speculative since there is no experimental evidence to support it.

If pinocytosis were the means of entry, the need for Ca^{++} would be clearer since Ca^{++} is required in other systems for pinocytosis to take place (Brandt and Freeman, 1967). Adsorption of the complex to the cell surface in the presence of Ca^{++} presumably would initiate the pinocytosis (MacKenzie and Donaldson, 1969). Gräsbeck (1967) suggested that the receptor site in the mucosa is part of a carrier that becomes complete and operative when the IF-B_{12} complex is attached to it. The complex in that way is transported through the membrane and into the cell.

If the vitamin B_{12} is absorbed alone, there must be a system at the receptor site that releases the vitamin from the complex for entrance into the cell. Herbert et al. (1964) suggested that a "releasing factor" probably exists. Such a factor may be specific for IF or it may be nonspecific acting on mucoproteins and mucopolysaccharides. Its postulated action is to split IF-B_{12} complex so that vitamin B_{12} can enter the cell and leave the IF behind. A "releasing factor" has been found in fish tapeworm. Infestation with fish tapeworm is reported to be common in Finland and when present produces a vitamin B_{12} deficiency (Nyberg, 1960). By releasing the vitamin B_{12} from the IF-B_{12} complex in the intestinal tract, the tapeworm ungraciously grabs the vitamin, and the host eventually develops a vitamin B_{12} deficiency and probably a variety of other nutrient deficiencies. For species other than tapeworms, however, there is no evidence for a "releasing factor."

Another intriguing suggestion for the entry of vitamin B_{12} into the mucosal cell has been offered by MacKenzie and Donaldson (1969) with the admission that there were no relevant experimental data to support it. They suggest that the IF-B_{12} complex on the surface of the cell might be digested to yield a small cobalt-containing "active fragment" of the vitamin that would readily pass through the microvillus membrane. The complete vitamin B_{12} molecule would then be resynthesized within the cell from the absorbed precursor in a manner analogous to the hydrolysis and resynthesis of triacylglycerols during lipid absorption.

Whatever the mechanism, there are just two choices: either the entire IF-B_{12} complex enters the cell, or the complex is split and vitamin B_{12} enters alone. If the complex enters the cell, there are again two choices: either the complex is split in the cell and vitamin B_{12} leaves alone, or the entire IF-B_{12} complex passes into the circulation. A molecule as large as IF-B_{12} would surely have to leave the cell via the lymphatics, but 95 percent of absorbed vitamin B_{12} has been shown to leave the mucosa via the portal vein and no IF has been found there (Boass and Wilson, 1964). It must be assumed, therefore, that IF is left behind, either at the mucosal barrier or in the cell. Regardless of whether the vitamin B_{12} is liberated before or after the complex enters the cell, once within the cell the vitamin combines with cell protein and is transported slowly across the cell for passage into both the blood and lymph. The vitamin B_{12}-binding protein in plasma, transcobalamin II, is an α_1-globulin, and it is in this form that the vitamin is transported perhaps in a manner analogous to the transport of iron as transferrin (Herbert et al., 1964).

It is apparent that many questions remain to be answered about the complex mechanism of vitamin B_{12} absorption. The unique gastric secretion responsible for delivering minute quantities of the vitamin to the absorption site has certain characteristics that invite speculation about the mechanism. IF chemically resembles the "fuzz" or cell coat that is mucopolysaccharide or mucopolypeptide material synthesized within the cell and extruded to its surface. (See Chapter 12.)

Particular carbohydrate groups in the cell coat function in recognition and adhesion, in selective passage through the membrane, and in provision of specific receptor sites. If the information carried by some proteins is enhanced by the addition of particular carbohydrate chains that confer different types of specificity, Whaley et al. (1972) suggest that such carbohydrate-containing materials on the surface of the cell would have particular informational characteristics that are capable of influencing a wide range of cellular activities. This concept, carried one step further, suggests the possibility of a "detachable" or "shuttle" form of cell coat synthesized and extruded by cells in the gastric mucosa. This cell coat recognizes and adheres to the surface of the ingested vitamin B_{12} molecule, and the IF-B_{12} complex detaches from the rest of the cell coat. The complex travels to the ileum where it recognizes specific receptor sites in the coat of the ileal cells, perhaps as an antibody recognizes an antigen, and adhesion takes place. Selective passage through the membrane follows. Simplistic? Perhaps. But often, and probably unavoidably, attempts to unravel a mechanism produce unnecessary and tangential complexities. The classic simplicity and elegance of many physiological phenomena become apparent only much later in time when conjecture yields to fact. The hypothesis we propose is entertaining, but we recall that the late A.J. Carlson of the University of Chicago warned his students that it was all right to entertain an hypothesis as long as the hypothesis doesn't entertain you.

For additional insight into the mechanism of vitamin B_{12} absorption, see Matthews (1974); Jacob et al. (1980).

Myoinositol.   The absorption of myoinositol from segments of hamster small intestine fulfills all the current criteria of active absorption: accumulation against a concentration gradient, energy-dependence, Na^+-dependence, and phlorizin sensitivity (Caspary and Crane, 1970). Phlorizin, a potent inhibitor of sugar entry into the cell (Lotspeich and Wheeler, 1962), acts at a superficial level in the mucosa (Parsons et al., 1958). It was shown to be a strictly competitive inhibitor for the sugar substrates (Alvarado and Crane, 1962) and was also shown to interact competitively with the myoinositol binding site (Caspary and Crane, 1970). However, the affinity for the myoinositol site was 10- to 100-fold less than it was for the common sugar-binding site. The pathway for myoinositol to cross into the mucosal cell was not the same as D-glucose but there was an interaction between the two at the level of translocation.

Whether the water-soluble vitamins or vitaminlike substances not discussed are absorbed by mechanisms other than simple diffusion is a moot question. Convincing evidence, as yet, is not available.

Fat-Soluble Vitamin Absorption
The fat-soluble vitamins are usually associated with the other lipids in the diet. Their absorption is assumed to depend on those conditions that favor lipid absorption, including the presence of bile. Only recently have some of the mechanisms of absorption become clear and, as is usually the case, the unraveling of the mechanisms illumined some links between the fat-soluble vitamins and other

nutrients. Relationships that had been the subjects of conjecture can now be explained on a more rational basis.

Vitamin A.   The absorption of vitamin A has been studied extensively in rats and chicks as well as in humans. Although some species differences have been shown, the similarities among species are striking. Absorption of both the provitamin, β-carotene, and preformed vitamin A occur primarily from the duodenum and the jejunum.

Cleavage of β-carotene to form vitamin A occurs mainly in the intestinal mucosa during absorption although some cleavage can occur in the liver in those species that can absorb some intact carotenoids. At either location, β-carotene is cleaved in a two-step process to form two molecules of retinaldehyde. The reaction depends on molecular oxygen reacting with the two central carbon atoms of β-carotene (Goodman and Huang, 1965). The enzyme involved is β-carotene-15-15^1 dioxygenase, the carotene cleavage enzyme (Olson and Hayaishi, 1965). In addition, a detergent-lipid mixture is necessary for the *in vitro* reaction (Goodman et al., 1967) suggesting that a bile-lipid combination is probably active under physiological conditions. Cleavage in the intestine is followed by the reduction of retinaldehyde to retinol in the mucosal wall. The enzyme involved in the rat is an aldehyde reductase that requires either NADH or NADPH and resembles the alcohol dehydrogenase enzymes isolated from many tissues (Fidge and Goodman, 1968). The retinol is then esterified to retinyl ester. The retinyl esters so formed from β-carotene are indistinguishable from those derived from preformed vitamin A (Goodman, 1969a), and travel in the lymph with them (see below). Although the rat cannot, the human being can absorb a small amount of dietary β-carotene unchanged (Goodman et al., 1966), and this also leaves the mucosal cell via the lymph.

See Olson and Lakshmanan (1970) for a review of the mechanisms of carotenoid cleavage.

Retinyl esters are the principal form in which preformed vitamin A is present in food. The hydrolysis of retinyl esters is a prerequisite for absorption and retinol is released through the action of pancreatic hydrolase (Mahadevan et al., 1963a; 1963b). Bile is essential for both the activation of the enzyme and the incorporation of the released retinol and remaining unhydrolyzed retinyl esters into micellar solution. The retinol and its esters are picked up from the micelle by the microvilli of the mucosal cell. The retinol passes directly into the cell but those retinyl esters that escape enzymatic hydrolysis in the lumen are met by a retinyl ester hydrolase oriented on the outer surface of the microvilli (David et al., 1966). The retinol so formed can then pass into the mucosal cell. Once inside the cell, reesterification takes place, preferentially with palmitic acid (Mahadevan and Ganguly, 1961), although some retinyl stearate, oleate, and linoleate also are formed (Goodman et al., 1966). The retinyl esters leave the mucosal cell as chylomicrons in the lymph. The fatty acid composition of chylomicrons and of lymphatic triacylglycerols and cholesterol esters usually reflects the composition of ingested fat. Retinyl esters, however, are unique in that both in humans and rats they are predominantly palmitates regardless of the type of dietary fat consumed (Mahadevan et al., 1963a; Goodman et al., 1966).

Retinaldehyde fed to rats appears in the tissues and blood, and as retinol and its esters in the mucosal cell (Deshmukh et al., 1965). *In vitro* studies with everted sacs from rat intestine incubated with retinaldehyde demonstrated the formation of large amounts of retinol, retinyl esters, and retinoic acid (Deshmukh et al., 1967). Since the alcohol and acid can diffuse out of the cell readily, Ganguly (1969) speculated that ester formation was either a trapping mechanism or a means to protect retinol from the retinol dehydrogenase in the mucosa.

Retinoic acid was not found in animal tissues after feeding and it was assumed, therefore, that it was not absorbed. This obviously was not the case since it was shown to promote growth in animals on a vitamin A-deficient diet (Arens and van Dorp, 1946) although it did not prevent blindness (Dowling and Wald, 1960). Further study revealed that retinoic acid could be detected in the blood of humans (Jurkowitz, 1962) and chicks (Krishnamurthy et al., 1963). It was then found to be absorbed by rats via the portal blood but rapidly removed from tissues (Deshmukh et al., 1964). When Fidge et al. (1968) fed labeled retinol or retinaldehyde the label was recovered in the lymph associated with retinol and its esters; but in the bile a significant portion was associated with retinoic acid. These data clearly indicated that retinoic acid could be absorbed and furthermore, that fed retinol and retinaldehyde could be oxidized in the mucosa to retinoic acid. The oxidation of retinol to retinoic acid, however, is not reversible.

The chylomicrons containing retinyl esters, and any β-carotene that was absorbed, enter the sytemic blood via the thoracic duct. The retinyl esters are in the hydrophobic core of the chylomicra and remain with the chylomicron remnants during the process of peripheral removal of triacylglycerol. The retinyl esters containing chylomicron remnants are cleared from the circulation by the parenchymal cells of the liver, the hepatocytes. Although the hepatocytes initially take up the newly absorbed vitamin A, some of the vitamin A can be transferred from the hepatocytes to other liver cells for long-term storage (Blomhoff et al., 1982). These cells have been called vitamin A storing cells, Ito cells, or Stellate cells. The significance of the Stellate cells in the overall metabolism of vitamin A remains to be established. Although the retinyl esters are hydrolzed betwen uptake and long-term storage, vitamin A is stored primarily in the form of retinyl esters in the lipid droplets of the liver. As in the intestine, hepatic vitamin A is esterified primarily with palmitic acid.

An enzyme, retinyl palmitate hydrolase, which produces retinol and free fatty acids, has been detected in rat liver (Prystowsky et al., 1981). The exact role of this enzyme has not been established; however, the liver retinyl esters are hydrolyzed before they are secreted into the plasma.

The transport of retinol is in conjunction with and dependent on two specific proteins: retinol-binding protein (RBP) and transthyretin (formerly called prealbumin or thyroxine-binding prealbumin). Both of these proteins are known to be synthesized in the hepatocytes.

The RBP has the characteristic electrophoretic mobility of an α_1-globulin, a molecular weight of 21,000, and a single binding site for retinol (Kanai et al., 1968). The usual concentration in plasma is in the range of 4 to 5 mg/dl (Goodman, 1969b). One molecule of RBP is complexed with one molecule of transthyretin and together the two proteins transport one molecule of retinol. The RBP interacts with retinol, a lipid-protein interaction, and with transthyretin, a protein-protein interaction (Goodman, 1970). This arrangement with transthyretin serves to stabilize and to protect the retinol-RBP complex. In addition, the transthyretin-RBP complex prevents the loss of the retinol-RBP through glomerular filtration because of the large size of the complex (Vahlquist et al., 1973).

Transthyretin binds thyroxine as well as RBP (Purdy et al., 1965; Oppenheimer et al., 1965). The binding sites are different and the presence of RBP does not affect the capacity or affinity of transthyretin for thyroxine, nor does the presence of thyroxine affect the affinity of transthyretin for RBP. Transthyretin is one of the most fully characterized human proteins. It is a symmetrical tetramer with four identical subunits and a molecular weight of 54,980 (Kanda et al., 1974). High resolution X-ray crystallography has been used to determine the full three-dimensional picture of transthyretin (Blake et al., 1978).

A summary of the related steps in vitamin A absorption from ingestion to transport in the systemic blood as retinol bound to RBP and transthyretin is shown in Fig. 6.17. For reviews of vitamin A absorption, see Ganguly (1969), and Olson and Lakshmanan (1970).

A relationship between marginal vitamin A status and the regulation of RBP secretion from the liver was demonstrated in the rat (Muto et al., 1972). With the development of vitamin A deficiency, serum vitamin A values decreased gradually to extremely low levels as did RBP. When vitamin A was administered to deficient rats a rapid increase in serum RBP level occurred within an hour (Smith and Goodman, 1979), indicating that a pool of previously formed RBP was present in the liver and was released into the serum when vitamin A became available. During vitamin A deficiency the synthesis of RBP continues at the normal rate (Soprano et al., 1982). Since RBP is not secreted from the livers of the deficient rats, this implies that the RBP is degraded in the liver (Smith et al., 1975). Vitamin A deficiency, however, does not affect the secretion of transthyretin (Navab et al., 1977).

The free RBP molecule is small enough to be filtered through the glomerulus of the kidney followed by tubular resorption and degradation. Patients with chronic renal disease accumulate high levels of RBP in the plasma (Smith and Goodman, 1971). The elevated RBP levels frequently are accompanied by elevated vitamin A. As a result, such patients may develop vitamin A toxicity with a vitamin A intake in the range of 10,000 I.U. per day.

The absorption of both the carotenoids and preformed vitamin A is promoted by the presence of bile salts in the intestinal lumen. The detergent properties of the bile acids contribute to the emulsification of lipids in the intestinal lumen and, in addition, to the activation of pancreatic hydrolases for digestion of complex lipid materials. A detergent-lipid mixture was implicated in the activity of the carotene cleavage enzyme (Goodman et al., 1967), and bile salts are probably

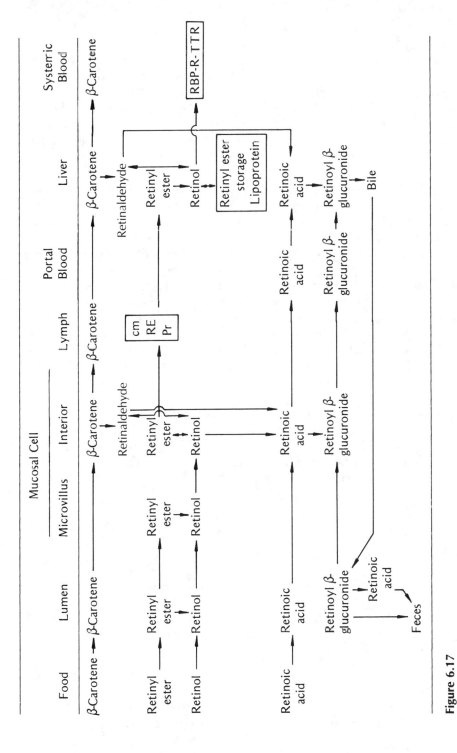

Figure 6.17
Summary of steps in vitamin A absorption in man. cm-RE-Pr = chylomicron containing retinyl ester and protein; RBP-R-TTR = retinol binding protein-retinol-transthyretin.

involved in the *in vivo* reaction. Bile salts also play a role in the formation of the micelles that participate in bringing retinol and its esters to the microvillus surface for transport into the mucosal cell.

It is the unique molecular structure of bile salts that enables them to behave in aqueous solutions as amphipathic molecules forming mixed micelles. Since solubilization into micelles facilitates the absorption of polar lipids and is a prerequisite step in the absorption of nonpolar lipids, the role of bile salts was studied in relation to the solubilization of polar retinol and of nonpolar β-carotene. The presence of polar lipids in complex micelles is known to enhance the solubilization of nonpolar solutes, and El-Gorab and Underwood (1973) presented *in vitro* data indicating the solubility of retinol to be approximately 7 to 9 times greater than that of β-carotene. They suggested that the two molecules are solubilized independently in different regions of the complex lipid-bile salt micelles and that this might be related to the size of the micelle formed. In a subsequent study, El-Gorab (1975) suggested that the polar retinol expands the size of the micelle by aggregating at the periphery and thereby increasing the inner volume of the complex. This increase in inner volume enables the nonpolar β-carotene to enter the center of the micelle and be carried to the membrane-binding sites for uptake (Fig. 6.18). Bile salts, therefore, are involved indirectly in vitamin A absorption through their role in lipid digestion and are more directly involved in vitamin A and carotene absorption through their participation in the formation of mixed micelles.

Low intakes of dietary fat have been associated with inefficient absorption of the carotenoids. This assumes great importance when the major portion of the vitamin A in the diet is in the form of the provitamin. In a vegetarian population in Central Africa, Roels et al. (1958) found that the carotene absorbed by children depended on the amount of fat that was consumed and not on the amount of

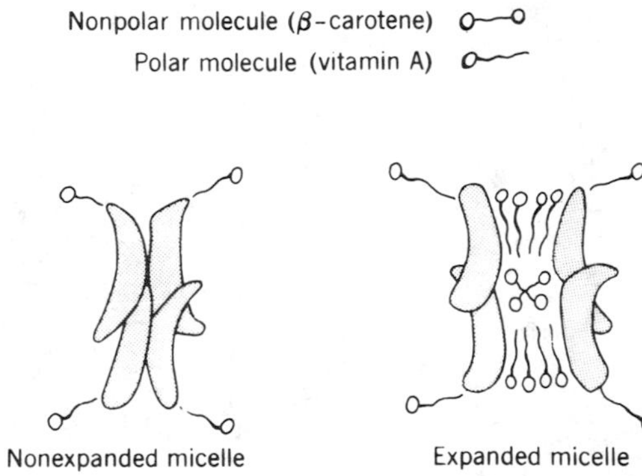

Nonpolar molecule (β-carotene)
Polar molecule (vitamin A)

Nonexpanded micelle   Expanded micelle

Figure 6.18
Expansion of the inner volume of a micelle by the aggregation of polar retinol at the periphery and of nonpolar β-carotene in the center. (By permission from M. El-Gorab.)

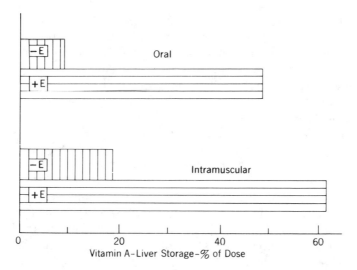

Figure 6.19
Effects of vitamin E and vitamin A utilization in vitamin E-deficient rats. (From S. R. Ames, *Am. J. Clin. Nutr.* 22:934, 1969.)

carotene in the diet. The addition of small amounts of fat to the diet improved
the absorption of carotene, increased serum vitamin A levels, and was associated
with a reduction of the symptoms of vitamin A deficiency. Furthermore, disturbances in fat absorption such as occurs in celiac disease interferes not only with
the absorption of carotene but also of vitamin A (Breeze and McCoord, 1939).
However, the effect on vitamin A is much less than on carotene. The incidence
of night blindness was reduced in a study group not with the addition of carotene
alone, but when both fat and carotene were added to the diet (Roels et al., 1963).

Another factor affecting vitamin A absorption is the state of vitamin E nutriture.
Vitamin A absorption is markedly impaired in vitamin E-deficient rats. When an
oral supplement of D-α-tocopherol was fed to vitamin E-deficient rats, absorption
of orally fed vitamin A increased approximately sixfold (Ames, 1969). An intramuscular injection of an emulsified form of vitamin A evoked no response in
vitamin E-deficient rats, but with the simultaneous injection of vitamin E the
response was marked (Fig. 6.19). Thus, the effect produced by vitamin E is not
solely in the lumen of the intestinal tract. The mechanism involved is not clear
but may be related to the action of vitamin E in preventing peroxidative destruction
of certain labile substances such as vitamin A both in the lumen and in the tissues.

A relationship between dietary protein deficiency and low plasma vitamin A
values was reported for children with protein-energy malnutrition (Trowell et al.,
1954; Arroyave et al., 1959; Gopalan et al., 1960). Since the dietary sources of
vitamin A were probably not different in children with and without protein-energy
malnutrition in the same population group, interference with utilization of vitamin

A was postulated. Smith et al. (1973) found that children with protein-energy malnutrition had markedly depressed levels of serum RBP and transthyretin as well as vitamin A. When these children received supplements of protein and calories, but not vitamin A, all the serum values returned to the normal range. These observations suggest that the inability to mobilize liver vitamin A reserves is related to the lowered production of RBP. It is not clear at this time if the lowered production of RBP is caused by a lack of necessary amino acids or if it represents a regulatory depression related to the lower vitamin A requirement of the growth-depressed children.

In addition, there is a reduction in the intestinal absorption of vitamin A related to the synthesis of the enzymes that hydrolyze retinyl esters. Periera et al. (1967) observed that interference with the absorption of naturally occurring vitamin A probably occurred at the level of hydrolysis and reesterification. They found that vitamin A, when fed as a water dispersion of vitamin A palmitate to children with protein-energy malnutrition, reached the plasma whereas vitamin A fed in oil did not. Absorption of vitamin A palmitate was slower in protein-deficient chicks, and the amount left in the intestinal tract was always higher. This was observed only when vitamin A was given as the ester and did not occur when retinol was fed. When absorption was bypassed by intravenous injection of vitamin A given as the palmitate, acetate, or alcohol, protein restriction had little effect on the rate of vitamin A disappearance from the blood or on liver storage. These data support the conclusion that the block occurs at the stage of hydrolysis in the intestinal lumen. Enzymes secreted by the pancreas are reduced in protein malnutrition (Scrimshaw et al., 1956) and a reduction in retinyl esterase may well be a rational explanation of the decreased vitamin A absorption accompanying protein deficiency.

Vitamin D.   The mechanism of vitamin D absorption from the intestinal lumen still is not clear. Avioli (1970) refers to the "vitamin D information gap," which has resulted from accelerated vitamin D research in animals and the knowledge of vitamin D activity in humans. Indeed, there is question as to whether it should even be called a vitamin; many believe its mode of action allies it more closely to the hormones. However, if vitamin D is present in or added to food, whether vitamin or hormone, it becomes available as a nutrient, only if it can penetrate the intestinal mucosa. *That* this occurs is not disputed, but *how* is still fairly vague and generalized. Only since the middle of the 1960s have specific data been forthcoming.

One of the first steps in attempting to ascertain how vitamin D was absorbed was to establish where in the intestinal tract absorption occurred. Establishing the location awaited methods and instruments capable of detecting very small quantities of vitamin D in tissues and fluids. Not until radioactive forms of the vitamin were available could serious work begin. Studies employing labeled vitamin D_3 fed to rats indicated that the primary site of absorption was the ileum (Norman and DeLuca, 1963; Callow et al., 1966). This was disputed by Schachter et al. (1964) who reported that the greatest capacity for absorbing vitamin D_2 was in the midsection of the jejunum although absorption was also observed in most of the proximal three-fourths of the small intestine. Kodicek (1960) fed labeled vitamin D_2 to infants and found that 13 to 23 percent appeared in the feces within three days. It was assumed that the rest was absorbed. A later report on human adults (Thompson et al., 1965) indicated that vitamin D could be absorbed efficiently even if only a small remnant of the jejunum remained after intestinal resection. Whether the jejunum was indeed the primary site of vitamin D absorption, or whether adaptation had occurred and absorption took place there because that section was all that remained, was not apparent.

Observations of conditions that led to defective absorption of vitamin D established the importance of bile salts. In obstructive jaundice bile was prevented from entering the small intestine; after intestinal resection bile salts could not be reabsorbed and recycled. In both conditions defective vitamin D absorption was reported (Schacter et al., 1964). Conditions that led to fecal excretion of fat, such as celiac disease (Thompson et al., 1966a), also were accompanied by malabsorption of tritiated vitamin D_3 as was partial gastrectomy even in the absence of steatorrhea (Thompson et al., 1966b).

By cannulating the thoracic duct and following the absorption of tritiated vitamin D_3 in man, Blomstrand and Forsgren (1967) demonstrated clearly that bile salts were essential for vitamin D absorption. Further, they established that the pathway for absorption in humans was through the lymph just as had been reported previously for rats (Schachter et al., 1964). From these data certain preliminary conclusions could be drawn: vitamin D probably is absorbed at the level of the jejunum; it is dependent on the presence of bile; and it is carried in the chylomicra of the lymph.

Although a small quantity of vitamin D esters have been detected both in lymph and blood, their significance is not understood (Fraser and Kodicek, 1968a; 1968b; 1968c). Most of the vitamin D in the lymph chylomicra is present as the free alcohol (Schachter et al., 1964). It is not clear if vitamin D remains with the chylomicron remnants as does vitamin A, or if extrahepatic tissues (muscle and adipose) remove vitamin D from the chylomicra along with triacylglycerol. Studies in both humans (Mawer et al., 1972) and rats (Rosenstreich et al., 1971) have shown that vitamin D deposits in muscle and especially in adipose tissue represent the major body stores of vitamin D.

The highest concentration of vitamin D is in the liver, but the larger mass of muscle and adipose tissue makes their total reserves much larger than the total vitamin D in the liver.

Although a substantial amount of vitamin D is present in blood, the vitamin D metabolite $25(OH)D_3$ accounts for more than half of the vitamin D activity in human plasma. The two metabolites that are produced in the kidneys, $1,25(OH)_2D_3$ and $24,25(OH)_2D_3$, are found at much lower levels.

Vitamin D and all of its metabolically active metabolites circulate in plasma bound to a specific transport protein called "the binding protein for vitamin D and its metabolites" or simply DBP. In 1976 three laboratories reported the isolation of human DBP (Bouillon et al., 1976; Haddad et al., 1976; Imawari et al., 1976). As suggested by Daiger et al. (1975) DBP was identical with the Group-specific component (Gc) protein. This protein had been studied extensively as a genetic marker protein before its function was identified. There is good agreement that DBP has a single binding site for vitamin D and its metabolites, and the estimates of its molecular weight range from 52,000 to 59,000. In humans, the normal plasma concentration of DBP ranges from 300 to 600 μg/ml. In contrast to RBP, the vitamin A transport protein that circulates in plasma highly saturated with retinol, only about 2 to 3 percent of the DBP circulates with bound vitamin D or 25 (OH)D_3. The large quantity of unbound DBP insures that DBP is always available to transport the vitamin metabolites. Even in hepatitis and cirrhosis when DBP drops to 60 percent of the normal level, the transport of vitamin D and its metabolites is not impeded (Imawari et al., 1979). The decrease in plasma DBP levels in liver disease reflects the fact that the liver is the sole site of synthesis of DBP (Prunier et al., 1964).

The cytosol fraction of all nucleated tissues contains DBP (Cooke et al., 1979). Van Baelen et al. (1980) reported that the cytosolic DBP is present as a 1:1 molar complex with actin. The function of DBP in these tissues is not clear.

Vitamin E.   The absorption of this vitamin is understood only in the most general terms. The superior biological activity of α-tocopherol over the other naturally occurring forms has been attributed in part to its more efficient intestinal absorption (Draper and Csallany, 1970). It is assumed that certain aspects of molecular structure may facilitate absorption but what these aspects are is not known (Bieri, 1970). Like other fat-soluble vitamins, vitamin E absorption from the intestinal lumen depends on the presence of both pancreatic secretions and bile (Greaves and Schmidt, 1937; Gallo-Torres, 1970b; MacMahon and Thompson, 1970). In humans, conditions of pancreatic insufficiency or biliary obstruction have been associated with malabsorption of vitamin E (Binder et al., 1965; MacMahon and Neale, 1970) and, in fact, malabsorption of vitamin E is more marked than that of dietary triacylglycerols (MacMahon and Neale, 1970). Pancreatic juice may supply a specific enzyme for the hydrolysis of vitamin E esters in the lumen and thereby account in part for malabsorption associated with pancreatic insufficiency (Gallo-Torres, 1970a). The essentiality of bile for vitamin E absorption is due to its role in formation of mixed micelles (MacMahon and Neale, 1970) which is more important in the absorption of nonpolar lipids such as α-tocopherol than for the absorption of polar lipids such as long chain fatty acids (MacMahon and Thompson, 1970).

The vitamin E that enters the mucosa apparently is not esterified and leaves unchanged via the lymph (Johnson and Pover, 1962). The lymphatic route has been clearly demonstrated by thoracic duct cannulation studies in rats (Gallo-Torres, 1970a; MacMahon and Thompson, 1970) and in humans (Forsgren, 1969). However, under abnormal conditions such as the absence of bile, a significant uptake of vitamin E can occur via the portal route (MacMahon et al., 1971). Losowsky et al. (1972) suggest that a previously demonstrated need for bile in the absorption of α-tocopherol may be secondary to its effect on the absorption of fat and, in fact, demonstrated that better absorption of fat occurred when long chain triacylglycerols were replaced by medium chain triacylglycerols. In each case the major pathway of α-tocopherol absorption paralleled fat absorption.

Although rats appear to have an alternate route for the absorption of vitamin E, in the human the formation of chylomicrons is essential for the normal delivery of vitamin E into the general circulation. Individuals with the condition called abetalipoproteinemia develop neurological symptoms that can be corrected by the administration of massive doses of α-tocopherol (Muller and Lloyd, 1982). Such individuals are unable to synthesize apo-B which is the major protein in chylomicra and which is essential for chylomicron formation. The intestinal mucosal cells of these individuals absorb lipids, but the cells retain the lipids since their normal release mechanism is not available. When the mucosal cells are sloughed off into the lumen of the intestine they are excreted in the feces along with the lipids they contain. As a result, individuals with abetalipoproteinemia become vitamin E-deficient.

Although investigators have been searching long and hard for an enzymatically active metabolite of vitamin E in animal tissues, thus far none has been found and the existence of such a form is doubted (Draper and Csallany 1969; 1970; Bieri, 1970; also see Chapter 4). One can only conclude that α-tocopherol in the diet is absorbed through the intestinal mucosal cell and normally is transported via the lymph to the liver and many other tissues where it can be stored. Whether the storage form is different from the form in which it enters and leaves the liver is not known, nor has a specific carrier protein for its transport in the plasma been identified. A dynamic equilibrium exists between the vitamin E in the plasma lipoprotein and that in the erythrocytes (Kayden and Bjornson, 1972). These are all problems awaiting a solution.

Vitamin K.   The vitamin K in the intestinal lumen is derived from two sources: that present in ingested food and that synthesized by the flora in the tract. Both sources are available for absorption. There is only general information concerning the passage of vitamin K from the intestinal lumen into the mucosal cell. Those factors that promote the absorption of fat, such as the presence of bile, are also important for the absorption of vitamin K; those conditions that lead to fat malabsorption will interfere with vitamin K absorption. In addition, because one source of intestinal vitamin K is that synthesized by intestinal flora, any condition that interferes with intestinal synthesis, such as oral administration of antibiotics, will affect vitamin K availability and absorption.

Blomstrand and Forsgren (1968) cannulated the thoracic lymph duct of four human subjects and studied the absorption of radioactive vitamin K_1. After an oral dose, 19 to 61 percent of the radioactivity was recovered in the lymph. Although essentially all of the radioactivity cochromatographed with vitamin K_1, only about 73 percent of the lymph radioactivity was associated with the chylomicra. In contrast, a patient with a bile obstruction absorbed less than 3 percent of the radioactive dose.

In studies with everted rat intestinal sacs, Hollander (1973) found greater vitamin K_1 uptake by the proximal small intestine than by the distal portion. The absorption by the proximal small intestine appeared to be an energy-mediated process, whereas uptake by the distal intestine appeared to be a passive process. In contrast, vitamin K_2 was absorbed by a passive process in all sections of the small intestine (Hollander and Rim, 1976). Vitamin K_2 of bacterial origin was also found to be passively absorbed in the rat colon. Hollander et al. (1976) suggested that the absorption of bacterially synthesized vitamin K_2 in the colon was sufficient to meet the daily requirement of the rat.

Only one limited study has been conducted on the plasma transport of vitamin K in humans. Vitamin K_1 was found to circulate in association with the lipoproteins (Shearer et al., 1970). No attempt was made to identify the specific lipoproteins. Research on vitamin K metabolism has been seriously hampered by the lack of simple and inexpensive assay methods.

Water and Electrolyte Absorption

The water and electrolytes in the lumen of the intestine represent both dietary intake and the endogenous water and electrolytes secreted into the lumen. The quantity of ingested water may amount to one to two liters per day. The endogenous secretions (gastric, pancreatic, and intestinal juices, plus bile) contribute an additional seven to eight liters or 80 percent of the water, as well as 80 percent of the sodium chloride and 50 percent of the potassium and calcium. Absorption from the gut reclaims the major portion of this secreted water. Only one to one and a half liters enter the colon and, of this, about 100 ml appear in the feces. At any one time, the amounts of fluid and electrolytes in the lumen are the consequence of the simultaneous fluxes from the lumen to the blood and from the blood to the lumen. Absorption then is defined as the net decrease in the amount of electrolyte or water in the lumen resulting from a flux out of the lumen that is greater than the flux into the lumen (Berger, 1960). These exchanges are referred to as "gastrointestinal circulation" (Bland, 1963).

In the upper part of the small intestine the concentration of sodium and chloride in the lumen is greater than in the mucosal cells and movement follows the gradient from the lumen to the cells. In addition, the active transport of glucose and amino acids, discussed above, is accompanied by the absorption of sodium and water. In the lower part of the small intestine, the concentration gradient toward the cells no longer exists and the reclamation of water and electrolytes from the lumen takes place through an active transport system. The sodium pump moves sodium from the lumen into the mucosal cells. Chloride and water are carried along passively, chloride to maintain electrical neutrality across the membrane and water to maintain osmotic balance.

Since the absorption of water is passive and accompanies the passage of its solutes, the rate and locus of its absorption depends on the solutes it accompanies. The major solute absorption takes place in the duodenum and upper jejunum which is, therefore, the site of the major water absorption. Because of the quantitites involved, any interference with absorption of water and electrolytes from the intestine results in diarrhea, dehydration, and electrolyte imbalance and can be extremely serious, particularly in very young, very old, or debilitated individuals.

For a detailed presentation of water and electrolyte absorption, see Schultz (1981a).

Mineral Absorption

In general, the absorption of divalent ions (Ca^{++}, Fe^{++}) is slower than that of monovalent ions (Na^+, K^+). Calcium, for example, is absorbed 50 times more slowly than sodium, yet its rate of absorption far exceeds that of iron, zinc, and manganese. (See Wilson, 1962.) The absorption of specific ions appears to be regulated by homeostatic mechanisms. For example, restricted absorption appears to be related to the organism's inadequacy in handling excretion or in coping with surplus; increased absorption occurs when the dietary supply or body stores are reduced. The absorption of calcium and iron, two minerals long known to be essential and apt to be in short supply, has been subjected to considerable study. In the past decade, absorption of trace minerals, such as zinc, copper, and selenium, has been studied extensively.

In addition to the intrinsic, homeostatic regulation, mineral absorption is influenced importantly by the health of the individual and by dietary factors. Diseases that alter the intestinal transit time (gastric surgery), the intraluminal pH (pancreatic insufficiency), or mucosal integrity (celiac sprue), have profound effects on the absorption of nutrients. Nonnutritive dietary compounds, such as insoluble phytates and dietary fiber present in whole grains, nuts, and beans, and tannins and oxalate in certain leaves and sprouts, inhibit the uptake of divalent minerals. Although high phytate intake initially inhibits calcium absorption, a certain degree of intestinal adaptation and compensation soon occurs. (See Irving, 1957.) Breast milk has certain properties that enhance the absorption of the calcium, iron, and zinc it contains. A general overview of factors that affect the biological availability of dietary minerals has been presented by Rosenberg and Solomons (1982) (Table 6.7). In the intestinal lumen, the chemical form of the mineral and its interactions with other dietary components can enhance or inhibit its uptake. In addition, factors within the mucosal cells or in the mesenteric circulation can also influence absorption.

The tempo of research, especially in the area of calcium absorption, has greatly accelerated as knowledge of vitamin D activity has unfolded. Many gaps in our knowledge of mineral absorption still exist, but they are becoming ever smaller.

Calcium. The presence of relatively large amounts of calcium in the feces led to the early suggestion that this was the pathway of calcium excretion. However, the calcium in the lumen of the small intestine is a combination of dietary calcium and the endogenous calcium secreted into the gut as a constituent of the digestive juices (Bronner and Harris, 1956). Since the quantity of endogenous calcium is difficult to ascertain, studies reported calcium absorption as the difference between intake and fecal excretion. Such metabolic studies estimating apparent absorption of dietary calcium indicated that normal individuals from preschool age through adulthood absorb 15 to 40 percent of ingested calcium (Leichsenring et al., 1951; Brine and Johnson, 1955; Nordin et al., 1979). The balance tech-

TABLE 6.7
Factors Affecting the Bioavailability of Minerals

I. Intraluminal Factors
  1. The chemical form of the metal/mineral
     a. Inorganic salts
     b. Valence
        Organometallic compounds
        Covalent complexes
        Noncovalent complexes
  2. Interaction in the lumen with:
     a. Proteins, peptides, amino acids
     b. Triglycerides, fatty acids
     c. Carbohydrates
        Monosaccharides
        Disaccharides
        Polysaccharides (including fiber)
     d. Anions and anionic substances
     e. Other metals/minerals

II. Intracellular and Post-cellular Factors
  1. At the intestinal membrane
     a. Competition for transport
     b. "Coadaptation"
  2. Intracellular binding
  3. Release and transport from the enterocyte
     a. Circulating binding proteins
     b. Endogenous mediators

Source: I.H. Rosenberg and N.W. Solomons, *Am. J. Clin. Nutr.* 35: 781–782, (1982).

nique, however, invariably underestimates the amount of calcium that is absorbed since the endogenous contribution of calcium to fecal output is in the range of 100 to 130 mg/day in the adult (Brine and Johnston, 1955; Heaney and Skillman, 1964).

With increased demand for calcium, as in infants (Benjamin et al., 1943) or calcium-depleted children (Nicholls and Nimalasuriya, 1939; Mills et al., 1940), up to 80 percent of luminal calcium is absorbed. Many factors including calcium nutriture, vitamin D status, pregnancy, lactation, age, and disease influence absorption of the calcium from the intestinal lumen even though it is in a soluble, and hence theoretically absorbable, form. This phenomonon was reported in early balance studies in children (Daniels et al., 1935) and adults (Steggerda and Mitchell, 1941).

Techniques other than balance studies indicated the relationship of metabolic need to calcium absorption. The adjustment to the increased need during pregnancy was observed in a study using everted sacs from rats. Sacs from rats in the third week of pregnancy transferred more calcium than did sacs from nonpregnant rats (Schachter et al., 1960). The effect of age was also an observed adaptation to increased need. Increased efficiency of calcium absorption during the stages when bone growth was most active indicated that young animals had a greater capacity to absorb Ca^{++} than adults. Active transport in old nongrowing rats was minimal (ibid). Similarly, Cannigia and coworkers (1964) found little difference in the time it took for radioactive calcium to appear and to reach its maximum level in venous blood in nongrowing human subjects ranging from 29 to 70 years of age.

Sites of calcium absorption.   The site of calcium absorption has been the subject of studies in both humans and laboratory animals. Calcium, like other minerals, must be released from complexes in food and made soluble before it can be absorbed. The acidic pH of the stomach assists in freeing calcium but often the process is not complete until the chyme is in the jejunum. Since calcium tends to precipitate at a pH higher than 6.0, it is theoretically in a more absorbable form in the duodenum and proximal jejunum, where the pH is less alkaline, than in the more distal intestine. In addition, calcium-binding protein (see below) which appears to play an important role in calcium absorption is abundant in the duodenum. Thus, the efficiency of calcium absorption, that is, the amount of calcium taken up per unit length of small intestine, is greater in the upper portions of the small intestine than in the more distal segments (Wensel et al., 1969).

The amount of time that chyme remains at a given level of the gastrointestinal tract is another important factor influencing the net uptake of calcium. Since chyme remains in the more distal segments of the intestine for a longer time than in the proximal, the net absorption of dietary calcium from a meal supplying abundant calcium is greater from the lower jejunum and ileum than from the duodenum (Birge et al., 1969). The colon traditionally is thought to be relatively inert with respect to the absorption or conservation of nutrients. However, evidence from both animals (Petith and Schedl, 1979) and humans (Hylander et al., 1980) suggests that the colon may play a physiological role in calcium absorption. It has even been suggested that colonic conservation of calcium is under the hormonal influence of vitamin D (Petith et al., 1979).

Absorption from the intestinal lumen involves the same three-step process for calcium as for all nutrients: 1) transfer through the microvillus membrane of the mucosal cell; 2) transport through the cell; and 3) exit from the cell across the basolateral membrane into the extracellular fluid and into the blood. Membrane transfer (see Chapter 9) can be passive (down a gradient with no expenditure of energy) or active (againt a gradient and requiring energy expenditure). When radioisotopes of calcium became available, studies were initiated to clarify the mechanisms involved in calcium absorption. Over the years, methods have become more sophisticated and investigations more intense, but as will become apparent, data often appear to be conflicting and the problem is far from being resolved.

Schachter and Rosen (1959), using everted gut sacs, were the first to report the movement of ^{45}Ca through the mucosal membrane against a concentration gradient, indicating active transport. This suggestion was reinforced by the observation that transport was depressed by inhibitors of oxidative metabolism. Active transport also was suggested by Kimberg et al. (1961) who showed that calcium transport from duodenal segments of rats was twice as great on low as on high calcium diets. The debate at the present time does not appear to be whether transport through the mucosal membrane is active or passive. Apparently both types occur and probably, at the mucosal membrane, it is predominantly passive when calcium is abundant.

Role of vitamin D in calcium absorption.   The relationship of vitamin D to calcium metabolism and bone formation was known long before specific actions of the vitamin could be explained. Greenberg (1945) showed that the presence of vitamin D increased the absorption of radiocalcium from the intestine of the rachitic rat. Harris et al. (1965), using ^{47}Ca, studied the response of rachitic children to vitamin D administration and concluded that a direct action of vitamin D on the intestinal mucosa improved absorption of both dietary and digestive juice calcium. That the effect of vitamin D on calcium absorption was not due to the simultaneous presence of the two nutrients in the gut became evident when a lag in response following vitamin D administration was reported (Williams et al., 1961). This lag effect suggested to some investigators that the action of vitamin D was not directly on the mucosal membrane, but that its role was a more fundamental one that might require protein synthesis. Early evidence, however, was conflicting (Zull et al., 1965; Norman, 1965).

One of the several physiologically active forms of vitamin D, $1,25(OH)_2D_3$, identified almost simultaneously by Holick et al. (1971a) in the United States and by Lawson et al. (1971) in England, was shown to increase the transport of calcium and phosphate through the intestinal mucosa (Garabedian et al., 1974). The mechanisms involved in the promotion of calcium transport by vitamin D action have been and are being studied intensively and remain the subject of considerable controversy. The development of various models and the contributions emanating from some of the principal laboratories investigating the role of vitamin D in the intestinal absorption of calcium follow.

A protein formed in chick mucosa after administration of vitamin D to a rachitic chick was identified by Wasserman and Taylor (1966) and designated *calcium-binding protein* (CaBP). CaBP was subsequently found in mucosal homogenates from rats (Schachter et al., 1967) and other species. (See Wasserman, 1970.) The fact that this protein was not found in the mucosa of rachitic chicks but appeared after vitamin D treatment suggested that it was induced by vitamin D (Wasserman and Taylor, 1966). Ebel et al. (1969) reported the appearance of CaBP in intestinal homogenates at the same time that an increase in calcium absorption due to vitamin D was observed. The capacity of CaBP to bind calcium and form a complex with it suggested that it was involved in the movement of calcium through the intestinal mucosa (Wasserman and Taylor, 1968; Taylor and Wasserman,

1969). Subsequent studies questioned a direct relationship between vitamin D-stimulated absorption of calcium and CaBP and suggested that other vitamin D-responsive mechanisms were probably involved as well, since increased calcium intake precedes the appearance of CaBP (Spencer et al., 1976; 1978).

Both DeLuca et al. (1982) and Bronner et al. (1982) support the thesis that calcium transport in response to $1,25(OH)_2D_3$ is due to nuclear activity leading to protein synthesis in the intestinal cell. The DeLuca group proposes that a receptor molecule present in the cytosol (or in the nucleus) interacts with the $1,25(OH)_2D_3$ delivered to the mucosal cell by the blood and is prerequisite to its action. Before calcium transport into the cell takes place $1,25(OH)_2D_3$ must appear in the nucleus for formation of mRNA leading to protein synthesis. The synthesized proteins stimulate calcium transport through the microvillus membrane. Since both rapid and slow responses to $1,25(OH)_2D_3$ are observed, DeLuca et al. (ibid) suggest that the rapid response is due to an effect on the nuclei of mature villus cells, and the slow response to an effect on the maturing crypt cells. The exact nature of the transport proteins, except for CaBP, is not known. Bronner's group (ibid) also stresses that the time and nature of the responses are dependent both on calcium intake and the vitamin D status of the animal.

Recently there have been suggestions that the action of vitamin D is through its effect on the architecture and lipid composition of the mucosal membrane. Rasmussen et al. (1982) propose that the entry of calcium into the mucosal cell stimulated by $1,25(OH)_2D_3$ is the result of specific alterations in the membrane. This suggestion is based on the finding that administration of $1,25(OH)_2D_3$ leads to synthesis of phosphatidylcholine, to its increased content in the membrane, and to change in membrane lipid structure that increases membrane fluidity and calcium transport into the cell. This entrance of calcium occurs without the synthesis of new protein. Once in the cell, the calcium binds to CaBP, the synthesis of which is also under the influence of $1,25(OH)_2D_3$. Schachter and Kowarski (1981; 1982) have identified an intestinal membrane calcium-binding protein (IMCal) in the cytosol that is clearly distinguishable from CaBP. They suggest that it is a likely component of the mechanism that controls entry of calcium into the cell. IMCal is an intrinsic membrane protein (see Chapter 9) with high affinity for calcium. It consists of ten subunits and could, therefore, form a calcium channel by interacting with other membrane components including membrane lipids.

Intracellular free calcium must be maintained at very low levels to avoid profound effects on cell metabolism, and there is evidence that this is accomplished by complexing the calcium with transport proteins and/or by sequestering it in cellular organelles. The role of mitochondria in regulating intracellular calcium uptake associated with fundamental intracellular functions has been known for a long time. (See Chapter 13.) Mitochondria were believed to be the major intracellular calcium transport system acting as buffers when calcium concentration in the cytosol became high (Carafoli and Crompton, 1978), but this role for mitochondria is now being questioned (Bikle et al., 1979). There are reports that calcium-binding proteins in the Golgi are vitamin D-dependent (Freedman et al.,

1977), which suggests that they, and perhaps other organelles, may play roles in the transport of calcium through the intestinal cell to the point of exit (Bronner et al., 1982).

The calcium that enters and moves through the cell involving transport proteins and cellular organelles, must then be extruded through the basolateral membrane to the extracellular fluid. The primary extrusion system appears to be a Ca-ATPase

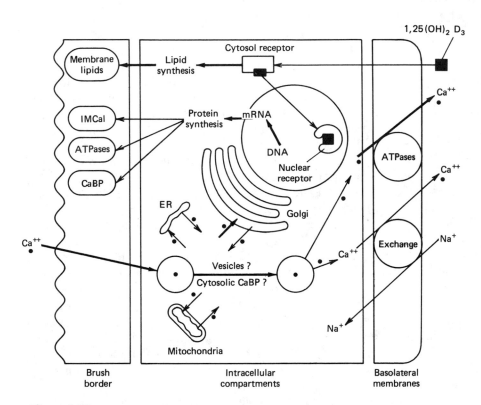

Figure 6.20
A composite of suggested mechanisms in the movement of calcium into, through, and out of the intestinal cell. Heavy arrows indicate events that appear to be vitamin D-dependent. $1,25(OH)_2D_3$ interacts with receptors in both the cytosol and nucleus leading to the sequence of events which results in the synthesis of membrane lipids and various membrane proteins that appear to be involved in entry of Ca^{++} from the lumen into the cell. Transport through the cell may be in association with vesicles or cytosolic CaBP. The Golgi and endoplasmic reticulum (ER) are involved in sequestering Ca^{++} to prevent cytosolic Ca^{++} from reaching toxic levels. The role of mitochondria in intracellular Ca^{++} regulation is now in dispute. Ca^{++} is extruded against a gradient through the basolateral membranes by a Ca^{++}-dependent ATPase. When this system reaches capacity at relatively high levels of intracellular Ca^{++}, a Na^+-Ca^{++} exchanger becomes operative. (Adapted from R. H. Wasserman and C. S. Fullmer, *Ann. Rev. Physiol.* 45:376, 1983.)

pump (Van Os et al., 1981). According to Carafoli (1981a), a second system, a Na^+-Ca^{++} exchanger, comes into play when the Ca-ATPase pump is working at capacity. Only after passage through this last membrane is calcium absorbed.

Figure 6.20 presents a composite of current models of intestinal absorption of calcium: entrance into the cell, passage through the cytosol, and exit through the basolateral membrane.

Factors affecting calcium absorption.   The association of calcium with lactose in milk and the observed beneficial effects of lactose on calcium absorption provide grist for the teleological mill. By design or not the two are associated and their simultaneous presence in the intestinal lumen was shown to improve the absorption of calcium (Greenwald and Gross, 1929; Lengemann et al., 1959). An early suggestion was that this was due to the effect of lactose on intestinal flora and the consequent lowering of the pH. It now appears that the enhancing effect of lactose is coupled to the absorption of monosaccharides since any metabolizable sugar instilled in the ileum enhances calcium absorption to some degree (Vaughan and Filer, 1960). Thus, the less efficient clearance of lactose from the upper intestinal lumen when the intralumenal concentration is high, and its persistence in the chyme in the ileal segment may explain its enhanced effect compared with other sugars. Inhibition of calcium absorption accompanying lactose malabsorption (see section on Carbohydrate Digestion) has been reported by some investigators (Condon et al., 1970; Kocian et al., 1973).

Individuals with pathological conditions accompanied by fat malabsorption excrete large amounts of calcium in their stools. In normal healthy individuals, however, the amount of fat does not affect calcium absorption. Diets with fat content varying from 32 percent to 1 percent but containing equal amounts of calcium resulted in identical calcium balance in healthy volunteers (Steggerda and Mitchell, 1951). There were no correlations between fecal fat excretion and calcium output in infants with different fat intakes (Filer et al., 1970; Shaw, 1976).

Certain plant components may affect calcium absorption. McCance and Widdowson (1942) first showed that the substitution of whole wheat flour for white flour in wartime England reduced calcium absorption in human subjects. Negative calcium balance is produced with high intakes of bran (Cummings et al., 1979). Both dietary fiber and phytic acid in whole wheat and bran contribute to the observed inhibition of calcium absorption by binding the calcium in the intestinal lumen in an insoluble form. Cellulose (Kelsay et al., 1979; Slavin and Marlett, 1980) and uronic acid (James et al., 1978) also bind calcium, but fermentation by flora in the colon may liberate a considerable amount of the calcium for absorption (see section on Colon Function and Fecal Composition). Oxalates bind calcium in green leaves and apparently make that calcium unavailable (Fincke and Sherman, 1935; Fairbanks and Mitchell, 1938; Johnston et al., 1952) but it is uncertain whether the oxalate in one food reduces the availability of the calcium in other foods.

For reviews of various aspects of calcium absorption, see Wasserman et al. (1980); Deluca (1981); Allen (1982); Bronner (1982); Levine et al. (1982); Wasserman and Fullmer (1983).

Iron.   The presence of relatively large amounts of iron in the feces and very small quantities in the urine led to the early obvious suggestion that iron, like calcium, was excreted into the lumen of the gastrointestinal tract. However, McCance and Widdowson (1937) clearly demonstrated that iron that was injected directly into the blood was not excreted either by way of the urine or feces. This work was subsequently confirmed by many investigators and by the use of radioactive iron tracers. It is now fairly well established that there is a unidirectional movement of iron across the intestinal mucosal cell with no satisfactory means of excretion either through the gut or kidney (Sheehan, 1977).

Excess iron that does enter by injection or by disruption of the normal regulation of iron absorptive processes has no means of exit and, as a result, accumulates in storage as ferritin or hemosiderin in the reticuloendothelial cells of the liver, spleen, and bone marrow. Normally the body mass of iron is maintained within relatively narrow limits and, with the demonstrated inability to cope with excess by excretion, the only logical means of explaining control is at the point of entry. That is, regulation must occur at one or more of the following steps: (1) uptake from the intestinal lumen by the mucosal cell, (2) transit through the cell, or (3) release from the cell to the blood. Various aspects of this movement of iron are under intensive investigation in laboratories in the United States and elsewhere in an effort to discover the mechanisms of control. Models, many of which overlap, have been proposed; some of these will be presented and discussed.

Early suggestions that ferritin was involved in the control of iron absorption (Hahn et al., 1939; 1943) and that divalent iron was more readily absorbed than trivalent (Moore et al., 1944) led Granick (1949; 1954) to propose the Mucosal Block Theory (Fig. 6.21). He postulated that the mechanism for regulation of iron absorption resided in the mucosal cell of the duodenum and upper jejunum and that control was exerted by the ferritin content of the cells. The suggested mechanism involved the change from ferric to ferrous iron in the intestinal lumen, reoxidation in the mucosal cell, and attachment to the apoferritin synthesized in the cell to form ferritin. In response to body need, iron was released from ferritin, reduced for passage through the serosal membrane, reoxidized, and attached to

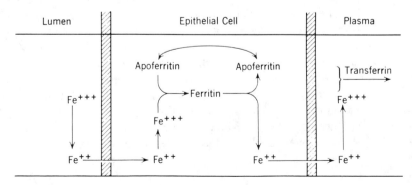

Figure 6.21
"Mucosal Block" hypothesis. (From S. Granick, *Bull N. Y. Acad. Med.* 30:81, 1954.)

the specific iron-binding β_1-globulin, transferrin. The apoferritin in the cell was continually broken down and resynthesized. Iron not needed to maintain the body mass of iron remained in the mucosal cell as ferritin and, according to Granick's theory, high levels of ferritin in the cells blocked further absorption of iron, whereas low levels permitted iron to enter. Granick's theory has more than served its purpose, that of providing a base for further investigation which more sophisticated laboratory procedures have made possible. However, the basic concept of control of iron absorption at the level of the mucosal cell is not questioned nor are certain aspects of the process, but exactly how and where control is exerted still is not clear. Discussion of postulated mechanisms of absorption will be presented first, followed by discussion of the factors affecting the availability of the kinds of food iron in the intestinal lumen.

Current investigations of the mechanisms of iron absorption fall into three main categories: (1) passage through the mucosal membrane, (2) the role of iron compounds in transit through, or storage in, the mucosal cell, and (3) passage through the serosal membrane and into the blood. The three phases of absorption could not be separated in early studies but this can be achieved now and, insofar as possible, these steps will be discussed separately.

Passage through the mucosal membrane. Using everted gut sacs of rat duodenum, Dowdle et al. (1960) demonstrated that the transfer of iron from the mucosa to the serosa was an active process against a concentration gradient and depended on phosphate bond energy. In subsequent *in vitro* studies by Manis and Schachter (1962; 1964), mucosal uptake and serosal transfer were shown to be distinct sequential processes. Mucosal uptake was more rapid and increased in proportion to the concentration of iron in the medium. Serosal transfer was slower and remained constant and maximal. They reported that both steps were energy-requiring, but appeared to operate independently. Both *in vitro* and *in vivo* work indicated that the second step, serosal transfer, had the greater dependence on oxidative metabolism. Similar results were reported in studies on humans (Hallberg and Sölvell, 1960a; 1960b; 1960c).

Conflicting data have been presented on the iron content of isolated mucosal cells in normal compared with iron-deficient or iron-loaded rats (Balcerzak and Greenberger, 1968), guinea pigs (Pollack and Campana, 1970), and humans (Allgood and Brown, 1967). However, Greenberger et al. (1969) found Fe^{++} bound to brush borders of mucosal cells of rats and reported that the quantity could be depressed by prior iron loading and increased by iron depletion. These investigators also reported that the mucosal transfer of iron did not require energy. They suggested that iron was adsorbed to receptor sites and that it was the iron in the brush border that was the regulator of transport. In studies using ^{59}Fe, Linder and Munro (1975) also suggested that some control of iron uptake is exerted at the mucosal cell surface and may be dependent on the number of receptors in the membrane. However, Linder et al. (1975) suggest that the process is one requiring energy, and that it is ionic iron that is transferred by the receptor. How information on the status of body iron is transmitted to govern the number of receptor sites is not known, but Linder et al. (ibid.) propose that it may be a hormone-related process regulating the rate of receptor synthesis.

Transit through or storage in the mucosal cell. Some investigators have suggested that iron enters the cell as chelates of sorbitol or fructose (Charley et al., 1963), of porphyrin (Weintraub et al., 1968) or of ascorbic acid and amino acids (Schade et al., 1968) and Helbock and Saltman (1967) reported that chelate formation was a necessary step. Linder et al. (1975) suggest that chelation with amino acids is more likely to occur following the release of ionic iron into the cytoplasm after transfer through the mucosal membrane, but Sheehan and Frenkel (1972) found no evidence of a soluble iron-chelating molecule within the mucosal cell.

The storage protein ferritin was isolated by Granick (1943) and was endowed by him with a key role in regulation of iron absorption. The presence of ferritin in mucosal and other cells is undisputed, but the significance of its role in regulation of iron absorption has undergone many revisions. An early modification of the suggested role for ferritin in iron absorption came about following increased understanding of the cell renewal process of the intestinal mucosa (see section on Mucosal Structure p. 217). Conrad and Crosby (1963) proposed that (1) the quantity of ferritin incorporated into mucosal cells at the time of their generation in the crypts of Leiberkühn reflects body iron status, (2) this "messenger iron" determines the receptivity of the cells to iron from the lumen, (3) high ferritin blocks further absorption but low ferritin promotes absorption, and (4) iron not transferred through the serosal membrane remains in the cell to be sloughed off with the cell from the tip of the villus.

With the use of radioactive tracers, Van Campen (1974) confirmed that body iron status is reflected in the amount of iron incorporated into crypt cells and that this iron determines the amount transferred from the lumen into mature villus cells. In addition, he proposed that iron in the mucosal cell is in two forms, storage iron and transit iron (Fig. 6.22). Before long, two iron-binding proteins that participate in the iron absorption process, ferritin and a transferrin-like protein, were isolated from mucosal cells in rats (Huebers, 1975), guinea pigs (Pollack and Lasky, 1975), and humans (Anand et al., 1976). Additional proteins have been isolated but may or may not be the result of contamination of the tissue fraction or of varying degrees of proteolysis (Linder and Munro, 1975).

A distinctive property of ferritin is its capacity to bind iron. The amount of iron that is bound ranges from none in the apoferritin to an amount one-quarter the weight of the protein (Harrison et al., 1974). The ferritin molecule accumulates and releases iron without disintegration (Mazur and Carleton, 1963). This information, newer methods available for isolating ferritin (Drysdale and Munro, 1965), and knowledge of the mechanisms regulating protein synthesis led Munro and his group to reinvestigate the role of iron in regulating the accumluation and turnover of ferritin protein in the cell. They showed unequivocally that iron administration leads to *de novo* synthesis of apoferritin (Drysdale and Munro, 1966) and that iron is preferentially incorporated into newly synthesized apoferritin as compared with older ferritin molecules already partially filled with iron. They showed further that iron incorporated into newly formed partially filled ferritin is more labile, and iron in filled and older ferritin molecules more inert (ibid). It follows, then, that large amounts of iron introduced into the cell fill ferritin mol-

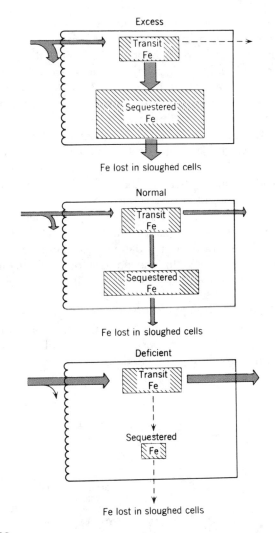

Figure 6.22

Effects of iron status on transport of iron across intestinal mucosal cells. After an oral dose of radioactive iron to rats with normal iron stores (center), radioactivity is concentrated in cells present and absorbing when the dose is given and remains in the cells until they are sloughed off into the lumen. Less radioactivity appears in cells formed later. No radioactivity appears in the villi of rats that were either iron-loaded (top) or iron-depleted (bottom). No absorption of radioactive iron occurs in iron-loaded rats. In iron-depleted rats, absorbed iron is transported through to the plasma. After an injected dose of radioactive iron, radioactivity appears in cells generated *after* iron administration in both normal and iron-loaded rats. No radioactivity appears in the villi of iron-depleted rats since all of the injected iron is used to correct the depletion and none is available for use as messenger iron. (From D. Van Campen, *Fed. Proc.* 33:100, 1974.)

ecules more rapidly and provide more of the relatively inert variety of ferritin. This was first studied in the liver cell and then in the intestinal mucosal cell where the same mechanism of regulation is operative (Smith et al., 1968).

The investigations of Munro's group led them to suggest that synthesis of apo-ferritin induced by iron is a cytoplasmic event. This fits in with the assumption that proteins synthesized for export are synthesized on membrane-attached ri-bosomes (see Chapter 11), whereas proteins retained within the cell are synthe-sized on polysomes free in the cytoplasm (Takagi and Ogata, 1968). Indeed, Hicks et al. (1969) showed that ferritin protein is formed by RNA located on free polysomes in the cell. Bédard et al. (1971) found most of the absorbed radioactive iron in the rough endoplasmic reticulum and in the ribosome-containing areas of the cytoplasm in their studies of iron absorption in mouse duodenum. Figure 6.23 presents the mechanism Munro and Drysdale (1970) proposed whereby available iron regulates both synthesis and breakdown of ferritin protein. The role of ferritin in the intestinal cell is one of accommodating excess iron, according to Linder and Munro (1975), and not part of the mechanism for regulating iron absorption. However, Savin and Cook (1980) attribute a more important role to ferritin (see below).

An interesting aspect of the work reported from Munro's laboratory (Drysdale and Munro, 1966) is the use of leucine-^{14}C to carry the label for ferritin protein, in contrast to most other studies that used an iron label. An iron label would indicate the total iron taken into the cell and not just the iron that is incorporated

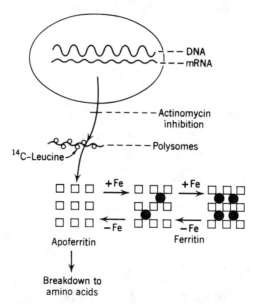

Figure 6.23
Suggested mechanism by which the availability of iron regulates both the synthesis and deg-radation of ferritin protein. (From H. N. Munro and J. W. Drysdale, *Fed. Proc.* 29:1469, 1970.)

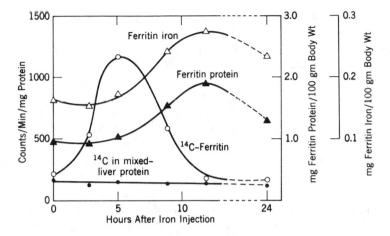

Figure 6.24
Uptake of leucine-^{14}C into liver ferritin and into mixed liver proteins
after a 2-hr pulse dose of leucine-^{14}C given to rats at various times
after injection of iron. Each rat received 400 μg of iron/100 gm of
body wt, followed at 1, 3, 7, 10, and 22 hr by 5 μC of leucine-
^{14}C/100 gm of body wt. The animals were killed 2 hr after injection
of leucine. (From J. W. Drysdale and H. N. Munro, *J. Biol. Chem.*
241:3630, 1966.)

into ferritin. The distribution of the label among the iron components of the cell
has been a point of controversy (Balcerzak and Greenberger, 1968; Greenberger
et al., 1969; Bédard et al., 1971; Sheehan and Frenkel, 1972). Leucine can, of
course, be incorporated into many cell proteins, and Drysdale and Munro (ibid.)
demonstrated a steady and low level of incorporation of leucine into mixed liver
protein after iron administration and a significant peak into ferritin (Fig. 6.24).
Because of the variable content of iron in the ferritin molecule, it seems that the
label appearing in the protein moiety more accurately signals the ferritin synthesis
induced by iron. The work reported from Munro's laboratory strongly suggests
that iron stimulates the formation of ferritin in the cell and that the lability of the
iron is related to the saturation of the ferritin. Furthermore, the stability of the
protein moiety depends on the presence of the iron, confirming an *in vitro* study
by Crichton (1969) that showed tryptic digestion of the protein apoferritin to be
2.5 times that of ferritin. When large quantities of iron are present in the lumen,
macrophages in the villi take up some of the excess iron into their lysosomes.
(See Chapter 14.) These iron-filled macrophages are capable of crossing the epithelium to carry this intercepted iron back into the lumen for excretion (Astaldi
et al., 1966). Since only the iron that penetrates the serosal membrane is "absorbed," the ferritin returned to the lumen in the sloughed off cells or sequestered
in lysosomes is iron that for one or another reason is not absorbed.

Passage through the serosal membrane. Transferrin, the other major iron-containing protein in the mucosal cell, is generally believed to be the intracellular

carrier in the iron absorption path through the cytosol (Huebers et al., 1971). Iron is carried to the membrane on the serosal side of the cell bound to transferrin. Penetration of the serosal membrane is the last step in the transfer of iron from the gut lumen to plasma, and Wheby and Crosby (1963) were the first to postulate serosal control of absorption. How this transfer through the membrane occurs and how it is controlled still is conjectural. Whether it is carrier-mediated and energy-dependent (Manis and Schachter, 1962) or involves receptors and is energy-independent (Linder and Munro, 1977) continues to be debated. Whatever the mechanism, iron must be released to the membrane on the intracellular side and picked up on the other side for transport through extracellular fluid to the blood. It seems likely that iron released to the membrane by cellular transferrin is picked up on the other side of the membrane by plasma transferrin. Plasma transferrin differs from mucosal cell transferrin in amino acid composition as well as immunologically (Huebers et al., 1976) and is distributed equally between plasma and extravascular fluids. The equivalent of the total plasma pool of transferrin enters and leaves the extravascular circulation each day (Morgan, 1974). According to Fletcher and Huehns (1968) and supported by Brown (1975), one of the two binding sites on the plasma transferrin molecule is particularly avid for iron from the intestinal mucosal cell. Further, Levine et al. (1972) found that cells from rat small intestine have a greater affinity for apotransferrin than for transferrin. If this is so, then iron delivered through the cytosol to the basal membrane most likely is oxidized (Gaber and Aisen, 1970) and picked up by plasma transferrin on the other side, completing the route from the intestinal lumen to plasma. The quantity of iron absorbed would then be related to the iron uptake from plasma transferrin by reticulocytes and other cells, but there is no firm evidence that this is more than one facet of the regulatory mechanism, especially since plasma transferrin is normally only 30 percent saturated with iron. For further details on the transferrins, see Aisen (1980).

The relationship of transferrin to ferritin in the mucosal cell has been suggested by Savin and Cook (1980) as the monitor of iron absorption. The ferritin compartment, a passive system, binds the iron not rapidly transported into the circulation and is closely related to body iron stores; that is, high ferritin levels accompany high body iron. In contrast, transferrin, the transport compartment, varies inversely with body stores; that is, high levels of transferrin accompany low body iron. Iron absorption observed in normal, iron-deficient, and iron-loaded rats by Savin and Cook (ibid) correlated better with the ratio of mucosal cell transferrin:ferritin than with either of the parameters separately (Fig. 6.25). They suggest that one parameter may be more sensitive to changes in iron absorption when stores are high, and the other when stores are low. Therefore, monitoring sensitivity at both ends of the spectrum of iron status, using the ratio of one to the other, provides a better correlate of iron absorption. According to this view, the mechanism regulating iron absorption resides within the mucosal cell and is related to the balance maintained between ferritin and transferrin synthesis. How the messages for synthesis are relayed to the mucosal cell when increased iron absorption is necessary remains conjectural. It is generally agreed that increased

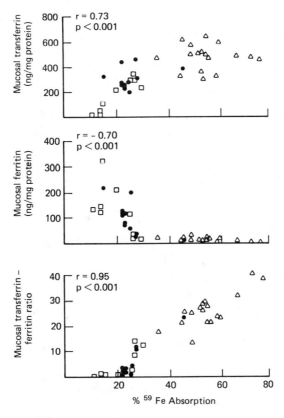

Figure 6.25
Relationship between iron absorption and mucosal transferrin (top), mucosal ferritin (middle), and transferrin:ferritin ratio (bottom). Results are plotted for normal (●), iron-deficient (△), and iron-loaded (□) rats. Correlation was significantly higher with transferrin:ferritin ratio than with either ferritin or transferrin concentration alone. (From M. A. Savin and J. D. Cook, *Blood* 56:1032, 1980.)

need for iron stimulated by pregnancy, growth, anemia, and hypoxia leads to increased erythrocyte formation and stimulates the sequence of events that leads to iron transfer across the intestinal mucosa into the plasma. But this is only a superficial statement of cause and effect that does little more than camouflage our ignorance. (Aspects of iron metabolism related to hematopoiesis will be discussed in Chapter 16).

A derangement in the regulation of iron absorption leading to siderosis has been observed in the Bantus, who consume up to 150 mg of iron per day (Walker and Arvidsson, 1973). This excessively high dietary iron comes from the iron utensils used in the preparation of both food and a fermented maize beer (Gillman et al., 1959). It appears that it is not the high intake of iron alone but its association with a high maize diet that is responsible for the siderosis. It has been shown that animals fed iron-enriched maize diets develop siderosis whereas those on enriched stock diets consuming twice as much iron do not (Kinney et al., 1949). Changes observed in the intestinal cells included disorganization of the endoplasmic reticulum and swelling of the mitochondria on high iron-high maize intakes. Whether these findings are analogous to those occurring in the Bantus is not known, nor is it known whether disproportionate amounts of other dietary constituents can produce disruption of intestinal mucosal cell structure and function.

A reduction in iron absorption of over 60 percent was observed in children during periods of fever (Beresford et al., 1971). Why this should occur is not clear. Schade et al. (1970) suggest that the block may be in the incorporation of iron into the ferritin molecule since cobalt, which is not incorporated into ferritin but shares the iron pathway in serosal transfer, is not reduced. The relationship of iron to fever may be somewhat more complex. Iron absorption is reduced during febrile episodes and susceptibility to infection is increased several-fold in iron deficiency (Chandra et al., 1977). One can speculate on whether the deficiency is primary and leads to decreased iron absorption, or whether prolonged fever and the accompanying reduction in iron absorption predisposes to iron deficiency.

For reviews of the postulated mechanisms of iron absorption, see Brozović (1975); Jacobs and Worwood (1981); Hallberg (1982); Charlton and Bothwell (1983).

Bioavailability of iron.   Iron absorption depends not only on a properly functioning mechanism regulating uptake of iron through the intestinal mucosa, but also on availability of the food iron. The quantity of iron in a food is no indication of the amount available for absorption; nor is the amount available for absorption an indication of how much will be absorbed when the food is part of a meal. Both the chemical nature of the iron in the food and the combination of foods in the meal affect the availability of the iron. In addition, the iron status of the individual influences the efficiency of absorption which undoubtedly is related to mechanisms of control rather than to bioavailability; but, according to Hallberg (1981a), bioavailability must be expressed in relation to the state of iron nutriture.

Dietary iron exists in two forms as far as mechanisms of absorption are concerned: *heme iron* and *nonheme iron*. Heme iron is the form within the porphyrin ring and found primarily in hemoglobin and myoglobin. About 40 percent of the iron in all animal tissues is heme iron and the remaining 60 percent mostly in the storage forms of ferritin and hemosiderin. All the iron in plant products is nonheme iron. In regions of the world where the diet is essentially vegetarian and cereal grains are the major source of iron, virtually all of the dietary iron may be nonheme.

Heme iron was thought to be unavailable to humans on the basis of animal studies (Elvehjem, 1932; Weintraub et al., 1965). The rat, mouse, and human all digest hemoglobin in the lumen, but the released heme polymerizes in the animal lumen and becomes unabsorbable. In the human, heme enters the mucosal cell (Calender et al., 1957; Turnbull et al., 1967) where the ring is split and the iron released (Weintraub et al., 1968). Dawson et al. (1970) suggested that the enzyme responsible for liberating the heme iron is xanthine oxidase, but Raffin et al. (1974) identified heme oxygenase as the enzyme in the mucosal cell responsible for the release of heme iron. It is apparent then that the iron from hemoglobin protected by the porphyrin ring until it reaches the confines of the cell is not subjected to the same hazards in the intestinal lumen as iron from other sources, nor is its absorption inhibited or enhanced by other constituents of the diet.

An understanding of the differential absorption of heme and nonheme dietary iron was achieved through the use of radioactive tracers of iron: ^{59}Fe and ^{55}Fe. In early experiments, the technique known as *intrinsic labeling* was used to tag the iron in specific foods. This biosynthetic labeling was accomplished by hydroponic cultivation of plant foods in media containing the iron isotope, and by injecting the radioisotope into animals several months prior to using animal products as a food source (eggs, milk, muscle meat). Moore and Dubach (1951) pioneered in the use of such labels in the study of iron absorption in humans and they reported that citrus fruit juice had a beneficial effect on the absorption of iron from egg. Schultz and Smith (1958) reported that less radioiron from egg was absorbed when given with a combination of orange juice, toast, and milk than when egg was given alone. Iron absorption from a test meal of iron-fortified bread was studied in subjects who served as their own controls (Callender and Warner, 1968). Both forms of iron commonly used in the fortification of bread, ferric ammonium citrate and reduced iron, were poorly absorbed even by subjects with quite severe iron deficiency and amounted to only one-tenth the amount absorbed from a dose of ferrous iron by the same subjects. Addition of orange juice to the meal almost doubled absorption of the iron from bread. Comparable results on the enhancement of iron absorption with orange juice were reported by Elwood et al. (1968), and with ascorbic acid by Steinkamp et al. (1955) and Kuhn et al. (1968). The subject of intraluminal effects became clouded further by data indicating that egg markedly inhibits absorption of iron salts (Callender et al., 1970), but apparently does not affect the absorption of wheat iron (Elwood et al., 1968).

Since foods are not normally eaten alone, the difference in iron absorption from foods consumed in different combinations prompted the use of a different radioisotope of iron in each of two foods consumed simultaneously to study the effect of food combinations on iron absorption. Layrisse et al. (1968) found that a certain proportion of animal food enhanced the absorption of iron from vegetable sources; however, less of the iron from the animal source was absorbed when combined with the vegetable source. A compilation of studies from different laboratories showed consistently higher absorption from animal foods that sometimes was even greater than absorption of a reference dose of ferrous ascorbate. (See Martinez-Torres and Layrisse, 1974.) Because of the infinite variety of food combinations and the tediousness and expense of intrinsic labeling, the prospect of obtaining practical data with this method appeared remote.

An idea for a method believed suitable for measuring iron absorption from a mixed meal evolved at a joint meeting of the International Atomic Energy Agency-World Health Organization (IAEA-WHO). The method was based on the premise that as far as absorption is concerned food iron is a two-pool system: heme and nonheme. Although an inorganic iron tracer cannot be used to measure heme absorption, it might be a valid measure of the absorption of nonheme iron due to partial isotopic exchange between the tracer and the food iron. If such an exchange occurs, mixing of the tracer in the preparation of the food should give a more reliable index of absorption than administration of the tracer as a drink along with the food. The method involved preparation of a food, such as maize, wheat, or eggs, containing an intrinsic label to which a trace amount of an iron salt labeled with another iron radioisotope (*extrinsic label*) was added during the food preparation. Absorption of the intrinsic and extrinsic labels was found to be the same, and the use of extrinsic labeling to ascertain absorption of nonheme iron was validated in several laboratories (Bjorn-Rasmussen et al., 1972; 1974; Cook et al., 1972). Since the absorption of nonheme iron from different foods consumed in a meal was the same, it is apparent that isotope exchange does indeed occur and that all the nonheme iron in a meal becomes part of a common nonheme iron pool. (See Cook, 1977.)

The use of extrinsic labels made it possible to explore how some foods inhibited and others enhanced the absorption of nonheme iron in a meal. Since the inhibitory action of one food depresses iron absorption from all foods taken at the same time and enhancing effects operate similarly, it is apparent that the effects are exerted on the pool of nonheme iron. Cook and Monsen (1975) developed a semisynthetic meal with the same total chemical composition as a standard meal and used extrinsic tags to measure nonheme iron absorption in a group of 32 women. Ten percent of the iron was absorbed from the standard meal but only 1.8 percent from the semisynthetic. The difference was explained by the enhancing effect of meat in the standard diet, an effect reported by Oldham et al. (1937) who, in balance studies, found consistently higher iron retention when beef was added to the diet of an infant. Cook and Monsen (ibid.) suggest the use of the semisynthetic diet for studying enhancers of iron absorption, and the standard diet for studying inhibitors.

All sources of animal protein are not equivalent in promoting the absorption of nonheme iron. An increase in absorption of two to four times was observed when beef, lamb, pork, liver, fish, or chicken were substituted for egg ovalbumin, but no increase when milk, egg, or cheese were substituted (Cook and Monsen, 1976). When Martinez-Torres et al. (1981) observed a doubling of nonheme iron absorption due to cysteine, an effect that mimics the enhancing effect of meat, they suggested that the mechanism of enhancement might be the same since animal protein and cysteine are the only enhancers of both heme and nonheme iron.

The enhancing effect of orange juice and ascorbic acid reported in early studies (see above) appears to be due to the ability of ascorbic acid to maintain iron in a reduced, more soluble form. Ascorbic acid also forms chelates with ferric iron in the stomach thereby maintaining solubility of the iron with increasing pH in the duodenum. Orange juice consumed with a meal can increase iron absorption from 5 to 20 percent and is an effective means of promoting iron absorption in vegetarian diets (Monsen and Balintfy, 1982). The pronounced effect of ascorbic acid in increasing absorption of nonheme iron suggests that fortification of a food with ascorbic acid may be more effective than fortification with iron. (See Cook, 1977.)

The availability of iron from human milk is approximately twice that from bovine milk (Saarinen et al., 1977). The only plausible suggestion so far for the differences in iron absorption from bovine, simulated human, and human milk comes from *in vitro* studies involving bovine and human lactoferrin (Cox et al., 1979). Lactoferrins are the specific proteins in milk that bind and deliver iron. Human intestinal mucosal cells transfer several times the amount of iron from human than from bovine lactoferrin, and this appears to be due to the affinity of human lactoferrin for receptors in the human enterocyte. Results of such *in vitro* tests cannot give the answer, but they do indicate where to look.

Many factors have been identified as inhibitors of nonheme iron absorption. Widdowson and McCance (1942), using chemical balance techniques, were first to report lower iron absorption of diets with brown rather than white bread. The effect was attributed to the bran or the phytate the brown bread contained. Later Bjorn-Rasmussen (1974), using double isotopes, studied the effect of bran on iron availability and found that iron absorption was decreased twofold when 7 percent bran was added to white flour. Similar results were obtained when brown and white rice were compared and the decrease in iron absorption was found to be proportional to the bran content. In a recent study involving 20 adults, McWhinnie and Mack (1982) found a significant decrease in absorption of a 300 mg therapeutic dose of ferrous sulfate when given with than without 7.5 gm of natural wheat bran. They suggest that interference with iron absorption is due to the phytate content of the bran, but they did not rule out other binding factors. However, evidence that phytate might not be the culprit in bran was obtained from human balance studies by Simpson et al. (1981) who separated dephytinized bran into a soluble phosphate-rich fraction and an insoluble high fiber fraction. They found the soluble fraction more inhibitory, indicating phosphates inhibit iron absorption more than fiber. Others (Hegsted et al., 1949; Cook et al., 1973) had implicated phosphates earlier. Nevertheless, fiber has not been absolved as an inhibitor of iron absorption. Reinhold et al. (1981) showed that when cereal intake is high, a high proportion of nonheme iron is unavailable unless the iron is released from the fiber by gastric acid or enhancers such as ascorbic acid, fruit juices, or cysteine. These investigators suggest that the lack of interference by fruit and vegetable fiber in the report by Kelsay et al. (1979) may have been due to the high ascorbic and citric acid contents.

Other inhibitors of nonheme iron absorption are tannates (Disler et al., 1974), antacids (Monsen et al., 1978) and, interestingly, fortification iron such as pyrophosphates, orthophosphates, and some preparations of reduced iron (Cook et al., 1973).

It is apparent that evaluation of the bioavailability of nonheme iron is complex and not entirely clear. However, sufficient data have been obtained to permit estimation of available iron, that is, how much iron is actually absorbed. A model for the calculation of available iron on a meal basis was proposed that involves the amounts of both heme and nonheme iron, the availability of each, and the content of enhancing factors in the meal such as ascorbic acid and meat (Monsen et al., 1978). A formula for such calculations has been reported and computer programs now are available (Monsen and Balintfy, 1982).

Human absorption studies are both difficult and costly. It is of interest, therefore, that Miller et al. (1981) developed an *in vitro* method for the estimation of iron availability in which a standard meal formulated and prepared to duplicate that of Cook and Monsen (1976) was used along with enhancers and inhibitors. A comparison of the *in vitro* data with the published human data of Cook and Monsen (ibid) indicated significant agreement (Schricker et al., 1981), and a more accurate indication of food iron availability to humans than did rat studies in which the same diet was used. It appears that this method could be of considerable value in preliminary trials of iron bioavailabiility.

For more extensive reviews of the bioavailability of iron, see Cook (1977); Hallberg (1981b;1982); Morris (1983).

Zinc.   In the past decade much has been learned about zinc absorption. It appears now that zinc absorption, like that of iron, is subject to control according to the requirement of the individual. Many components of this regulatory system currently are being defined. The biological availability of zinc depends on its release from complexes in food (Solomons, 1982). Once in a soluble form, it can cross the membrane into the mucosal cell, but it is subject to binding or chelation by food components such as phytates and tannins (ibid). In addition, it appears that iron and perhaps calcium and tin compete with zinc in some way for the pathways of absorption or otherwise reduce its uptake (Solomons and Jacob, 1981). Zinc absorption is enhanced by meat (Shah and Belonje, 1981), breast milk (Casey et al., 1981), and wine (McDonald and Margen, 1980).

The pancreas appears to play an important role in the absorption of zinc. Studies by some investigators (Evans et al., 1975), not confirmed by others (Antonson et al., 1979), have shown that ligation of the pancreatic duct reduces the uptake of ^{65}Zn in experimental animals. This finding suggests that a substance, present in pancreatic secretions, is important in the absorption of dietary zinc. No such compound has been identified but picolinic acid (Evans, 1980) and citric acid (Lönnerdal et al., 1980) have been mentioned as candidates for the physiologically important zinc-binding ligand, presumably present in pancreatic secretion. Since zinc is an important component of one of the main endocrine secretions of the pancreas, insulin, it is interesting that pancreatic exocrine secretion should play a role in insuring zinc absorption from the intestinal lumen.

In addition, Spencer et al. (1965) showed that pancreatic secretion is the dominant pathway for the excretion of endogenous zinc. Thus, each time a meal is consumed and pancreatic secretion is stimulated by the arrival of food in the duodenum, an additional amount of zinc is released into the intestinal lumen. The elegant perfusion studies of Matseshe et al. (1980) demonstrated that endogenous zinc from such secretions is usually equivalent to or greater than that consumed in a meal. By the time chyme passes through the middle portion of the jejunum, about the same amount of zinc originally present in the meal is taken up by the intestine (Matseshe et al., 1980). An excess of inhibitory factors in a meal may not only reduce the absorption of the zinc in the food, but may prevent the recovery of endogenous zinc and thus precipitate the depletion of zinc stores. Thus it appears that the distal jejunum and the ileum may have an important role in the absorption of zinc if positive zinc balance is to be maintained. In fact, Antonson et al. (1979) reported that in *in vivo* perfusion studies in rats absorption from the duodenum and jejunum were equal but that three times as much zinc was absorbed in the ileum.

Evidence has accumulated that the level of body zinc is homeostatically reg-ulated both by the magnitude of excretion of excess zinc into the gastrointestinal tract (Weigand and Kirchgessner, 1980) and by mucosal cell control of zinc uptake and its passage into the blood (Cousins, 1979). The elements of this mucosal regulation are illustrated in Fig. 6.26. There is a bidirectional flux of zinc from mucosal to serosal and from serosal to mucosal surfaces of the cell, but the intestine is capable of transporting zinc against a concentration gradient, sug-gesting active transport. Zinc within the cell has four possible destinies: (1) it can move back into the lumen, (2) it can function within the enterocyte, (3) it can move into the blood, or (4) it can become trapped within the cell bound to metallothionein. The important features in the regulation of the mucosal to serosal flow of zinc represent another example of "mucosal block."

High levels of zinc can induce the transcription of mRNA for the synthesis of metallothionein (see Fig. 6.26). Metallothionein is a small protein (6,000 to 8,000 daltons) with large numbers of exposed sulfhydryl groups capable of chelating

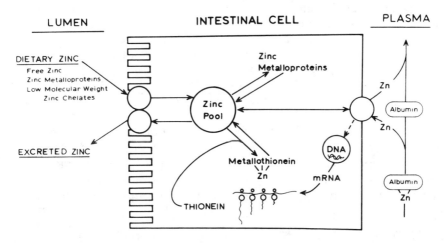

Figure 6.26
Regulatory pathway of dietary zinc processing by intestinal cells. (From C. J. Cous-ins, *Nutr. Rev.* 37:98, 1979.)

divalent cations. When zinc encounters excess amounts of this intracellular binding protein, it is bound and immobilized, and excreted into the lumen in the normal course of mucosal cell turnover and exfoliation (Cousins, 1979). Recent evidence also suggests that the brush border membrane of the mucosal cell is selectively permeable to zinc (Menard et al., 1983). This too might represent a physiologically relevant mechanism for the control of entry of zinc into the body. There is controversy as to which circulating plasma protein transfers zinc from the serosal side of the mucosa into the blood. Both transferrin (Evans, 1976) and albumin (Smith et al., 1978) have been suggested as the transport protein for recently absorbed zinc.

Other Minerals.   *Magnesium* is absorbed primarily by passive diffusion and the efficiency of the process is conditioned by the dietary concentration of magnesium and the nutritional needs of the individual.

   Copper absorption has several unique features. If it arrives in the stomach in a soluble form, as in a beverage, it can be absorbed through the gastric mucosa (Van Berge Henegouwen, 1977). The absorption of copper is not influenced greatly by phytate or fiber (Sandstead, 1982), but high levels of dietary zinc can interfere with copper absorption and result in copper deficiency anemia (Prasad et al., 1978). The presumed mechanism is the induction of metallothionein by zinc, which traps not only zinc but also copper in the intestinal mucosa (Fischer et al., 1981). The primary route of copper excretion is through the bile. The reabsorption of biliary copper is poor, presumably due to the chemical form of copper in bile (Solomons, 1980). Whether casual mixing of dietary copper with bile in the duodenum influences the bioavailability of the metal is not known.

   Selenium absorption is dependent on the chemical form found in food. Dietary selenium is present as inorganic selenium (selenium salts) and selenomethionine. The latter compound is in organic form, in which selenium substitutes for sulfur in the amino acid, methionine.

$$CH_3-Se-CH_2-CH_2-\underset{\underset{NH_2}{|}}{CH}-COOH$$

Selenomethionine

Young et al. (1982) speculate that the absorption of selenium in this chemical form is similar to that of sulfur amino acids. Selenium exists in many valence states, and it appears that the more reduced forms have superior biological availability. Thus, dietary reducing agents, such as ascorbic acid, may improve the absorption of inorganic forms of dietary selenium (Combs and Pesti, 1976).

CONCLUSION

The plasma membrane of the intestinal mucosal cell is only the first of the barriers through which nutrients must pass from the environment of the organism to the

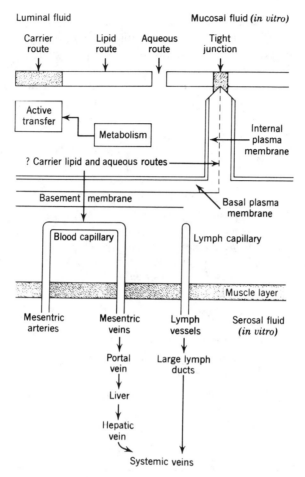

Luminal fluid   Mucosal fluid *(in vitro)*

Carrier   Lipid   Aqueous   Tight
route   route   route   junction

Active
transfer   Internal
                                                   plasma
          Metabolism   membrane

? Carrier lipid and aqueous routes

Basement | membrane   Basal plasma
                                       membrane

Blood capillary   Lymph capillary

Muscle layer

Mesentric   Mesentric   Lymph   Serosal fluid
arteries   veins   vessels   *(in vitro)*

                Portal   Large lymph
                 vein   ducts
                Liver
               Hepatic
                vein
                   Systemic veins

Figure 6.27
Diagrammatic representation of the gut wall to show
the various pathways available to the absorbed nutrients both *in vivo* and *in vitro*. (From D. H. Smith,
Transport Across the Intestine, W. L. Burland and P.
D. Samuel, eds., Churchill Livingstone, Edinburgh,
1972, p. 3.)

environment of its constituent cells. Fig. 6.27 indicates the series of additional
membranes and compartments through which passage must occur. After leaving
the mucosal cell through its lateral or basal plasma membrane, nutrients must
then penetrate the glycoprotein of the basement membrane, enter the extracellular
fluid compartment, and pass through the capillary or lacteal wall for delivery to
the systemic circulation either by way of the liver or the lymphatics. For delivery

to the cells, nutrients leave the circulation through capillary walls and enter the extracellular fluid before entering a cell. This activity and the distance traveled, accompanied by a considerable expenditure of energy, is all preamble to nutrient function.

The following tribute seems a fitting farewell to the role of the small intestine:

THE SUPERBOWEL

I think that I shall never see
A tract more alimentary.
A tube whose velvet villi sway
Absorbing food along the way.
Whose surface folded and striate
Does rapidly regenerate.

A magic carpet whose fuzzy nap
Miniscule molecules entrap.
Then, microvilli with enzymes replete
The last hydrolyses complete.

A tunnel studded with protection
Against abrasion and infection
(Goblet cells their mucus spill
While lymphoid cells the microbes kill).

To top things off, it should be noted,
This Grand Canal is sugar coated!*

George J. Fruhman

Perspect. Biol. Med.17:66(1973).

Colon Function and Fecal Composition

It seems logical at this point to follow the relatively small volume of material that leaves the small intestine and enters the colon before following the products of digestion that leave through the intestinal mucosal cells.

The fluid contents remaining in the ileum are propelled through the ileocecal valve into the cecum and thence to the colon. The total volume constitutes a mere one-twentieth of the secreted and ingested fluid, or 400–500 ml, the remainder having been absorbed through the mucosal membrane higher in the tract. The fluid entering the colon contains sodium and chloride in approximately the same concentrations as extracellular fluid and potassium in somewhat higher concentration. During passage through the colon, water and sodium are absorbed from the lumen but potassium is secreted into it. The 75–170 gm of feces formed

---

*The surface coat of the small intestine, also known as the fuzzy coat, is particularly well developed over the microvilli. It is glycoprotein in nature and gives a positive acid-Schiff reaction.

per day contain approximately 100 ml of water, 2–5 mEq of sodium, and 8–13 mEq of potassium. The difficulties in maintaining water and electrolyte balance in any condition that speeds the passage of the intestinal contents, as in severe diarrhea, becomes readily apparent. For a review of ion transport by the large intestine, see Schultz (1981b).

Only a small part of the organic material in the colon is the fibrous matter from plant cell walls that cannot be digested by enzymes in the tract. The major portion of the material that eventually appears in the feces is composed of desquamated cells, mucus, digestive secretions and bacteria, yeast, and fungi. The bacteria have been estimated at about 1×10^{11} per gm wet weight, or the excretion of about 1.2×10^{13} cells per day (Stephan and Cummins, 1980).

Much has been written about the influence of the intestinal bacteria on the nutrient economy of the organism. Only in the case of vitamins, required in such small quantities, did it seem likely that subtraction from or addition to the nutrient intake of the host could be of consequence. Since bacteria synthesize the vitamins essential for their own growth, it had been suggested that these products of bacterial synthesis could be absorbed through the intestinal mucosa and provide a convenient source of supply for the host. However, since dietary deficiency of vitamins can produce disorders in laboratory animals and in humans, absorption is minimal if it occurs at all. Only in the case of vitamin K are we beholden to the intestinal flora. The newborn infant with a sterile tract lacks the vitamin K essential for prothrombin formation until the establishment of flora in the tract, after which synthesis and absorption of vitamin K occurs.

Some of the difficulties inherent in a quantitative appraisal of the give and take between bacteria and host are readily apparent, but the development of techniques for growing germ-free animals has helped to elucidate some aspects of the complex role of intestinal flora. Barnes and his group (1963) have shown that the dietary requirements of the rat for the micronutrients can be altered considerably by the synthetic activity of the intestinal bacteria. However, the rat can benefit from intestinal synthesis only if the feces are recycled through the tract. This normally occurs in the rat unless efforts are made to prevent coprophagy. Since the effects on growth rate could be observed only when the feces were consumed directly from the anus, it is presumed that anaerobiosis must be maintained. Daft et al. (1963) have shown that coprophagy is essential to protect against symptoms of pantothenic acid deficiency but that folic acid, which is not normally required in the diet of the rat, is obtained in sufficient amounts from bacteria in the intestine tract without coprophagy.

Intestinal bacterial synthesis in the rat, under specific conditions, can provide vitamin K and the B-vitamins to the host. However, Levensen and Tennant (1963) found that conventional guinea pigs developed scurvy more quickly than germ-free animals, which suggests that the flora in the intestine may be robbing the host of available tissue ascorbic acid. Early work by Parsons et al. (1945) showed that consumption of live yeast deprived the host of B-vitamins available for absorption. These results raise questions concerning utilization of nutrients by flora in the human tract and the effects this may have in estimating requirements.

During the last decade there has been renewed interest in the relationship of diet to the human intestinal ecosystem and the relationship of this ecosystem to human health. The maintenance of the vast and varied population of bacteria in the colon is dependent on the kinds and amounts of undigested fiber, gastrointestinal secretions, mucus, bile salts, electrolytes and fluid, as well as the pH of the contents and the motility of the tract. With so many variables, it is not surprising that the bacterial population varies from individual to individual under the same conditions and in the same individual when conditions change (Speck, 1976; Flynn et al., 1977).

The dependence of ruminants on the microbial ecosystem in the rumen for the fermentation of the consumed food to short-chain volatile fatty acids has been studied extensively. Only recently has microbial fermentation been studied in humans. Cellulose, hemicellulose, and pectins, as well as the polysaccharides of endogenous mucins and those from consumed meat, reach the colon undigested (Salyers, 1979). There is, in addition, the vast quantity of sloughed off cells from the intestinal epithelium (see above). Enzymes produced by bacteria present in the colon hydrolyze all these materials. The hydrolyzed products can then be fermented by the same or other of the microflora (Holloway et al., 1978). The products of this fermentation are similar to those produced in the rumen: acetate, propionate, butyrate, methane, hydrogen, and carbon dioxide (Miller and Wolin, 1979). Since the calculated quantity of very short chain fatty acids produced by fermentation in humans far exceeds the quantity excreted in the feces, it is assumed that most enter the blood and are metabolized. The amount of metabolizable energy available from this source can be sizable in individuals who regularly consume large amounts of plant fiber. Most of the methane and hydrogen produced is absorbed into the blood, removed in the lungs, and exhaled. The hydrogen in the breath resulting from the fermentation of lactose was discussed above as a method for the screening of individuals with lactose intolerance.

For a review of fermentation in the rumen and the human large intestine, see Wolin (1981); Wolin and Miller (1983). See Connell (1981) for a review of the physiological effects of dietary fiber.

How bacterial flora affect the nutrient assortment available to the host is, undoubtedly, more complex than originally supposed. It is very likely that nutritional requirements, as they are now studied in the human, are distorted by the give and take of the bacterial population in the colon. However, the extent and importance of this intervention to the total organism is still far from clear. Since diet may affect the fecal flora composition and there are suggestions that fecal flora and the products of their metabolism may play a role in human health and disease, extensive research in this area can be expected. (See Hentges, 1980; Talbot, 1981; Ulrich et al., 1981.) It is conceivable that a population of flora could be established that would provide an optimal contribution to both the nutrition of the host and the host's resistance to disease.

For extensive and detailed coverage of the physiology of the gastrointestinal tract, see Johnson (1981).

Epilogue

Whatever the nutritional potential of a food, its contribution is nonexistent if it does not pass the test of absorption. Those nutrients that have not been transferred through the intestinal mucosal cell to enter the circulation have, for all nutritional intent and purpose, never been eaten. The variety of nutrients from the organism's environment that have been made available by absorption must be transported through the circulatory system to the aqueous microenvironment of the cells. There, they serve their ultimate purpose: participation in the metabolic activities in the cells on which the life of the total organism depends.

chapter 7

transport and exchange

1. Pathways
   a. The "Internal Environment" and Concept of Homeostasis
   b. Route to the Cells
   c. Control of Plasma Constituents
      (1) Fluid compartments
      (2) Metabolic pools
      (3) Storage and reserves
      (4) Normal values
2. Mechanisms
   a. Microcirculation
   b. Ion Distribution
   c. Fluid Movement
   d. Renal Controls
      (1) Water and Sodium
      (2) Nutrient Conservation
      (3) Nitrogen Excretion
      (4) Regulation of Plasma pH
   e. Intracellular pH Regulation
3. Coda

"All the vital mechanisms, however varied they may be, have always but one goal, to maintain the uniformity of the conditions of life in the internal environment.

Claude Bernard, 1878a

"The word (homeostasis) does not imply something set and immobile, a stagnation. It means a condition—a condition which may vary, but which is relatively constant."

Walter B. Cannon, 1929

Pathways

The assortment and concentration of each nutrient in the plasma depend not only on the quantity arriving through the intestinal mucosa but also on the integrated regulatory mechanisms that are the means of fine adjustment of supply to demand. Despite variation in the nutrient assortment presented to the plasma by the dietary intake, intricate control mechanisms operate to maintain circulating concentrations of many nutrients and synthesized constituents within rather narrow ranges. The enormity of the task and the dynamism inherent in it become evident with the realization that each of the myriad cells is constantly removing from its individual environment all of the nutrients essential for its metabolic needs and returning to this environment both products of synthesis and catabolism. *Homeostasis* is maintained despite constant change. If this is interpreted as maintaining the status quo, it is the achieving of constancy through rapid, purposeful, orderly change; the maintenance of a steady state by means of rapid flux. The overall logistics are illustrated in Fig. 7.1. It is by means of the plasma that the materials of metabolism move, but it is within cells and subcellular units that the purposeful change is engineered.

THE "INTERNAL ENVIRONMENT" AND THE CONCEPT OF HOMEOSTASIS

Claude Bernard (1878b) in his prescience developed the concept that the living organism exists

> . . . in the liquid *milieu intérieur* formed by the circulating organic liquid which surrounds and bathes all the tissue elements; this is the lymph or plasma, the liquid part of the blood which in the higher animals is diffused through the tissues and forms the ensemble of the intracellular liquids and is the basis of all local nutrition and the common factor of all elementary exchanges.

Thus, the extracellular fluid was recognized by Bernard 150 years ago as the "internal environment," the medium in which nutrients were brought to the cells. If Bernard's laboratory instruments had been able to expand his vision of what he called "the tissue elements," he would probably have anticipated the additional necessary steps to reach the "internal environment." This environment whose precise maintenance is critical to the life of the organism now is envisioned as the intracellular fluid, the environment of the subcellular units or organelles. It is at this level that the coordinated physiological reactions, the homeostatic mechanisms postulated by Cannon (1929), must take place. How this occurs raises many questions, some answered, some still to be answered, and some yet to be posed. Claude Bernard conceived the concept of the constancy of the internal environment to life, and Cannon coined the word homeostasis to describe that steady state. Since that time scientists have been probing to discover the regulatory mechanisms involved. A likely mechanism of control appears to be mediated by protein molecules that undergo conformational changes (Umbarger, 1964). Such conformational changes operate within cells in metabolic regulation, between

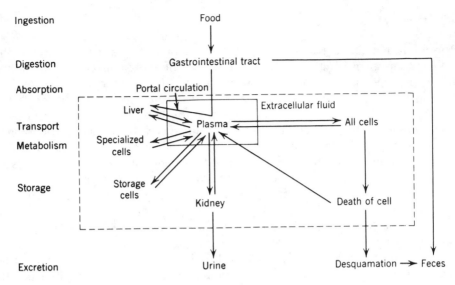

Figure 7.1
The pathways through which the nutrients in food become available and are transported to the individual cells in humans.

cells in hormonal and neural signals, and between cells and the environment in sensory receptors. Thus, mechanisms that operate in sensing and regulation in biological systems are similar (Koshland et al., 1982). Knox (1976) suggested that the discovery of regulatory mechanisms at the molecular level during the past several decades indicates a need for a new and grand conceptual scheme that would integrate what some know as homeostasis with the related but newer molecular discoveries of regulation and control.

ROUTE TO THE CELLS

The plasma is the extracellular fluid of blood in which the cellular constituents of the blood are suspended. The plasma constitutes about half the total blood volume from which the cells can be readily separated by centrifugation. Over 90 percent of the plasma is water that readily exchanges with the interstitital fluid surrounding the cells of all tissues in the body. Plasma water functions not only as the solvent or carrier for all of the materials transported but also in maintaining the water balance of body compartments. That part of the plasma which is not water—8 to 9 percent—contains, by extremely conservative estimates, from 150 to 200 different kinds of molecules. These include electrolytes, lipids, carbohydrates, organic acids, proteins, amino acids and other nonprotein nitrogenous molecules, vitamins, hormones, and enzymes (Table 7.1). Because methods and instruments continually improve, more precise separations of components are likely to be made. For example, the plasma globulins were first separated into α_1 and α_2. Now it is estimated that there are 14 different fractions comprising the

α_2 group alone. The same is true of most of the plasma proteins, lipoproteins, and other complex molecules. Estimation of some components, such as certain enzymes and hormones, is hampered by their transitory appearance in the plasma, ease of destruction, and inadequacy of methods for detecting ultramicro quantities.

The plasma, functioning as the transport medium in the organism, must carry in it: (1) any nutrient required by a cell, (2) any excretory product released by a cell, and (3) any synthetic product exported by a cell. The plasma carrying materials from and to the external environment of the organism is the liaison with the external environment of the cells. It must have in it, readily available and in proper concentration, every nutrient required by the cells. And, since the demands of each cell however centrally or remotely located in the body must be met continuously, an extremely sensitive and controlled information system must be in effect to maintain the concentrations of the multitude of constituents in the plasma and tissue fluids within suitable limits. These may vary according to the requirements of specific tissues.

The plasma, then, operates as a highly effective transport route in which all essentials for both cellular metabolism and regulation are provided and by means of which all products of metabolism are removed. To reach the cells, solutes in the plasma leave the capillary and enter the interstitial fluid that, together with the plasma, constitutes the extracellular fluid. The interstitial fluid is the moat between the capillary membrane and the cell membrane and is the immediate external environment of the cells. Materials transported to the interstitial fluid can be selectively taken up by the cell membrane and transported into the cell's interior.

Transport into the cell interior until recently had been considered of primary importance since the life of the cell depends on the successful exchange of nutrients and metabolites across the cellular membrane into and out of the cell. However, as our knowledge of cell function increases, it is apparent that still other sets of membranes must be considered. Intracellular fluid surrounds the subcellular structures (the organelles) each of which has its own distinct internal medium influenced by and influencing the intracellular fluid that surrounds it. The subcellular compartments possibly account for the major portion of the intracellular fluid but how this volume is distributed within the various organelles is an area still to be explored. Intramitochondrial volume changes, for example, are associated with uptake and release of metabolites involved in mitochondrial function (see Chapter 13) but quantification of such changes is still beyond even our most advanced laboratory methods. Some of the fundamental mechanisms responsible for the homeostasis of the organism are controlled by regulatory molecules that travel the plasma route to receptor sites on subcellular membranes and affect organelle function in a specific way.

Constituents of the plasma participate in controlled but dynamic exchange with materials in the other extracellular fluid compartments and, ultimately, with all cells including those specialized cells that form the boundary with the organism's external environment: the cells lining the intestinal lumen and those comprising the kidney tubules and lung alveoli. Nutrients that the body cannot accumulate,

TABLE 7.1
Some Reported Plasma Constituents in Humans

Minerals	Carbohydrates	Proteins	Lipids
Aluminum	Fructose	Prealbumin	Cephalin
Bicarbonate	Glucosamine	Albumin	Cerebrosides
Bromine	Acetyl glucosamine	Angiotensinogen	Cholesterol
Calcium	Glucose	Calmodulin	Free
Chloride	Glucuronic acid	Ferritin	Ester
Chromium	Glycogen	α_1 Acid glycoprotein	Cholic acid
Cobalt	Heparin	α_1 Glycoprotein	Chylomicrons
Copper	Lactose	α_1 Lipoproteins	Fat, neutral
Fluorine	Pentose	α_2 Glycoproteins	Fatty acids
Iodine	Polysaccharides	Ceruloplasmin	Glyceride-
Iron	Nonglucosamine	Haptoglobins	Phospholipid-
Lead	Protein-bound	α_2 Macroglobulins	Saturated
Magnesium		Prothrombin	Lecithin
Manganese		β glycoproteins	Phospholipids
Molybdenum		Transferrin	Prostaglandins
Nickel		β_2 Globulin	Sphingomyelin
Phosphate		Fibrinogen	Triacylglycerols
Phosphorus		Isoagglutinin	
Inorganic P		Kininogens	
Organic P		Plasminogen	
Adenosine triphosphate P		β_1 Lipoproteins	
Glycerophosphate P		β_2 Globulins	
Hexosephosphate P		γ Globulins	
Lipid P			
Nucleic acid P			
Potassium			
Rubidium			
Selenium			
Silicon			
Sodium			
Sulfate			
Sulfur			
Tin			
Vanadium			
Zinc			

TABLE 7.1 (continued)

Nonprotein Nitrogenous Substances	Vitamins	Enzymes	Hormones
Allantoin	Vitamin A	Adenosine poly-	Acetylcholine
Amino acids	Carotenes	phosphatases	Adrenocorticotropin
Alanine	Thiamin	Aldolase	Aldosterone
Aminobutyric acid	Riboflavin	Amylase	Androgens
Arginine	Nicotinic acid	Angiotensinase	Angiotensins
Asparagine	Pyridoxine	Catalase	Bradykinin
Aspartic acid	Pantothenic acid	Cathepsins	Corticosteroids
Citrulline	Folacin	Cholinesterase	Calcitonin
Cysteine	Vitamin B_{12}	Converting enzyme	Cholecalciferols
Cystine	Ascorbic acid	Dehydropeptidase	Cholecystokinin
Glutamic acid	Vitamin D	B-glucuronidase	Endorphins
Glutamine	Tocopherols	Histaminase	Epinephrine
Glycine	Biotin	Kallikreins	Erythropoietin
Histidine	Choline	Kininases	Estrogens
Isoleucine	Inositol	Lactic dehydrogenase	Follicle-stimulating
Leucine		Lipases	hormone
Lysine		Pepsinogens	Gastrin
Methionine		Phenolsulfatase	Glucagon
1-Methylhistidine		Phosphatases	Glucocorticoids
3-Methylhistidine		Phosphoglucose	Gonadotropins
Ornithine		isomerase	Growth hormone
Phenylalanine		Plasmin (fibrinolysin)	Insulin
Proline		Prekallikrein activators	Interferons
Serine		Profibrinolysin	Luteinizing
Taurine		Renin	hormone
Threonine		Transaminases	Melatonin
Tryptophan			Norepinephrine
Tyrosine			Oxytocin
Valine			Parathyroid hormone
Bilirubin			Progastrin
Creatine			Progesterone
Creatinine			Proinsulin
Histamine			Prolactin
Imidazoles			Relaxin
Indican			Releasing factors
Urea			Secretin
Uric acid			Serotonin
Ammonia N			Somatomedin
Polypeptide N			Testosterone
			Thrombopoietin
			Thyroxine
			Triiodothyronine
			Vasopressin

and products of metabolism that it cannot tolerate, must be transported between the cells and the external environment of the organism unceasingly, as in the case of oxygen and carbon dioxide. Other nutrients or products of metabolism such as vitamin A and fat, both of which can be stored in large quantities will, if and when needed, travel in the plasma between depots and cells. Estimations of plasma level of nutrients, therefore, may not be at all indicative of the state of body nutriture since they are the immediate currency for metabolism and will be reduced only when stores and reserves can no longer maintain nutrient levels. The greater the storage of a nutrient the smaller the chance that plasma levels will fall below the normal range. However, when such a nutrient does fall in the plasma the situation is likely to be critical.

Two-way movement of nutrients and metabolites between the external environment of the organism and the innermost units of the cell are illustrated in Fig. 7.2.

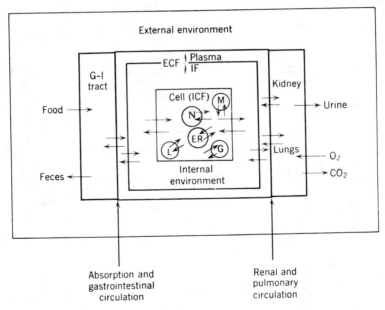

Figure 7.2
Exchanges of nutrients and metabolites between body fluid compartments showing relationship of the external environment to the internal environment in a complex organism. Within the cell, fluid compartments within each organelle influence and are influenced by the intracellular fluid and the enveloping layers of extracellular environments. Extracellular fluid (ECF), interstitial fluid (IF), intracellular fluid (ICF), endoplasmic reticulum (ER), Golgi (G), lysosome (L), mitochondrion (M), nucleus (N).

CONTROL OF PLASMA CONSTITUENTS

The relative constancy of plasma constituents indicates that the nutrients constantly being withdrawn are counterbalanced by like quantities being sent into
the plasma. Variability of dietary intake would make that source too precarious
to depend on for any real control of supply. When absorption from the small
intestine provides more than is required to compensate for current use, the excess,
depending on the nutrient, either is circulated to become part of storage or reserves
or, for those water-soluble nutrients that do not accumulate, is excreted by the
kidney that acts as the regulatory organ controlling overflow. (Kidney threshholds
will be discussed in the section on renal function.) If the quantity of a nutrient
being absorbed is too small to compensate for uptake by the tissues, the deficit
in plasma content is made up from storage or reserves as long as these supplies
are available.

Fluid Compartments

Body fluid compartments as shown in Fig. 7.3 represent an overall and oversimplified view of fluid volume relationships. (For methods of measuring volume in
the several compartments and variation with age and sex, see Chapter 22.) Reference to either the intracellular area or the interstitium as "fluid" compartments
tends to be misleading if fluid is envisioned as a pourable liquid. The interstitial
fluid that lies outside the blood vessels and lymphatics and between the cells is
enmeshed in a fibrous mat composed of bundles of collagen fibers. Much smaller
reticular filaments fill the spaces between the collagen fibers. The reticular fila-

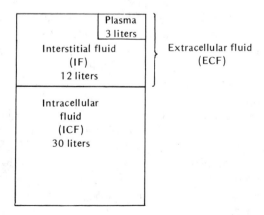

Figure 7.3
Body fluid compartments.

ments are composed of mucopolysaccharides, the most important constituent of which is hyaluronic acid. The polymerized hyaluronic acid molecules are large and fluffy and trapped in the collagen mat so that virtually all of the space is occupied. It is in this occupied space that the interstitial fluid is held. The mucopolysaccharides, by preventing free flow of fluid, protect us from what could be a devastating effect of gravity. However, they do permit slow fluid movement in the short distances between blood and lymph capillaries and offer virtually no impediment to the diffusion that carries materials to and from the cells (Guyton et al., 1979).

It has become quite apparent that this extravascular-extracellular fluid compartment, the interstitium, is not a single compartment with a homogeneous fluid but, in all probability, a series of compartments and fluids that vary from tissue to tissue. The view of three fluid compartments, one plasma, one extracellular fluid, and one intracellular fluid is patently false according to Neuman (1969) who suggests that every organ system may regulate the composition of its own fluid medium, and gives as an example the differences observed between extracellular fluid in bone and other extracellular fluid. He suggests that this can be explained only in terms of compartmentalization by a functional membrane that regulates passage between general extracellular fluid and bone extracellular fluid. In other words, an additional membrane barrier is interposed between general interstitial fluid and the discrete and controlled interstitial fluid in specific organ systems.

Andersson (1971) discusses compartmentalization of the extracellular fluids (ECF) of the brain (Fig. 7.4). The capillaries in brain tissue appear less permeable to solutes and ions than other capillaries. For this reason direct transfer from the plasma to brain tissue is either prevented or delayed. This allows a more stable fluid environment to be maintained. Cerebrospinal fluid (CSF) is secreted by the cells of the choroid plexus and this fluid is different in ionic composition from plasma. The CSF is continuously transported through the ventricles, drained out into the blood in the subarachnoid space, but replaced by secretion. A barrier between CSF and brain ECF is created by the epithlial cell layer lining the walls of the brain ventricles, thereby delaying exchange between these two fluids despite the fact that in most instances their ionic composition appears to be almost identical. However, Bito (1969) observed that the ECF of mammalian cerebral cortex had lower K^+ and higher Mg^{++} concentrations than were present in the plasma or even the CSF, and he postulated an active transport system across the blood-brain barrier. Because of the barrier to free exchange between plasma and the ECF of brain tissue by the interposition of the CSF compartment, a more stable cellular environment can be maintained. In this way, the brain is protected from variations in plasma composition that might be acceptable to other less discriminating tissues (Davson, 1976). Neuron function is so completely dependent on the ionic composition of surrounding fluids (see Chapter 19) that even slight variations can have far-reaching effects. Similar mechanisms of compartmentalization of ECF appear to be present in other tissues, for example, the humors of the eye and the synovial fluid of joints. The distinctiveness of compartments is

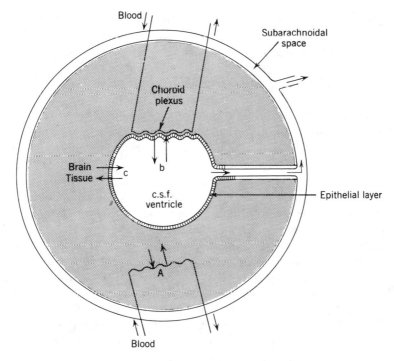

Figure 7.4
Compartmentalization of extracellular fluid in the brain. (a) The blood-brain barrier. (b) The blood-cerebrospinal fluid (CSF) barrier. (c) The cerebrospinal fluid-brain barrier. (From B. Andersson, *Am. Sci.* 59:411, 1971).

dependent on the functioning cells and subcellular units *within* each compartment. An understanding of the controlled environmental conditions of various organs and tissues will lead to better understanding of the intricacies of their functions.

Metabolic Pools
Early investigators suggested a separation in metabolism of those materials coming from outside, exogenous metabolism, and those of the body substance, endogenous metabolism (Folin, 1905). The revolutionary studies presented by Schoenheimer (1942), now ranked with the classics of biochemical literature, clearly demonstrated that (1) such segregation does not exist in metabolism, (2) all constituents of living matter, structural and functional, are in a steady state of rapid flux, and (3) fragments derived from complex molecules in the body merge indistinguishably with fragments derived from food sources to form *metabolic pools*.

A pool, then, is the quantity of a specific substance that is in a state of active turnover. It should be readily apparent that this kind of pool cannot be located in any one particular place. It is, in fact, illustrated by the two-directional arrows in the box depicting transport, metabolism, and storage in Fig. 7.1. It represents available labile nutrients in dynamic flux.

Pool size can be measured by administering a radioactive isotope and determining its dilution. The size of the pool can be small for some substances and larger for others. However, in a small pool the turnover can be quite enormous, as it is in the case of ATP which the human produces in an equivalent to his body weight (70 kg) every 24 hours (Karlson, 1968). Steele (1964) defined a pool of material in steady-state turnover as "a collection of identical molecules from which deletions are made at a constant rate, along with simultaneous addition of new identical molecules at the same rate, the total pool size remaining unchanged." Such turnover was first reported by Schoenheimer (1942), who showed that even adipose tissue was far from static and that 44 percent of an administered tracer dose was in the depots at the end of eight days although the total body fat of the animal had not changed. Similar pool exchanges were observed when labeled amino acids were administered. With these studies Schoenheimer established the concept of the dynamic state of the body's metabolism. Pools are everchanging and dynamic. They do not constitute storage that, although in a dynamic state, is localized and expendable; but they are fed by and feed into metabolizing cells, storage, and reserves.

Storage and Reserves

Storage, as the term generally applies, is an extra supply of a substance collected in specific cells or tissues that is available when and if needed. Withdrawal from the store in no way interferes with the function of the storage area or with the metabolic activity of the organism. Fat storage is the most obvious and increase or reduction in the quantity stored occurs only when the energy expenditure of the organism is not balanced with intake. Less obvious than fat storage is the far more extensive vitamin A storage in the liver of a well-nourished individual which may be large enough to last for a period of 1–2 years. Table 7.2 illustrates the extreme variation in the normal body content of some of the major and minor nutrients with the resulting extremes in survival time that range from 2 days–20 years.

Reserves for a nutrient such as protein differ from stores in that they do not have a specific locus but are instead all protein tissue that can be reversibly depleted and repleted. The most extensive and most labile protein reserves are in liver and muscle both of which are composed mainly of protein. Much of liver and muscle protein is broken down and resynthesized at a rapid rate. Amino acids released by the protein breakdown are recycled within the cell or are transported to enter protein anabolic pathways at other sites. Such recycling is part of normal amino acid economy and its extent is related to protein and energy intake. (See Chapter 23.)

TABLE 7.2
Normal Stores or Reserves in the Human Body

	Total Body Content	Permissible Total Loss	Possible Daily Loss	Survival Time
Fat (gm)	9000	6500	150[a]	6–7 weeks
Protein (gm)	11,000	2400[b]	60[c]	6–7 weeks
Carbohydrate (gm)	500	150	—	a few hours
Water (gm)	40,000	4000	1000[d]	4 days
Sodium (mEq)	2600	800[e]	320[f]	2–3 days
Potassium (mEq)	3500	300	260[g]	1–2 days
Calcium (gm)	1500	500[h]	0.1[i]	10–20 years
Iron (mg)	4000	3000[j]	23[k]	4–5 months
Vitamin A (I.U.)	500,000[l]		1000[m]	1–2 years
Vitamin B$_{12}$ (μg)	5000[n]		1[o]	10–20 years
Vitamin B$_1$ (mg)	25[p]		0.35[q]	2–3 months

Source: From R. Passmore, in *Human Body Composition,* J. Brozek, ed., Pergamon Press, Oxford, 1965, pp.124–125.

Note: The figures given for total body content are representative values for a normal person living on a good diet. In many parts of the world, where the daily diet is unsatisfactory, the reserves will be much less. The figures for possible daily losses are such as might occur with dietary restrictions or in various diseases as explained in the notes. The figures for survival time may vary greatly, but the orders of magnitude in which they are given are correct.

[a]Equivalent to 1400 kcal.

[b]Wasting of tissue, predominantly muscle, amounting to 20 percent of total protein.

[c]Providing 240 kcal. With 150 gm of fat this will supply 1640 kcal, enough to meet the needs of a starving person.

[d]Under the best possible conditions a person unable to take in water will lose 800 gm by evaporation from the skin and lungs and 400 gm in the urine. Against this about 200 gm of metabolic water must be offset.

[e]A reduction of the extracellular fluid from 15 liters (Na 140 mEq/liter)—13 liters (Na 123 mEq/liter) and a loss of 300 mEq of sodium from bone.

[f]Sweating at the rate of 4.1 liters/day with a sweat content of 80 mEq/liter.

[g]Severe diarrhea and vomiting.

[h]Assuming clinical osteoporosis does not occur until one-third of the bone mineral is lost.

[i]A substantial figure for a continued negative calcium balance.

[j]A reduction in hemoglobin to 20 percent and a loss of 1 gm of iron, previously stored as ferritin.

[k]Assuming a daily loss of 50 ml of blood from a chronic hemorrhage plus a physiological loss of 1 mg/day and partly offset by increased absorption of 3 mg/day.

[l]A normal content of the liver for the people of the United Kingdom.

[m]A high estimate. Many adults in Southeast Asia live on diets providing much less and with no obvious evidence of vitamin A deficiency.

[n]Almost all in the liver.

[o]This amount of the vitamin will bring about a remission in most patients with pernicious anemia. The daily physiological requirement may be even less.

[p]Assuming about 0.5 μg/gm in skeletal muscle and 1.0 μg/gm in the principal viscera.

[q]Assuming a daily minimum need of 0.7 mg and diet of polished rice providing only 0.35 mg.

Tissues that lose protein most rapidly, such as liver, intestinal epithelium, and kidney, probably are the reserves that supply most of the amino acids required during postabsorptive intervals and during early stages of deprivation; in later stages and in prolonged starvation amino acid needs are provided primarily by muscle (Mortimore, 1982). Because of the size of the muscle mass and the lability of its protein, skeletal muscle can maintain not only circulating levels of amino acids but glucose level (through gluconeogenesis) as well (Daniel et al., 1977).

When a diet is deficient in either protein or energy but not both, the amino acids released by muscle breakdown are available for other tissues because there is an immediate and sustained fall in the rate of muscle protein synthesis. Under these conditions, no protein is lost by the organism. This recycling of amino acids appears to be a regulatory, and probably hormonal, response to a nutritional state (Millward and Waterlow, 1978). With continued protein deficiency, protein loss occurs even though the muscle breakdown rate may be reduced by half. When both protein and energy are deficient, as in starvation, protein breakdown is greater and protein loss occurs (Fig. 7.5). Young and Munro (1978) reported similar results using 3-methylhistidine excretion as an indicator of protein breakdown.

Allison and his group (1963) reported that tissue RNA and the RNA/DNA ratio are closely correlated with protein synthesis. On a protein-free diet or during starvation, the RNA/DNA ratio falls in tissues that contribute to protein reserves but the ratio does not fall in a resistant tissue such as brain (Fig. 7.6). Recently, Millward and Waterlow (1978) observed that diurnal changes occur in muscle RNA in meal-fed rats and that there is an immediate muscle RNA loss in fasted rats.

The storage, metabolic, and homeostatic activities of skeletal muscle suggested to Daniel et al. (1977) that these activities were almost as vital as the role muscle performs in maintaining posture and providing the power for movement. Taking this idea a step further, one could suggest that these functions are probably interrelated, since during growth muscle protein breakdown is stimulated by muscle protein synthesis. This paradox has been related to the remodeling and proliferation of muscle during growth (Millward et al., 1980).

For discussion of the mechanisms involved in regulating cellular protein synthesis and breakdown, as a means of providing protein reserves, see Mortimore (1982); Ballard and Gunn (1982).

Normal Values

The concept of normality, while comforting, is an illusion arrived at by computation. The definition of normality, while useful, is arbitrary since normality, like beauty, is in the eyes of the beholder. If it is understood and appreciated for what it is, it has meaning; if misunderstood or abused, it may be insidious.

The mass of tables available that catalog and present "normal values" for constituents of plasma, for example, suggest a stability that far exceeds reality and a standard of reference that implies perfection or an ideal. These tables are enormously important and valuable as long as they are properly understood. They

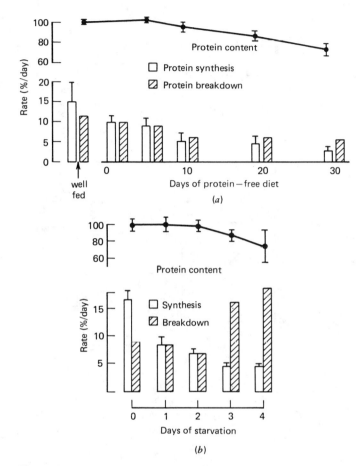

Figure 7.5

(a) Effect of protein deficiency on muscle protein turnover. Protein-free diet initially suppresses growth by depressing protein synthesis; then induces a progressive reduction in synthesis rate. Rate of protein breakdown also falls initially so that little protein is lost during the first 10 days. Then, because protein synthesis falls to a lower rate than breakdown, net breakdown results and protein is lost. (b). Effect of starvation on muscle protein breakdown. Initial response to starvation is the same as response to protein deficiency. After 2 days, protein breakdown increases to higher than initial values inducing a rapid loss of protein. (From D. J. Millward and J. C. Waterlow, Fed. Proc. 37:2283, 1978.)

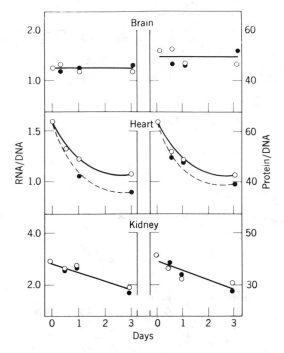

Figure 7.6
Effect of protein-free diet (open circles) or starvation (closed circles) for various times on the RNA-
DNA ratio and protein-DNA ratio of brain, heart,
and kidney. (From J. B. Allison et al., *Fed. Proc.*
22:1126, 1963.)

are, in fact, a compilation of findings that can be quantitatively measured. They
are obtained from a random sampling of a population judged to be representative
of a general population and based on the assumption that they fall into a distribution pattern described as a normal curve. In some cases the figure in the table
may have been derived from a large and representative sample; in other cases,
for a variety of reasons, the sample may have been small and the figure of
questionable validity if it is used as a norm for a general population. The figures
presented, for example, in the *Biology Data Book* published by FASEB (Altman
and Dittmer, 1964) indicate where values for 95 percent of the population would
be expected to lie (Fig. 7.7). This excludes the 2.5 percent at either extreme of
the normal curve and therefore, by definition, 5 percent of the so-called normal
population is outside the limits that are then prescribed as normal. Moreover, the
values obtained for any one individual attain a distribution pattern or normal
curve established through time; yet the "normal values" for a population are
obtained from a compilation of single random values in the continuum of values

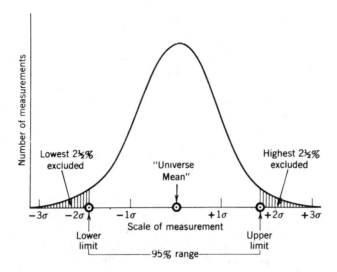

Figure 7.7
Normal frequency distribution curve. (From *Biology Data Book*, "Introduction," P. L. Altman and D. S. Dittmer, eds., FASEB, 1964, p.xvii.)

for the individuals who comprise the randomly derived sample of a population. It becomes clear that there are, in fact, no "normal values" but normal *ranges* of values, and that even ranges, in some cases, may be too narrow or too wide to be diagnostically useful (McCammon, 1966).

The line between normal and abnormal is an arbitrary one, and what is normal for an individual at a specific moment in time may be abnormal at other times (McCammon, 1966; Thomas, 1966); moreover, what is normal for one individual may be abnormal for others (Widdowson, 1962). Some of the difficulties inherent in establishing normal limits are illustrated by Simonson (1966) and emphasize the fact that the normal limits as they are used are no more than a prediction of the probability of being normal (Fig. 7.8). Only through an understanding of human variation and adaptation can one appreciate why under controlled experimental conditions the minimum requirement for a nutrient, for example, may differ among subjects by 100 percent or more; or why under identical conditions some individuals may develop a disorder and others may not (Boyd, 1966).

The visible aspects of human variation are expected and accepted, and their determinants are both genetic and environmental. Some of the hidden aspects of variation such as individual differences in metabolic response were studied in great detail by Keys and his co-workers (1950). The concept of biochemical individuality was delineated by Williams (1956) who has suggested that each organism possesses a complex and unique metabolic pattern that encompasses

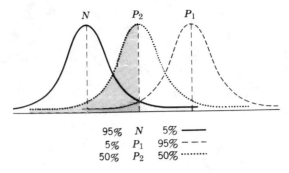

$$
\begin{array}{ccc}
95\% & N & 5\% \; \text{———} \\
5\% & P_1 & 95\% \; \text{– – –} \\
50\% & P_2 & 50\% \; \text{·········}
\end{array}
$$

Figure 7.8
Frequency distribution of a hypothetical normal sample (N) and two samples of patients (P_1 and P_2) representing two different types of disease for a hypothetical item. The dividing line for 5 percent at the upper end of the normal distribution coincides with that for 95 percent of the patients in group P_1 and for 50 percent (median) in group P_2. The areas of overlap are shaded (From E. Simonson, *Ann. N.Y. Acad. Sci.* 134:541, 1966.)

every aspect of the individual's biochemistry. Others explored various aspects of physiological individuality (Sargent and Weinman, 1966; Garn, 1966). The relationship between individual genetic and therefore metabolic traits and disease symptomatology has led to special diagnostic procedures (Hsia, 1966; Friedmann, 1971). Pauling (1968) suggests that individual variation in the optimal concentration of specific nutrients for metabolism of specific organs may be considerable and lead to greatly increased requirements for proper metabolic activity in those individuals.

Certainly, acceptance of the idea that there is genetic control of all biochemical reactions must have as its corollary that individual variations are to be expected and that they may be substantial. "Book values" are useful but only if used judiciously.

Mechanisms

The basic function of the circulatory system is to bring the blood close enough to each cell to permit rapid exchange of nutrients and removal of products of metabolism. The mechanisms regulating exchange between the cell and its immediate environment involve both active and passive transfer (discussed in Chapter 9). Exchange between the plasma and interstitial fluid is a function of the composition of the fluids and the overall dynamics of the body fluid system.

Although pressure relationships between capillary and interstitial fluid may account for some exchange, a more realistic description of the mechanisms by which the nutrients in the circulatory system are brought close enough to each cell to permit rapid exchange involve branching and local control exerted in the capillary bed. The major vessels in the arterial system branch into smaller and smaller arteries, arterioles, and finally into the extremely large number of capillaries in close association with the individual cells. Because the same volume of blood per minute carried by the aorta under pressure is diverted through capillaries that have 500 to 600 times the cross-sectional area, there is a drastic reduction of pressure and a corresponding reduction in rate of flow when the blood reaches the capillary bed (Fig. 7.9). It is the flow through the capillary bed, or the microcirculation, that is the most important function of the cardiovascular system. Indeed, the primary purpose of the heart and major vessels is to maintain flow through the capillary bed and thereby provide an effective environment for the individual cells.

MICROCIRCULATION

The network of approximately 60,000 miles of capillary has been described as the microcirculation. The arrangement of these capillaries that connect arterioles and venules differ from tissue to tissue but the general plan is similar and is one that facilitates control of blood flow. Control of the volume and direction of blood flow in the microcirculation is dependent on the two specialized components described by Zweifach (1961), the thoroughfare channels and the true capillaries. Blood flows from the arteriole into the *thoroughfare channel* or *metarteriole*. This is the *preferential channel* and the main pathway. Sparsely distributed smooth muscle cells in the walls of these vessels control the rate of flow toward a secondary network of *true capillaries*. At the origin of the true capillary there is a precapillary sphincter, usually a single smooth muscle cell, which controls the flow into the capillary. Precapillary sphincters open and close periodically permitting flow through different parts of the microsystem. Closing of the precapillary sphincter restricts blood flow to the thoroughfare channel in what could be considered a shortcut to the venous system. Additional shortcuts are provided by arteriovenous anastomoses which are short connections between arterioles or metarterioles and venules (Fig. 7.10). The basic characteristics are the same in all tissues: a thoroughfare channel whose muscle cells, though sparsely distributed, control the rate of flow into a secondary network of true capillaries where flow is controlled by precapillary sphincters. So widely spaced are the muscle cells along the thoroughfare channels that they are almost indistinguishable from the true capillaries. The structure or complexity of the network depends on the needs of the tissue. Tissues with changing metabolic needs, such as striated muscle, have a large number of small channels that, when opened, can supply the greatly increased needs of the cells during activity. Secretory cells, with more modest demands,

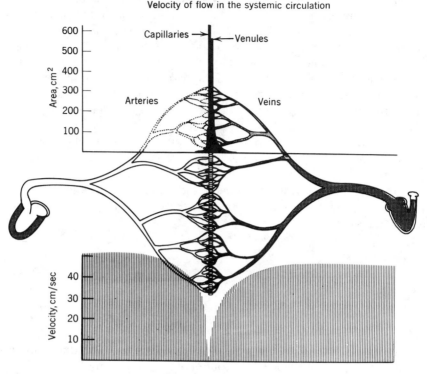

Figure 7.9
At each successive branching of the arterial system, the cross-sectional area increases slightly. The terminal branches of the arterial system greatly increase the total cross-sectional area of the arterioles to some 125 times and capillaries about 600 times that of the aorta. The velocity of blood flow through the vessels diminishes as the cross-sectional area increases. (From R. F. Rushmer, *Cardiovascular Dynamics,* 2nd ed., W. B. Saunders Co., Philadelphia, 1961, p. 5.)

may have few true capillary branches from the thoroughfare channels. The dependence of the rapidly metabolizing cell on a correspondingly rapid exchange of nutrients is illustrated by the effects of interruption of blood flow to the brain, which can lead to unconsciousness in about seven seconds.

The control of the muscle cells in the capillary bed is not clear. There is no obvious or direct innervation that would indicate control through the nervous system. There is, however, direct contact with the interstitial fluid surrounding the cells served by the capillary bed. Changes in the concentration of specific substances in the interstitial fluid or specific metabolic products released into the fluid by the cells might well exert the necessary control. Therefore, it appears

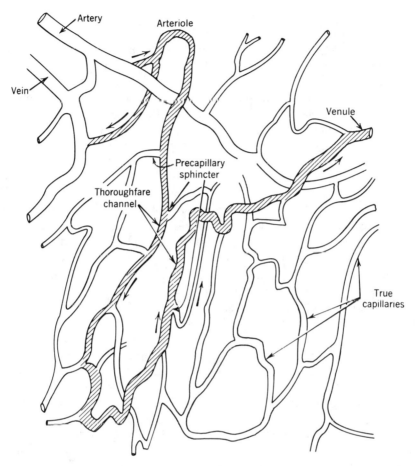

Figure 7.10
Schematized tracing of capillary bed indicating terminology for different
structural components. The preferential pathway for the microcirculation is
shaded. Also indicated is a direct anastomosis between a small artery and
its adjacent vein. (From B. W. Zweifach, *Functional Behavior of Microcirculation,* Charles C Thomas, Springfield, Illinois, 1961, p. 10.)

most likely that control of blood flow in the microcirculation is exerted by nutrients
and metabolites in the local fluid environment (Haddy and Scott, 1968).

In addition, the capillary bed exhibits extreme sensitivity to chemical stimuli.
These facts suggested to Zweifach (1961) that control might well be maintained
jointly by hormonal factors and specific products of tissue metabolism, and he
mentioned norepinephrine as a possible candidate for the role of maintaining
tone in the microcirculation. The effects of norepinephrine mediated through the
action of cAMP have been shown in a variety of tissues (Sutherland, 1972). Triner

et al. (1971) reported that increased formation of cAMP is associated with decreased contractility of vascular smooth muscle; conversely, decreased cAMP leads to increased contractility. The intimate relationship of the capillary muscle cells to the plasma and interstitial fluid of the tissue supplied by the capillary strongly suggests that increased blood flow through the capillary bed may be in response to some factor in cellular metabolism. As either a direct or indirect result, increased adenyl cyclase and cAMP decrease the contractility or tonus of the thoroughfare channel. Cheung (1972) suggests that the action of cAMP might be explained on the basis of a versatile allosteric effector and that the different effects of cAMP could be explained by the kinds of protein with which it interacts. He also indicates how cAMP might act as a unidirectional "off" switch for the effective termination of the action of hormones. If so, the norepinephrine effect might be involved. It almost seems as though the available threads of information about the control of microcirculation involving norepinephrine, cAMP, and the distinctive location of the effector site are just waiting to be woven into whole cloth.

The movement of fluid from the microcirculation into and out of the interstitial space, except for such sequestered spaces as cerebrospinal fluid, occurs at rates of exchange as high as 50–100 times per minute in areas immediately adjacent to the capillaries. The rate slows down to once every 1–10 minutes at distances of 50–100 μ away from the capillary. (See Guyton, 1975, p. 10.) The volume of fluid that diffuses out of the capillaries and into the interstitial space may be difficult to comprehend: 80,000 liters each day (Pappenheimer, 1953). Obviously, a like amount must return to the capillaries. Nutrients move with the fluid and, for example, 20,000 gm of glucose per day diffuse in both directions across the capillary wall. The margin of safety is great since this is probably 50 times the quantity needed by the cells. An estimated capillary surface area of 60 m^2 accommodates this vast movement. Transfers of such magnitude and such importance are precisely controlled. The role played by the microcirculation is of primary importance in this control.

ION DISTRIBUTION

The protein concentration of the plasma is approximately 7.5 gm/dl and the protein concentration of interstitial fluid is only about 1.0 gm/dl. The difference in concentration is maintained, in part, by the fact that the capillary membrane which separates the two comparments is impermeable to plasma proteins. (The relatively small amount of protein that does penetrate the membrane formerly referred to as leakage, now is regarded as a normal physiological process. The quantity involved amounts to 80–200 gm/day and its return to plasma through the lymph will be discussed in the next section.) The protein held within the capillary imposes restraints on the free exchange of ions between the capillary and interstitial fluid. This restraint is due to the negative charge carried by most protein molecules. The presence of nondiffusable protein anions on one side of the capillary membrane that is permeable to all other ions causes an unequal distribution of diffusable ions on the two sides of the membrane. The distribution is referred to as the *Gibbs-Donnan Equilibrium.*

According to the Gibbs-Donnan Equilibrium, in which the permeating particles are influenced by simple passive forces, the ionic distribution on the two sides of the capillary membrane must satisfy three requirements: (1) the sum of all the cations must equal the sum of all the anions on each side of the membrane, (2) on the side lacking protein, diffusable anions must be present in greater concentrations than on the side containing protein so that electroneutrality is maintained, and (3) osmotic pressure on the side containing protein must be balanced to prevent transfer of fluid and this is effected by the greater hydrostatic pressure in the capillary. The Gibbs-Donnan distribution, then, accounts for the lower concentration of diffusable anions and slightly higher concentration of diffusable cations in the plasma than in the interstitial fluid. It also accounts for the higher osmotic pressure within the capillary and helps to explain how disturbances in ionic distribution occur when plasma protein concentrations are reduced.

FLUID MOVEMENT

The movement of fluid from the capillary lumen into the interstitial space and back into the capillary was described by Starling (1896). His hypothesis suggested that the higher hydrostatic pressure at the arterial end of the capillary overcomes the osmotic pressure within the capillary which is due to plasma protein content and which forces an ultrafiltrate into the interstitial space. The hydrostatic pressure falls as the remaining fluid moves through the capillary. At the venous end the osmotic pressure within the capillary is greater than the opposing hydrostatic pressure; thus fluid is drawn back into the capillary lumen from the interstitial space. Starling's concept soon will have its centennial yet it remains the basis for understanding the forces responsible for maintaining fluid balance between the capillary circulation and the interstitium.

When Starling's hypothesis was formulated, the gel-like organization of collagen and mucopolysaccharides in the interstitial space was not understood. The transfer of protein to the interstitial space was regarded as "leakage" rather than a normal process. In addition, maintenance of slightly negative pressure in the interstitial fluid had not been established. (See Guyton et al., 1979.) In fact, the concept of subatmospheric pressure is still being debated by some. (For arguments on both sides of the issue, see Aukland and Nicolaysen, 1981; Brace, 1981; Taylor, 1981.) Nevertheless, mechanisms regulating fluid movement still can be explained according to Starling's principles.

Three different pressures are involved in moving fluid out of the arterial end of the capillary: the hydrostatic or capillary pressure, the negative interstitial fluid pressure, and the colloid osmotic pressure of the interstitial fluid. Only the colloid osmotic pressure of the plasma tends to move fluid into the capillary. The relationships among these pressures are illustrated in Fig. 7.11. Net pressure responsible for movement of fluid from the capillary to the interstitial space is obtained by adding the three pressures involved in moving fluid out (24 + 6.2 + 4.5 mm Hg) and subtracting the sum from the colloid osmotic pressure (28 mm Hg) which exerts its effect in the opposite direction. The resulting net pressure of 6.7 mm Hg is responsible for moving fluid out of the arterial end of the capillary into the interstitial space. Fluid is returned to the capillary at the venous end due primarily to the considerable decrease in hydrostatic pressure in the capillary (from 24–10 mm Hg). The colloid osmotic pressure within the capillary, which pulls the fluid in, overbalances the sum of the pressures that exert effect in the opposite direction by a net absorption pressure of 6.1 mm Hg. Fluid and the nutrients and metabolites it contains thus circulate out at the arterial end, through the interstitial space, and in at the venous end of the capillary.

Some of the fluid that leaves the capillary along with the protein that enters the interstitial space is returned to the circulation by way of the lymph. This movement is depicted in Fig. 7.11 by the arrow to the lymph capillary. Flow into the lymph capillary takes place because of both the negative pressure inside the capillary and the closing of flaps which prevent return to interstitial space of fluid that has entered the lymph capillary. Contractile action of the endothelial cells of the lymph capillary wall returns the lymph to the major lymph ducts and eventually to the blood.

Under normal conditions, pressure, volume, and protein content of interstitial fluid are maintained within rather narrow bounds. As long as the interstitial fluid pressure remains subatmospheric, fluid diffusing to the interstitial space equals the fluid returned to the circulation and the interstitial fluid volume remains constant. Should excess fluid begin to collect in the interstitium, the increase in fluid pressure leads to a rapid increase in lymph flow preventing accumulation of the excess fluid. This is a built-in safety factor against edema. However, operation of the lymph flow safety factor ceases when pressure in interstitial space rises to the atmospheric level.

The amount of protein that sieves through the capillary wall into the interstitium normally is balanced by the amount returned to the circulation by the lymph. Should permeability of the capillary wall increase and excessive amounts of protein accumulate in the interstitium, an increased amount of fluid is brought in by osmosis and interstitial fluid pressure rises. Since the increased pressure leads to increased lymph flow, high concentration of interstitial fluid protein results in a rapid return of protein to the circulation and edema will not develop.

A significant decrease in plasma protein concentration results in a drop in the colloid pressure within the capillary and a consequent drop in net absorption pressure. This leads to edema if the drop in pressure is excessive (Guyton et al., 1979). A variety of conditions that can produce a plasma protein deficit and an associated edema are of importance to the nutritionist: malnutrition or starvation, malabsorption syndromes, excessive and prolonged bleeding, significant and prolonged proteinuria, massive surface burns, plasma dilution by infused fluid, and increased capillary permeability.

The dynamic mechanisms regulating fluid movement from the capillary to interstitial space and back to the capillary, as well as the role of the lymphatics

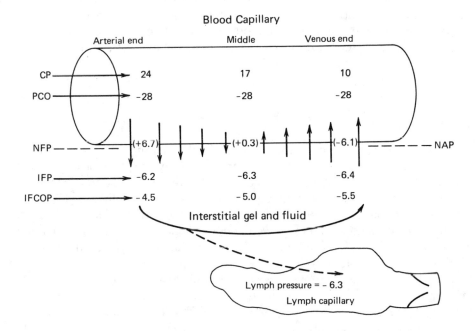

Figure 7.11
Dynamics of pressure equilibria and fluid flow through the capillary membrane, through the gel-filled tissue spaces, and into the lymph capillary. Capillary pressure (CP), plasma colloid osmotic pressure (PCOP), net filtration pressure (NFP), interstitial fluid pressure (IFP), interstitial fluid colloid osmotic pressure (IFCOP), net absorption pressure (NAP). (From A. C. Guyton et al., *Circulatory Physiology II: Dynamics and Control of the Body Fluids*, W. B. Saunders Co., Philadelphia, 1975, p. 102.)

in returning fluid and protein to circulation, are being clarified but still are not fully understood. Recent active research in this area is directed not only to details of the mechanisms involved and to development of more precise methods of measurement but, more importantly, toward developing a concept integrating all body fluids into a dynamically functioning system.

If proper fluid and ionic exchanges occur between the plasma and interstitial fluid, the cell has placed in its immediate environment the nutrients essential for its metabolism. Similar exchanges occur across the cell membrane between the interstitial fluid and the fluid inside the cell, before the nutrients essential for metabolism are at the final membrane crossings: the membranes of the various organelles. Through the series of intercompartmental exchanges, nutrients are delivered from the gut to the plasma and to the intracellular environment, and the products of cellular metabolism are removed. The products of metabolism that leave the cell and enter the plasma are transported to other locations for use in metabolic or regulatory processes or for excretion. The major control of body fluid volume and composition lies in the ability of the kidneys to regulate precisely not only the volume of fluid excreted, but also the solutes that the fluid contains.

For a detailed presentation of the logical pattern of mechanisms for control of body fluids, see Guyton et al. (1975).

RENAL CONTROLS

The kidney provides the chief means whereby the chemical homeostasis of all body fluid is maintained. Each minute approximately one liter of blood or 20 percent of the cardiac output courses through the renal circulation. Of this liter, 120 ml/min of ultrafiltrate pass through the glomeruli and into the tubules, which together constitute over one million nephrons in each human kidney. The total filtration surface is estimated to be well over one square meter. If the 120 ml/min of ultrafiltrate escaped into the urine, the extracellular spaces would be drained of everything but protein in 25 minutes, a rapid road to desiccation. Or, if the organism were obliged to replace this catastrophic loss, it would require approximately 173 liters of fluid per day plus adequate quantitites of all of the solutes that the filtrate contains: glucose, vitamins, amino acids, electrolytes, hormones, and so forth. Normal kidney function averts the need for such imbibing. Of the original 120 ml/min, only 1 ml/min appears in the bladder as urine, or approximately 1.5 liters per day. It is during the passage through the nephron that the volume and composition of the filtrate are altered, water and essential solutes are returned to the circulation, and end products of metabolism and dietary surplus (exclusive of the calorie-yielding variety and other materials that can be stored) become urinary constituents. It is of more than passing interest that the enormous filtration job performed by the glomeruli requires no energy on the part of the kidney since the requisite energy is imparted by the pressure of the blood entering the glomeruli. However, work is performed in the active reabsorption of the filtrate constituents through the tubular cells for their return to the circulation. The kidneys' job classified on this and other bases is one of conservation and regulation rather than excretion. The quantitative aspects of the conservation of body water and electrolytes are illustrated in Table 7.3. For details of nephron structure and function, see Gottschalk and Lassiter (1980).

Water and Sodium

Water is freely diffusable between the intra- and extracellular fluid compartments but cell membranes act as though they are relatively impermeable to Na^+. This, then, makes the relation between the two compartments dependent on the Na^+ concentration in the ECF that, along with total water content, is maintained within rather narrow limits in the adult mammal. Deviation from the normal distribution stimulates restoration of normal water content through stimulation of thirst or adjustment in the secretion of vasopressin (antidiuretic hormone, ADH) and through

TABLE 7.3
Electrolyte and Water Conservation: Comparison of Levels in Plasma, 24-Hour Filtrate, and Urine[a]

Substance	Plasma mEq/liter	Filtered mEq/24 hr	Reabsorbed mEq/24 hr	Excreted mEq/liter	Reabsorbed percent
Sodium	140	25,200	25,099	101	99.6
Chloride	105	18,540	18,430	110	99.4
Potassium	5	900	833	47	92.6
Bicarbonate	27	4860	4858	2	99.9+
Phosphate	2	360	326	34	95[b]
Sulfate	1	180	126	54	70[b]
Water	940 ml/liter	169,200 ml	168,000 ml	1200 ml	99.3

[a]Based on filtration of 180 liters/24 hr.
[b]Varies.

restoration of Na^+ mediated by angiotensin and aldosterone. The operation of these compensatory mechanisms in adjusting and maintaining body fluid distribution and composition is under intensive investigation in many research and clinical laboratories. Changes in body fluid distribution and composition accompanying shifts in water and salt balances are illustrated in Fig. 7.12.

The role of the kidney in maintaining the volume and tonicity of the extracellular fluid is accomplished by the coordination of neural and hormonal stimuli with the reabsorptive capacity of the kidney tubules. One model includes the concept of "osmoreceptors" in the brain and was postulated by Verney (1947). He suggested that stimulus to ADH secretion resulted from change in composition of the ECF leading to cellular dehydration and reduction in volume of the osmoreceptors. Jewel and Verney (1957) localized the osmoreceptors in the hypothalamus and demonstrated that these receptors responded to the hydration level of the organism. They proposed that dehydration of the receptor cells stimulated both the thirst mechanism and the secretion of ADH leading to increased water intake, decreased excretion and, consequently, rehydration.

Data presented by Andersson and his colleagues (Andersson et al., 1967; 1969) challenged the concept of osmoregulation. Their data obtained from goats suggested that Na^+-sensitive receptors inside the blood-brain barrier responded to the Na^+ concentration in the CSF. In a critical evaluation of these and other data, Thrasher (1982) finds little to support either the idea of Na^+ receptors or their location inside the blood-brain barrier. However, he does present data from his own and other laboratories and from a variety of animals supporting the role of osmoreceptors in the homeostatic mechanisms responsible for the stimulation of thirst and ADH secretion. He suggests that these receptors are located in areas

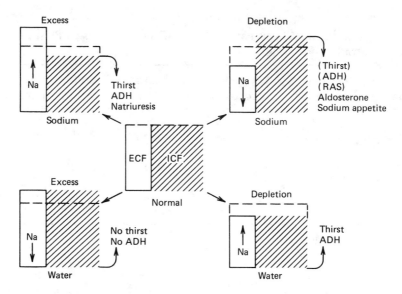

Figure 7.12
Diagram of changes in body fluid distribution and extracellular Na$^+$ concentration during positive and negative sodium and water balance. Compensatory factors indicated to the right of each diagram. Antidiuretic hormone (ADH), extracellular fluid compartment (ECF), intracellular fluid compartment (ICF), renin-angiotensin system (RAS). (From B. Andersson et al., *Ann. Rev. Nutr.* 2:75, 1982.)

surrounding the ventricles, outside the blood-brain barrier. Many details in the monitoring of ADH secretion and stimulation of thirst in response to dehydration remain unresolved. For a review of the role of osmoreceptors and vasopressin, see Bie (1980).

The action of ADH following its release occurs in the kidney tubule and Orloff and Handler (1967) suggested that ADH action was mediated by cAMP. This suggestion was supported by the demonstration of receptors binding ADH molecules coupled to adenyl cyclase in cell membrane fractions from kidney medulla (Bockaert et al., 1973). The activation of the cAMP-dependent system and the increase in cell cAMP increases the permeability of the plasma membrane to water but how this occurs is not yet known (Handler and Orloff, 1981).

Work in other laboratories centered on the role of the renin-angiotensin system in the induction of thirst (as well as the way it affects aldosterone secretion and Na$^+$ reabsorption which will be discussed below). As long ago as 1969, it was observed that stimulation of the renin-angiotensin system also stimulated the thirst mechanism (Fitzsimons, 1969) and that injection of angiotensin into the blood of the rat produced drinking (Fitzsimons and Simons, 1969; Epstein et al., 1969). These investigators suggested that angiotensin either stimulated the brain directly or increased the sensitivity of the receptors in the brain. Bonjour and Malvin (1970) showed that angiotensin stimulated both the thirst mechanism and the release of ADH, and later Brooks and Malvin (1979) demonstrated that endogenous angiotensin plays a physiological role in the control of thirst and the release of ADH. They suggested that the conversion of angiotensin I to the active angiotensin II might occur in the brain.

The brain renin-angiotensin system has been the subject of extensive research in recent years. Some investigators, although not ruling it out, do not believe that the evidence for the presence of a brain system independent of the one in the kidney is convincing (Reid, 1979; Share, 1979). Other investigators (Ganong, 1977; Phillips et al., 1979) argue that the brain has an intrinsic renin-angiotensin system that activates thirst. They suggest that the brain system probably parallels the system in the kidney and possibly could take over when needed.

The renal renin-angiotensin system is of primary importance in the regulation of sodium and water intake and excretion. Receptors in the juxtaglomerular apparatus in the kidney sensistive to a decrease in plasma volume and/or pressure stimulate the secretion of renin (Skinner et al., 1964). Renin secretion is also stimulated by a decrease in the plasma Na^+ concentration (Vander and Miller, 1964). Released renin acts on a circulating α_2-globulin, renin substrate synthesized by liver cells, to release angiotensin I, an inactive decapeptide (Fig. 7.13). An enzyme known simply as converting enzyme, a glycoprotein bound to plasma membranes in tissues such as lung and kidney, splits two amino acids from angiotensin I to yield angiotensin II close to the sites where it acts (Erdös, 1977). In addition to its powerful and rapid vasoconstrictor effect, angiotensin II also increases blood volume by increasing Na^+ and fluid retention through action on the adrenals and the brain. The adrenal response is the increased synthesis and secretion of aldosterone which stimulates the kidney tubules to increase the reabsorption of Na^+. The response in the brain, discussed above in relation to the brain renin-angiotensin system, is through stimulation of thirst and ADH secretion. A negative feedback mechanism acts on the juxtaglomerular cells either by way of pressure- or Na^+-sensitive receptors to cut off the renin secretion that started the cycle (Laragh et al., 1972). A model of these relationships is shown in Fig. 7.14.

In addition to angiotensins I and II, the heptapeptide angiotensin III appears to be active in this system. Angiotensin III is formed by the action of a plasma aminopeptidase that removes aspartate from the N-terminal of angiotensin II (see Fig. 7.14). Angiotensin III is more potent than angiotensin II in its aldosterone-stimulating activity but has only about half the pressor activity of angiotensin II (Davis and Freeman, 1977). It has been suggested that angiotensin III is the aldosterone-stimulating peptide and angiotensin II the pressor peptide (Freeman et al., 1977).

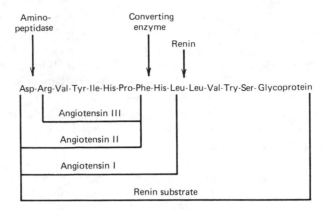

Figure 7.13
Successive cleavages of renin substrate to yield angiotensins I, II, and III. The proteolytic enzyme renin splits angiotensin I from renin substrate, a plasma α_2-globulin. Converting enzyme, a dipeptidyl-carboxypeptidase, removes a dipeptide to yield angiotensin II. An aminopeptidase removes one amino acid from the N-terminal of the peptide resulting in the formation of angiotensin III, [des-Asp^1] angiotensin II.

For reviews of various aspects of the renin-angiotensin-aldosterone mechanism, see Vander (1967); Reid et al. (1978); Fitzsimons (1978); Freeman and Davis (1979); Levens et al. (1981); Phillips et al. (1982).

Nutrient Conservation
Under normal circumstances all of the nutrients in the filtrate are returned to the plasma by the tubular cell, but the quantity returned varies with both the nutrient and the plasma level. Nutrients that are maintained in the plasma by dynamic regulatory mechanisms such as glucose, amino acids, and sodium have high renal thresholds and are returned almost completely; those nutrients for which plasma concentrations are a reflection of dietary intake, such as the water-soluble vitamins, have low renal thresholds. For example, plasma levels of water-soluble vitamins reach a maximum point as dietary intake is increased, and any further loading is reflected in markedly increased urinary excretion. Whether this is because of the inability of tissues to store these vitamins or to the inability of the kidney to reabsorb them is an interesting question. (See Chapter 15.)

The conservation of nutrients by the renal tubule is accomplished primarily by active transport. (See Chapter 9.) Competition may exist for both shared carriers and transport energy. Glucose, for example, shares a carrier with xylose, fructose, and galactose, but glucose has the highest affinity for the carrier and its reabsorption takes preference. Glucose passes through the membrane of the kidney

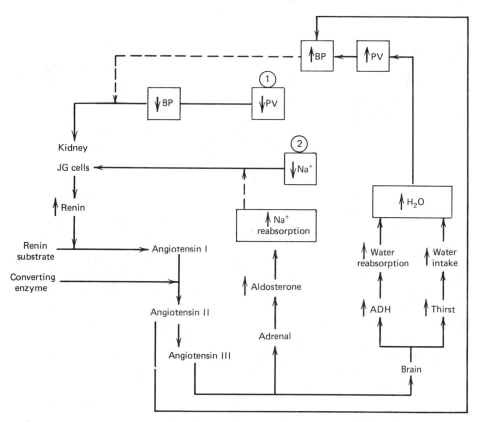

Figure 7.14
A model of the renin-angiotensin-aldosterone system regulating sodium and water intake
and reabsorption in the control of ① plasma volume (PV) and ② plasma Na^+ concentration. Receptors sensitive to a decrease in PV or plasma Na^+ concentration stimulate the juxtaglomerular (JG) cells of the kidney to secrete renin leading to the release
of the angiotensins. Angiotensin II exerts a direct pressor effect. Angiotensin III stimulates
aldosterone and antidiuretic hormone (ADH) secretion leading to reabsorption of Na^+
and water, and also stimulates the thirst mechanism. The dotted lines indicate feedback
control.

tubule coupled to Na^+ and the Na^+ gradient is the driving force. The gradient
is created and maintained across the membrane by Na^+-K^+ATPase. Na^+ is
pumped out of the cell but glucose leaves the cell passively for return to the
circulation. (See Ullrich, 1979.) If the quantity of glucose presented for reabsorption greatly exceeds the carrier capacity or renal threshold, which is approximately 180 mg/dl, the excess glucose will appear in the urine. In uncontrolled
diabetes, plasma glucose and, therefore, the level of glucose in the filtrate can
be two or more times above the renal threshhold and the amount of glucose
appearing in the urine can be exceedingly high.

The amino acids in the plasma and in the tubular filtrate are in dynamic equilibrium with the amino acids in all cells, including those of the tubule, and thereby constitute a portion of the amino acid pool of the body. Under normal circumstances approximately 99 percent of the filtered amino acids are reabsorbed from the proximal tubule. Amino acid absorption, like glucose absorption, is coupled with Na^+ and is dependent on Na^+-K^+ATPase for maintaining the Na^+ gradient across the tubule membrane. (See Ullrich, 1979.) The transport receptors for amino acids are highly stereospecific and, at present, there appear to be at least seven different transport systems for naturally occurring amino acids. They are for (1) neutral amino acids, (2) acidic amino acids, (3) basic amino acids, (4) imino acids, high affinity, (5) imino acids, low affinity shared by glycine and neutral amino acids, (6) glycine shared by neutral amino acids, and (7) β amino acids (Silbernagl et al., 1975).

The cells of the renal tubules are concerned with more than conservation and transport of amino acids. They are active also in transamination, deamination, and the formation of urea and ammonia and therefore are critical in the maintenance of normal protein metabolism.

In addition to the cotransport of Na^+ into the tubular cell with glucose and amino acids, and its extrusion as part of a Na^+-K^+ exchange pump, Na^+ from the filtrate also diffuses into the tubular cell and is pumped into the interstitium by an electrogenic Na^+ pump. This pump helps to maintain the electronegative state of the cell interior by extruding the positive Na^+. Cl^- moves out of the cell passively with the Na^+ and is replenished by Cl^- which diffuses into the cell from the tubule.

The mechanisms regulating K^+ reabsorption are somewhat more complicated. About 90 percent of the filtered K^+ is actively reabsorbed before the filtrate reaches the distal segment of the nephron. Adjustments in the amount of K^+ excreted are made in the distal segment where K^+ may be secreted into, as well as reabsorbed from, the tubule. Secretion of K^+ into the distal segment is usually inversely related to the concentration of H^+, and both K^+ and H^+ secretion depend on the availability of Na^+ for reabsorption. Some of the complexities operating to maintain K^+ exchange in the kidney are discussed by Wright (1981) and O'Neil (1981).

Only about 50 percent of plasma calcium appears in the kidney filtrate since only that much is in the form of free ions. The remainder of plasma calcium is protein-bound and therefore unable to penetrate the glomerular membrane. Of the Ca^{++} in the filtrate, 99 percent is actively reabsorbed. Just as Na^+ is regulated by the secretion of aldosterone, Ca^{++} reabsorption is under the influence of parathyroid hormone. (See Chapters 5 and 17.)

About 80 percent of the filtered phosphate is reabsorbed. Although this may occur in any part of the tubule, most of the reabsorption occurs through active transport in the proximal segment. Phosphate, like Ca^{++}, is influenced by parathyroid hormone and, in addition, is highly dependent on Na^+, but the mechanism is not clear. For a review of the renal handling of both calcium and phosphate, see Dennis et al. (1979).

Nitrogen Excretion

In the process of metabolism the disposal of any carbon, hydrogen, or oxygen as carbon dioxide or water is no problem; nitrogen, however, requires the formation of ammonia, uric acid, or urea. An organism's position on the evolutionary ladder and its habitat give a fair indication of its mode of nitrogen excretion. The toxicity of ammonia makes it a suitable excretory product only for marine animals who have no trouble diluting it and losing it in a watery environment. To embryos that develop within hard shells, ammonia would be lethal; these organisms excrete uric acid, which is quite insoluble and therefore harmless. This change during evolution appears to have been an adaptation to land life. Although mammals excrete some uric acid, the major means of eliminating nitrogen is by the formation of urea which has the virtue of being nontoxic and soluble. The formation of urea will be described in Chapter 15. The presence of urea in the plasma and therefore in the tubular filtrate is directly related to the quantity of protein consumed and the rate of protein catabolism. Tubular reabsorption of urea is passive and closely proportional to the amounts filtered. At normal rates of urine flow, approximately 60 percent of the urea remains in the tubule to be excreted in the urine; but at low rates of urine flow, the amount excreted may be only 10–20 percent of the amount filtered. The increased reabsorption when flow rates are low is due to the increased opportunity for the passive diffusion to take place. Reabsorbed urea collects in the interstitium of the renal medulla and its concentration is kept high in the area surrounding the collecting ducts. As a result, there is a relatively low concentration gradient between the fluid inside and outside the collecting ducts, less urea diffuses out, and more remains to be excreted. The level of urea in the plasma is dependent, then, not only on its rate of synthesis, but also on the ability of the kidney to excrete a suitable proportion of the quantity presented to it. For discussion of the renal countercurrent mechanism, particulary as it is involved in the tubular exchanges of urea, water, and Na^+, see Gottschalk and Lassiter (1980); and Jamison (1983).

The uric acid concentration of the plasma is approximately 4 mg/dl and is derived from the breakdown of purines. About 5 percent of urinary nitrogen is in the form of uric acid. Although it is filtered freely, approximately 98 percent of the uric acid in the filtrate is reabsorbed. However, uric acid is also secreted into the proximal tubules and about 1 gram per 24 hours appears in the urine. How the reabsorption and secretion of uric acid is controlled is not clear, nor is it certain whether the quantity appearing in the urine is the result of incomplete reabsorption or excessive secretion into the tubules. Uric acid levels in the plasma and urine are of concern only in individuals with gout and in such cases a variety of drugs can be administered to increase uric acid excretion.

One product of metabolism present in the tubular filtrate and rejected completely by the tubular cells for reabsorption is creatinine, the end product of creatine metabolism. The amount of creatinine appearing in the 24-hour urine of a given individual remains relatively constant and often is used in metabolic studies to identify a cheating or forgetful research subject.

The renal functions that have been discussed are regulatory in the sense that they operate to adjust and maintain the chemical composition of the plasma and thereby the chemical composition of the extracellular environment in the entire organism. In this sense, the excretory functions of the kidney are also regulatory in that they insure the removal from the body fluids of molecules present in excess of the body's need or beyond its capacity to manage. A prerequisite for renal disposal of such a plethora is, of course, its presence in the glomerular ultrafiltrate. This prerequisite explains the inability to excrete iron or lipids in the urine. Since iron is present in the plasma as transferrin and lipids as lipoproteins, they, along with all other macromolecules, never get through to the renal tubule. The ability of molecules to penetrate the glomerular membrane was believed to be dependent solely on molecular size. Recently, however, molecular charge and shape (Rennke and Venkatachalam, 1977) as well as certain hemodynamic factors (Deen et al., 1977) have been shown to be important also in determining the selectivity of the glomerular membrane.

Regulation of Plasma pH

Related to the renal control of water balance and nutrient conservation is the control of blood pH. The maintenance of near neutrality of the blood is accomplished by the buffering systems of the blood itself, by respiratory exchange in the lungs involving regulation of carbonic acid, and by regulation of the bicarbonate ion by the kidney tubules. Rapid but incomplete adjustments are made in the lungs; slower but more complete adjustments in the kidneys. When all controls act in concert, blood pH is maintained at 7.4 by the buffering systems. Only renal control will be discussed here.

The kidney can increase or decrease blood pH by stabilizing the bicarbonate level of the plasma. This involves almost complete reabsorption of the quantities normally filtered. If an excess of bicarbonate gains entrance to the body, its excretion will be controlled by the tubules. Depletion of bicarbonate reserves is arrested by excretion of titratable acid and ammonia. In the formation of titratable acid, hydrogen ions are exchanged for sodium; in the formation of ammonia, the amino group from the deamination of amino acids or deamidation of glutamine diffuses into the tubule and is trapped as the ammonium ion. The operation of this ion exchange is illustrated in Fig. 7.15. For a more complete discussion, see Gottschalk and Lassiter (1980).

INTRACELLULAR pH REGULATION

If the true internal environment is the fluid matrix inside the cell and its organelles, biological regulation must occur at that level. The composition of the plasma then must depend on regulatory processes within cellular and subcellular units. Thus, the plasma may be considered a regulated buffer region that acts as the first line of defense in maintaining the fixity of the intracellular environment (Robin, 1977). In this context, it becomes apparent that the pH of the blood, however important and rigorously controlled, is of less consequence than the pH of the intracellular

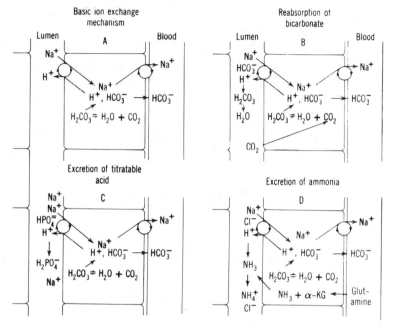

Figure 7.15
Role of the exchange of cellular H^+ ions for Na^+ ions of tubular fluid in the reabsorption of bicarbonate and in the urinary excretion of titratable acid and ammonia. (From R. F. Pitts, *Physiology of the Kidney and Body Fluids*, 2nd ed., Year Book Medical Publishers Inc., Chicago, 1968, p. 210.)

fluid where conditions for enzymatic functions must be meticulously protected. Indeed, the cells defend their internal pH which has been shown to be different from that of the blood (see below). It is intracellular pH that ultimately determines the blood pH which the lungs and kidneys then keep constant. In still another instance, it appears that the blood is relegated to a role subservient to the true internal environment which lies within the membrane of the cell. The interesting development of the newer concepts of pH regulation follow.

"The voice of the turtle is heard in our land,"[1] and it was most specifically heard by Robin (1962). He observed that a blood pH of 7.4, the then accepted norm for acid-base regulation in all animals, was not maintained by the turtle. The pH of turtle blood changed with changes in temperature. This unexpected finding was confirmed in other cold-blooded vertebrates and an inverse relationship was observed between blood pH and temperature (Howell et al., 1970). A series of studies established that the acid-base status of a cold-blooded animal should be evaluated in terms of the constancy of the OH^-/H^+ ratio of the blood and not at a particular pH. Rahn and Howell (1978), in presenting the OH^-/H^+

[1]Song of Solomon, II, 12

theory, acknowledge that their presentation was the fourth reincarnation of this concept and cite Santayana (1905–1906) who said, "Those who cannot remember the past are condemned to repeat it." Apparently the previous investigators were concerned with the acid-base balance of an animal at a fixed temperature.

At 37°C, the normal body temperature for humans, the pH of blood, and intracellular fluid are the same for humans and turtles. These findings turn out to be more far-reaching than turtle-talk and led Reeves (1972) to suggest that the α-imidazole group of histidine is responsible for the acid-base regulation of all vertebrates. Histidine is the only amino acid that dissociates in the neutral pH range. It is this characteristic that allows certain histidine residues to play important roles in catalytic activities of some enzymes (Conn and Stumpf, 1972, p. 72). In fact, Rahn et al. (1975) suggested that the intra- and extracellular buffer system involving the imidazole of histidine is a "fossil" protein selected in the evolutionary history of animals, since the response of blood as a function of temperature is similar in all present day invertebrates and vertebrates. There are, in fact, several "fossil" molecules in which the imidazole ring of histidine participates. Some of these are hemoglobin, myoglobin, cytochromes, hemocyanin, and chlorophyll, all involved in the most basic aspects of metabolic activity in plants and animals: oxygen transport, electron transport, and photosynthesis. (See Chapter 16.)

The pH of intracellular fluid parallels that of blood in both cold- and warm-blooded animals. The intracellular compartment is maintained close to neutrality and the blood is 0.6 pH units higher. At a body temperature of 37°C, intracellular pH is 6.8 and blood pH is 7.4 (Rahn, 1979). Regulatory mechanisms in the cells defend their internal pH, and the internal pH in key cells, such as cells in the brain and kidney, ultimately determine changes in the pH of the plasma (Robin, 1977).

Regulatory processes within the cell maintain an intracellular environment compatible with cell function; but cell function actually occurs within the organelles. It seems reasonable to assume that mechanisms within the organelles regulate their internal environment. Indeed, this has been demonstrated in brain mitochondria by Robin and his colleagues (see Robin, 1979) who observed autoregulatory responses to changes in osmolality in brain mitochondria. Although the mechanisms of regulation are not known, the evidence is clear that intramitochondrial environment is maintained despite changes in the composition of intracellular (extramitochondrial) fluid. The mitochondrion is another site for "fossil" enzymes, such as the cytochromes, that function so importantly in chloroplasts as well as mitochondria. The environment of our enzymes tells much about our history.

Claude Bernard's environment moves inward, and Cannon's homeostatic mechanisms become more delicately tuned.

Coda

The complex of processes by which food is digested and its constituent nutrients enter the body and reach the locus for metabolic activity is dependent on the coordinated and synchronized activities of the total organism. Just as in music it is the integration of the composer's score, the musician's skill, and the conductor's interpretation that expresses in totality what no one of them could convey alone, so, too, is understanding and appreciation of the physiological aspects of nutrition (which only to some may be more mundane than a symphony) an exquisite blend of written description of fact, skillful interpretation, and knowledgeable integration. Pathways and mechanisms are not just roadmaps; they must be linked, combined, coordinated, and developed into the metabolic scheme. By seeing individual roles, meaning is imparted to the whole; but the symphony, too, is far more than a sequence of individual themes. Breakdown and analysis followed by interpretation and resynthesis serve equally well in understanding and appreciating symphonies and science.

part three

the cell

Cells are highly individual. There are infinite variations not only in unicellular life, but in the variety of cells that make up complex organisms. However, all cells have certain structural constituents in common; since these constituents are orderly interrelated arrangements of macromolecules, and the macromolecules have various constituent molecules in common, these points of likeness have given rise to the concept of the *typical cell*. The typical cell, like the so-called average person, is an image arrived at by extrapolation, a statistical creation that does not actually exist. Nevertheless, it is a convenient point of departure and, if accepted in that sense, provides the Utopian norm: visionary, nonexistent, and impossibly ideal.

chapter 8

orientation to cellular nutrition

1. **Rationale**
2. **Historical Aspects**
3. **Instruments and Techniques**
   a. **Microscopy**
      (1) Light Microscopy
      (2) Electron Microscopy
      (3) Anhydrous Preparation Methods
      (4) The Electron Microprobe
      (5) Radioautography
   b. **Biochemical and Physical Methods**
      (1) Differential Ultracentrifugation
      (2) x-Ray Diffraction
      (3) Electrophoresis and Chromatography
      (4) Immunochemical Technique
      (5) Nuclear Magnetic Resonance
   c. **Tissue Culture**
   d. **Summary**
4. **Problems Inherent in Studying Cells**
5. **Rewards Resulting from Studying Cells**
6. **Geography of the Cell**

". . . Exploration (of cells) used to be dominated by the microscopic study of fixed and stained tissue specimens. Cells were distinguished by the visual appearance of their embalmed mummies, which contributed neither less nor more to the understanding of the living cell than does the study of the ruins of an ancient city tell of the life of its people. Life is process in time. No static image can reflect that time dimension. Microscopic anatomy thus tended to freeze our concepts of the cell: the cell's incessant variation in response to a continuously changing environment escaped attention. Knowledge was hemmed in by limitations of technique. In order to enlarge the scope and content of our knowledge, we must rely on the technical advances."

Paul A. Weiss, 1971

"Thus the things of our world are simple or complex, according to the techniques that we select for studying them. In fact, functional simplicity always corresponds to a complex substratum. This is a primary datum of observation, which must be accepted just as it is."

Alexis Carrel, 1935

Rationale

Understanding biological activity depends on an understanding of the fundamental unit of activity: the cell. According to Ham (1969), "a cell is the smallest organized unit of living material capable of existing independently in a suitable nonliving environment, replacing its own substance as necessary by synthesizing new components from nutritives absorbed from its environment." It becomes apparent that proper nutrition is a primary requisite for the existence of the cell. The nutrients are the source of the cell's energy and of the materials for its syntheses. Without suitable nutrient supplies the cell cannot exist.

To understand this fundamental biological unit, its structural composition and molecular organization must be related to its functions. Operations within any of its subunits are related to the operation of the unit as a whole, to other units with which it is associated and, in a coordinated complex of cells, to the total organism and the environment in which it exists. The cell can be viewed from the outside looking in or from the inside looking out; but any attempt to extrapolate what might occur at one level of operation from observations at another level can be hazardous. The behavior of a molecule in solution in a test tube is not the same as its operation in an intact organism; but the *in vitro* behavior can give important information on how it *might* behave *in vivo*. Similarly, organelles in isolation do not operate as they do in cells; however, observations of both structure and function can give insight into their likely activities when they are subjected to the interrelated and coordinated functions of other organelles within the cell. Nor do cells in culture function as they do in an intact organism where they are subjected to the influence of other cells and organs; but cell cultures give some indication of specific capabilities and attributes of the constituent cells.

Historical Aspects

All the spectacular advances of today are completely dependent on and inseparable from the advances made all though the long history of science. The hesitating steps and wrong turns, as well as the great leaps, have added to our scientific knowledge. Today's hindsight can thoughtlessly tarnish or spoil the brilliance of yesterday's foresight, but without the discoveries of all of the yesterdays, today's world, its aspirations and dreams, its science and technology would not exist. We could not be studying cell organelles had not the powerful electron microscope been developed; nor cells without the light microscope; nor microscopes if Galileo and those before him had not been interested in lenses; nor lenses had not the ancient Egyptians discovered how to make glass. To paraphrase Macbeth, all our yesterdays have lighted the way to the scientific creativity of today.

An unknown and miniature world came into view with the construction of the first compound microscope by Zacharias Janssen in 1590. In 1665 Robert Hooke, observing cork through a microscope, used the word cell for the first time as a biologically descriptive term. He described cork as a tissue that was made up of "little boxes or cells." This may have been an accurate description for cork tissue as Hooke observed it, but this word, carried over from the descriptions of the seventeenth-century botanists, came into use to designate the ultimate particle of living matter. For the seventeenth century, this *was* the ultimate unit of structure; nothing smaller could be seen or, perhaps, imagined. It was during that century, too, that the atom was described as a body so small as to be incapable of further division, and it was assumed to be the ultimate particle in which matter existed. For both the cell and the atom, technology eventually provided the means for going beyond what was thought then to be ultimate. Ferreting out and understanding the substructure within the cell is the biological counterpart of the physical study of atomic particles.

Instruments and Techniques

The sophisticated methods employed in studying cellular morphology and physiology are the direct outgrowth of an increasingly sophisticated technology. Advances in biological probing, like advances in atomic or cosmic probing, have been closely tied to progress in optics, electronics, and engineering. Many similar laboratory instruments are used today in studying the nutrition of the cell, the composition of moon rocks, and the identity of atmospheric pollutants. The hands and senses of the nutritional scientist are probably limited more often by vision than by the availability of instrumental means. The acceleration of analytical work, recording, and calculating are the combined contributions of automation and computer science. Some of the available techniques are discussed below.

MICROSCOPY

Twenty years after Hooke's observations on cork, Anton van Leeuwenhoek ground and polished high power lenses that enabled him to see objects 100 times smaller than could be observed by the naked eye. He was the first to observe the existence of unicellular life. Remarkable insight was gained by the careful studies of eighteenth century microscopists.

Light Microscopy
Today's light microscopes can magnify 1,000 times or more and permit observation of some cellular detail. Development of special optical techniques has

permitted the study of living cells. Use of *phase contrast* and *interference microscopy* are based on the fact that biological structures, which are highly transparent to visible light, can cause phase changes in transmitted radiations. These result from small differences in the refractive index and thickness of different parts of the structure. Phase microscopy has permitted study of living cells using time-lapse motion pictures to record cell division, phagocytosis, formation of membranes, and other structure-related processes of living. Interference microscopy, based on the same principles as phase microscopy can, in addition, give quantitative data; for example, simultaneous determination of the thickness of an object, concentration of dry matter, and water content.

Electron Microscopy

More specific knowledge of cell structure and the structure of organelles within the cell is the result of the development of the *electron microscope* by Knoll and Ruska in 1933. This instrument, which became available for general research about 1940, permits magnifications of 150,000–300,000 times and greater, revealing intimate details of cell structure. Electron microscopy has permitted visualization of cellular structures down to molecular dimensions. It has revealed that macromolecules are arranged in strict and orderly patterns and constitute the substructures or organelles of the cell.

The transparence of tissue in visible light makes it necessary to utilize techniques to increase contrast. For light microscopy, biological stains that react with specific molecules in the cell are used. In electron microscopy, heavy atoms such as lead and osmium form dense derivative compounds with cellular material and, in effect, are electron stains. The use of any foreign material reacting with the molecular material of the cell can, and does, produce artifacts. Cytologists suggest that some of the details clearly observed in electron microscopy may, in fact, be the result of such interactions between the molecular components of the cell and the heavy atoms rather than actual details of cell structure.

The *scanning electron microscope* uses secondary electrons produced by the scanning beam to give a lifelike, almost three-dimensional, image of the surface of the specimen being scanned. The magnification can be from 10–100,000 times or more which means that it overlaps the hand lens, the light microscope, and the electron microscope. In addition to the wide range of magnification, it also extends the range and quality of the electron micrograph. The image is not only larger than life, but it seems twice as real. The scanning electron microscope permits in depth visualization of microfeatures, a topological picture, giving actual spatial relationships. (See Fig. 20.1.)

Anhydrous Preparation Methods

To visualize the cell and its constituents in a close-to-living form, various anhydrous methods have been developed. *Freeze-etching* permits study of membranes and organelles from unfixed cells. Tissue is frozen in a coolant chilled by liquid nitrogen and then fractured under vacuum along natural cleavage planes with a sharp blade. The splintered preparation is etched by sublimation. Platinum and carbon are deposited along the fracture surface. This replica is then mounted for electron microscope study. It is believed that electron micrographs prepared in this way give images of cell structures that closely approximate the normal condition since no chemical fixatives and dehydrating agents are used and since a rapid freezing method is employed. Due to the etching and shadowing the view is somewhat three dimensional (Fig. 8.1).

It is also possible to cut ultrathin sections from rapidly frozen tissue samples. The sections can be viewed in a hydrated or freeze-dried state, depending on the design of the electron microscope. Alternatively, rapidly frozen tissue can be freeze-dried and embedded in anhydrous resins prior to sectioning. These methods provide a means of retaining soluble tissue constituents. Such preparations can then be *low-temperature ashed* for visualization of metallic substances within cells. Organic matter is selectively removed with a stream of very reactive, excited oxygen. The remaining ash represents the mineral/metallic ultrastructure of cells (Hohman and Schraer, 1972).

The Electron Microprobe

This instrument provides a means of determining subcellular elemental composition in tissue sections at the spatial resolution of the electron microscope and is capable of detecting 10^{-19} grams of material. When a section is bombarded with electrons in the electron microscope, a specturm of x-rays is produced. Each element present can be recognized by its own x-ray which has a specific energy. The amount of x-rays given off is directly proportional to the concentration of elements present. Depending on the concentration of elements, a volume as small as a ribosome can be analyzed. All elements with an atomic number of 11 (sodium) and above can be detected simultaneously.

Radioautography

A radioactive label incorporated into metabolizing tissue can be detected after the tissue is fixed and prepared for microscopy since the radioactive products in the section emit electrons that affect photographic emulsions. The prepared slides are permitted to develop in a light-proof box for a period of time during which each minute amount of isotope is a source of radiation hitting the photographic emulsion. After a suitable period of time, the preparations are developed just as photographic negatives are developed. In the developed radioautographic preparation, areas of radiation in the tissue below show as black dots indicating where the administered isotope was incorporated into the cell. Isotopic labels attached to specific molecules used in cellular syntheses can be traced into final products through radioautography. Through the use of suitable techniques, tissue can be prepared for study by either light or electron microscopy.

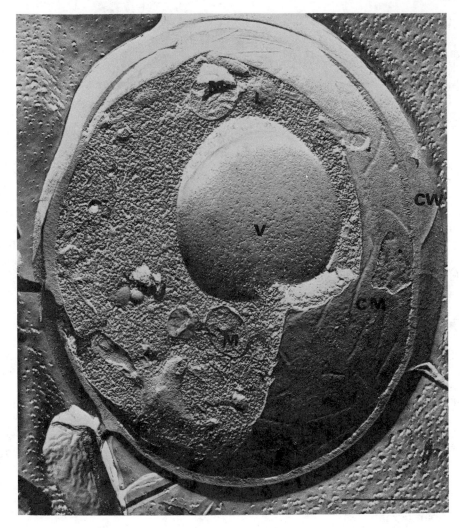

Figure 8.1
Freeze-etch electron micrograph of yeast cell, *Saccharomyces cerevisiae*, showing cell wall (CW) and cell membrane (CM), mitochondria (M), lipid granule (L), and large cytoplasmic vacuole (V). Marker bar = 1μ. Shadow direction from bottom to top. Magnification 32,500. (Courtesy of Thomas E. Rucinsky.)

BIOCHEMICAL AND PHYSICAL METHODS

Although structural patterns can be observed visually, the function of the organelles and of their constituent chemical components is dependent on the development and use of other instruments and techniques. Svedberg's interest in colloids led him to develop the first centrifuge to give quantitative data on sedimentation rates. This instrument, developed in 1924, whirled at 10,000 rpm and produced a centrifugal force 5,000 times gravity. Ultracentrifuges are now obtainable that can generate centrifugal forces in excess of 500,000 × g. The ultracentrifuge permitted the estimation of molecular weights and confirmed the existence of giant molecules.

Differential Ultracentrifugation

This permits biochemical study of organelles and of their functional attributes. Cells placed in a suitable medium, usually sucrose, are disrupted mechanically or sonically, and the homogenate is subjected to successive centrifugations (Fig. 8.2). The size, density, and shape of the particles determine their movement in the centrifugal field, and this forms the basis for differential ultracentrifugation. At a given force, large, heavy, and dense structures sediment most rapidly and, with increasing force, successive fractions are obtained. Some organelles, nuclei and mitochondria, for example, come down essentially intact; however, the fraction designated as the microsomes is composed mostly of fragmented bits of endoplasmic reticulum and plasma membrane. There are, of course, no organelles called microsomes. Isolated cell fractions can be subjected to full biochemical and physical analyses.

Various refinements in technique and use of the analytical ultracentrifuge permit further separation of materials into macromolecular layers. In this way, the relationship of the structural units, or organelles, of the cell can be related to molecular constituents and to function.

x-Ray Diffraction

This technique has wide application in the study of the configuration of molecules. Collimated x-rays traverse the material to be analyzed, and the diffraction pattern is recorded on a photographic plate. Through a complex mathematical process a three-dimensional representation of the object can be constructed.

Electrophoresis and Chromatography

These are the principal tools for separating and characterizing macromolecules. The basis of electrophoresis is that charged molecules such as DNA, RNA, and proteins move in an electric field because of their charge. *Two-dimensional gel electrophoresis* has been refined to the point that on the order of 5,000 proteins in a mixture can be resolved. Chromatographic separations are dependent on molecular size.

Immunochemical Techniques

These are being applied in increasing frequencies at the molecular and cellular levels. The major reasons are the extraordinarily high resolutions that can be achieved. For example, by *radioimmunoassay* any substance to which an antibody can be made is detectable in 10^{-11}–10^{-9} gram quantities. Antibodies can also be labeled with fluorescent or electron-dense molecules and applied to sections for microscopic localization.

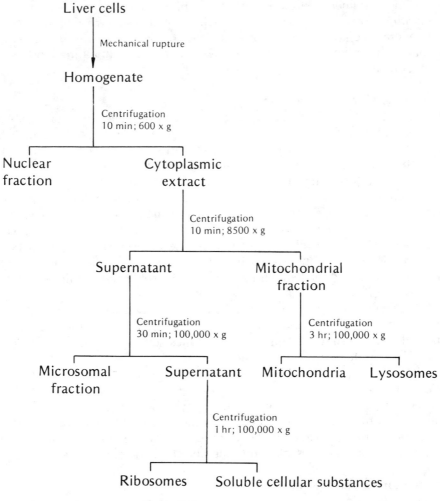

Figure 8.2
Differential ultracentrifugation.

Nuclear Magnetic Resonance

Perhaps one of the most exciting recent technological developments for appli-cation to biological problems is nuclear magnetic resonance. It is a type of ad-sorption spectroscopy and is based on the fact that some atomic nuclei possess a net spin and will resonate at a characteristic frequency in an appropriately directed magnetic field. The intracellular concentrations of various metabolites, ions, and other compounds, as well as pH, have been detected in living cells. Membrane transport kinetics and steady state fluxes of metabolites also have been studied. Applications of the technique have been reviewed recently by Radda and Seely (1979); Gadian and Radda (1981); and Shulman (1983).

TISSUE CULTURE

Tissue culture techniques permit the study of living cells grown in a suitable medium that contains the nutrients and oxygen essential for growth. Nutritional requirements of specific cells and organs can be studied under a variety of experimental conditions. Tissues in culture will grow and divide behaving to some degree as they do in the total organism. They are of value also in studying particular attributes of cell membranes in a living cell through the use of phase microscopy and nuclear magnetic resonance. Synthetic media for organ culture permit the study of growing bone and endocrine glands under a variety of experimental conditions.

SUMMARY

Neither biochemical nor morphological studies of cells tell the full story, but they complement each other in providing an understanding of relationships of structure to function and in suggesting mechanisms of operation within the living cell. Furthermore, knowledge of the living cell suggests mechanisms of operation and understanding of relationships existing in the total organism. The complementary effects of various avenues of study at any level of biological organization is illustrated in Fig. 8.3.

For further discussion of methods employed in the study of cell structure and function, see Branton and Deamer (1972); Giese (1973); Cooper (1977); DeRobertis and DeRobertis (1980); Nicolini (1982).

Problems Inherent in Studying Cells

When tissues are prepared for histological or cytological study, activity or life is stopped abruptly at a moment in time. Such cells are as representative of the "true" or living appearance of the cell as a photograph is of a living person. Moreover, distortions are imposed by (1) the fixative that coagulates the protein and hardens the tissue, (2) dehydration, (3) infiltration with paraffin or resin, and (4) sectioning and staining. The objective in preparation is, of course, to permit as little distortion as possible but deviations from the live state are inevitable. An additional difficulty is that of studying a three-dimensional object in two dimensions and then interpreting and visualizing it in three dimensions. Finally, the differences in the appearances of a structure resulting from the plane of sectioning compounds the problem (Fig. 8.4) and has perpetuated errors (Elias, 1971).

Preparative methods for biochemical studies of cellular organelles involve procedures as drastic as those in microscopy. Maceration of the tissues prior to centrifugation permits loss of soluble enzymes and enzyme systems from specific loci in the cell to the cytosol. Fractions that contain only one organelle are extremely difficult to obtain and must be checked by electron microscopy. The

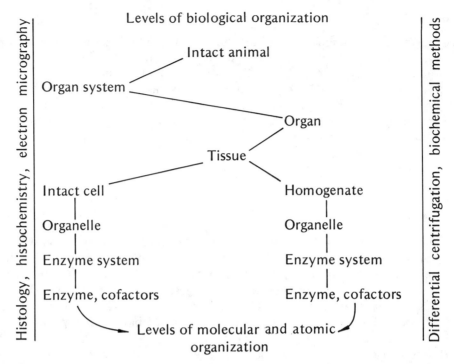

Figure 8.3
Levels of biological organization. Morphological and biochemical studies of the cell complement each other, and events at any level may be involved in observations at any other level. (From J. Tepperman, *Metabolic and Endocrine Physiology*, 2nd ed., Year Book Medical Publishers, Chicago, 1968.)

cytosol which contains what is referred to as the soluble fraction has in it enzymes and enzyme systems that were originally in, but pulled from, organelle fractions.

Rewards Resulting from Studying Cells

The instruments and methods developed during the last decade or so have provided the means for the essential communication between cytologist and biochemist. Previously the cytologist was restricted to studying static images of the living cell through fixed and stained preparations, and the biochemist was limited to studying composition and chemical activity in disrupted cell fragments. The cytologist lost sight of the dynamics of the cell, and the biochemist lost sight of the understanding of the correlative organization that is implicit in living material. In a sense, advancement in techniques and instruments were able to merge the focus of the biochemist and cytologist, and a new field of study—called biochemical cytology, cellular physiology, or molecular biology—evolved. This new

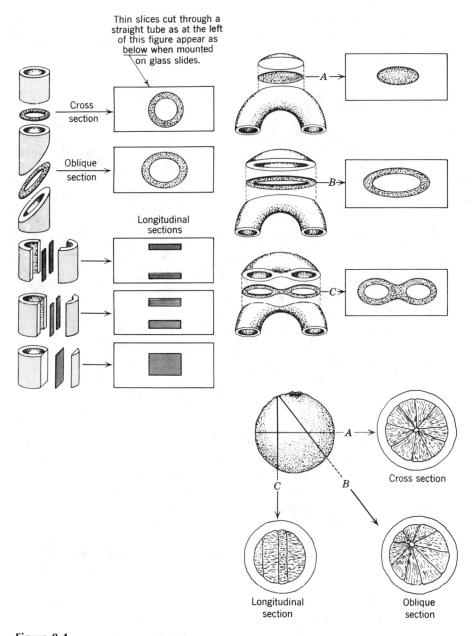

Thin slices cut through a straight tube as at the left of this figure appear as below when mounted on glass slides.

Cross section

Oblique section

Longitudinal sections

A

B

C

Cross section

Longitudinal section

Oblique section

Figure 8.4
Diagrams showing different appearances of sections cut in different planes. (From A. W. Ham, *Histology*, 6th ed., J. B. Lippincott Co., Philadelphia, 1969, p. 29.)

branch of science is concerned with the relationship of subcellular structure to biochemical function and therefore to a basic understanding of the fundamental activities in the nutrition of the cell.

Geography of the Cell

Cells occur in a wide assortment of shapes and sizes. Most cells range in diameter from 0.5–20 μ but some may be huge, such as the ostrich egg; and some, such as nerve cells, may be several feet long. The architecture and chemical components of different cells may be very different, and the variety of specialized functions they perform quite diverse, but all cells have certain basic similarities: each has a limiting membrane; all have or had a nucleus; most contain varying amounts of endoplasmic reticulum, ribosomes, mitochondria, and Golgi apparatus (Fig. 8.5).

The limiting membrane, or *plasma membrane,* separates the cell from its environment yet permits it to maintain contact with that environment on which it depends. The membrane is capable of performing a variety of specialized functions such as absorption, secretion, and fluid transport. It also can establish and maintain contact with other cells. Certain structural characteristics enhance these capabilities. For example, outfoldings or microvilli greatly extend the surface area; infoldings facilitate transport of fluids and develop into pinocytotic vesicles which are the surface invaginations that pinch off and become free in the cytoplasm. Flagellae and cilia are motile specializations on the membrane surface.

The *nucleus,* the most conspicuous component of the cell, is separated from the rest of the cell by its own membrane that, like the plasma membrane, both maintains separation and permits contact with the rest of the cell. The nucleus contains practically all of the cell's DNA and is the site of both replication of DNA and its transcription to RNA. The DNA because of its affinity for biological stains was originally called chromatin, and the concentrated areas of RNA are referred to as *nucleoli.* The nuclear membrane is continuous with the endoplasmic reticulum of the cell.

The *endoplasmic reticulum,* an interconnected system of membraneous channels, appears to be a means for channeling substances through the cell. The rough endoplasmic reticulum is studded with *ribosomes* that are composed of RNA and protein which complex with messenger RNA to form polysomes. Protein synthesis takes place on the polysomes, and the proteins enter the channels of the endoplasmic reticulum to be transported to different parts of the cell. Some ribosomes are free in the cell matrix and these, too, are concerned with protein syntheses. Another type of reticulum that is continuous with the rough endoplasmic reticulum is smooth endoplasmic reticulum. It is involved in synthesis of steroids and other lipids.

The *Golgi apparatus,* usually between the nucleus and the apex of the cell consists of a stack of flat sacs and vesicles of different sizes. It is the area where synthesized materials are concentrated and packaged in membrane-limited ves-

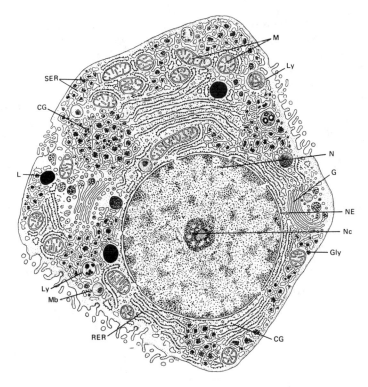

Figure 8.5
Drawing showing fine structure of hepatocyte. PM, plasma membrane; M, mitochondrion; Ly, lysosome; SER, smooth endoplasmic reticulum; RER, rough endoplasmic reticulum; N, nucleus; NE, nuclear envelope; Nc, nucleolus; G, golgi complex; Mb, microbody; CG, cisternae of endoplasmic reticulum; L, lipid droplet; Gly, glycogen. (From T. L. Lentz, *Cell Fine Structure*, W. B. Saunders Co., Philadelphia, 1971.)

icles for export from the cell. The Golgi are also responsible for the synthesis of complex carbohydrates.

Mitochondria are the site of cellular respiration. Cells that are metabolically active may contain as many as 1,000 mitochondria; other cells may contain only a few. They are usually located in the region of the cell's greatest metabolic activity. Some nonnuclear DNA is contained in mitochondria and is probably responsible for coding for specific mitochondrial proteins.

Lysosomes are membrane-limited bodies that contain a variety of hydrolytic enzymes that function in the breakdown of materials taken into the cell by phagocytosis. Because of their function, their appearances are quite diverse. Some lysosomes containing indigestible remnants are called residual bodies.

Cell inclusions are the inactive storage forms of cell products and include lipid droplets, glycogen granules, and pigment granules.

The *cytoplasmic matrix* has embedded in it all of the structures and organelles of the cell. It consists of water, ions, soluble metabolites and proteins, and the components of the *cytoskeleton*. The soluble phase of the matrix is thought to be structureless, but instruments providing greater magnification and resolution may in the future disclose some structural characteristics.

The aim of this overview of the cell and its contents is only to provide some points of reference. Detailed study of structure and function of the organelles in the chapters that follow then can be understood as part of the integrated whole.

chapter 9

the plasma membrane

All cells are units separated from their environment by a membrane. This is a barrier whose presence determines the shape and encloses the substance of the cell. Despite the variability and potential hostility of the outside environment, it is the membrane on which the constancy of the internal chemistry of the cell is dependent. The discharge of this responsibility is made possible by the ability of the membrane to discriminate among those organic and inorganic molecules in the surrounding medium, permitting entrance to some and rebuffing others. This is a truly vital task since either mass invasion of potentially toxic materials or rejection of essential nutrients can lead to cellular death by asphyxiation, hydration, desiccation, poisoning, starvation, or other equally effective means. The cell, thus dependent on the external environment for all the raw materials from which it is made and with which it operates, by means of the membrane barrier and its fastidious selectivity, can enjoy a distinct and separate existence.

A cell in equilibrium with its environment is a dead cell. One of the fundamental attributes of a living cell therefore is the ability to prevent the establishment of an equilibrium between its cytoplasm and the extracellular fluid. The differences in concentration of ions and molecules between these two compartments are maintained by the diligent and persistent management of movement through a barrier. The specific barrier is the innermost section of the cell membrane, the *plasma membrane*. Many cells may have protecting or supporting membranes exterior to the plasma membrane, but it is this innermost section of the membrane that exerts the dominant role in the viability of the cell and maintains the dynamic relationship between the cell and its environment. To achieve such a relationship, selected nutrients must constantly flow in and reaction products must flow out through the boundary of the system in a controlled manner. A congested or ungoverned traffic pattern would be as devastating to the cell as it would be to a busy highway.

Incoming nutrients provide the materials on which the life of the cell and its substance depend: carbohydrates, proteins, lipids, minerals, and vitamins. These nutrients are of value to the living cell, whether it be a protist or each of the millions in a complex organism, only after they have passed the hurdle of the plasma membrane. Once inside the cell, the nutrient may play any of its defined roles. In this fundamental way the unicellular and multicellular organisms in both the plant and animal kingdoms are identical. The hurdles leading up to the final barrier of the plasma membrane may range from a simple protective membrane in a free-living cell to the complexities of mammalian digestive and transport systems through which nutrients must pass. In the long voyage to each of the cells, membranes must be traversed: from the lumen of the digestive tract into and out of the cells of the intestinal mucosa and then into and out of the vascular system. Finally, the nutrients can be presented to the plasma membranes of each of the individual cells in the complex multicellular organism. After passing this final barrier, the nutrients can participate in the metabolic processes which release energy and provide the constituents for synthesis of both the cell's own substance and its secretory or other products. *It is for these purposes, and at this level of organization, that food is essential for life.*

Role

The complex processes involved in the acceptance and utilization of nutrients presented to the cell are dynamic, interrelated, and cyclic. The presentation of nutrients to the outer surface of the plasma membrane is but the first step and does not insure passage. If cellular work is required to transport the molecules across the membrane, this work is supported by energy provided by nutrients previously admitted to the cell. Essential nutrients supplied by the environment, transmitted through the membrane, and presented to the cellular organelles, permit the synthetic processes and the supporting energy-yielding catabolic activities to be carried on. A cell, any cell, deprived of nutrients to yield the energy to synthesize its substance cannot survive.

Although any starting point is arbitrary in describing as cyclic an activity as cellular nutrition, life begins—or ends—with the capacity of the plasma membrane of an existing and functioning cell to properly perform its specific functions. Molecular pathologies may arise, however, that interrupt membrane function.

For example, in the untreated diabetic, glucose entry into the cell is impaired due, in some cases, to defective insulin receptors within the plasma membrane. In other cases, insulin insufficiency is the problem. Normal carbohydrate metabolism is interrupted and the classic symptoms of diabetes develop.

The exact manner in which the plasma membrane discharges its fundamental responsibility remains an enigma. Some of the details of the membrane architecture have been revealed, others are conjectural. What is known is that the intracellular environment is meticulously maintained and this, presumably, is effected by the systematic arrangement and functional capabilities of the macromolecules synthesized by the cell. However, the performance of the plasma membrane is dependent not only on its own capabilities and the supporting cellular activity but also on the degree of stress imposed on it by its environment.

Structure

The cell membrane is actually a group of membranes only one section of which, the boundary or *plasma membrane,* is essential for the life of the cell. Damage to the plasma membrane is as lethal to the cell as damage to the nucleus itself. The plasma membrane lies closest to the cytoplasm and the layers exterior to it are supporting or protecting membranes.

EARLY STUDIES

The structure of the plasma membrane was first described decades before it was ever seen. Using a light microscope, one could easily see the discrete cell distinct from its environment. However, the nature of the demarcation between the cytoplasm of the cell and the extracellular sphere under such magnification could only be deduced from knowledge of its functional role. As early as 1895 Overton suggested that the cell was covered with lipid since it was preferentially permeable to lipid-soluble substances. Knowledge of the manner in which fatty acid molecules behave at a water interface provided a basis for defining membrane structure and permeability behavior (Fig. 9.1). The reason for the tidy alignment of fatty acid molecules resides in the properties of the molecules themselves. Fatty acids contain a carboxyl group that is *hydrophilic,* or freely miscible in water, and a hydrocarbon chain that is *hydrophobic,* or incompatible with water. It is for this reason that fatty acids orient themselves at an oil-water interface so that the hydrocarbon chain is in the oil and the carboxyl or *polar* group is in the water. The polar, or charged, groups are freely miscible in water because they dissociate and form hydrogen bonds to water molecules. Such molecules are called *amphipathic,* that is, they are structurally asymmetric with one highly polar and one nonpolar end. The lipid portions of living membranes are made up of phospholipids, cerebrosides, and cholesterol. The hydrocarbon chains of these lipids are the hydrophobic groups. The polar groups, in the case of the phospholipids, are the charged phosphate and various other ionic groups characteristic of phospho-

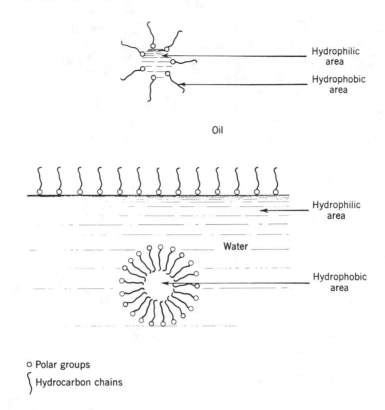

Oil

Water

○ Polar groups
} Hydrocarbon chains

Figure 9.1
Model of polar lipids at oil-water interface. (From V. Luzzati et al.,
Farad. Soc. Disc., No. 25, 43, 1958.)

lipids. (See Chapter 2.) The single hydroxyl group of cholesterol makes it weakly
hydrophilic.

DEVELOPMENT OF THE UNIT MEMBRANE CONCEPT

Lipid extracted from red blood cell membranes indicated that there was enough
lipid for a double layer (Gorter and Grendel, 1925). Since both the internal and
external environments of the cell are aqueous and since the membrane is freely
permeable to lipid-soluble substances, it was reasonable to postulate a double
layer of lipid, oriented so that polar groups formed the inner and outer boundaries
with the two rows of hydrocarbon forming the core (Fig. 9.2). Such reasoning
and knowledge of the physiological properties of membranes led to the deductions
made by Danielli and Davson (1935). They based their structural model on certain
fundamental properties of cell membranes: preferential permeability to lipid-soluble substances, existence of a low surface tension, and high electrical resistance.
From these properties they deduced that there must exist a continuous layer of

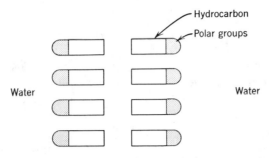

Figure 9.2
Model of red cell membrane. (From E. Gorter
and F. Grendel, *J. Exp. Med.* 41:439, 1925.)

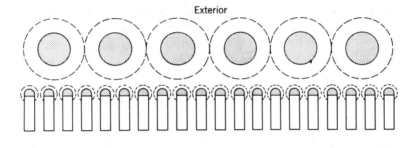

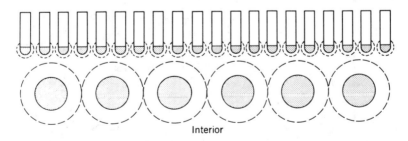

Figure 9.3
Conception of cell membrane structure according to J. F. Danielli and H.
Davson (*J. Cell. Comp. Physiol.* 5:495, 1935). The membrane is represented
by a layer of lipoid of indefinite thickness with polar surfaces oriented
toward both the exterior and interior of the cell. These polar surfaces are
shown covered by monolayers of globular protein molecules. (From J. D.
Robertson, *Prog. Biophys. and Biophys. Chem.* 10:343, 1960.)

lipid molecules, such as phosphatides, sterols, and fats, with their polar groups oriented toward both the exterior and interior of the cell, and that on these polar surfaces were adsorbed a single layer of protein molecules (Fig. 9.3). They suggested that the protein layer consisted of polypeptide chains, or meshworks of such chains, lying in the plane of the interface with the hydrocarbon portions of the amino acid residues dissolved in the lipid layer and the polar groups in the aqueous phase. The elasticity and the relatively great mechanical strength of the membrane were attributed to the polypeptide chains.

Twenty-five years after the Danielli and Davson proposal, during which time membranes were studied by electron microscopy, x-ray diffraction, and chemical techniques, Robertson (1959) presented a model of the *unit membrane* that corresponded to the one proposed by Danielli and Davson although it was based on different lines of evidence. Robertson described the structure as a central core of a bimolecular leaflet of lipid bounded on either side by protein or other hydrophilic monolayers of nonlipid material (Fig. 9.4). Examination of cell membranes from a great variety of tissues from many species of plants and animals led Robertson (1960) to postulate that this structure was probably universally present in all animal and possibly all plant cells, and it was for this reason that he called it the unit membrane. The unit membrane was thought to be not only the barrier between the cell and its environment but also between the cell organelles and the cell matrix.

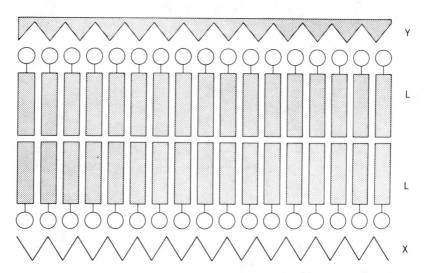

Figure 9.4
Model of unit membrane. A highly schematic diagram of a unit membrane showing two monolayers of lipid molecules (L) and two fully spread monolayers of nonlipid designated by the letters X and Y. Different letters are used for the nonlipid monolayers to indicate that they are chemically different, even though the exact nature is as yet unknown. X borders cytoplasm. (From J. D. Robertson, *Ann. N. Y. Acad. Sci.* 94:339, 1961.)

MODIFICATION OF THE UNIT MEMBRANE CONCEPT

The concept of the universality of the unit membrane was later amended on the basis of evidence that all plasma membranes were not symmetrical structures and that the layers on either side of the lipid core differed in chemical reactivity. Information obtained from the use of a variety of fixatives in the preparation of sections for electron microscopy led Robertson to suggest that the lipid core might be bounded on one side by a protein monolayer and on the other side by a carbohydrate-containing monolayer.

Objections to the concept of a unit membrane common for all structures were based on the fact that Robertson's theory was derived from the study of myelin (Fig. 9.5), and generalizations drawn from such a specialized membrane seemed unwarranted (Korn, 1966; 1969). Furthermore, the unit membrane theory presupposed sufficient lipid to cover the surface area of the membrane with a bimolecular leaflet. This idea was based on data from the erythrocyte membrane and seemed reasonable at the time. However, protein-lipid ratios of membranes have since been shown to vary, as do the fatty acid compositions, so it must be assumed that a wide spectrum of membrane components exists with myelin at one end of the spectrum. Although there is reasonable but not conclusive evidence to support the bimolecular leaflet of phospholipid and protein as the structure of myelin, there is little basis for extending this concept to biological membranes in general (Korn, 1966; Sjöstrand, 1968). The specialized function of myelin is that of an electrical insulator for which it is well adapted with its repeating layers of lipids. However, the diversified functions of membranes suggest that such a single structure is rather unlikely. (For further discussion of myelin, see Chapter 19.)

CURRENT MEMBRANE MODELS

Other investigators proposed models with globular micelles of lipid in dynamic equilibrium with the bimolecular leaflet and indicated either globules of proteins to account for the enzymes known to be in membranes (Lucy, 1968) or repeating globular lipoprotein subunits associated to form a two-dimensional membrane (Benson, 1966; Green and Tzagoloff, 1966). A model proposed by Lenard and Singer (1966), and subsequently extended (Glaser and Singer, 1971; Singer, 1971; 1972), has the formidable name of the *lipid-globular protein mosaic*. This model has a great number of adherents. It shows the lipid arranged in a discontinuous bilayer alternating with the globular proteins. The interspersed proteins are arranged with their ionic and highly polar groups exposed at the exterior surfaces of the membranes. Singer and Nicolson (1972) suggest that it can be best thought of as a two-dimensional oriented viscous solution, in other words, a *fluid mosaic* as it is sometimes called. A schematic cross-sectional view is presented in Fig. 9.6. The folded polypeptide chains of the globular proteins may be partially embedded in the phospholipid bilayer or may extend through the bilayer protruding from each surface and maintaining contact with the aqueous solvent on both sides of the membrane. In each case, the ionic residues of the protein are on the protruding surfaces and the nonpolar residues are in the embedded parts.

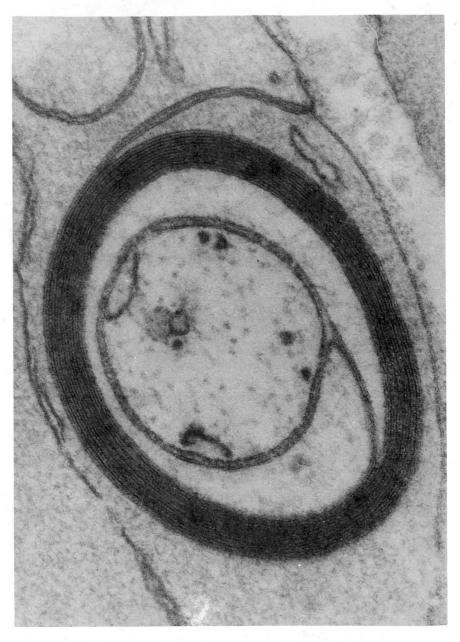

Figure 9.5
Concentric organization of unit membranes forming a myelin sheath. Mouse sciatic nerve. Magnification 135,000. (Courtesy of Dr. J. David Robertson.)

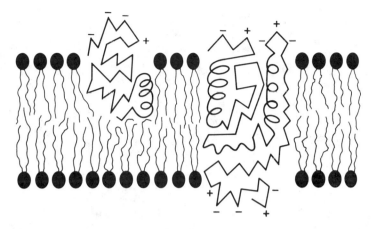

Figure 9.6
The lipid-globular protein mosaic model of membrane structure:
schematic cross-sectional view. The phospholipids are arranged as
a discontinuous bilayer with their ionic and polar heads in contact
with water. The integral proteins, with the heavy lines representing
the folded polypeptide chains, are shown as globular molecules
partially embedded in, and partially protruding from, the membrane. The protruding parts have on their surfaces the ionic residues
($-$ and $+$) of the protein, whereas the nonpolar residues are largely
in the embedded parts; accordingly, the protein molecules are amphipathic. The degree to which the integral proteins are embedded
and, in particular, whether they span the entire membrane thickness
depend on the size and structure of the molecules. (From S. J. Singer
and G. L. Nicolson, *Science,* 175:720, 1972.)

The extent to which any protein is embedded in the membrane is determined by
the size and structure of the molecule. The fact that different proteins can be
integral parts of the membrane helps to explain the variety of functional membranes. The three-dimensional model of the lipid-globular protein mosaic (Fig.
9.7) shows the large irregular globular proteins embedded to various degrees in
the phospholipid matrix. The embedded proteins are the *intrinsic* or *integral*
proteins of the membrane. They may extend partly or all the way through the
lipid bilayer thereby forming an integral part of the membrane continuum. The
extrinsic or *peripheral* proteins are associated with the exposed surfaces of the
membrane and can be easily dissociated from the membrane as molecularly intact
proteins free of lipid and relatively soluble. The extrinsic proteins are not critical
to the structural integrity of the membrane (Singer and Nicholson, 1972; Capaldi,
1974). Although no proteins or polypeptide subunits in the membrane serve purely
structural purposes, proteins unique to particular membranes and associated with
their functions can also serve a structural role (Dreyer et al., 1972). In fact,

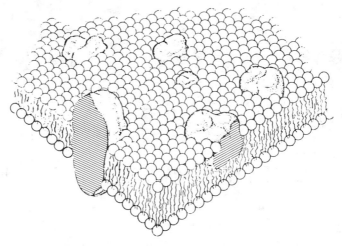

Figure 9.7
The lipid-globular protein mosaic model with a lipid matrix
(the fluid mosaic model); schematic three-dimensional and
cross-sectional views. The solid bodies with stippled surfaces
represent the globular integral proteins, which at long range
are randomly distributed in the plane of the membrane. At
short range, some may form specific aggregates, as shown.
(From S. J. Singer and G. L. Nicolson, *Science,* 175:720, 1972.)

membrane function depends on how the membrane proteins are linked in the
membrane structure.

The matrix in which the protein is embedded is fluid under physiological conditions and therefore dynamic: that is, the membrane appears to be a two-dimensional viscous solution that permits the protein components to maintain mobility and enables carrier mechanisms to operate. The fluidity of the phospholipid
matrix is determined by the structure and relative proportion of the unsaturated
fatty acids and by ambient temperature (Fox, 1972). At body temperature, phospholipids with only saturated fatty acids are arranged in an orderly and rigid
crystalline fashion. Mixtures of saturated and unsaturated fatty acids provide a
less orderly arrangement and are, therefore, more fluid. This occurs because the
double bonds lead to structural deformation and disturb ordered stacking. The
greater the degree of unsaturation of the fatty acids in the phospholipids, and the
greater the proportion of unsaturated to saturated fatty acids, the more fluid the
membrane.

Mammalian cell membranes contain a considerable portion of unsaturated fatty
acids and, therefore, the melting or *transition temperature* for the lipid bilayer is
below normal mammalian body temperature, permitting relatively free movement
of the fatty acid tails. The combination of unsaturation and temperature gives the
whole lipid bilayer the consistency of a light oil, and the lipid and protein mol-

ecules are free to move, mostly from side to side (Capaldi, 1974). Independent movement of the lipid and protein molecules has also been demonstrated in red cell membranes by Glaser et al. (1970), adding support to the suggestion for organization in a mosaic. The main constituents of the membrane appear to be held in place by noncovalent interactions, making fluid motion possible.

In eukaryotes, membrane fluidity is influenced, even regulated, by both fatty acid saturation and by cholesterol content. Cholesterol fits between fatty acids and prevents the crystallization, or solidification, of the membrane and thus leads to increased fluidity. Cholesterol also has the opposite effect since it blocks lateral movement by steric hindrance.

The Singer-Nicholson fluid-mosaic model is supported by a wide variety of experimental observations and is now widely accepted. One of the major reasons for acceptance comes from freeze-fracture studies. Such studies have provided direct evidence that particles (proteins) are intercalated within the membrane. Further, it has been found that lipids and some proteins can diffuse laterally within the plasma membrane an average distance of 2 μm in one second. A red blood cell is about 6 μm in diameter.

MEMBRANE ASYMMETRY

Membranes are both structurally and, as will be discussed later, functionally asymmetric. As depicted in Fig. 9.8, the outermost surface consists of carbohydrate chains attached to lipids or to proteins. The carbohydrate chains constitute the *cell surface coat*. Proteins are inserted asymmetrically and the outer half of

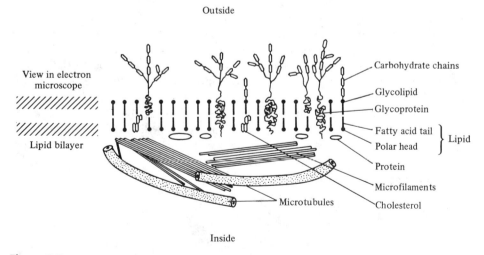

Figure 9.8
Diagram illustrating the asymmetrical molecular structure of the cell membrane. (From A. W. Ham and D. H. Cormack, *Histology*, 8th ed., J. B. Lippincott Co., Philadelphia, 1979 p. 112.)

the membrane contains various *receptors* which interact with specific molcules in the cell's environment. Protein pumps such as the $Na^+ - K^+$ ATPase pump are oriented so that Na^+ is transported out of the cell and K^+ in. Lipids are also distributed unevenly. In the case of red blood cells, sphingomyelin and phosphatidyl choline are more concentrated in the outer half and phosphatidyl ethanolamine and phosphatidyl serine in the inner half. Various proteins are associated with the inner face of the membrane, including globular proteins, microfilaments, and microtubules. For a review on membrane asymmetry, see Rothman and Lenard (1977).

MEMBRANE INTEGRITY

The lipid-protein complexes that form the plasma membranes, and the complexes with a relatively greater amount of phospholipid containing polyunsaturated fatty acids that form the membranes of organelles, are particularly susceptible to peroxidation. The membrane containing unsaturated fatty acid tails is predisposed to disruption which occurs through the chain reactions associated with the generation of free radicals. Demopoulos (1973) indicates that drastic effects should be expected also on membrane proteins and membrane-associated structures such as attached ribosomes, surface glycoproteins, and various complex receptor sites as a result of lipid peroxidation. Such peroxidative changes undoubtedly play a significant role in cellular pathology (Pryor, 1973). Often, powerful catalysts that initiate lipid peroxidation, such as coordinated iron and hemoproteins, are located in close proximity to polyunsaturated membrane lipids. The damage that ensues involves changes in the membrane proteins resulting from polymerization, polypeptide chain scission, and chemical changes in individual amino acids (Tappel, 1973). The polymerization or cross-linking of enzymes can wreak particular havoc to a cell and its organelle membranes completely disrupting the precise arrangement of molecules responsible for the integration of structure and function. Among the amino acids most readily susceptible to the effects of lipid peroxidation are methionine, histidine, cystine, and lysine (Tappel, 1973). If the membrane subjected to lipid peroxidation and rupture is a lysosomal membrane, the release of the enzymes normally contained within the confines of the organelle initiates random hydrolyses within the cell, further damaging structure and function.

The generally accepted mechanism of peroxide formation involves the formation of a free radical ($R^{.}$) by a polyunsaturated fatty acid (RH), followed by the addition of oxygen to form a peroxide ($ROO^{.}$):

$$RH \longrightarrow R^{.} + H^+$$
$$R^{.} + O_2 \longrightarrow ROO^{.}$$
$$ROO^{.} + RH \longrightarrow ROOH + R^{.}$$

A chain is propagated by the reaction of the peroxide with another polyunsaturated fatty acid to produce another free radical. (See Uri, 1961.) A chain reaction such as this can be inhibited either by replacing or depleting one of the substrates.

Vitamin E exerts a protective action in preventing lipid peroxidation and in so doing is fundamental to the structural and functional integrity of cell membranes and, therefore, the cell itself. It should come as no surprise that the function of vitamin E in membrane protection is closely related to its position in membrane structure. Vitamin E interdigitates with the phospholipids, cholesterol, and tri-acylglycerols in the plasma membrane and in the membranes of the mitochondria, lysosomes, and endoplasmic reticulum. In mitochondrial membranes, the ratio in vitamin E to the polyunsaturated fatty acids in membrane phospholipids, whose unsaturated state the vitamin E protects, is about 1:1000. From its vantage point within the membrane structure, vitamin E is in an ideal position to capture free radicals.

Vitamin E functions as an antioxidant (AH) by replacing a fatty acid as substrate for the oxidation and thereby breaking the chain of free radical formation. This mechanism is referred to as hydrogen abstraction:

$$ROO^{\cdot} + AH \longrightarrow ROOH + A^{\cdot}$$

Thus, the close association of vitamin E and fat *in vivo* is propitious. (However, the relationship can present a problem to the investigator who wishes to prepare a vitamin E-free ration since the vitamin E must be stripped from fats or oils.) Tappel and Zalkin (1959) showed *in vivo* lipid peroxidation in the mitochondrial and microsome fractions from livers of vitamin E-deficient rabbits. Zalkin and Tappel (1960) concluded that vitamin E functions solely to stabilize cellular un-saturated lipids against oxidative deterioration, thereby maintaining structural and functional integrity at the subcellular level. Vitamin E functions in maintaining membrane integrity by interacting with free radicals that are generated during certain types of oxidoreductase activities (McCay et al., 1972). In the process, α-tocopherol is converted to a polar lipid. Inadequate membrane protection may be the explanation for the fragility of erythrocyte membranes and for alterations in the structure of hepatocyte membranes in vitamin E deficiency (Machada et al., 1971). The hemolytic anemia that occurs in premature infants also appears to be due to vitamin E deficiency. In this instance, fragility of the erythrocyte membranes is due to inadequate absorption of the vitamin through the immature intestinal mucosal cells (Gross and Melhorn, 1972). It is probable that the fragility and spontaneous hemolysis of blood stored in blood banks for periods longer than two to three weeks are due to peroxide generation from red cell lipid, which is enhanced by heme and produces a reduction of vitamin E in the erythrocyte. György (1962) suggests that vitamin E repeatedly added to blood might permit longer storage.

Although the precise molecular mechanisms remain unknown, recent studies indicate that lipid peroxidation leads to a loss of membrane phospholipid, inhibition of certain membrane-associated enzymes, and increased membrane rigidity (Hochstein and Jain, 1981). Clearly, lipid peroxidation is an important problem and has to be dealt with many times in the life of a cell. Understanding the extent to which it occurs under physiological conditions is still very much in the investigative phase (McCay, 1981).

In addition to vitamin E, small amounts of sulfhydryl compounds such as glutathione, sulfhydryl proteins, cysteine, and methionine also react as free radical scavengers and peroxide decomposers (Tappel, 1973). Glutathione peroxidase, a selenium-requiring enzyme located in the plasma membrane of red blood cells, is also important in defending against peroxidation. (See Flohé et al., 1976.)

Vitamin D has been found to alter the synthesis of lipids by the duodenal mucosal cell (Rasmussen et al., 1982). An increased amount of phosphatidyl choline results in increased membrane fluidity. The way increased fluidity leads to increased calcium transport is thought to be related to an increased mobility of calcium transport proteins. (See Chapter 6.)

OTHER GENERAL STRUCTURAL CHARACTERISTICS

Glycocalyx or Cell Coat

What originally was thought to be an extraneous coat or "fuzz" covering the plasma membrane has recently been shown to have fine structure and histochemical properties to indicate that it is syntheiszed by the cell whose free surface it covers. This cell coat or *glycocalyx* is an integral part of the membrane and glycoprotein in nature. It appears to be a dynamic surface component and requires the intact cell not only for its synthesis but also for its maintenance (Ito, 1969). It appears to be filamentous and inseparable from the cell as long as the cell maintains its integrity; however, the fine structure of the glycocalyx tends to vary with different preparative procedures. The functions of the glycocalyx will be discussed in a subsequent section; its synthesis by the Golgi apparatus in Chapter 12.

Membrane Pores

A characteristic of membrane structure, postulated by some investigators as perhaps fundamental to certain aspects of permeability, is the presence of membrane pores. Danielli first suggested that groups of protein molecules, oriented radially with their polar groups directed toward the interior, formed pores that he called *polar pores*. Solomon (1960) estimated that about 0.06 percent of the red blood cell surface is occupied by pores.

There is now considerable evidence showing the transmembrane-protein nature of at least some pores: For example, the $Na^+ - K^+$ transport system and $Ca^{++} - ATPase$ have been purified separately; when reinserted into artificial lipid membranes they are functional. This experimental approach provides a powerful research tool. Further discussion is included in the section on function.

Cell Junctions

Membranes of adjacent cells in a tissue may run straight and parallel to each other or may have tortuous interdigitations (Fig. 9.9). Not only does the membrane form the boundary for the individual cell but it also participates in the formation of specialized junctions between cells that are important in cell to cell transport

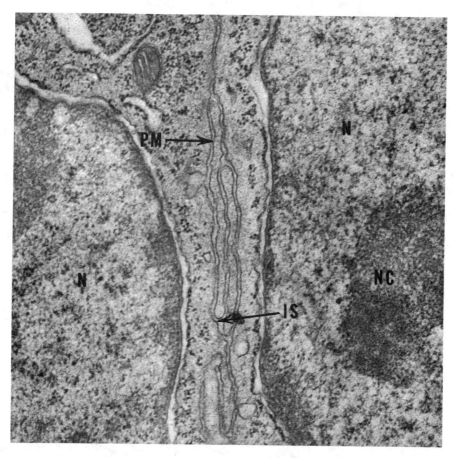

Figure 9.9
Interdigitating plasma membranes (PM) with intercellular space (IS) between. N =
nucleus, Nc = nucleolus. Gland cells of uterine mucosa of Japanese quail. Magnification 40,000. (Courtesy of Dr. Harald Schraer.)

mechanisms. Cell junctions are composed of four elements: the *zona occludens*
or *tight junction, zona adherens* or *intermediate junction,* the *macula adherens*
or *desmosome,* and the *gap junction* or *nexus.* These zones appear structurally
distinguishable and functionally distinct. Fig. 9.10 illustrates the junctional complex in intestinal epithelial cells. The zona occludens begins close to the lumen
at the junction of neighboring cells where the surface plasma membrane is de-
flected inward. There is fusion of the two straight and parallel adjacent plasma
membranes and no intercellular space. This area encircles the cell in a ribbonlike
fashion, thereby sealing off the lumen from the rest of the intercellular space. The
membranes then diverge and are separated by an intercellular space to form the
zona adherens. This area, too, runs around the perimeter of the cell. The area

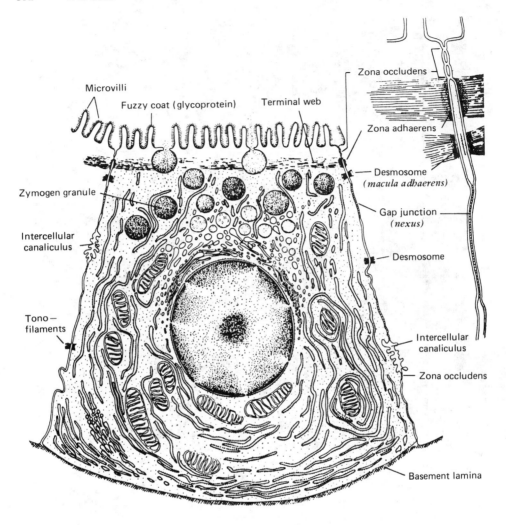

Figure 9.10
Diagram illustrating the junctional complex of a columnar epithelial cell. (From E. D. Hay, *Histology,* 4th ed, L. Weis and R. O. Greep, eds., McGraw-Hill, New York, 1977, p. 129.)

between the membranes is filled with a material of low electron density and may be glycocalyx material. Dense patches of fine filaments are arranged on the cytoplasmic sides of the membranes. The desmosome (Fig. 9.11) is extremely dense in electron micrographs where an ordered system of cytoplasmic fibrils converge on the cytoplasmic sides of the two cells to form a supporting structure. The cells appear neither to be fused nor in direct contact. The dark line in the center of the area is thought to be merged glycocalyx from the two cells. The desmosomes are not continuous around the cell but occur only at discrete points. Approximately 15 proteins have been identified in desmosomes. Gap junctions are aqueous

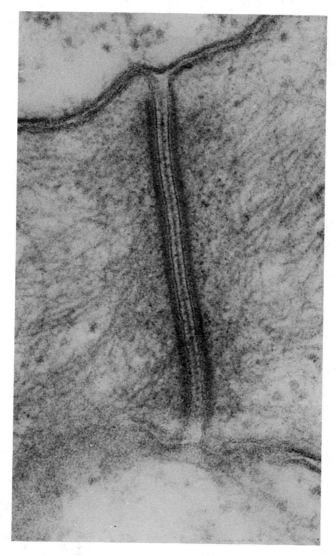

Figure 9.11
Desmosome from the skin of the frog, Rana pipiens. Magnification 120,000. (Courtesy of Dr. Joan Borysenko.)

channels that form between cells of such organized tissue as heart, liver, and epithelium. The walls of the gap junction are comprised of protein which appears to have six subunits (Fig. 9.12). The size of the channels has been determined to be about 20 nm long and 1 nm in diameter on the basis of electron microscopy, electrical measurements, and by the diffusion of tracers. Polar molecules having a molecular weight of about 1,900 or less can pass through the channels (Simpson

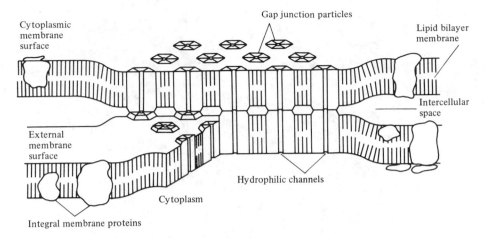

Figure 9.12
Diagrammatic reconstruction of a gap junction. (From L. A. Staehlin, *Int. Rev. Cytol.*
39:249, 1974.)

et al., 1977). Gap junctions form within seconds when certain cells are in contact
with each other. Thus it appears that they are formed from proteins already in
existence in the plasma membrane. For a review of gap junction literature, see
Gilula (1977).

The roles of the junctional complex in the attachment of cells to each other in
tissue and in cell to cell transport mechanisms will be discussed in the section
on function.

For reviews of membrane structure see Bretscher (1973), Capaldi (1974), and
Rothman and Lenard (1977).

Function

The concept of diversity in structure is consonant with the diversity in function
that is known to exist. The capacity of the cell membrane to act as both barrier
and gateway is undoubtedly a function of its molecular structure and of the size
and character of the molecules seeking passage. Above and beyond the preferential admission of nutrients to the cell, membranes exert a selectivity leading to
localization and concentration of specific nutrients in certain organelles, cells,
and tissues. Such selectivity is inextricably related to specialized function. That
the membrane is not a static barrier will be apparent: neither size nor concentration
gradient nor chemical resemblance is itself sufficient to insure acceptance of
unwanted molecules. It is reasonable to suspect that the physiological diversities
may be attributable to (1) the assortment of lipid constituents, (2) the character
of the globular proteins interspersed in the lipid matrix, and (3) the chemical
specificty of different sections of a continuous membrane and its glycocalyx.

GENERAL CHARACTERISTICS

All membranes have in common the characteristic of *selective permeability*. A membrane that is selectively permeable permits one material to pass more easily than another; this is different from a semipermeable membrane that is permeable to the solvent only. The characteristic of selective permeability enables the membrane to maintain a balance between the osmotic pressure of the intracellular fluid and that of the interstitial fluid. It also enables a difference in the ionic concentration between the cell and extracellular fluid to be maintained, and this leads to an electrical potential across the membrane. These characteristics associated with diffusion, plus the mechanisms that require energy generally described as active transport, account for the major exchanges across membranes.

The structure of the membrane also contributes to its characteristics of selective permeability. Although it is practically impermeable to intracellular protein and related anions, it is freely permeable to water and to sodium, potassium, and chloride. These differences in permeability create the chemical and electrical gradients existing between the cell and its environment. The cell maintains a high concentration of potassium along with a high concentration of protein and related anions. It has a low concentration of sodium and chloride. The environment surrounding the cell on the other side of the membrane has a low concentration of potassium and a high concentration of sodium. Unrestrained cation movement would be along the gradient: sodium moving into the cell and potassium moving out. It is obvious that such movement along the concentration gradients is either counterbalanced or impeded since all cells maintain high ratios of potassium to sodium in an environment with a reverse ratio. Sodium does diffuse into the cell and potassium does diffuse out, but the passive diffusion along the concentration gradients are counterbalanced by active transport. In effect, the emigrating potassium ions are returned to the cell and the emigrating sodium ions to the environment. Current hypotheses explaining this mechanism will be discussed in detail in a later section.

The counterbalancing effect of ion diffusion is supported by the favorable electrical gradient which tends to retain potassium within the cell. The concentration of anions within the cell attracts and holds the positively charged potassium creating an electrical gradient from the outside in. Disruption of this favorable electrical gradient by chloride, which diffuses freely, is prevented because the chloride ions that enter are repelled by the concentration of anions within the cell. A balance is thus achieved with more potassium ions inside the cell and more chloride outside. The active extrusion of sodium is also a major factor in the maintenance of this potential difference. Because some potassium does passively diffuse out of the cell and some chloride in, an electrical potential is created across the membrane. The membrane is said to be polarized with the cytoplasm negative to the extracellular fluid. In other words, there are more positive charges on the outer surface and more negative charges along the inner surface. This is true of most membranes. The transient reversal of this state of polarization in nerve and muscle cells explains their physiological action and will be discussed in Chapters 18 and 19.

TRANSPORT

Passive Transport

There are three major categories of passive transport: *simple diffusion, facilitated diffusion*, and *exchange diffusion*. Although these will be discussed individually, it will become apparent that these mechanisms are not rigidly defined and, in fact, do overlap.

Simple Diffusion.   Simple diffusion along a concentration gradient or an electrical gradient occurs from a high concentration or potential to a lower one. It is always in a downhill direction, and no energy is required for the process (Fig. 9.13). However, in some instances, a revolving door policy is established and an intruding molecule that has diffused in may be escorted out again. The planned exit is an active, energy-requiring process against the gradient and is discussed in the section on active transport. Passive diffusion, of course, could not be the only mechanism in the maintenance of the relationship between the cell and its environment since, unrestricted and unchecked, an equilibrium would ultimately be established leading to the death of the cell.

The major deterrent to penetration by diffusing molecules is in the lipoprotein character of the membrane itself. Brown and Danielli (1964) suggest that the membrane resistance is tripartite: (1) resistance encountered in passing from the aqueous phase of the environment into the membrane, (2) resistance encountered in diffusing through the membrane, and (3) resistance encountered in passing from the membrane into the watery milieu of the cell's interior. Each of these may be the limiting step, depending on the diffusing molecule.

If a molecule is passing from the water phase of the environment into the membrane, all the hydrogen bonds to the water must be broken simultaneously if entrance into the lipid phase is gained. If there are three or more polar groups in the molecule, this step is likely to be the one that limits the rate of entry.

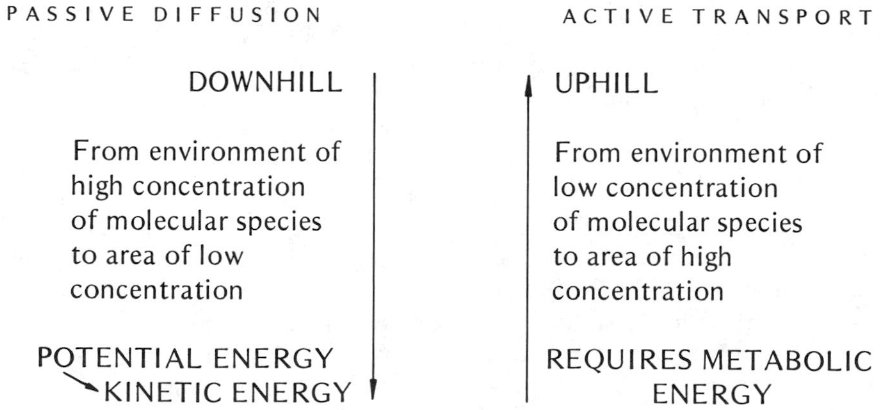

PASSIVE DIFFUSION	ACTIVE TRANSPORT
DOWNHILL	UPHILL
From environment of high concentration of molecular species to area of low concentration	From environment of low concentration of molecular species to area of high concentration
POTENTIAL ENERGY KINETIC ENERGY	REQUIRES METABOLIC ENERGY

Figure 9.13
Contrast of passive diffusion and active transport.

Thus the entry of predominantly polar molecules such as sugars, glycerol, and glycogen would be slow.

If the molecule seeking entrance is predominantly nonpolar, the rate-limiting factor is the diffusion from the membrane to the watery interior. The longer the hydrocarbon chain, the slower is the penetration. A considerable amount of kinetic energy is required to transfer each CH_2— group from the lipid to water, and all these groups in the molecule must be transferred simultaneously if the molecule is not to be partly trapped in the lipid phase. However, Danielli has suggested that trapped lipid may be "squeezed out" into the aqueous phase by force exerted on the plasma membrane by cytoplasmic movement. Molecules such as vitamin A, cholesterol, and fats are therefore slow to diffuse.

Some molecules have many polar and many nonpolar groups and the difficulties of diffusion are compounded: there is the need to break the hydrogen bonds for entry into the lipid phase followed by the movement of the nonpolar groups from the lipid to the water phase. Diffusion would therefore be slow for proteins and is probably an unlikely means of passage.

Studies of the kinetics of diffusion indicate that many different nonelectrolytes, as indicated above, can penetrate a lipoprotein membrane by simple diffusion. However, it is evident that other more selective and rapid means of entry into a cell must occur if the required broad assortment of nutrients are to enter and if the cell is to maintain its discriminating position in an environment on which it is totally dependent.

Facilitated Diffusion.   One means of facilitating the passage of solutes across the plasma membrane is by the provision of a carrier to link with the solute and carry it across. This type of transport, facilitated diffusion, does not require an expenditure of energy by the cell and proceeds downhill along the concentration gradient. The molecule being transported is temporarily bound to a membrane constituent at one surface of the membrane, diffused through as a complex, and released at the opposite side. Presumably the carrier returns to pick up another molecule or ion (Fig. 9.14). This type of diffusion can proceed as long as carriers

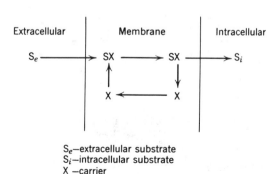

S_e—extracellular substrate
S_i—intracellular substrate
X —carrier

Figure 9.14
Model of facilitated diffusion.

are available; that is, up to the point where the carrier system becomes saturated. The differential rates of sugar transport, for example, are probably due to competition for carrier molecules. The order of decreasing affinities to transport—glucose, mannose, xylose, galactose, arabinose, sorbose, fructose—suggests that success in competition for a position on the carrier is affected by the configuration of the molecule. (See Chapter 6.) A transport protein for glucose has now been isolated and purified. (See Baldwin and Lienhard, 1981.)

Facilitated diffusion does not alter the final equilibrium that could be attained even if the carrier were not present; but it does alter the speed with which the equilbrium is attained.

Exchange Diffusion.   Another type of carrier-dependent transport that has been shown to operate in the passage of certain ions and amino acids is exchange diffusion. For each molecule transported through the membrane in one direction, a similar molecule must be transported on the return trip (Fig. 9.15). Because of the dependence on the carrier molecule, the rate of transport is independent of the solute concentration but limited by the number of carrier molecules. This type of diffusion is responsible for the major exchange of labeled for nonlabeled ions and amino acids. A sodium for a sodium or a glycine for a glycine is termed autoexchange. What purpose this type of equal exchange may serve is not clear. Some heteroexchange may also take place but is very specific for carrier substrates.

Active Transport
When a substance must be moved against a concentration or electrochemical gradient, work is required. The source of the energy for this work is metabolically

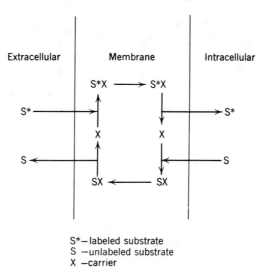

S*—labeled substrate
S —unlabeled substrate
X —carrier

Figure 9.15
Model of exchange diffusion. (From D. B. Tower, S. A. Luse, and H. Grundfest, *Properties of Membranes,* Springer Publishing Co., New York, 1961.)

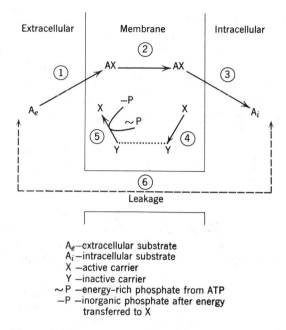

A_e—extracellular substrate
A_i—intracellular substrate
X —active carrier
Y —inactive carrier
~P —energy-rich phosphate from ATP
—P —inorganic phosphate after energy
transferred to X

Figure 9.16
Model of active transport. (From E. Heinz and P.
M. Walsh, *J. Biol. Chem.* 233:1492, 1958.)

derived and the movement is called active transport. Active transport is carrier-mediated, and the carrier is a specific transport protein that is an integral part of the membrane to be traversed. A carrier works by binding the substance, carrying out translocation, and then releasing it (Pardee, 1968). Carriers involved in any type of transport can become saturated with the substance to be transported; each has specificity for the substance it transports; and each is subject to specific inhibition by molecules that can compete for the specific binding site.

An early model of active transport (Fig. 9.16) incorporated the characteristics of the simpler transport systems with the addition of an energy-rich phosphate from ATP to activate the carrier. The model proposed that the activated carrier released the molecule it transported, reverted to an inactive form, and subsequently was reactivated by ATP as it returned through the membrane. Since active or energy-dependent transport was often compared to a pumping system, such as that required to carry water from a lower to a higher level, models appeared that described the active transport of sodium and were referred to as the *sodium pump*. Energy derived from cellular metabolism was depicted as driving the pump or, more specifically, of energizing the carrier to transport sodium out of and potassium into the cell. The release of the sodium to the outside was presumed to convert the carrier by enzymatic action to one which carried potassium to the inside. Net transport of the two ions results because the rate of active transport exceeds the rates of leakage along the gradients in the opposite direction.

Isolation of an enzyme system activated by sodium and potassium ions and dependent on the presence of both ATP and Mg^{++} was shown to be capable of hydrolyzing ATP at a rate that depended on the concentration of sodium inside the cell and of potassium outside (Skou, 1965). The enzyme, Na, K-adenosine triphosphatase (Na,K-ATPase), was shown to be in the membranes of all cells that had a coupled transport mechanism for sodium and potassium. It was suggested that this enzyme system was the one involved in the active transport of sodium and potassium across cell membranes.

Increased insight into membrane structure and the isolation of this enzyme system led to intensified work on the nature and operation of the sodium-potassium pump. Because all cells maintain low levels of sodium and high levels of potassium, the Na-K pump is probably the most ubiquitous transport system in nature. It has been shown that the cation that activates the ATPase is on the side of the membrane from which it is transported; that is, the concentration of sodium activates from the inside and the concentration of potassium from the outside. The hydrolysis of the substrate Mg-ATP takes place inside the cell, and the rate of active transport and the rate of enzyme activity regulate each other. The main features of the pump are (1) it is a protein that appears to consist of four subunits, two large and two small, (2) ATP is hydrolyzed in such a way that the products of hydrolysis stay inside the cell, (3) the splitting occurs only when sodium is on the inside and potassium is on the outside, (4) the ions are moved as part of the vectorial reaction[1], (5) sodium is required to permit the substrate, Mg-ATP, to attach to the enzyme, and (6) a phosphate intermediate is formed and then broken down by the potassium on the outside. Based on these and other data, it is suggested that the enzyme, Na,K-ATPase, in the membrane can assume two conformations: one shape when sodium facilitates attachment of Mg-ATP to the enzyme forming a phosphate intermediate; the other after hydrolysis occurs as a result of the external potassium. This second change is associated with the movement of the ions, and the enzyme reassumes its original conformation. This type of enzyme is *allosteric,* one with two or more distinct binding sites where the binding to one site affects the conformation of the protein and, therefore, the binding to the second site.

Although many features of the Na-K pump have been identified, the precise structure and the mechanism of action of the pump have not yet been elucidated. Several models have been proposed (Jardetzky, 1966; Whittam, 1967; Stein et al., 1974). Fig. 9.17 shows the net reaction.

The directional transport of glucose and of amino acids into the cell accompanied by the sodium ion may well be part of a similar system. In both cases the carrier protein also has a binding site for sodium and is not active unless both the sodium and the glucose (or amino acid) sites are filled. Sodium enters the cell along a downward gradient carrying the glucose (or amino acid) along with it against their respective gradients. The downward gradient of sodium is main-

---

[1]A vectorial reaction is one that is directional because one of the components (ATPase) is fixed in space (the membrane), and the two sides can be distinguished (either Na or K affinity).

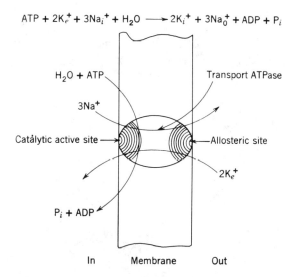

$$ATP + 2K_e^+ + 3Na_i^+ + H_2O \longrightarrow 2K_i^+ + 3Na_0^+ + ADP + P_i$$

Figure 9.17
Net enzyme reaction of active transport. (From R. Whittam, *The Neurosciences,* the Rockefeller Institute, New York, 1967, p. 313.)

tained by its active extrusion from the cells it has thus entered. According to Crane (1965) the sodium and glucose entry and the sodium extrusion are independent, and this is thought to be true also for amino acid transport. Such transport is *noncoupled transport* in contrast to the *coupled transport* of sodium and potassium.

Bulk Transport
Although active or passive transport through the cell membrane may be viewed as polite tasting and sipping of what the environment has to offer, gorging and gulping also occur. A distinction is made between the gorging of solids, *phagocytosis,* and the gulping of liquids, *pinocytosis.* In both cases the material is encircled and taken into the cell. De Duve (1963a) has suggested that the general term *endocytosis* designate the introduction of any foreign materials into the cytoplasm completely surrounded by a membrane and therefore segregated from the cytoplasm itself. In the process of engulfing, the cell membrane sends out pseudopod-like projections that surround and trap the desired material. The encircling membrane then separates from the inner surface and becomes a small membrane-enclosed vesicle within the cell, called a phagosome or a pinosome. The phagosome may be one of the precursors of the lysosome, the cellular digestive system to be discussed in Chapter 14.

Recent evidence indicates that macromolecules are endocytosed by eukaryotic cells by a complex receptor-mediated process (Fig. 9.18). The molecule binds with high specificity to a receptor on the cell surface. The receptors are located in *coated pits.* After binding occurs, the pits bud into the cytoplasm and pinch

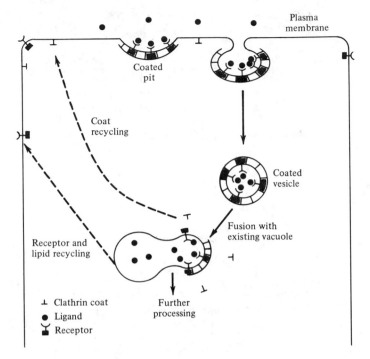

Figure 9.18
Diagrammatic representation of a cycle of coated vesicles. Subsequent fates of the internalized molecules might be: inclusion in
specialized storage vacuoles, digestion in lysosomes, or transfer
intact across the cell and secretion from the opposite cell surface.
At the same time other members of the coated vesicle population
may be engaged in the delivery of newly synthesized molecules to
appropriate compartments (e.g., receptors, proteins for export, and
perhaps lysosomal enzymes). (From B. Pease, *Trends Biochem. Sci.*
5:131, 1980.)

off to form a vesicle. Within seconds the vesicle sheds its coat of clathrin molecules. (Clathrin, a 180,000 m.w. protein, is an important factor, possibly in
recognition, in the shuttling of vesicles between membranes.) Eventually the membrane is cycled back to the plasma membrane while the endocytosed material is
channeled, for example, into lysosomes. Receptor-mediated endocytosis and
membrane recycling have been reviewed recently by Goldstein et al. (1979) and
Pearse and Bretscher (1981).

It is not clear whether endocytosis is a characteristic of all cells, but it would
appear to be a rather general phenomenon and probably retained in most, if not
all, animal cells. Classic examples of mammalian cells generally involved in
endocytosis are the granular leucocytes, the macrophages of the reticuloendothelial system, and the endothelial cells lining the sinusoids of the liver, among
others.

The amoeba, which is both accessible and photogenic, suggests that endocytosis is discriminatory and that there is something of the gourmet about cells that partake in this way. The amoeba will not drink plain water or water to which sugar or other carbohydrate has been added, but when given protein, or amino acids and salts, all restraint is lost. The amoeba becomes an unabashed glutton, drinking to exhaustion and consuming within 30 minutes an amount equivalent to 25 percent of its total mass. The exhaustion is not fatigue on the part of the cell but rather the depletion of available membrane for invagination (Holter, 1961). The ability of certain substances to induce endocytosis, or the predilection of the membrane for these substances, may be presumed to be due to an affinity or binding between the substance and the membrane. This first step appears to be the essential prelude to consumption and may, indeed, be an important *mechanism of cell nutrition* as suggested by Lewis in 1931 when he first observed the process and coined the term *pinocytosis* to describe it.

Bulk transport occurs also in reverse, not into but out of cells. Evidence is accumulating that secretion from endocrine as well as exocrine and nerve cells occurs by the process called *exocytosis* or *emiocytosis*. Morphological evidence for this process was difficult to obtain in thin electron micrograph sections, but recently, use of the freeze-fracture technique has shown the extent of exocytosis in stimulated cells of the adrenal medulla. Visual evidence of attachment and fusion to the plasma membrane followed by extrusion of vesicle contents and retrieval of vesicle membrane has been obtained (Smith et al., 1973). A similar series of events on the cell surface of the stimulated β cells of the pancreas has indicated that this is also the means for insulin release (Orci et al., 1973a; 1973b), although the authors do not rule out the possibility of other mechanisms as well, leading to concomitant release of the hormone.

An important step beginning to be investigated is the mechanism that permits fusion between pinocytotic vesicles and plasma membrane but prevents fusion between intracellular membrane-bound organelles and the membrane. This mechanism is being studied in endothelial cells and applies also to exocytotic vesicles. Dempsey et al. (1973) present evidence suggesting that the polarity of the vesicle membrane may lead to its preferential fusion with the plasma membrane. Some means of recognition of the desired direction of membrane traffic is, of course, of fundamental importance to the cell and the organism of which it is a part.

COMMUNICATION BETWEEN CELLS

Cells functioning together as part of an organized tissue are joined through the membrane junctional complexes described under the section entitled "Structure." The junctional complexes were originally thought to be solely for the purpose of adhesion and organization of the independent cellular units, areas containing the hypothetical intercellular cement. The junctional complexes are, instead, important functional areas in a tissue. Sections of the junctional complex have been found to effectively seal off certain areas of membrane and to provide a means for intercellular communication through other areas.

The zona occludens (see Fig. 9.10) provides a strong and effective seal between adjacent cells and between the lumen and the intercellular space. In the intestinal tract this zone effectively seals off the lumen and prevents its contents from mixing with the intercellular fluid.

The desmosome that is separated from the zona occludens by the zona adherens forms another seal. This one, however, provides only localized restriction to diffusion. The cells at this point are not in direct contact although there is the suggestion that fibril bridges may cross the intercellular space. The function of the desmosome appears to be primarily to promote strong adhesion.

The area that permits real communication of cell contents among the cells comprising the epithelial tissues is the gap junction. Molecules at this part of the junctional complex pass from cytoplasm of one cell to that of the next. Each individual cell functions along with all the others as a unit. As described by Palay (1967): "The cells, more or less alike and bound together by the junctional complexes . . . carry out similar functions, each unit repeating what its neighbors do with the monotonous regularity required by the functions of the epithelium as an organ." This means of communicating makes the group of cells a coordinated tissue rather than a collection of isolated and individual units. The permeability of the gap junction channel is regulated by calcium. As intracellular calcium rises above $10^{-7}M$, the channels close. This is thought to provide a mechanism for the regulation of intracellular communication. (See Loewenstein, 1977.) In addition, it provides a means of sealing off healthy cells from damaged ones. In some tissues, notably heart, ion flow through gap junctions provides electrical coupling so that synchronous contraction occurs. The coupling between cells is also metabolic. Small molecules such as vitamins, sugars, amino acids, nucleotides, and other metabolites flow from cell to cell. This is an essential source of nutrients for cells distant from blood vessels. It is interesting to note that gap junctions are not present in rat myometrium during pregnancy but appear immediately prior to delivery (Garfield et al., 1977). Their appearance may lead to the termination of pregnancy.

An interesting observation reported by Loewenstein and Kanno (1967) was that growth-controlling substances appeared to be transmitted through junctions in normal tissues but that no communication was detectable among certain types of cancer cells or between cancer and normal cells. This suggests that communication through junctional complexes has an unusual potential in developmental processes where information concerning a cell community's finite number, shape, and position of cells must be conveyed. The production of defective junctional connections with the consequent noncoupling and uncontrolled growth as a result of a genetic defect continues to be investigated.

SPECIALIZATION AND CONTROL

Function in all cell membranes depends on the structural characteristics that determine the selectivity of the membrane. The passage of materials into and out of the cell is coordinated with the activity of the cell and of the organelles within it. For example, specialized membrane receptors provide the thyroid cell with a special affinity for iodine; liver and fat cells for insulin; ileal cells for the vitamin B_{12}-IF complex. In the lumen of the small intestine the glycocalyx of cell membranes is provided with disaccharidases, dipeptidases, proteases, and a variety of other enzymes synthesized within the cell that are important in the membrane phase of digestion. (See Chapter 6.) In other words, the membrane structure and function depend on the synthetic capacities of the cell, and the synthetic capacities of the cell, in turn, depend on membrane structure and function. Understanding of the interrelated dependence of cellular function and membrane integrity helps to clarify the far-reaching effects of specific nutrients.

Cells that are sensitive to and respond to stimuli evoked by hormones, metallic ions, or other specific molecules must be recognized by the stimulatory agent and then must interact with it to initiate a specific sequence of events. In the case of insulin, the "receptor" is comprised of molecules not only capable of recognizing insulin, but also possessing the ability to convey the existence of the "recognition" to other structures, thereby eliciting a biologically significant event (Cuatrecasas, 1973). Tissues that are responsive to insulin include skeletal and cardiac muscle, fat cells, liver, white blood cells, mammary glands, bone, skin, lens, pituitary, peripheral nerve, and aorta. Red blood cells, gonads, intestinal mucosa, and brain are unresponsive. The membrane-bound receptor responds to insulin exclusively and leads to the specific insulin effect evoked in that cell. The precise effect is suggested to be the result of conformational changes in membrane molecules brought about by the interaction of insulin and receptor. Insulin plays a key role in the integration of cell utilization of nutrients. It promotes anabolic processes and inhibits catabolic ones. It increases the rate of synthesis of glycogen, fatty acids, and proteins and stimulates glycolysis as well. These functions of insulin are mediated, at least in part, by activation of glucose and amino acid transport across the plasma membrane following the binding of insulin to its receptor. The intracellular messengers mediating these changes have not been identified, but they appear *not* to be cAMP. Insulin receptors occupy only about 0.001 percent of the cell surface. For a recent review, see Czech (1977).

Many hormones do appear to utilize cAMP as a second messenger, including calcitonin, chorionic gonadotrophin, corticotropin, epinephrine, follicle-stimulating hormone, glucagon, luteinizing hormone, lipotropin, melanocyte-stimulating hormone, norepinephrine, parathyroid hormone, thyroid-stimulating hormone, and vasopressin. For a review of the biochemical properties of hormone-sensitive adenylate cyclase, see Ross and Gilman (1980).

Evidence presented by Rodbell (1973) suggests that a membrane receptor for glucagon acts through allosteric regulation to produce the glucagon effect. The hormone-receptor interaction is envisioned as triggering one or more allosteric transformations of membrane proteins thereby leading to the activation of adenyl cylcase in the membrane. (See Tepperman, 1973.) According to the concept enunciated by Sutherland and Robison (1966), the hormone, or first messenger, interacts with a membrane receptor to stimulate adenyl cyclase which, in turn, produces an increase (or in some cases a decrease) in cAMP, or second messenger, from the intracellular ATP.

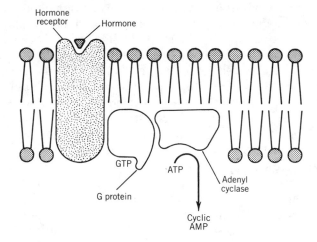

Figure 9.19
Diagram of the relationship of a hormone receptor in the
plasma membrane and its effector enzyme, adenylate
cyclase. (From L. Stryer, *Biochemistry*, 2nd ed, W. H.
Freeman and Co., San Francisco, 1981, p. 844.)

Considerable research effort has been placed on elucidating molecular mechanisms of adenyl cyclase since Sutherland and his colleagues (Sutherland et al.,
1962) uncovered the existence of cAMP in the early 60s. The current model is
shown in Fig. 9.19. When a hormone binds to the receptor, a conformational
change occurs which leads to a change in the G-protein. The G-protein can now
bind GTP and having done so can activate adenyl cyclase. The sequence of events
stops when GTP is hydrolyzed by the protein to which it is attached. Thus, there
is a built-in device for self-regulation. In some cells, adenyl cyclase also depends
on calcium. In this case the calcium-binding protein, calmodulin, is also a part
of the whole complex. In fact, many of the cellular effects of calcium appear to
be exerted through calmodulin-regulated enzymes (Cheung, 1980).

It is the fluid, dynamic, ever-changing membrane that has the capacity to retain
its own integrity, specificity, and unique characteristics that is responsible
not only for the cell it surrounds but also for the widespread effects that radiate
to the total organism. In some cases an obvious relationship exists: a membrane
enzyme such as lactase is defective or missing from the intestinal mucosal cell
membrane; or an unresponsive insulin receptor in the fat cell membrane prevents
glucose entry into the cell. (See Chapter 20.) In other cases the relationship may
be less clear, perhaps merely suspected; in still other instances, not even suspected. According to Christensen (1981), biochemical reactions, when examined
in detail, are usually transport processes. It is obvious that a nutrient or metabolite
cannot influence the course of cell metabolism nor the cell influence the metabolism of the total organism if the gates to the arena are barred.

Summary

The discriminatory role the plasma membrane plays is not only the basis for the very existence of the cell, its uniqueness and individuality, but for whatever specialized capabilities it may possess. The membrane is, of course, a product of the genetic endowment of the cell: its structure depends on molecular syntheses within the cell, its function on the specificity of the carriers it synthesizes. The exquisitely engineered membrane becomes dynamic only by being coordinated with intracellular activity. An adequate supply of nutrients in the environment of the cell insures adequate nutrition only if the molecules presented to the membrane can be selectively transported. The selectivity demands syntheses that fall within the scope and control of nuclear and ribosomal activity and availability of high energy phosphate that the mitochondria have trapped in ATP in the course of intermediary metabolism. The integration of structure and function and of syntheses and degradations in the single-celled independent organism or in a single cell of the liver, intestine, muscle, or gland of a complex mammal are all inextricably linked to the plasma membrane.

chapter 10

the nucleus

The nucleus is the keeper of the keys to the cell's genetic archives. It is within the nucleus that the plans for construction of all of the cell's proteins are filed in the form of deoxyribonucleic acid (DNA), which the nucleus can duplicate for the endowment of daughter cells and for the continuity of the species. It can also transcribe this genetic information into ribonucleic acids (RNA) that, acting as emissaries from the nucleus, appear in the cell matrix and translate the message into cell protein. Since all cellular function depends on enzyme systems, and since enzymes are proteins, it is obvious that the life of the cell and of the species depend on this nuclear capability.

When the nucleus was first observed by early cytologists, the christening was probably easy since it was usually in the central part of the cell, surrounded by the rest of the cellular material. As observations on the cell became more detailed, the early cytologists as well as today's molecular biologists surely agree that the name *nucleus* was prophetic. As we observe it today, the nucleus may not fulfill the original geometric conditions of location; but of far more consequence is the applicability of the name to the central and coordinating role played by the nucleus in the organization, operation, and perpetuation of the cell. The nucleus is, indeed, the central part of the cell and, as such, central to its life. The cell without a nucleus is in even worse straits than the proverbial ship without a rudder. At least the ship can survive, albeit without direction, if the environmental conditions are favorable. The cell without a nucleus, in the most favorable of environments, will slow down and die.

The nucleus of the cell was at first thought to contain all of the DNA which was replicated during cell division, thereby insuring continuation of its kind. It is now apparent that some genetic material resides in the mitochondria as mitochondrial DNA. The significance and function of this DNA which apparently is specific for certain mitochondrial coding will be discussed in Chapter 13. Nuclear DNA however can still be considered the repository for the information required for the preponderance of protein syntheses. It is protein synthesis on which, ultimately, all other cellular reactions depend, since cellular reactions require enzymes, and enzymes are proteins. The coded information in DNA reproduced in the form of RNA for transmission to the cytoplasm is the prerequisite of protein synthesis. The miniaturization of the mechanism is apparent from the calculation that the DNA containing all of the genetic information of mankind would weigh roughly 20 mg (Dobzhansky, 1964).

The replication of DNA and its transcription into RNA require, in addition to specific enzymes, the presence of the nucleotide components of these complex, yet so simple, polymers. The cell can synthesize the fundamental ring structure of the purines and pyrimidines from simple sources of carbon and nitrogen. These are joined with the sugar and phosphate to make the nucleotides of the nucleic acids. It is this stroke of synthetic genius that permitted life to evolve on this planet.

Structure and Composition

The structure of the nucleus refers to what can be seen; the composition to what can be separated out and analyzed. Integration of these procedures at micro- and ultramicro levels has been the means of probing into the nucleus.

The size of the nucleus varies with cell type and function. For example, the nucleus of liver cells constitutes 10 to 18 percent of cell mass, but the nucleus of the sperm cell is almost the entire cell. The nucleus also varies with the stage in the cell's life cycle. Every cell has essentially two periods: *interphase,* the period of nondivision, and *division,* which produces two daughter cells. The cycle is repeated each cell generation, but the length of the cycle varies greatly among cells. Some cells such as the intestinal mucosal cells have a very short life span and others, like the nerve cell, may have a life-span that matches that of the organism. For details of the changes that occur in nuclear structure and composition during division, see DeRobertis and DeRobertis (1980).

Most cells are mononucleate, but there are binucleated cells such as some liver and some cartilage cells, and polynucleated cells such as the osteoclasts. (See Chapter 17.) Certain tissues appear as a large protoplasmic mass called *syncytium* in which cell boundaries are not apparent and the nuclei are extremely abundant; striated muscle is such a tissue. (See Chapter 18.) The location of the nucleus in the geometric center of the cell occurs only in embryonic cells. As differentiation takes place, the nucleus assumes a characteritic position for the type of cell; in gland cells, for example, the nucleus is located in the basal portion of the cell.

The structures visible in the nucleus vary with the type of cell, the preparation of the specimen and the magnification. Generally, in electron micrographs the following are visible: (1) a *nuclear membrane* or *nuclear envelope,* which provides a clear demarcation on both the nuclear and cytoplasmic sides, (2) *nucleoli,* spheroidal bodies that are often quite large, and often multiple, which are regions of condensed chromatin that vary in ribonucleoprotein content and, therefore, in prominence in stained preparations, (3) *chromatin,* which is in the form of filaments distributed throughout the nuclear sap and in clumps near the nuclear envelope in the interphase nucleus. It is composed of deoxyribonucleoprotiens and is the material that forms the chromosomes during division, and (4) *the nuclear sap* or *nuclear matrix,* which fills the space between other nuclear components.

NUCLEAR MEMBRANE OR NUCLEAR ENVELOPE

The nuclear envelope is revealed through electron microscopy as two concentric membranes separated by the perinuclear space. Most descriptions of the membranes have indicated their similarity to other cellular membranes (Franke, 1966). The membranes that make up the nuclear envelope appear to be dynamic structures intimately involved in exchange of information between nucleus and cytoplasm. The arrangement provides continuity of the channel between the two nuclear membranes with those of the endoplasmic reticulum. (See Chapter 11.) In this way, materials in the extracellular environment can enter, pass through the channels of the endoplasmic recitulum, and reach the envelope surrounding the nucleus. It would therefore be possible to obtain entry to the nucleus without passing through the cytoplasmic matrix. It is conceivable that certain materials denied transport through the plasma membrane may reach and be selectively absorbed through the specialized nuclear membrane.

Fusion of the inner and outer membranes of the nuclear envelope occurs at irregular intervals forming *nuclear pores.* The number of pores varies with the species and cell type and may account for 10–30 percent of the envelope. According to Franke and Scheer (1970a; 1970b) a universal structure exists for the pore complex (Fig. 10.1). This pore complex model consists of a ringlike structure, the *annulus,* plus the pore itself around which are spaced eight granules on both the nuclear and cytoplasmic sides. One to three central granules of variable shape and dimensions appear to be in the process of going through the pore, and Franke (1970) has interpreted this to mean that the central granules are ribonucleoprotein particles and, if so, are not structural components of the nuclear pore. Models of the pore complex have also been proposed by Gall (1967) and Vivier (1967) among others. The pore complex appears to restrict free communciation between the nucleus and cytoplasm and Afzelius (1955) suggested that the annulus might function as a diaphragm. The presence of a structural element on the inner surface of the nuclear envelope led Fawcett (1966) to suggest that this was a septum or diaphragm with an easily discernible flange (Fig. 10.2). Such covered pores would not act as fixed canals but, it is presumed, would react to conditions on either side of the membrane and thus be involved in nucleocytoplasmic exchanges. The dense areas of chromatin near the nuclear envelope with distinct interchromatin channels leading to the nuclear pores also suggest an arrangement for exchange between the nucleus and the cytoplasm.

For further details on the nuclear envelope, see Feldherr (1971) and Wischnitzer (1974).

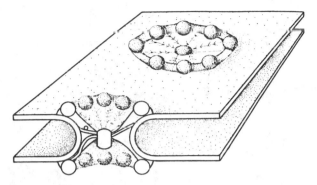

Figure 10.1
Diagrammatic representation of the pore complex. (From
W. W. Franke, *A. Z. Zellforsch.* 105:405, 1970, in C. M.
Feldherr, *Adv. Cell Molec. Biol.* 2:273, 1972.)

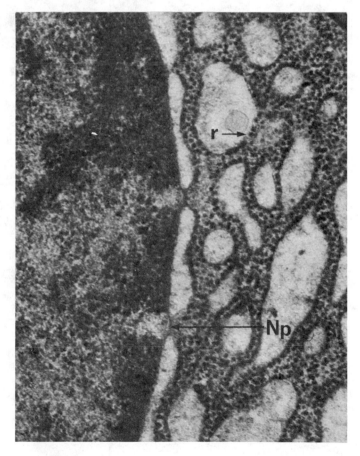

Figure 10.2
Nuclear pores (Np) between nucleus and endoplasmic reticulum
containing ribosomes (r). Pancreatic acinar cell from rat. Magnification 59,000. (Courtesy of Dr. Harald Schraer.)

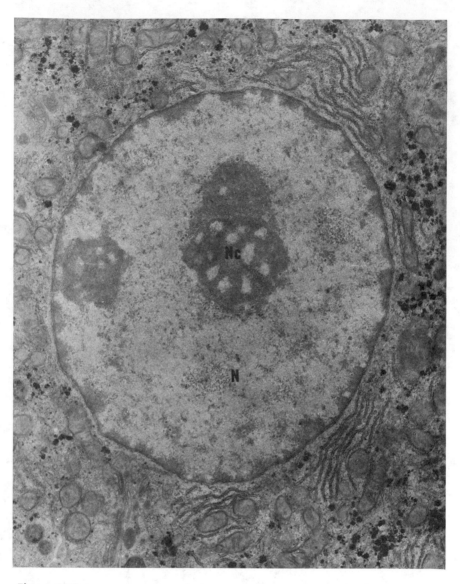

Figure 10.3
Dense area of nucleolus (Nc) within the nucleus (N). Nuclear membrane separates nucleus from cytoplasmic material but no membrane separates nucleolus from the rest of the nucleus. Mouse liver cell. Magnification 11,600. (Courtesy of Dr. Harald Schraer.)

NUCLEOLUS

The nucleolus is readily observable, even by light microscopy, as a dense area within the nucleus. However, there was little information assembled concerning the nucleolus until the 1960s when improved fixation and embedding techniques permitted better preservation of ultrastructure and analysis of nucleolar organization. It was found that the architecture of the nucleolus varied with the physiological state of the cell and with cell type. Detailed observation with the electron microscope revealed that this dense structure has no membrane to separate it from the rest of the nucleus (Fig. 10.3). There is therefore no barrier limiting the interactions between the nucleolus and the other nuclear material.

The nucleolus is not visible during certain stages of cell division but, when division is completed, a new nucleolus is formed at particular locations on the chromosomes. It is conspicuous in highly active cells such as nerve cells and secretory cells and, in some cases, multiple nucleoli are observed. The nucleolus contains fine coiled material in an amorphous background.

Four principal components of the nucleolus have been recognized: (1) a network of closely packed fibrils, (2) granules along and between the strands of the fibrillar network, (3) amorphous matrix material, and (4) nucleolar-associated chromatin surrounding the nucleolus. (See Bernhard and Granboulan, 1968.) It was shown that the nucleolar fibrils and granules contained RNA, and that these RNA fibrils represented the origin of the ribonucleoprotein (RNP) granules, precursors of ribosomal RNA (rRNA). The fibrils also contain DNA.

Although there are many morphological indications that ribonucleoproteins pass into the cytoplasm through the nuclear pores, there is no biochemical evidence to support this concept (Franke, 1974). Nucleolar proteins make up the amorphous matrix within the nucleolus, and studies with ^{3}H-leucine indicate that the synthesis of these proteins takes place in the nucleolus. Their chemical nature, however, has not been clarified. The nucleolar-associated chromatin and the intranucleolar chromatin form a single system, and the indications are that a very large quantity of nucleolar DNA could operate as a template for nucleolar RNA synthesis. All biochemical, genetic, and cytological findings agree that the nucleolar RNA is the precursor of the rRNA; and it is generally believed that the nucleolus is the locus where very active RNA synthesis from a DNA template takes place with the resulting accumulation of ribosomes as a visible electron-dense mass.

CHROMATIN

Chromatin is a complex structure that contains, in addition to DNA, large amounts of histone and nonhistone proteins and small amounts of RNA (Stein et al., 1974). (For a review of the structure of both DNA and histones, see Chapter 2.) When a cell undergoes division the chromatin becomes condensed into chromosomes which are clearly visible in the light microscope. The chromatin fiber is made of repeating units of DNA surrounding a core of histone proteins. The units are

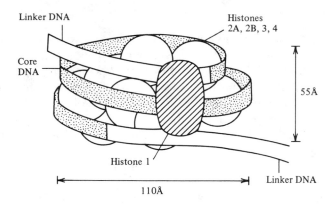

Figure 10.4
Schematic diagram of a nucleosome. The DNA double helix
is wound around an octamer of histones (two molecules each
of 2A, 2B, 3, and 4). Histone 1 binds to the outside of this
core particle and to the linker DNA. (After *DNA Replication*
by A. Kornberg. W. H. Freeman and Co. Copyright © 1980.)

known as nucleosomes and are linked together by a strand of DNA. Two of each
of four kinds of histones comprise the core (McGhee and Felsenfeld, 1980). A
single molecule of a fifth type of histone is thought to bind to the nucleosome so
that the DNA entering and exiting is fixed into position, thus stabilizing the
nucleosome (Thoma et al., 1979) (Fig. 10.4).

The total chromosomal DNA of any cell is its *genome*. Radioautographic studies
with *Drosophila* have shown that the chromosome contains a single molecule of
DNA (Kavenoff et al., 1973). The amount of DNA is constant in all diploid cells
of the individual and for the species since the DNA is related to the number of
chromosome sets in the nucleus. Therefore, determination of the total DNA content
permits calculation of the number of nuclei in a given tissue. (See Chapter 21.)
This calculation does not hold for cells containing two or more nuclei; in most
cases, however, it can be used for the number of cells. The weight of the nucleus
can be calculated from the total weight of the tissue divided by the number of
nuclei. The weight per nucleus varies with cell size and can be used, therefore,
as a means of distinguishing *hypertrophy*, increase in cell size, from *hyperplasia*,
increase in cell number.

The *genes* are functionally defined segments of the DNA molecule that code
for specific polypeptide chains. Most genes contain from 600–1800 nucleotides
that would code for 200–600 amino acids in a polypeptide chain. In a chromosome, the distance between one gene and the next may be very short, perhaps
only a few nucleotides. The evidence is strong that adjacent genes in a chromosome
are related in function; however, they are not necessarily arranged according to
the order in which the respective enzymes participate in a biosynthetic pathway.

NUCLEAR MATRIX

Completely filling the space between the other components of the nucleus is what had been referred to as the nuclear sap or nucleoplasm. These are old terms that appear to have outlived their usefulness. They were a means of acknowledging that the space was occupied by a clear fluid or transparent gel in which the stainable portions of the nucleus were suspended. *Nuclear matrix* is probably a better term to identify this area that is occupied by dispersed chromatin and all the other soluble and insoluble materials essential for the activity of the nucleus. A great deal of activity must go on in this matrix, and it must account for the nuclear constituents revealed in chemical analysis that have not been assigned to known nuclear sites. For example, in addition to the residual protein that appears to be part of the chromosome structure, there are the enzymes that are also nonhistone proteins as well as loosely bound histones and other proteins. A variety of enzymes have, in fact, been identified in the nucleus, and these could be components of the colloid matrix and participate in many of the nuclear synthetic activities. There are DNA polymerases, RNA polymerases, exonucleases, ligases, NAD synthetase, nucleoside triphosphatases, and various other enzymes concerne with purine and nucleoside metabolism as well as with protein metabolism.

In many of the types of nuclei studied, all of the enzymes necessary for glycolysis were present suggesting that the nucleus uses glycolysis as the main source of energy. Two substrate-linked oxidative phosphorylations that provide a source of nuclear ATP were identified, and a great increase in nuclear glycolysis was noted when nuclear activity increased. An unsuspected finding was a complete TCA cycle in calf thymus nuclei. Several enzymes and substrates in the TCA cycle also have been isolated from nuclei of liver, kidney, and brain cells. Further, there is a high concentration of the pyridine nucloetide coenzymes, and the nucleus is the main site of NAD bisynthesis. In thymus nuclei, electrons are transferred from NADH or (NADPH) to flavin coenzymes. These cells appear to contain a complete cytochrome sequence and are also capable of aerobic phosphorylation. Evidence has been obtained as well for the presence of enzymes of the hexose monophosphate shunt. (See Allfrey, 1970; also see Chapters 11 and 13.)

There is some speculation that ATP is transferred into the nucleus from the mitochdonria since mitochdonrial membranes and nuclear membranes have often been observed in very close proximity to each other. However, the ability of the nucleus to synthesize some of its own requirements locally is accepted.

Calcium and magnesium are both present in the nucleus. Calcium is firmly held to the protein, and magnesium appears to be bound to both DNA and a mononucleotide, probably at the phosphate groups. Sodium was thought at one time to be higher in concentration in the nucleus than in the cytoplasm (Naora et al., 1962) and to be actively transported across the nuclear envelope (Goldstein, 1964). However, evidence indicates that sodium concentration is higher in the cytoplasm than in the nucleus (Riemann et al., 1969; Century et al., 1970). It is generally assumed that the sodium in the nucleus enters as part of the active transport of amino acids through the nuclear membrane, a process that also requires ATP. The concentration of potassium also is higher in the nucleus than in the cytoplasm and may be related to a higher concentration of nuclear water (Horowitz and Fenichel, 1970). The high phosphate content of the nucleolus suggests that it may serve as the precursor of the RNA phosphorus (Tandler and Sirlin, 1962).

Function

It is fast becoming axiomatic that the replication of DNA in cell division is the basis for the continuity of the species. On cursory examination, DNA replication does not appear to be of any concern to the nutritionist, although it is, of course, of primary concern to the species. Lederberg (1960) stated in his Nobel lecture, "If species are delimited by their genes, then genes must control the biosynthetic steps which are reflected in nutritional patterns." These nutritional patterns therefore reflect the limitations of the biochemical capability of the cell. In other words, genes dictate which substances the cell can synthesize for itself and which substances it must obtain from its environment as food. For example, all mammals with the exception of the human, monkey, and the guinea pig have the capacity for synthesizing ascorbic acid and therefore do not require a dietary source. The human, monkey, and the guinea pig, in the course of evolutionary development, have lost this capability and, for them, ascorbic acid is an essential nutrient.

Of extraordinary interest is the fundamental similarity in nutrient needs among all living cells, and this similarity far overshadows the differences. But, as for all characteristics and attributes, the differences among species and individuals provide the spice. It was the observation and study of the differences in nutrient needs of strains of red bread mold, *Neurospora,* that opened up the entire field of biochemical genetics. Although nutritionally speaking, there is little difference among molds and mice and men, both scientist and layman, for diverse reasons, can say *vive la difference!*

Biologists have long known that the nucleus contains the chromosomes and that the chromosomes contain the genes. It has also been known that there is a linear splitting of the chromosomes during cell division, providing each daughter cell with identical halves of the chromosome material. These established facts are compatible with more recently accumulated data and accompanying theory.

The ability of the double-stranded DNA polymer to replicate provides the way that the genetic information encoded in the cell is divided and passed on to daughter cells during cell division, thereby providing for continuity of a species. However, this equal division of the parental genetic legacy is negotiable only if the coded message it contains can be transcribed into a form that can be used in protein synthesis. The transcription is carried out in the nucleus through the synthesis of the several forms of RNA: messenger RNA (mRNA), ribosomal RNA (rRNA), and transfer RNA (tRNA). These molecules leave the nucleus for the endoplasmic reticulum where they are finally translated into polypeptide chains. (See Chapter 11.) Fig. 10.5 indicates these fundamental functions of DNA.

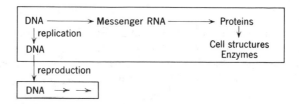

Figure 10.5
Functions of DNA.

REPLICATION

The Watson-Crick model of the double helical structure of DNA provided a neat means of postulating replication since the two strands were complementary; separation of the strands would permit each to attract a complementary strand resulting in two daughter DNA molecules (Fig. 10.6). Each of the new molecules would then contain one of the parental strands. This is referred to as *semiconservative replication,* and was proved to be the means of replication by Meselson and Stahl (1958). One would assume that this was what occurred in mitosis when each of the chromosomes was observed to split longitudinally to form two chromatids, which in turn became the chromosomes in the daughter cells, each identical to the parental chromosomes.

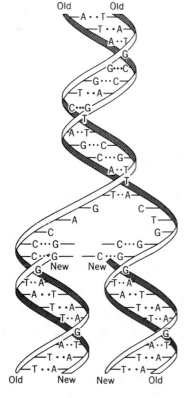

Figure 10.6
The replication of DNA. (From J. D. Watson, *Molecular Biology of the Gene,* 2nd ed., W. A. Benjamin, New York, 1970, p. 267.)

Several problems arise concerning the mechanism of replication. The manner in which the parent strands go through the process of sequential unwinding and rewinding of the helix about each other during replication is still not clear. It has been estimated that the 1,000 μ-long DNA molecule of E. coli has approximately 300,000 twists, and since it replicates in 30 minutes it must participate in an untwisting process that can operate continuously at 10,000 rpm! Evidence to date appears to indicate that the unwinding of the parent strands and the rewinding of the daughter strands occur simultaneously forming a *replication fork* in which all three strands are spinning rapidly along their own axes, the unwinding in front and the rewinding following.

A problem in DNA replication not covered by the Watson-Crick model arose from the fact that DNA polymerase functions in polymerization only in one direction, from the 5' end to the 3' end. When the strands unwind, the 5' end of one is opposite the 3' end of the other, and the question of how both chains could be replicated simultaneously presented a problem. The observation of numbers of DNA fragments in rapidly growing E. coli cells suggested a means of simultaneous replication of the two antiparallel strands (Okazaki et al., 1968). According to this model, one strand of the double helix is synthesized continuously in a 5' to 3' direction, but the other strand is synthesized in short segments that are later linked together. Support for this idea was provided by Sugimoto et al. (1968) who found that fragments accumulated in a mutant E. coli had defective polynucleotide ligase. These findings, along with those of Kornberg (1969), that DNA polymerase binds duplex DNA only at nicks, led to the following model for DNA replication (Fig. 10.7) that involves three enzymes, DNA polymerase, DNA ligase, and a endodeoxyribonuclease, which operate as follows:

1. Replication starts when a nick is made in one strand of the duplex DNA by the action of the endonuclease.
2. DNA polymerase then catalyzes the addition of successive nucleotides to the one strand growing from the 5' to the 3' direction. The other antiparallel strand peels away.
3. After the DNA polymerase has catalyzed the addition of a number of nucleotides to the one chain, it switches, or jumps, to the other strand at the fork where the two strands separate. The enzyme then proceeds to add nucleotides in the 5' to 3' direction down this strand until it is replicated.
4. The endonuclease then nicks the newly formed strand at the fork, and the polymerase proceeds up along the one strand and down the other as before.
5. A ligase joins the newly formed broken fragments on the loose template.
6. The entire process starts again with the endonuclease cleaving at the fork.

In this manner with three enzymes—an endonuclease, a polymerase, and a ligase—the DNA is replicated in successive stages, always in the 5' to 3' direction, first up along one strand and then down the other in repeating cycles.

For discussion of some of the complexities of the multienzyme systems involved in replication, see Schekman et al., (1974).

1. DNA polymerase binds to nick on strand *b*.

5'   Nick in
3'   *b* strand

a *b*

2. Strand *a* is replicated while nicked strand *b* is peeled back.

3'   5'

3. DNA polymerase jumps from strand *a* to strand *b* and replicates the latter in the 5' → 3' direction.

5'
3'

4. The newly formed strand is nicked at the fork by an endonuclease.

5'
5'
3'

5. DNA polymerase now returns and resumes replication of strand *a* at 3' end. At the fork, it jumps to strand *b* and replicates it until earlier fragment is reached.

3'
5' 5'
3'

6. DNA ligase joins the two fragments complementary to strand *b*. Endonuclease nicks new strand at the fork and a new cycle begins. In this fashion both strands are replicated in short lengths, with the polymerase replicating always in the 5' → 3' direction. The new strand which is complementary to strand *b* is formed by joining the fragments through the action of DNA ligase.

3'
5'
5'
3'

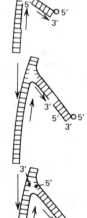

Figure 10.7

Hypothesis of Kornberg for the replication of both strands of antiparallel duplex DNA by DNA polymerase. (From A. L. Lehninger, *Biochemistry*, Worth Publishers, New York, 1970, p. 674.)

Mutations

Any mistake in the sequence of base pairing would be carried to the daughter cells and, if it were not a lethal mistake, would appear in all progeny. This is a mutation. Gene mutations can also occur by substitution of nucleotide pairs, by deletion of one or more units, or by insertion of units (Fig. 10.8). In this way, the so-called inborn errors of metabolism arise and are transmitted.

Since the genetic code is read linearly starting from one end, either deletion or insertion of one or more nucleotides generally leads to completely nonfunctional genes. However, if there is substitution of a single nucleotide in the sequence, the result is referred to as a "leaky gene" in which the resultant mutant protein has partial enzymatic activity. There is no reason to believe that all nucleotide substitutions result in functional changes in the corresponding proteins (Yanofsky, 1967). It is the location of the substitution and consequently of the amino acid in the synthesized polypeptide that determines the effect. If the aberrant amino acid is at a critical point in the molecule, the resulting change in the properties of the polypeptide chain could lead to complete interference with the activity. Such a single nucleotide change resulting in the substitution of valine for glutamic acid in one of the chains of hemoglobin is responsible for sickle cell anemia. In this condition the characteristics of the molecule are so altered that the entire erythrocyte form is changed, and it is much less effective in transporting oxygen. Other changes in polypeptide sequence resulting from substitution of a single nucleotide in the gene coding for hemoglobin chains may or may not give rise to pathological conditions. Over 120 abnormal human hemoglobins have been detected through electrophoretic analysis but many show no deviation from normal functional properties.

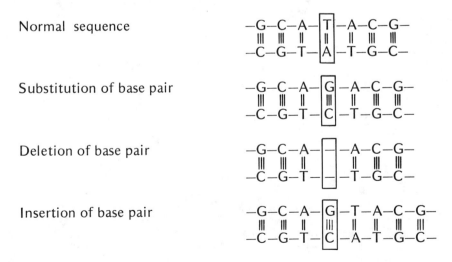

Figure 10.8
Development of mutations due to changes in sequence of base pairing.

All of the so-called inborn errors of metabolism, or genetic disorders, are the result of mutation, a change in the nucleotide sequence that is reflected in a changed polypeptide chain and expressed as a defective or nonfunctional enzyme. It is a change at this level that is responsible for the occurrence of phenylketonuria, hemophilia, albinism, and other known, inherited enzyme defects, as well as other disorders with heritable tendencies such as diabetes, certain cardiovascular disorders, pernicious anemia, hemoglobinopathies, and others. Spontaneous mutations probably take place frequently in all living cells, but only the indifferent or superior ones are likely to be retained. Stable inferior mutations are lost in natural selection, some being lethal mistakes. In addition, mutations may also occur as the result of high energy radiation and a variety of chemical agents that react with DNA (Auerbach, 1967).

Repair Synthesis
The chances that a mutation will occur are not nearly as impressive as the apparent stability of the DNA molecule. However, it is clear that changes in DNA have occurred that, along with natural selection, have led to evolutionary change. Without mutagenesis, evolution could not have occurred, and such a contingency would have eliminated this discussion. Genetic stability, then, is not the result of infallibility but the result of a fallible error-correcting mechanism, one that has permitted some "mistakes" to remain whereas others were corrected.

According to Hanawalt (1972), there are three ways in which an organism can respond to damaged DNA: (1) repair the damage *in situ,* (2) replace the damaged portion, or (3) bypass the damage. A specific type of repair process was discovered by accident following ultraviolet irradiation of bacteria. Ultraviolet light causes thymine dimers to be produced; that is, it causes fusion of two adjoining thymine molecules in the nucleotide chain. The discovery of a bacterial strain that was resistant to ultraviolet irradiation was the first inkling of a molecular mechanism for repair. Setlow and Carrier (1964) found that the resistant strain was able to release the dimers and this led to the repair model suggested by Pettijohn and Hanawalt (1964) called *excision repair* or, more familiarly, *cut and patch.* A model of the postulated steps in excision repair (Fig. 10.9) involves a specific endonuclease, DNA polymerase I, and polynucleotide ligase, functioning as follows:

1. Upon recognition of the damaged DNA strand, a specific endonuclease makes an incision in the parent DNA strand.
2. DNA polymerase I, which possesses a 5' to 3' exonuclease activity, specifically releases the damaged or mismatched sequence from the DNA while concurrently adding nucleotides complementary to the good strand at the initial incision (Kelly et al., 1969).
3. Polynucleotide ligase forms the last 3' to 5' phosphodiester bond. (For discussion of the structure and function of DNA ligase in repair as well as replication, see Lehman, 1974.) Therefore, under the aegis of three enzymes, the damage is located, excised, and repaired. Cleaver (1968) has shown that

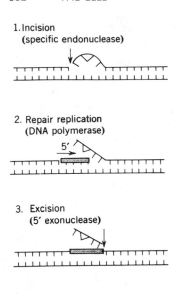

1. Incision
   (specific endonuclease)

2. Repair replication
   (DNA polymerase)

3. Excision
   (5' exonuclease)

4. Rejoining
   (polynucleotide ligase)

Figure 10.9
The postulated steps in excision repair. The repair patch is shown as a heavy line. The vertical arrows indicate the locations of nuclease cuts in the damaged parental strand and the horizontal arrow indicates the direction of repair replication, beginning at a 3'OH end of the parental strand. (From P. C. Hanawalt, *Endeavor* XXXI(113):83, 1972.)

the absence of the normal repair system in skin fibroblasts in man following ultraviolet irradiation is responsible for a type of skin cancer.

Another type of repair system, *genetic recombination,* was proposed by Rupp and Howard-Flanders (1968). This model suggests that gaps are left in daughter strands where dimers occur and replication proceeds again after the interruption. This leads to smaller strands (Fig. 10.10). The gaps are filled subsequently with the correct nucleotides "borrowed" from the other parental strand. These nucleotides join the smaller broken strands (Rupp et al., 1971). The dimer is not removed from the parent strand, and a similar correction is required each time around, but the corrected daughter strand serves each time as the template for replication. Hanawalt (1972) suggests that the same DNA polymerases may be used as in the excision-repair process.

Another type of repair that is rather like a "quality-control" has been postulated by Brutlag and Kornberg (1972). This may have an editing role *in vivo* by correcting base pairing errors produced in the course of normal replication. This repair mechanism has a 3' to 5' exonuclease that removes mismatched nucleotides from the 3' OH end of a growing DNA strand.

TRANSCRIPTION

The genetic information replicated by DNA to insure continuation of the species contains all of the specific information required by the cell for the synthesis of proteins. Since cell activity can function only in the presence and under the

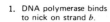

1. DNA polymerase binds to nick on strand *b*.

5'
Nick in
3'
b strand

a ☐ *b*

2. Strand *a* is replicated while nicked strand *b* is peeled back.

3' 5'

3. DNA polymerase jumps from strand *a* to strand *b* and replicates the latter in the 5' → 3' direction.

5'
3'

4. The newly formed strand is nicked at the fork by an endonuclease.

5' 5'
3'

5. DNA polymerase now returns and resumes replication of strand *a* at 3' end. At the fork, it jumps to strand *b* and replicates it until earlier fragment is reached.

3'
5' 5'
3'

6. DNA ligase joins the two fragments complementary to strand *b*. Endonuclease nicks new strand at the fork and a new cycle begins. In this fashion both strands are replicated in short lengths, with the polymerase replicating always in the 5' → 3' direction. The new strand which is complementary to strand *b* is formed by joining the fragments through the action of DNA ligase.

3'
5'
5'
3'

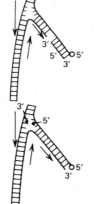

Figure 10.10

A postulated model for postreplication recombinational repair. Normal replication proceeds, but leaves gaps opposite distorted regions of the parental strand. After replication the other parental strand provides the missing nucleotide sequence to fill the gaps. A DNA polymerase fills in gaps remaining opposite undamaged strands of either parental or daughter strands. Some of the double-strand templates for the next round of normal replication contain no damage. The damaged DNA strands are gradually "diluted out," but the damage is never removed from those strands. (From P. C. Hanawalt, *Endeavor* XXXI(113):83, 1972.)

influence of the protein enzymes, the existence of the cell is dependent on the transcription of the genetic code to a form that can direct protein synthesis. The formation of RNA fulfills this second fundamental function of the nucleus. The discharge of this function is dependent on the translation of the four-letter code of polynucleotides into the 20-odd unit language of proteins. In this way RNA provides the link between the information coded in the DNA in the nucleus and the protein synthesis that takes place in the cytoplasm. The regulation and separation of the two kinds of DNA template activity is undoubtedly under the control of specific mechanisms, since they must and do occur at different times and therefore, one would guess, under different auspices. Only precise control, suavely administered, could prevent schizophrenic DNA.

The chemical similarity of RNA to DNA has been discussed in Chapter 2. Despite the differences that do exist, RNA molecules are also capable of forming complementary helical structures similar to those formed by DNA; however, most RNA exists as single polyribonucleotide strands. In mammalian cells about 10 percent of the cellular RNA is in the nucleus. Of this, about 20 percent is present in the dense nucleolar material and the remainder in the nucleoplasm or matrix. However, the quantity in a cell varies markedly with the condition of the cell and its nutritional state. For example, during starvation, when catabolic processes take precedence and protein synthesis is limited, nuclear RNA may be drastically reduced. Apparently this is a result of the depressed activity of RNA polymerase observed in starvation (Onishi, 1970). It is generally found that cells active in protein synthesis have RNA-rich nuclei and those performing little synthetic activity have RNA-poor nuclei. Nuclear RNA has a high turnover rate and except for what is needed for the synthesis of nuclear protein, all the RNA molecules synthesized in the nucleus migrate to the cytoplasmic matrix.

Regulation of Gene Action
Since the DNA of each cell in a multicellular organism appears to be the same, this means that various cell types use the information contained in this DNA differently. In fact, most of the DNA in the nucleus does not function in transcription, and much of the cell RNA is coded by less than 1 percent of the genome or chromosomal DNA. This includes both the rRNA and tRNA. The amount of DNA that codes for mRNA and for other types of nuclear and cytoplasmic RNAs amounts to less than 5 percent of the cellular DNA. Therefore, most of the DNA of the genome is nonfunctional at a given time. Specific regulatory mechanisms must, therefore, be available for activating and inactivating particular regions of the genome for RNA synthesis depending on the requirements of the cell.

A model to explain the mechanism that promotes DNA transcription to a specific mRNA for subsequent protein synthesis was proposed by Jacob and Monod (1961) and earned its orginators a Nobel Prize in 1965. It is based on the concept of the *operon* that, together with a *regulatory gene,* an *operator,* a *promoter,* and a *repressor protein,* can explain both induction and repression of mRNA synthesis (Fig. 10.11). The operon according to this model is a section of DNA consisting of adjacent and related genes that function together. These structural genes are

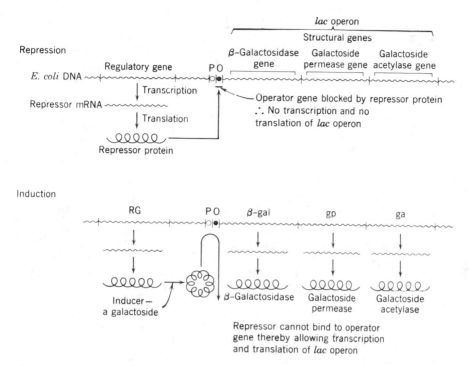

Figure 10.11

Regulation of gene action as postulated by Jacob and Monod, illustrating repression and induction of enzyme synthesis by the lactose operon in *E. coli*. (From E. E. Conn and P. K. Stumpf, *Outlines of Biochemistry*, 3rd ed., John Wiley, New York, 1972, p. 481.)

responsible for transcription to mRNA and are under joint control of the operator and a regulatory gene. The promoter, which is next to the operator, is the attachment site for the RNA polymerase. Transcription of the structural genes is initiated here. According to this model, the regulatory gene codes for the mRNA which is the template for the repressor protein. The repressor protein binds to the operator and blocks the attachment of RNA polymerase to the promoter so that transcription of the structural genes is prevented. For induction of mRNA synthesis by the structural genes (leading, in turn, to induction of enzyme synthesis) the repressor must be blocked. This occurs if an inducer is present that combines with the repressor at a specific binding site to form a *repressor-inducer complex*. This complex is unable to bind to the operator and, therefore, transcription of the structural genes takes place and is normally followed by their migration to the endoplasmic reticulum for translation to specific polypeptides. (See Chapter 11.) The repressor molecule is envisioned as one with two binding sites, one for the inducer and one for the operator. When one site is filled, the other becomes inoperable.

The operon-regulator gene hypothesis of Jacob and Monod has been extended also to explain some aspects of differentiation during development. All cells of higher organisms are believed to contain the entire genome for that organism; that is, each cell contains the full book of genes, but much of the genome in any one cell is repressed. Differentiation is thought to take place by what is termed *programmed derepression* of different operons. This area of study has been named *epigenetics*. An example of programmed derepression is the rapid rise in lactase activity in the intestinal mucosa just prior to birth. Its fall in postweaning years is coupled with the rise in maltase and sucrase. (See Chapter 6.) The shift from the prenatal hemoglobin, Hb-F, to the adult form, Hb-A, is another example of programmed derepression. Each of the hemoglobin chains is under separate genetic control. During recovery from some types of anemia, there is temporary induction of Hb-F synthesis followed by its repression and the induction of Hb-A. (See Chapter 16.)

The mechanism for control in the regulation of transcription in the Jacob and Monod model is still largely conjectural. Histones have been reported to inhibit the ability of DNA to serve as a template for RNA synthesis (Huang and Bonner, 1962; Allfrey et al., 1963). The histones in the cell nucleus, present in the form of deoxyribonucleohistone complexes, have been implicated in the more permanent type of repressor in the nucleus that undergoes derepression primarily during differentiation. The fact that histones are not present in cells that do not differentiate and are conspicuous in cells that do, has suggested their implication in this process. When the histones are removed from metaphase chromosomes, a scaffold of nonhistone protein remains with a shape similar to the intact chromosome. The histone-free DNA appears to be attached to this protein (Fig. 10.12).

There is also provocative evidence suggesting the intervention of nonhistone chromosomal proteins in the regulation of specific gene transcription. These proteins are made in the cytoplasm (Stein and Baserga, 1971) and are more actively synthesized and turned over than histones (Hancock, 1969; Holoubek and Crocker, 1969). Synthesis of specific classes of these nonhistone proteins is associated with the induction of gene activity (Teng and Hamilton, 1969). It has been established also that nonhistone chromosomal proteins interact with DNA and modify transcription in a way that is characteristic of the tissue from which they have been derived (Stein et al., 1974). They are highly heterogeneous and possess both tissue and species specificity. It was speculated originally that nonhistone chromosomal proteins displaced the inhibitory histones from the DNA-histone complex thereby permitting the DNA to become active as a template for RNA synthesis. Histones have been shown to stimulate the phosphorylation of the nonhistone chromosomal proteins (Kaplowitz et al., 1971). Stein et al. (1974) suggest that this could release histone from the DNA double helix thereby allowing gene transcription to take place.

One important unresolved question is how specific genes are recognized. A suggested possibility is that phosphorylation may be involved in the recognition of the promoter site for transcription, a function performed by the sigma factor

Figure 10.12
Electron micrograph showing histone-depleted DNA attached to a central protein scaffold. Histones were removed from metaphase chromosomes of HeLa cells by treating them with polyanions. (Courtesy of Dr. Ulrich Laemmli.)

associated with RNA polymerase. (See following section on RNA synthesis.) The sigma factor can be phosphorylated (Stein et al., 1974), but whether this is related to or dependent on the phosphorylation of either histones or nonhistone chromosomal proteins, or both, is entirely speculative. Nevertheless, it appears that the nonhistone chromosomal proteins play a role in the regulation of gene activation and that phosphorylation is somehow involved. What the specific mechanism is that initiates, modifies, or augments the transcription of specific mRNA molecues encoded in the cell's DNA is still far from clear. If phosphorylation does regulate transcription, then a major question is, "What regulates the phosphorylation?"

Mechanisms involving induction of enzyme systems at the level of mRNA translation into protein are discussed in Chapter 11.

RNA Synthesis

Synthesis of RNA is fundamentally very similar to the synthesis of DNA. Nucleotide triphosphates are the precursors, and the synthetic reaction is catalyzed by a single enzyme, RNA polymerase in the presence of Mg^{++}, for all four possible nucleotides. Although only one of the two DNA strands is transcribed, double-stranded DNA is required as the template, and the synthesis of many RNA chains takes place simultaneously from a single gene. The base composition of the RNA is complementary to the DNA template with uracil as the complement to adenine instead of thymine as in DNA. RNA transcription is probably as accurate as DNA replication. However, if errors occur there is no need for correction since the mistake dies with the molecule; RNA is not self-replicating. (See below for exception.)

RNA polymerase, responsible for the synthesis of RNA from the DNA template, is a much more complicated enzyme than is DNA polymerase, which is a single polypeptide chain. RNA polymerase contains five different polypeptide chains with a molecular weight of over 500,000. For RNA polymerase to function properly it must have associated with it the sigma (σ) factor. This factor is one of the polypeptide chains that readily dissociates from the rest of the enzyme after it has recognized the specific nucleotide sequence for starting an RNA chain. Speculation of how this recognition takes place was discussed in the preceding section. The released σ repeats its function with another core RNA polymerase. Synthesis of all chains starts with either adenine or guanine, depending on the start signal in the DNA template. As in replication, transcription proceeds in the 5' to 3' direction. A stop signal at a specific nucleotide sequence identifies the conclusion of the chain that always ends with a triphosphate group. The stop signal is not part of RNA polymerase but is a separate factor called the rho (ρ) factor. How this factor operates also is not at all clear. A summary of RNA transcription is illustrated in Fig. 10.13.

It appears that there is but a single DNA-directed RNA polymerase for the synthesis of mRNA, rRNA, and tRNA. These three RNAs are in reality three different classes of RNA since there are three types of rRNA, about 60 tRNAs, and an extremely large number of mRNAs in every cell. Ribosomal RNAs, composed of a large and a small RNA molecule associated in the ribosomes with protein chains, contain approximately 6,000 nucleotides compared with the tRNAs,

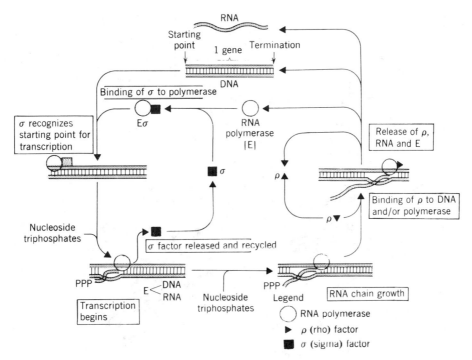

Figure 10.13
RNA synthesis-outline diagram. (From J. D. Watson, *Molecular Biology of the Gene,* 3rd ed., W. A. Benjamin, New York, 1973, p. 299.)

which are the smallest of the natural nucleic acid molecules and contain some 80 nucleotides. Each of the tRNAs has a specificity for a given amino acid, and there is a similarity of structure and dimensions, the advantage of which becomes readily apparent as these molecules participate in protein synthesis. Messenger RNA, which carries the information from nuclear DNA to the protein-synthesizing ribosomes, is extremely variable in length since it takes three nucleotides for each of the amino acids in the chain to be synthesized. Rarely do polypeptide chains contain fewer than 100 amino acids, which means that mRNA molecules must contain at least 300 nucleotides and may contain far more. In addition, 1 mRNA frequently codes for the synthesis of several different polypeptide chains with related functions, and the nucleotide count may go beyond 10,000. The structural characteristics of each of the classes of RNA will be discussed in relationship to their function in Chapter 11.

Visualization of the process of RNA formation is possible in the giant chromosomes located in the giant cells of the salivary glands of the fruit fly *Drosophila.* These chromosomes are almost 100 times thicker and 10 times longer than chromosomes of typical cells. Beermann and Clever (1964) found puffs scattered along these chromosomes and found that puffing was associated with RNA production (Fig. 10.14). Edstrom and Beermann (1962) demonstrated that different puffs

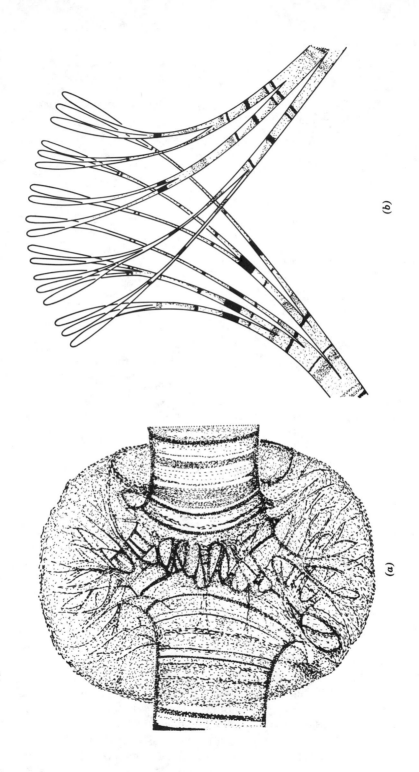

(b)

(a)

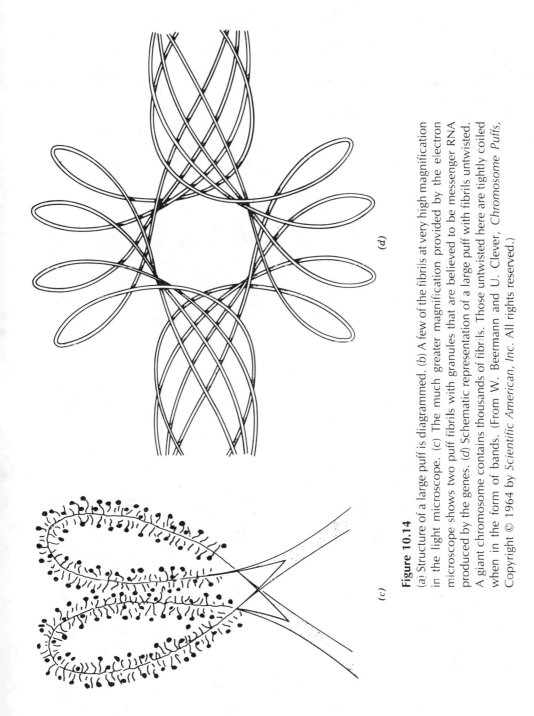

(c)

(d)

Figure 10.14

(a) Structure of a large puff is diagrammed. (b) A few of the fibrils at very high magnification in the light microscope. (c) The much greater magnification provided by the electron microscope shows two puff fibrils with granules that are believed to be messenger RNA produced by the genes. (d) Schematic representation of a large puff with fibrils untwisted. A giant chromosome contains thousands of fibrils. Those untwisted here are tightly coiled when in the form of bands. (From W. Beermann and U. Clever, *Chromosome Puffs*, Copyright © 1964 by *Scientific American, Inc.* All rights reserved.)

produced different kinds of RNA and that the RNA produced represented the activity of only one of the DNA strands. The biochemical activities associated with puff formation were studied through cytochemical and autoradiographic techniques. A clear association was established between a puff and a specific cellular product thus demonstrating that a definite relation exists between certain puffed genes and certain cell functions. Swelling or looping out of the puff appeared before RNA synthesis (Berendes, 1968) and was associated with the accumulation of acid proteins that were not synthesized in the puff. Later Stein and Baserga (1971) showed that synthesis of these proteins occurred in the cytoplasm. With the increase in acidic protein there was a relative fall in the basic histone although the ratio of histone to DNA remained constant. When RNA synthesis started, the puff attained maximum size. In some instances, the puff size was related to the amount of RNA that was synthesized.

The puffing of one strand of the DNA is interpreted as reasonable and visible evidence of mRNA synthesis (Beermann and Clever, 1964) since only one of the two possible RNA copies of the double-stranded DNA serves as a template. Movement of particles in the nuclear matrix has been observed. It is presumed that the particles carrying mRNA pass through the nuclear pores and, in association with the ribosomes that also are synthesized in the nucleus, participate in protein synthesis.

REVERSE TRANSCRIPTION

The *central dogma* of molecular biology first formulated by Crick (1970) states that once information has passed into protein it cannot get out again; that is, genetic information can be transferred from DNA to DNA or from DNA to RNA to protein, but the reverse cannot take place. Work reported by Temin (1972) indicates that what had been referred to as *reverse transcription* can take place. Information can be transcribed from RNA into DNA. This occurs under the influence of *RNA-directed DNA polymerase*. The suggestion is that all DNA polymerases are capable, under appropriate conditions, of transcribing information from RNA into DNA. Temin (1972) suggests that this may occur in normal cellular processes such as those involved in embryonic differentiation of cells. He calls this the *protovirus hypothesis,* which states that there are regions of DNA in normal cells that serve as templates of RNA and that this RNA, in turn, serves as a template for the synthesis of DNA, which then becomes integrated with the cellular DNA. By this process certain portions of DNA become amplified and changes introduced into the DNA of some cells can be different from the DNA of other cells. This has been shown to occur in tumor-causing viruses but may have far greater implications.

NUCLEAR PROTEIN SYNTHESIS

In addition to the synthesis of DNA and the RNAs, the nucleus also synthesizes ATP and other nucleotide triphosphates, ribonucleoprotein, and various other proteins and enzymes. The histones, for example, which represent up to 32 percent of the nucleolar proteins, are reported to be synthesized in the nucleolus (Flamm and Birnstiel, 1964). In the sperm cell protamines are substituted for histones and these, too, may be synthesized in the nucleus. The details of protein synthesis will be discussed in Chapter 11 since the major portion of cellular protein synthesis occurs in the endoplasmic reticulum and the mechanisms in the nucleus are believed to be comparable.

Conclusion

The nucleus, separated from the cytoplasm of the cell by a double membrane, is the repository of the cell's genetic information, DNA. Replication of DNA is a prerequisite to cell division for it is only in this way that the encoded information which determines all the nuclear and cytoplasmic characteristics of the cell is made available to daughter cells for continuity of the cell species. Transcription of DNA to RNA translates the code to forms usable for protein synthesis in the cytoplasmic portion of the cell. The control over what the cell can synthesize determines what nutrients must be acquired from the environment.

The activities of the nucleus are continually dependent on and responsive to the activities of the other organelles in the cell and on the demands of the total organism and its environment. Allfrey (1970) points out that the scope of nuclear involvement and responsibility is slighted when it is simplistically stated that the nucleus is responsible for the DNA that makes RNA that makes protein.

chapter 11

the cytoplasmic matrix and endoplasmic reticulum

The cytoplasmic matrix is that part of the cell that holds within it or surrounds all the membrane-enclosed bodies in the cytoplasm including the endoplasmic reticulum, the mitochondria, lysosomes, and nucleus. In addition, there are lipid droplets, vacuoles, filaments, microtubules, and the many dense particles rich in RNA, the ribosomes, which are closely associated with the continuous membranes of the endoplasmic reticulum. The endoplasmic reticulum is the complicated and organized system of membranes within the cytoplasmic area of the cell. The endoplasmic reticulum and the surrounding matrix are not only areas for specific metabolic activities, but they also provide the means of communication among the external, nuclear, and organelle environments.

Light microscopy could give only the barest hints of the organization that was present in the cytoplasmic area of the cell. Although some structures had been identified, such as the Golgi apparatus and the mitochondria, the revelation of the complex organization of the cytoplasmic components of the cell awaited the development of the electron microscope. The reticular character of the endoplasmic portion of the cell was first noted by Porter et al. (1945) and they proposed that it be called the *endoplasmic reticulum*. Palade defined the endoplasmic reticulum and discovered the ribosome, the particle associated with it. For this work and his identification of the ribosome with protein synthesis, he was a Nobel prize recipient in 1974. This ramification of channels constituting the endoplasmic reticulum extends through the cell and is separated by the channel membrane from the *cytoplasmic matrix* or cytosol. The cytoplasmic matrix surrounds all of the organelles within the cell; it is the colloidal sea that supports them.

The Cytoplasmic Matrix or Cytosol and the Cytoskeleton

The cytoplasmic matrix, the continuous phase of the cytoplasm, is the true internal environment of the cell. Under the light microscope it appears homogeneous or finely granular, but the apparent lack of fine structure may be due only to the limitation of instruments and techniques. The cytosol contains the soluble proteins and other substances, including the subunits of structural materials for the cytoskeleton and the small molecules and ions which are important in maintaining appropriate intra- and extracellular environments. The cytoplasmic matrix contains a meshwork of microtubules and a variety of microfilaments collectively termed the *cytoskeleton*. The different components of the cytoskeleton are now under intense investigation which has resulted in a much clearer understanding of how the shape and movement of cells are related to structures in the cytoplasm and of how organelles and other cell components may be translocated.

MICROTUBULES

Microtubules were observed as filamentous structures with the light microscope especially when they were organized to form the mitotic apparatus in dividing cells. With the advent of the electron microscope and improved methods of tissue preservation and preparation (Sabatini et al., 1963) they have been observed routinely. Microtubules are distributed in the cytoplasm of all kinds of cells except bacteria and some algae. They are about 24 nm in diameter and vary in length. A microtubule consists of 13 protein subunits visible in cross section. The protein, tubulin, is in the form of dimers. Brain tissue is most commonly used as a source of tubulin. When tubulin is extracted from brain small amounts of other proteins are associated with it and are known as microtubule-associated proteins (MAPS). The MAPS may be involved in the assembly of microtubules (Murphy and Borisy,

1975). The sites of microtubule initiation in cells are thought to be the centrioles, basal bodies, and centromeres. Certain organelles such as cilia, flagella, and basal bodies have special arrangements of microtubules as a major feature of their structure.

Microtubules maintain the characteristic shape of a cell, have a role in cell motility, and appear to facilitate the transport of particles within the cell. For example, microtubules in the axons of nerve cells provide support and may also direct the flow of material synthesized near the nucleus toward the extremity of the axon. A very readable account of the history and biology of microtubules was written by Dustin (1978).

MICROFILAMENTS

To paraphrase Brinkley (1982) ". . . the recognition of major musclelike proteins in the cytoplasm of nonmuscle cells is one of the most significant episodes in modern cell biology." These contractile proteins are in the form of threadlike structures in the cytoplasmic matrix and are known as microfilaments. They are found in a wide variety of cells. The protein is called actin which is very similar to the actin found in muscle. (See Chapter 18.) Actin microfilaments are from 4–6 nm in diameter and are present mainly in the cytoplasmic zone adjacent to the cell membrane. Myosin is another contractile protein which is found in muscle and nonmuscle cells. Myosin filaments vary in width and, with actin, are involved in changes of shape and in contractile movements of cells.

Although they can be observed with the electron microscope, microfilaments also are readily seen by fluorescent immunochemical localization in the light microscope (Fig. 11.1). An interesting example of microfilament architecture and function is the brush border of the intestinal epithelium (Fig. 11.2). The cores of the microvilli contain actin filaments which seem to be attached to a dense material at the apical end, and to the lateral membranes by protein bridges. The microfilaments extend into the terminal web region which contains actin and myosin filaments. Interaction of the actin and myosin filaments with filaments emanating from the zonula adherens of the junctional complex (Hull and Staehelin, 1979) may be the basis of the motile action of the brush border (Burgess and Prum, 1982).

INTERMEDIATE FILAMENTS

Another group of filaments, the intermediate filaments, are included in the cytoskeleton. They are about 10 nm in diameter and may be divided into five subclasses based on biochemical and immunological criteria. Keratin filaments are found in epithelial cells; desmin is found mainly in muscle cells; vimentin filaments are found in most differentiating cells and cells grown in tissue culture; glial filaments have been detected only in glial cells; and neurofilaments have been detected in neurons (Lazarides, 1982). The function of the intermediate filaments appears to be mechanical integration of cellular space.

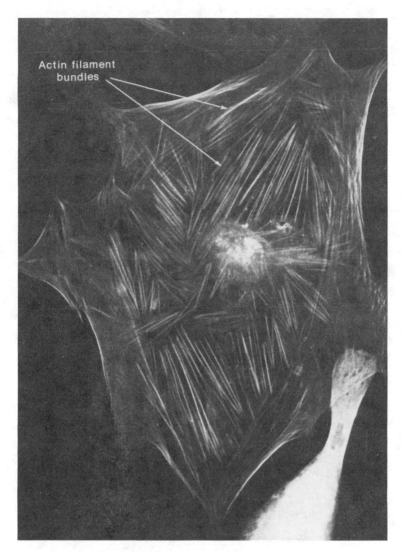

Figure 11.1
Indirect immunofluorescence with actin and tropomyosin antibodies. The photograph shows immunofluorescent staining of human skin fibroblasts with these antibodies. (From E. Lazarides, *J. Cell Biol.* 65:549, 1975.)

Endoplasmic Reticulum

The channels comprising the endoplasmic reticulum (Fig. 11.3) are, in reality, part of the larger cytoplasmic vacuolar system that includes the nuclear envelope (Chapter 10 and below) and the Golgi complex (Chapter 12). This system, divided

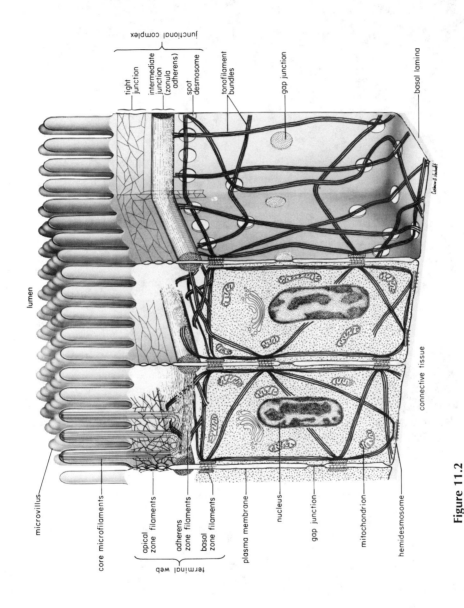

Figure 11.2

Organization of the cytoplasmic filaments in columnar epithelial cells of the intestine. This diagram illustrates the association of the filaments with tight junctions, intermediate junctions (zonulae adherentes), spot desmosomes, and hemidesmosomes. (From B. E. Hull and L. A. Staehlin, *J. Cell Biol.* 81:80, 1979.)

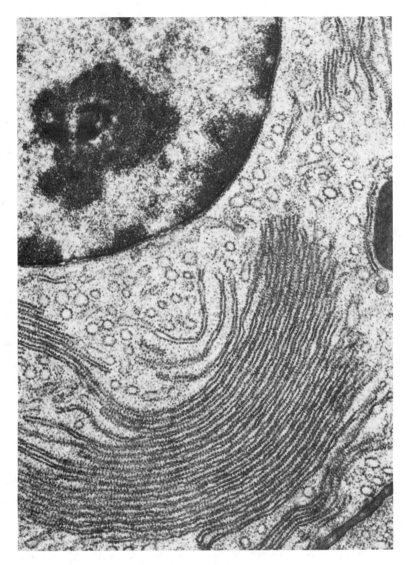

Figure 11.3
Electron micrograph of acinar cell from the pancreas of the bat, *Myotis lucifugus*. The membranes of the endoplasmic reticulum are studded with ribosomes and the area is designated as the rough endoplasmic reticulum. (From D. W. Fawcett, *The Cell*, W. B. Saunders Co., Philadelphia, 1981.)

into compartments that can function independently, is a continuous system that synthesizes, circulates, and packages materials absorbed by the cell or synthesized within it.

The membranous channels constituting the endoplasmic reticulum occur in all cells of higher plants and animals with the exception of the mature erythrocyte, which in mammals has neither a nucleus nor endoplasmic reticulum. The complexity of the reticulum appears to vary directly with the degree of protein synthesis that takes place within the cells, being well developed, therefore, in secretory cells particularly in those secreting a protein-rich product. The absence of both the nucleus and endoplasmic reticulum in the erythrocytes readily explains the inability of these cells to synthesize enzymes since, with the lack of nuclear RNA and of the endoplasmic reticulum, both management and assembly line for protein synthesis are missing. (See Chapter 16.) The liver cell, in contrast, has a well-developed endoplasmic reticulum. The total surface of the endoplasmic reticulum contained in 1 ml of liver tissue has been calculated by Weibel et al. (1969) to be approximately 11 m², two-thirds of which is granular and one-third smooth. (See Chapter 15.)

Granular or *rough endoplasmic reticulum,* abundant in growing cells and in others engaged in protein synthesis, is easily recognized. Along the outer surfaces of the membranous channels facing the cytoplasmic matrix are dense particles of uniform size, the *ribosomes.* These may be arranged in close proximity to each other or may be spread out along the surface. The greater the protein synthetic activity, the denser the ribosomal population. It is this type of reticulum that forms the outer membrane of the nuclear envelope.

Agranular or *smooth endoplasmic reticulum,* as the name implies, does not have the ribosomal studding along the outer membrane and therefore gives a smooth appearance. In other respects it appears similar to the granular form and is continuous with it and with the Golgi complex. It is found (1) in cells that synthesize steroids, (2) in liver cells where it is associated with detoxification functions and with lipid and cholesterol metabolism, (3) in the small intestine where it is associated with lipid absorption and transport, and (4) in skeletal muscle where it participates in excitation-contraction coupling. The specialized endoplasmic reticulum in skeletal muscle is called sarcoplasmic reticulum and will be discussed in Chapter 18.

STRUCTURE

The endoplasmic reticulum is a membranous system of channels that leads from the plasma membrane to the nuclear membrane (Fig. 11.3). In a sense, it provides an extracellular environment deep within the structure of the cell and surrounding the nucleus, thereby providing a means of communication between the extracellular and intranuclear environments.

A three-dimensional view of the continuously folded membranous channels shows cavities of varying sizes and shapes appearing as vesicles and tubules and flattened sacs (Fig. 11.4). The variety in the shape and size of the areas enclosed by the membrane is due both to the folding and to the plane of the sectioning. A three-dimensional reconstruction of serial sections reveals the interconnections and tortuous winding of the channels. This should be easy to reconstruct mentally if one imagines a long piece of rubber tubing folded back and forth and placed in a box which is then cut through the middle. The cut tubing would appear as circles, ellipses, and long tubules, depending on the angle of the cutting edge. The picture can be further complicated by enclosing several lengths of tubing,

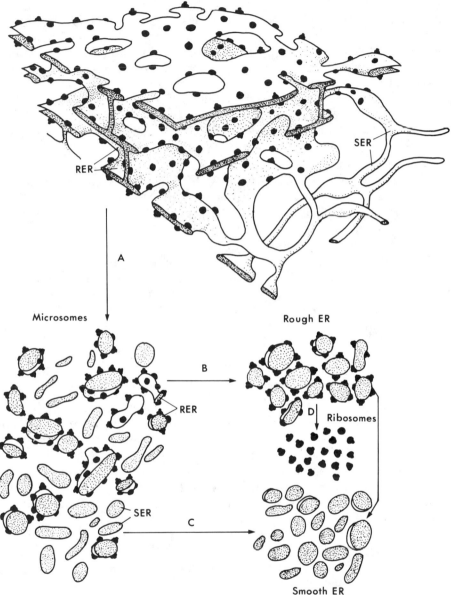

Endomembrane System

RER

SER

A

Microsomes

Rough ER

B

RER

D

Ribosomes

SER

C

Smooth ER

Figure 11.4
Three-dimensional diagram of the endomembrane system. A, isolation of microsomes by homogenization and differential centrifugation; B and C, separation of rough and smooth vesicles of the endoplasmic reticulum; D, separation of ribosomes from the RER. RER, rough endoplasmic reticulum; SER, smooth endoplasmic reticulum. (From E. D. P. DeRobertis and E. M. F. DeRobertis, *Cell and Molecular Biology*, 7th ed., W. B. Saunders Co., Philadelphia, 1980.)

all folded but all with one end at the edge of the box and the other in the center. This latter picture would probably be a closer representation of the channels in the cell and a better explanation for the appearance of tissue sections.

The structure of the endoplasmic reticulum can only be studied by electron microscopy of the intact cell. It cannot be separated out by centrifugation and subsequently studied as can certain of the other organelles because centrifugation breaks up the membranes and they appear as fragments. This fraction referred to as the microsomal layer is an artefact of homogenization and includes fragments of the endoplasmic reticulum, Golgi complex, and of the plasma membrane. In some cases the ribosomes are also part of the fraction although they can be separated out. Such preparations have been used extensively for biochemical studies of both composition and function.

The membrane of the endoplasmic reticulum, like the plasma membrane and all other membranes of the cell, was first described in terms of the unit membrane theory of Robertson (1959). Sjöstrand (1964) suggested that functional advantages would accrue if there was discontinuity in the lipid layer and in the arrangement of the protein to form septa connecting the two surface layers. Despite the teleological overtones, the discussion of membrane structure in Chapter 9 indicates that current models of membranes suggest such arrangements of the protein and lipid constituents. In the chapter on the Golgi complex, the membraneous system within the cell will be presented as a product of its own synthesis. It is subjected to modifications in composition and structure during the process of membrane flow. (See Chapter 12.)

In tissue sections, the *nuclear envelope* appears as a large cisternal unit of the granular endoplasmic reticulum that surrounds the nucleus and is separated from the nuclear membrane by a space that, according to Porter (1961b), resembles a moat. At intervals, the inner and outer membranes are joined, forming pores (see Chapter 10) that are continuous with the cytoplasmic phase of the endoplasmic reticulum (Fig. 11.5). Some investigators suggest that the pore is an open structure permitting passage of molecules from the nuclear contents to the cytoplasmic matrix (Moses, 1964); and others, that it is plugged or covered (Merriam et al., 1961), but, one would presume, opened when traffic warranted. In the discussion on protein synthesis that follows, it is evident that mRNA, tRNA, and ribosomes must pass from within the nucleus to the cytoplasmic matrix. In the case of these and other macromolecules, the pores in the nucleus are likely to be the only pathway to the cytoplasm. Feldherr (1972) suggests that the annular material of the pore complex is able to limit the size of the particles that can penetrate and can also select and concentrate substances for passage. There is the possibility that this may be an energy-requiring process since Klein and Afzelius (1966) found that the pore complex material contained ATPase activity.

In addition to the emigration of molecules from the nucleus to the cytoplasmic phase of the cell, there would have to be passage of all of the nutrients required to support the major biosynthetic activities that occur in the nucleus from both the extra- and intracellular environments. (See Chapter 10.)

The channels of the endoplasmic reticulum, from the plasma membrane to the nuclear envelope, provide contact with the extracellular environment; the nuclear

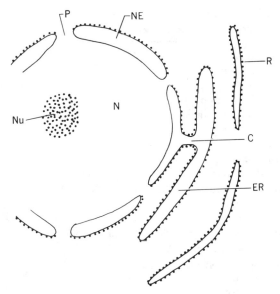

Figure 11.5
Nuclear envelope (NE) showing nucleolus (Nu), pores
(P), granular endoplasmic reticulum (FR) with ribosomes (R) attached, and channel (C) from nucleus (N)
to ER. (From G. H. Haggis et al., *Introduction to
Molecular Biology*, John Wiley, New York, 1964, p.
145.)

pores provide continuity with the cytoplasmic matrix. One must assume that two-
way traffic prevails on both routes.

The suggestion has been offered that the endoplasmic reticulum may develop
by evagination from the nuclear envelop (Porter, 1961), however, there is evidence that the converse actually occurs: the nuclear envelope is reformed after
cell division by the vesicles of the endoplasmic reticulum (Barer et al., 1959).
Cytochemical study suggested the identical composition of these two membranes
(Essner and Novikoff, 1962) but biochemical analyses indicate that, despite general similarity, specific differences are apparent in lipid content (Kleinig, 1970),
protein content (Franke et al., 1970), and enzymatic activity (Kasper, 1971).
Kasper (ibid) suggests that the outer leaflet of the nuclear envelope may represent
an undifferentiated segment of the endoplasmic reticulum. This is consonant with
the findings of Morré and his group (see Chapter 12) who showed the direction
of development to be from the nuclear membrane to the plasma membrane.

COMPOSITION

In the fractionation of cell homogenates, the microsomal fraction usually constitutes
about 15–20 percent of the cell. The protein component of the fraction is 40–60
percent, the lipid from 30–50 percent, and there is some RNA even after the
ribosomal portion is removed. Siekevitz (1963) found that the RNA content after

TABLE 11.1
Some Microsomal Enzyme Activities

Synthesis of glycerides
    Triacylglycerols
    Phosphatides
    Glycolipids and plasmalogens
Metabolism of plasmalogens
Fatty acid synthesis
Steroid biosynthesis
    Cholesterol biosynthesis
    Steroid hydrogenation of unsaturated bonds
$NADPH_2 + O_2$-requiring steroid transformations
    Aromatization
    Hydroxylation
$NADPH_2 + O_2$-requiring drug detoxification
    Aromatic hydroxylations
    Side-chain oxidation
    Deamination
    Thio-ether oxidation
    Desulfuration
L-Ascorbic acid synthesis
UDP-uronic acid metabolism
UDP-glucose dephosphorylation
Aryl- and steroid-sulfatase

Source: Modified from J. Rothschild, *Biochem. Soc. Symp.* 22:4 (1963).

ribosomal removal still constituted about 10 percent of the total dry weight of the membranes. The protein has been described as partly structural and partly enzymatic, but there is question concerning such distinctions and the suggestion is that the enzymatic protein component of membrane performs a dual role. (See Chapter 9.) The lipid is predominantly phospholipid, most of which is lecithin, but there are also cephalins, inositides, and cholesterol and its esters. The enzyme composition reflects the variety of metabolic activities (Table 11.1), some of which will be discussed in a later section.

FUNCTION

The specialized functions of the endoplasmic reticulum are localized among the various structural subdivisions. There are, however, the general functions such as mechanical support, transport, and exchange.

Mechanical Support

By compartmentalizing the intracellular fluid, the complex membranous channels provide supplementary mechanical support for the colloidal structure of the cytoplasmic matrix. This, undoubtedly, is of great importance since the integration of structure and function presumes a complex organization of molecules in space as prerequisite to organization of function.

Transport and Exchange

It is evident that both nutrients and products of metabolism move not only in and out of the cell but also from one area of the cell to another. A molecule of glucose that enters the cell and is phosphorylated may be metabolized to pyruvic acid in the cytoplasmic matrix, may become a part of the TCA cycle in the mitochondria, and through oxidative phosphorylation may have its potential energy trapped in ATP. Some of the trapped ATP in the mitochondria must be released into the matrix for activation of the amino acids transported there for protein synthesis. Some of the synthesized proteins are the enzymes which participate in all of the foregoing processes, and they therefore must be transported to their sites of action through the various membranes along the route. All aspects of membrane transfer discussed in Chapter 9 are pertinent for the membranes of the endoplasmic reticulum and other organelles.

A further complicating factor is the change of locus during synthesis of a particular metabolite that may involve shuttling of intermediates through membranes from organelles to matrix and back again in varying orderly pathways. Following the synthetic pathway of one protein or one steroid hormone can be fascinating and will be presented later in this chapter; following the concurrent activities within the cell becomes too staggering to comprehend. Inability to comprehend, however, should not preclude our attempts to apprehend the complexity of a problem that future students may be expected to grasp.

Protein Synthesis

A general acceptance of the idea that genes controlled protein and, therefore, enzyme synthesis developed early in the twentieth century with the work of Garrod (1902) who described alkaptonuria as an "inborn error of metabolism," that is, a defect in biochemical function due to a defective gene. The work of Pauling et al. (1949) provided clear evidence that a gene determines the structure of a protein, and it soon was demonstrated that it is the single polypeptide chain that the gene controls. How the genes exert such control was not known but with the announcement of the Watson-Crick model of DNA (Watson and Crick, 1953) came the tremendous impetus in research into the mechanism of genetic control of polypeptide synthesis.

Genetic Code. Crick et al. (1961) set forth a group of assumptions based on the then current thought and slim empirical evidence. They asserted that the genetic code was in the form of nucleotide triplets; was not overlapping; was read from a fixed starting point with no special "commas"; and was probably degenerate, that is, one amino acid could be coded by several triplets. Crick and his colleages then proceeded to put these assumptions to experimental test. Perhaps this group was prescient since other groups were arguing in favor of either two letter (Sinsheimer, 1959) or four letter codes (Gamow, 1959), overlapping codes (Wall, 1962) as well as other variations, all of which were being tested by statistical and other means. Just about this time, Nirenberg and Matthaei (1961) reported that they had induced the synthesis of polypeptides by adding ribonucleic acid to a cell-free system. They had synthesized a nucleotide containing only uridylic acid, poly U, which led to the production of a monotonous polypeptide containing only phenylalanine units. They found also that poly C, or CCC, carried the message for proline. This work, together with the work from Crick's laboratory, was taken to mean that the triplet UUU was the code or *codon* signifying phenylalanine and CCC, proline. This development was a major landmark in accelerating the understanding of the genetic code and protein synthesis since it provided an *in vitro* system for investigating what otherwise would have to be studied by genetic methods involving the effects of amino acid replacements and the effects of mutagenic agents, a far more tedious and time-consuming procedure.

Nirenberg et al. (1962) next showed that phenylalanine-tRNA was an intermediate in the synthesis of polyphenylalanine and then that poly U associated rapidly with ribosomes (Barondes and Nirenberg, 1962). These findings were in accord with the concept that had been proposed by Jacob and Monod (1961) that RNA was an intermediate in the transfer of information from DNA to protein and that this "messenger RNA" had a short half-life. Soon, other investigations indicated that the code for lysine was AAA (Ochoa, 1963). This work was followed

TABLE 11.2
RNA-Amino Acid Code

		SECOND BASE OF CODON					
		U	**C**	**A**	**G**		
FIRST BASE OF CODON	**U**	UUU UUC } Phe UUA UUG } Leu	UCU UCC UCA UCG } Ser	UAU UAC } Tyr UAA UAG }	UGU UGC } Cys UGA UGG Try	U C A G	THIRD BASE OF CODON
	C	CUU CUC CUA CUG } Leu	CCU CCC CCA CCG } Pro	CAU CAC } His CAA CAG } GluN	CGU CGC CGA CGG } Arg	U C A G	
	A	AUU AUC } Ileu AUA AUG Met	ACU ACC ACA ACG } Thr	AAU AAC } AspN AAA AAG } Lys	AGU AGC } Ser AGA AGG } Arg	U C A G	
	G	GUU GUC GUA GUG } Val	GCU GCC GCA GCG } Ala	GAU GAC } Asp GAA GAG } Glu	GGU GGC GGA GGG } Gly	U C A G	

Source: From A. S. Spirin and L. P. Gavrilova, *The Ribosome,* Springer Verlag, New York., 1969, p. 9.

by the use of polynucleotides having more than one kind of base. Most of the work on coding was carried on in the laboratories of Nirenberg and Ochoa and within a year 54 random codons were assigned, all but 8 of which were correct (Nirenberg, 1963). From this work it became fully apparent that the code was indeed a triplet code and that it was degenerate (two or more codons coding for the same amino acid).

The now completed dictionary of accepted codon assignments is shown in Table 11.2. Several features are apparent: all codons are triplets and the code is highly degenerate, but the degeneracy has a pattern, one that was first deduced by Eck (1963). The codons for each amino acid consist of two bases that are characteristic of the amino acid; and the third base is read only as a purine, a pyrimidine, or merely as a base. Three exceptions—leucine, serine, and arginine—have two sets of base pairs that are characteristic for them. Methionine and tryptophan have only one set, or a single codon. Two nonsense codons, not assigned to any amino acid, appeared to act as punctuation.

The universality of the code, at least for bacteria and protozoa, at first became evident from detailed consideration of the relations between DNA and protein compositions (Sueoka, 1961a; 1961b). Studies of amino acid replacements due to single base changes in the code were next studied in a plant virus, bacterium, and mammal. The discovery of sickle cell hemoglobin by Pauling et al. (1949) had been shown to be due to substitution of a normal valine by a glutamic acid in one position in the β chain of hemoglobin (Ingram, 1957; Hunt and Ingram, 1959). Other human abnormal hemoglobins also had been shown to be due to single amino acid replacements. All the amino acid replacements in the hemoglobin mutations proved to be compatible with the code (Table 11.3).

Punctuation.   Since the code is read sequentially, the matter of punctuation, or where to start and where to stop, is crucial. Using three of the simplest codes—poly U, poly A, and poly C—it will become obvious that a wrong start drastically changes the meaning. Fig. 11.6 shows how a one-nucleotide shift in the starting position changes the codons and, therefore, designates a different sequence of amino acids providing, of course, that the codons are valid. Crick (1963) showed that the message is read starting with a constant fixed point at one end of the nucleotide chain and reading in successive triplets from there.

If the triplet sequence in mRNA contains the message or the template for the construction of a polypeptide chain, the next big question was how the amino acids recognized their codes or call numbers. It certainly was not a random, hit-or-miss, come-when-you-can invitation to the amino acids. If the message is read as Braille from one end to the other without interruption, then the required amino acids must be delivered into their proper positions sequentially. The direction of the assembly of ribonucleotides by addition to the 3'-OH group of the end ribonucleotide was established in an *in vitro* system of RNA polymerase primed with DNA (Maitra and Hurwitz, 1965). The initial residue remained as a triphosphate. The assembly of protein was clearly demonstrated to be sequential (Dintzis, 1961; Naughton and Dintzis, 1962). Tritium-labeled leucine was added to suspensions of reticulocytes that were actively synthesizing hemoglobin but

TABLE 11.3
Examples of Possible Codon Changes Underlying Some Amino Acid Replacements in the Mutant Hemoglobins

Amino Acid in Normal Hemoglobin		Amino Acid in Mutant Hemoglobin	
Lysine (AAA)	$\longrightarrow$	Glutamic acid (GAA)	A → G
Glutamic acid (GAA)	$\longrightarrow$	Glutamine (CAA)	G → C
Glycine (GGU)	$\longrightarrow$	Aspartic acid (GAU)	G → A
Histidine (CAU)	$\longrightarrow$	Tyrosine (UAU)	C → U
Asparagine (AAU)	$\longrightarrow$	Lysine (AAA)	U → A
Glutamic acid (GAA)	$\longrightarrow$	Valine (GUA)	A → U
Glutamic acid (GAA)	$\longrightarrow$	Lysine (AAA)	G → A
Glutamic acid (GAA)	$\longrightarrow$	Glycine (GGA)	A → G

Source: From J. D. Watson, *Molecular Biology of the Gene,* 2nd ed., W. A. Benjamin Inc., New York, 1970, p. 418.

that were being retarded by low temperature. Samples were taken at intervals and plotted to show the specific activity of the leucine-containing peptides whose positions were known in the hemoglobin chain. In the first samples, only the leucine-containing peptides from the COOH-terminal ends of the α and β chains were labeled. Longer exposure to the ^{3}H-leucine led to a gradual increase in the number of labeled peptides proceeding toward the NH$_2$ terminus. After 60 minutes all were labeled (Fig. 11.7). Clearly, polypeptides grow by stepwise addition of

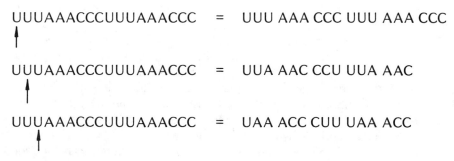

Figure 11.6
How a one-nucleotide shift in the initiation point changes the code.

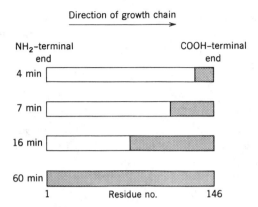

Figure 11.7
Addition of labeled leucine residues to the
COOH-terminal end of a polypeptide chain.
The dark portions of the bars indicate the relative radioactivity of leucine residues along the
a chain of hemoglobin following addition of
^{3}H-leucine to reticulocytes. At 4 min, only a
few leucine residues at the COOH-terminal end
were labeled; by 60 min, the entire chain was
labeled. (From H. M. Dintzis, *Proc. Natl. Acad.
Sci. U. S.*, 47:247, 1961.)

single amino acids starting with the amino terminal and ending with the carboxyl
terminal. Any interference in the continuity of assembly for lack of a required
amino acid halts synthesis completely and the polypeptide chain is not formed.
(Here is the fundamental explanation for the dictum established by nutritionists
over two decades ago: *the time factor in protein synthesis.* On the basis of animal
feeding experiments it was established that protein synthesis could take place
only if all of the necessary amino acids were present in the proper amounts at
the same time (Geiger, 1950). The mechanisms involved in protein synthesis
worked out jointly by geneticists and biochemists now explain why.)

The need for punctuation that had been postulated became even more apparent
when Jacob and Monod (1961) reported that one mRNA carried the code for a
series of separate proteins. The codons signifying *N*-terminal punctuation, or the
starting amino acid, *N*-formyl methionine in bacterial systems and methionine in
animal systems (Petermann, 1971), turned out to be AUG and GUG. These are
ambiguous codons in the sense that they can be read both as internal amino acids
and as *N*-terminal methionine. The way they are read depends on whether they
are preceded by C-terminal punctuation or the codon for another amino acid.
The C-terminal punctuation appears to be provided by termination signals, also
called nonsense codons, that is, codons that do not specify any amino acid. The
termination codons, UAA, UAG, and UGA, in the sequence of nucleotides indicate the C-terminal, or stop signal. When the ribosome reaches a termination

signal the completed polypeptide is released. The details of *how* this works are not entirely clear, but there is substantial evidence to support the fact that it *does* work. The suggestion is that these codons are read by specific proteins, the releasing factors (see below).

The Adaptor Hypothesis. In order for the code to be translated into amino acids, there must be some means whereby amino acids recognize specific codons. It became apparent early that RNA could not be a direct template and Crick (1966a), in reviewing early history, reports his suggestion in 1957 of an RNA molecule acting as an adaptor between the template and the amino acid. It soon became evident that the adaptors were the relatively small molecules of transfer RNA (tRNA). Like all other cellular RNA, tRNA is specified by a base sequence in DNA. The tRNAs for the 20 different amino acids are different, yet alike in certain respects. Each contains approximately 80 nucleotides in a single chain, the 3' end of which always reads CCA and the 5' end is usually an unpaired guanine.

Alanine-tRNA (Fig. 11.8) was the first to have its nucleotide sequence worked out (Holley et al., 1965). Only after the nucleotide sequences in several other tRNAs had been determined was it realized that there were certain sequences common to all; the configurations that led to the maximal number of base pairings led to a common shape, that of the cloverleaf (Fig. 11.9). Each tRNA has its characteristic *anticodon* that pairs with the codon on the template mRNA. The anticodon is antiparallel, that is, it reads in the 3' to the 5' direction. When it became evident that a highly purified specific tRNA could recognize several codons, and that inosine often replaced one of the four common bases in the anticodon, Crick (1966b) proposed the *wobble hypothesis*. Since the third base in a codon could vary without changing meaning, he suggested that this might occur also in the anticodon with the two bases at the 3' end of the anticodon quite specific for an amino acid, but the one at the 5' end not as confined spatially, that is, it could wobble and form hydrogen bonds with bases other than those in standard base pairs.

The evidence was clear that the adaptor was tRNA and that this nucleotide was the intermediary through which the code was translated into amino acids. For more details on tRNA, see von Ehrenstein (1970).

A recitation of the rapid rate of discoveries leading to an understanding of the genetic code and its translation has the advantages bestowed by hindsight. The literature from 1961 on is filled with reports on all conceivable aspects of the coding problem and of attempts to arrive at a solution. Various systems of coding were postulated and became dogma, only to be discarded. For an extensive and thorough history of biological coding, see Yĉas (1969). For briefer views, see Woese (1967) and Nirenberg (1970).

The Ribosomes. The ribosomes are the ribonucleoprotein particles in which the protein synthesis takes place. They consist almost entirely of ribosomal RNA and ribosomal protein. The RNA molecules during synthesis in the nucleolus are complexed with protein that is synthesized in the cytoplasm and transported into the nucleus (Miller, 1973). The ribosome is synthesized as a large precursor

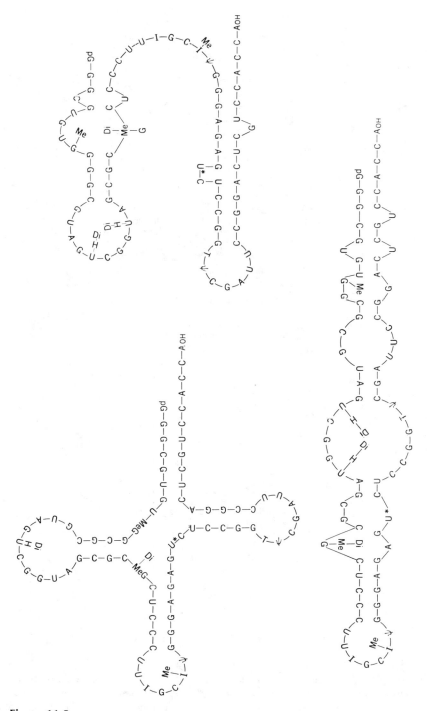

Figure 11.8
Schematic representation of three conformations of the alanine RNA with short, double-stranded regions. (From R. W. Holley et al., *Science* 147:1462, 1965.)

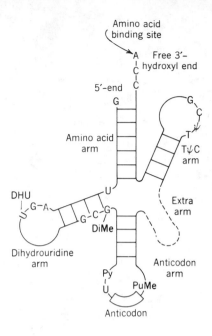

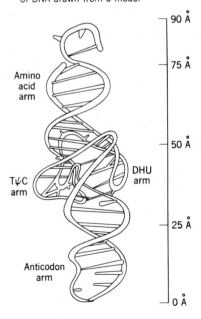

The three-dimentional conformation
of DNA drawn from a model

Figure 11.9
Structure of tRNA. The common features in the structure of tRNAs (see text). Some tRNAs, such as those for serine, have an extra arm of varying length. Maximal intrachain H-bonding yields the cloverleaf structure shown. X-ray evidence suggests, however, that the lateral arms are folded closely alongside the vertical arms. The anticodon is always demarcated by the neighboring bases shown. The symbols are ψ, pseudouridine; Py, pyrimidine; Pu, purine; Me, methyl; DiMe, dimethyl; DHU, dihydrouridine. (From A. L. Lehninger, *Biochemistry*, Worth Publishers, Inc. New York, 1970, p. 695.)

molecule that is cleaved in the nucleolus to form the two subunits that leave the nucleus. The subunits reassociate in the cytoplasm (but not necessarily as units from the same precursors) to form the complete ribosome. In bacteria the ribosome has a sedimentation coefficient of 70 Svedberg units and is commonly referred to as the 70S ribosome, with a 30S and 50S subunit (Tissiers and Watson, 1958). In higher plants and animals the ribosome is 80S (Tashiro and Siekevitz, 1965) with subunits of approximately 60S and 40S. Since the bacterial ribosome has been studied much more extensively, reference here will be mostly to the 70S ribosome and its component parts.

The 30S subunit contains about 20 different proteins each of which appears to have an individual role in the structure or function of the ribosome (Nomura, 1970); the 50S subunits contain 30–36 individual proteins (Petermann, 1971). The association of the subunits into the ribosome is stable only in solvents that contain enough Mg^{++} to saturate the RNA phosphate groups. When the Mg^{++} is reduced and two-thirds dissociates from the ribosome, the two subunits of the ribosome separate. In some cases Ca^{++} has also been found associated with the ribosome (Ts'o et al., 1958) and has been shown to be able to replace Mg^{++} to some degree (Chao, 1957; Elson, 1959; 1961). Stabilizing roles have also been attributed to Mn^{++} and Co^{++} (Lyttleton, 1960; 1962; Abdul-Nour and Webster, 1960).

Under physiological conditions, ribosomes bound to endoplasmic reticulum membranes in the eukaryotic cell are in the form of polysomes, that is, groups of ribosomes. The binding of the mRNA to the ribosome involves the small subunit, whereas the binding of the ribosome to the membrane involves the large subunit (Sabatini et al., 1971). Each 70S or 80S ribosome contains two sites into which tRNA can be inserted: the peptidyl or *P site*, and the aminoacyl or *A site*. These ribosomal sites can accept any aminoacyl tRNA since the ribosome binds to an unspecific part of the tRNA molecule. It is only the codon-bound surface of the tRNA that is specific. The growing polypeptide chain is always terminated by a tRNA and it is the binding of this terminal tRNA to either the P site or the A site of the ribosome that is the main force holding the growing chain to the ribosome.

Electron microscopic observations on isolated membrane from microsomal fractions (Sabatini et al., 1966; Florendo, 1969) show that the groove separating the ribosomal subunits of a membrane-bound ribosome lies parallel to the membrane surface (Fig. 11.10).

To explain the process whereby protein is transferred across the membrane of the endoplasmic reticulum the "signal hypothesis" was proposed by Blobel and his colleagues. (See Blobel, 1977.) The current version of this hypothesis proposes that all mRNAs for secretory proteins contain "signal codons" localized on the 3' side of the AUG initiation codon. Translation of the signal codons to initiate protein synthesis takes place on free ribosomes. When the nascent polypeptide chain containing the signal sequence emerges from the channel in the large ribosomal subunit, it interacts with the membrane of the endoplasmic reticulum so that the ribosome is attached to the membrane. The signal sequence causes several ribosome receptor proteins to interact and form a tunnel through the

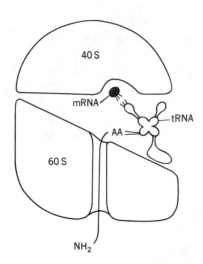

Figure 11.10
Diagram of a ribosome showing the two subunits and the probable position of the messenger RNA and the transfer RNA. The nascent polypeptide chain passes through a kind of funnel within the large subunit. (From E. D. P. DeRobertis, W. W. Nowinski, and F. A. Saez, *Cell Biology*, 5th ed., W. B. Saunders Co., Philadelphia, 1970, p. 401.)

membrane. The tunnel on the large ribosomal subunit is brought into alignment with the tunnel on the membrane. When the signal sequence on the lengthening polypeptide chain moves into the interior of the lumen of the endoplasmic reticulum a "signal peptidase" is thought to cleave it from the uncompleted nascent chain. The polypeptide continues to grow until chain termination and release occur. The protein is now segregated in the cisternal space and the ribosome is then detached from the membrane. The tunnel in the membrane is obliterated by diffusion of the ribosome receptor protein in the plane of the membrane. A scheme of the signal hypothesis is shown in Fig. 11.11. This mechanism operates in cells synthesizing protein such as hormones, milk, and certain enzymes for export. Passage through the channels of the endoplasmic reticulum is followed

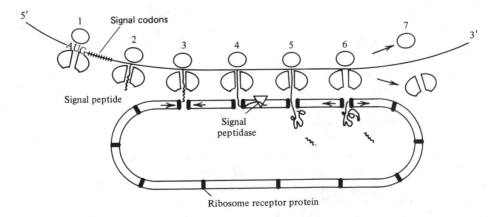

Figure 11.11
Schematic illustration of the signal hypothesis. (From G. Blobel, in *International Cell Biology*, B. R. Brinkley and K. R. Porter, eds., The Rockefeller University Press, New York, 1977, p. 320.)

by packaging in the Golgi complex prior to discharge. (See Chapter 12.) Proteins that are synthesized for internal use are synthesized by the free polysomes in the cytoplasmic matrix. In this category are the enzymes maintained in the cytoplasmic matrix for cellular metabolism as well as those required for such specialized protein syntheses as hemoglobin in the erythrocyte.

For more detailed reviews on ribosomes, see Spirin and Gavrilova (1969); Nomura (1969); Petermann (1971); Miller (1973); Wool (1979).

Building a Polypeptide.   For polypeptide synthesis to take place in the endoplasmic reticulum mRNA, rRNA and ribonucleoproteins, tRNAs, and the required enzymes must be assembled in the cytoplasmic matrix where the amino acids, cations, and energy sources are all simultaneously available.

Several other factors that play specific roles in the synthetic process have been identified: three specific protein-initiation factors identified as F1, F2, and F3 were isolated and characterized in Ochoa's laboratory (Thach et al., 1966; Iwasaki et al., 1968; Revel et al., 1968). These appear to interact with and stabilize the 30S subunit complex. Peptidyl transferase factors, TF1 and TF2, active in the elongation of the polypeptide chain, were isolated in Lipmann's laboratory (Nishizuka and Lipmann, 1966; Ertel et al., 1968). TF2 is sometimes referred to as translocase.

For protein synthesis to proceed, there first must be activation of the amino acids through formation of an amino acid adenylate (Hoagland, 1955; Hoagland et al., 1956):

1. AA + ATP $- - -\rightarrow$ AMP $\sim$ AA + PP

followed by transfer, or transacetylation of the amino acids to tRNA (Allen et al., 1960):

2. AMP $\sim$ AA + tRNA $- - -\rightarrow$ AA $\sim$ tRNA + AMP

Steps 1 and 2 are both catalyzed by the same enzyme, aminoacyl synthetase. The amino acids are transferred to the terminal adenylic acid of tRNA, each of which has a 3' terminus reading CCA.

Since the same activating enzyme binds to a given amino acid and to its tRNA, the enzyme must have two different binding sites. Each tRNA also must have two binding sites, one for the activating enzyme, and the other for a specific group of template nucleotides. This latter site carries the anticodon for each of the amino acids and, therefore, determines the specificity of the tRNAs for the various amino acids (Berg and Ofengand, 1958).

The process of polypeptide synthesis can be divided into three steps: *initiation, elongation,* and *termination.* In the initiation step, a free 30S ribosomal subunit binds to the mRNA at the specific initiation site that reads AUG. Protein factor F3 is required for the binding. The 30S-mRNA complex binds the starting aminoacyl tRNA, which is met-tRNA in animals and F-met-tRNA in bacteria. An amino peptidase has been identified that subsequently removes the terminal methionine from many of the completed chains (Clark and Marker, 1968). The 50S-ribosomal subunit joins the complex. Whether entry of the met-tRNA complex to the 50S-ribosomal subunit is made at the A site or directly to the P site is not known, but with the starting complex at the P site, the ribosome becomes functional. Figure 11.12 illustrates the geography of a functional ribosome with the starting aminoacyl-tRNA in place.

A second aminoacyl-tRNA with an anticodon that complements the second codon on the mRNA joins the complex and occupies the A site on the 50S ribosome. Peptide bond formation then occurs by a reaction between the amino group of the aminoacyl-tRNA and the carboxylic group of the peptidyl-tRNA. This reaction is catalyzed by the enzyme peptidyl transferase and requires GTP (Fig. 11.13).

After the formation of the peptide bond, the peptidyl-tRNA and the now-elongating chain are part of the complex on the A site and must be translocated to the P site before the next aminoacyl-tRNA can bind at the A site. Simultaneously, the deacylated tRNA leaves the P site, and the mRNA moves along three nucleotides so that the next nucleotide triplet codon is in the correct position at the A site.

After the full complement of amino acids is thus added, termination of the chain is activated by the stop codons, UAG, UAA, UGA. The stop codon causes termination of the chain with the amino acid on the codon just prior to it. The stop codon is recognized by the protein release factors that act enzymatically splitting off the terminal tRNA (Siekevitz and Palade, 1960). The polypeptide that has probably assumed its three-dimensional configuration is released directly into the channel of the endoplasmic reticulum if it is a secretory protein, or into the cytoplasmic matrix by free polysomes. The released ribosome is dissociated into the 30S and 50S subunits that become available for reuse, as is the free tRNA that delivered the carboxyl terminal amino acid (Fig. 11.14).

The synthesis of many polypeptide chains occurs on the succession of ribosomes that form the polysome associated with one mRNA. Each ribosome functions independently of the others and a relatively short mRNA may be read simultaneously by 6 or so ribosomes constituting the polysome, whereas an mRNA that codes for a long polypeptide chain of perhaps 1,500 amino acids might accommodate a polysome of up to 100 ribosomes simultaneously reading the 4,500 nucleotide mRNA tape.

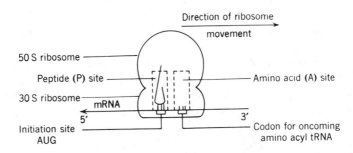

Figure 11.12
Geography of a functional ribosome with starting aminoacyl-tRNA in place.

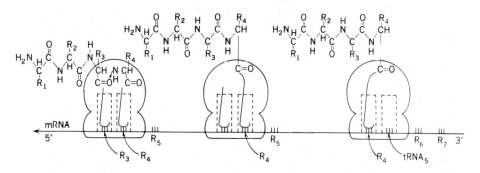

Figure 11.13
Peptide bond formation between the carboxyl group of the peptidyl-tRNA and the amino group of the aminoacyl-tRNA followed by translocation of the aminoacyl-tRNA carrying the polypeptide chain to the P site.

For further reading on polypeptide synthesis, see Lipmann (1969); Nirenberg (1970).

Regulation of Protein Synthesis

All cells synthesize protein for their own internal need, that is, complex molecules for structural components and enzymes for cell functions. In addition, many cells synthesize specific products for export: digestive enzymes from mucosal cells and pancreatic cells, plasma proteins from liver cells, collagen from fibroblasts, antibodies from plasma cells, and hormones from various endocrine cells, to name

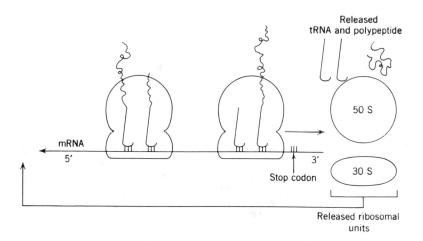

Figure 11.14
Termination of polypeptide chain by the stop codon. The polypeptide release is accompanied by release of tRNA and the dissociated ribosomes that are available for reuse.

some examples. Proteins synthesized for internal use are assembled on free ribosomes in the cytoplasmic matrix. (Some protein synthesis for internal use also takes place in the mitochondria and will be discussed in Chapter 13.) The protein for export, as indicated earlier, is released directly into the channels of the endoplasmic reticulum and passes through the Golgi apparatus for additions of complex carbohydrate, lipid, sulfate, or other molecules prior to concentration, storage, and release.

Since all metabolic processes depend on enzyme action, and since all enzymes are proteins, the life of the cell depends on its protein synthetic capacity. The only cell deprived of the ability to synthesize protein is the mature erythrocyte since it loses its nucleus during maturation and therefore loses the required DNA for RNA production. This cell exists and functions only as long as its RNA and package of enzymes lasts. (See Chapter 16.) When these have been used up, since they cannot be replaced, the erythrocyte lifespan is completed. In other cells, ifthe DNA in the nucleus is induced to produce the requisite RNA and if the necessary nutrients for synthesis are available, the cell will synthesize the enzymes or other proteins it requires for its structure and function.

There is a constant turnover of cellular protein, that is, synthesis and degradation within the cell. The turnover rates vary not only among cells but also among organelles and specific proteins within the cells. For example, the half-life of the protein of the endoplasmic reticulum is approximately two days, whereas that of mitochondria is almost seven days. Some enzymes have a half-life of two to four days and others just a few hours.

The protein production schedule for any cell must, of necessity, be very carefully organized and controlled if the proper amounts of each of the multitude of enzymes required for cell function are to come off the assembly line at the proper time. In addition, there must be careful allocation and precise regulation of the common precursors, as well as energy, necessary for the cell's countless functions. Syntheses must be started, and they must be stopped, and both the initiation and termination of each synthesis is part of the overall program. The surviving cell is proof of successful regulation.

Initiation of the synthesis of a protein involved in a metabolic reaction in the cell may occur when the substrate is introduced. This is called *enzyme induction* and the enzymes themselves are said to be *inducible enzymes*. This type of response has been studied in bacterial cultures but is also implicated as a type of control in mammalian metabolism. For example, introduction of lactose as the sole source of carbon to bacterial culture will induce the synthesis of β-galactosidase that will continue as long as lactose is the carbon source. If glucose is provided, the enzyme β-galactosidase will no longer be induced. Some investigators have suggested that a similar type of enzyme induction might be the mechanism responsible for the lactose tolerance observed in adult Caucasians. (See Chapter 6.)

Inhibition of Protein Synthesis.   From what has been discussed in Chapter 10 it is evident that DNA transcription is normally believed to be in an "off" position. According to the Jacob and Monod model, the regulatory gene codes for the mRNA that is the template for the repressor protein. The repressor protein generally functions to block the operator gene so that transcription does not take place. However, when the inhibition is counteracted by an inducer that combines with the repressor to form a repressor-inducer complex, transcription to mRNA occurs leading to protein synthesis. Once started, however, there must be ways to get it stopped, and several mechanisms have been suggested to explain what the procedure might be.

Product and Feedback Inhibition.   If a cell is supplied with a product it normally synthesizes, it will frugally cut off its own production by repressing synthesis of the enzymes involved. Such a cutoff stimulated by the end product is called *product inhibition* or *enzyme repression* and is usually the result of a mass action effect.

When the synthesis of a product is the result of a series of enzyme actions, accumulation of the end product triggers a regulating mechanism that sets up the inhibition at the point of the first enzymatic reaction in the chain, thereby preventing further production of that metabolite and of its immediate precursors in the synthetic pathway. This is called *feedback inhibition* and is one of the common means of controlling metabolic pathways (Fig. 11.15). In feedback inhibition, the enzyme responsive to the block is also referred to as the *pacemaker* or *regulatory enzyme*. Enzymes exerting this type of regulation are usually allosteric, that is, they will have one site promoting the reaction and another site responsive to the end product leading to inhibition of the reaction. Through this type of regulation there can be continual adjustment in the rate of enzyme synthesis to fulfill the demands of the cell. Increased demand delays both product and feedback inhibition, whereas a decrease in demand leads to a cut-off in synthesis. Many variations of feedback inhibition have been described to account for control of metabolic pathways of varying complexities. (See Conn and Stumpf, 1972, p. 471.)

Repression of Protein Synthesis.   The model of Jacob and Monod accounts for the repression exerted by the biosynthetic end product by postulating that the repressor molecule does not act by itself in a feedback inhibition but must have a *corepressor*. The corepressor is usually a small molecule that may be an end product in the metabolic pathway. It becomes the repressing metabolite and forms the *repressor-corepressor complex*, which then combines with the operator gene to prevent transcription.

Several other types of data have been forthcoming to provide support for the Jacob-Monod hypothesis. Two repressor proteins have been isolated: the galactosidase repressor (Gilbert and Müller-Hill, 1966) and the repressor protein for the *lac* operon (Ptashne, 1967). It was mentioned previously that lactose supplied

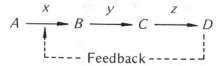

Figure 11.15
Feedback inhibition. Accumulation of product *D* inhibits enzyme x required for reaction A→B.

as the only source of carbon for *E. coli* induced synthesis of enzymes for its metabolism. The repression of these enzymes effected by the addition of glucose is called *catabolite repression,* and its action has recently been linked to cAMP. Pastan and Perlman (1968) have demonstrated that the mechanism involves binding of cAMP to the *receptor protein* followed by association of *cAMP-receptor protein* with a specific binding site in the *lac* genome. This promotes the binding of RNA polymerase to DNA thereby increasing the rate of synthesis of the enzymes essential for lactose metabolism. The addition of glucose to the medium decreases the concentration of cAMP and interferes with this binding (Fig. 11.16).

The presence of receptor sites in plasma membranes that operate through an associated adenyl cyclase site to stimulate the formation of cAMP was discussed in Chapter 9. Similarly associated receptor and adenyl cyclase sites are present in the membranes of the endoplasmic reticulum and mitochondria. Several mechanisms involving selective induction of enzyme synthesis by cAMP have been proposed.

The exquisite sensitivity with which the selective induction of hepatic enzymes occurs following stimulation by various hormones has been attributed to cAMP (Wicks, 1971; Wicks et al., 1974). In both glycogenesis and glycogenolysis there is elegantly coordinated control of the involved enzymes which is mediated by hormones through cAMP. The biochemical pathways will be discussed in subsequent sections; the mechanisms of enzyme activation and control are pertinent here. The same cAMP-dependent protein kinase controls *phosphorylase activation* and *glycogen synthetase inactivation.* This clearly permits the right hand to know what the left hand is doing in making glucose available or sequestering it as glycogen. The action of cAMP in activating protein kinase simultaneously converts inactive phosphorylase b kinase to the active form and active glycogen synthetase to the inactive form. This leads through a cascade of events to the stimulation of glycogenolysis and the inhibition of glycogenesis (Fig. 11.17).

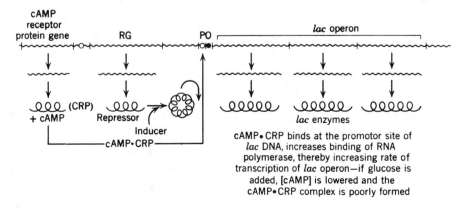

Figure 11.16
Catabolite repression indicating effect of cAMP. (From E. E. Conn and P. K. Stumpf, *Outlines of Biochemistry,* 3rd ed., John Wiley, New York 1972, p. 483.)

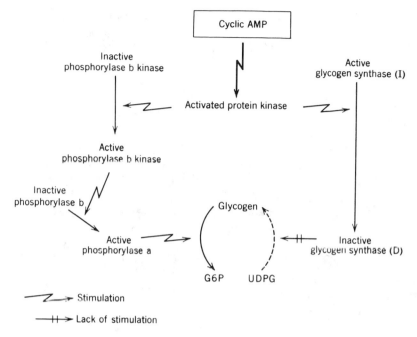

Figure 11.17
Coordinate stimulation of glycogenolysis and inhibition of glycogenesis. (From
J. Tepperman, *Metabolic and Endocrine Physiology,* 3rd ed., Year Book
Medical Publishers, 1973, p. 28.)

Garren et al. (1971) have postulated that ACTH acts through cAMP to regulate
adrenal function by modulating protein synthesis at the level of translation of
mRNA. They propose that the binding of cAMP to the inhibitory receptor protein
causes it to dissociate from the protein kinase activating the enzyme. The activated
enzyme then catalyzes the transfer of phosphate from ATP to ribosomal protein.
This action of cAMP, releasing the inhibition of the protein kinase, appears to be
a general phenomenon and not limited to the adrenal cortex. Tao (1971) reported
a similar mechanism in rabbit reticulocytes and Kuman et al. (1970) in liver.
These observations are consistent with the finding that protein kinase is composed
of two subunits that together form an inactive enzyme. By binding with one
subunit, cAMP causes the release of the other subunit, which is the active kinase.
Two suggested models are depicted in Fig. 11.18.

It may well be that the general mechanism of hormone action starts with the
activation of adenyl cyclase in the cell membrane leading to formation of cAMP,
the second messenger, that in turn releases active protein kinase. Protein kinase
may be involved in most of the effects of cAMP (Sutherland, 1972). It may activate
another enzyme and produce a rapid response; or it may influence the binding
of RNA polymerase and thereby the rate of transcription and enzyme synthesis
in the slower type of hormone response. Cheung (1972) suggests that cAMP
functions as a versatile allosteric effector and that the different effects of cAMP

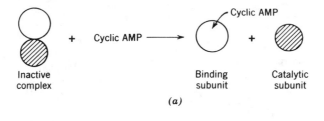

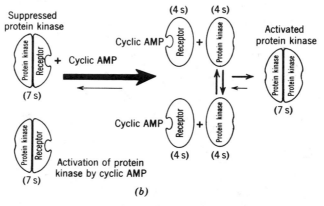

Figure 11.18
Two models of protein kinase activation by cAMP. (a) A model
for the mechanism of activation of kinase 1 by cyclic AMP. (From
M. Tao, *Ann. N. Y. Acad. Sci.* 185:227, 1971.) (b) Hypothetical
model for the activation of protein kinase by cAMP. (From T. A.
Langan, *Ann. N. Y. Acad. Sci.* 185:166, 1971.)

are explained by the kinds of proteins with which it interacts and, it could be
added, by the kind of proteins it represses or induces.

Glycolysis

A fundamental role of the cytoplasmic matrix is the preparatory degradation of
carbohydrate units to pyruvic acid which enters the mitochondria and there is
further oxidized for the release of energy. *Glycolysis* is the term used to describe
this initial stage of carbohydrate metabolism and refers to the breakdown of
glucose or glycogen to pyruvic acid.

Glucose enters the cell from the interstitial fluid in the free state and is transported across most cell membranes under the influence of the hormone insulin.
The membranes of some cells, however, such as intestinal mucosa and brain, do
not require insulin for glucose transport. This function of insulin accounts for
many of the aberrations in carbohydrate metabolism observed in the diabetic state
but does not explain other apparently direct effects of the hormone, such as the
effects on fatty acid and protein synthesis.

The passage of the somewhat polar glucose molecule is facilitated by specific
carrier proteins in the membrane. The carrier in the liver functions without any

known controls; glucose rapidly equilibrates between the liver cytosol and the extracellular fluid. Brain has a transport capacity well in excess of demand unless blood glucose concentrations drop to low levels. Transport into heart, skeletal and smooth muscle, and adipose tissue is tightly regulated by insulin concentration. Little glucose moves into resting msucle unless insulin is present; the uptake of glucose is increased by an unknown mechanism when the muscle is excited to contract.

Free glucose cannot enter into cellular metabolic activity; thus, upon entrance into the cell, it is immediately phosphorylated, a process that requires ATP and which results in the formation of glucose-6-phosphate. Glucose enters into the glycolytic pathway by phosphorylation to glucose-6-phosphate. A molecule of ATP is used to trap the glucose as glucose-6-phosphate, which will not freely pass the membrane. Phosphorylation serves to maintain the concentration gradient by keeping the concentration of free glucose low inside the cell so that glucose will continue to enter the cell without expenditure of energy. This reaction is accomplished by the enzyme hexokinase and by an additional enzyme in liver, glucokinase, which is inducible. Hexokinase has a high affinity (low K_m) for glucose and is inhibited by its product, glucose-6-phosphate; glucokinase has a low affinity (high K_m) and is not inhibited by its product.

Three chief pathways are open to the phosphorylated glucose: glycolysis, glycogenesis (formation of glycogen), or metabolism by way of the pentose phosphate shunt. The pathway followed is determined by the metabolic state existing within the cell; primarily, the available amounts of glucose, ATP, NADP, and oxygen determine the pathway of glucose degradation.

Glycolysis has been studied most in muscle and nerve tissues but occurs actively in liver cells and undoubtedly occurs in cells of all tissues. The metabolic scheme is known as the Embden-Meyerhof glycolytic pathway in honor of two of the scientists whose work contributed most to elaboration of the reactions involved. Glycolysis may proceed from either free glucose or glycogen, but in either instance the formation of the active metabolite, glucose-6-phosphate, is essential. Phosphorylation of free glucose, however, requires the high energy of ATP, whereas phosphorylation of a glucose unit from glycogen is accomplished by phosphorolysis, a reaction utilizing inorganic phosphate and which, therefore, does not require the expenditure of high energy. The difference in initial energy expenditure affects the final net yield of energy from glycolysis depending on whether the starting point is glucose or glycogen.

The principle reactions involved in the Embden-Meyerhof scheme are shown in Fig. 11.19 and are described as follows:

1. Glucose-6-phosphate is formed either by phosphorylation of free glucose that has just entered the cell or phosphorolysis of glycogen with glucose-1-phosphate as an intermediate.
2. Glucose-6-phosphate is isomerized to the phosphorylated keto hexose, fructose-6-phosphate.
3. Fructose-6-phosphate is further phosphorylated by ATP at the first carbon to form fructose-1,6-bisphosphate. The reverse reaction involving fructose-1,6-

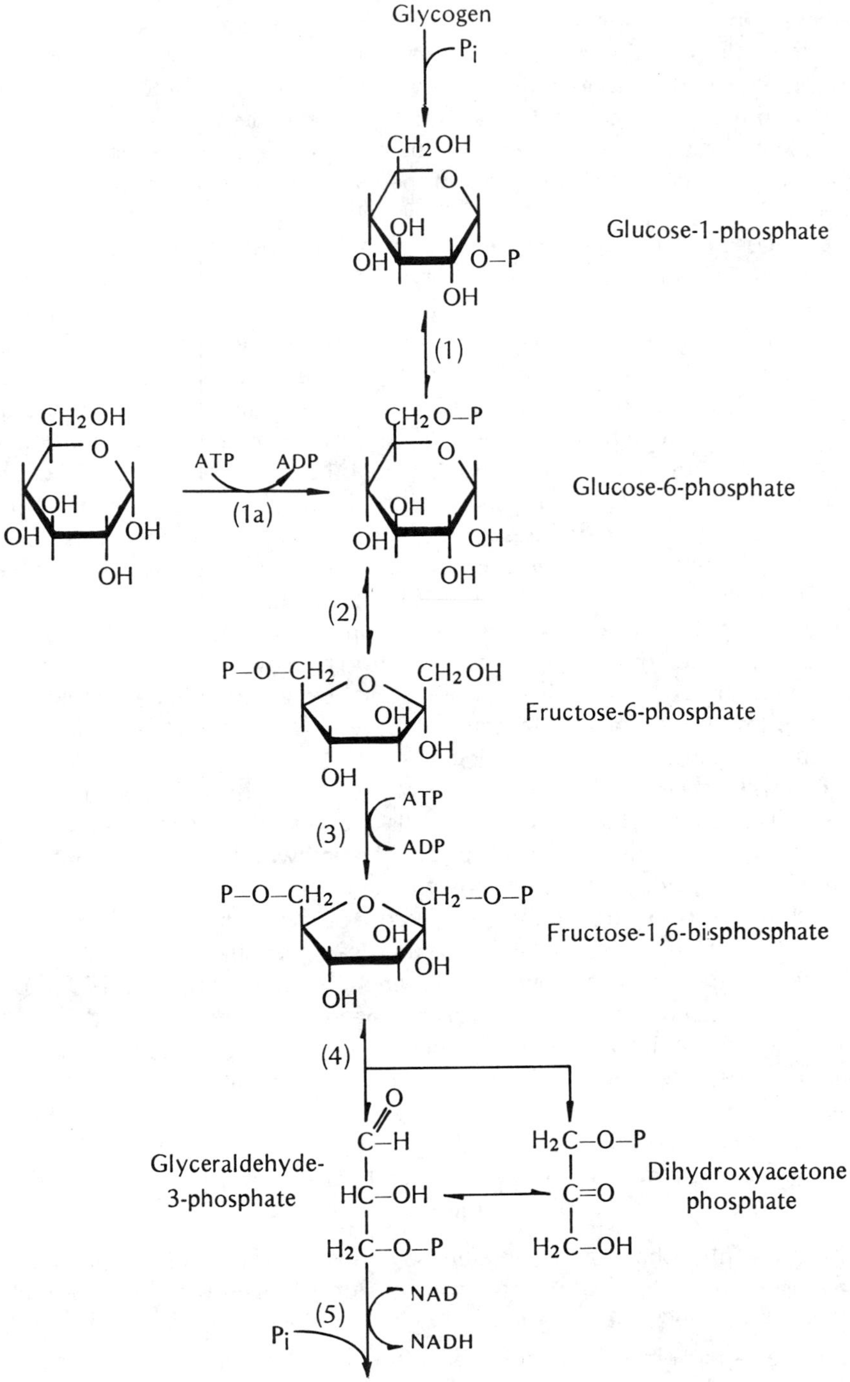

Glycogen

$\overset{\displaystyle\frown}{}P_i$

Glucose-1-phosphate

(1)

CH$_2$OH

ATP   ADP

(1a)

CH$_2$O–P

Glucose-6-phosphate

(2)

P–O–CH$_2$ CH$_2$OH

Fructose-6-phosphate

(3)   ATP

ADP

P–O–CH$_2$ CH$_2$–O–P

Fructose-1,6-bisphosphate

(4)

Glyceraldehyde-3-phosphate

$$\underset{\text{H}_2\text{C-O-P}}{\overset{\overset{\text{O}}{\parallel}}{\text{C–H}}}$$

HC–OH

Dihydroxyacetone phosphate

H$_2$C–O–P

C=O

H$_2$C–OH

(5)   NAD

P$_i$

NADH

424

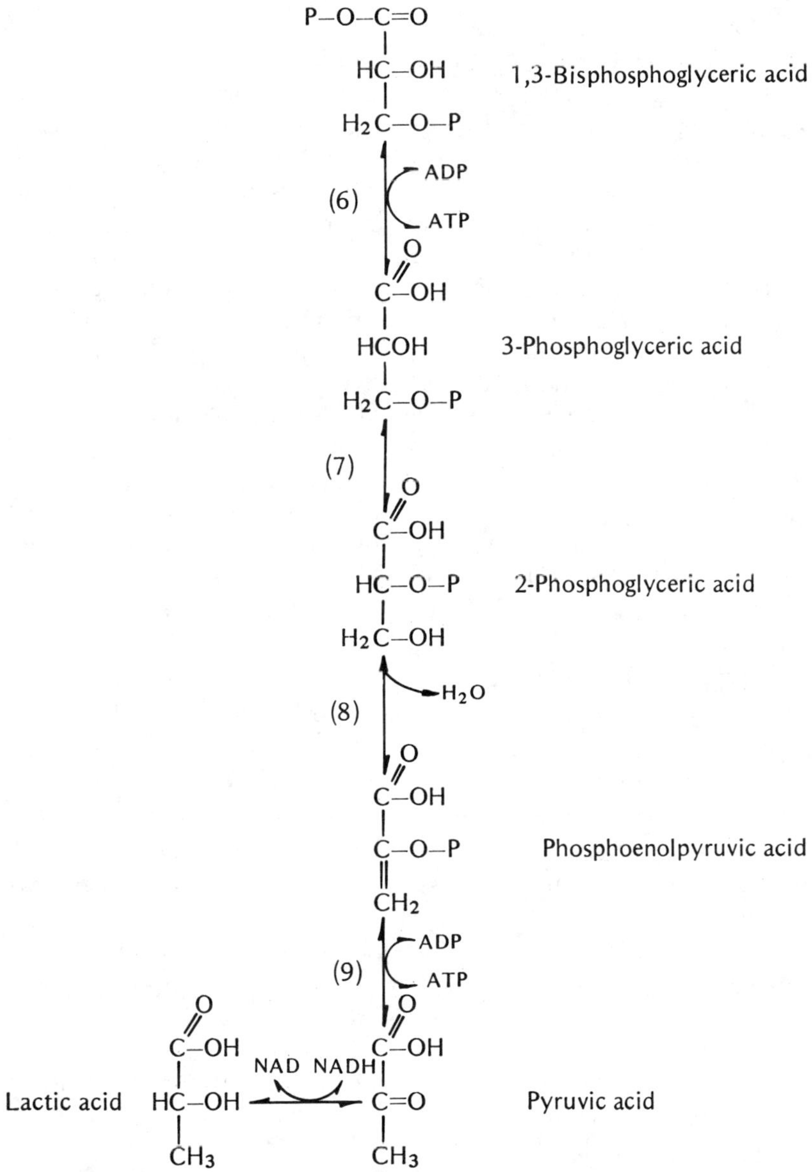

P—O—C=O
|
HC—OH   1,3-Bisphosphoglyceric acid
|
H_2C—O—P

(6) ⤵ ADP
     ⤴ ATP

O
‖
C—OH
|
HCOH   3-Phosphoglyceric acid
|
H_2C—O—P

(7)

O
‖
C—OH
|
HC—O—P   2-Phosphoglyceric acid
|
H_2C—OH

(8) → H_2O

O
‖
C—OH
|
C—O—P   Phosphoenolpyruvic acid
‖
CH_2

(9) ⤵ ADP
     ⤴ ATP

O   O
‖   ‖
C—OH   NAD NADH   C—OH
| |
Lactic acid   HC—OH ⟶   C=O   Pyruvic acid
| |
CH_3 CH_3

Figure 11.19
Embden-Meyerhof glycolytic pathway. Enzymes are (1) phosphoglucomutase, (1a) glucokinase, (2) phosphoglucoisomerase, (3) phosphofructokinase, (4) fructose bisphosphate aldolase, (5) glyceraldehyde-3-phosphate dehydrogenase, (6) phosphoglyceryl kinase, (7) phosphoglycerol mutase, (8) enolase, and (9) pyruvic kinase.

bisphosphatase utilized in gluconeogenesis does not yield a molecule of high energy phosphate, that is, generation of ATP.

4. Fructose-1,6-bisphosphate is cleaved in the middle to form two molecules of triose phosphates. The reaction is catalyzed by the enzyme fructosebisphosphate aldolase and generates glyceraldehyde-3-phosphate and dihydroxyacetone phosphate. The two triose phosphates are isomers and can be interconverted by the enzyme triose phosphate isomerase. Dihydroxyacetone phosphate may be utilized to form the glycerol portion of the triacylglycerol molecule (triglycerides), particularly in adipose tissue and muscle, and thus provides a link between carbohydrate metabolism and fat metabolism. From this point, carbohydrate metabolism proceeds from glyceraldehyde-3-phosphate, but, because this compound and dihydroxyacetone phosphate are interconvertible, in effect, two molecules of glyceraldehyde-3-phosphate are formed from one hexose unit.

5. The first step in the triose stage of glycolysis is the oxidation of glyceraldehyde-3-phosphate to 1,3-bisphosphoglycerate. The hydrogen thus released is taken up by NAD, which may be reoxidized by the mitochondrial electron transport system leading to the synthesis of three moles of ATP. (See Chapter 13.) In the absence of oxygen (anaerobic glycolysis), NADH is utilized in the formation of lactic acid (reaction 9).

6. The high energy phosphate in 1,3-bisphosphoglycerate (the 1-phosphate anhydride is a high energy bond) is transferred to ADP forming ATP and releasing 3-phosphoglycerate.

7. The phosphate group is reversibly transferred from C3 to C2 of glycerate, a reaction catalyzed by phosphoglyceromutase.

8. The 2-phosphoglycerate is subsequently dehydrated by the action of the enzyme, enolase, to form phosphoenolpyruvate, a high energy phosphate compound.

9. The final reaction of the Embden-Meyerhof pathway to pyruvate is the transfer of the high energy phosphate from phosphoenolpyruvate to ADP forming ATP. The enzyme responsible for catalysis is pyruvate kinase.

Pyruvic acid, thus formed, enters the mitochondrion for further oxidation. When the oxygen supply is low, as in prolonged muscular activity, pyruvic acid may be used to oxidize NADH, forming NAD and lactic acid. The reaction is catalyzed by the enzyme lactic dehydrogenase (LDH) and is coupled with the NADH-forming reaction between glyceraldehyde-3-phosphate and 1,3-bisphosphoglycerate, as shown below.

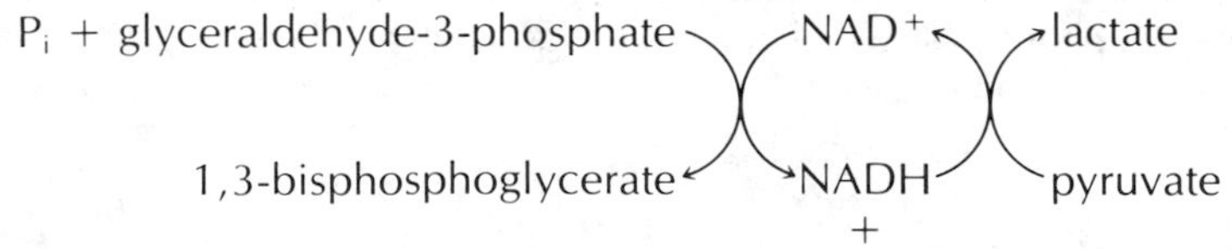

$$P_i + \text{glyceraldehyde-3-phosphate} \quad NAD^+ \quad \text{lactate}$$

$$\text{1,3-bisphosphoglycerate} \quad NADH + H^+ \quad \text{pyruvate}$$

Lactic dehydrogenase occurs in several molecular forms, or isozymes. At least five different isozymes are known to occur in animal tissues. The enzyme in heart (H_4) and the enzyme in skeletal muscle (M_4) have been shown to have very different kinetic properties that are, however, beautifully consistent with the functions of the two tissues. The heart enzyme is inhibited by pyruvate and is active only at low levels of pyruvate. This property assures a steady supply of necessary energy from the complete oxidation of pyruvate by way of the TCA cycle. In contrast, muscle LDH does not operate at maximum rate until pyruvate concentrations are quite high and, unlike the heart, energy demands can be supplied for short periods of time by anaerobic glycolysis in which ATP is generated. (See Fig. 11.19, reactions 6 and 9.) Thus LDH isozymes may operate in highly aerobic (H_4) or anaerobic (M_4) environments. Other forms of LDH (M_3H_1, M_2H_2, and M_1H_3) occur in tissues in which the metabolic activity is intermediate between these two extremes.

Furthermore, when the oxygen supply is low and large amounts of lactic acid are formed, the lactic acid, so produced, is transported to the liver for resynthesis to glycogen. (See Chapter 15.) This step is necessary since there is no enzymatic mechanism in muscle cells for the conversion of lactate to glucose. The cycling of lactic acid formed from anaerobic glycolysis in muscle to the liver for glycogen synthesis was first described by Carl and Gerti Cori and is known as the Cori Cycle. (See Cori, 1931.)

Although glycolysis may proceed in the presence or absence of oxygen, from the standpoint of energy yield to the cell aerobic glycolysis is the more efficient mechanism. The energy yield of anaerobic glycolysis is low. Two ATP are formed in the substrate level phosphorylation of reactions 6 and 9, a total of four ATP from one hexose unit yielding two triose units. Assuming glucose as the starting point, two ATP are used up in the phosphorylation of glucose and of fructose-6-phosphate and therefore must be subtracted from the total ATP produced. The net gain in ATP thus is only 2 moles.

When the oxygen supply is high, lactic acid is not formed and NADH synthesized in reaction 5 may be oxidized through the mitochondrial electron transport system. Six additional moles of ATP then are formed, three for each pair of electrons, assuming two triose units for each hexose. The total energy yield for aerobic glycolysis thus is eight ATP, exactly four times that of anaerobic glycolysis (Chapter 13).

If the starting point of glycolysis is glycogen rather than free glucose, which requires high energy phosphate, the energy yield is increased by one ATP for either aerobic or anerobic glycolysis.

Pentose Phosphate Shunt

The pentose phosphate shunt, sometimes called the hexose monophosphate shunt, is a significant alternative pathway for glucose oxidation. This pathway is active in liver, adipose tissue, adrenal cortex, thyroid, erythrocytes, testis, and lactating mammary gland. It is not active in nonlactating mammary gland, and activity is low in skeletal muscle. A major function of the pentose phosphate shunt is the provision of NADPH and ribose. Most of the tissues in which the shunt is active use the NADPH in the synthesis of fatty acids or steroids. The pentose phosphate shunt also provides pentoses for nucleotide and nucleic acid synthesis. Within the erythrocyte, NADPH is used for the reduction of oxidized glutathione, a reaction catalyzed by glutathione reductase. The reduced glutathione is used in the destruction of hydrogen peroxide by glutathione peroxidase, an essential reaction to prevent the oxidation of hemoglobin to methemoglobin by the H_2O_2.

The outline shown in Table 11.4 is simplified and is intended chiefly to point up reactions of special interest and significance in the total metabolic scheme. Six moles of glucose-6-phosphate enter into the chain of reactions during which 1 mole of glucose is oxidized completely by the shunt mechanism. The oxidation is accomplished entirely in reactions 1-3 in which $NADP^+$ is reduced to NADPH, CO_2 is released, and 6 moles of ribulose-5-phosphate are formed. The rest of the series results in the rearrangement of molecules to form compounds with 5, 7, 3, 4, and 6 carbon atoms in the chain leading ultimately to the final formation of 5 moles of glucose-6-phosphate, which can then reenter the cycle.

The overall reaction may be written as follows:

$$6 \text{ Glucose-6-phosphate} + 12 \text{ NADP}^+ \rightarrow$$
$$5 \text{ Glucose-6-phosphate} + 6 \text{ CO}_2 + 12 \text{ NADPH} + 12 \text{ H}^+ + \text{P}_i$$

The individual reactions are shown in Table 11.4 and are described below.

Reaction 1, 2, and 3

In two separate oxidation steps, NADP is hydrogen acceptor. NADPH, thus formed, may be oxidized by way of the electron transport system after

TABLE 11.4
Pentose Phosphate Shunt

1. Glucose-6-phosphate + $NADP^+$ $\xrightarrow{\text{glucose-6-phosphate dehydrogenase}}$ 6-Phosphogluconolactone

2. 6-Phosphogluconolactone + H_2O $\xrightarrow{\text{gluconolactonase}}$ 6-Phosphogluconate + H^+

3. 6-Phosphogluconate + $NADP^+$ $\xrightarrow{\text{6-phosphogluconate dehydrogenase}}$ Ribulose-5-phsophate + CO_2 + NADPH

4. Ribulose-5-phosphate $\xrightleftharpoons{\text{phosphoriboisomerase}}$ Ribose-5-phosphate

5. Ribulose-5-phosphate $\xrightleftharpoons{\text{ribulose-phosphate 3-epimerase}}$ Xylulose-5-phosphate

6. Xylulose-5-phosphate + ribose-5-phosphate $\xrightleftharpoons{\text{transketolase}}$ Glyceraldehyde-3-phosphate + Sedoheptulose-7-phosphate

7. Sedoheptulose-7-phosphate + Glyceraldehyde-3-phosphate $\xrightarrow{\text{transaldolase}}$ Fructose-6-phosphate + Erythrose-4-phosphate

8. Erythrose-4-phosphate + Xylulose-5-phosphate $\xrightleftharpoons{\text{transketolase}}$ Fructose-6-phosphate + Glyceraldehyde-3-phosphate

passing on its electrons to NAD (Chapter 13). There is no built-in system in this series of reactions for reoxidation of NADPH, such as occurs when NADH is reoxidized in the formation of lactic acid in the Embden-Meyerhof pathway. Highly significant, however, is the specific requirement for NADPH in certain cellular reactions such as synthesis of fatty acids and cholesterol, conversion of phenylalanine to tyrosine, and reduction of dihydrofolic acid to tetrahydrofolic acid. These specific requirements are met in large part by the pentose phosphate shunt production of NADPH.

Reaction 4

Ribose formed by isomerization of ribulose-5-phosphate may be utilized directly in synthesis of ribonucleic acid and nucleotides such as NAD, ATP, and UTP.

Reaction 5 and 6

Ribulose-5-phosphate may also isomerize to form the 5-carbon keto sugar, xylulose-5-phosphate, which in turn may react with ribose-5-phosphate, an aldo sugar, to form the 7-carbon sedoheptulose and the 3-carbon glyceraldehyde-3-phosphate. The reaction is one of a general group catalyzed by the enzyme, *transketolase*, which catalyzes the transfer of a ketol grouping

$$\begin{pmatrix} CH_2\!-\!OH \\ | \\ C\!=\!O \\ | \end{pmatrix} \text{ to an aldehyde acceptor } H \begin{pmatrix} H \\ | \\ C\!=\!O \\ | \end{pmatrix} \text{ and}$$

which requires thiamin pyrophosphate (TPP) and Mg^{++} as cofactors. The transketolase enzyme may also catalyze the transfer of a ketol group from xylulose-5-phosphate to erythrose-4-phosphate to form fructose-6-phosphate and glyceraldehyde-3-phosphate **(reaction 8).** The importance of the transketolase reaction in the study of thiamin deficiency will be dealt with in a later section (Chapter 24).

Reaction 7

The reaction between sedoheptulose-7-phosphate and glyceraldehyde-3-phosphate is not a transketolase reaction, but is catalyzed by a transaldolase enzyme involving the transfer of a dihydroxyacetone grouping

$$\begin{pmatrix} CH_2OH \\ | \\ C\!=\!O \\ | \\ HOCH \\ | \end{pmatrix}$$

to an aldose acceptor. This reaction does not require TPP as a coenzyme.

Glycogenesis

The formation of glycogen, *glycogenesis*, involves the addition of a glucose unit to an already existing glycogen chain. Since the glycogen molecule is not a stable structure, but constantly changes as glucose units are added or removed, glycogen may be designated for convenience as comprised of n glucose units. The first step in the addition of a glucose residue to the glycogen molecule is the conversion of glucose-6-phosphate to glucose-1-phosphate, catalyzed by phosphoglucomutase. The glucose-1-phosphate then reacts with a nucleotide, uridine triphosphate (UTP), to yield uridine diphosphateglucose (UDPG) and inorganic pyrophosphate. The UDPG donates glucose residues used for extending the terminal branches of glycogen in a reaction catalyzed by glycogen synthase; a molecule of UDP is released for each glucosyl residue added. UTP may be regenerated by transfer of a high energy phosphate from ATP (ATP + UDP $\rightleftharpoons$ ADP + UTP). These reactions are depicted in Fig. 11.20.

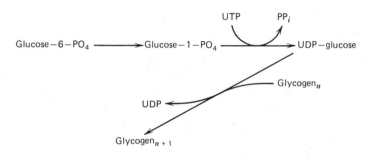

Figure 11.20
Glycogenesis.

As the additions of glucosyl residues simply extend the 1,4 chain, only long amylose chains would be made by the reactions utilizing glycogen synthase. Glycogen is normally highly branched; therefore, a mechanism is required for this addition. Cells storing glycogen also have a branching enzyme, glycosyl-4:6-transferase, which catalyzes the transfer of a segment of an amylose chain to the C6 hydroxyl of a neighboring chain. This enzyme transfers a block of approximately seven 1,4-residues from a chain at least 11 residues in length and transfers it to another segment of amylose chain at a point 4 residues removed from the nearest branch.

Fatty Acid Synthesis

Fatty acids may be synthesized by at least two pathways: (1) elongation of existing fatty acid chains by addition of two-carbon acetyl CoA units, such as the conversion of palmitic to stearic acid, and (2) *de novo* synthesis from acetyl CoA, that is, the formation of a fatty acid from two-carbon units only. The former pathway is a function of the cytoplasm and the mitochondria (Chapter 13); the latter pathway appears to be limited to the soluble fraction of the cytoplasm.

The key compound in *de novo* synthesis of fatty acids is not acetyl CoA but a compound derived from the acetyl unit, malonyl CoA. The discovery by Wakil (1958) of malonyl CoA as an intermediate in fatty acid biosynthesis was a major contribution to the understanding of the process involved. *De novo* synthesis is referred to as the palmitate-synthesizing system and converts acetyl CoA to long chain fatty acids. The reactions involved require ATP, HCO_3^- (as a source of CO_2), Mn^{++}, and NADPH.

There appear to be two types of fatty acid synthase systems in the soluble portion of the cell. In bacteria, plants, and some single cell organisms, the individual enzymes of the system may be separate and the acyl groups are found in combination with a protein called acyl carrier protein. However, in mammals, the synthase is a multienzyme complex that cannot be subdivided without loss of activity and acyl carrier protein is part of this complex. Acyl carrier protein contains a 4'-phosphopantetheinyl residue (which is derived from the vitamin pantothenic acid) and it is to the sulfhydryl group of the 4'-phosphopantetheinyl residue that the acyl groups are linked through a thio-ester linkage. (see chapter 3.)

The first step in fatty acid synthesis is the formation of malonyl CoA from acetyl CoA. The reaction is catalyzed by acetyl CoA carboxylase, a biotin-containing enzyme, which requires Mn^{++} as a cofactor. The reaction is shown below:

$$CH_3CO-SCoA + HCO_3^- + ATP \xrightarrow{Mn^{++}} {}^-OOCCH_2CO-SCoA + ADP + P_i$$
Acetyl CoA   **Malonyl CoA**

The synthesis of fatty acids begins with the binding of an acetyl or butyryl group (from acetyl CoA or butyryl CoA) to the sulfhydryl group of the 4'-phosphopan-

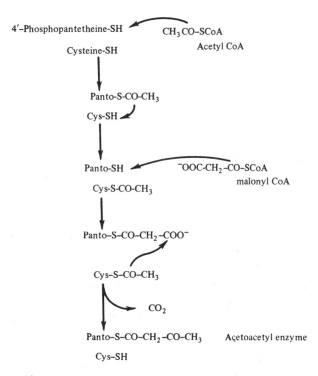

Figure 11.21
Assembly of the carbon chain in fatty acid synthesis.

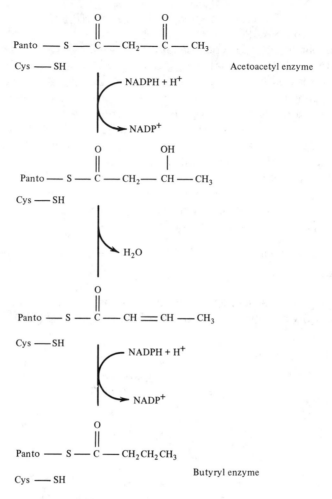

Figure 11.22
Reduction of the β-ketoacyl group to a saturated acyl group during fatty acid synthesis.

tetheinyl residue. (Acetyl groups are used as starter molecules by mammalian adipose tissue; butyryl groups are used by mammalian liver and mammary glands). (See Volpe and Vagelos, 1976.) The acyl group is then transferred to a cysteine residue of the synthase enzyme and a malonyl group is now bound to the 4'-phosphopantetheine. The malonyl group then moves into the proximity of the acyl group, and the groups condense. The condensation involves transfer of the acyl group to the malonyl group which is simultaneously decarboxylated, as shown in Fig. 11.21.

The next steps convert the 3-keto acyl group to the corresponding saturated acyl group. The compound is first reduced to the D-(−)-β-hydroxyacyl group

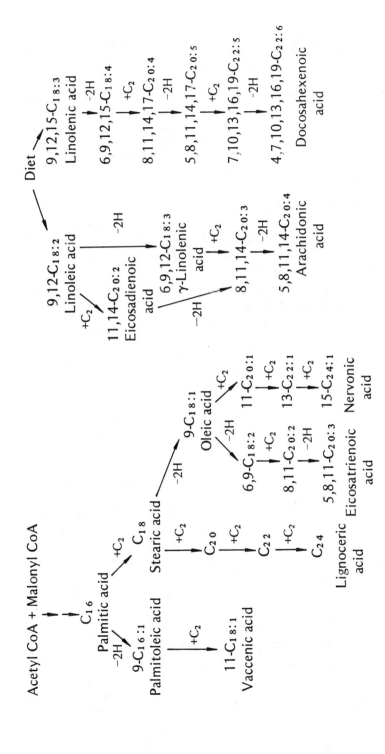

Figure 11.23
Biosynthesis of some fatty acids in mammals. The numbers in boldface indicate the position of the double bonds; the subscripts indicate the number of carbon atoms, with the number of double bonds to the right of the colon. See text on p. 434. (From A. White et al., *Principles of Biochemistry*, 5th ed., McGraw Hill, New York, 1973, p. 567).

which is subsequently dehydrated to form the α,β-unsaturated acyl group. This group is then reduced again to form the fully saturated acyl group still bound to the 4'-phosphopantetheine residue. Both reductions are accomplished by NADPH. (See Fig. 11.22.)

The acyl group, so formed, is then transferred to the cysteine residue, the phosphopantetheine residue loaded with a malonyl group from malonyl CoA and the reactions are repeated as described in Figs. 11.21 and 11.22. The chain continues to grow until a 16-carbon residue (palmitoyl group) is generated, at which point the chain is released as palmitic acid. The palmitate is converted to palmitoyl CoA and may then be elongated by reactions exactly analagous to those detailed above, but which are accomplished on the endoplasmic reticulum.

Synthesis of Unsaturated Fatty Acids

Of the various unsaturated fatty acids present in animal tissues only one series of compounds can be synthesized in the animal body. These unsaturated fatty acids contain double bonds only between the carboxyl group and the seventh carbon from the terminal methyl group (Chapter 2) and derive from the palmityl synthesizing system. The various fatty acids are subsequently produced by alternate desaturation and elongation of the carbon chains (Fig. 11.23). The latter reactions occur to a greater extent in liver than in other tissues.

The essential fatty acids all contain one or more double bonds within the terminal seven carbons of the fatty acid chain. For this reason they cannot be synthesized by the body and must be supplied in the diet. These acids also undergo alternate desaturation and elongation resulting in the formation of other more unsaturated fatty acids of longer chain length. (See Fig. 11.23.)

Conclusion

The endoplasmic reticulum is part of the continuous and dynamic membrane structure of the cell. It not only provides mechanical support for the cytoplasmic contents of the cell but also provides its transport lanes. The concentration of membranous endoplasmic reticulum varies with the synthetic activity of the cell, sparse in those cells in which synthesis is limited to internal needs, and extremely dense in those that are active in synthesizing proteins for export. The cytoplasmic matrix is the transport medium in which all nutrients and metabolites are carried on their way from one organelle to another. It also is the medium in which specific metabolic reactions take place. The reticulum and the matrix, therefore, provide the lanes of communication within the cell and to the exterior. In this way, they contribute both to the movement of metabolites and to their temporary sequestration.

chapter 12

the golgi apparatus

The Golgi apparatus was barely mentioned in the first edition of this book beyond noting its presence and indicating its function. Details of how it performed its suggested assembly-line function of packaging synthesized products for export were not sufficiently deciphered to warrant more extended treatment. Now the status of the Golgi apparatus as an organelle of consequence is fully established. No longer are there disbelievers in its existence. It is known to occupy a key position in the transport system of the cell and, according to Northcote (1971), "acts like a valve in controlling the distribution of cellular material."

In 1898 Golgi discovered a structure in the cell close to the nucleus that he called the internal reticular apparatus. Many cytologists thought this was an artifact attributable to his staining technique since it could not be seen in the living cell nor with routine stains. Not until the 1950s and the advent of the electron microscope was it finally established that, skeptics notwithstanding, such an organelle did exist as Golgi had indicated. Further, this organelle, now called the *Golgi apparatus* or *Golgi complex*, can be found in almost all mammalian cells. In fact, it has come to be one of the readily identifiable components of the cell in electron micrographs (Fig. 12.1).

Structure

The Golgi complex consists mainly of smooth surfaced membranes that, in electron micrographs, appear as a stack of more or less flattened vesicles that are variously called *cisternae, lamellae,* or *saccules*. These stacks may appear singly or, in secretory cells, several may appear together. They vary in size and usually contain from five to eight lamellae but may contain many more in a slightly curved stack (Fig. 12.2). The stack is the *dictyosome*. The location and size of the dic-

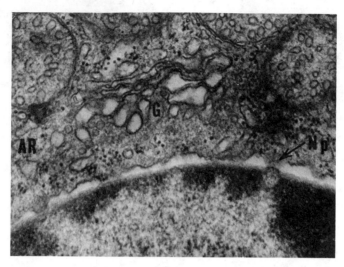

Figure 12.1
Golgi complex (G) showing flattened sacs and clusters of vacuoles. The reticulum (AR) is the smooth or agranular type. Mitochondria show the tubular cristae seen in adrenal cortical cells.
NP = nuclear pore. Adrenal cortex of rat. Magnification ×
56,800. (Courtesy of Dr. Harald Schraer.)

tyosome varies among cell types and also with the physiological state of the cell.
Generally, the dictyosomes are polarized so that one pole is associated with the
endoplasmic reticulum or the nuclear envelope. This is the proximal pole and is
the *forming face* or *immature face*. These cisternae are usually flat and appear
empty, and the membranes are similar in structure and enzyme composition to
those of the endoplasmic reticulum. The opposite pole is concave and is closer
to the plasma membrane. This is the distal pole or *maturing face*. In secretory
cells the distal pole faces the apex of the cell through which the secretory product
is delivered. The ends of the cisternae in this part of the complex are often bulbous
and swollen in appearance. Dictyosomes are surrounded by regions of differentiated cytoplasm that are nearly devoid of other cell components. This is referred
to as the zone of exclusion (Mollenhauer, 1965).

Transfer vesicles bud off from the transitional elements of the rough endoplasmic
reticulum which lacks polysomes on the membrane adjacent to the forming face
of the Golgi stack. Jamieson and Palade (1966) suggest that transfer vesicles act
as "shuttle" vesicles. They fuse with the Golgi lamellae bringing with them the
enclosed quantities of material synthesized by the rough endoplasmic reticulum.
In this way membrane is continuously added to the forming face of the Golgi
stack. This membrane resembles that of the endoplasmic reticulum in thickness
and staining characteristics (Grove et al., 1968; Morré et al., 1970).

Condensing vacuoles that are large and light appear at the mature face of the

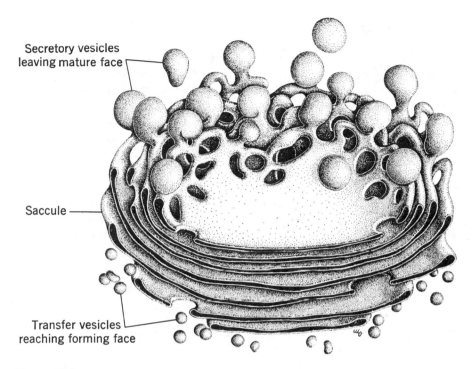

Secretory vesicles
leaving mature face

Saccule

Transfer vesicles
reaching forming face

Figure 12.2
Drawing depicting the Golgi apparatus of a secretory cell in three dimensions. The
transfer vesicles shown below are in this instance small enough to be termed micro-
vesicles, but in some kinds of cells they are larger. The transfer vesicles bud off from
rough-surfaced endoplasmic reticulum, which would be below. The secretory vesicles
that bud off from saccules on the mature face become, in the instance of acinar cells,
the so-called zymogen granules. (From A. W. Ham and D. H. Cormack, *Histology*,
8th ed., J. B. Lippincott, Philadelphia, 1979, p. 131.)

stack. These, like the transfer vesicles, sometimes appear to be continuous with
the lamellae. The vacuoles pinch off from the ovoid, swollen ends of the lamellae
and carry away the secretion. After becoming progressively smaller and denser,
they are often called *zymogen granules*. They move toward the plasma membrane
or apex of the secretory cell and discharge their contents by exocytosis. In the
process, the membrane of the vacuole, which by now resembles the plasma
membrane in thickness and staining intensity, fuses with it (Dalton, 1961; Grove
et al., 1968; Morré et al., 1970). This membrane leaving the stack balances that
brought to the forming face by the transfer vesicles.

The entire membranous complex of the Golgi apparatus is in a dynamic state,
constantly being renewed. The vesicle merges with the lamellae at the forming
face and the vacuole pinches off or "blebs" at the mature surface to migrate to
the plasma membrane (Morré et al., 1971b). This renewal is part of a larger system

of renewal designated as membrane flow that will be discussed in the section on function.

From work on Golgi lamellae in tissue culture cells, Takagi et al. (1965) found that these were flexible and elastic structures. The gradient they exhibit in morphology, from endoplasmic reticulumlike to plasma membranelike, results from either difference in chemical composition or the arrangement of molecules within the membrane (Morré et al., 1971a). In the transformation of endoplasmic reticulum membrane into Golgi membrane, enzymatic activities and prosthetic groups are progressively lost. The lecithin content of Golgi membranes and the chemical lipoprotein composition is intermediate between that of endoplasmic reticulum and plasma membrane (Keenan and Morré, 1970; Yunghans et al., 1970). Gel electrophoresis patterns are intermediate between plasma membrane and endoplasmic reticulum as far as appearance and number and position of the bands but resemble more closely the pattern of endoplasmic reticulum (Yunghans et al., 1970).

Concentrated in the Golgi complex are ADPase, Mg^{++}ATPase, CTPase, TPPase, and acid phosphatase. In addition, there are high concentrations of UDP-*N*-acetylglycosamine transferase and galactosyl transferase, but glucose-6-phosphatase, which is characteristic of the endoplasmic reticulum, is in low concentration in the Golgi complex (DeRobertis and DeRobertis, 1980). Enzyme activities change when endoplasmic reticulum membranes are incorporated into Golgi saccules (Novikoff et al., 1962). In cells where TPPase is not present in the endoplasmic reticulum, the Golgi membrane acquires it or, if the endoplasmic reticulum had such activity, it becomes higher in the Golgi. Then, when the vacuoles leave the Golgi complex, they lose the TPPase activity (Novikoff, 1962). Another change observed is the loss of nucleoside diphosphatase activity from the endoplasmic reticulum to the saccule (Novikoff, ibid.).

How the Golgi complex originates has not been established. It is clear that it multiplies in some way since there is no decrease in number after cell divisions (Morré et al., 1971c). How multiplication occurs is far from clear but over the years several suggestions have been made including *de novo* formation (Flickinger, 1969); derivation from preexisting Golgi material by division (Whaley, 1966) or fragmentation (Mollenhauer and Morré, 1966); and derivation from another membrane system of the cell. (See Beams and Kessel, 1968.) The arguments are not strong for *de novo* synthesis and studies of dividing cells have shown fragmentation of the Golgi complex followed by a quantitative separation between the two daughter cells. Opinion concerning division has not changed in over 50 years since Bowen (1926) stated that the Golgi complex maintained itself through a process of mass division that was much like fragmentation and had nothing in common with the precise division observed for nuclear material.

According to Morré et al. (1971c) the Golgi apparatus appears to be formed from dictyosomes that arise one cisterna at a time. Fig. 12.3 summarizes the series of postulated stages leading up to dictyosome formation, one cisterna at a time, by what appears to be fusion of vesicles in a cytoplasmic zone of exclusion.

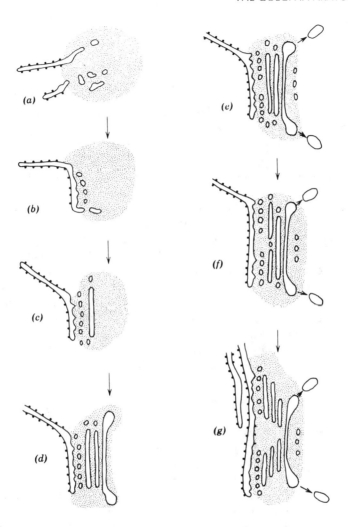

Figure 12.3
Hypothetical scheme relating observations concerning the origin and continuity of Golgi apparatus. (a→d) In the absence of preexisting dictyosomes, cisternae are presumed to arise from small groups of vesicles associated with the endoplasmic reticulum or nuclear envelope. Further differentiation gives rise to flattened platelike cisternae. Additional cisternae form by multiplication of this process. (e→g) Multiplication of Golgi apparatus suggested by formation of two sets of shorter cisternae where there was previously one longer cisterna. Continued separation leads to formation of two daughter stacks. (From D. J. Morré et al., *Origin and Continuity of Cell Organelles*, Vol. 2, Springer-Verlag, New York, 1971, p. 82.)

Function

MEMBRANE FLOW

An important function of the Golgi complex alluded to in the section on structure is the role it plays in *membrane flow*. Biochemical and morphological studies both indicate that plasma membranes are derived from the nuclear membranes or endoplasmic reticulum via the Golgi complex, and that this occurs through a process of membrane flow and differentiation. Morré and Ovtracht (1977) describe this concept as one in which membranes move along a chain of cell components that serve as a developmental pathway. As the membranes move along this path they are transformed. This membrane flow and change is apparent from the endoplasmic reticulum to the plasma membrane via the Golgi apparatus.

Kinetic evidence of membrane flow was obtained from short-time labeling studies with rat liver cells (Morré et al., 1971a). Fractions obtained from liver cells of rats injected with ^{14}C-arginine were assayed for the marker. The order of the labeling was endoplasmic reticulum or nucleus, Golgi apparatus, and plasma membrane. Radioactivity increased steadily in the plasma membrane and decreased rapidly in the endoplasmic reticulum and Golgi apparatus. Morré and Ovtracht (1977) conclude that membrane differentiation coupled with membrane flow account for the origin of the plasma membrane from the endoplasmic reticulum, with the Golgi apparatus acting as the mediator (Fig. 12.4).

Membranes of secretory vesicles are morphologically similar to plasma membranes and fuse with plasma membranes when the product is extruded (Sjöstrand, 1963; Helminen and Ericsson, 1968). Jamieson (1971) suggests that the cell probably reuses its intracellular membranes extensively during the course of transport and discharge of secretory proteins. In addition, the discharge of the secretory product requires respiratory energy, and this may be related to the membrane fusion process involved in zymogen discharge. Similarly, the membrane of a phagocytosed particle is plasma membrane, and this is replaced by flow through the synthetic assembly maintained by the Golgi complex.

There are suggestions, also, that the Golgi complex may function in the formation of "new" membrane since the assembly of lamellae or cisternal envelopes increases substantially under some conditions, and the Golgi apparatus is the logical place for this activity to occur (Whaley et al., 1971). Fawcett (1962) postulated that membrane components might be withdrawn from the plasma membrane and then reassembled in the Golgi region. Hokin (1968) suggested that membrane subunits are transferred to the endoplasmic reticulum and to the Golgi complex for reassembly (Fig. 12.5). In either case, on leaving the Golgi complex the membrane may function as plasma membrane, membrane bounding vesicles, vacuoles, or some other intracytoplasmic membrane system. There is no doubt that an important function of the Golgi complex is in the assembly of membrane, its differentiation in both structure and enzyme constituents, and its transfer to other membrane-bound organelles such as lysosomes (Whaley, 1968).

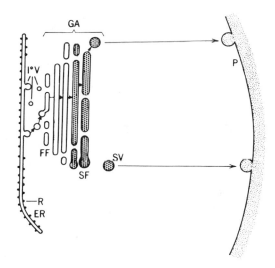

Figure 12.4
Diagrammatic representation of Golgi apparatus functioning in membrane flow and differentiation. ER, endoplasmic reticulum; R, ribosome; GA, Golgi apparatus; FF, forming
face; SF, secreting face; 1°, primary vesicle; SV, secretory vesicle; PM, plasma membrane.
Direction of membrane flow and vesicle migration denoted by arrows. (From D. J. Morré
et al., *Biomembranes*, Vol. 2, Plenum Press, New York, 1971, p. 95.)

In order to function in this manner, it is clear that there must be integration of
function among cellular organelles and recycling of the membrane constituents.

CELL SURFACE MATERIALS

Associated with the role of the Golgi apparatus in membrane flow is its role in
providing the cell with materials that confer surface specificity to membranes.
These materials are either on the outer surface of the membrane, the *cell coat*
(*glycocalyx*), components of the plasma membrane itself, or cell surface-associ-
ated materials. The surface specificity provides for selective uptake of materials
through adhesion characteristics, receptor sites, ion permeability, antigen specificity, and the like. Such cell surface information plays a role in interactions
between cells and between an individual cell and its environment; in gamete
recognition; in cell differentiation during development; in development of tissue
structure; in specialized function of intestinal microvilli including enzyme content
and specific receptor sites; and other similar functions dependent on recognition
phenomena. Many of the macromolecules that confer such specificity have carbohydrate moieties, and it is the Golgi apparatus that functions in the synthesis
of these polysaccharides and attaches them to the protein moiety in the formation
of such substances as glycoproteins and mucopolysaccharides. Genetic control

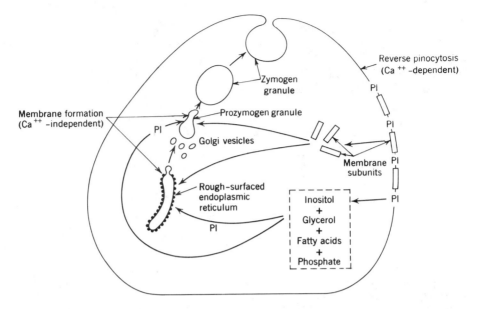

Figure 12.5
A possible mechanism of membrane circulation based on subunit relocation. Membrane added to the plasma membrane following coalescence of a zymogen granule is broken down into subunits and released back into the cytoplasm. The breakdown into subunits possibly is due to hydrolysis of phosphatidylinositol (PI) postulated to link subunits together. In this way, membrane lost from the endoplasmic reticulum and Golgi apparatus in the formation of zymogen granules is replaced by reassembly of subunits in these organelles through the resynthesis of phosphatidylinositol to join them together. (From C. E. Hokin, *Internatl. Rev. Cytol.* 23:187, 1968.)

is exerted through the enzymes present in the membranes of the Golgi complex for the synthesis of the particular carbohydrate components. It is the specific carbohydrate component linked to the specific protein material that provides the informational properties. Through membrane flow and recycling of the surface materials, changes in information can be provided (Whaley and Dauwalder, 1979).

The relationship between the polysaccharide synthesis in the Golgi complex and its localization at the cell surface has been established through a variety of staining procedures (Rambourg and Leblond, 1967; Rambourg et al., 1969). Further evidence has been obtained through radioautographic techniques indicating the uptake of labeled sugars directly into the Golgi complex and their subsequent secretion as part of a surface macromolecule (Ito, 1969; Bennett, 1970; Bennett and Leblond, 1970). Revel and Ito (1967) postulated that this mechanism is similar to other secretory mechanisms except that the Golgi-synthesized material remains attached to the membrane when the membrane is exteriorized.

SECRETION

The Golgi apparatus is highly developed in secretory cells, especially those cells secreting protein or complex polysaccharides. The secretory mechanism in each case has been followed by autoradiography as well as through fractionation procedures. Using leucine-^{14}C and following its incorporation into chymotrypsinogen by pancreatic acinar cells, Siekevitz and Palade (1958) observed rapid uptake by the ribosomes and endoplasmic reticulum, followed later by the transfer of the label to the Golgi apparatus and related vesicles and then into zymogen granules for export from the cell. From this and other related studies they described the secretory cycle that is now well defined: (1) incorporation of amino acids into polypeptides by the rough endoplasmic reticulum, (2) transfer of the nascent proteins into the cisternae of the endoplasmic reticulum, (3) intracellular transport to the Golgi apparatus for packaging into zymogen granules, and (4) migration of zymogen granules in the vacuoles toward the apex of the cell for discharge into the lumen of the gland (Fig. 12.6). The procedure is rapid, and Caro and Palade (1964) showed with the use of leucine-^{3}H that within 5 minutes after injection the label appeared in the rough endoplasmic reticulum; by 20 minutes, in the Golgi complex; and after 60 minutes the label was in the zymogen granules. It has since been established that the smooth surfaced vesicles are the means of transport from the rough endoplasmic reticulum to the Golgi complex (Jamieson and Palade, 1965; 1966; 1967a; 1967b); that the secretory protein is carried from the Golgi complex by the condensing vacuoles; and that progressive concentration occurs in the vacuoles in the formation of zymogen granules.

In many cells the synthesis of complex carbohydrates, such as glycoproteins, mucopolysaccharides, and glycolipids, takes place in the Golgi complex. This was demonstrated in the mucus-secreting goblet cells of rat colon. Using radioautographic techniques, Neutra and Leblond (1966) found that 5 minutes after the injection of ^{3}H-glucose the label was in the cisternae of the Golgi complex; at 20 minutes both the cisternae and mucinigen granules were labeled; by 40 minutes all the label was in the mucinigen; and within 1–4 hours the labeled granules had migrated from the region of the Golgi complex to the apex of the cell for extrusion. From this it was concluded that the Golgi complex is the area for the synthesis of the complex carbohydrate that is joined to protein delivered to it from the endoplasmic reticulum to form the glycoprotein of the mucus (Fig. 12.7). Neutra and Leblond (1966) estimated that one distended saccule was transformed into mucigen granules and released by each Golgi stack every 2–4 minutes. This is indicative of a rapid renewal of the Golgi stack by addition to the immature face. The entire Golgi apparatus in the mucus-secreting goblet cells of the colon was estimated to be formed and re-formed within 20–40 minutes.

The Golgi complex is also the site of sulfonation of the carbohydrates of mucus (Berlin, 1967) and for the addition of sulfate to chondroitin in collagen formation (Neutra and Leblond, 1969).

Many cell products are known to be packaged and transported through the Golgi apparatus and its associated vesicles. Many of these are polysaccharides,

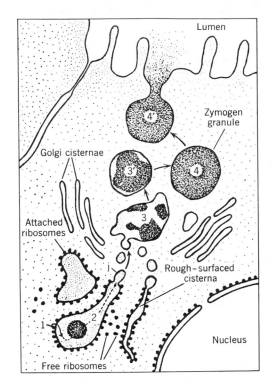

Figure 12.6
Diagram summarizing events in elaboration of the enzyme secretion in the pancreatic acinar cell. (1) Synthesis of the secretory protein on the ribosomes and into the channel of the endoplasmic reticulum. (2) Transfer of the nascent protein out of the endoplasmic reticulum into transfer vesicles formed by blebbing of the wall. (3) Fusion of isolated vesicles with condensing vacuoles of Golgi complex. (4) Conversion into zymogen granules and release from cell. (From G. E. Palade et al., *Ciba Foundation Symposium on Exocrine Pancreas, Normal and Abnormal Functions,* A. V. S. Rueck and M. P. Cameron, eds., Churchill, London, 1962, p. 23.)

or they are proteins or lipids that acquire carbohydrate moieties to become glycoproteins or glycolipoproteins in the membranes of the Golgi apparatus. In fact, Northcote (1971) speculates that conjugation with carbohydrate may be a prerequisite for subsequent transport of materials across the plasma membrane. If indeed this is so, the role of the Golgi apparatus takes on even greater significance.

Only the complex carbohydrates attached to protein and destined for secretion are synthesized in the Golgi complex. Glycogen is not synthesized there but in the cytoplasm instead. (See Chapter 11.)

For further discussion of Golgi complex involvement in the synthesis of complex carbohydrate, see Neutra and Leblond (1969).

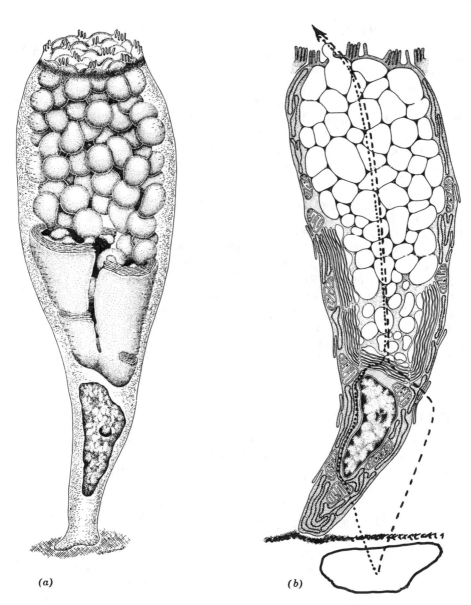

(a)   (b)

Figure 12.7
(a) Diagram illustrating the relationship of the Golgi complex and mucigen granules in colonic goblet cells. (b) This illustrates the activity within the goblet cell based on the radioautographic studies of Neutra and Leblond (1966). This diagram indicates the entrance of amino acids into the goblet cells from a capillary where they are synthesized into protein in association with the endoplasmic reticulum. The newly synthesized proteins are transported to the Golgi complex which synthesizes carbohydrate. The carbohydrate is added to the incoming protein, both materials being packaged in the Golgi region and released. The mucigen granules then migrate to the apical end of the cell and are released to the exterior. (Courtesy of Dr. C. P. Leblond.)

LYSOSOME FORMATION

The formation of lysosomes by the Golgi apparatus is analogous to the synthesis of protein secretion granules and is discussed in detail in Chapter 14. This role of the Golgi apparatus may be considered synthesis of catabolic agents; that is, synthesis of enzymes into vesicles whose membranes have the capacity to fuse with endocytotic vesicles or the plasma membrane itself for catabolic purposes. The informational characteristics of the lysosomal membrane, incorporated into it in the Golgi complex during synthesis, endow it with the capacity to ferret out only specific membranes with which to merge and to shun all others.

PHOSPHOLIPID SYNTHESIS

Membrane phospholipids may be synthesized by a variety of cell components including both rough and smooth endoplasmic reticulum (Stein and Stein, 1969). However, if the Golgi complex is implicated in changing endoplasmic reticulum-like to plasma membranelike membranes, this involves a change in lipid composition (Morré et al., 1971a). In the transition toward the plasma membrane type, there is an increase in the proportion of sphingomyelin and sterols with a corresponding decrease in the proportion of phosphatidyl choline (lecithin). In Golgi apparatus fractions from rat liver, Morré et al. (1970) found choline kinase and phosphorylcholinecytidyl transferase important in lecithin and sphingomyelin metabolism.

LIPOPROTEIN SYNTHESIS

The synthesis and transport of lipoprotein particles in liver cells studied by Morré and his group (Morré et al., 1971b) illustrate the multistep, continuous process in which lipids, sterols, and polysaccharides are added to the protein component (Fig. 12.8). During the process the protein particles migrate from their area of origin in the rough endoplasmic reticulum through what appears to be smooth endoplasmic reticulum to the transfer vesicles of the Golgi complex. The integration of structure and function is apparent from the associated changes in membrane type with change in activity as the synthetic process proceeds through the cisternal channels to the secretory vacuoles. The enzyme complement in the Golgi complex membranes may well serve both in the synthesis of membrane components and of products synthesized for export.

Nyquist et al. (1971) suggested that the involvement of the Golgi apparatus of liver cells in lipoprotein transport may be but one aspect of a broader function that could include the fat-soluble vitamins, particularly vitamin A. The vitamin A content of the Golgi complex fraction of liver cells was found to parallel the vitamin A status of the animal, and no vitamin A was detected in the fraction from vitamin A-deficient rats. A role for the Golgi complex in the mobilization and transport of vitamin A compounds was suggested. Alternative, or possibly additional, roles of vitamin A might be related to its function in changing the

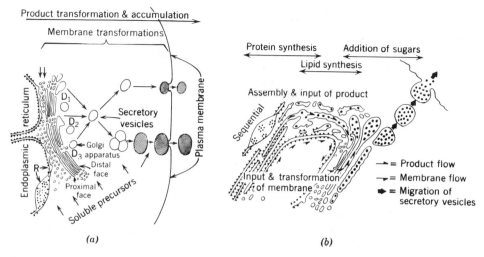

Figure 12.8
Summary of the structural and functional relationships among Golgi apparatus, endoplasmic reticulum, secretory vesicles, and the plasma membrane. The common function
of the Golgi complex in the different cell types appears to be the transformation of membranes from endoplasmic reticulumlike to plasma membranelike. (a) In polysaccharide-
or mucopolysaccharide-secreting cells, product formation is associated with progressive
changes in both cisternal and vesicle contents. (b) In hepatocytes the synthesis and transport
of lipoprotein particles (solid black dots) is visualized as a continuous multistep process
with the addition of lipids, sterols, and polysaccharides to the protein component. At the
same time the particles migrate from the point of origin to the secretory vesicles. (From
D. J. Morré et al., *Origin and Continuity of Cell Organelles*, Vol. 2, Springer-Verlag, New
York, 1971, p. 82.)

properties of cytoplasmic and lysosomal membranes (Dingle and Lucy, 1965),
and in mucopolysaccharide synthesis.

HORMONE SYNTHESIS AND SECRETION

In general, the Golgi complex in cells of endocrine glands secreting protein and
peptide hormones is the area where the product is concentrated and formed into
droplets enclosed in a membrane. Usually after a period of storage the secretory
product is released through the plasma membrane through exocytosis.

The role of the Golgi complex in the thyroid gland is somewhat different since
there is no storage of the secretion within the cell. Instead, the secretion is stored
in a follicle as the colloid thyroglobulin. It is believed that the carbohydrate moiety
of thyroglobulin is added to the secretion before it is transported into the follicular
lumen for storage. When the gland is stimulated to secrete, the colloid is taken
from the follicle into the cell by endocytosis, and the hormone is released through

lysosomal action. (See Chapter 14.) Since the lysosomes originate in the Golgi apparatus, this is another aspect of the role of this organelle in thyroid function. The lysosomes release thyroxine from thyroglobulin prior to its secretion from the cell into the perifollicular capillaries.

Steroid-secreting cells have prominent Golgi complexes that become enlarged when the cells are stimulated. The role of the Golgi apparatus is baffling since storage granules that would indicate involvement in packaging are not visible in the cells. Sulfation of protein-polysaccharide complexes is known to take place in the Golgi complex and, since it is believed that steroids are secreted as sulfates, Fawcett et al. (1969) suggest that steroid sulfates may be formed in the Golgi prior to release.

The catecholamines, epinephrine and norepinephrine (secreted by the cells of the adrenal medulla), and other neurosecretory hormones held in synaptic vesicles (see Chapter 19) are packaged in granules enclosed by a smooth-surfaced membrane. This suggests involvement of the Golgi complex.

For further discussion of Golgi complex function, see Jamieson and Palade (1977), Leblond and Bennett (1977), and Whaley and Dauwalder (1979).

MILK SYNTHESIS

Lactogenesis, or the synthesis and secretion of milk, depends on hormonal action for its initiation. Before synthesis can take place, changes occur in the mammary cells and their constituent organelles. These are induced by estrogen and progesterone as well as by prolactin, the lactogenic hormone from the pituitary. The Golgi apparatus is specifically involved in the secretion of prolactin in the pituitary cells. Smith and Farquhar (1970) have shown, in addition, that enzymes—primarily phosphatases derived from the Golgi—are packaged in the secretory granule containing prolactin.

In the mammary cells there is extensive proliferation of the rough endoplasmic reticulum in the basal portion of the cell for the synthesis of milk protein. The protein is delivered in transfer vesicles to the saccules on the forming face of the Golgi apparatus located on the lumen side of the cell. Passage of the secretory product through the Golgi apparatus in the mammary cell is probably similar to that of other secretory cells such as the exocrine pancreas. According to Patton (1969), it is reasonable to assume that α-lactalbumin, the B protein of lactose synthetase, joins the A protein in the Golgi apparatus. This allows the synthesis of lactose to take place in the Golgi prior to the packaging of the lactose, milk protein, and other constituents of milk serum for secretion. The protein in the vacuoles of the Golgi has the appearance of casein micelles in electron micrographs. Patton (ibid.) suggests that other proteins may be present also and that the vacuoles must carry some of the fluid of milk and may provide the vehicle for the secretion of milk serum constituents such as lactose.

In mammary cells, as in other cells, the lipid is synthesized in the cytoplasmic matrix. The lipid droplets are extruded from the cell into the lumen by what appears to be reverse pinocytosis.

Conclusion

Despite the list of functions attributed to the Golgi complex, it should be apparent that these could be consolidated into two categories: (1) membrane synthesis and recycling, and (2) compartmentalization of synthesized products. One could even suggest the single all-encompassing function of membrane synthesis since compartmentalization can occur only if membrane boundaries are established. Membranes are, without doubt, primary and indispensable units of biological structure and function. It would seem, therefore, that the membranes that synthesize membranes should occupy a position of prestige in the hierarchy of organelles. However, the Golgi complex as the synthesizer of membranes performs only one role in the closely integrated collaboration controlling the dynamic yet disciplined character of cellular function. Only the most shortsighted view would suggest an inequality of roles among the organelles. In the long view, each shares equally in the ultimate responsibility for the life or death of the cell, a responsibility that can be fulfilled successfully only when assured by the nutrient content of the extracellular environment.

chapter 13

the mitochondria

The mitochondrion is the "powerhouse of the cell" and is responsible for transforming the chemical bond energy of nutrients into the phosphate bonds of ATP. A proton gradient transmits the energy. There may be 50–2,500 of these organs of respiration in a single cell, each containing 500–10,000 complete sets of oxidative enzymes. Each enzyme assembly contains 15 or more active molecules in a highly ordered arrangement which is an integral part of the organelle structure. All the activities of the cell that are necessary for both its survival and specialized functions are completely dependent on the ability of the mitochondria to release the potential energy in a nutrient molecule and transduce that energy into a form of cellular work: osmotic, mechanical, electrical, chemical.

The development of molecular biology probably received its greatest impetus when the granules that the cytologists called mitochondria were first isolated by differential centrifugation and found by the biochemists to be capable of carrying out the oxidation of all the Krebs tricarboxylic acid (TCA) cycle intermediates. The transformations of energy that are accomplished by this series of integrated enzymatically controlled reactions end in a chemical trap: the formation of ATP, the universal intracellular carrier of chemical energy. The locus for this activity in all cells, from the single cell of the protist to each of the myriad cells in the complex organism, is the mitochondrion. It is the discharge of this function on which the continuing supply of energy for all other mitochondrial and cellular functions depend. There are other mitochondrial functions that may vie with, but can never overshadow, the primacy of this process of oxidative phosphorylation. This should in no way depreciate the ability of the mitochondrion to synthesize fatty acids, synthesize and catabolize proteins, form amino acids, perform carboxylations, participate in ionic regulation in the cell, and change the permeability of its membranes to make new substrate available. Nor can the presence of the only extranuclear supply of DNA so far discovered be easily subordinated. However, these processes could not progress far without the requisite energy that the mitochondrion releases for itself and for all the activities of the organelles of the cell.

Location and Number

Mitochondria are found in all aerobic respiring cells except bacteria. Although they appear to be distributed rather generally throughout the cytoplasmic matrix, their locations within the cell are related to their function. They may be located close to the source of fuel; in liver cells of fasting rats they have been found clustered around lipid droplets. More often, according to Lehninger (1967), they are found near the structure that will receive their end product, the ATP molecules. The locations in different cell types is frequently characteristic: in muscle cells, they are aligned in rows along the sacromeres (Chapter 18); in axon endings, near where transmitter substances are synthesized (Chapter 19); in acinar cells of the pancreas, they are in and near the rough endoplasmic reticulum where active enzyme synthesis is taking place. Generally, in secretory cells their orientation is along the secretory axis.

The number of mitochondria in a cell varies enormously with the cell type. Liver cells may contain 1–2,000 and renal tubule cells about 300. Sperm cells have as few as 20 mitochondria and, never underestimate the power of the female, oocytes may contain up to 300,000 mitochondria per cell (Lehninger, 1964; 1967).

Structure

Mitochondria were first discovered in the late 1800s by Altman who predicted that these organelles would be associated with cellular oxidation. It was the study of enzymes essential for oxidative phosphorylation in mitochondrial fragments that led to the first truly collaborative efforts of cytologists and biochemists. In suspensions of disrupted mitochondria Kennedy and Lehninger (1949), Schneider and Potter (1948), and Green et al. (1948) identified the enzymes of the Krebs cycle in the soluble portion, and the electron transport mechanism in the lipoprotein moiety of the cristae membrane. All efforts to separate the enzyme activity from the membrane were unsuccessful and it became evident that the enzymes were, in fact, an integral part of the membrane structure.

There is a striking similarity in the fundamental structure of mitochondria found in all forms from protozoa to primates. Palade (1952) was first to describe the complex and highly differentiated ultrastructure of the mitochondrion revealed by the electron microscope (Fig. 13.1). From his early description and later from more detailed studies, the mitochondrion was revealed as a double-membraned structure, one sac enclosing another (Fig. 13.2).

The two membranes are quite different in structure and in their biochemical and physical properties. The outer membrane is smooth and the inner one has infoldings or invaginations, often shelflike, that extend into the lumen. These are the *cristae* or *mitochondrial crests*. The number of cristae and the surface area of their membranes vary directly with the respiratory activity of the cell. In some cells the cristae may be short and relatively few in number but in cells having intense activity they are very numerous and regularly arranged. For example, in a cell with a moderate rate of respiration, such as the liver cell, the area has been estimated to be 40 m^2/gm protein (Mitchell, 1966), but muscle mitochondria may comprise ten times that area. A most complex arrangement of cristae, which is practically a crystallinelike lattice, has been found in the heart muscle of the canary, which beats at a rate of 1,000 per minute (Slautterback, 1965).

The outer membrane is separated from the inner membrane by a space that is referred to as the outer compartment. The inner membrane bounds the inner compartment, which is the larger of the two chambers, and contains the mito-chondrial matrix. The matrix is a proteinaceous gel and appears granular and generally homogeneous, but filaments have been observed (DeRobertis and Franco Raffo, 1957). Electron-dense granules are observed in the inner compartment, free in the matrix, and often close to the inner membrane. The granules are believed to be sites for binding divalent cations such as Ca^{++} and Mg^{++}. The matrix can take up enormous amounts of calcium phosphate, as shown in Fig. 13.3. The inner and outer mitochondrial membranes are physically separated, probably by repulsion of the negatively charged surfaces, except at *contact sites*. As many as 100 contact sites exist between the membranes in rat liver mito-chondria (Hackenbrock, 1968). The sites appear to contain a high density of fixed anionic charges and are probably sialoglycoproteins (Hackenbrock and Miller, 1975). The function of the contact sites is unknown. However, cytoplasmic ri-bosomes, which translate polypeptides destined for mitochondria, are anchored at the contact sites (Butow et al., 1975). Further, polypeptides synthesized in the mitochondria first appear at the contact sites (Werner and Neupert, 1972). It is possible that cooperative assembly of mitochondrial proteins, such as cytochrome oxidase, which derive from both cytoplasmic and mitochondrial polypeptides, occurs at the contact sites.

The structure of outer and inner mitochondrial membranes is distinctly different and the structure of the inner membrane, in particular, has been the subject of controversy for nearly two decades. The inner surface of the inner membrane is covered with thousands of small particles that were referred to by Green and Hatefi (1961) as the electron transport particles and which are now termed the F_1-ATPase. Fernandez-Moran (1962), by electron microscopy, showed them to

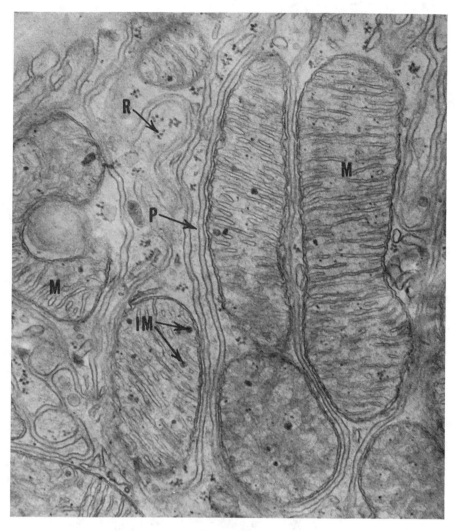

Figure 13.1
Mitochondria (M) showing double membrane structure and transverse cristae. IM
= intramitochondrial granules, P = plasma membrane, R = ribosomes. Rat kidney
proximal tubule. Magnification × 42,000. (Courtesy of Dr. Harold Schraer.)

be connected by narrow stalks to the core of the membrane. Smith (1963) estimated that there were about 4,000 particles/μ^2 of membrane surface. Thus, a
mitochondrion has as many as 10^5 F_1-particles. Stoeckenius (1963; 1966) suggested that the particles of Fernandez-Moran (1962) and of Green (1964) might
be large ATPase molecules. In preparations of submitochondrial fractions studied
biochemically and electron microscopically, Racker (1967; 1968) reported that
the so-called elementary particles do not represent the electron transport enzymes

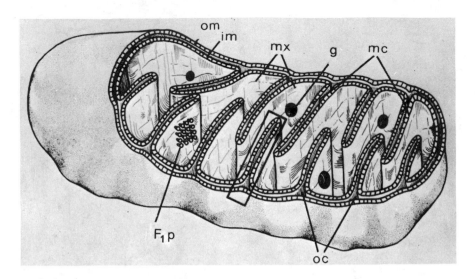

Figure 13.2
A three-dimensional diagram of a mitochondrion showing the outer membrane (om),
the inner membrane (im), cristae membranes (mc), the space occupied by the mitochondrial matrix (mx), the granules (g) present in the matrix which contain calcium,
magnesium, phosphates, and carbonates. The outer chamber (oc), between the
membranes, and the F_1 particles (F_1p) are also indicated. An entire mitochondrial
crest is delineated by the rectangle. (From E. D. P. De Robertis et al., *Cell Biology*,
5th ed., W. B. Saunders Co., Philadelphia, 1970, p. 203.)

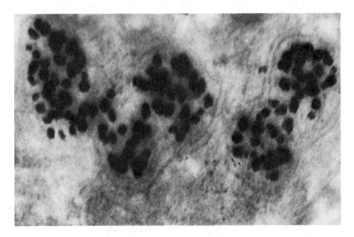

Figure 13.3
Numerous calcium phosphate granules can be found in mitochondria such as these when anhydrous methods are used. Unstained frozen thin-section. (Courtesy of Dr. Carol V. Gay.)

since rapid oxidation of NADH occurred in the absence of the particles. The precise location of the ATPase within (or on) the inner mitochondrial membrane was at the heart of the controversy. Technological advances in electron microscopy, such as freeze-fracturing and freeze-etching, indicate that the F_1- ATPase protrudes from the surface.

It is now generally agreed, as reviewed by De Pierre and Ernster (1977), that the mitochondrial ATPase is a structurally complex molecule having three distinguishable parts. (1) The F_1 particle is a soluble 85Å ATPase headpiece which projects from the matrix side of the cristae (Fig. 13.2). F_1 has a molecular weight of 360 kilodaltons. It is comprised of five subunits ranging in size from 7–53 kilodaltons. (2) A less well characterized, very hydrophobic proteolipid complex, termed F_0, is localized in the inner membrane lipid bilayer. (3) F_1 and F_0 are connected by a stalk that confers oligomycin sensitivity onto the complex. Several other subunits with less well-defined functions have also been identified.

Composition

The exquisite precision with which the mitochondrion performs the intricate biochemical procedures, particularly those involved in oxidative phosphorylation, implies a corresponding precision in organization. Such coordinated and efficient function could not occur by random meeting of enzymes and substrates.

In cells with high mitochondrial counts, the mitochondria may account for over 20 percent of the cytoplasmic volume and for 30–35 percent of the total protein of the cell. Of the mitochondrial protein, approximately 4 percent is in the outer membrane, 21 percent in the inner membrane, 67 percent accounted for by the matrix, and the remainder in the intermembrane space (Sottocasa et al., 1967; Schnaitman and Greenawalt, 1968). More than 70 enzymes and coenzymes have been identified in mitochondria. Numerous cofactors and metals are also essential for mitochondrial function. At least 23 percent of the protein in the inner membrane is made up of catabolically active proteins. About 70 percent of the inner membrane protein is integrated, or spans the membrane (Harmon et al., 1974), so that even though the inner membrane is largely protein (75%) about two-thirds of its two surfaces is occupied by the lipid bilayer (Vanderkooi, 1974).

Although a contractile protein similar to myosin had been reported by Ohnishi and Ohnishi (1962a; 1962b), and Lehninger (1962; 1964), and referred to as mitochondrial actomyosin, Conover and Bárány (1966) have since suggested that such a factor was due to contamination. Bemis et al. (1968) report that mitochondria do not contain a contractile protein and that change in shape is due to the flexibility of the membranes and the passive consequence of ion-pumping coupled to electron transport.

Glycoproteins have been identified in liver mitochondria (Sottocasa et al., 1972) and appear to be located in the outer compartment. Swelling of the mitochondria leads to the release of some 30 percent of the total mitochondrial protein.

The lipid content of all mitochondria is approximately the same, 27 percent, with phospholipid accounting for 90 percent of the lipid fraction (Fleischer et al., 1967). The phospholipids present in all mitochondria are phosphatidyl choline, phosphatidyl ethanolamine, and cardiolipin. Phosphatidyl choline and phosphatidyl ethanolamine are present in approximately equal amounts comprising 76–78 percent of the total phospholipid present, and cardiolipin 20 percent. There is a very high degree of unsaturation found in the fatty acyl chains, but chain length and chain unsaturation vary within wide limits among both species and organs and are thought to be influenced by both dietary and environmental factors (Chapman and Leslie, 1970). A comparative study on the effect of diet on mitochondrial lipid patterns (Richardson et al., 1961; 1962) showed a higher degree of unsaturation in fish and fish-eating animals, but whether this is due to possible dietary or environmental temperature effects among the species could not be ascertained. Fish mitochondria were found to have little or no linoleic, linolenic, and very little arachidonic acid in contrast to those of the rat. Richardson and Tappel (1962) suggest that some of the very highly unsaturated lipids (22:5 and 22:6) in fish mitochondria are associated with their ability to function at lower temperatures. Vos et al. (1972) found that the total number of membrane-bound fatty acyl chain double bonds was lowered in vitamin E deficiency and that the effect was much more obvious in the inner mitochondrial membranes than in the microsomal membranes.

Separation of the inner and outer mitochondrial membranes has been effected by exposing mitochondria to swelling agents or detergents and subjecting them to density centrifugation (Sottocasa et al., 1967; Schnaitman and Greenawalt, 1968). This has permitted a clear demonstration that the two membranes differ considerably in chemical composition, enzyme content, and ultrastructure (Table 13.1). The most distinguishing feature is the lipid distribution between the inner and outer membranes (Stoffel and Schiefer, 1968). The inner membrane is 80 percent protein and only 20 percent lipid. These relative proportions are very different from the outer and most other membranes, which are approximately 60 percent protein and 40 percent lipid. The large protein-lipid ratio of the inner membrane indicates a large degree of insertion of protein into the lipid bilayer. (See the fluid model of membrane structure, Chapter 9.) This concept of structural organization has been borne out by freeze-fracture studies (Melnick and Packer, 1971). Qualitative differences in the phospholipid composition are striking particularly with respect to cardiolipin, which is predominantly, if not exclusively, in the inner membrane and phosphatidyl inositol, which is mostly in the outer membrane. (See Ernster and Kuylenstierna, 1970.) In both cases, the outer membrane of the mitochondrion resembles that of endoplasmic reticulum. Most of the cholesterol is in the outer membrane giving a molar ratio of cholesterol to phospholipid of 1:9, whereas the ratio for the inner membrane is 1:53 (Levy and Sauner, 1968). The presence of any cholesterol in the inner membrane of liver mitochondria is questioned by Neupert et al. (1972), but they do suggest that sterols in general are essential components of the outer mitochondrial membranes; in *Neurospora* there is an extremely high concentration of ergosterol; in liver, it is cholesterol.

TABLE 13.1
Localization of Some Liver Mitochondrial Enzymes

Outer Membrane	Intermembrane Space	Inner Membrane	Matrix
Rotenone-insensitive NADH-Cyt b_5 reductase	Adenylate kinase[a]	Cytochrome b, c, c_1, a, a_3	Malic dehydrogenase[a]
	Nucleoside diphosphokinase		Isocitric dehydrogenase
		β-Hydroxybutyrate dehydrogenase	
Monoamine oxidase[a]		Ferrochelatase	Glutamic dehydrogenase
Kynurenine hydroxylase		δ-Amino levulinic synthetase	Glutamic-aspartic-transaminase
ATP-dependent fatty acyl CoA synthetase		Carnitine palmityl transferase	Citrate synthase
Glycerophosphate acyl transferase		—	Aconitase
Lysophosphatidate acyl transferase			Fumarase[a]
		Fatty acid elongation enzymes	Pyruvic carboxylase
Lysolecithin acyl transferase		Respiratory chain-linked phosphorylation enzymes	Protein synthesis enzymes
Phosphocholine transferase		Succinic dehydrogenase	Fatty acyl CoA dehydrogenase
Phosphatidate phosphatase		Cytochrome a_3 oxidase[a]	Nucleic acid polymerases
Nucleoside diphosphokinase		Mitochondrial DNA polymerase	ATP-dependent fatty acyl CoA synthetase
Fatty acid elongating system C_{14} - C_{16}			GTP-dependent fatty acyl CoA synthetase

Source: Adapted from L. Ernster and B. Kuylenstierna, *Membranes of Mitochondria and Chloroplasts*, E. Racker, ed., Van Nostrand Reinhold Co., New York, 1970, p. 196. The location and properties of 117 mitochondrial enzymes have been tabulated by P. L. Altman and D. D. Katz, eds., *Biological Handbooks I: Cell Biology. Fed. Am. Soc. Exp. Biol.*, Bethesda, Md.: 143–230 (1976).

[a]Marker enzymes.

With improved biochemical techniques that permit analysis of each of the membranes, coupled with electron microscopic analyses, a molecular picture of the organization of the inner membrane has been formulated. Both surfaces of the inner mitochondrial membrane are now experimentally accessible. The outer membrane can be stripped away, exposing the inner. Next, inside-out vesicles of the inner membrane can be made by sonication. By the use of specific anti-bodies, proteolytic enzymes, lectins, and other membrane probes, the approximate arrangement of the respiratory chain proteins has emerged. (See section on electron transport and oxidative phosphorylation.) In a single liver mitochondrion there are estimated to be about 15,000 electron carrier molecules and about 50,000 in a heart mitochondrion. Calculations indicate that one respiratory assembly occupies an area equivalent to a square 200 Å on a side. In all types of mito-chondria in all species the respiratory assembly is similar with the result that the number of respiratory assemblies per mitochondrion and the area of the inner membrane are proportional.

Mitochondrial Compartments

Most of the important metabolic activities for which the mitochondrion is re-sponsible take place within the inner compartment. The outer membrane is freely permeable to water, simple electrolytes, sucrose, and molecules as large as 10,000 daltons, including some polypeptides. The unusually high permeability of the outer membrane is partly conferred by its high cholesterol content. The inner membrane is permeable to water and to certain small molecules such as urea, glycerol, and short chain fatty acids. However, it is not permeable to lipid-insoluble nonelectrolytes with a molecular weight greater than 100–150, nor simple charged ions. Flavoproteins, nucleosides, mono-, di-, or triphosphates, and CoA and its esters also do not permeate the inner membrane. Thus, the innermost compartment of mitochondria contains an internal pool of these mol-ecules that is separate and distinct from the cytoplasmic pool. All of the respiratory substrates must enter the inner compartment for oxidation; ADP and phosphate must enter if ATP is to be formed and, of course, the ATP must be able to cross the membrane to leave the mitochondrion. A diagram of the metabolic traffic is shown in Fig. 13.4. The mechanisms controlling the mitochondrial membrane traffic are of considerable interest. Two mechanisms that appear to be involved are (1) substrate-specific carrier systems that are probably membrane proteins or lipoproteins, and (2) shuttle systems that employ mobile, relatively low molecular weight molecules, such as small proteins, as carriers.

Specific carriers in the inner mitochondrial membrane are believed to function by facilitated diffusion. The best characterized carrier is the one for ATP and ADP (Riccio et al., 1975). The ATP-ADP carrier, which works in close conjunction with the phosphate carrier system, operates on an exchange basis, and a molecule of ADP can enter the inner compartment only if a molecule of ATP leaves. A 29,000

Metabolic exchanges across the mitochondrial membranes

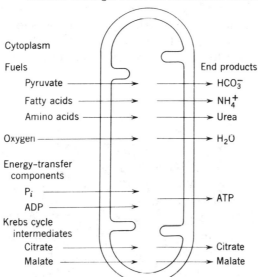

Figure 13.4
The metabolic traffic across the mitochondrial membrane. (From A. L. Lehninger, *Adv. Cytopharmacol.* 1:199, 1971a.)

dalton ATP-ADP carrier has been isolated (Klingenberg et al., 1976). There is strong evidence that carriers also exist for succinate or malate, isocitrate, glutamic acid, and bicarbonate (Lehninger, 1971b). Lehninger (1969) also presented evidence of a carrier specific for Ca^{++}, Mn^{++}, or Sr^{++}. Since the electrical charge must be balanced on either side of the membrane, Pfaff and Klingenberg (1968) suggest that the carriers are electrically integrated.

The Ca^{++} carrier has been extensively studied. It is a protein that is different from the calcium-binding protein found in the intestine (Wasserman et al., 1968a). This carrier may be involved in rapid reversible segregation of ionic Ca^{++} in mitochondria during muscular activity as well as during calcification changes in bone. (See Chapters 17 and 18.) Carafoli et al. (1972) have isolated mitochondrial fractions capable of binding Ca^{++} and have found that a component common to the binding factors is sialic acid and that the purified glycoprotein also contains hexosamines and neutral sugars.

Two additional mitochondrial shuttle systems of importance, which will be discussed in a subsequent section, are the α-glycerophosphate shuttle of liver and muscle and the acylcarnitine transferase system. The latter system enables transfer from extramitochondrial CoA to intramitochondrial CoA. Studies utilizing scanning calorimetry (Edidin, 1974) and freeze-fracture technology (Hackenbrock, 1977; Schneider et al., 1980; Sowers and Hackenbrock, 1981) clearly demonstrate the occurrence of lateral and transverse diffusion of proteins in the membrane. The inner membrane of calorigenically responsive mitochondria, for example from liver, kidney, muscle, and adipose tissue, also appears to contain a receptor for thyroid hormone (Stirling et al., 1978). This finding has physiological relevance since thyroxine is known to stimulate oxidative phosphorylation (Stirling et al., 1977).

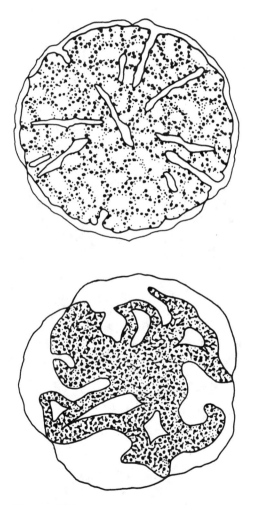

Figure 13.5
The conformation states of rat liver mito-chondria. Top: orthodox conformation ob-served in absence of ADP. Bottom: con-densed conformation observed in presence of ADP. (From A. L. Lehninger, *Adv. Cy-topharmocol.* 1:199, 1971a.)

Conformational Changes

The ability of the mitochondrial membrane to swell or to contract was observed and was believed to depend on the oxidation-reduction state of the enzymes in the membranes (Lehninger, 1962).

It was demonstrated through electron microscopy (Hackenbrock, 1966; 1968) that liver mitochondria reversibly oscillate between two states: the classical or *orthodox* state observed in the absence of ADP, and the *condensed* state that occurs with the addition of ADP and the stimulation of respiration (Fig. 13.5). In the condensed state the inner compartment is contracted with a 50 percent decrease in volume. With phosphorylation of all the ADP the mitochondria return to the orthodox state. The concentration of proteins in the matrix is about 56 percent (Hackenbrock, 1968) and when the matrix condenses, during respiration, the concentration increases further. Thus, even though the enzymes (e.g., Krebs cycle enzymes) present in the matrix are soluble, they must be packed together very closely. Srere (1980) points out that the close packing will profoundly influence the kinetic behavior of the enzymes involved. The structure-function relationships of the matrix components within intact mitochondria are poorly understood. The development of noninvasive methods such as nuclear magnetic resonance spectroscopy will entice investigation along this avenue of research.

Function

In order to understand the mechanisms by which the mitochondrion traps energy in ATP for subsequent use in cellular processes and becomes, thereby, the powerhouse of the cell, many accepted generalities, scientific clichés, and terms of convenience must be unveiled and then scrutinized, comprehended, and redefined. Only then will the scientific colloquialisms acquire meaning and the concepts become lucid.

The law of conservation of energy can be mouthed by almost any schoolboy. What concepts does it encompass? Does it include the utter dependence of animal life on the photosynthetic trap in the chloroplasts of the plant cell? Does it point to the uniqueness of the photosynthetic process in utilizing quanta of light as the energy source? Does it recognize that only the plant cell of all living things possesses the capacity to absorb solar energy[1] and to convert and trap it as chemical energy? Does it clarify why plant life had to precede animal life on this planet? Does it explain why food for all animal cells comes ultimately from plants and that food is the sole source of energy on which animal life depends? Does

---

[1]We do not intend to ignore, or even minimize, the capacity of photoreceptor cells, such as those found in the retina, to absorb light energy nor the photoactivation of 7-dehydrocholesterol in the cells of the skin. However, except in these specialized cases, the capacity to use light energy appears to be nonexistent in animal cells.

it humble sophisticated man who comes to realize his complete subordination to the genius of the grass on which he treads?

The foodstuffs, carbohydrate, protein, and fat, are the fuel that the animal cell is capable of converting into mechanical, chemical, electrical, osmotic, sonic, light, or heat energy. The measurement or quantitation of these forms of energy can be made in any convenient unit and the unit may vary with the kind of energy measured and the ease of measurement: ergs, electron volts, kilowatt hours, millimeters of mercury, or decibels. The potential energy of foodstuffs is measured as heat and, since other forms of energy are easily expressed in heat units, the *kilocalorie* (kcal) has until recently been the accepted unit of measurement in nutritional studies. A kilocalorie is defined as the amount of heat required to raise the temperature of one kilogram of water from 14.5–15.5°C. (The kilocalorie is to be distinguished from the calorie that is used later in this chapter in calculating the energy yield of metabolic oxidation. The calorie is the amount of heat required to raise the temperature of one gram of water from 14.5°–15.5°C.)

The kilojoule (kJ) is now the international unit of energy and is defined as the energy expended when 1 kilogram is moved 1 meter (m) by a force of 1 newton (N). Conversion of kilocalories to kilojoules is accomplished by multiplying by a factor of 4.2. Because of the large amounts of energy involved in some nutritional calculations, the megajoule (mJ) is sometimes preferred. For purposes of comparison some of the data presented in Chapter 23 will be expressed in terms of both kilocalories and kilo- or megajoules.

The conversion, then, of the potential energy supplied by the cell's food to chemical bond energy in ATP is measured in calories. This conversion is the primary function of the mitochondria. The manner in which the mitochondria accomplish this ultimate goal involves a series of reactions in which intermediary products in the metabolism of carbohydrates, fats, and proteins are broken down in a succession of steps and merge in a common oxidative pathway, the TCA cycle. This oxidative pathway leads to the release of carbon dioxide and hydrogen. The carbon dioxide is quickly removed from the cell as a noxious and potentially dangerous waste product. It is cycled through the bicarbonate buffer system, the major buffer of the body. The rapidity of removal of CO_2 is facilitated by the action of the zinc-containing enzyme, carbonic anhydrase, which is in the cytoplasm of the cell (Enns, 1967). The hydrogen (H^+ and electron) is carried along a chain of reactors, eventually combining with molecular oxygen to form water. In this process, the energy released by the transfer of electrons along the respiratory chain is captured by ADP and inorganic phosphate to form ATP. This coupling of the oxidation of foodstuffs (oxidation being a loss of electrons) with the formation of ATP, aptly described by Szent-Györgyi as the *energy currency* of the cell, is known as *oxidative phosphorylation*. Oxidation in a living cell thus proceeds in an orderly step-by-step fashion enabling the cell to harness efficiently the energy released from food, the energy requisite for its existence.

Carbohydrates, fats, and proteins enter the mitochondria as their breakdown products: pyruvic acid, fatty acids, and amino acids. The general pathway of these metabolites to their common oxidative fate, the TCA cycle, is depicted in Fig. 13.6. Pyruvic acid and fatty acids are degraded to the two-carbon acetate

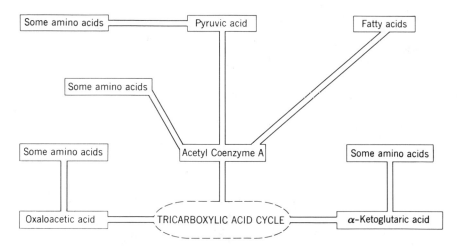

Figure 13.6
Oxidation of foodstuffs in mitochondria.

and enter the cycle joined to the pantothenic acid-containing CoA. Amino acids undergo a variety of changes: some are converted to pyruvic acid, some to acetyl CoA, and others to the TCA cycle intermediaries oxaloacetic acid and α-keto-glutaric acid. This diagrammatic representation is, of course, grossly oversimplified. Each step involves a series of reactions and requires a number of enzymes, coenzymes, and other factors. The purpose of the following sections is to add to a general understanding of these processes. No attempt will be made to present the detailed intricacies of the enzymatic machinery involved.

OXIDATION OF FATTY ACIDS

The oxidation of fatty acids to acetyl CoA involves a series of reactions by which two-carbon fragments are split off a fragment at a time. This process may be depicted as a spiral (Fig. 13.7). The loss of each two-carbon fragment involves five separate reactions in which CoA-acyl derivatives are formed. The oxidation of 1 mole of stearic acid (C_{18}), for example, would necessitate at least 45 separate reactions leading to the formation of 9 moles of acetyl CoA.

The steps in the oxidation of fatty acids are given below and correspond to the numbers in Fig. 13.7. ATP is required to prime the reaction, to provide the energy of activation.

1. Activation of the fatty acid by formation of a corresponding fatty acid CoA ester. The products are fatty acid CoA ester, AMP, and inorganic pyrophosphate (PP_i) which may be further degraded to the monophosphate (P_i).

$$R{-}CH_2{-}CH_2{-}COOH + ATP + CoA \xrightarrow{Mg^{++}K^+}$$

$$R{-}CH_2{-}CH_2\overset{O}{\overset{\|}{C}}{-}SCoA + AMP + PP_i$$

2. Dehydrogenation of the fatty acid CoA ester to form the α-β-unsaturated acyl CoA. The enzymes involved in this reaction contain FAD and copper or iron.

$$R{-}CH_2{-}CH_2C\overset{O}{\underset{}{\|}}{-}SCoA \underset{+2H^+}{\overset{-2H^+}{\rightleftharpoons}} R{-}CH{=}CHC\overset{O}{\underset{}{\|}}{-}SCoA$$

3. Hydration of the α-β-unsaturated acyl CoA ester to form β-hydroxyacyl CoA. The unsaturated bond becomes hydrated.

$$R{-}CH{=}CHC\overset{O}{\underset{}{\|}}{-}SCoA + H_2O \rightleftharpoons R{-}CHOHCH_2C\overset{O}{\underset{}{\|}}{-}SCoA$$

4. Dehydrogenation of the β-hydroxy acyl CoA to form β-keto acyl CoA. NAD is the hydrogen acceptor.

$$R{-}CHOHCH_2C\overset{O}{\underset{}{\|}}{-}SCoA + NAD \underset{-2H}{\overset{+2H}{\rightleftharpoons}} R{-}C\overset{O}{\underset{}{\|}}{-}CH_2{-}C\overset{O}{\underset{}{\|}}{-}SCoA + NADH_2$$

5. Thiolytic cleavage of the β-keto acyl CoA to yield acetyl CoA and a fatty acyl CoA having 2 fewer carbon atoms.

$$R{-}C\overset{O}{\underset{}{\|}}{-}CH_2{-}C\overset{O}{\underset{}{\|}}{-}SCoA + CoASH \rightleftharpoons R{-}C\overset{O}{\underset{}{\|}}{-}SCoA + CH_3C\overset{O}{\underset{}{\|}}{-}SCoA$$

The cycle, then, is repeated as indicated by the spiral representing subsequent removal of two carbon fragments as acetyl CoA. Rapid changes in the synthesis of CoA are among the mechanisms controlling the synthesis and oxidation of fatty acids in mitochondria (Smith, 1978; Smith et al., 1978).

OXIDATION OF PYRUVIC ACID

Pyruvic acid, the converging point for the oxidation of glucose and of the amino acids alanine, serine, and cysteine, enters the TCA cycle as acetyl CoA. The oxidation of pyruvate to acetyl CoA is an oxidative decarboxylation and involves a sequence of reactions requiring TPP, lipoic acid, CoA, NAD, Mg^{++}, and a large complex of enzymes known as the pyruvic dehydrogenase complex. Four vitamins, thiamin, pantothenic acid, riboflavin, and nicotinic acid, participate in pyruvate oxidation. The overall reaction can be summed up briefly as:

$$Pyruvate + CoA + NAD \xrightarrow[\text{Lipoic acid}]{\substack{FAD \\ TPP}} Acetyl\ CoA + CO_2 + NADH_2$$

A more detailed but still incomplete representation (Fig. 13.8) illustrates one way in which these four vitamins virtually control a key reaction in cellular metabolism.

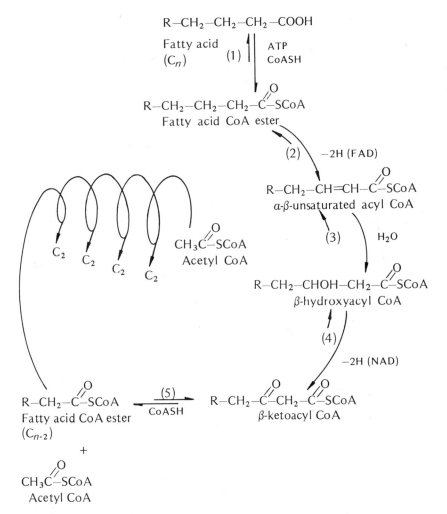

Figure 13.7
Fatty acid oxidation. Enzymes are (1) acyl CoA synthetase, (2) acyl CoA dehydrogenase, (3) enoyl CoA hydrase, (4) β-hydroxyacyl CoA dehydrogenase, and (5) β-ketoacyl thiolase.

Each acts independently; yet a lack of any one of these vitamins will interfere with the coordinated flow of the reaction.

The steps in pyruvate oxidation are as follows:

1. Pyruvic acid is decarboxylated after it becomes attached to the thiazole ring of TPP. This reaction requires Mg^{++}. Protonation then yields hydroxyethyl TPP. The reaction is catalyzed by the pyruvate dehydrogenase component of the multi-enzyme complex.

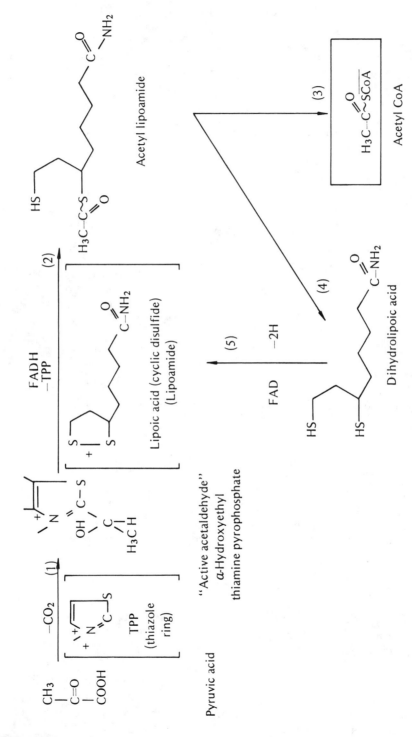

Figure 13.8
Oxidative decarboxylation of pyruvate.

2. The hydroxyethyl group is oxidized to an acetyl group which is transferred to lipoamide, splitting off TPP. Lipoamide is reduced, breaking the disulfide ring. A sulfhydryl group is formed at one sulfur and the acetyl group is attached to the other sulfur in a thioester linkage. This and the following step are catalyzed by dihydrolipoyl transacetylase.
3. The acetyl group, now in the form of a thioester, is transferred to CoA to form acetyl CoA.
4 and 5. Reduced lipoic acid, or dihydrolipamide, remains after removal of the acetyl group and is oxidized back to the active cyclic disulfide form with NAD as the hydrogen acceptor. Dihydrolipoyl dehydrogenase, with FAD as its prosthetic group, catalyzes the reaction.

The loss of hydrogens in Reaction 5 and subsequent release of energy by way of the electron transport system results in the formation of 3 moles of ATP. Acetyl CoA formed in the oxidative decarboxylation of pyruvate may condense with oxaloacetate for further degradation by way of the TCA cycle, or it may be diverted to other cellular processes for which it is required, such as fatty acid oxidation and synthesis.

TRICARBOXYLIC ACID CYCLE (KREBS CYCLE, CITRIC ACID CYCLE)

The TCA cycle is described as the final pathway in the oxidation of carbohydrates, fats, and proteins. In a quantitative sense, this cycle is also the most important phase in the oxidation of foodstuffs, since approximately 90 percent of the energy released from food is the result of TCA cycle oxidation.

Although metabolites may enter the cycle at any point, the cycle usually is visualized as beginning with the condensation of acetyl CoA with oxaloacetate to form citric acid. The subsequent series of reactions comprising the cycle uses up 2 moles of H_2O and results in the release of 2 moles of CO_2 and 4 pairs of hydrogens and electrons. The overall reaction in the degradation of acetate may be expressed as:

$$CH_3COOH + 2H_2O \rightarrow 2CO_2 + 8H^+$$

The individual reactions are depicted diagrammatically in Fig. 13.9. A description of the reactions corresponding to numbers in the diagram follows:

Product Released	Reaction	
	1.	Condensation of oxaloacetate and acetyl CoA to form citrate. CoA is split off hydrolytically in the process and is recycled.
	2 and 3.	Isomerization of citrate to yield isocitrate. Cis-aconitate may be formed as an intermediary. Water assists in the isomerization but is not used up in the process.

$2H^+$		4.	Dehydrogenation of isocitrate to form oxalosuccinate (not shown). NAD or NADP may serve as hydrogen acceptor.
CO_2		5.	Decarboxylation of oxalosuccinate to α-ketoglutarate. Loss of CO_2 results in first shortening of the carbon chain.
CO_2	$2H^+$	6.	Oxidative decarboxylation of α-ketoglutarate to form succinyl CoA. This reaction requires TPP, Mg^{++}, NAD, FAD, lipoic acid, and CoA as cofactors and is analogous to the oxidative decarboxylation of pyruvate. NAD is the hydrogen acceptor. The loss of a second CO_2 molecule results in a four-carbon chain.
		7.	Utilization of high energy bond from succinyl CoA to form succinic acid and donation of high energy phosphate bond to GDP to form GTP. The high energy phosphate is transferred to ADP to form ATP. This is the only reaction in the TCA cycle that directly yields a high energy phosphate bond. All others are formed during electron transport, as will be discussed presently.
$2H^+$		8.	Dehydrogenation of succinate to form fumarate. FAD is the hydrogen acceptor.
		9.	Addition of water to fumarate to form malate.
$2H^+$		10.	Dehydrogenation of malate to form oxaloacetate.

Oxaloacetate now is available to condense with another mole of acetyl CoA and thus to repeat the cycle. This is not an obligatory reaction, however. Oxaloacetate can contribute to other cellular processes such as synthesis of glucose and certain amino acids by the loss of carbon dioxide and formation of phosphoenolpyruvate. The reverse of this reaction is a means of providing oxaloacetate when the supply is limited. Decreased formation of oxaloacetate might occur, for example, if TCA cycle intermediates are diverted to other reactions and, in a very loose sense, leave the cycle.

Acetyl CoA arises through the degradation of fatty acids and certain amino acids as well as from carbohydrate, and its oxidation is dependent on a ready supply of oxaloacetate. The oxidation of acetyl CoA produces no *net* increase in oxaloacetate or other cycle intermediaries; therefore if additional oxaloacetate is needed, it must be provided from other sources. One such source is the conversion from phosphoenolpyruvate. Pyruvate also may give rise indirectly to oxaloacetate; this reaction involves the addition of carbon dioxide to form malate which then

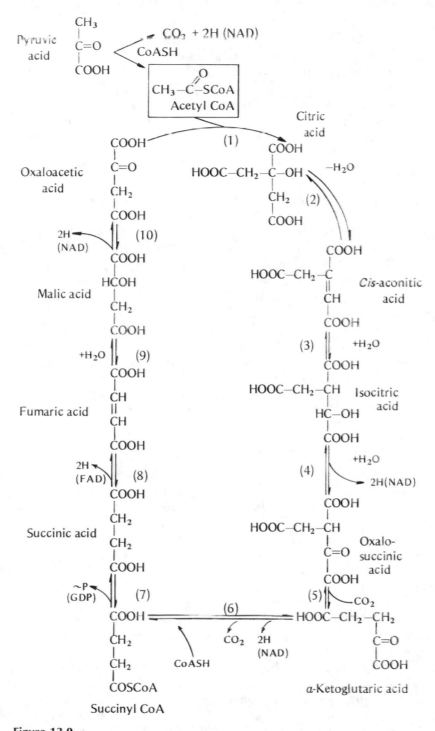

Figure 13.9
Tricarboxylic acid cycle. Enzymes are (1) citrate synthase (formerly condensing enzyme), (2) and (3) aconitase, (4) and (5) isocitrate dehydrogenase, (6) α-ketoglutarate dehydrogenase, (7) succinyl CoA synthetase, (8) succinic dehydrogenase, (9) fumarase, and (10) malate dehydrogenase.

is dehydrogenated to oxaloacetate. The conversion of carbohydrate metabolites to oxaloacetate may account, in part, for the ameliorative effect of carbohydrate feeding when ketosis develops as a consequence of a predominantly fatty acid metabolism as, for example, occurs during fasting.

All of the enzymes and coenzymes necessary for TCA metabolism are located either in the inner membrane or in the inner matrix of the mitochondrion. As indicated in Chapter 11, pyruvate produced by anaerobic metabolism of carbohydrate in cytoplasm must enter the mitochondrion to be oxidized via the TCA cycle.

Certain other TCA cycle intermediates also permeate the mitochondrial membrane in either direction by an exchange mechanism involving other compounds within or outside the mitochondrion (Fig. 13.10). Malate, succinate, citrate, and isocitrate enter in exchange for an equivalent amount of inorganic phosphate. α-Ketoglutarate does not cross the mitochondrial membrane as such but is converted first to glutamate that, after traversing the membrane barrier, is reconverted to the keto acid. Fumarate and oxaloacetate, however, cannot cross the mitochondrial membrane in either direction.

Biosynthetic and degradative processes often utilize two-carbon units. However, a mechanism for handling one-carbon compounds exists. Such transfers are mediated by protein-bound tetrafolic acid, an extramitochondrial process. Recently, a folic acid-binding protein has been identified in the cytosol and partially characterized in mitochondria (Wittwer and Wagner, 1981a; 1981b). This protein is believed to be important in the transfer of one-carbon units into mitochondria.

OXIDATION OF AMINO ACIDS

Although some synthesis of protein apparently takes place in the mitochondrion, it is generally believed that amino acids traverse the mitochondrial membrane chiefly to be oxidized via the TCA cycle. In order for oxidation to take place, an amino acid first must lose its amino group. The keto acid so formed may be oxidized through the cycle or converted by a series of reactions to an oxidizable substrate.

Fig. 13.11 indicates that amino acids enter the TCA cycle through at least three avenues: pyruvic acid, TCA cycle intermediaries, and acetyl CoA. The term *glycogenic* is used to designate amino acids that give rise to TCA cycle intermediates or pyruvate, resulting in net synthesis of glucose. *Ketogenic* refers to amino acids that give rise to ketone bodies through acetyl CoA and consequently are potential fatty acid and acetoacetate producers.

The diagrammatic representation in Fig. 13.11 obviously is oversimplified. Only three amino acids—alanine, aspartic acid, and glutamic acid—are converted directly to keto acids that are intermediaries in the main oxidative scheme. These keto acids are pyruvate, oxaloacetate, and α-ketoglutarate. Other amino acids must undergo a series of reactions before they are converted to substances that can be oxidized through the TCA cycle. In the degradation of phenylalanine and

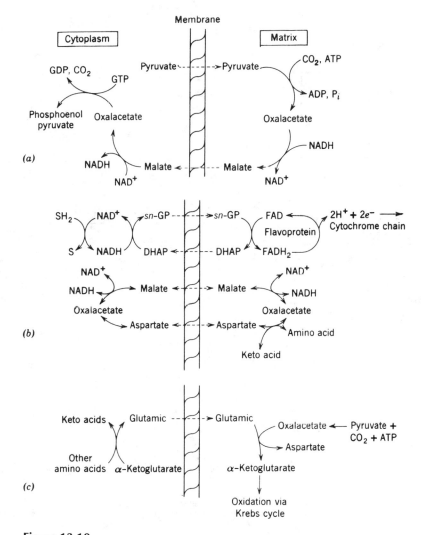

Figure 13.10
Four shuttle systems operating across the mitochondrial inner membrane. (a) System required to convert pyruvate (or lactate) to phosphoenol pyruvate in gluconeogenesis. (b) The unidirectional sn-glycerol phosphate (sn-GP) and dihydroxyacetophosphate (DHAP) shuttle that transports reducing equivalents only *into* the mitochondrial matrix. (c) The reversible malate-oxalacetate-aspartate shuttle for reducing equivalents. (d) The glutamate shuttle for transport of amino nitrogen. (From E. E. Conn, and P. R. Stumpf, *Outlines of Biochemistry*, 4th ed., John Wiley, New York, 1976, p. 402.)

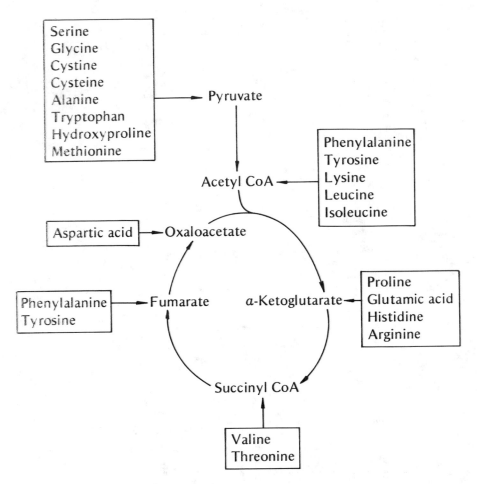

Figure 13.11
Oxidative pathways of amino acids.

tyrosine, for example, the molecule splits, forming two oxidizable substances: fumarate and acetoacetate. The mechanisms by which amino acids are degraded vary in complexity, depending on the amino acid involved. All, however, share the initial step; that is, removal of the amino group.

The most common method for biological removal of amino groups is *transamination*. This reaction requires both an amino acid and an α-keto acid. The amino and keto groups are exchanged, forming a new amino acid and a new keto acid. Transamination requires the vitamin B_6 coenzyme, pyridoxal phosphate, and a variety of specific enzymes known appropriately as transaminases.

The classic examples of transamination are the alanine-pyruvate, aspartate-oxaloacetate, and glutamate-α-ketoglutarate systems. However, all amino acids participate in transamination; and, with the exception of lysine and threonine, the reactions are reversible. In most or in all transaminations, glutamate and α-ketoglutarate are involved. A typical example is as follows:

| Tyrosine | α-Ketoglutaric Acid | Phenylhydroxy Pyruvic Acid | Glutamic Acid |

Another method for removing amino groups is *oxidative deamination*. Although theoretically all amino acids can be deaminated by this method, apparently the only such reaction of physiological importance is that involving glutamic acid. The initial reaction is a dehydrogenation with NAD or NADP as hydrogen acceptor, followed by hydrolysis yielding α-ketoglutarate and ammonia. This reaction also requires pyridoxal phosphate as a coenzyme.

$$\text{Glutamic acid} + \text{NAD} + H_2O \rightarrow \alpha\text{-Ketoglutaric acid} + NH_3 + NADH_2$$

Deamination of glutamate is significant chiefly as a means of disposing of amino groups transferred from other amino acids to α-ketoglutarate in transamination reactions. Ammonia formed by this process can be converted to urea.

ELECTRON TRANSPORT AND OXIDATIVE PHOSPHORYLATION

The process of *oxidative phosphorylation* is not only the primary goal of mitochondrial activity, but it is also the fundamental device at the command of the cell for trapping energy in a manner compatible with life and in a form that can be utilized efficiently by the cell. The oxidation of carbohydrates, fats, and proteins via the TCA cycle is the common pathway in the conversion of the energy of foodstuffs to a form that the cell can use. This usable form of energy is contained in ATP, the *currency of the cell*. The energy-yielding system is the electron transport system or respiratory chain that couples the oxidation of TCA cycle substrates with the formation of ATP, thus transforming the energy of oxidation into the phosphate bond energy necessary for cellular processes.

The components of the electron transport system are proteins with prosthetic groups, usually a heme, which are capable of alternate reduction and oxidation. A general scheme showing the electron carriers and sites of ATP formation is shown in Fig. 13.12.

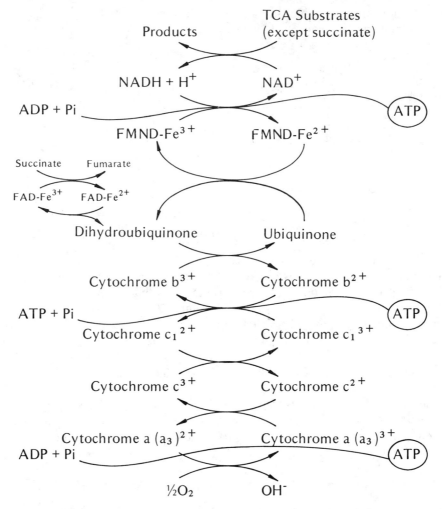

Figure 13.12
Electron transport and oxidative phosphorylation.

Electrons from oxidized TCA substrates, with the exception of succinate, are transferred to NAD. NADH and NAD do not permeate mitochondria. Only the electrons from NADH are shuttled across the membrane by a carrier such as glycerol 3-phosphate (Fig. 13.13). Other shuttles appear in Fig. 13.10.

Electrons are also donated to NAD from pyruvate and α-ketoglutarate dehydrogenase by way of the flavoproteins associated with these enzyme complexes. Electrons from succinate oxidation are donated to FAD. Ubiquinone, or coenzyme Q, serves as the electron carrier between the flavoproteins (FMN, FAD) and the cytochromes. Since ubiquinone has a highly nonpolar isoprenoid tail it diffuses rapidly in the hydrocarbon phase of the inner membrane. Cytochrome c is the only other component of the respiratory assembly that appears to be mobile.

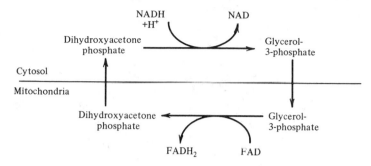

Figure 13.13
Glycerol phosphate shuttle.

The cytochromes are reduced when ubiquinone is reoxidized. Each quinone can provide two electrons for the reduction of cytochrome. Therefore, two molecules of cytochrome are required to react with one molecule of reduced ubiquinone. In this way two protons ($2H^+$) are released into the surrounding medium, and the electrons are transferred to the iron-containing cytochromes ultimately to be accepted by oxygen. The excitation of oxygen by electrons permits it to join with the hydrogen ions to form water.

Reactions transferring hydrogen directly to oxygen liberate much more energy than that required for the formation of a high energy phosphate bond; therefore a one-step reaction would be wasteful and perhaps disastrous to the cell. Much of the energy would be lost as heat that, in addition to being uneconomical, would strain the homeostatic mechanisms involved in maintaining body temperature.

The step-by-step transfer of two pairs of electrons along the respiratory chain results in the formation of 2 or 3 moles of ATP depending on whether succinate or other TCA cycle substitutes are oxidized. In this manner, potential energy is transformed gradually into the form of chemical energy useful to the cell. The three approximate sites for coupling of the oxidation process with the formation of ATP are shown in Figs. 13.12 and 13.14.

The respiratory chain and phosphorylating system (see Fig. 13.14) represent about 35 percent of the inner membrane protein. The remainder of the proteins are carriers of various ions and metabolites and/or are structural proteins. A number of laboratories have contributed to the isolation and characterization of the four main complexes of the respiratory chain, namely NADH-Q reductase, succinate-Q reductase, QH_2-cytochrome reductase, and cytochrome-c reductase. These enzymes hold the iron-containing cytochromes. When these are mixed in the appropriate stoichiometry, a functional electron transport chain can be reconstituted. (See Racker, 1980.) Imagine the excitement in the laboratory at such a success! Some of the characteristics of the respiratory chain complexes that have been identified are molecular weight, number of protein subunits, attendant prosthetic groups, surface topology of active sites in relation to the membrane, and relationships to each other (Table 13.2). There is biochemical evidence for all the details of Fig. 13.13. Reviews by De Pierre and Ernster (1977) and Racker (1980) are recommended.

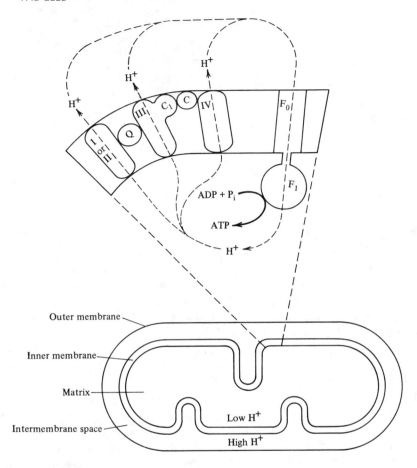

Figure 13.14
Diagram of the inner mitochondrial membrane which delineates a possible
organization of the respiratory chain, ATPase, and the directions of proton
movement which result in the formation of ATP. Compare with Table 13.2.

The manner of electron transfer between respiratory chain components is beginning to be understood. Because cytochrome c is soluble it has now been
isolated, purified, and its three-dimensional structure well characterized (Dickerson, 1972). It has a diameter of 34 Å, slightly less than half the thickness of a
typical membrane. Its amino acid residues surround the charged central heme
group in such a way that the heme group is held less than 8 Å from the heme of
the adjacent chain components, making direct heme-heme electron transport a
likely possibility. Cytochrome c appears to first recognize QH_2-cytochrome-c
reductase, then the cytochrome oxidase through the arrangement of charged
lysines on the face of the molecule. This highly successful system for electron
transfer evolved over 1.5 billion years ago and has been highly conserved, with
26 of the 104 residues being invariant. Thus, wheat germ cytochrome c will

TABLE 13.2

Composition and Topology of the Inner Mitochondrial Membrane Electron-Transport Chain

Enzyme Complex	Molecular Weight	Electron Accepting Centers	Position of Catalytic Sites		
			M-side	Center	C-side
I. NADH-Q reductase	850,000	FMN FeS	NADH	Q	
II. Succinate-Q reductase	97,000	FAD FeS	Succinate	Q	
III. QH$_2$-cyto-chrome-c reductase	280,000	b heme c$_1$ heme FeS		Q	cyto c
Cytochrome c	13,000	c heme			cyto c$_1$ cyto a
IV. Cytochrome-c oxidase	200,000	a heme a$_3$ heme Cu	O$_2$(?)		cyto c

Source: From J. De Pierre and L. Ernster, *Ann. Rev. Biochem. 46:* 215 (1977). The Roman numerals designate the complex. M-side and C-side are matrix and cytoplasmic sides, respectively.

transfer electrons to human cytochrome oxidase! For recent accounts, see Salemme (1977) and Dickerson (1980).

It was believed that the rate of the respiratory chain was controlled solely by the availability of reduced substrate and the ATP/ADP ratio. Recently, however, it has been demonstrated that glucagon stimulates the respiratory chain between cytochrome c$_1$ and c (Halestrap, 1978). Thus, this effect of glucagon suggests that mitochondrial metabolism is even more highly integrated with cell metabolism than was once thought.

The mode of coupling NADH oxidation to ATP synthesis remained an enigma for many years. Numerous investigators searched for an activated protein or high-energy intermediate that could serve as a precursor to ATP. In 1961, Peter Mitchell proposed a totally different mechanism, the *chemiosmotic hypothesis*. The proposal is that ATP synthesis and electron transport (which begins with NADH oxidation) are coupled by a proton gradient. The energy given up as electrons travels along the respiratory chain and drives the pumping of protons across the inner mitochondrial membrane to the intermembrane space against a gradient. The gradient is formed and maintained because the inner membrane is impermeable to hydrogen ions. Because of the gradient, commonly referred to as the *proton motive force*, hydrogen ions will tend to move from regions of high concentration to low, from intermembrane space to matrix. Protons (H$^+$), returning to the matrix through the ATPase, force the ATPase to operate in reverse. ATP is synthesized (Mitchell, 1976).

The electrochemical potential gradient of protons can also be utilized as the energy source for a number of processes, including transport of metabolites and calcium into mitochondria, transfer of electrons from NADH to NADPH, and various active transport processes. Articles in the primary literature documenting the chemiosmotic process are discussed from an historical perspective by Racker (1980).

Although the chemiosmotic hypothesis has become widely accepted, a number of controversies and unsolved mysteries still remain. For instance, the precise mechanism, on a molecular basis, of the proton translocations, first across or through the three sites in the electron transport chain, and then through the ATPase, is not known. Currently research is under way to characterize the proton channels (Wikström et al., 1981).

ENERGY YIELD

Oxidative Phosphorylation

The energy yield from TCA cycle oxidations can be estimated from the moles of ATP produced (Table 13.3). Those reactions giving rise to NADH lead to the formation of 3 moles of ATP and include all but two of the energy-yielding reactions of the cycle. An additional high-energy phosphate is formed from the conversion of succinyl CoA to succinate in a complex reaction involving the enzyme succinate thiokinase in which the coenzymes are guanosine di- and triphosphate. The oxidation of succinate to fumarate bypasses the NAD step and therefore yields only 2 moles of ATP. The total yield in high-energy phosphate from the TCA cycle totals the equivalent of 15 moles of ATP.

Similarly the high-energy phosphate yield from the complete oxidation of glucose also can be estimated. The degradation of glucose to pyruvate results in the formation of 2 moles of ATP from substrate level phosphorylations. (See Chapter 11.) Since 1 mole of glucose yields 2 moles of pyruvate, the total via the TCA cycle then is 30 moles of ATP. The total yield from the oxidation of 1 mole of glucose then is at least 32 moles of high-energy phosphate. In addition, 6 moles of high-energy phosphate may be added to the total of 32 moles of ATP if pyruvate

TABLE 13.3
Energy Yield from Pyruvate Oxidation via the TCA Cycle

Reaction	Coenzyme	ATP Yield
Pyruvate→ acetyl CoA	NAD	3
Isocitrate → α-ketoglutarate	NAD	3
α-Ketoglutarate → succinyl CoA	NAD	3
Succinyl CoA + ADP + P_i → succinate + ATP	GDP	1
Succinate → fumarate	FAD	2
Malate → oxaloacetate	NAD	3
		15

is not reduced to lactate. In this case, 2 moles of NADH remain in the cytoplasm to be accounted for and, although oxidation is not obligatory, in tissues actively oxidizing glucose completely to CO_2 and H_2O these 2 molecules could be oxidized by the electron transport chain to produce 6 moles of ATP. Thus, a total of 38 moles of ATP conceivably could be produced from the complete oxidation of glucose.

Complete Oxidation of Glucose

As noted in the previous section, the efficiency of energy transformations in biological systems is approximately 40 percent. This is a relatively high rate since the best man-made devices are only about 30 percent efficient. The theoretical yield for oxidation of glucose from calorimetric data is $-686,000$ cal. If there were no mechanism for harnessing this energy, all of it would be lost as heat. In biological systems, however, the coupling of energy released to ATP formation conserves the amount of energy equivalent to a maximum of 38 moles of ATP. Since each mole of ATP is equivalent to $-7,300$ cal, the total amount of energy conserved is $-277,000$ cal ($38 \times -7,300$). The efficiency of the total reaction, thus, is 40 percent ($-277,000/-686,000 \times 100$).

Fatty Acid Oxidation

The oxidation of fatty acids yields acetyl CoA and the reduced coenzymes, NADH and $FADH_2$. The latter are oxidized by the electron transport system to yield 5 moles of ATP for each mole of oxygen used for the production of acetyl CoA. Oxidation of acetyl CoA via the TCA cycle yields another 12 moles of energy-rich phosphate for each mole of acetyl CoA. As an example, the β-oxidation of stearate yields 148 moles of high-energy phosphate. Stearate yields 9 acetyl CoA ($9 \times 12 = 108$). Eight moles of O_2 are required since the terminal acetyl does not require oxygen. Thus, NADH and $FADH_2$ give rise to an additional 40 moles of high-energy phosphate. Assuming an energy worth of $-7,300$ cal/mole of ATP under physiological circumstances, this represents a yield of about 1,080,400 cal, which is about half the energy released when 1 mole of stearate is oxidized in a bomb calorimeter.

SYNTHESIS

Fatty Acids

Although fatty acid synthesis apparently proceeds more efficiently in cytoplasm and the endoplasmic reticulum (Chapter 11), mitochondria contain an enzyme system capable of catalyzing the elongation of preformed saturated or unsaturated fatty acids by the successive additions of acetyl CoA. The mitochondrial system requires both NADH and NADPH. The fatty acids formed are primarily C_{18}, C_{20}, C_{22}, and C_{24} fatty acids.

The mitochondrial system does not require CO_2 fixation and the reactions leading to elongation of existing fatty acids apparently are at least partially a reverse of β-oxidation.

Protein

Until quite recently it was believed that the cell's entire complement of DNA was in the nucleus. When small amounts of DNA appeared in mitochondrial fractions it was ascribed at first to contamination. However, Nass and Nass (1963) showed that the fiberlike inclusions in the mitochondria of normal chick embryos were DNA by specifically removing them from ultra-thin sections with DNAase. When it was shown that the DNA in intact mitochondria was not susceptible to DNAase, the intramitochondrial locus of DNA was substantiated (Luck and Reich, 1964).

Mitochondrial DNA differs from the nuclear DNA in the same cell in size and base composition. Like the DNA of certain viruses, it is a circular and hypertwisted double strand (Van Bruggen et al., 1966). A typical mitochondrial DNA molecule from an animal cell has a molecular weight of approximately 11 million, enough DNA to represent about 10–25 average-sized genes (Goodenough and Levine, 1970). Each mitochondrion may contain 2–6 DNA circles. Mitochondrial DNA is located in the matrix compartment and is probably attached to the inner membrane at the site where replication begins. The initiator of replication is not known. It is estimated that the DNA in a single bovine heart mitochondrion can maximally code for about 70 polypeptides (Schatz, 1970). The genetic role for mitochondrial DNA is supported by the fact that both RNA synthesis and amino acid incorporation are blocked by actinomycin, which is a specific inhibitor of DNA transcription.

Mitochondrial DNA does not carry a sufficient amount of genetic information to code for all the proteins and enzymes present in the mitochondrion. Mitochondrial DNA codes for mitochondrial ribosomal RNA, for at least 19 tRNAs, for mRNAs of 20 proteins, and for some highly hydrophobic proteins. Beattie (1971) estimates that less than 10 percent of total mitochondrial protein is directed by mitochondrial DNA and that most of it is localized in the inner membrane. The remainder of the protein in the inner membrane, and the protein of the outer membrane and the matrix are synthesized outside the mitochondrion and transferred in. (See Grivell, 1983.)

The protein synthesis within the mitochondrion presumes both a transcription and translation system. Conclusive proof of mitochondrial tRNA distinct from cytoplasmic tRNA was reported by Barnett and coworkers (Barnett and Epler, 1966; Barnett and Brown, 1967; Barnett et al., 1967). Mitochondrial ribosomes that are smaller than cytoplasmic ribosomes have been identified by André and Marinozzi (1965). Mitochondrial rRNA is unquestionably coded for in the mitochondrion, yet most if not all of the ribosomal proteins are coded for by the nucleus and synthesized on cytoplasmic ribosomes. Several inner membrane proteins consist of polypeptides of both cytoplasmic and mitochondrial origin. These include cytochrome oxidase, cytochrome b, and ATPase with approximately half of the subunits of mitochondrial origin. (See Wickner, 1979.) The molecular mechanism of this intricate process of protein synthesis remains to be elucidated. Mitochondrial ribosomal proteins are quite distinct from cytoplasmic ribosomal proteins (Raff and Mahler, 1972).

For a recent review of mitochondrial protein synthesis, see Kreil (1981).

CALCIUM TRANSPORT

Mitochondria have the capacity to accumulate Ca^{++}. *In vitro* studies have indicated that the accumulation can be quite massive and can progress to the extent that no Ca^{++} is left in the reaction medium (Vasington and Murphy, 1962). DeLuca and Engstrom (1961) and DeLuca et al. (1962) reported similar results. This uptake of calcium and of other divalent cations (Mn^{++}, Mg^{++}, and Sr^{++}) were shown to be coupled with electron flow and will be discussed in a subsequent section. However, about 50 percent of the total calcium transport in mitochondria is energy-independent and of considerable physiological interest (Carafoli and Rossi, 1971).

The data assembled by Carafoli and his colleagues (Patriarca and Carafoli, 1968; Carafoli et al., 1969) indicate the role of mitochondrial calcium transport in the contraction and relaxation of the heart. Heart muscle, in contrast to skeletal muscle, is rich in mitochondria and the segregation of Ca^{++} in the mitochondria instead of the sarcoplasmic reticulum returns the muscle to the resting state. In an *in vitro* study on energy-linked calcium transport in hearts from genetically myopathic hamsters with advanced degree of heart failure, Sulakhe and Dhalla (1973) demonstrated a decrease in calcium binding and uptake by the mitochondrial and heavy microsomal fractions of hearts. Their results suggest alterations in the membranes of cardiac mitochondria in heart failure. The reduced ability of the subcellular particles from the failing heart to bind and accumulate calcium was conceived to interfere with the process of relaxation of the cardiac muscle. Such impairment is considered to result in decreasing the intracellular stores of calcium thereby making less calcium available for release on depolarization of the failing heart cell.

Carafoli and Rossi (1971) suggest that many other cellular reactions may depend on mitochondrial calcium transport. There have been suggestions of mitochondrial intervention in biological mineralization and demineralization. Gonzales and Karnowski (1961) observed many electron-dense masses in mitochondria of osteoclasts in healing bone fractures, and DeLuca et al. (1962) reported that calcium uptake by mitochondria was influenced by parathyroid hormone. Rasmussen and Nagata (1970) reported a rise in free plasma calcium concentration after parathyroid hormone administration; and Borle (1973) suggests that mitochondria respond also to the influences of calcitonin and vitamin D. In vitamin D-deficient rats complete disappearance of calcium granules in the mitochondria of the intestinal cells was reported (Sampson et al., 1970). This was followed by an immediate and dramatic increase in number and density of granules after vitamin D administration. Borle (1973) postulated that mitochondria may be the main regulators of cytoplasmic calcium activity and calcium transport. His suggestion is that mitochondria function as an ion buffer, as a calcium trap, and as the main regulator of the concentration of free calcium in the cytoplasm. He further suggests that vitamin D may be essential for the uptake of calcium by mitochondria and that mitochondria control cell calcium metabolism. In vitamin D deficiency the mitochondrial buffer system would be slowly depleted and cease to function, and the calcium activity of the mitochondria and consequently the free calcium in the cytoplasm would fall, leading to a decreased efflux and transport of calcium across the intestinal epithelium.

Investigations reported by Schraer et al. (1973) on both *in vivo* and *in vitro* response to calcium by the mitochondria of avian shell gland and liver strongly support the concept that the mitochondrion is involved in the cellular transport of calcium. The propensity for mitochondria to accumulate calcium led to speculation about their role in biological calcification. In the shell gland of the hen the observation was made that there was more calcium in the endoplasmic reticulum than in the mitochondria when calcification was taking place; but there was more in the mitochondria when calcification was not taking place (Hohman and Schraer, 1966). This was interpreted to mean that during shell formation calcium moved from the mitochondria through the endoplasmic reticulum to the cell exterior for deposition as calcium carbonate. When shell formation was not occurring, calcium moved into the mitochondria from the cytoplasm with the consequent decrease in the endoplasmic reticulum. Similarly, Lehninger (1970) postulated that during bone calcification calcium moves through the mitochondrial membrane to the cytosol and then to bone matrix. However, the evidence implicating mitochondria in bone calcification is less clearly established than in shell gland.

For further discussion of the interrelated roles of parathyroid hormone, calcitonin, and vitamin D on calcium metabolism, see Chapter 17.

The precise manner in which mitochondria regulate intracellular calcium is still not known. However, a considerable amount of evidence indicates that there are two calcium transport systems in the inner mitochondrial membrane. Influx, through a unidirectional carrier, is down the electrochemical gradient. Efflux utilizes a second carrier and requires energy, as it is against the electrochemical gradient. The energy appears to be supplied by the membrane potential since altering the membrane potential reduces efflux.

The transport cycle of calcium provides control of cytoplasmic calcium and can be finely regulated. Finely tuned calcium regulation is an important feature of cell metabolism because a number of enzymes are stimulated or inhibited by calcium. Because mitochondrial dehydrogenases are affected, intramitochondrial calcium concentration may regulate oxidative metabolism and hence, indirectly, ATP production. (See Nicholls and Crompton, 1980; Denton and McCormack, 1981.)

Biogenesis of Mitochondria

The origin of mitochondria with their full complement of enzymes has been the subject of both speculation and investigation. Three major hypotheses have been presented concerning their biogenesis: (1) formation from other intracellular structures, (2) *de novo* formation, and (3) growth and division of preexisting mitochondria.

Almost every cellular organelle has been implicated at one time or another in mitochondrial biogenesis. It has been suggested that they are formed from the existing plasma membrane (Robertson, 1961), the nucleus (Hoffmann and Grigg, 1958), the nucleolus (Ehret and Powers, 1955), and the Golgi complex (Lever, 1956a; 1956b). As techniques improved in electron microscopy, and these were correlated with biochemical procedures, some of the apparent similarities in structure and composition gave way to obvious differences. With the identification of DNA in mitochondria (Wildman et al., 1962; Luck 1963a; 1963b; Gibor and Granick, 1964) and the presence of RNA (Rendi, 1959) it became more and more difficult to postulate mitochondrial origin from other cellular organelles. However, it is apparent that the endoplasmic reticulum does synthesize most of the mito- chondrial proteins (Beattie, 1971) and probably some of the lipids, but this occurs also for other organelles and their membranes.

The data that have recently been assembled provide evidence of the existence of a specific mitochondrial genetic system and make it difficult to support the suggestion that *de novo* synthesis occurs. It is unlikely that there are many who are willing to strongly support such an hypothesis.

The formation of mitochondria by growth and division of existing mitochondria has for a long time been intriguing to many investigators. Observations of dumb- bell-shaped mitochondria in many tissues were presented as evidence of incipient division (Lafontaine and Allard, 1964; Fawcett, 1955). When Luck (1963b) in- corporated labeled choline in phosphatidyl choline of mitochondrial membranes of *Neurospora*, and observed that when the number of mitochondria increased all contained labeled phospholipid, he concluded that most, if not all, of the mitochondria formed had arisen by growth and division of preexisting mitochon- dria. Gibor and Granick (1964) postulated that a DNA unit that is self-duplicating and serves as a code for RNA is the basic hereditary unit of each mitochondrion. Current evidence is strong enough to no longer question the fact that mitochondria are capable of growth and division and that this is probably the manner in which mitochondrial multiplication occurs. There are interactions between mitochondria and other cytoplasmic organelles and substantial evidence that some of the mi- tochondrial protein arises through synthesis by the endoplasmic reticulum. This suggests that mitochondria are biochemically integrated with other organelles in the cell. Probably most of the outer membrane and many of the enzymatically active proteins are synthesized extramitochondrially (Neupert et al., 1972) and under the direction of nuclear DNA. However, the mitochondrion is unique, as far as is now known, in that it does contain genetic capability, even though somewhat limited, that permits it to synthesize a small, but essential, portion of its own substance. Many investigators have drawn analogies between mitochon- dria and chloroplasts and between these organelles and procaryotic organisms and suggest that these organelles had their origins as independent organisms (Raven, 1970; Goodenough and Levine, 1970; Raff and Mahler, 1972; Schwartz and Dayhoff, 1978).

For a more detailed presentation on the origin and evolution of mitochondria, see Gillham (1978); Frederick (1981).

Conclusion

The exquisite precision with which the mitochondrion performs its intricate bio-chemical procedures implies a corresponding precision in organization. Such coordinated and efficient function could not occur by random meeting of enzymes and substrates; it could only occur with an architectural design elegantly integrated with function. It is quite apparent now that the mechanisms of energy transfer associated with respiration and oxidative phosphorylation are but one facet of the functional capability of the mitochondrion. However, it is the ATP made available by mitochondrial activity that provides the power for all the energy-requiring activities of the cell: synthesis of large molecules, mechanochemical work of contraction, and osmotic work involved in active transport.

The nutritionist ascertaining the energy expenditure or metabolic rate of the whole organism is, in effect, estimating very indirectly the total amount of ATP trapped by the prodigious number of mitochondria (approximately 10^{17} in the adult human) that function at quite disparate rates in oxidizing the cells' food. The metabolic rate of the whole organism is, in reality, the sum of the metabolic rates in the incomprehensively large total mitochondrial population of its constituent cells.

chapter 14

the lysosomes and microbodies

The lysosome is the cell's cup of hemlock or, as de Duve described it, the "suicide bag," a term that he deplores now as "unfortunately catchy," since the lysosome's active role in cell life is of greater import than its role associated with cell death. This organelle is present in cells in varying numbers, being particularly large and abundant in cells that perform digestive functions such as the macrophages and white blood cells. It is a membrane enclosing three dozen or so powerful enzymes capable of breaking down complex nutrients. As long as the membrane remains intact, the lysosome can and does function as the digestive organ of the cell. However, disruption of the membrane frees the enzymes and the cell then digests itself. The disruption of a cell by a lysosome is obviously catastrophic in the life of a single cell organism but in complex organisms, the death of individual cells and their replacement by new young cells occurs in the normal course of events and is characteristic of certain tissues.

Identification of Lysosomes

The *lysosome* was identified and named by de Duve et al. (1955). The relatively tardy recognition of its existence was undoubtedly due, in part, to its heterogeneity in appearance and its small size when seen in electron photomicrographs. The lack of structural conformity made it extremely difficult for cytologists to identify lysosomes as specific organelles on the basis of appearance, and their recognition was the result of the complementary efforts of cytologists and biochemists. Collaborative studies revealed that certain cytoplasmic particles appeared to be associated with a group of hydrolytic enzymes, all of which showed an acid pH optimum. This association of the particles and enzymes led de Duve to suggest the name lysosome, which means lytic body. For his work on the identification of lysosomes, de Duve was one of the recipients of a Nobel prize in 1974.

Lysosomes are present in greatest number in kidney cells, certain white blood cells with macrophagic function, thymus, and spleen, but they occur in all animal cells except red blood cells. The high concentration of lysosomes in the macrophages is associated with the phagocytic function of these cells since one aspect of lysosomal function is the role it plays in the processing and digestion of extracellular materials.

Some of the difficulties encountered in the isolation and identification of lysosomes were due to the fact that early methods of centrifugal fractionation put the particles containing the hydrolases in both the mitochondrial fraction and in the fraction containing microsomes, the fragmented portions of the endoplasmic reticulum. It was through de Duve's critical standardization of fractionation techniques that the lysosomal fraction was separated from other cell fractions (see Chapter 7), and the morphological studies of Novikoff et al. (1956) that led to the lysosomal concept. Novikoff identified the so-called dense bodies, surrounded by a single lipoprotein membrane, as the structures containing the histochemically detectable acid phosphatase, one of the characteristic lysosomal enzymes. This was the first time that such a sequence in the identification of an organelle, first biochemical and then visual, had occurred.

The lysosomes were first described as membrane-bound granules containing five acid hydrolases in latent form (de Duve et al., 1955). The list of enzymes quickly increased to 12. By 1976 the number of hydrolytic enzymes associated with lysosomes stood at 57 (Altmann and Katz, 1976, p. 318). This spectrum of enzymes acts in an acid pH and is capable of splitting important biological compounds such as proteins, nucleic acids, polysaccharides, and phospholipids. Such a powerful arsenal is potentially lethal to the cell unless it is contained, controlled, and channeled for proper use. The existence of such a stockpile of potential danger in a functioning cell indicates that some barrier must exist to unrestrained hydrolytic activity. Yet if these enzymes perform a digestive function for the cell, the substrates for their activity must be presented within the confines of the organelle barrier. This line of reasoning led de Duve to present a model of the lysosomes as a biochemical concept (Fig. 14.1) that visualizes the intact lysosome surrounded by a lipoprotein membrane making the enzymes inaccessible to the rest of the cell. Injury to the membrane, however, by known abnormal situations, such as freezing and thawing, sonic vibrations, fat solvents, and detergents or by inadequate osmotic protection or drastic changes in cellular pH or temperature, could liberate the contained enzymes into the cell contents. The meeting of lysosomal enzymes and the substrates within the cell would lead to

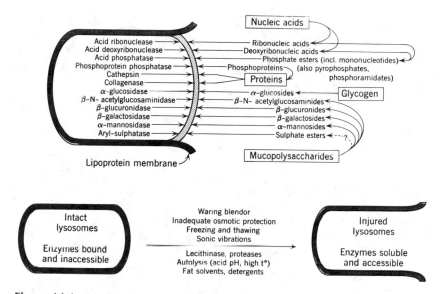

Figure 14.1

Lysosomes as a biochemical concept. The model shown applies to rat liver lysosomes. Additional enzymes identified in lysosomes include lysozyme, phospholipase, phosphatidic acid phosphatase, esterases, and hyaluronidase. (From C. de Duve, *Ciba Foundation Symposium on Lysosomes*, A. V. S. de Rueck and M. P. Cameron, eds., Little, Brown and Co., Boston, 1963, p.2.)

the digestion of the cell. Such a seemingly catastrophic situation might be the sequence in a normal developmental process or in a pathological situation. Examples of both processes will be discussed.

For an interesting view of the lysosome in retrospect and the work leading to the current concept of the lysosome as part of a cell system, see de Duve (1969a).

Structure

The heterogeniety of lysosomes with respect to size, form, function, and origin can be more readily understood now that lysosomes have been identified as part of a complex system of great importance to the physiology of the cell, rather than merely as a digestive and waste-disposal system.

Lysosomes are so varied in structural appearance and so lacking in unique morphological characteristics that their identification without combined biochemical or cytochemical methods is extremely difficult. They possess no aspects of fine structure that could categorize them unmistakably as do the constant features found in mitochondria, nuclei, or endoplasmic reticulum (Fig. 14.2). The appearance of lysosomes depends on their functional state. There are, however,

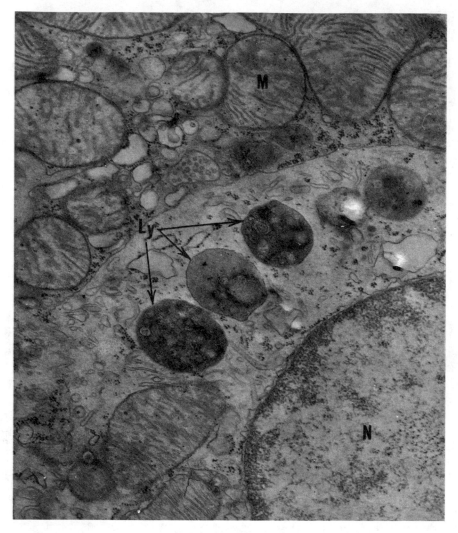

Figure 14.2
Variations in the fine structure of lysosomes in a cell from rat kidney proximal tubule.
Lysosomes (Ly), nucleus (N), mitochondrion (M). Magnification × 21,200. (Courtesy
of Dr. Harald Schraer.)

certain characteristics that they have in common. They have a single limiting
membrane that, like the membrane of the Golgi vesicles, is 25 percent thicker
than the membranes of mitochondria, rough endoplasmic reticulum, and Golgi
lamellae (Yamamoto, 1963). Another characteristic of lysosomes is the *halo*, a
clear electron-lucid rim just inside the limiting membrane and between it and the
dense matrix (Maunsbach, 1966a). In addition to these structural features, histochemical tests for acid phosphatase are characteristic of lysosomes, as is their

ability to accumulate exogenous material. In this last respect, they are unique among cytoplasmic organelles (de Duve, 1963).

MEMBRANE CHARACTERISTICS

The membrane of the lysosome, which forms the barrier between the cytoplasm and the arsenal of enzymes within, functions as the semipermeable membrane of an osmotic system. The simplest model of such a system would be the enzyme-containing bag first suggested by de Duve. This model does not imply that the contents are devoid of fine structure, but it does indicate that the hydrolases have freedom of movement when the barrier is broken (de Duve, 1963). The demonstration of the mobility of the enzymes by de Duve's laboratory and of the elution of the enzymes from lysosomal membranes by Tappel and his group (1963) suggested at that time that the enzymes were not closely bound in either the inner structure of the lysosome or in the lipoprotein of the membrane. However, present biochemical evidence suggests that some of the lysosomal enzymes are constituents of the membrane itself and, furthermore, that a portion of the soluble enzymes are bound to the membrane and possibly form a protective lining. Three lysosomal enzymes have been identified as constituent parts of the membrane: β-N-acetylglucosaminidase, α-glucosidase, and sialidase. Other enzymes have been shown, under experimental conditions, to be bound to membranes. Although lysosomes contain a variety of proteases, the enzymes that are part of or bound to membranes appear stable and quite resistant to the proteolytic enzymes (Tappel, 1969). The lysosomal membrane, therefore, must differ from that of other organelles since the membranes of mitochondria and endoplasmic reticulum are hydrolyzed within the confines of the lysosome.

Despite the content of highly active hydrolytic enzymes, autolysis does not usually occur in the cell, and this has been attributed to what de Duve calls *structure-linked latency* of the lysosomal hydrolases. In other words, the extralysosomal cytoplasm remains intact because any heterolytic digestive action of the lysosome takes place only after a substrate has come within the confines of the lysosomal membrane. It follows that a break in the membrane must precede any autolytic activity. It is the membrane shield or the *structure* that is responsible for and *linked* to the inactive presence or *latency* of the enzymes. The integrity of the membrane was thought to be secured by the fact that neither lipases nor phospholipases had been identified, but no longer can this be a comfort since it appears that lysosomes have a complete complement of hydrolytic enzymes for the breakdown of lipids (Tappel, 1969), along with the enzymes acting on proteins, glycogen, nucleic acids, and mucopolysaccharides.

De Duve (1963) suggested the membrane was responsible for the latency of the enzymes and that the lysosome may be comparable to a bag of fluid in which the enzymes are suspended or dissolved. Since then a number of nonenzymatic constituents have been identified in lysosomes, including histamine, cationic protein, several phospholipids and glycosphingolipids, and cholesterol (Altman and Katz, 1976). Koenig and Jibril (1962) suggested that the lysosomes may be solid complexes and that the latency depends on ionic binding of the enzymes to acidic glycolipids, which renders them inactive. This is the *matrix binding theory*, in which the lysosome is regarded as a membrane-limited polyanionic lipoprotein granule. According to this model (Koenig, 1969), the hydrolytic enzymes within the lysosome are in an inert state by electrostatic binding to the acidic groups of the lipoprotein matrix. The active sites of the hydrolases are unavailable to react with their substrates because of ionic linkage to the lysosomal matrix. The acidic lipoprotein acts as an inhibitor of lysosomal enzymes, and the membraneous envelope serves mainly to limit the freedom of the enzyme-lipoprotein complex. Studies with phospholipase C indicate that the phosphoryl groups of the lipoprotein phospholipids play an important role in the structural latency of the lysosomal enzymes. Fig. 14.3 shows how the phosphoryl groups probably serve as binding sites for the acid hydrolases. The remaining phospholipid phos-

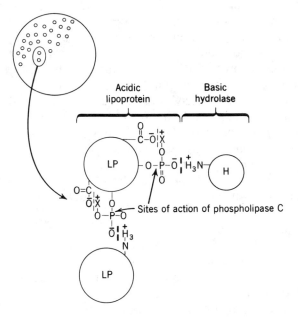

Figure 14.3
Matrix binding theory of the lysosome. The basic groups of the phospholipid are represented as being internally neutralized through electrostatic interaction with adjacent carboxylic groups of the lipoprotein, leaving the negatively charged phosphoryl group free for binding the cationic hydrolases or other lipoprotein macromolecules. (From H. Koenig, in *Lysosomes in Biology and Pathology*, Vol. 2, J. T. Dingle and H. B. Fell, eds., Wiley-Interscience, New York, 1969, p. 142.)

phate, which is less accessible to the action of the enzyme, according to Koenig (1969), seems to be essential for the maintenance of the structural integrity of the lysosomal particle.

Whether or not there is a fine structure to the interior of the lysosome is yet to be revealed. The disclosure of details of an internal structure may help to pinpoint the responsibility for latency. It may also indicate whether a nonenzymatic constituent of lysosomes that gives a histochemical reaction indicating the presence of mucopolysaccharide or glycolipid is a part of the membrane or, possibly, a part of the still undiscovered fine structure.

MEMBRANE STABILIZERS AND LABILIZERS

The stability of the membrane defining the lysosome and holding its package of potentially powerful hydrolytic enzymes is of major importance in the normal physiology of the cell. Those agents that favor the maintenance of lysosomal membrane integrity have been termed *stabilizers*. In contrast, agents that disturb cellular pH, osmotic relations, chemical stability, or perhaps electrical charge of the membrane are all potentially disruptive and can promote the liberation of the contained enzymes into the cellular contents. Such agents are *labilizers* of the lysosomal membrane. An intact lysosomal membrane would be dependent on the counterbalancing influences of membrane stabilizers over membrane labilizers. Just as the cell is dependent on the nutrients coming in from its environment, so are the organelles dependent on and affected by the nutrients available in the intracellular environment. It should come as no surprise that specific nutrients have been shown to exert either stabilizing or labilizing influences on the lysosomal membrane.

Vitamin A was reported to be an extremely effective labilizer of the lysosomal membrane. Several investigators, including Dingle (1963) and Weissmann and Thomas (1963), showed in *in vivo* and *in vitro* studies that vitamin A alcohol or acid acted directly on lysosomes releasing the confined enzymes. Tissues from hypervitaminotic A animals consistently released more enzymes than control tissues. It was suggested that a reaction occurs between the lipoprotein membrane of the lysosome and the vitamin in which the vitamin penetrates the membrane and causes expansion of the lipoprotein components, thus leading to instability of the membrane and the consequent release of enzymes. Fell (1965) suggested that spontaneous fractures observed as a result of excess dosage of vitamin A are due to the release of lysosomal enzymes from cartilage and bone cells into the extracellular environment. One could speculate that this capacity of vitamin A to labilize lysosomal membranes and release the confined enzymes is also a specific mechanism employed in normal bone growth, perhaps triggered by growth hormone or thyrotropin.

The labilizing effect attributed to vitamin A became confused when Roels et al. (1964) demonstrated that vitamin A deficiency in rats also led to a considerable degree of lability of liver lysosomes. However, administration of oral retinyl acetate restored lysosomal fragility to normal. No conclusion could be reached whether the effect was a specific one due to vitamin A deficiency or to the general tissue degeneration accompanying the advanced deficiency state (Roels, 1969). Here was an instance where both a plethora and a deficiency of vitamin A had a labilizing effect on lysosomal membranes. Vitamin A has also been shown to be teratogenic in both deficiency and in excess, and Lloyd and Beck (1969) suggest that the effect of excess may be due to lysosomal rupture. They indicate that the teratogenicity of vitamin A deficiency could be due to action of vitamin A on biological membranes although the exact mechanism is not clear.

Other labilizers of the lysosomal membrane are ultraviolet light and ionizing radiation, both of which are extremely effective in disrupting the membrane and causing the enzymes to leak out into the surrounding area. The effect is due to the sensitivity of the membrane to damage by free radicals. Free radicals are produced when ionizing radiations hitting the cells are absorbed by the water in the cell, ionizing and decomposing the water. Hydroxyl and perhydroxyl radicals are formed as well as oxidizing compounds such as hydrogen peroxide and organic peroxides. These can be extremely toxic to tissue, leading to blistering and other more serious symptoms such as those observed in severe sunburn and x-ray burn. This effect of free peroxide can only be counteracted by the action of the iron-containing enzyme catalase, which can decompose hydrogen peroxide to water and oxygen. When free radical generation exceeds the capacity of the catalase reaction, the toxic effects become evident.

Vitamin E acts as a membrane stabilizer since its antioxidant properties prevent lipid peroxidation and the consequent generation of a free radical system (Tappel, 1972) leading to the disruption of the lysosomal membrane. (See Chapter 9.) However, there is controversy as to whether the antioxidant theory of vitamin E action is sufficient to explain its role in maintaining membrane stability. According to Green (1972), the role of vitamin E at membrane sites has yet to be clarified.

Some of the conflicting reports on the effects of vitamin E on lysosomal membrane stability apparently are due to the levels of the vitamin used. When small quantities were employed in *in vitro* work (Guha and Roels, 1965), there was stabilization of lysosomal membranes; but when large doses were employed (de Duve et al., 1962), labilization of the membrane occurred. Roels (1969) concludes that the *in vitro* effect of vitamin E on lysosomes greatly depends on the quantity: doses in the physiological range tend to stabilize the membrane, whereas large amounts tend to produce labilization.

When the interaction of vitamins A and E on lysosomes was studied in rat liver (Roels et al., 1965; Guha and Roels, 1965), it was concluded that vitamin A appeared to regulate the stability of lysosomal membranes and that its effect was dependent on the level of α-tocopherol in the diet. In vitamin A-deficient rats, increasing amounts of α-tocopherol had an increasingly stabilizing effect on the lysosomal membrane.

An interaction was also observed between vitamin E and selenium (Brown and Pollack, 1972). Using low levels of selenium and vitamin E, a potentiating effect was observed; that is, the combination of the two nutrients produced stabilization of lysosomal membranes at levels that neither could do alone. However, if vitamin

E and selenium were given in the same ratio but at 100 times the level, labilization of lysosomal membranes was observed.

Zinc markedly stabilizes lysosomal membranes and its effect appears to be at the surface of the membrane. Since cadmium and lead are also effective, although less so than zinc, the suggested action is one of interfering with oxidation of membrane components (Chvapil et al., 1972).

The lysosomal membrane depends for its successful functioning on controlled instability, that is, sufficient lability to permit it to function in endo- and exocytosis, secondary lysosome formation, and other kinds of membrane fusion (Lucy, 1972). The relationships between the stabilizers and labilizers of the membrane structure, therefore, must in some way participate in jointly establishing that control. How this occurs remains the lysosomes' secret.

Origin, Development, and Fate of Lysosomes

The *primary lysosome* is believed to develop in the cell through the combined activities of the endoplasmic reticulum and the Golgi complex. Lysosome formation has been studied in granular leucocytes of the rabbit since these cells permit ease of identification of primary lysosomes, that is, *storage granules*, whose enzymes participate in digestion after phagocytosis. Using tritiated lysine in both *in vivo* and *in vitro* studies, Fedorko and Hirsh (1966) followed its incorporation in the formation of the granules in the membrane-bound primary lysosome. Within 5–10 minutes after the pulse, the label was highest (71 percent) over the rough endoplasmic reticulum and cytoplasmic matrix, fell to 50 percent and was maintained at that level. Label over the Golgi complex was 11 percent at 10 minutes, increased to 37 percent by 30 minutes, and then fell back to 11 percent by 180 minutes. The label over the cytoplasmic granules rose steadily to 37 percent by 180 minutes. From this and other studies, it was concluded that the Golgi complex receives the newly formed protein from the endoplasmic reticulum and packages it in membrane-bound cytoplasmic granules.

The process of primary lysosome formation from the Golgi apparatus (see Chapter 12) and from the Golgi-endoplasmic reticulum-lysosome complex (GERL) is depicted in Fig. 14.4. This same system synthesizes proteins for secretion. The manner in which the secretory proteins and hydrolytic enzymes are sorted out for packaging is a fascinating aspect of cell function and is receiving appropriate attention in research laboratories (Hasilik, 1980). Sugar groups on the protein chains appear to play a decisive role in the sorting. It may be that, in addition to the traditional pathway of synthesis in the endoplasmic reticulum followed by intracellular transfer to the lysosomes, the enzymes are first secreted, then taken up from the extracellular milieu. This hypothesis has been termed secretion-reuptake. (See Neufeld, 1977.) Figure 14.4 also shows the relationship of primary lysosomes to secondary lysosomes and the plasma membrane. Not surprisingly, all the lysosomal transformations indicated in Fig. 14.4 do not occur in the same cell.

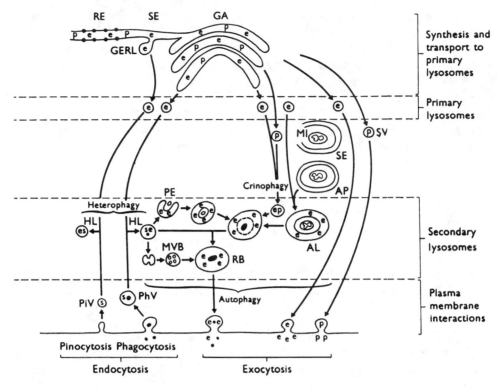

Figure 14.4
Diagram of the synthesis of lysosomal enzymes, the formation of primary lysosomes, their fusion with a variety of intracellular substances to form secondary lysosomes, and the types of interactions that occur with the plasma membrane. Within membranes: lysosomal enzymes (e), secretory proteins (p), soluble substrates for lysosomal digestion (s), particulate substrates are represented as solid areas. Outside membranes: rough endoplasmic reticulum (RE), smooth endoplasmic reticulum (SE), Golgi apparatus (GA), Golgi-endoplasmic reticulum-lysosome complex (GERL), secretory vesicle (SV), autophagosome (AP), autolysosome (AL), peroxisome (PE), multivesicular body (MVB), residual body (RB), pinocytic vesicle (PiV), phagocytic vacuole (PhV), heterolysosome (HL), mitochondrion (M). (From R. T. Dean, *Lysosomes*, Edward Arnold Publishers, London, 1977, p. 27.)

The formation of *secondary lysosomes* was studied in cultured macrophages by time-lapse cinematography (Cohn and Benson, 1965). Pinocytotic vesicles were formed at the peripheral membrane and migrated toward the cell interior with some fusing to form larger vesicles or *heterophagosomes*. Close to the Golgi complex they became smaller and denser. The actual fusion of the pinocytotic vesicles and the vesicle containing the granules that budded off from the Golgi saccule (the primary lysosome) just prior to the increase in density and decrease in size was observed by Hirsh et al. (1970). At this stage the test for acid phosphatase, the characteristic enzyme of lysosomes, was strongly positive. Since these contained both environmental molecules and newly synthesized hydrolases, they are identified as *secondary lysosomes*, or *heterolysosomes*. Had they evolved from a merger of intracellular material, an *autophagosome*, and lysosome, they would be *autolysosomes*. A form of heterolysosome is the *multivesicular body*, which results from the penetration of intact Golgi vesicles through heteropha-gosome membranes (Novikoff et al., 1964). These form physiological time bombs, according to Beck and Lloyd (1969), since they are in a position to release hydrolytic enzymes at any time after penetration into the phagosome. It is generally assumed that the contents of the lysosome are emptied into the phagosome after lysosome-phagosome fusion and that the fusion itself is due to *fusion compatability* between these membranes compared to an incompatability between the lysosome and other intact organelles. The membrane of the secondary lysosome that is thus formed is partly plasma membrane that originally surrounded the phagosome and partly lysosomal membrane. (See Daems et al., 1969.)

After the first fusion of a pinocytotic vesicle with the primary lysosome to form the secondary lysosome, additional fusions with vesicles can occur leading to successive acts of digestion and the piling up of residues (de Duve and Wattiaux, 1966). Eventually sufficient residue is accumulated in the lysosomes and they can no longer pick up materials ingested by the cell (Daems et al., 1969). De Duve and Wattiaux (1966) suggest that these filled secondary lysosomes develop into *telolysosomes*, which develop lipofuscin granules as they age. According to Daems et al. (1969), telolysosomes are the secondary lysosomes that have reached their maximum loading capacity and no longer accumulate material nor renew their enzymes. Finally, a structure that is functionally and enzymatically inactive is formed that consists solely of digestive residues, the *residual body*. The residual bodies have an accumulation of electron-dense pigments, lipid droplets, amor-phous masses, and degraded membrane fragments that appear as dense swirls in electron micrographs and are called myelin figures (Fig. 14.5).

It has been suggested that the accumulated material in the residual bodies can leave the cell by defecation (Ericsson et al., 1965) but the fact that pigment accumulation occurs in liver cells in jaundice (Novikoff et al., 1964) and that storage is progressive in pathological storage diseases suggests that a defecation mechanism, if it does exist, is not very efficient.

The discharge of some of the products of digestion by the lysosome into the cytoplasm of the cell certainly occurs in protists that depend on the lysosome as the source of digested materials for metabolism. It is assumed also that this occurs in cells of higher organisms without affecting the integrity of the lysosomal mem-brane; for example, the breakdown of colloid in thyroid cells leading to the release of thyroxin from thyroglobulin (Seljelid, 1967), and the release of iron from eryth-rocytes that have been engulfed by lysosomes (Daems, 1969). Both of these examples will be discussed in a later section.

With very slight modifications, de Duve's representation of the lysosomal forms and their interrelationships (Fig. 14.6) is still applicable. In fact, it clearly depicts the birth, life, and death of this organelle. For further detail on the formation and fate of lysosomes, see Dean and Barrett (1976) and Holtzmann (1976).

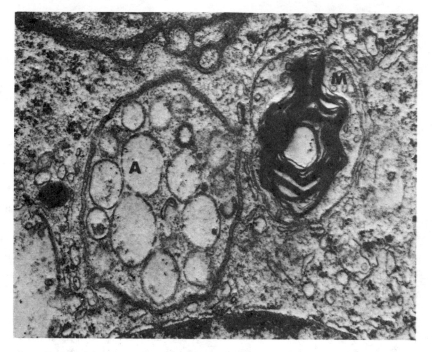

Figure 14.5
Autophagic vacuole (A) and myelin figure (M) indicating degeneration of cellular organelles. Zona glomerulosa cell of the adrenal cortex of a pregnant rat fed a low sodium diet. Degenerative changes attributed to cellular exhaustion as a consequence of the inability of the cell to cope with the excessive demand for aldosterone secretion. Magnification × 30,000. (Courtesy of Dr. Helen Smiciklas-Wright.)

Function of Lysosomes

The presence within a membrane-enclosed structure of a collection of acid hydrolases suggested to de Duve (1963) only one function: acid digestion. Since pinocytosis is a phenomenon that probably occurs in all cells, and since the pinocytotic invagination becomes the membrane-enclosed phagosome, de Duve postulated the merging of the enzyme-containing lysosome and the substrate-containing phagosome. This merger would enable the digestive process to occur entirely within the confines of an enclosing membrane. Residual materials could either be retained within the membrane-enclosed area in the cell or released from the cell by a process which could be called *exocytosis* or defecation. Such a progressive digestive process could account for the diversity in appearance of the lysosomes and, in addition, make this characteristic understandable in terms of

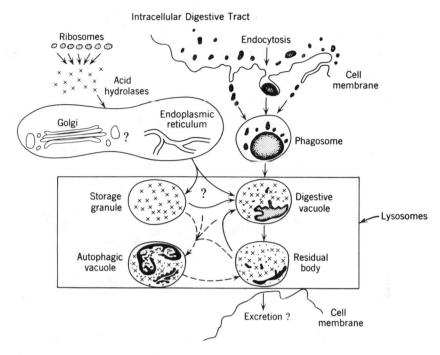

Figure 14.6
Diagrammatic representation of the four functional forms covered by the lysosome concept and of their interrelationships. (From C. de Duve, *Ciba Foundation Symposium on Lysosomes*, A. V. S. de Rueck and M. P. Cameron, eds., Little, Brown and Co., Boston, 1963a, p. 20.)

organelle function. Further, it could explain the mechanism involved in the phagocytic function of the specialized cells found in the blood, liver, spleen, and other tissues. Since few cell types in higher organisms are able to eliminate their digestive residues, de Duve (1963) suggested the possibility that accumulated residues in the cells may play an important part in the phenomenon of aging.

The fusion of heterophagosomes with the plasma membrane, depicted in Fig. 14.4, suggests that the amount of plasma membrane could change with cell activity. In fact, despite the continual fusing of membranes, the membrane surface area remains remarkably constant. This has led Palade (1975) to postulate that membranes translocated during the secretory process are recycled. Some evidence has been garnered by using membrane markers, such as cationized ferritin. It has been possible to follow the movement of membranes from one organelle to another, supporting the concept of membrane recycling.

In the years following the description of lysosomes as discrete biological entities, they have been shown to be as much a part of the cell's dynamic state as the mitochondria and polysomes. The lysosome system is, in fact, crucial in the interactions between the cell and its environment. Lysosomal sensitivity to both the intra- and extracellular environment is either directly or indirectly involved in many physiological and pathological processes.

De Duve's (1969a) concept of lysosomes describes five basic functions. (1) The simplest function of the lysosome is *storage* both of biosynthetic products within zymogen granules and other secretion granules in the primary lysosomes and of materials brought in by endocytosis. (2) Related to storage is the *exocytotic discharge* of stored materials. If the stored products were secretory materials, the process is called *secretion*; if the products had previously been taken in by endocytosis and are returned to the space from which they came, it is *regurgitation*; or, if they are released to another space, it is *transcellular transport*. (3) Another fundamental function results from the merger of the phagosome and a lysosome that results in the *digestion* of the material in the phagosome. (4) *Cellular autophagy* is still another function. It is a process whereby an autophagic vacuole fuses with a lysosome and enables the cell to rid itself of cytoplasmic fragments and damaged or worn out organelles. (5) The *release of storage material* either by defecation or exocytosis. The process may be excretory or secretory. Continued accumulation in storage without the mechanism of release leads to interference with normal cell function.

In the sections that follow, specific lysosomal activities will be discussed. In each case, one or more of the basic functions of this organelle system are involved.

LYSOSOMES AND KIDNEY FUNCTION

Although lysosomal function has been studied in different sections of the nephron, the role in the proximal tubule is best known. Following careful differential centrifugation, several species of lysosomes that vary in fine structure have been identified in proximal tubule cells. It is assumed that different ultrastructural characteristics are associated with differences in function. Of particular interest is the evidence that cells of the proximal tubules have the ability to absorb proteins from the glomerular filtrate (Latta et al., 1967; Straus, 1967). This could be of importance in pathological conditions, but there is evidence that small amounts of protein, primarily albumin, are normally present in the filtrate of mammals (Dirks et al., 1964). This albumin is reabsorbed into the proximal tubule cell and catabolized there (Schultze and Heremans, 1966). The albumin first appears in the cells in endocytotic vacuoles that fuse with each other and then with lysosomes (Maunsbach, 1966a; 1966b). There is no evidence that the absorbed protein molecules are extruded from the cells. However, *in vitro* studies on purified lysosomes (Maunsbach, 1969) have indicated the presence of several albumin-degrading enzymes. He has proposed that the proximal tubule cell lysosomes function in protein catabolism. In animals with experimental proteinuria, increased protein breakdown was shown to occur in the kidney tubules (Katz et al., 1963; 1964). The suggestion is that under such conditions, or in human disorders in which proteinuria is heavy, the normal albumin absorption process is accelerated, and the lysosomes in the tubular cells are responsible for the increased protein catabolism.

There is evidence that all proteins are not handled as albumin and, indeed, that foreign proteins may become localized in particles that resemble lysosomes (Novikoff, 1963; Graham and Karnovsky, 1966). Allergic reactions initiated by antibodies to foreign protein and leading to lysosomal enzyme release have been impugned in various disorders including glomerulonephritis (Coombs and Fell, 1969).

MACROPHAGES AND OTHER PHAGOCYTES

One of the principal functions of macrophages is the uptake of substances by endocytosis. An actively endocytosing macrophage appears to recycle its entire surface area once every half hour. Lymphoid macrophages, part of the reticulo-endothelial system, operate in the first line of defense for the removal of deleterious substances by sequestering them in their lysosomes. What happens to these substances subsequently depends on the lysosome. Those materials susceptible to lysosomal enzyme attack are digested; inert substances accumulate. The accumulations may be relatively harmless, as the dust collected in the lung cells; or painful, as the accumulations of uric acid crystals in gout; or seriously injurious, as the accumulation of asbestos and silica by lung macrophages (Allison, 1967). Although the accumulation of uric acid crystals appears to cause release of lysosomal enzymes and the subsequent inflammation and pain in the joints, silica and asbestos accumulated by macrophages in the lungs are far more damaging. These materials apparently react with the lysosomal membrane rendering it unstable and ultimately causing release of its hydrolytic enzymes. The silica or asbestos particles are released only to be reengulfed. This leads to further damage each time the cycle repeats and produces further necrosis and eventual fibrosis (Slater, 1969).

An active physiological process in which the macrophages participate is erythrophagocytosis (Daems, 1969), or the phagocytic action on the worn-out erythrocytes pulled into the spleen (Bowers, 1969). Whole erythrocytes have been observed inside lysosomes in electron micrographs of guinea pig macrophages in culture (North, 1966). Erythrocytes in various stages of digestion have been observed and the salvage of iron is important in the body's iron economy. (See Chapter 16.)

Another macrophage function that is part of a normal repair process involves white blood cells that migrate from the vascular system to the tissue involved. In wound healing, the lysosomes of the macrophages play an important role. The neutrophils, one of the group of granular leucocytes in the blood, phagocytose invading bacteria and subject them to lysosomal digestion. However, if no bacteria are there for the eating, the deprived neutrophil appears to succumb and, with the rupture of its cell membrane, it releases enzyme-containing granules into the wound site where they act on the cellular debris. Invasion of the wound by monocytes from the blood is next, and they complete the removal and digestion of tissue debris. This, too, is due to the activity of lysosomes (Ross, 1969). Only after this phagocytic activity can other cells move in for the synthesis of collagen, scar formation, and tissue synthesis in the process of healing.

HORMONE SECRETION AND REGULATION

The thyroid hormones, thyroxine and triiodothyronine, are synthesized in the thyroid gland linked to the protein, thyroglobulin. This is subsequently stored as colloid in the follicle of the gland. When the gland is stimulated to release the thyroid hormones, the thyroglobulin moves from the follicle back into the cell where the protein is hydrolyzed by the action of lysosomal enzymes before the hormones can be released.

Passage of thyroglobulin into the cell from the follicle occurs by endocytosis (Fig. 14.7). Pseudopods engulf large colloid droplets that are taken into the cell. They are found within 5 minutes after stimulation with thyroid-stimulating hormone (TSH), and the number of droplets increases progressively (Shishiba et al., 1967). As the colloid droplets migrate toward the base of the cell they merge with dense granules, primary lysosomes, that migrate toward them carrying the necessary hydrolytic enzymes (Wetzel et al., 1965; Seljelid, 1967). The fusion appears to be rapid and hydrolysis of the thyroglobulin follows. Thyroxine and triiodothyronine are released, first to the cytoplasm of the thyroid cell, then to the blood (Fig. 14.7). Probably mono- and diiodotyrosine are liberated in the cell, but they are deiodinated and the iodide reused (Greer and Grimm, 1968). Whether the thyroglobulin is hydrolyzed to amino acids or partially hydrolyzed to a "core" that is reused in synthesis is not known. For a detailed account of the secretion of thyroid hormones, see Wollman (1969); Herzog (1981).

The adrenal medulla synthesizes and stores the catecholamine hormones, epinephrine and norepinephrine, as chromaffin granules. Some of the cells in the medulla are specialized to secrete epinephrine and some, norepinephrine. (Synthesis of these hormones is discussed in Chapter 19.) The granules are formed in the Golgi region of the medullary cell (Holtzmann, 1967) as are the enzyme constituents of the lysosomes. An interesting observation is that mature chromaffin granules are rich in lysolecithin, but neither lysolecithin nor the enzyme responsible for its formation from lecithin is present in early granules (Winkler et al., 1967). The enzyme responsible for the formation of 1-acyl lysolecithin is phospholipase A_2, which is found in the adrenal medulla only as a lysosomal enzyme. Smith and Winkler (1969) postulate that the phospholipase A_2, which is incorporated into the lysosomes in the Golgi region, may also be used at that locus to form the lysolecithin in the membranes that ultimately surround the chromaffin granules. (For discussion of the role of the Golgi in altering membrane enzyme content, see Chapter 12.)

If hormones are synthesized and stored as granules in the cells prior to secretion, some mechanism must exist to dispose of the accumulated secretory products. Farquhar (1969) reported on the role played by the lysosomes in degrading the undischarged granules. This was studied in the pituitary cell that secretes the lactogenic hormone. The normal sequence of events seems to be the synthesis

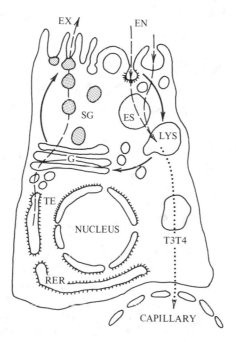

Figure 14.7
Diagram of a thyroid cell showing bidirectional
transport of thyroglobulin (thin broken lines) and
concomitant distal membrane interactions (thick
arrows). Newly synthesized thyroglobulin is
transported from the rough endoplasmic reticulum (RER) via transitional elements (TE) to the
Golgi apparatus (G), packaged in secretion granules (SG), and released by exocytosis (EX). During endocytosis (EN), thyroglobulin is internalized and transferred to lysosomes (LYS) via a
prelysosomal compartment, the endosome (ES).
Although thyroid hormones (T3, T4) are liberated
from thyroglobulin by lysosomal enzymes (dotted line), some membrane appears to pinch off
the lysosomal surface and to be recovered by
insertion into the membranes of Golgi cisternae.
(From V. Herzog, *Trends Biochem. Sci.* 6:319,
1981.)

of the hormone by the endoplasmic reticulum, passage through the Golgi complex, and release as the secretory granules. The granules coalesce and during
active secretion they fuse with the cell membrane and leave the cell by exocytosis.
However, when secretory activity is suppressed, the excess stored hormone does
not fuse with the membrane but, instead, fuses with existing lysosomes in the
cell. This is followed by lysosomal digestion until only a lipid droplet and a
residual body can be observed (Fig. 14.8).

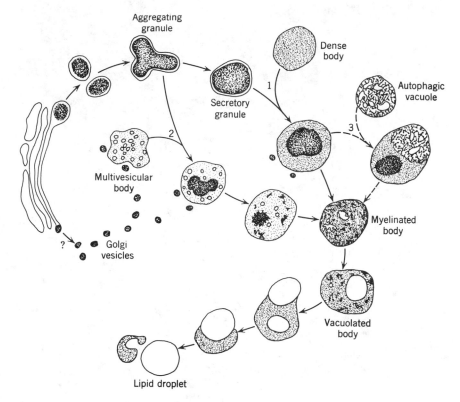

Figure 14.8
Diagram to illustrate lysosomal digestion of stored lactogenic hormone in the anterior pituitary cell following suppression of secretion. Mature secretory granules are incorporated into dense bodies (arrow 1) and immature or aggregating granules into multivesicular bodies (arrow 2). Rough endoplasmic reticulum and ribosomes are sequestered in autophagic vacuoles which can merge with dense bodies (arrow 3). This last path is not obligatory but takes place primarily when there is pronounced cellular involution. In subsequent steps the material entering the lysosomal system through all three pathways is progressively degraded to yield a vacuolated dense body. The vacuole is shown successively protruding from and eventually separating from the peripheral dense rim, leaving a free lipid droplet and a residual dense body. (From M. G. Farquhar, *Lysosomes in Biology and Pathology*, Vol. 2, J. T. Dingle and H. B. Fell, eds., Wiley-Interscience, New York, 1969, p. 471.)

BONE RESORPTION

Osteoclasts, cells responsible for eroding bone during development and throughout life to provide for the finely regulated levels of calcium in the blood, operate in association with acid phosphatase and other lysosomal enzymes. Electron photomicrographs of osteoclasts show vacuoles in the cytoplasm and no conspicuous endoplasmic reticulum. Specialized invaginations of the plasma membrane, termed the ruffled border, are associated with the cytoplasmic vacuoles and debris of the resorption process. The ultrastructure of an osteoclast is shown in Fig. 14.9.

The presence of lysosomes in bone cells has been clearly shown through biochemical studies. Nine acid hydrolases were found associated with the lysosomal fraction of bone homogenates (Vaes, 1965; Vaes and Jacques, 1965). Ultrastructural histochemistry has revealed numerous acid phosphatase-rich structures which are presumably lysosomes (Lucht, 1971; Göthlin and Ericsson, 1972). Furthermore, the presence of dense bodies similar to lysosomes was observed in the cytoplasm close to the ruffled border of osteoclasts (Scott, 1967) and the cartilage-resorbing chondroclasts (Schenk et al., 1967).

For bone resorption to occur, both collagen and mineral must be dissolved. It seems reasonable to assume that the mineral must be removed before enzymatic action on the remaining collagen can occur. Ham (1979) suggests that an acid environment created by the osteoclast at the bone surface dissolves the mineral, and that lysosomal enzymes are liberated to the surface to digest the remaining

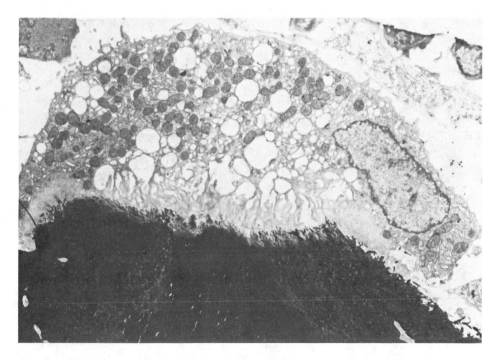

Figure 14.9
Electron micrograph of an osteoclast showing the ruffled border (RB) beneath which resorption occurs. The resorbing region is sealed by the clear zone (CZ) at the cell periphery. Numerous digestive vacuoles and smaller lysosomes are present along with many mitochondria. Only one nucleus is present in the plane of the section. Magnification × 3,000. (From R. Schenk, *Verh. Dtsch. Ges. Path.* 58:72, 1974.)

collagen fibers. Although some investigators suggest that intracellular digestion by lysosomal enzymes occurs after the material is brought in by pinocytosis (Scott, 1967), Vaes (1968) proposes that the acid hydrolases of the lysosomes are excreted in bulk through exocytosis into the resorption zone and that an eroding action occurs on the organic components of the bone matrix. This can proceed because of stimulation of the synthesis of lysosomal enzymes in the cells. Vaes (1969) postulated that acid excreted into the resorption zones as a result of aerobic glycolysis within the osteoclast permits solubilization of the mineral component of the matrix and favors the action of the acid hydrolases. Alternatively, the acid assumed to be secreted may be a result of carbonic anhydrase action. This enzyme has been localized in osteoclasts by ultrastructural immunocytochemistry (Anderson et al., 1982). The enzyme is present in the cytoplasm and, when the cell is actively resorbing bone, it is also associated with the plasma membrane. Fragments of matrix released by this extracellular resorption are taken up into the osteoclasts by pinocytosis for further digestion intracellularly by lysosomal enzymes and H^+ ions. The observation that some of the large vacuoles at the ruffled surface are open to the extracellular resorbing zone suggests that there is continuous mixing of substrates and enzymes through endocytosis and exocytosis in which the pinocytotic vacuoles, the lysosomes, and the extracellular fluid participate (Vaes, 1969). A suggested mechanism of bone resorption is shown in Fig. 14.10. For further discussion, see Vaes (1969, 1980); see also Chapter 17.

Since a lack of vitamin A has been shown to arrest bone growth, one might question whether this arrest is due to interference with the continuous destruction of cartilage and bone, which must take place as bones increase in length and shaft diameter. Is this effect of vitamin A deficiency due to an inability to labilize lysosomal membranes in the osteoclasts? Is the spontaneous fracturing that is a manifestation of vitamin A toxicity due to excessive labilization of the lysosomal membrane? These are interesting questions for nutritionists.

CELLULAR AUTOPHAGY

Not all materials destined for lysosomal digestion come from outside the cell. The formation of an autophagic vacuole in the cell may provide a neat procedure for the disposal of worn-out or damaged subcellular organelles as well as constituents of such organelles that are replaced at fairly constant rates. This "turnover" varies with the tissue, the organelle, and the chemical constituent. The turnover of whole organelles—such as mitochondria—by autophagy and involving lysosomes is supported by evidence from electron microscopic studies (de Duve and Wattiaux, 1966). Autophagic activity under normal conditions rids the cell of worn-out organelles and pieces of cytoplasm without losing the constituent chemical components that can be reutilized by the cell. Since the half-life of liver mitochondria is approximately 10 days, and the half-life of the liver cell is about 150 days, the mitochondrial population of each liver cell is renewed about 15 times during the cell's lifetime (Ericsson, 1969). It has been estimated that 10^9

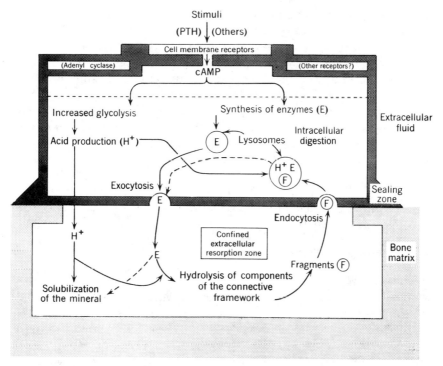

Figure 14.10

Presumed mechanism of the osteoclastic bone resorption: a working hypothesis. Membrane receptors (adenyl cyclase, ion transport systems, receptors for endocytosis, etc.), stimulated by parathyroid hormone (PTH), release intracytoplasmic messengers (cyclic AMP, ions, endocytosis vesicles, etc.) which, directly or indirectly, cause the various metabolic and cytological transformations leading ultimately to bone resorption: stimulation of glycolysis and of acid excretion, increased synthesis and exocytosis of lysosomal enzymes, extracellular digestion of the bone matrix, endocytosis and intracellular digestion of fragments in the lysosomal system. Some stimuli (dibutyryl cyclic AMP, possibly vitamin A, and excess oxygen) may however directly penetrate through the plasma membrane of the cell into the cytoplasm, and exert there themselves, either directly or indirectly, alterations leading to the same end-result. (From G. Vaes, *Lysosomes in Biology and Pathology*, Vol. 1, J. T. Dingle and H. G. Fell, eds., Wiley-Interscience, New York, 1969, p. 244.)

mitochondria per gram of liver tissue are destroyed per hour. What is true for mitochondria is probably true for other cellular components.

Cellular autophagy also plays a role in the disposal of whole organs that have outlived their usefulness. Examples are the regression of the tadpole tail in the metamorphosis of the frog (Weber, 1963; 1969) and regression of the Müllerian ducts in the male chick embryo (Scheib, 1963). In addition, normal involutionary changes occur in the mammary glands on cessation of lactation (Helminen and

Ericsson, 1968), in skin keratinization (Farquhar and Palade, 1965), in thymus involution (Gad and Clark, 1968), and in bone due to the action of parathyroid hormone and $1,25(OH)_2D_3$. (See above and Chapter 17.)

Another role for cellular autophagy is that of providing a survival mechanism in times of emergency. Through digestion of dispensable cellular contents, essential nutrients can be provided for high priority functions in the cell. Such an autolytic procedure during a period of starvation, when the cell decreases in volume, appears to be an important mechanism in the mobilization of proteins from liver and muscle for release of amino acids to the blood for essential syntheses at other body sites. The precisely controlled proteolytic process appears to be regulated by glucagon (Mortimore and Ward, 1976). During a 24-hour fast, rat liver loses 20–40 percent of its protein (Soberon and Sanchez, 1961).

When cell injury occurs, augmented autophagy is a sequel and appears to be a mechanism that prevents spread of the insult to other parts of the cytoplasm.

LYSOSOMES AND DISEASE

Storage Diseases

Interference with a normal hydrolytic process within the cell may occur if the requisite lysosomal enzyme is missing or defective. Hers (1963) suggested that the inability to attack glycogen molecules, due to a lack of α-glucosidase in the complement of lysosomal enzymes, was the fundamental defect in the genetic disorder, Type II Glycogen Storage disease. This glycogenosis was the first disease to be clearly attributed to a missing lysosomal hydrolase. Electron microscopic examination of liver (Baudhuin et al., 1965) and other tissues (Hers and Van Hoof, 1969) indicated accumulation of glycogen in vacuoles, surrounded by one membrane, which were in fact enlarged lysosomes. Since there is also evidence of some glycogen in the cell outside the lysosome, such patients are not hypoglycemic since the glycogen dispersed in the cytoplasm can be mobilized for metabolism. The glycogen in the vacuole, however, is not available. The death of the patient results from muscle destruction due to disruption of the engorged lysosome followed by proteolytic destruction of the muscle (Hers and Van Hoof, 1969).

Other storage diseases in which genetic lysosomal enzyme defects have been implicated (see Hers and Van Hoof, 1969; Kint et al., 1973) result in excessive storage of mucopolysaccharides (Hurler syndrome), gangliosides (Tay-Sachs disease), glucocerebrosides (Gaucher disease), and sphingomyelin (Niemann-Pick disease).

For further details, see Callahan and Lowden (1981).

Muscular Dystrophies and Vitamin E Deficiency

The characteristic muscular dystrophy of vitamin E-deficient rabbits and chicks and of genetically dystrophic mice appears to be due to injury to the lysosomal membrane of muscle cells. Large quantities of at least four lysosomal enzymes have been detected in muscle cells from dystrophic animals. For further discussion of lysosomal involvement in muscular dystrophies, see Weinstock and Iodice (1969).

The brain damage in vitamin E deficiency according to Kummerow (1964) occurs because the antioxidant effect of the vitamin is missing and the peroxides alter the structure of the cell membrane, perhaps deactivating specific enzyme systems. Since prompt administration of vitamin E will reverse such changes, and since vitamin E is a stabilizer of most intracellular membranes including that of the lysosome, it is tempting to think that the later irreversible brain damage that occurs is due not to the deactivating of enzymes but rather to the rupture of the lysosome, the release of enzymes, and the consequent digesting of surrounding intracellular material including some mitochondria and parts of the endoplasmic reticulum.

Rheumatoid Arthritis

Suggestions have been offered concerning the role of lysosomes in rheumatoid arthritis (Weissmann, 1972). The primary reason for implicating lysosomes is that the local lesions of human disease can develop in laboratory animals injected with lysates of purified lysosomes. Histochemical and ultrastructural studies of synovial tissues of arthritic individuals have indicated abnormalities in lysosomes indicating that they may be more permeable to substrate (Hamerman, 1968). Weissmann (1972) proposed that macrophages crowd the inflamed synovial lining and that phagosomes still open at the external surface merge with lysosomes permitting "regurgitation during feeding." The lysosomal contents entering the synovial fluid and surrounding tissues lead to the local lesions. It is doubtful that acid hydrolases will be active outside the synovial cells. However, neutral proteases, which are also present in lysosomes, are likely candidates for the destruction that occurs.

It is also argued that arthritis may be associated with incomplete cellular autolysis, implying failure of lysosomal enzymes to perform their function of digesting dead cells and debris (Lack, 1969). Joint damage in rheumatoid arthritis involving both membrane and cartilage is mainly caused by lysosomal enzymes released from the cells of the synovial lining by infecting organisms. These organisms are normally phagocytosed by macrophages from the blood. If the scavenger mechanisms are defective, possibly because of enzyme deficiencies, this would allow an abnormal persistence of debris. This debris would subsequently be enveloped by fibrous tissue, a defense strategy employed by cells that isolate what cannot easily be digested.

For further discussion, see Page-Thomas (1969), Lack (1969), and Krane et al. (1981)

Microbodies or Peroxisomes

Another group of cell components, the *microbodies* or *peroxisomes*, share with lysosomes the characteristic single limiting membrane. However, microbodies differ from lysosomes in that they can be identified morphologically. They possess a moderately dense matrix that is finely granular and usually shows a denser core with a lattice structure varying in composition from one species to another (Baud-huin et al., 1965; Afzelius, 1965; Ericsson and Trump, 1966). Evidence that microbodies are different from lysosomes is based on the absence of acid phosphatase in microbodies (Miller and Palade, 1964); on the fact that they do not accumulate materials through pinocytosis (Shnitka, 1965); and on their characteristic enzymes that include catalase, urate oxidase, L-α-hydroxy acid oxidase, and D-amino acid oxidase. (See de Duve and Baudhuin, 1966.) They are usually found in close association with the smooth endoplasmic reticulum from which they appear to form by budding (de Duve, 1973).

On the basis of the association of urate oxidase, xanthine dehydrogenase, and allantoinase with peroxisomes, Scott et al. (1969) concluded that they play a role in the degradation of purines. The suggestion has been made also that microbodies are important sites of hydrogen peroxide metabolism. β-oxidation appears to be established as a major function of peroxisomes in some tissues (Tolbert, 1981). The biological significance of microbodies has been questioned because of duplication of metabolic pathways in other parts of the cell. Recently, however, a fatal cerebrohepatorenal syndrome in infants has been associated with the absence of lysosomes in liver and kidney cells (Goldfischer, 1979).

De Duve (1969b) speculated on the origin and evolution of peroxisomes and suggested that such thoughts might contribute to an understanding of their biological significance. The evolutionary survival of these organelles and their presence in large numbers in certain mammalian cells with high mitochondrial and gluconeogenetic activity have suggested that one common functional property of peroxisomes in various plants and microorganisms is gluconeogenesis. Another constant component of all peroxisomes and in remarkably high concentrations is catalase, suggesting that these microbodies may be vestiges of early respiratory mechanisms characteristic of primitive aerobes, and that they appeared in response to hydrogen peroxide formation that arose either spontaneously or by catalysis. The possibility that this enzyme might be involved in some yet unsuspected role is also suggested. The D-amino acid oxidase and L-α-hydroxy acid oxidase are not vitally important, and de Duve (1969b) suggested that if these enzymes perform the sole functions of microbodies in higher organisms, then microbodies decrease in importance as we go up the evolutionary scale. Perhaps, according to de Duve, the peroxisome is a dying organelle, at least in animals.

For further details, see Tolbert (1981); de Duve (1983).

Conclusion

The lysosome functions as a digestive organ by making soluble and available the nutrients from phagocytosed particles; as a protective organ by engulfing and killing bacteria or foreign particles; as a site for mobilizing protein for the release of needed amino acids; as the assassin of worn-out cells; as a means of disposing of embarrassing appendages in the process of metamorphosis; and as an essential participant in processes such as bone growth. These are all normal physiological functions and, it is presumed, that precise and balanced mechanisms such as hormonal stimulation and nutrient supply would trigger the lysosomes into action at the proper time, thereby avoiding the untimely and disastrous activity of the hydrolytic enzymes. The role of many microbodies in animal cells seems to be β-oxidation of fatty acids.

Experimental evidence suggests that excess or deficit of certain nutrients may, by action on the lysosomal membrane, lead to widespread pathological manifestations. Such findings serve to emphasize that the effects of nutrient adequacy or potential toxicity must eventually be appraised at the cellular level.

part four

specialized cells

In a sense, all cells are specialized since the "typical cell" does not exist. The kind and degree of specialization of a cell or an organism is related to the life it leads, whether it is a free-living entity in a specific kind of environment or one of a myriad of highly specialized cells that function together as part of a unit, or organ, in a complex organism. The basic machinery with which the cell functions is present, with modifications, in practically all cells: nucleus, mitochondria, endoplasmic reticulum, plasma membrane. When a cell's capability to perform a specific function becomes enhanced through differentiation, it usually sacrifices the ability to carry out some other functions. However, certain metabolic processes essential to life continue: selective transport through the plasma membrane, synthesis of protein (although this, too, may be lost as in the mature erythrocyte that no longer has a nucleus), release of energy from cellular nutrients, and the trapping of this energy in ATP. Specialization often is accompanied by distinctive adjustments in nutrient needs, some of which are determined by morphological features and others by physiological characteristics.

When the fertilized ovum enters into a series of divisions they are, at first, quantitative; that is, there is an increase in number but not in kind. The resulting group of similar cells form the hollow ball or blastula stage in embryonic development which is followed by gastrulation and the formation of the germinal layers. (See Grobstein, 1959.) It is at this stage that differentiation begins and proceeds into the development of specialized tissues and organs. The tissues arising from the three germinal layers are both similar and diverse in their biochemical characteristics. From the one cell comes approximately 10^{14} cells that comprise a man, each identical insofar as its chromosomal endowment, or the coded information in its DNA is concerned; yet they are different in that certain potentialities have been accentuated and others repressed or lost. For example, hemoglobin is synthesized only by the erythrocyte, insulin by the beta cell of the pancreas, hydrochloric acid by the parietal cell in the gastric mucosa. Extreme differences are also apparent in the way specialized structure is adapted to the specialized function: the long, insulated nerve fiber is irritable and has the capacity to conduct and transmit; the muscle, by virtue of the arrangement of its protein molecules, can adjust its length; the bone's affinity for calcareous matter and the arrangement of the mineral in spicules along the lines of force give the skeleton strength and rigidity. In each instance, a particular capability has been exploited and, as a result, the cell and its cytoplasmic proteins possess characteristics that differentiate it from other cells. It follows, then, that only a small fraction of the genes carried by any one cell are functional, that is, transmit their information by forming messenger RNA. The basic questions yet to be answered unequivocally: "What determines which of the genes in a particular cell are to be operative" or, "Which molecules of the DNA are to be transcribed into RNA?" were discussed in Chapter 10.

Despite the illusiveness of the mechanism, the process of specialization nonetheless occurs and is probably operative at the level of the gene. In a sense, the cells are what they synthesize. However, Grobstein (1964) points out clearly that in the multicellular organism the differentiations of individual cells are linked into a total pattern that "makes sense." It is therefore evident that intracellular controls operate to make the integrated whole.

Specialization and the consequent division of labor in a complex multicellular organism lead to a loss of independence. Each specialized cell becomes dependent on other specialized cells for the performance of functions essential for the survival of the total organism. This interdependence is taken for granted when function proceeds undisturbed, but it becomes manifest, often strikingly, when there is interruption or interference with normal function. The total organism carries with it a great deal of insurance in the form of extra cells of all kinds. Rarely is the total number of like cells required for any specific function. However, when a sufficient number of cells specialized to perform unique functions can no longer operate, the effects will be spread throughout the functioning whole. The effects that we recognize we call disease.

Of all the cells in an organism the only ones that possess the ability to develop into any one of the specialized cells of the body are the *totipotent* germ cells such as the fertilized ovum. During development this totipotentiality is sequestered only in germ cells and not into the other cell types into which they differentiate.

Some cells are so highly specialized that soon after birth they lose all ability to reproduce. There is no way of replacing such cells when they have become worn out or destroyed. Such is the fate of nerve cells and, as a consequence, the total organism may be affected.

Some cells that are highly specialized and unable to reproduce have very short life spans due to wearing out or the sloughing off from surfaces. A steady population of such cells is maintained by cells called *stem cells* that have differentiated only so far as to become one of the family of cells. Steady reproduction of stem cells provides a supply of cells that can be stimulated to differentiate further to replace and maintain the cell population. Cell populations of this type that undergo continuous replacement from a pool of stem cells are the mucosal cells lining the gastrointestinal tract which last for only a few days, and the erythrocytes that have a span of about 120 days.

Some highly differentiated cells with long life spans that normally do not reproduce after full growth of the organ is attained can, under extraordinary circumstances, start to reproduce again. A description of such an event comes from Greek mythology: "Jupiter had him (Prometheus) chained to a rock on Mount Caucasus, where a vulture preyed on his liver, which was renewed as fast as devoured."[1] It seems unlikely that mere mortals can work quite that fast today, but the laboratory rat after two-thirds of its liver is removed can regenerate it fully within days through cell divisions of the remaining third. The liver which is indispensable is also resourceful. A protein factor in serum of rats found 12 hours after partial hepatectomy is capable of stimulating DNA synthesis specifically in livers (Morley and Kingdon, 1973). There is at present only a suggestion, but it appears to be released from the remaining portion of liver (Morley, 1974).

Cell specialization, however important in a multicellular society, carries with it the defects of its virtues.

---

[1]*Bullfinch's Mythology, The Age of Fable*, Chapter 2, p. 20, First Modern Library Edition, 1934.

chapter 15

hepatocytes

The size of the liver and its prominence in the abdominal cavity was undoubtedly a factor in the importance that the ancient Babylonians ascribed to it. The liver was used in medical diagnosis, but interestingly, it was not the patient's liver but that of a sheep into whose nose the patient had breathed. The liver from the slaughtered sheep was compared with a clay liver which priests had carefully zoned into regions to indicate the nature of the disease. In a sense, the Babylonians could be considered prescient in the importance they placed on liver function and appearance; but many centuries passed before the central role of the liver in the total metabolic scheme was recognized.

The structural plan of the liver is adapted to the diversity of hepatocyte function. Every cell is oriented so that the plasma membrane is adjacent on one side to the sinusoids that receive blood from both the portal and arterial circulation and on the other side to the bile canaliculi that form a communicating and collecting system for the bile synthesized by the liver cells. The cells thus form a narrow wall between the blood on one side and the bile on the other. The architectural plan of the liver showing a continuous mass of cells in the form of anastamosing trabeculae of hepatocytes is illustrated in Fig. 15.1. These trabeculae must be at least two cells thick or two cells wide so that a bile canaliculus is formed between them. All of the spaces between the trabeculae of hepatocytes are the blood sinusoids into which the individual hepatocytes deliver their synthetic products, except for the exocrine secretion, bile. Bile is delivered into the bile canaliculi, the spaces between the cells. The arrangement provides for close contact and exchange between the hepatocytes and both the blood and the exocrine ducts that carry the bile. In that way the hepatocytes can respond quickly to the demands of the total organism they serve.

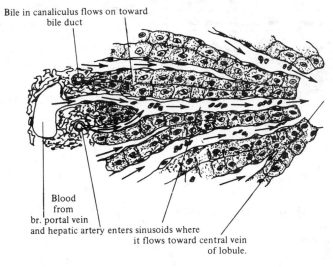

Bile in canaliculus flows on toward
bile duct

Blood
from
br. portal vein
and hepatic artery enters sinusoids where
it flows toward central vein
of lobule.

Figure 15.1
Diagram illustrating how blood from branches of the portal vein
and hepatic artery (left) flows into sinusoids that lie between trabeculae and empty into a central vein (right). The way bile travels
in the opposite direction in canaliculi to empty into bile ducts in
portal areas is also shown. (From A. W. Ham and D. H. Cormack,
Histology, 8th ed., J. B. Lippincott, Philadelphia, 1979.)

Of the blood entering the liver, 65–75 percent comes via the portal vein and
carries in it all of the nutrients absorbed into the blood from the small intestine;
the remaining 25–35 percent is arterial blood that enters through the hepatic
artery. The nutrients absorbed into the lymph from the small intestine arrive at
the liver cell with the arterial blood. The liver sinusoids, therefore, bring to the
cells simultaneously arterial blood and all of the products of intestinal digestion.
In a sense, the liver cells are transfer or nutrient redistribution centers that, under
the influence of hormonal regulatory mechanisms, can store or metabolize nutrients and then transfer the metabolic products to the hepatic vein or the bile
canaliculi.

Structure

The liver cell, or hepatocyte, displays no strikingly unique morphological characteristics. It contains a large nucleus, sometimes two nuclei, well developed
rough and smooth endoplasmic reticulum, Golgi complexes, many discernable
lysosomes, numerous and well developed mitochondria, and a variety of inclusions such as aggregates of glycogen granules, lipid droplets, and pigment.

Specialized Functions

The unspectacular appearance of the liver cell belies the diversity of specialization of its metabolic pathways. Most cells metabolize the major foodstuffs, synthesize ATP, and are self-sufficient in the sense that they synthesize the enzymes required both for their intracellular metabolic activity and for specialized export products. However, the magnitude of the liver's participation in such synthetic activities is probably its most characteristic attribute. The scope and variety of vital functions performed is variously estimated from 100 to perhaps over 500. Practically all the reactions of intermediary metabolism can take place in the liver, and some reactions occur in no other place. For example, the liver is primarily responsible for the synthesis of urea, creatine, plasma proteins, triacylglycerols, phospholipids, and bile acids. Because of the scope of metabolic pathways open in the liver cell, it has the capability of performing integrated regulatory functions not possible in other cells, and upon which homeostasis depends in the complex multicellular organism as, for example, the fine regulation of the blood sugar concentration and the maintenance of plasma protein levels. The scope of liver synthetic function both in terms of products for export and enzymes for intra-hepatocyte synthesis indicates that these cells have the capability of synthesizing unique types of RNA; that is, in these cells mechanisms must exist which permit the reading of more specific DNA regions of the genes than are read in other cells.

REGULATION OF BLOOD GLUCOSE LEVEL

The maintenance of the normal blood glucose concentration is a coordinated process in which the rate of glucose entry into the blood is balanced by its rate of withdrawal. The liver cell, responding to hormonal and various other influences during plethora, can withdraw glucose from the blood for the synthesis of glycogen for storage; or, in times of shortage, can supply glucose derived from its readily available store of glycogen through glycogenolysis. Since liver glycogen capacity is rather limited, the hepatocyte is equipped to tap more extensive sources of ultimate glucose such as amino acids, lactate, the glycerol moiety of fats, and propionyl-CoA from the oxidation of odd-chain fatty acids. (See Seifter and Englard, 1982.)

In a postabsorptive state, blood glucose concentrations are maintained within the normal range of 80–100 mg/dl by the glycogenolysis and gluconeogenesis in the liver cell to counterbalance the glucose that is constantly withdrawn from the circulation for oxidative and synthetic activities of all of the other cells of the complex organism. The efficiency and rapidity of regulation in the normal individual are such that despite periods of fasting or overeating, blood glucose levels remain remarkably constant ranging from 60–160 mg/dl. Unger (1981) suggests that perhaps evolutionary success required staunch defense of the range of blood sugar since exceeding the limits at either end produces dire consequences. Normal brain function requires approximately 6 gm of glucose per hour which can be delivered only if arterial blood contains over 50 mg/dl. At the other end of the range, normal control of glycosylation, which conveys structural and functional characteristics to certain proteins (for example, lens protein), requires a blood sugar level that does not exceed 180 mg/dl. Increased glycosylation associated with hyperglycemia may be responsible for the changes in the eyes of uncontrolled diabetics (Stevens et al., 1978).

Major control of blood glucose levels is achieved through the actions of the antagonistic pancreatic hormones, glucagon and insulin. For example, the slightest rise in plasma glucose leads to a decrease in glucagon secretion and an increase in insulin secretion whereas the reverse occurs when plasma glucose falls. Other factors also play important roles in a glucose homeostasis. For the effect of nutrients and gastrointestinal hormones on glucagon and insulin secretion, see Bloom (1981) and Dobbs (1981); for neural control of pancreatic secretions, see Palmer and Porte (1981).

Hepatocytes maintain normal blood sugar levels by responding to the complex of neural and hormonal stimuli. There are specific receptors in the hepatocyte membrane not only for glucagon and insulin, but also for catecholamines, growth hormone, secretin, vasoactive intestinal peptide, prostaglandins, and others. Receptors, like other membrane proteins, are continually synthesized and degraded, and receptor concentration in the target cell is an important factor in the response to hormone levels. In the case of insulin, the receptor concentration is controlled by the hormone itself and is associated with what is called "down regulation," that is, high levels of plasma insulin lead to a decreased concentration of insulin receptors thereby reducing the number of molecules that can bind to the membrane. Low plasma insulin levels, in contrast, are associated with an increased concentration of membrane receptors. Recent evidence suggests that the insulin receptor in the hepatocyte membrane is a protein kinase (Roth and Cassell, 1983). However, it is not clear whether the kinase activity of the receptor explains all of the effects of insulin. The regulation of glucagon receptor concentration is less well understood, but an inverse relationship between plasma glucagon and the number of glucagon receptors in hepatocyte membranes in the rat has been reported (Freeman et al., 1977).

The most vital function of glucagon is to maintain plasma glucose at a level adequate for the function of the CNS regardless of energy intake or expenditure. This function is carried out through regulation of the amount of glucose produced by the hepatocytes. In the fasting state about 75 percent of hepatic glucose production is glucagon-mediated (Liljenquist et al., 1977). Glucagon binds to its specific receptors in the hepatocyte membrane to initiate its regulatory action. Until recently this binding was believed to lead directly to the activation of adenylate cyclase for the generation of cAMP (Levey, 1975). However, studies by Rodbell and his co-workers (see Rodbell, 1981) indicate that a nucleotide regulatory protein comes between the receptor and the enzyme and is essential for the activation process. It is not clear whether the regulatory protein is an intrinsic membrane protein. What is clear is that the regulatory protein reacts with guanine nucleotide (GTP). According to Rodbell (ibid.) glucagon acts on the hepatocyte membrane from the outside and GTP from the inside with the nucleotide regulatory protein as the crucial connecting link in the activation process which also requires metal ions. The result of this activation is the generation of cAMP within the cell. The cAMP activates protein kinases which in turn phosphorylate other regulatory proteins in the cell. The effects of glucagon on glycogenolysis clearly are due to the cAMP-mediated phosphorylation of the inactive glycogen phosphorylase$_b$ to the active form, glycogen phosphorylase$_a$. (See Hers, 1976.) Effects of glucagon on the gluconeogenic mechanism are incompletely understood. (See Exton, 1981; also see Chapter 11.)

To defend against hyperglycemia, insulin binds to the hepatocyte membrane and produces specific cellular responses (see below). In addition, insulin-receptor complexes have been identified within the cell suggesting "internalization" of insulin. Autoradiography and sophisticated video techniques have shown that following membrane binding, penetration into the cell is mediated through clathrin-coated pits which may then fuse with a lysosome. Whether this endocytotic process is associated with degradation of the hormone or the so-called "down regulation" of hormone receptors, or with some other physiological effect is unclear. (See De Meyts and Hanoune, 1982.)

Insulin's major action in the hepatocyte is the inhibition of glucagon-mediated activity by (1) blocking glycogenolysis and gluconeogenesis and (2) removing the glucagon block on liver glycogen synthase (Hostmark, 1973). The exact mechanisms of action have not been resolved but the effect of insulin is attributed mainly to inhibition of cAMP production and the consequent blocking of glycogenolysis. (See Exton, 1981.) In addition, increased conversion of glycogen synthase to its active (nonphosphorylated) form explains at least a part of the known effect of insulin on glucose uptake by the liver cell (Villar-Palasi et al., 1971).

Another action of insulin is induction of the activity of glucokinase thereby increasing the uptake of glucose by the liver when plasma glucose levels are elevated. (See Czech, 1980.) Insulin also appears to increase glycolytic activity through an increase in phosphofructokinase and pyruvate kinase, as well as pentose phosphate shunt activity through an increase in 6-phosphogluconate dehydrogenase. All these actions increase utilization of glucose by the liver and thus maintain plasma glucose concentrations in the normal range following an influx of carbohydrate. For a review of insulin action, see Czech (1981); see Chapter 9 for details of insulin action on the hepatocyte membrane.

In addition to the regulation of glucose production by the actions of glucagon and insulin upon the hepatocyte, epinephrine and norepinephrine, by activating the splanchnic sympathetic nerves, may induce hepatic glycogenolysis. These hormones also may inhibit insulin output by the β cells of the pancreas. Glucocorticoids, particularly cortisol, also tend to increase glucose production by the liver cell and decrease glucose utilization in both muscle and fat cells. All these actions, in effect, counteract the effects of insulin and tend to increase blood glucose concentration. For discussion of the effects of counterregulatory hormones on the feedback loop of glucagon and insulin, see Porte and Halter (1981).

Hepatocytes are subject also to direct control by both sympathetic and parasympathetic nerves. Sympathetic nerves control glycogenolysis by increasing phosphorylase activity and activating glucose-6-phosphatase. The important and glycogenolytic activity essential for response to stress is the result of hypothalamic coordination of three separate sympathetic mechanisms: (1) direct innervation of the hepatocyte, (2) release of epinephrine from the adrenal medulla, and (3) release of glucagon from the pancreas. In contrast, parasympathetic nerves directly influence glycogenesis in the liver cell through activation of glycogen synthase and this activity, too, is part of hypothalamic coordination of liver glycogen metabolism and glucose homeostasis (Shimazu, 1981). For a review of CNS peptides and glucoregulation, see Frohman (1983).

The hepatocyte, like all other cells, is responsive to the availability of substrate. However, the liver cell's response appears to be of a broader nature in that its metabolic environment mirrors that of the total organism, and it functions in the homeostasis of that total metabolic environment to a far greater extent than other cells. Substrates arriving at the plasma membrane of the hepatocyte are accepted, metabolized, stored, or replenished according to the needs of the total organism. Control mediated through the endocrine glands and coordination through the CNS results in appropriately timed modifications in hormonal, hepatic, and peripheral tissue metabolic activities. Only through such a highly coordinated and finely tuned mechanism can the rapid adaptation to metabolic change essential for glucose homeostasis be achieved. Figure 15.2 illustrates the basal feedback loop for the regulation of plasma glucose and the modifying effects of the other factors that ultimately determine blood sugar level.

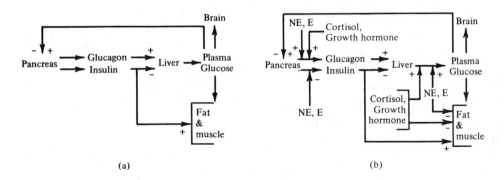

(a)   (b)

Figure 15.2
(a) Basal feedback loop for the regulation of plasma glucose. Glucose regulates insulin and glucagon secretion which, in turn, control hepatic glucose production. Glucose production is matched by glucose uptake in muscle and adipose tissue and insulin-independent glucose uptake in brain to close the loop. (b) Counterregulatory hormone modulation of the basal feedback loop. Final plasma glucose is determined by these and all other factors that influence the liver, pancreas, and peripheral tissues. (From S. C. Woods et al., *Handbook of Diabetes Mellitus*, Vol. 3, M. Brownlee, ed., Garland STPM Press, New York, 1981, pp. 232; 234).

GLUCONEOGENESIS

Gluconeogenesis is the synthesis of glucose from noncarbohydrate sources: lactate, pyruvate, glycerol, and certain amino acids. The liver is the major site of gluconeogenesis but under certain circumstances, such as starvation, the kidney is equally as important as liver in this process. Gluconeogenesis is a primary source of providing glucose to body cells when carbohydrate intake is limited and body glycogen stores are depleted. This process further provides for the recycling of lactate (the Cori cycle) and glycerol when these compounds accumulate in muscle tissues, such as occurs following heavy exercise. When amino acids are degraded in normal metabolism or when excessive amounts are degraded, as occurs during starvation, a major pathway is the formation of glucose or glycogen. In prolonged starvation, the ammonia thus released, is significant in counteracting acidosis. Almost all amino acids are potentially glucogenic; only leucine cannot contribute to the generation of glucose by the body (Goldberg and Chang, 1978).

An alanine cycle has been identified (Mallette et al., 1969; Felig et al., 1970) that is somewhat analagous to the lactate cycle and involves the conversion of alanine to glucose and reconversion to alanine. Pyruvate derived from glucose oxidation in muscle is transaminated to form alanine, which is transported to the liver where its carbon skeleton is reconverted to glucose (Fig. 15.3). The cycle

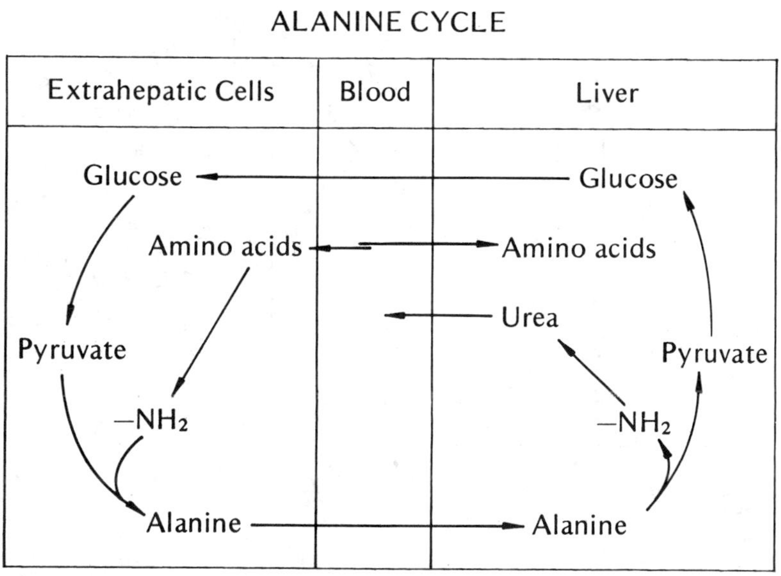

ALANINE CYCLE

Figure 15.3
Diagrammatic representation of the postulated role of alanine in the transfer of amino groups from extrahepatic tissues to the liver. (From L. E. Mallette et al., *J. Biol. Chem.* 244:5712, 1969.

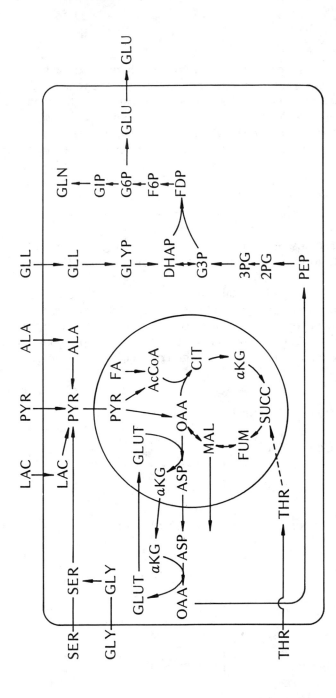

Figure 15.4

Gluconeogenesis in the liver cell. Rectangle represents the plasma membrane; circle, a mitochondrion. Abbreviations are LAC, lactate; PYR, pyruvate; ALA alanine; SER, serine; GLY, glycine; FA, fatty acid; AcCoA, acetyl CoA; CIT, citrate; α-KG, α-ketoglutarate; SUCC, succinate; FUM, fumarate; MAL, malate; OAA, oxalacetate; ASP, aspartate; GLUT, glutamate; THR, threonine; PEP, P-enol pyruvate; 2PG, 2-P-glycerate; 3PG, 3-P-glycerate; G3P, glyceraldehyde-3-P; DHAP dihydroxyacetone-P; GLYP, glycerol-1-P; GLL, glycerol; FDP, fructose-1, 6-di-P; F6P, fructose-6-P; G6P, glucose-6-P; GLU, glucose; G1P, glucose-1-P; GLN, glycogen. (From J. H. Exton, *Metabolism* 21:945, 1972.)

is important in gluconeogenesis as a source of glucose when exogenous supply is low and when metabolic demands for oxidizable substrate, as in exercise, are high. The cycle also is important in nitrogen metabolism since, in transferring amino groups from muscle to liver, alanine acts as a nontoxic alternative to ammonia. For a detailed discussion of the alanine cycle, see Felig and Wahren (1974).

Figure 15.4 shows the pathways by which glucose and glycogen are formed from various other noncarbohydrate sources.

ACETOACETYL CoA AND KETONE BODY FORMATION

Normally fatty acid oxidation does not result in any significant accumulation of intermediary metabolites. However, under certain conditions, acetoacetyl CoA is formed by reversal of the β-ketoacyl thiolase reaction resulting from condensation of 2 moles of acetyl CoA. Acetoacetyl CoA subsequently gives rise to free acetoacetic acid, β-hydroxybutyric acid, and acetone. These three compounds are referred to as *ketone bodies*.

In order to form free acetoacetate, acetoacetyl CoA must be converted in the liver to 3-hydroxy-3-methyl glutaryl CoA (HMG), an important intermediate in the biosynthesis of cholesterol. Cleavage of 3-hydroxy-3-methyl glutarate yields acetoacetic acid and acetyl CoA. These reactions are shown as follows:

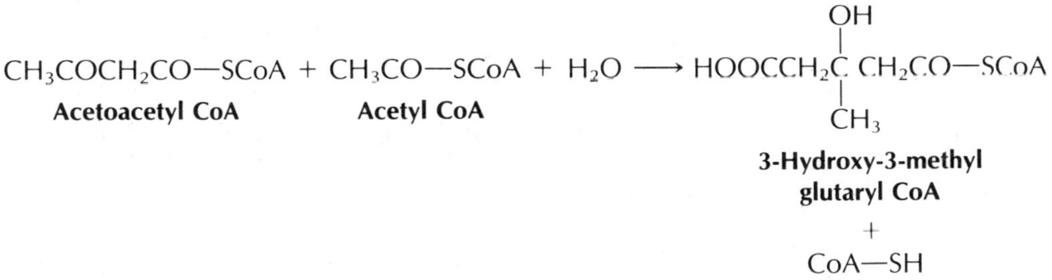

$$CH_3COCH_2CO\text{—}SCoA + CH_3CO\text{—}SCoA + H_2O \longrightarrow HOOCCH_2\overset{\overset{\textstyle OH}{|}}{C}CH_2CO\text{—}SCoA$$

Acetoacetyl CoA   **Acetyl CoA**

3-Hydroxy-3-methyl glutaryl CoA

$+$

CoA—SH

3-Hydroxy-3-methyl glutaryl CoA $\longrightarrow CH_3COCH_2COOH + CH_3CO\text{—}SCoA$

Acetoacetic acid   **Acetyl CoA**

Figure 15.5 illustrates the pathway of ketogenesis in the liver cell. Acetoacetate, thus formed, may be reduced to form β-hydroxybutyrate in a reversible reaction or decarboxylated to form acetone.

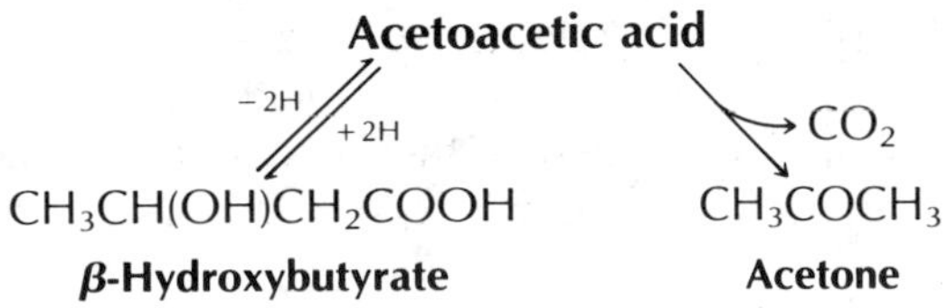

Acetoacetic acid

$-2H$ / $+2H$ $\rightarrow CO_2$

$CH_3CH(OH)CH_2COOH$ CH_3COCH_3
β-Hydroxybutyrate   **Acetone**

PATHWAY OF KETOGENESIS

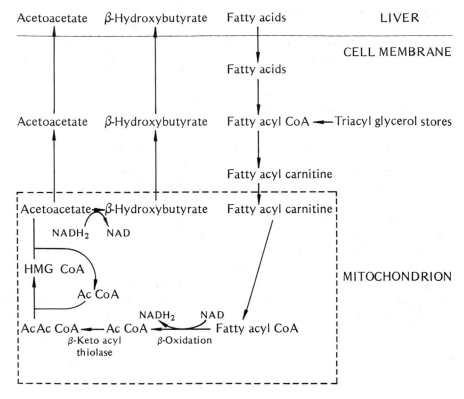

Figure 15.5
Diagram of the pathways of ketogenesis from fatty acids in the liver. (From *Best and Taylor's Physiological Basis of Medical Practice,* J. B. Brobeck, ed., 9th ed., Williams and Wilkins Co., Baltimore, 1973, pp. 7–140.)

The reversible reaction between acetoacetate and β-hydroxybutyrate, catalyzed by β-hydroxybutyrate dehydrogenase, is determined by the ratio of NADH to NAD in the mitochondria. The formation of the β-hydroxybutyrate is, in effect, withdrawing electrons from the mitochondria to make a more reduced substrate. Later oxidation of the compound in the peripheral tissue can produce more high energy phosphate than does the oxidation of acetoacetate.

Liver mitochondria are incapable of oxidizing ketone bodies. Mitochondria of various extrahepatic tissues such as muscle and brain, however, readily oxidize acetoacetate via the TCA cycle. β-hydroxybutyrate is converted to acetoacetate in extrahepatic mitochondria by an NAD-coupled β-hydroxybutyrate dehydrogenase. The acetoacetate so formed is then converted to acetoacetyl CoA by transfer of the CoA group from succinyl CoA.

$$\beta\text{-Hydroxybutyrate} \underset{\text{NAD} \quad \text{NADPH}+\text{H}}{\rightleftharpoons} \text{acetoacetate} \quad \text{succinyl CoA}$$

$$2 \text{ Acetyl CoA} \longleftarrow \text{acetoacetyl CoA} \quad \text{succinate}$$

The resultant acetoacetyl CoA is split by a thiolase enzyme to form 2 acetyl CoA groups which may then enter the TCA cycle.

Acetoacetate is continually undergoing spontaneous decarboxylation to form acetone. The reaction is slow, but if the concentration of acetoacetate is high enough, the odor of acetone may be detectable in the breath. Acetone is difficult to oxidize *in vivo*.

Under certain conditions, such as markedly increased fat catabolism (as in the fasting state) and relatively decreased carbohydrate catabolism, acetoacetate is formed at a faster rate than it can be oxidized. This leads to the accumulation of ketone bodies in blood (ketonemia). If the blood level exceeds the renal threshold for these compounds, ketone bodies are excreted in large amounts in the urine (ketonuria). This condition (ketonuria and ketonemia) is known as ketosis. The exact mechanism precipitating ketosis is not understood. It is clear, however, that under normal conditions ketone bodies are produced and oxidized and, moreover, under certain conditions ketone bodies may supply a major source of energy to the cell. Such a condition prevails in the fasting state. The brain, which normally utilizes glucose as its source of energy, shifts to a predominantly ketone body metabolism as fasting progresses (Fig. 15.6). Other tissues also use ketone bodies to a limited extent during fasting but rely chiefly on fatty acids as a source of energy. Thus, ketone bodies are a source of fuel for the body and function in the same way as glucose and fatty acids.

PLASMA PROTEIN SYNTHESIS

The early work of Whipple and his associates (Madden and Whipple, 1940) suggested that the liver was the specific site for synthesis of plasma proteins. Although a number of the plasma proteins are synthesized, in part, by extrahepatic tissues, the great preponderance of the plasma proteins are indeed synthesized by the liver.

Albumin is by far the most abundant of the plasma proteins. Normally 150–250 mg albumin/kg body weight are synthesized daily in the adult human. (See Rothschild et al., 1969.) The turnover rate of albumin is high as is that of all plasma proteins. The synthesis and release of one albumin molecule requires about 30 minutes in humans and in the rabbit (Peters, 1962), and some of the newly synthesized albumin probably stays within the cell for a short time. Peters (ibid.) has shown that the bulk of albumin is attached to the endoplasmic reticulum. About half as much is found in mitochondria, and traces appear in nuclei and lysosomes.

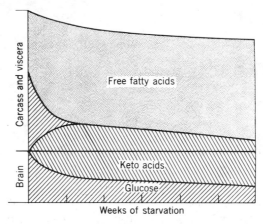

Figure 15.6
Substrate oxidation in fasting man. Schematic
representation of the transition from glucose to
fatty acid utilization by the carcass and viscera
and from glucose to ketoacids by the brain. (From
G. F. Cahill, Jr. et al., *Adipose Tissue, Regulation
and Metabolic Function*, B. Jeanrenaud and D.
Hepp, eds., Academic Press, New York, 1970,
p. 181.

   The synthesis of albumin is markedly lowered as a result of fasting or malnutrition. In children suffering from protein-calorie malnutrition, albumin synthesis
ranges between 100–148 mg/kg/day as compared with 222–233 mg/kg/day in
well nourished children (James and Hay, 1968). Studies with perfused livers from
fasted rabbits have indicated that in the fasting state albumin synthesis was stimulated by tryptophan and, to a lesser extent, by isoleucine. No increase in synthesis
occurred as a result of perfusion with methionine, lysine, leucine, valine, or
threonine (Rothschild et al., 1969). Thus, albumin synthesis is determined not
only by the available supply of amino acids but under some conditions may be
responsive to specific amino acids.

CREATINE SYNTHESIS

The synthesis of creatine is a function of liver and of kidney cells. The amino
acids—glycine, arginine, and methionine—each contribute a part of the molecule
(Fig. 15.7). The synthesis begins with the reversible transfer of the guanidine
moiety of arginine to glycine, a transamidination reaction catalyzed by the enzyme, transamidinase. The products of the reaction are guanidoacetic acid and
ornithine. The final reaction is the methylation of guanidinoacetic acid to form
creatine under the influence of the enzyme guanidinoacetate methyltransferase.
The methyl group is donated by s-adenosylmethionine, which is formed from

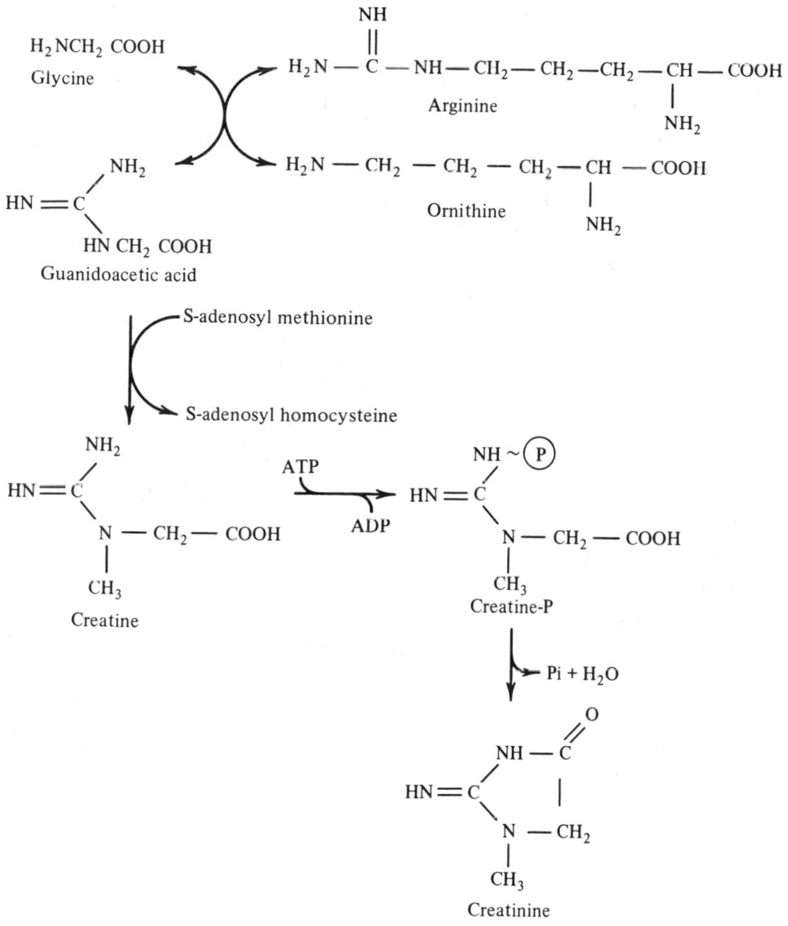

Figure 15.7
Creatine and creatinine synthesis.

methionine and ATP. As a result of the transmethylation, s-adenosyl homocysteine and creatine are formed.

Creatine may be converted to phosphocreatine in muscle in a reaction catalyzed by creatine kinase. Phosphocreatine is a store of high energy phosphate which can be used to generate more ATP when ATP is being hydrolyzed by muscular contraction. (See Chapter 18.) At times of rest, phosphate is transferred to creatine, thereby rebuilding the stores of phosphocreatine. Phosphocreatine spontaneously cyclizes at a slow rate to form creatinine, which cannot be metabolized further and is excreted in the urine. The rate of loss is dependent largely on the phosphocreatine content and therefore is relatively constant from day to day in a given individual. Other factors that affect creatinine excretion are discussed in Chapter 22.

UREA SYNTHESIS

A major and critical function of the liver is the synthesis of urea; this synthesis is the most significant pathway for disposal of ammonia arising from the deamination of amino acids and of amines, such as histamine and glutamine, and from absorbed ammonia synthesized by intestinal bacteria from urea and other sources.

All amino acids except lysine participate in transaminations and thereby may lose amino groups to form glutamic acid from α-ketoglutarate. Some amino acids lose their amino groups predominantly by other pathways, however. Histidine may undergo direct deamination to form urocanate; serine and threonine are deaminated by dehydration; and the amide groups of glutamine and asparagine are lost by hydrolytic deamination. Direct oxidative deamination is limited chiefly to deamination of glutamic acid through a reaction catalyzed by glutamate dehydrogenase and provides a route for making ammonium ions from many of the amino acids by way of the amino transferase reactions. The ammonium ions are toxic at even modest concentrations; the formation of urea, which can be tolerated in much higher concentrations, thus represents a detoxication mechanism in which the liver is the chief participant.

The mechanism of urea synthesis, first proposed by Krebs and Henseleit (1932), was based on *in vitro* experiments in which formation of urea in liver slices was observed to increase when either arginine, ornithine, or citrulline were added to the reaction medium. On the basis of these experiments, coupled with results of earlier isolated studies reported in the literature, they proposed that formation of urea is a cyclic process accomplished through the breakdown and resynthesis of arginine. The scheme shown in Fig. 15.8 is only slightly different from the original Krebs-Henseleit proposal. They assumed that both atoms of urea nitrogen came from ammonia; now it is known that one nitrogen atom comes from ammonia and one from aspartic acid. The hydrolysis of arginine is the final step in the formation of urea; this reaction is catalyzed by the enzyme arginase. Borsook and Keighley (1933) established that urea synthesis, like most biosynthetic mechanisms, is an energy-requiring process. The ATP requirement for urea synthesis has been cited by Krebs (1964) as one factor contributing to the greater heat production following protein ingestion and will be discussed in a later section on the calorigenic effect of food. (See Chapter 23.)

Although urea formation is the chief means of disposing of ammonia, it is not the only mechanism. Ammonia may be used also in the synthesis of glutamine, the acid amide of glutamic acid, which then may give up its ammonia for synthesis of urea or other nitrogenous compounds, such as purines. Glutamine appears to serve as a major transport form for amino groups from the peripheral tissues to the liver.

PLASMA LIPID SYNTHESIS

Although liver appears to be no more important than other tissues in the synthesis of fatty acids, it is the principal site of synthesis of the plasma triacylglycerols and phospholipids and of their incorporation into lipoproteins that are fractions of the α-, pre-β-, and β-globulins. The key compound for the formation of both the

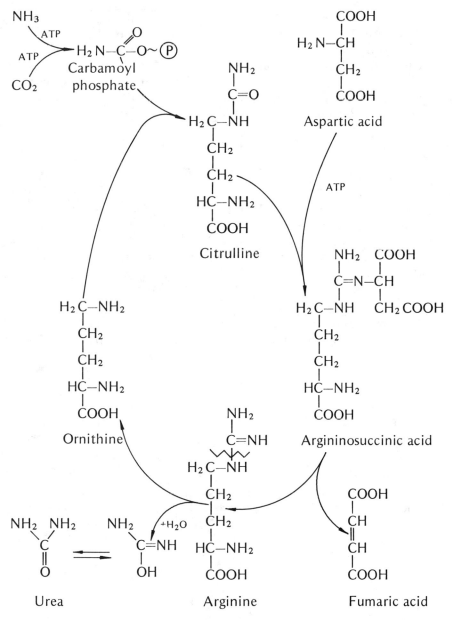

Figure 15.8
Synthesis of urea.

triacylglycerols and the phospholipids is phosphatidic acid. This compound can be synthesized in liver from either glycerol-3-phosphate or dihydroxyacetone phosphate.

   The synthesis of phosphatidic acid via glycerol-3-phosphate occurs in both liver and adipose cells. Glycerol-3-phosphate is formed in the liver from the phosphorylation of free glycerol by glycerokinase and ATP, or by the reduction of dihydroxyacetone phosphate.

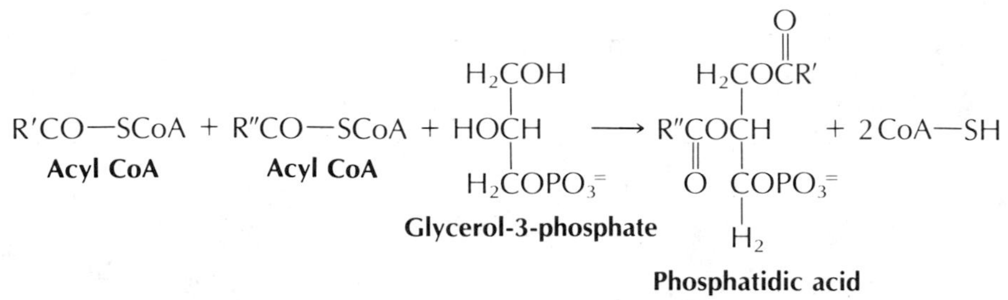

$$
\underset{\textbf{Acyl CoA}}{R'CO\!-\!SCoA} + \underset{\textbf{Acyl CoA}}{R''CO\!-\!SCoA} + \underset{\textbf{Glycerol-3-phosphate}}{\begin{array}{c} H_2COH \\ | \\ HOCH \\ | \\ H_2COPO_3^= \end{array}} \longrightarrow \underset{\textbf{Phosphatidic acid}}{\begin{array}{c} \overset{O}{\overset{\|}{H_2COCR'}} \\ | \\ R''COCH \\ \| \;\;\; | \\ O \;\; COPO_3^= \\ | \\ H_2 \end{array}} + 2\,CoA\!-\!SH
$$

Dihydroxyacetone phosphate can lead to the formation of phosphatidic acid, however, without being converted to glycerol-3-phosphate. The pathway is shown below.

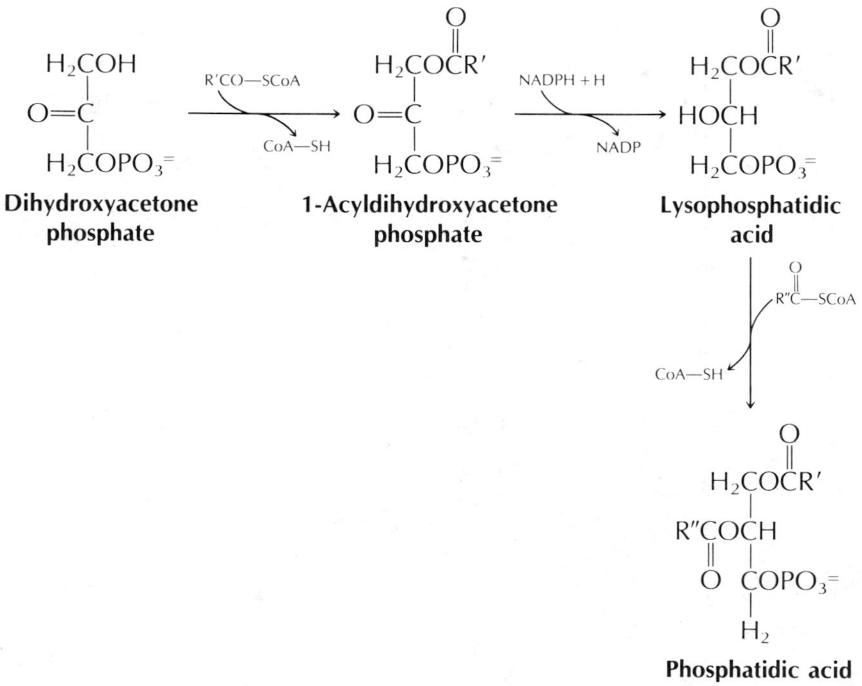

$$
\underset{\substack{\textbf{Dihydroxyacetone}\\\textbf{phosphate}}}{\begin{array}{c} H_2COH \\ | \\ O\!=\!C \\ | \\ H_2COPO_3^= \end{array}} \xrightarrow[\text{CoA}-\text{SH}]{\text{R'CO}-\text{SCoA}} \underset{\substack{\textbf{1-Acyldihydroxyacetone}\\\textbf{phosphate}}}{\begin{array}{c} \overset{O}{\overset{\|}{H_2COCR'}} \\ | \\ O\!=\!C \\ | \\ H_2COPO_3^= \end{array}} \xrightarrow[\text{NADP}]{\text{NADPH}+\text{H}} \underset{\substack{\textbf{Lysophosphatidic}\\\textbf{acid}}}{\begin{array}{c} \overset{O}{\overset{\|}{H_2COCR'}} \\ | \\ HOCH \\ | \\ H_2COPO_3^= \end{array}}
$$

$$
\xrightarrow[\text{CoA}-\text{SH}]{\overset{O}{\overset{\|}{R''C}}-\text{SCoA}}
\underset{\textbf{Phosphatidic acid}}{\begin{array}{c} \overset{O}{\overset{\|}{H_2COCR'}} \\ | \\ R''COCH \\ \| \;\;\; | \\ O \;\; COPO_3^= \\ | \\ H_2 \end{array}}
$$

The formation of 1-acyldihydroxyacetone phosphate is catalyzed by an acyl transferase which is present in mitochondria and microsomes and is specific for saturated fatty acids. The reduction of this compound to lysophosphatidic acid is catalyzed by a microsomal enzyme. The second acylation resulting in the formation of phosphatidic acid is accomplished also by a microsomal enzyme which is preferential for unsaturated fatty acyl CoA esters.

The synthesis of triacylglycerols and some phospholipids proceeds from phosphatidic acid which is hydrolyzed by a specific phosphatase to yield 1,2 diacyl-

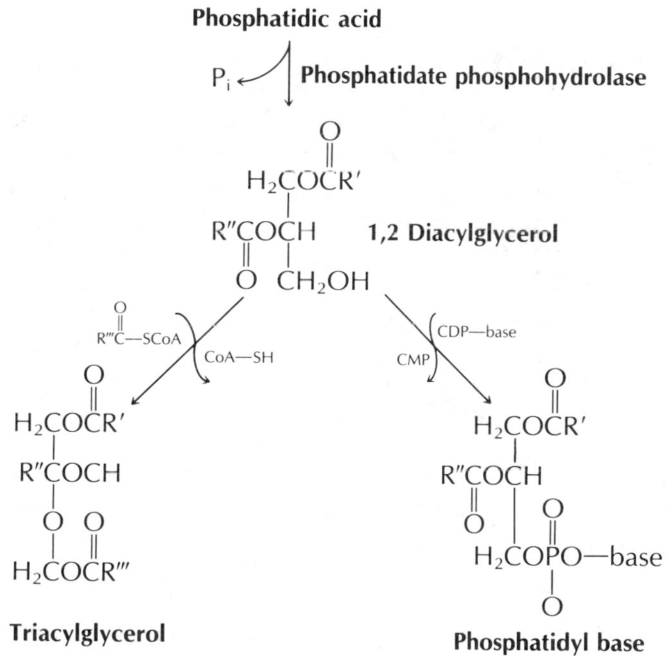

Phosphatidic acid

P_i ⤺⟋| **Phosphatidate phosphohydrolase**

$$
\begin{array}{c}
O \\
\parallel \\
H_2COCR' \\
| \\
R''COCH \qquad \text{1,2 Diacylglycerol} \\
\parallel \; | \\
O \; CH_2OH
\end{array}
$$

R'''C—SCoA ⟍ CoA—SH   CDP—base ⟍ CMP

Triacylglycerol

$$
\begin{array}{c}
O \\
\parallel \\
H_2COCR' \\
| \\
R''COCH \\
\parallel \\
O \quad O \\
| \quad \parallel \\
H_2COCR'''
\end{array}
$$

Phosphatidyl base

$$
\begin{array}{c}
O \\
\parallel \\
H_2COCR' \\
| \\
R''COCH \\
\parallel \quad \quad O \\
O \quad | \quad \parallel \\
H_2COPO\text{—base} \\
| \\
O
\end{array}
$$

glycerol. Finally, as shown below, the diacylglycerol is fully acylated to yield a triacylglycerol or reacts with a cytidine diphosphate base (choline, serine, or ethanolamine) to form a phospholipid.

The liver is also the site of plasma lipoprotein synthesis (with the exception of the chylomicrons which are synthesized in the intestinal epithelium). The various fractions of lipoprotein function in the transport of triacylglycerols, phospholipids, and cholesterol esters. (See Chapter 6.)

CHOLESTEROL SYNTHESIS AND DEGRADATION

Virtually all tissues containing nucleated cells are capable of synthesizing cholesterol, but the principal tissues for cholesterol synthesis are the liver, adrenal cortex, skin, intestine, testis, and aorta. The liver plays a major role in the synthesis, catabolism, and excretion of cholesterol.

All of the carbon atoms of cholesterol are derived from acetyl CoA. At least 26 steps are known to be involved in the biosynthesis of cholesterol; a gross outline of the major steps is shown in Fig. 15.9. The synthetic pathway can be thought of as occurring in three stages. In the first stage, 3 moles of acetyl CoA are converted to a six-carbon thioester intermediate, 3-hydroxy-3-methylglutaryl CoA (HMG CoA). These initial reactions occur in the cytoplasmic matrix. (HMG is also an intermediate in ketone body formation, a reaction that takes place in the mitochondria.)

The second stage involves the conversion of HMG CoA to squalene, an acyclic hydrocarbon containing 30 carbon atoms. The first step in this stage of cholesterol biosynthesis involves the reduction of HMG CoA to mevalonate, a reaction catalyzed by HMG CoA reductase and utilizing 2 moles of NADPH as the reducing agent. This reaction is the rate-limiting step in cholesterol biosynthesis and occurs in the microsomal fraction. (See Rodwell et al., 1973.)

The final stage of cholesterol biosynthesis is the conversion of squalene to cholesterol. The squalene molecule is converted to cyclized intermediates which are eventually transformed into cholesterol; the reactions occur while the intermediates are bound to a specific cytoplasmic protein, sterol carrier protein.

The extent of cholesterol synthesis appears to be regulated by the amount in the body and therefore is influenced by the quantity in the diet both in experimental animals (Morris and Chaikoff, 1959) and humans (Bhattathiry and Siperstein, 1963). The effect of dietary cholesterol in suppressing cholesterol biosynthesis was first shown by Siperstein and Guest (1960) to be exerted at the HMG CoA reductase step establishing that this enzyme, in effect, controls cholesterol synthesis. As total body cholesterol increases, synthesis tends to decrease. The suppression of cholesterol biosynthesis by dietary cholesterol seems to be confined to synthesis in the liver and does not affect synthesis in other tissues to any great extent. The effect of suppression of cholesterol biosynthesis on the overall economy of cholesterol metabolism varies with the amount absorbed. When high levels of the sterol are ingested the decrease in synthesis is not sufficient to prevent an increase in the total body pool of cholesterol.

Cholesterol synthesis also is regulated (or affected) by a number of factors: caloric intake, certain hormones, bile acids, and the degree of saturation of the fatty acids in the diet. Reduced caloric intake decreases synthesis of cholesterol by decreasing the concentration of various necessary substrates or reactants such as acetyl CoA, ATP, and NADPH. Bile acids have a direct inhibitory effect on cholesterol synthesis in the intestinal mucosa. (See Rodwell et al., 1973.) The mechanism by which dietary unsaturated fatty acids reduce plasma cholesterol concentrations remains unknown.

Dietary cholesterol does not inhibit cholesterol synthesis in the intestine, but does have a strong feedback inhibitory effect on synthesis in the liver. This inhibition in liver is accomplished by a reduction in the synthesis of the HMG CoA

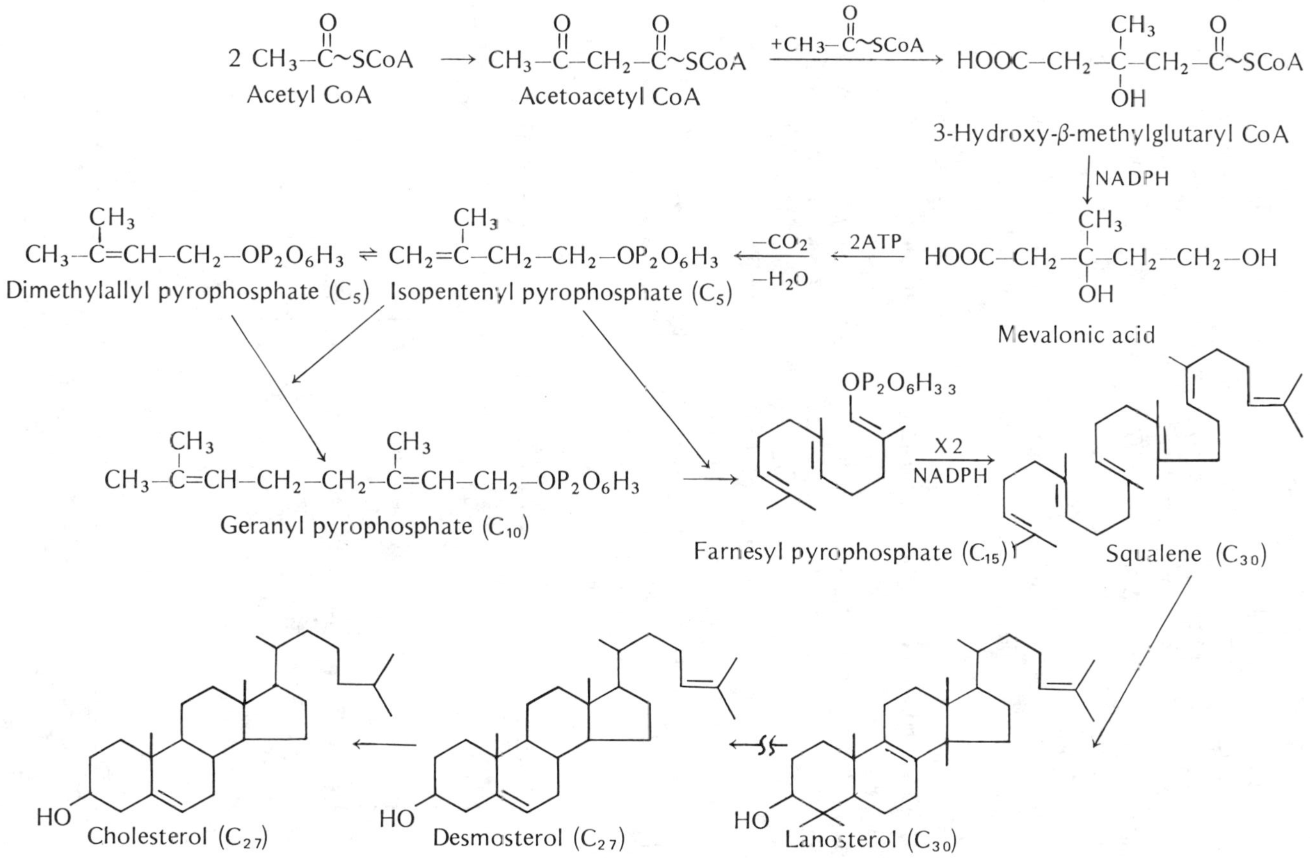

Figure 15.9
Biosynthesis of cholesterol.

reductase enzyme, not by feedback inhibition of the enzyme activity. (See Rodwell et al., 1973.) It is important to note, however, that although hepatic feedback inhibition occurs, it does not appear to be able to compensate completely for dietary modifications. In humans, if large quantities of cholesterol are ingested, about 60 percent of plasma cholesterol still is derived from biosynthesis, and plasma concentrations are elevated from 10–25 percent; if fed a cholesterol-free diet, there is a 10–25 percent decrease in plasma concentrations. (See Montgomery et al., 1980.)

HMG CoA reductase also is regulated by phosphorylation and dephosphorylation. The enzyme is inactivated by phosphorylation; the kinase responsible is present in both cytosol and microsomes of the liver. A phosphatase found in the cytosol reactivates the enzyme. Both the kinase and phosphatase are themselves regulated by phosphorylation and dephosphorylation in reactions involving the generation of cAMP. (See Chapter 11.) Thus increased levels of cAMP decrease enzyme activity whereas insulin and triiodothyronine (which lower cAMP) are associated with increased activity of the HMG CoA reductase (Beg et al., 1978).

The regulation of blood cholesterol level depends not only on the rate of synthesis, but also on the rate of degradation and excretion of cholesterol. Cholesterol is delivered from the liver into the intestine in the bile and is excreted in the feces. Additional amounts are derived from sloughed intestinal mucosal cells. Some of the cholesterol in the large intestine is acted on by intestinal bacteria

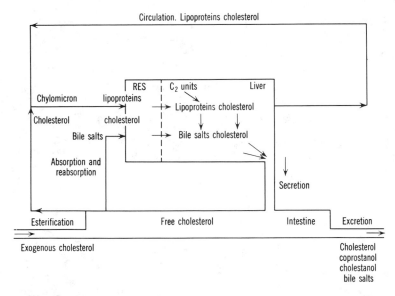

Figure 15.10
Role of the liver in cholesterol metabolism. (From P. Favarger, *The Liver*, Vol. 1, Ch. Rouiller, ed., Academic Press, New York, 1963, p. 587.)

and converted to various neutral sterols such as coprostanol, cholestanone, and cholestanol before excretion. Most of the cholesterol, however, is converted by the liver to the various bile acids. As shown in Fig. 15.10, regulation of blood cholesterol level is the net result of cholesterol absorption, synthesis, uptake by the liver, and subsequent oxidation and excretion from the body. Factors that tend to lower serum cholesterol, therefore, may operate at any one of these points.

BILE ACID SYNTHESIS

The bile acids, cholic and chenodeoxycholic acids, are the most important secretory products of the liver cell. The bile acids may be condensed with either glycine or taurine in the liver to form glyco- or tauro-conjugated bile acids. Both glycine and taurine are joined in amide linkage with the terminal carboxyl group of the bile acids. Bile acid biosynthesis is regulated by the amount of bile acid that is returned from the intestine to the liver: bile acid production equals bile acid losses.

Bile salts are of particular importance in the formation of micelles (Fig. 15.11) which promote solubilization of lipid and lipid-soluble materials for absorption through the mucosal membrane of the small intestine. (See Chapter 6.)

BILE PIGMENT FORMATION

Another major constituent of bile is the pigment derived from heme breakdown. Damaged and senescent red blood cells are removed by various elements of the reticuloendothelial system, especially the spleen. During catabolism, the ring system of hemoglobin is ruptured at the methene bond, the iron atom is removed,

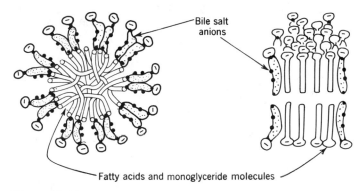

Figure 15.11
Two proposed models for the bile salt-polar lipid micelle. The aggregate on the left is spherical; that on the right is disc-shaped. (From A. F. Hofmann, *Medium Chain Triglycerides*, J. R. Senior, ed., University of Pennsylvania, 1968, p. 14.)

and the globin molecule is detached and hydrolyzed by intracellular proteases. The residue of the degraded porphyrin ring is known as biliverdin which is a dark green pigment. Reduction of the central methene bond of biliverdin produces bilirubin, an orange-yellow pigment. Bilirubin is transported bound to albumin from the reticuloendothelial cell to the liver. Within the liver, the bilirubin is modified by formation of a diglucuronide derivative. In the normal liver, most of the daily bilirubin production is collected in the bile and sent to the digestive tract. Action of the intestinal microorganisms converts most of the bilirubin to urobilinogen, a portion of which may be reabsorbed and excreted in the urine. The remainder of the urobilinogen passes to the lower portions of the large intestine where continued microbial action converts it to stercobilin, a deeply pigmented material that gives much of the characteristic color to feces.

When the blood contains excessive amounts of bilirubin (hyperbilirubinemia), the whites of the eyes and skin appear yellowish in color, a condition known as jaundice. This can occur for a variety of reasons: (1) excessive breakdown of red blood cells leading to greater levels of bilirubin than the liver can metabolize efficiently, (2) damage or necrosis of the liver (as in hepatitis or cirrhosis) which impairs the clearance of bilirubin from plasma or the ability to form the diglucuronide, and (3) posthepatic jaundice in which delivery of bilirubin to the intestinal tract is impaired. For a review, see Haslewood (1978).

Conclusion

The appearance of the hepatocyte does not proclaim its exploitation of some specific function as do the specialized cells in the chapters that follow. Its capabilities, nevertheless, are unique, its versatility awesome, and its competence unquestioned; yet its design is amazingly undistorted. It is, perhaps, the Leonardo of cells, with an innate genius for authoritative expression.

erythrocytes

"Aren't these erythrocytes, as you call them, simply what are known as red blood cells?" he asked, stretching out beside Dr. Streets on the soft, velvety surface.

"Exactly so," was the answer. "In fact, erythros means 'red' in Greek. The material which gives them that bright red color is known as hemoglobin and is a complicated chemical substance possessing great affinity for oxygen. When the blood stream passes through the lungs, these red blood cells adsorb large amounts of oxygen and carry it along to various cell colonies in the body. In fact, although erythrocytes occupy less than fifty percent of the volume of the blood fluid, they can adsorb seventy-five times more oxygen than can possibly be dissolved in the plasma itself."

"Must be a tricky substance," said Mr. Tompkins thoughtfully.

"So it is," agreed Dr. Streets. "And, as a matter of fact, biochemists have had to work hard to learn its exact composition."

George Gamow and Martynas Yčas, 1967

Blood is a connective tissue that differs from other types of connective tissue in that its intercellular substance is liquid. It constitutes a sizable mass, comprising one-eleventh to one-twelfth of body weight. Another distinctive feature of this tissue is the extremely rapid turnover of its cellular constituents. It has been estimated that 2.5 million erythrocytes, 20,000 white cells, and 5 million platelets are sent into the circulation *each second* (Bessis, 1961). Since the total number of cells in circulation remains fairly constant, one must assume that the number entering is balanced by an equal number of cells that are withdrawn from circulation. The successful execution of so relentless a task and one of such enormity is dependent on precise cues, skillful coordination, and conservation of resources.

A Cell Renewal System

The existence of a cell renewal system depends on the replacement of its relatively short-lived cells by proliferation and differentiation of less specialized precursor cells (Patt and Quastler, 1963). The three main lines of hematopoietic cells— erythroid, granulocytic, and thrombocytic—all arise in the bone marrow. They have certain characteristics in common: most of the cells in any one class are mature and highly differentiated; most of the mature cells have a relatively short life span of days or weeks; and all appear to be "end cells," that is, they cannot proliferate, and in the case of the erythrocyte and platelet, this is carried to the extreme in that the mature form in mammals even lacks a nucleus. In a cell renewal system such as that present in the epithelium of the intestinal villi, a progression in the renewal can be observed starting with cell generation in the crypt, to increasing maturity as the cell migrates up along the villus, to death in the lumen. In the blood, the mature cells circulate freely and independently with no obvious connections to their immediate ancestors that do not circulate.

It has long been debated as to whether there was one common ancestral cell from which all blood cells stemmed, a so-called pluripotential stem cell giving rise to several specialized lines of development; or whether each cell line has its own stem cell. As so often happens, both suggestions may turn out to be partially true. It appears that when cell lineages are traced back they seem to merge at the earliest stage. The *stem cell* has all options open to it. It can undergo a reversible transition from a state of rest to one of division (McCulloch, 1970), and it can serve as the target for control mechanisms to give rise to specific *precursor* or *progenitor cells* (Morse and Stohlman, 1966; Moore and Metcalf, 1970). Such progenitor cells are irreversibly *committed* to develop along a specific line leading to the mature cell at the end of that line (Fig. 16.1). It has been suggested that the bulk of the pluripotential stem cell compartment is in a steady state; that is, when cells are stimulated to differentiate, thereby decreasing the pluripotential stem cell compartment size, the remaining cells undergo mitosis and return the compartment to its original size (Stohlman, 1971). A negative feedback system is implied but no details are known of the feedback relationships between the pluripotential stem cells and the progenitor cell compartments.

The only external regulator of blood cell differentiation identified in humans thus far is erythropoietin, which is responsible for stimulating the differentiation of the committed erythroid stem cell. Vitamin E appears to be an erythropoietic

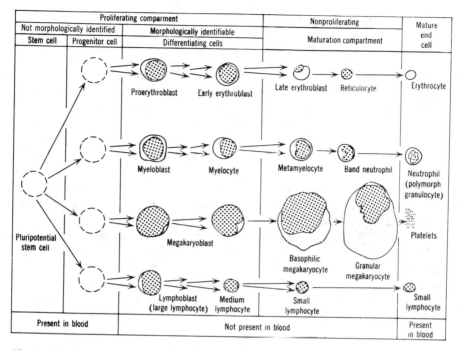

Proliferating compartment			Nonproliferating	Mature end cell
Not morphologically identified		Morphologically identifiable	Maturation compartment	
Stem cell	Progenitor cell	Differentiating cells		

Figure 16.1
Schematic diagram indicating the nomenclature, morphology, and some properties of the various blood cells. (From D. Metcalf and M. A. S. Moore, *Haemopoietic Cells,* North-Holland Publishing Company, Amsterdam, 1971, p. 3.)

factor in nonhuman primates and pigs and may be a potential factor in humans (Drake and Fitch, 1980). Similar regulators have been postulated for the other stem lines. In the material that follows, only the line committed to erythropoiesis and responsive to erythropoietin will be discussed.

Erythropoietin

The erythropoiesis-stimulating factor, *erythropoietin,* is a hormone that increases the total number and total volume of red blood cells in the circulation of normal animals. Its existence was postulated and effects attributed to it were demonstrated in 1906 by Carnot and Déflandre who called it *hématopoïétine.* (See Fisher, 1968.) Almost 50 years elapsed before there was verification of this original work. This was done by exposing one of a pair of parabiotic rats to air with lowered oxygen tension and its partner to normal air (Reissmann, 1950). The stimulation of erythropoiesis in both animals clearly indicated that a hormonal factor was involved. When Erslev (1953) injected an animal with plasma from an anemic animal and found that erythropoiesis was stimulated, the search began in earnest.

CHARACTERISTICS AND ORIGIN

Erythropoietin is a glycoprotein containing sialic acid, galactose, mannose, glucose, and glucosamine. There are at least 17 or 18 amino acids in a single polypeptide chain. The molecular weight, by different modes of estimation, ranges from 46,000–61,800 for human erythropoietin and 27,000–60,000 for the sheep hormone (Goldwasser, 1975). The chief difficulties in determining precise chemical structure and molecular weight are that the hormone is relatively unstable, the purification procedure is time-consuming and results in low yields, the bioassay is difficult to perform, and a rich source of hormone had not, until recently, been discovered.

Plasma was used in the first demonstrations of the existence of erythropoietin. In order to determine its source, plasma erythropoietin was assayed after organ resections and a dramatic fall in erythropoietin levels was found after nephrectomy (Jacobson et al., 1957). Although this evidence strongly suggested that the kidney was the sole source of erythropoietin, it was soon found that some of the hormone could be produced even in the absence of the kidneys (Mirand et al., 1959). Anephric mice and rats have approximately ten percent of their original capacity to produce erythropoietin. The extrarenal site of synthesis appears to be the liver, as several lines of evidence indicate. (See Graber and Krantz, 1978.)

Early attempts at obtaining erythropoietin from kidneys were unsuccessful. Consequently a number of hypotheses were proposed to account for the appearance of erythropoietin in plasma although the tissue of presumed origin seemingly lacked the hormone. These hypotheses are recounted in the review by Graber and Krantz (1978).

Recently a method has been devised, utilizing ion-exchange chromatography, to extract substantial amounts of erythropoietin from kidneys of several animal species (Sherwood and Goldwasser, 1978). The specific cells that synthesize erythropoietin seem to be the mesangial cells of the glomerulus since these cells in culture produce a substance that stimulates erythropoiesis (Kurtz et al., 1982).

Hypoxia or ischemia stimulates erythropoietin production, a process that appears to be mediated by increases first in renal prostaglandin, followed by cAMP levels (Rodgers et al., 1975). Evidence further suggests that the cAMP activates a protein kinase which, in turn, by phosphorylation, converts a precursor molecule to erythropoietin (Martelo et al., 1976).

The ability of cobalt to stimulate erythropoiesis is also mediated through a rise in kidney cAMP (Rodgers et al., 1972).

MECHANISM OF ACTION

The model of hematopoiesis (Fig. 16.2) suggested by Stohlman (1970a) shows the pluripotential stem cell giving rise to three lines of committed cells. The continuous accumulation of committed stem cells is prevented by the death of some that do not continue to differentiate. A feedback relationship appears to exist since depletion of the committed cell compartment leads to its replenishment

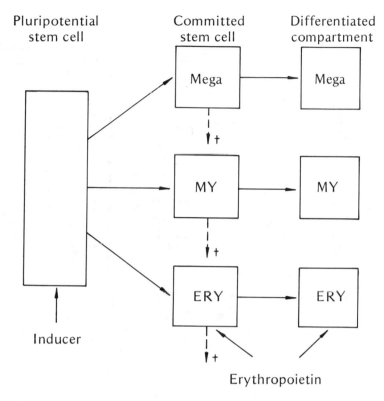

Figure 16.2
Schematic model of hematopoiesis. Mega, megakaryocytic; MY, Mye-
locytic; ERY, erythropoietic. Dashed line and cross indicate cell death.
(From F. Stohlman, Jr., *Regulation of Hematopoiesis*, A. S. Gordon,
ed., Vol. I, Appleton-Century-Crofts, New York, 1970, p. 317.

from the pluripotential compartment. Although the pluripotential stem cell may
not be directly affected by erythropoietin, both the committed stem cells and the
differentiated compartment cells are sensitive to the hormone.

The specific action of erythropoietin on the committed stem cell appears to be
initiation of hemoglobin synthesis. At the molecular level, this effect appears to
be mediated by the interaction of erythropoietin with an unidentified membrane
protein receptor followed by activation of a cytoplasmic factor which transfers
the hormonal message to the genome (Goldwasser and Inana, 1978). At the
nuclear level a repressor may be derepressed, thereby permitting the transcription
of mRNA for hemoglobin synthesis. In addition, erythropoietin also appears to
govern the rate of hemoglobin synthesis. A model (Fig. 16.3) of the kinetics of
erythropoiesis suggests that the cytoplasmic concentration of hemoglobin constitutes a negative feedback and terminates RNA synthesis and cell division. Stohlman (1964) suggested that a critical level for hemoglobin concentration in the

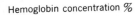

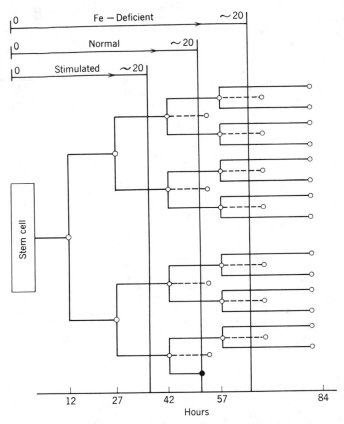

Figure 16.3
Model of kinetics of erythropoiesis postulates that when
hemoglobin concentration of ~20 percent is achieved, further nucleic acid synthesis and division cease. (From F.
Stohlman, Jr. et al., *Ann. N. Y. Acad. Sci.* 149:156, 1968.)

cell was perhaps about 20 percent. Since the interval between cell divisions
appears fixed (Stohlman, 1970b), if nucleic acid synthesis is cut off when a critical
level of hemoglobin is reached, then the rate of hemoglobin synthesis becomes
the factor determining the number of divisions between differentiation and the
final cell division. It follows, therefore, that an accelerated rate of hemoglobin
synthesis would cause fewer divisions to take place before the critical level was
reached and the cells would be larger; whereas in iron deficiency, rate of hemoglobin synthesis would be decreased, and more divisions could take place before
the critical concentration of hemoglobin was attained and microcytic cells would
be formed. In the case of iron deficiency anemia, Conrad and Crosby (1962)
showed that microcytosis precedes hypochromia. Support for such a model was

provided when the response to varying doses of iron in animals and humans with iron deficiency anemia were observed (Stohlman et al., 1963; Leventhal and Stohlman, 1966). When doses were high and iron was no longer rate-limiting, macrocytes were produced; but when doses of iron were low, although restoration to normal hemoglobin was attained, microcytes continued to be produced. If hypoxia is assumed to be the original stimulus to erythropoietin production, then erythropoietin action initiating and controlling the rate of hemoglobin synthesis would produce an increase in red blood cell mass and hemoglobin concentration in circulation. This would increase the oxygen-carrying power of the blood, relieve the hypoxia, and act as a feedback mechanism in cutting off the stimulus to erythropoietin production.

For the sake of clarity, the discussions of erythrocyte maturation and hemoglobin synthesis will be presented separately although, in fact, these two processes are inextricably linked and proceed simultaneously.

Erythrocyte Maturation

The progression of change in the committed stem cell under the influence of erythropoietin leads to the chemical and structural specialization observed in the mature erythrocyte carrying its characteristic load of hemoglobin. The erythroid precursor cells start to proliferate and over a period of four to seven days pass through several identifiable morphological stages, the first of which is the *proerythroblast,* also called *pronormoblast.* After three to four mitotic divisions, each primitive nucleated cell finally gives rise to eight or sixteen anucleate erythrocytes. The cells first appear in the circulation as *reticulocytes,* and after one to two days of further maturation become erythrocytes, remarkably uniform in size, shape, and life span. (See Hillman, 1970.)

Although the normal sequence of differentiation, proliferation, and maturation is fairly steady under normal conditions, the time can be speeded up to three to five days with erythropoietin stimulation. However, the time and maturation schedule is predicated on the presence of an adequate nutrient supply. Limitation of folic acid or vitamin B_{12} interferes with DNA replication and the number of cell divisions during maturation. This leads to fewer but larger and less mature cells, megaloblasts. Limitation of iron, by interfering with the attainment of the critical amount of hemoglobin to curtail cell division, leads to smaller or microcytic cells. With progression of an iron deficiency, synthesis of hemoglobin is further restricted, and the microcytic cells become hypochromic as well. In a cell renewal system of such magnitude any nutrient can interfere with cell proliferation when it becomes the limiting nutrient.

Tracing the earliest changes in development is complicated by the fact that the cells are not recognizably erythroid. Indeed, it has taken both morphological and biochemical sleuthing to discover which cells were destined to become mature erythrocytes. The earliest changes in the progression were presumed to be biochemical, and Krantz and Goldwasser (1965) were able to show that an erythrocyte-stimulating factor (ESF) added to an *in vitro* preparation of bone marrow cells produced an increase in RNA synthesis. Then, in an electron microscopic autoradiographic study, Orlic et al. (1968) were able to identify ESF-sensitive stem cells by their almost immediate incorporation of ^{3}H-thymidine indicating DNA synthesis, and of ^{3}H-uridine indicating RNA synthesis. These cells had numerous ribosomes, sparse endoplasmic reticulum and mitochondria. Nucleoli were seen from 4–12 hours after activation, and these remained prominent in the maturation which followed. At 12–24 hours the cells developed into proerythroblasts, the earliest recognizable erythroid cell, and into erythroblasts at 48–72 hours of maturation, still showing a portion of the original tritium label. Originally in 1–4 cells, by 48 hours the radioactive material was diluted into 18–36 erythroblasts. The ^{3}H-uridine taken up at 5.5 hours after activation was still present 42 hours later suggesting its incorporation into a stable RNA fraction. Many reticulocytes emerged with the uridine label. This was consistent with the knowledge that the rRNA and mRNA for directing hemoglobin synthesis are stable and that synthesis of hemoglobin continues to occur after nuclear extrusion and reticulocyte maturation are completed. A schematic summary is presented in Fig. 16.4.

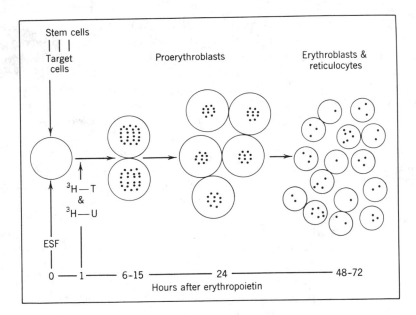

Figure 16.4
The incorporation of ^{3}H-nucleic acid precursors is represented by black dots (silver grains) over cells of the erythroid series. Both ^{3}H-thymidine and ^{3}H-uridine are incorporated within 1 hour after administration of erythropoietin, and ^{3}H-uridine uptake continues at 1.5, 3.5, and 5.5 hours. After exposures (three months), erythroblast autoradiograms indicated greatly reduced numbers of silver grains per cell compared with the total found in proerythroblast autoradiograms exposed for shorter times (three to four weeks). This dilution of label appears to occur through cell division. (From D. Orlic et al., *Ann. N. Y. Acad. Sci.* 149:198, 1968.)

From this and subsequent data, Orlic (1970) suggested that if ESF was, in fact, a derepressor of genes controlling the production of a specific erythroid substance (Krantz and Goldwasser, 1965), then its action was likely during the replication of DNA in cycling stem cells. Orlic (1970) also suggested, on the basis of ultra-structural observations, that the ribosomes were already present in the cytoplasm of the stem cells and that the cells need only acquire specific mRNA molecules to begin undergoing erythroid changes. This, he suggested, was in accord with Krantz and Goldwasser's (1965) hypothesis that the primary regulating event in ESF-induced differentiation of stem cells was synthesis of mRNA coded for hemoglobin.

Well developed nucleoli are observed in the proerythroblasts, and these presumably are responsible for the synthesis of nearly all the erythroid-specifying RNA that is transcribed later during hemoglobin synthesis (Orlic, 1970). As the cells develop, there is nuclear condensation which continues until there are only a few small areas of chromatin material. How the nucleus is finally extruded is not well understood. It takes only about ten minutes, as demonstrated by cinematography (Fig. 16.5), and the extruded nuclei are phagocytosed by macrophages in the marrow (Orlic, 1970). The cells never reach this stage in folic acid or vitamin B_{12} deficiency states.

The reticulocytes usually remain in the marrow for another one to two days during which time they synthesize additional hemoglobin. After penetrating the vascular lining cells, they enter the blood where, after another one to two days, they mature into biconcave discs devoid of all organelles but filled instead with hemoglobin. These cells are specialized to perform one major function, that of transporting oxygen. The biconcavity increases the surface area and permits more rapid absorption and release of the gases. The loss of all organelles provides optimum space for hemoglobin and makes the cell more efficient per unit volume. The physical structure of the hemoglobin protein and the shape of the cells provide pliability and resiliency and keep them from being prematurely shattered during their frenzied trips through the turbulent vascular system. Defects in hemoglobin protein may be responsible for the excessive fragmentation of erythrocytes as, for example, in sickle cell anemia.

Despite the lack of standard organelle equipment, the mature erythrocyte is far

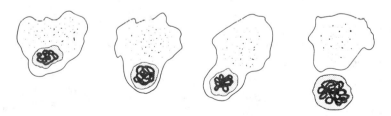

Figure 16.5
Loss of nucleus from erythroblast taken from film sequence. (Redrawn from M. Bessis, *The Cell*, Vol. V, J. Brachet and A. E. Mirsky, eds., Academic Press, New York, 1961, p. 183.)

from inert. It is a metabolizing cell that depends on glycolysis for its energy to maintain the high concentration of intracellular potassium and the functional state of reversible deoxygenation in hemoglobin. However, the major function of the erythrocyte requires no expenditure of energy. Both oxygen and carbon dioxide are transported through the plasma membrane by passive diffusion. The mature cell emerges from the bone marrow into the circulation with a supply of lipid, protein, lipoprotein, carbohydrate, ATP, and enzymes in addition to the extremely concentrated solution of hemoglobin, approximately 33 percent, which is just below the point of crystallization. Having lost its capacity for synthetic activity, its stockpile of nutrients and enzymes cannot be replenished. As the cells age, therefore, the complement of enzymes and available ATP decline, and electron-dense material called Heinz bodies, which are thought to be aggregations of denatured hemoglobin, accumulate. The cells that entered the circulation as trim, biconcave discs full of energy, become old and more spheroidal, worn out, and depleted. After about 120 days they are destroyed. Although the specific signal has not been identified, it seems likely that phagocytosis of aged cells is somehow initiated by their reduced deformability caused, in part, by lipid peroxidation (see Chapter 9) and polymerization of membrane proteins (Teitel, 1977; Hochstein and Jain, 1981). Probably some cells also are lost by fragmentation, hemolysis, or some combination of these causes.

For more detailed description of the development of erythrocytes, see Metcalf and Moore (1971); Golde et al. (1978); Ham and Cormack (1979).

Hemoglobin Synthesis

A single red blood cell contains about 280 million molecules of hemoglobin, each of which has a molecular weight of 64,500. Hemoglobin contains 10,000 atoms, four of which are iron firmly chelated to protoporphyrin. It is the iron-containing protoporphyrin, or heme group (Fig. 16.6a), that provides the oxygen-binding capacity of hemoglobin. The heme is attached to a 574 amino acid polypeptide chain (Fig. 16.6b). Four heme-globin subunits fit together in such a way that the hemes are nearly equidistant from each other at the surface of the molecule. Nine positions in each primary amino acid chain are highly conserved and are particularly important for maintaining the shape and function of the hemoglobin molecule. The amino acids at these positions are histidine, phenylalanine, leucine, glycine, proline, tyrosine, and threonine. The protoporphyrin portion of the molecule is a key compound in many types of cells from different species and functions in photosynthesis (chlorophyll), oxygen transport (hemoglobin and myoglobin), and electron transport (cytochromes). The synthesis of protoporphyrin comes about through a series of reactions starting with the ubiquitous succinyl CoA and glycine which condense in the presence of pyridoxal phosphate, the enzyme δ-aminolevulinic acid synthetase (ALA-S) and possibly iron (Brown, 1958), to form δ-aminolevulinic acid (ALA) (Fig. 16.7). This reaction takes place in the mitochondria where succinyl CoA is readily available through the TCA cycle. The condensation of two molecules of ALA yields porphobilinogen

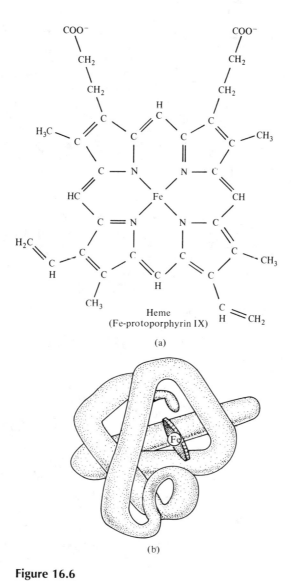

(a)

(b)

Figure 16.6
(a) Heme or Fe-protoporphyrin IX. (b) One of the four globin chains that constitute hemoglobin. (Adapted from R. E. Dickinson and I. Geis, *The Structure and Action of Proteins,* W. A. Benjamin, Inc., Menlo Park, California, 1969.)

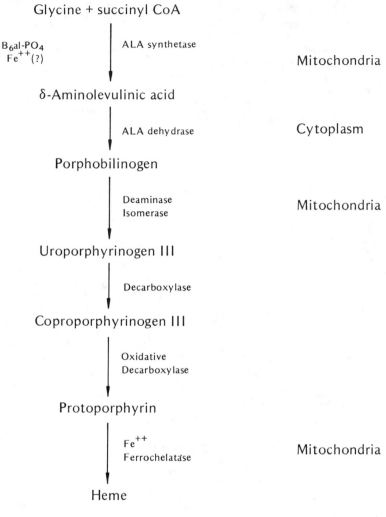

Figure 16.7
Synthesis of heme.

and is catalyzed by ALA dehydrase which is located in the cytoplasm. ALA dehydrase depends on free sulfhydryl groups for its activity, as does the enzyme in the final formation of heme from iron and protoporphyrin. The inhibitory effect of lead at these two points in hemoglobin synthesis has been reported (Chisolm, 1971). The inhibition of ferrochelatase activity probably is responsible for the anemia of lead intoxication. Lamola and Yamane (1974) recently reported that in the anemias of both lead intoxication and severe iron deficiency, Zn^{++} binds to the globin moieties and produces a fluorescent porphyrin. According to these investigators, this provides a simple and specific screening test for lead intoxication.

Recently, vitamin E deficiency, which has been associated with anemia in primates (Dinning and Day, 1957), was shown to produce a decrease in the activity of ALA dehydrase (Nair et al., 1972). From porphobilinogen, under the influence of a deaminase and an isomerase in the mitochondria, one of four possible isomers of uroporphyrinogen is synthesized, uroporphyrinogen III. A series of decarboxylations and oxidations follow to give protoporphyrin IX. A ferrochelatase in the mitochondria next inserts a ferrous ion into the tetrapyrrole ring to form heme. The main point of control in the synthetic pathway appears to be at ALA-S where heme exerts both a feedback control and a repression control. The second point of control appears to be at the level of ALA dehydrase. (See Nair, 1972.)

Caasi et al. (1972) showed that the defect in heme synthesis in vitamin E deficiency in the rat is at a site identical to that of ALA-dehydrase. The iron toxicity that develops in vitamin E deficiency is perhaps caused by the decrease in protoporphyrin IX which otherwise would be available for the acceptance of iron (Nair, 1972).

Iron Delivery

Approximately 1 percent of the red cell mass is replaced each day by the hematopoietic tissue and the iron required for the synthesis of that amount of hemoglobin is about 25 mg. This iron must be readily available to the developing erythron. Ultrastructural studies have indicated that within a few hours after erythropoietin activation, stem cells start to accumulate ferritin (Orlic et al., 1965). Others have shown ferritin adhering to specialized areas in the glycocalyx of the maturing erythrocyte, which then appeared to invaginate, pinch off, and form vesicles that move through the cytoplasm (Bessis, 1961; Fawcett, 1966; Lentz, 1971). There now is considerable doubt that this is the way the iron is presented to the mass of developing red cells although a small portion entering this way may be derived from catabolism of some erythrocytes in the marrow. Evidence that ferritin iron is the precursor of heme iron has been challenged. Primosigh and Thomas (1968) found that only a small and relatively fixed portion of iron that enters the cell is ferritin. The immature erythron appears to be able to obtain all the iron it requires for hemoglobin synthesis directly from the circulating iron-transferrin complex (Katz, 1970). Transferrin molecules bind at specific receptor sites on the surface of the immature red cells. There are about 500,000 receptors per cell (Octave et al., 1982). The iron is transferred to the interior of the cell, possibly by endocytosis (see Chapter 9) of the transferrin-iron complex (ibid). The site then receives another iron-transferrin complex and the process is repeated (Morgan et al., 1966). The entire process from the initial binding of iron by the cell surface receptors until its incorporation into hemoglobin requires only six to eight minutes (Allen and Jandl, 1960). The iron transfer peaks at the earlier stages of maturation with less taken up by the reticulocyte and none by the mature cell. How this attraction between the cell membrane and transferrin operates is not known, but iron-transferrin has greater affinity for the receptor sites than apotransferrin indicating that the iron plays a part in the "fit." It may also be worth-

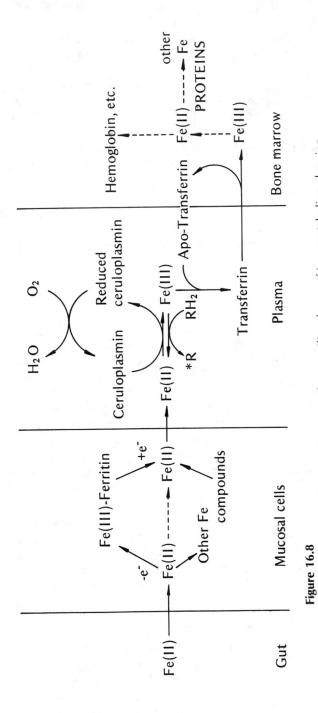

Figure 16.8
Summary of some of the initial aspects of a prevailing theory of iron metabolism showing the possible role of ceruloplasmin promoting iron utilization. (From S. Osaki et al., *J. Biol. Chem.* 241:2746, 1966.)

while recalling that transferrin is a glycoprotein, and this may endow it with a certain capacity for recognition of and affinity for the specific site on the membrane surface of the developing red cell.

It had long been recognized that copper was involved in some way in iron metabolism. The report of Osaki et al. (1966) established that the oxidase activity of ceruloplasmin, the copper-containing enzyme in the serum, is a controlling element in iron metabolism. In the absence of ceruloplasmin neither the rate of iron entry into the plasma nor its rate of oxidation are sufficient to meet the demands of the developing marrow or other tissues for iron. The presence of unsaturated transferrin (apotransferrin) in the serum is responsible for trapping the ferric ion and incorporating it into the transferrin complex. The mechanism postulated for this action is shown in Fig. 16.8. (See also Fig. 5.1.)

The release of ferric iron from ferritin apparently depends on a ferritin reductase system since iron must go through the ferrous state to be mobilized, only to be reconverted to ferric iron for every step in iron metabolism including storage, transport, biosyntheses, and degradation. A system has been found in liver for the reductive release of iron from ferritin that requires NADH and FMN (Frieden, 1973).

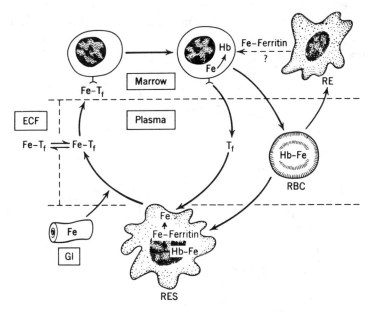

Figure 16.9
Diagrammatic representation of cyclic mechanisms of iron delivery to bone marrow. Not illustrated is uptake of iron by other tissues or feedback of iron from the so-called labile pool, both of which may involve transferrin binding to membrane receptors. T_f, transferrin; RE, reticuloendothelial cells; RES, reticuloendothelial system; Hb, hemoglobin. (From J. H. Katz, *Ser. Haemat.* 6:15, 1965.)

The release of the transferrin iron for the formation of hemoglobin in the developing erythrocytes involves a ferrochelatase, an enzyme that has been found in vertebrate liver and erythrocytes (Frieden, 1973). Iron uptake, however, is not regulated solely by the rate of hemoglobin synthesis since developing cells remove iron from transferrin before hemoglobin synthesis starts. All erythroid cells can synthesize ferritin (Primosigh and Thomas, 1968), and this may occur when the iron is in excess of immediate needs. Myhre (1964) and Noyes et al. (1964) have shown that up to 90 percent of the iron entering the intact marrow is converted into heme within one hour. A diagrammatic representation of the mechanisms of iron delivery to developing red cells in the marrow is shown in Fig. 16.9. For a review of heme synthesis, see Finch (1968); Kaplan (1970); Maines and Kappas (1977).

Globin Synthesis

During development there is a change in the type of hemoglobin chains that are synthesized and this seems to be correlated with the source of the oxygen that the hemoglobin carries. The embryonic hemoglobin, Hb-Gower 1, the more common one, and Hb-Gower 2 circulate during the earliest stages of gestation when the source of oxygen is from maternal interstitial fluid. These chains are replaced by Hb-F by the tenth week of gestation when oxygen uptake is via the

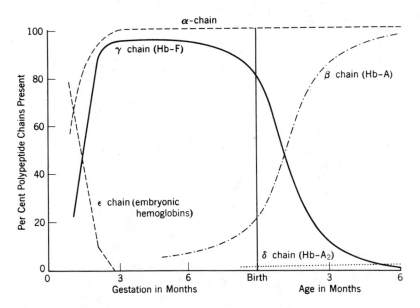

Figure 16.10
The developmental changes in human hemoglobin chains. (From E. R. Huehns and G. H. Beaven, *The Biochemistry of Development*, P. Benson, ed., J. B. Lippincott, Philadelphia, 1971, p. 177.)

placenta. From the newborn period onward, oxygen is obtained through the lungs, and Hb-F is replaced by Hb-A during the first six months of life (Fig. 16.10).

Studies on human embryonic hemoglobins, such as by Huehns et al. (1964), have shown that the ϵ chain is specific to the embryonic period and Hb-Gower 1 is probably made of four chains; Hb-Gower 2 has a structure of Hb-$\alpha_2\epsilon_2$. The α and ϵ globin chains differ from one another by several amino acid substitutions. The α chains in both fetal and adult type Hb are identical; the non-α chains, γ chains in Hb-F and β chains in Hb-A, are alike in structure and consist of 146 amino acids, 39 of which are different.

The synthesis of each of the polypeptide chains is under separate genetic control and characterization of the DNA specifically responsible for the synthesis of globin is the subject of intense investigation. One reason for this is that globin genes provide an excellent model for studies of genes that switch on and off during different times of development. Although the major events of globin synthesis are regulated at the level of transcription and subsequent RNA processing, the subcellular events that are responsible for the gradual, orderly change from γ chain synthesis to β chain synthesis in late fetal and early postnatal life remain unclear. It appears that both Hb-A and Hb-F coexist in the same cells during the period of switching. Preterm newborn infants were studied to determine if the transition of Hb-F to Hb-A synthesis was influenced by the birth process. The results indicated that the slow transition to Hb-A synthesis accelerates as the preterm infant approaches the 38th week of postconceptional age. At the postconceptional age corresponding to term, there is no statistical difference between the early preterm-born group and the full term newborn group. The rate of transition from Hb-F to Hb-A appears species-specific, and the switchover is related to the rate of biological maturation and is not affected in humans by a precocious exposure to extrauterine life (Bard, 1973).

The persistence of Hb-F, which has a greater capacity for oxygen than adult hemoglobins, or its reappearance in adult life, occurs in certain hemolytic disorders. In cases where erythropoiesis is stimulated by anemic hypoxia, Hb-F appears to provide a survival advantage to the erythrocyte containing it; in other cases, this explanation does not hold and no explanation can be offered for reversion to Hb-F (Bertles, 1970). A comprehensive treatise on human hemoglobin has been provided by Bunn et al. (1977).

Comprehension of the logistics involved in the intricate coordination of globin chain synthesis and heme synthesis with the velocity of the maturation schedule of the mass-produced erythrocytes appears at once impossible and intriguing.

Degradation of Erythrocytes

The 120-day life span of the erythrocytes is exceedingly long compared with that of some of the white blood cells, which may remain in the circulation for only 30 minutes, or the platelets that circulate for three to eight days. One can only be astounded at the magnitude and speed of the hematopoietic activity.

When the erythrocytes are withdrawn from the circulation they are taken up by the reticulum cells in the spleen, liver, and bone marrow and their digestion takes about five to ten minutes (Bessis, 1961). Around the fragments of the phagocytosed red cell, granules of ferritin or larger masses of hemosiderin are visible in electron micrographs. Bessis (1961) suggests that the ferritin observed in the reticulum cells may come directly from phagocytosed red cells or may be the iron carried to the cell by transferrin and stored there as ferritin for use in the synthesis of hemoglobin in the developing cells. More likely, the ferritin iron is released to transferrin and circulated to the marrow for incorporation into the developing erythrocytes. Approximately 90 percent of the iron in new hemoglobin is obtained from such recycling. The appearance in the plasma of catabolized heme iron bound to transferrin is rapid (Garby and Noyes, 1959; Noyes et al., 1960). The protein of the hemoglobin molecule is also released, and these amino acids become part of the amino acid content of the cell. The porphyrin portion of the hemoglobin molecule is degraded by the reticuloendothelial cells of the liver, spleen, and bone marrow. The first step involves opening of the pyrrole ring to form biliverdin, the first of the bile pigments. This is readily reduced to bilirubin by bilirubin reductase (Singleton and Laster, 1965). The bilirubin circulates in the plasma associated with albumin, and in the liver it conjugates with glucuronic acid catalyzed by glucuronyl transferase. The now water-soluble bilirubin is excreted with the bile into the intestinal lumen. In the colon, bilirubin is released from the glucuronide and undergoes progressive reduction by enzymes derived mostly from the anaerobic flora in the tract and eventually appears in the feces as stercobilin and urobilin (Watson, 1969; Lightner et al., 1969).

A method utilizing measurement of labeled serum bilirubin for the determination of mean red blood cell life span has been reported that can be used clinically. The method also gives information about the capacity of the liver to clear the plasma of bilirubin and thus is useful in diagnosis of liver disease (Berk et al., 1970).

Conclusion

A cell renewal system of the magnitude required for the maintenance of the circulating erythrocytes, or one of even greater magnitude such as required for the mucosa of the gastrointestinal tract, can function only if the nutrients supplied to the generating tissues are adequate. Any limiting nutrient will affect the total system. The more fundamental the metabolic role of the nutrient in the cell renewal process, the more severe will be the effect. It becomes apparent why the effects of vitamin B_{12} and folic acid deficiencies are so dramatic in both the gastrointestinal tract and the blood. If the enzymes involved in nucleotide synthesis are blocked, cell division is blocked. If cell division is blocked, there can be no cell renewal.

chapter 17

bone cells

"The mineral in the human skeleton is an integral part of a large calcium phosphate cycle which courses throughout the earth's biosphere. . . . Over eons of time the extended leaching of . . . primary rocks by the earth's waters made calcium and phosphate (as well as other ions) available for mineralogical and/or biological redisposition throughout the world. Thus, the oceans, rivers, and lakes move calcium and phosphate through the earth just as the blood system in man moves these ions in solution to the desired locus of mineral formation."

A. S. Posner, 1973

Bone as a Connective Tissue

Bone, like blood, is a connective tissue, and the intercellular substance is its most distinguishing characteristic. Whereas in blood the intercellular substance is liquid and the tissue itself is composed almost entirely of cells, other connective tissues consist almost entirely of intercellular material and have relatively few cells. The differences between types of connective tissue are due to modifications of the intercellular material that consists of fibers and the amorphous ground substance in between. The fibers are the fibrous proteins, collagen and elastin; the ground substance in which they are embedded consists primarily of proteoglycans. Other noncollagenous proteins such as osteonectin, osteocalcin, and phosphoproteins are also part of the organic matrix. The interstitial or intercellular substance in bone is impregnated with mineral but, in the case of hyaline cartilage, it is a firm gel. However, bone is not calcified cartilage. Because of the character of the

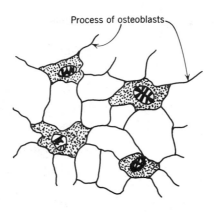

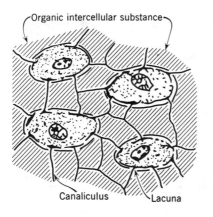
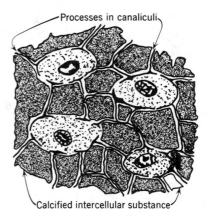

Figure 17.1
The osteoblasts secrete the organic intercellular substance of bone both around their cell bodies and around the cytoplasmic arms that extend from the cell bodies. The cytoplasmic arms serve as molds for tiny passageways called canaliculi which remain to provide communication between adjacent osteoblasts and the surface on which the bone is forming. When the osteoblasts are completely surrounded by the intercellular substance they have secreted, they are termed osteocytes. The organic intercellular substance then becomes impregnated with calcium salts. The canaliculi provide a means whereby materials can be transported between surfaces and the cells buried in the calcified intercellular substance. (From A. W. Ham and D. H. Cormack, *Histology,* 8th ed., J. B. Lippincott Company, Philadelphia, 1979, p. 381.)

interstitial substance in cartilage, nutrients diffuse through it to the cells; but if calcification occurs, diffusion stops and the cells die. Calcification in bone develops differently. The bone cells are in spaces called lacunae and have access to nutrient supplies through cytoplasmic processes that extend into the canaliculi and, therefore, they are metabolizing cells (Fig. 17.1). These cells are so arranged that they are never more than a fraction of a millimeter from a capillary carrying the blood supply which flows through the bone at an estimated rate of 200–400 ml/min.

Bone and other connective tissue cells, like blood cells, develop from a pool of common stem cells that, under appropriate circumstances, can differentiate along different lines. In the material that follows, only those stem cells that differentiate into *osteogenic cells,* also called *osteoprogenitor cells,* will be discussed. Osteogenic cells normally cover and line all bone surfaces, and they are the cells that eventually lead to the production of bone. They develop into *osteoblasts* that secrete organic intercellular substances around themselves and become *osteocytes.* The osteocyte has less cytoplasmic material since it no longer synthesizes and secretes protein and proteoglycans. The calcification of the surrounding organic intercellular material that began when the cell was an osteoblast continues until the matrix is solidly impregnated with mineral. The nutritional and physiological aspects of bone will be discussed below but the student is referred to Bloom and Fawcett (1968) or Ham and Cormack (1979) for details of morphological development.

Intercellular Substance

The osteoblasts of developing bone are similar to the fibroblasts of other connective tissues in their ability to synthesize and secrete intercellular substances such as collagen and proteoglycans.

COLLAGEN SYNTHESIS

Collagen, a connective tissue protein, constitutes one-third of the total protein of the body and 57 percent of it is in bone. Collagen differs from most other proteins in that it is fibrous and it contains an unusual assortment of amino acids. One-third of its amino acid content is glycine, which occurs in every third position in the polypeptide chains. It is also rich in proline and lysine (Fig. 17.2). Collagen contains no tryptophan and no cysteine. A biochemical puzzle was revealed when it was reported that labeled hydroxyproline was not incorporated into collagen and that free proline served as the source of both the proline and hydroxyproline in the molecule (Stetten and Schoenheimer, 1944; Stetten, 1949). Later it was shown that during collagen synthesis the polypeptide rich in proline and lysine was assembled and subsequently hydroxylated to hydroxyproline and hydroxylysine by the enzymes peptidyl proline hydroxylase and peptidyl lysine hydroxylase. Both enzymes are dependent on molecular oxygen rather than water

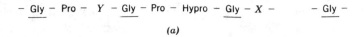

(a)

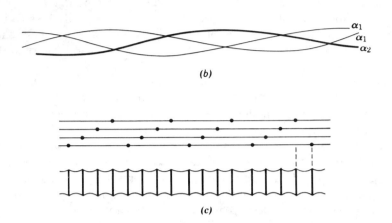

(b)

(c)

Figure 17.2
(a) Typical amino acid sequence in collagen. X and Y are any amino
acid other than Gly, Pro, Hypro, Lys, or Hylys. (b) Triple helix of
tropocollagen showing two α_1-chains and one α_2-chain. (c) Staggered
alignment of tropocollagen molecules accounting for the periodicity
of the collagen fibril.

as the source of the hydroxyl molecule (Fujimoto and Tamiya, 1962; Prockop et
al., 1963). Other requirements are α-ketoglutarate as co-substrate (Hutton et al.,
1967; Rhoads and Udenfriend, 1968), nonheme ferrous iron (Prockop and Juva,
1965; Prockop, 1971), and ascorbic acid (Stone and Meister, 1962). The nonheme
iron in the enzyme is loosely bound (Pankalainen and Kivirikko, 1970) and activates the enzyme (Bhatnagar et al., 1972). Ascorbic acid had been considered
a reducing agent in the reactions (Hutton et al., 1967), but recent evidence
suggests that, in addition, it may be implicated in the conversion of the inactive
precursor form of the enzyme to the active enzyme (Stassen et al., 1973). These
reactions appear to occur in the rough endoplasmic reticulum or in the cytoplasmic matrix.

It is assumed that immediately following hydroxylation, and while the chains
are still on the polyribosomes, helix formation occurs. The alignment of the three
individual chains into helix formation is thought to be aided by a number of extra
amino acid sequences at the amino terminals of the procollagen chains. The
removal of the amino-terminal extensions by procollagen peptidase (Bornstein et
al., 1972) occurs subsequent to the attachment of the carbohydrate moiety, galactose or glucose, by the galactosyl or glucosyl transferases which are in the
membranes of the Golgi complex (Weinstock and Leblond, 1974). The glycosylated procollagen in the secretory vacuoles from which the amino-terminal

sequences have been removed is *tropocollagen,* which leaves the cell by exocytosis. Miller and Matukas (1974) suggest that the microtubule system in the cell
plays a role in guiding the vacuoles to the membrane of the cell for secretion. A
summary of the steps in biosynthesis is shown in Fig. 17.3.

Following extrusion from the cell, there is alignment of the monomers side to
side and end to end in a staggered arrangement followed by cross-linking through
interchain hydrogen bonds and through covalent bonds between the ranks of the
monomers. (See Fig. 17.2.) Bone collagen is cross-linked rapidly and extensively,
and it is suggested that this is a means of stabilizing the tissue prior to and during

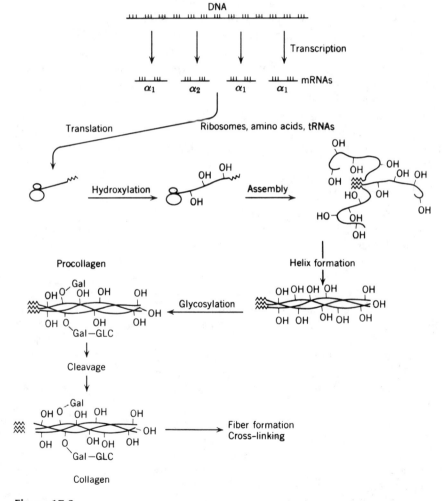

Figure 17.3
Schematic diagram illustrating the steps involved in biosynthesis of the monomer
collagen molecule. (From E. J. Miller and V. J. Matukas, *Fed. Proc.* 33:1197,
1974.)

mineralization (Miller, 1969). Although the primary structure of collagen from different tissues is similar, there may be unique although still unknown modification of the collagen in calcified tissues (ibid).

Interference with collagen synthesis has been demonstrated at various steps and attributed to the involvement of various nutrients. Feeding the sweetpea (*Lathyrus odoratus*) to growing rats causes connective tissue defects including costochondral junction enlargement and scoliosis. The molecular basis for the disease known as Lathyrism is a deficiency in the cross-linking of collagen and elastin due to the inhibition of lysyl oxidase by lathyrogens (Gallup and Paz, 1975). The compound that causes this disorder is β-aminoproprionitrile. Decreased uptake and hydroxylation of proline were reported in vitamin D deficiency in chicks (Canas et al., 1969). Since this effect preceded any changes in plasma calcium by 12 hours, the vitamin D effect on collagen synthesis was assumed to be direct and not dependent on changes in plasma calcium concentration. Decreased uptake and hydroxylation of proline were reported in zinc deficiency (Lema and Sandstead, 1970), but the role of zinc in collagen formation is not clear (Westmoreland, 1971). There is evidence of decreased structural stability of collagen in copper deficiency which is attributed to decreased cross-linkage of the polypeptide chains (Carnes, 1971). Vitamin E deficiency also has been implicated in the defective cross-linking of collagen (Brown et al., 1967).

PROTEOGLYCAN SYNTHESIS

Ground substance is the extracellular, interfibrillar component of all connective tissues. It provides the intercellular material that acts as a cement substance in which the collagenic fibrils are embedded, and it is probable that it also cements the microfibrils together to form the fibrils. Synthesis of ground substance, like that of collagen, is the responsibility of the osteoblasts.

Ground substance is chemically characterized by its glycosaminoglycans (formerly called mucopolysaccharides) which are composed of linear chains of alternating units of uronic acids and hexosamines. The hexosamines are usually N-acetylated and may have an ester-sulfate group at the 4 or 6 position. The glycosaminoglycans are linked together into larger aggregates called proteoglycans. Chondroitin 4-sulfate is a major glycosaminoglycan in bone. It is a polymer of glucuronic acid alternating with N-acetyl galactosamine in which the hydroxyl group on carbon-4 is sulfated. (See Chapter 2.) Synthesis of the sulfated proteoglycans takes place in the well developed Golgi apparatus of the osteoblasts (Leblond and Weinstock, 1976). As the osteoblasts mature into osteocytes and become embedded in the mineralized matrix, synthetic activity is devoted mainly to maintenance of the bone matrix and is reflected morphologically by less prominent endoplasmic reticulum and Golgi apparatus.

The essentiality of manganese in proteoglycan synthesis was revealed through study of the bone abnormalities in manganese-deficient chicks (Leach and Muenster, 1962; Leach, 1967). Manganese deficiency was found to interfere with the activity of the glycosyltransferase enzymes involved in chondroitin sulfate synthesis (Leach et al., 1969; Leach, 1971). Decreased sulfate uptake was reported in zinc deficiency in rats (Lema and Sandstead, 1971) and chicks (Neilson and Ziporin, 1969). The poor control of calcification observed in these animals was attributed to the decrease in sulfate groups in the matrix (Westmoreland, 1971). Alkaline phosphatases are zinc metalloenzymes and these, too, have been implicated in matrix formation (Miller et al., 1965).

MINERAL DEPOSITION

The process of calcification begins soon after the organic intercellular matrix is formed by osteoblasts. The ions that form the bone mineral are derived from the blood. Bone mineral deposition is initiated a short distance away from the osteoblasts which surround themselves with bone matrix to become osteocytes enclosed in lacunae. The bone mineral is believed to be an hydroxyapatite, the basic formation of which is $Ca_{10}(PO_4)_6(OH)_2$. The exact chemical composition is not accurately known because of a mixture of transition forms that are present as the bone matures and because of the various substitutions and exchanges of ions that occur in the crystal structure. It is well established that the mineral in bone is precipitated first as an amorphous material that is converted to a crystalline precipitate and then eventually to the final crystal (Eanes et al., 1967; Posner, 1973). In mature compact bone, about 40 percent of the total mineral is present in the form of a nonapatite component, and the percentage is higher in young bone. The amorphous phase is lower in Ca/P and, with the addition of calcium as the bone matures, the ratio rises (Posner, 1967). The concept of bone maturation may be clearer if the young crystal is viewed with calcium ions missing at random throughout the crystal structure and maturation as a process of filling in the calcium. It is this process of maturation of the apatite that is disturbed in bones of vitamin D-deficient animals whose bones contain a higher amorphous content than do normal bones of the same age (Muller et al., 1966).

There are three zones in the crystal lattice: crystal interior, crystal surface, and hydration shell, all of which are involved in exchanges of ions. Ions at the interior have the slowest rate of turnover, and this is the site for the sequestration of strontium, radium, and lead for which bone has an affinity. These minerals replace calcium in the crystal lattice. Fluoride produces changes in the bone crystal by replacing the hydroxyl ion which leads to growth and stabilization of the apatite crystal. Since larger crystals react more slowly than smaller ones, fluoride substitution produces more stable bone mineral (Posner, 1969). There is rapid turnover of ions at the crystal surface, and sodium, magnesium, citrate, and carbonate can be held by adsorption to the surface or by substitution on the surface. The hydration shell of the crystal allows diffusion of all the ions mentioned plus potassium and chloride. With age, the amount of water in bone decreases and the ions of bone salt are less accessible for exchange.

Bone crystals are ultramicroscopic in size and rodlike with a diameter averaging 50 Å. The surface area of the crystal is large in proportion to the mass; a single gram is reported to have a surface area in excess of 100 m². On this basis, McLean and Urist (1968) calculate that the total surface area of the bone crystals in the skeleton of a 70 kg man exceeds 100 acres, all of which is bathed by a few liters of bone fluid!

Normally one may view the ions on the surface of the crystals as being in equilibrium with those in the fluid bathing the bone. The entire system is a very dynamic one. However, bone fluid has been shown to differ markedly in composition from general extracellular fluids (Neuman, 1969). This is explained in terms of compartmentalization, presumably by a functional membrane that regulates the flow of cations. Rasmussen et al. (1970) strongly support the view that osteoblasts constitute an effective membrane separating the general extracellular fluids and the bone extracellular fluid. These cells control matrix synthesis and, in addition, regulate the exchange of ions between the general extracellular fluid and those of mineralizing bone matrix.

In addition to the physical process of ion exchange, there are hormonal factors involved in controlling deposition and release of mineral associated with bone metabolism and growth which will be discussed in a later section.

The canaliculi provide the means whereby nutrients and oxygen required by the cells can be transported from the bone surface, where the capillaries are situated, to the cell bodies embedded in the calcified intercellular substance. Such a system is obviously less proficient than one in which the plasma membrane of an individual cell lies in the aqueous nutrient medium. However, the proximity of the osteocytes to the capillary permits the system to operate efficiently.

Bone Growth

Most bones of the skeleton exist in embryonic life as cartilage models, and in development and growth the cartilage is gradually replaced by bone, due to the activity of invading osteoblasts. The skeleton of a fetus becomes the skeleton of an adult through a series of coordinated processes in which new bone is formed on the preexisting outer bone surfaces and resorbed from the preexisting inner surfaces. These two processes of formation and resorption are balanced so that as new bone is added to the outside of a bone shaft during growth bone is resorbed from the inner surface of the shaft to make the marrow cavity wider (Fig. 17.4). Resorption includes the processes necessary to put into solution the complicated structure of bone, and its component parts then can enter the circulation. The cells responsible for the resorption process are the *osteoclasts,* large cells often containing 15–20 nuclei.

The question of the origin of osteoclasts has long been in contention among bone biologists; however, in recent years the consensus is that osteoclasts are derived from macrophages and not from an osteogenic cell line. (See Ham and Cormack, 1979.) The manner in which the osteoclasts participate in bone resorption has not been clarified, but their direct involvement has been demonstrated by time-lapse motion pictures (Chambers and Magnus, 1982). According to McLean and Urist (1968) the organic and inorganic constituents of bone are

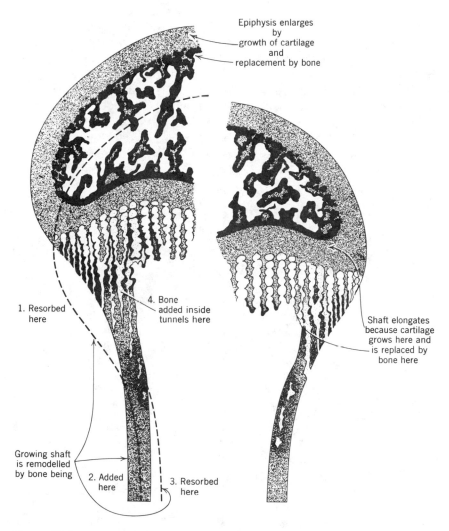

Epiphysis enlarges
by
growth of cartilage
and
replacement by bone

1. Resorbed
here

4. Bone
added inside
tunnels here

Shaft elongates
because cartilage
grows here and
is replaced by
bone here

Growing shaft
is remodelled
by bone being

2. Added
here

3. Resorbed
here

Figure 17.4
Diagram showing surfaces on which bone is deposited and resorbed to account
for the remodeling that takes place at the ends of growing long bones that have
flared extremities. (From A. W. Ham, *J. Bone Joint Surg.* 34 A:701, 1952.)

resorbed at the same time. This synchrony requires that there be a continuous
application to the inner resorbing surface of the bone of a solution that will
depolymerize proteoglycans, digest collagen, and hold calcium in solution. These
effects could be accomplished by the combined action of an enzyme such as
hyaluronidase, a protease, and a chelating agent, all of which can function at
the pH of body fluids. Such a hypothesis could be formulated which is not in
conflict with known facts but neither are there facts to support it (McLean and

Urist, 1968). It will be recalled that involvement of lysosomes has been suggested (see Chapter 14), and there is evidence that lysosomes contain a collagenase, proteases, and organic acids that could help to solubilize bone. Ham and Cormack (1979) question the possibility of osteoclasts breaking down collagen when it is encased by mineral and suggest that first osteoclasts create an acid environment beside a bone surface that favors mineral removal. The formation of an acid environment is then followed by enzymatic digestion of the collagen fibrils that remain on the surface of the resorbing bone by lysosomal enzymes liberated by osteoclasts. Mueller et al. (1973) present evidence indicating that osteoclastic bone resorption in laying hens is associated with release of hydrogen ions. Carbonic anhydrase has been localized in osteoclasts in physiologically significant quantities, which suggests that it may play a major role in bone resorption (Anderson et al., 1982). A link for carbonic anhydrase into the web of agents implicated in the maintenance of calcium homeostasis has been provided by Waite (1972). He found that bone resorption in rats stimulated by parathyroid secretion is mediated through the activity of carbonic anhydrase which produces carbonic acid.

Although growth in size of bone ceases in the mature individual, bone tissue formation and destruction continue within the framework of the skeleton. The unit of structure of bone is the Haversian system or *osteon*. When fully formed, this is a thick-walled cylindrical branching structure with a narrow lumen carrying one or several capillaries or venules. The osteons are usually oriented along the long axis of a bone and the walls consist of concentric layers of *lamellae* containing large numbers of lacunae in which are found the osteocytes. The interconnections among the osteocytes, the canaliculi, and lumen of the osteon canal provide the circulatory system of the hard tissue and the means by which nutrients in the blood are transported to the bone cells (Fig. 17.5). For a more detailed discussion of bone structure, formation, and growth, see McLean and Urist (1968); Ham and Cormack (1979); Urist et al. (1983).

When skeletal mass is increasing, bone formation predominates over resorption, whereas in old age, resorption may predominate. In the normal adult, formation and resorption tend to balance each other. The overall balance between the formation of bone and its resorption is reflected in the difference between calcium intake and calcium excretion, provided the extraskeletal calcium content of the body does not change. Since the body does not normally tolerate large changes in the extraskeletal calcium, which accounts for approximately 1 percent of total body calcium, the calcium balance is usually positive when bone formation dominates, negative when resorption dominates, and equilibrium exists when formation and resorption balance. Calcium balance, then, is an indication *solely* of the relationship between the rates of formation and resorption of bone and in no way indicates the level of metabolic activity. The simple illustration from Bauer et al. (1961) in Fig. 17.6 clearly shows that bone formation and resorption may proceed at equal rates under conditions of widely different metabolic activity. In each instance calcium equilibrium is attained, but calcium balance, as nitrogen balance, can be attained at many different levels of intake. (See Chapter 23.)

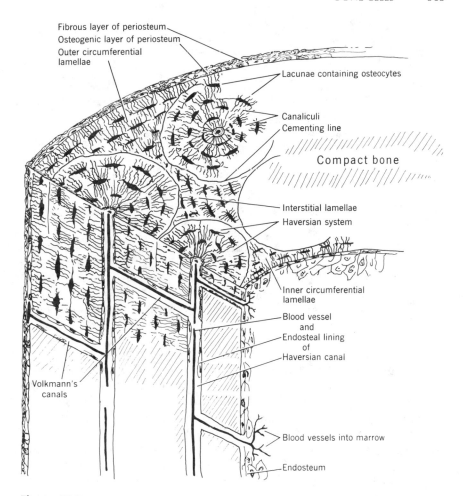

Fibrous layer of periosteum
Osteogenic layer of periosteum
Outer circumferential lamellae
Lacunae containing osteocytes
Canaliculi
Cementing line
Compact bone
Interstitial lamellae
Haversian system
Inner circumferential lamellae
Blood vessel and
Endosteal lining of
Haversian canal
Volkmann's canals
Blood vessels into marrow
Endosteum

Figure 17.5
A three-dimensional diagram showing the appearance of both a cross and a longitudinal section of the various components that enter into the structure of the cortex of the shaft of a long bone. (From A. W. Ham and D. H. Cormack, *Histology*, 8th ed., J. B. Lippincott Company, Philadelphia, 1979, p. 440.)

Bone Loss

Adult bone loss is a general phenomonon beginning at the fifth decade and progressing twice as fast in the female as in the male (Garn, 1967). Certain factors, such as small stature, hasten bone loss whereas less bone loss occurs in taller individuals. A larger skeletal mass attained by the fourth decade has been associated with slower evidence of bone loss in later life. At present, there is no satisfactory evidence to show that bone loss is due to low calcium intakes or that protection is afforded by high intakes. It is estimated that adult women lose

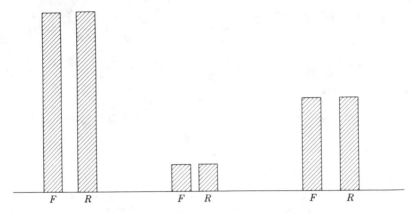

Figure 17.6
A simple illustration of three levels of calcium balance. In each case bone formation (F) and resorption (R) proceed at equal rates and the calcium balance is zero; metabolic activity, however, is vastly different. (From G. C. H. Bauer et al., *Mineral Metabolism*, Vol. I, Part B, C. F. Comar and F. Bronner, eds., 1961, p. 617).

approximately 30 mg of calcium per day or 900 mg per month, and intakes of even 1,000 to 1,500 mg/day do not prevent the loss (Garn, 1967; Heaney,1978). The meaning of calcium balance as usually measured is, therefore, questioned. Hegsted (1967) also suggests that concern with calcium balance in attempts to control bone loss may be misdirected and that attention should be centered on relationships between calcium and other nutrients.

A soluble factor was found in supernatant fluid from cultures of blood lymphocytes which stimulates osteoclast formation and activity (Horton et al., 1972). This factor has tentatively been named the osteoclast-activating factor, and its activity is comparable to maximally effective doses of parathyroid hormone (PTH) in culture. The authors suggest that the ability of lymphocytes to secrete a factor that promotes bone resorption may play a role in the pathogenesis of bone loss near areas of chronic inflammation such as might occur in rheumatoid arthritis or periodontal disease.

The one most significant relationship discovered to date in preventing bone loss is fluoride consumption. Relatively high levels of fluoride intake have been associated with substantial reductions in osteoporosis in women (Bernstein et al., 1966). Schraer et al. (1962) showed that fluoride increases bone crystallinity and decreases metabolic exchange of calcium. The mechanism of fluoride action postulated by Rich and Feist (1970), is that the absorbed fluoride is concentrated into bone crystals of newly formed bone at bone surfaces and along borders of osteocyte lacunae and canaliculi. The concentration of fluoride in extracellular fluid surrounding the osteocytes is low when bone is not being resorbed and high during bone resorption. High fluoride inhibits bone resorption because of its toxicity to the cells, and this inhibition leads to a compensatory increase in PTH just sufficient to maintain plasma calcium within normal range. There is evidence that fluoride stimulates osteoblastic differentiation within a few weeks of its administration (Reutter et al., 1970). Osteoblasts engaged in matrix production are less affected by fluoride in crystals at the surfaces of bone. Only when concentration of fluoride in extracellular fluid rises to a toxic level would osteoblastic function be altered. Therefore, bone formation proceeds and bone resorption is inhibited. For reviews of the role of fluoride in bone structure, see Gedalia and Zipkin (1973) and Eanes and Reddi (1979).

Calcium Homeostasis

Calcium in the blood and extracellular fluid is probably the best regulated ion in the body (Copp, 1960). About 65 percent of the calcium in normal plasma is present in the ionized form (Neuman and Neuman, 1958) and most of the remainder is protein bound. A third form—diffusable, nonionized calcium—is present only to the extent of 0.5–1 mg/dl. It is the ionized calcium concentration that controls and is controlled by the parathyroid secretion. This is the fraction involved in all aspects of calcium metabolism including muscle contraction (Imai and Takeda, 1967), nerve excitation (Koketsu and Miyamoto, 1961), and maintenance of the integrity of cell membranes (Streffer and Williamson, 1965). The constancy of blood calcium is maintained by absorption of calcium from the intestinal tract or that released by bone, counterbalanced by that deposited in the bone and excreted in the urine and feces. Maintenance of blood levels appears to depend on the integrated action of PTH, vitamin D, and thyrocalcitonin. The action of each of these will be discussed separately before an attempt is made to clarify their interrelationships.

PARATHYROID HORMONE

Parathyroid hormone (PTH) is a single chain polypeptide containing 84 amino acid residues and having a molecular weight of 8,500. The complete amino acid sequence of bovine (Brewer and Ronan, 1970; Niall et al., 1970), porcine (Sauer et al., 1974), and human (Brewer et al., 1972) parathyroid hormone have been determined. The structure of the bovine hormone is shown in Fig. 17.7. A synthetic peptide consisting of the first 34 amino acids from the amino terminus in the naturally occurring hormone was shown to have biologic effects identical to those of the natural hormone (Potts et al., 1971).

The primary action of PTH has been debated for many years. Collip and his coworkers suggested that the primary action of the hormone on the bone led to the release of calcium and phosphorus and this, in turn, led to the increased urinary excretion of these ions (Collip et al., 1934). Albright and Reifenstein (1948) contended that the primary action was on the kidney causing the increased excretion of phosphate which, by lowering of plasma phosphate, led to increased bone resorption. The debate has continued with MacIntyre (1970) lending support

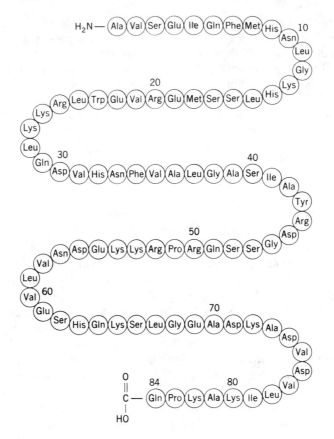

Figure 17.7
Structure of parathyroid hormone: a linear polypeptide of
84 amino acids. The physiologic activities of the peptide
on both skeletal and renal tissues are contained within the
34 amino acids counting from the amino terminal end of
the molecule. (From H. A. Harper, *Review of Physiological
Chemistry*, Lange Medical Publishers, Los Altos, California,
1971, p. 423.)

to the primacy of bone action, and suggesting that the action occurred under the
aegis of cAMP. The kidney as the principal target of PTH action received the
support of Nordin and Peacock (1970) who suggested the action led to tubular
calcium reabsorption. Fourman and Royer (1968) and McLean and Urist (1968)
diplomatically state that the bone and renal actions are independent effects of
the same hormone directed toward elevating plasma calcium concentrations without a concomitant elevation of plasma phosphate. The action of PTH on kidney
(Chase and Aurbach, 1968) and bone (Chase et al., 1969) have both been associated with the accumulation of cAMP. The investigations of this group (Aurbach
and Chase, 1970; Aurbach et al., 1971) led them to suggest that the activation

of adenyl cyclase constitutes the true primary action of PTH. In each of the target tissues the hormone binds to specific sites on the plasma membrane and then stimulates adenyl cyclase which is either an integral part of the binding site or next to it. The cAMP formed intracellularly activates specific processes within each tissue that account for the diverse physiological effects of PTH. The controversy that has existed from the early days of PTH research appears settled with cAMP as the arbiter, and both sides were right.

The activity of the parathyroid glands is directly related to the calcium ion concentration in the plasma to which it responds. The level of PTH secretion plays a decisive role in the homeostatic regulation of plasma calcium. By means of a system of negative feedback, the plasma calcium activates the regulatory mechanism: a shift toward hypocalcemia stimulates PTH secretion, which mobilizes calcium ions and elevates the plasma level; this, in turn, cuts off the stimulating effect. Such control regularly maintains the plasma level at approximately 10 mg/dl by stimulating osteoclastic activity and releasing calcium from stable bone mineral. This relatively slow action is responsible for the hour-to-hour and day-to-day adjustments, but the constancy of the plasma calcium level is maintained despite extremely rapid movement of calcium ions in and out of the blood. It has been estimated that one out of every four ions leaves the blood of the human adult every minute, and in a young animal there may be a 100 percent exchange every minute (McLean and Budy, 1961). Rasmussen et al. (1970) suggest that the minute-to-minute plasma calcium regulation depends on the osteocytes that form functional units of bone and that are vitally concerned with calcium homeostasis. The osteocytes, according to these investigators, form a functional syncytium of membranes covering the bone surface and separate the general extracellular fluid and bone extracellular fluid. This concept is elaborated further by the presentation of a model (Fig. 17.8) that indicates regulation of calcium exchange through a membrane between a specialized compartment of the extracellular fluids (gastrointestinal fluids, bone extracellular fluid, and glomerular filtrate) and general extracellular fluids. In this view the osteoclasts are conceived as being primarily involved in skeletal homeostasis or bone remodeling, and only secondarily involved in mineral homeostasis. They become important in mineral homeostasis only in abnormal situations such as hyperparathyroidism.

McLean and Urist (1968) introduced the concept of a dual mechanism of control to account for the rapid calcium turnover in both directions between plasma and bone (Fig. 17.9). The slow acting part of the mechanism is mediated by the parathyroid glands and depends on their control of osteoclastic activity. When plasma calcium falls below 10 mg/dl, the parathyroids are stimulated and calcium is released from the stable hydroxyapatite crystals of bone. This is a feedback mechanism and, therefore, self-regulatory. If the parathyroid glands are removed, plasma calcium concentration falls to approximately 7 mg/dl but is then maintained at that level by the other part of the dual mechanism which is independent of the parathyroids. This part of the action is rapid and maintains an equilibrium between the labile or reactive bone mineral and the ions in the surrounding bone fluid. If calcium is removed from the blood, calcium ions are transferred from

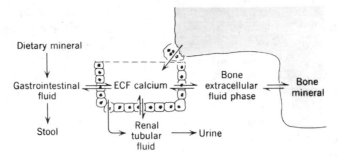

Figure 17.8

Schematic representation of the regulation of blood and extracellular fluid calcium. Calcium homeostasis is achieved
by regulating calcium exchange between the bulk extracellular fluids, and three specialized extracellular fluids (ECF):
(1) gastrointestinal fluids, (2) renal tubular fluid, and (3) bone
extracellular fluids. In addition, osteoclastic reabsorption
contributes directly to the bulk extracellular fluids. In the case
of both intestine and kidney, an epithelial membrane separates the special compartment from the bulk ECF, but in the
case of bone the membrane is a syncytium of mesenchymal
cells consisting primarily of resting osteoblasts and osteocytes, and so the present scheme is a highly stylized representation of the situation of bone. (From H. Rasmussen et
al., *Fed. Proc.* 29:1190, 1970.)

the surrounding bone fluid to the blood to restore the level. Calcium ions will
then move from the labile bone mineral to the surrounding bone fluid to reestablish
equilibrium. In contrast, addition of calcium to the blood leads to transfer of
calcium ions to the labile stores. The dual mechanism postulated by McLean and
Urist effects calcium transfer by ion exchange from the labile fraction of bone
and by bone resorption from the stable hydroxyapatite crystals of bone. For reviews
of PTH action, see Parsons (1976); Gudmundsson and Woodhouse (1976).

Recent evidence suggests that PTH influences all bone cells. For example, in
addition to being a stimulator of osteoclastic activity (Chambers and Magnus,
1982), PTH also was observed to bind to osteoblastlike cells and osteoprogenitor
cells but not to osteoclasts or osteocytes (Silve et al., 1982). These findings support
the hypothesis of Rodan and Martin (1981) that PTH induces osteoblasts to change
their shape, thus exposing the bone matrix to osteoclasts which then proceed
with resorption.

THYROCALCITONIN

A hypocalcemic factor released by the thyroid and parathyroid glands of dogs
perfused with blood high in calcium was demonstrated by Copp et al. (1962).

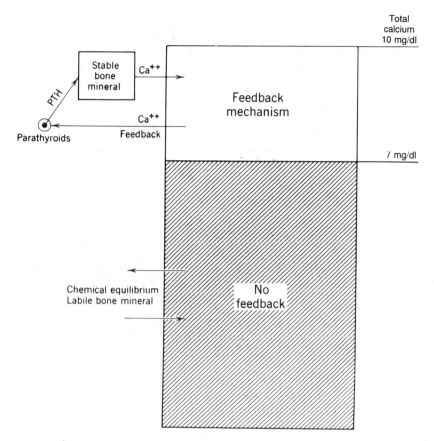

Figure 17.9
Diagram to illustrate mechanism of exchange of calcium between blood plasma and bones. Chemical equilibrium with labile fraction of bone mineral is independent of parathyroid glands and is adequate to maintain plasma calcium level at 7 mg/dl. Parathyroid activity is under control of feedback from Ca^{++} concentration in plasma and regulates release of calcium from stable hydroxyapatite crystals of bone mineral. This results in maintenance of plasma calcium at normal level of 10 mg/dl. (From F. C. McLean and M. R. Urist, *Bone: Fundamentals of the Physiology of Skeletal Tissue*, 3rd ed., University of Chicago Press, Chicago, 1968, p. 143.)

They postulated that the effect was due to a hormone released by the parathyroids that they named *calcitonin*. Others (Hirsch et al., 1963; Foster et al., 1964) attributed hypocalcemic activity to a hormone released by the thyroid gland and called it *thyrocalcitonin*. Although both names are used, the polypeptide hormone secreted by the C-cells of the mammalian thyroid is generally called thyrocalcitonin and that from the ultimobranchial glands of lower vertebrates is referred to as calcitonin.

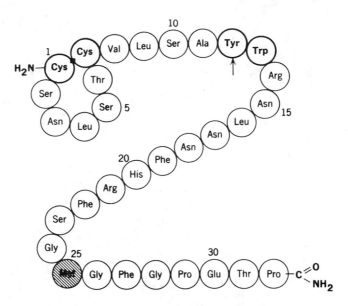

Figure 17.10
Schematic representation of the covalent structure of porcine calcitonin. Residues important for biological activity are indicated in boldface and heavy circles. Methionine (shaded), residue 25, is not essential for biological activity. (From J. T. Potts, Jr., et al., *Parathyroid Hormone and Thyrocalcitonin (Calcitonin),* R. V. Talmage and L. F. Belanger, eds., Excerpta Medica Foundation, Amsterdam, 1968, p. 65.)

The calcitonins of various species are polypeptides containing 32 amino acids. The complete amino acid sequence (Fig. 17.10) was determined independently by several groups (Potts et al., 1968; Neher et al., 1968; Bell et al., 1968). There is a homology in only a portion of the amino terminus among the calcitonins from different species (Fig. 17.11). Only 18 of the 32 amino acids in the human hormone correspond to the porcine hormone. However, in each instance the whole molecule appears to be necessary for biological activity. An unexpectedly high potency calcitonin was found in salmon (Guttmann et al., 1970). Despite having 16 of the amino acids different from the human hormone, it is particularly potent when assayed in comparison with other calcitonins. The potency of salmon calcitonin has been related to a longer half-life *in vivo* and resistance to degradation by plasma and tissue extracts (Habener et al., 1972; DeLuise et al., 1972). Marx et al. (1972), however, presented additional evidence that salmon calcitonin has high affinity for specific tissue receptors in kidney and bone and that this is important in contributing to its potency.

Thyrocalcitonin acts as a physiological antagonist to parathyroid hormone. The concentration of thyrocalcitonin is directly proportional to plasma calcium concentration whereas PTH is inversely proportional. These relationships are shown

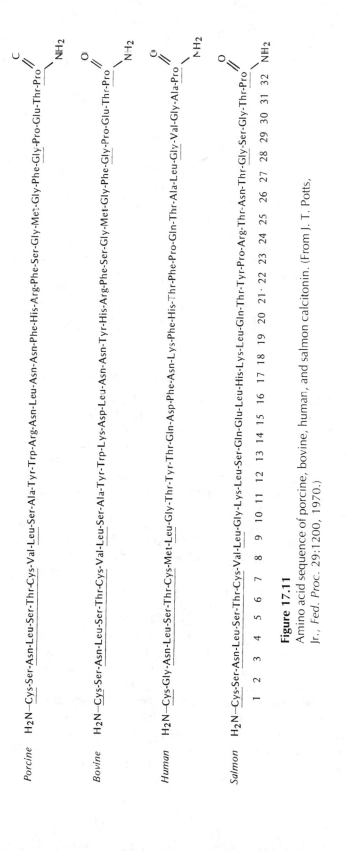

Figure 17.11
Amino acid sequence of porcine, bovine, human, and salmon calcitonin. (From J. T. Potts, Jr., *Fed. Proc.* 29:1200, 1970.)

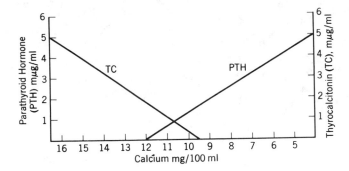

Figure 17.12
Effects of changes in serum calcium on the concentration of parathyroid hormone and thyrocalcitonin in peripheral blood. The concentration of thyrocalcitonin is directly proportional to calcium concentraion; the concentration of parathyroid hormone is inversely proportional to calcium concentration. (From J. T. Potts, Jr., *Ann. Intern. Med.* 70:1251, 1969.)

in Fig. 17.12. The rates of secretion of these two hormones are controlled by plasma calcium in a direct feedback mechanism (Potts, 1970). The response of the thyroid gland to very small increments in plasma calcium by releasing thyrocalcitonin to the circulation protects against hypercalcemia. The rise in plasma calcium due to intestinal absorption is postulated to stimulate the release of thyrocalcitonin which, by inhibiting calcium resorption from bone, reduces the plasma calcium toward normal. This response to absorption would conserve calcium by diminishing calcium loss from the plasma through the urine and preventing resorption of skeletal calcium (Gray and Munson, 1969). Munson and Gray (1970) suggest that this is the physiological mechanism protecting against hypercalcemia during calcium absorption from the intestinal tract. The presence of calcium in the gastrointestinal tract was postulated to cause the secretion of a gastrointestinal hormone which, in turn, signals the thyroid gland to secrete thyrocalcitonin (Cooper et al., 1971). Using pentagastrin, a synthetic pentapeptide containing the biologically active portion of the hormone gastrin, a marked, rapid, and transitory increase in thyrocalcitonin secretion was observed in the pig (ibid).

It was suggested that gastrin or a related gastrointestinal hormone, in concert with plasma calcium concentration, may be important in the physiological regulation of thyrocalcitonin secretion. There is circumstantial evidence that the secretion of thyrocalcitonin is increased by activation of adenyl cyclase in the C-cells (Care et al., 1971). How this activation might operate is not clear, but the suggestion is presented that cAMP can increase the permeability of cell membranes to calcium ions and thus increase the intracellular concentration of calcium. This action might then cause a release of thyrocalcitonin stored as granules within the C-cells.

The thyrocalcitonin-produced hypocalcemia results from the inhibition of bone resorption brought about by the action of the hormone on osteoclasts. This concept is strongly supported by the work of Warshawsky et al. (1980) who demonstrated specific calcitonin receptor sites on the surface membranes of osteoclasts.

For a review of thyrocalcitonin action, see Gudmundsson and Woodhouse (1976).

VITAMIN D

The effect of vitamin D on absorption of calcium from the small intestine is well established, and the postulated mechanism of action has been presented. (See Chapter 6.) Vitamin D also has a direct effect on the bone and, in the absence of vitamin D, bone resorption is impaired and plasma calcium levels fall (Rasmussen et al., 1963). It was found that vitamin D_3 did not stimulate bone resorption in culture but that $25(OH)D_3$ was effective (Blunt et al., 1969). This finding led to the work that demonstrated liver involvement in vitamin D_3 hydroxylation to $25(OH)D_3$ and the greater activity following a second hydroxylation to $1,25(OH)_2D_3$ in the kidney. A second dihydroxy derivative also produced in the kidney, $24,25(OH)_2D_3$, may be as effective in bone mineralization as $1,25(OH)_2D_3$; however, this is disputed (DeLuca, 1981).

The role of inorganic phosphorus, long implicated in the functional relationship between vitamin D and calcium, is now being elucidated. Data presented by Tanaka and DeLuca (1973) suggested that inorganic phosphorus regulates whether the second hydroxylation in the kidney is at the 1- or 24-position. They showed in work with rats that when the level of serum inorganic phosphorus is greater than 8 mg/dl the production of $24,25(OH)_2D_3$ is favored; when the level is less than 8 mg/dl, $1,25(OH)_2D_3$ is formed. Holick et al. (1972) had previously found that the 1,25-dihydroxy form predominated in hypocalcemia and the 24,25-dihydroxy form in normo- or hypercalcemia. Popovtzer et al. (1974) observed that $25(OH)D_3$ enhanced the tubular absorption of phosphorus in rats only in the presence of PTH. This PTH-dependent action, however, was unrelated to the formation of $1,25(OH)_2D_3$ since the latter failed to effect tubular reabsorption of phosphorus in parathyroidectomized rats. These reports helped to explain observations made half a century earlier, soon after the discovery of vitamin D, that both low calcium and high phosphorus diets contribute to the development of rickets in rats.

The depressing effects of certain minerals on bone mineralization, for example cadmium, appears to be due to interference with the synthesis of $1,25(OH)_2D_3$ by the kidney (Feldman and Cousins, 1973).

In addition to the physiologic effect of vitamin D_3 on bone resorption, Canas et al. (1969) observed an increased incorporation of ^3H-proline into the ^3H-hydroxyproline fraction of rachitic chicks after vitamin D_3 treatment. Since the effect on proline incorporation preceded changes in serum calcium by 12 hours, these investigators concluded that vitamin D has a direct effect on collagen synthesis and that it is not secondary to changes in plasma calcium concentration. A related observation after vitamin D treatment to osteomalacic patients was increased urinary excretion of hydroxyproline which also was interpreted as an indication of a direct effect of vitamin D on collagen metabolism (Smith and Dick, 1968). Whether these findings are directly related to the monohydroxylated form of vitamin D_3 or to one or both of the dihydroxylated forms is not known.

Additional evidence for an effect of vitamin D on bone growth is the pattern of intramitochondrial granules in chondrocytes. In normal rats, a gradient of distribution was observed along the epiphyseal plate that is the area of active bone growth, whereas in vitamin D-deficient rats, the granules were mostly in the area of provisional calcification. The normal growth pattern was assumed when vitamin D was added to the diet (Matthews et al., 1970). Evidence supporting the concept that mitochondria in mineralizing tissue accumulate Ca^{++} that is later released and then appears in the extracellular matrix vesicles has been summarized by Wuthier (1982). For a review of the involvement of vitamin D in bone metabolism, see Kodicek (1974); Hausler and McCain (1977); DeLuca (1981).

INTERRELATIONSHIPS AMONG PTH, THYROCALCITONIN, AND VITAMIN D

The tight control on the plasma calcium and phosphate levels and, therefore, on the metabolism of bone cells, depends on the interaction of PTH, thyrocalcitonin, and vitamin D. The responsiveness of parathyroids and of the C-cells of the thyroid to the level of plasma calcium brings about a precise minute-to-minute regulation of plasma calcium concentration. This control depends on the ability of PTH to mobilize calcium from bone when plasma calcium falls below 10 mg/dl and on the inhibition of bone mobilization by thyrocalcitonin when plasma calcium rises above this level. The presence of vitamin D is required for the bone mobilization effect of PTH and, conversely, the presence of PTH is required for the physiologic action of vitamin D in bone mobilization. The amount of vitamin D required for PTH action is very small, and the effect of the two together appears to be synergistic in stimulating bone resorption, that is, the response to vitamin D_3 and PTH together is effective at levels at which neither of them could be effective alone. The reason becomes clear with the knowledge that PTH stimulates the activity of the kidney enzyme responsible for the conversion of $25(OH)D_3$ to $1,25(OH)_2D_3$ (Rasmussen et al., 1972; Garabedian et al., 1972).

In contrast, the action of thyrocalcitonin does not require vitamin D_3, and thyrocalcitonin can reduce bone mobilization both in vitamin D deficiency and in PTH deficiency. Furthermore, thyrocalcitonin inhibits formation of $1,25(OH)_2D_3$ in the kidney, and its secretion is stimulated by conditions for which PTH is not required—that is, hypercalcemia and hypophosphatemia—both of which favor the synthesis of $24,25(OH)_2D_3$. Thyrocalcitonin can decrease bone mobilization induced by either vitamin D_3 or by PTH and, in addition, depress bone mobilization even when both these factors are absent.

In a vitamin D_3 deficiency, that part of the reduction in bone mobilization produced by thyrocalcitonin can be prevented by PTH (Morii and DeLuca, 1967); but when the vitamin is present, both PTH and thyrocalcitonin have their expected effects. For a review of the interrelationships among PTH, thyrocalcitonin and vitamin D, see Aurbach et al. (1981).

Vitamin D Toxicity

It has long been known that excessive vitamin D causes withdrawal of calcium from bone and a consequent hypercalcemia (Shelling, 1932). This effect appears to be an intensification of the normal physiologic action of the vitamin on bone (Lindquist, 1952) and is presumed to be responsible for the hypercalcemia and bone destruction in vitamin D intoxication (Carlsson and Lindquist, 1955). The therapeutic use of large doses of vitamin D in certain types of arthritis successfully removed calcium deposits but, unfortunately, led to deposition of calcium in soft tissues such as cardiac muscle.

Moderate overdose of vitamin D (1,800–6,300 I.U.) to infants was reported by Jeans and Stearns (1938) to have an adverse effect on linear bone growth. However, Fomon et al. (1966) report no effect on either bone growth or plasma calcium levels in infants receiving 400 or 1,600 units of vitamin D when compared with breast-fed infants who received a 200 unit supplement.

Other Factors Affecting Bone Metabolism

With all the synthetic activity accompanying growing bone, it becomes obvious that the growth pattern will be affected by any metabolic alterations that interfere with (1) cell multiplication, (2) the formation of intercellular substance, or (3) the mineralization of the organic matrix. The need for protein, calcium, and vitamin D has been emphasized repeatedly. Mineralization of bone, however, can take place only after a suitable matrix has been established.

Despite the fact that no disturbance exists in the mechanism of calcification, the abnormal matrix resulting from defective collagen in scorbutic animals is not normally calcifiable; the intercellular substance that does form, however, becomes heavily calcified. The retardation of ossification by the abnormal matrix is accompanied by the continuation of the resorptive process in bone with the result that the shaft of the growing bone becomes thin and porous, leading to spontaneous fractures. Piling up of calcified cartilage at the costochondral junctions is responsible for the so-called scorbutic rosary and pigeon breast. These lesions characteristic of ascorbic acid deficiency, but grossly similar to those of vitamin D deficiency, occur only in growing bone.

In a vitamin A deficiency the cartilage cells do not follow the normal pattern of growth, maturation, and degeneration and, as a result, bone formation ceases and abnormalities in shape appear. These effects are associated with diminished uptake of sulfur in the formation of chondroitin sulfate (Dziewiatkowski, 1954) and apparently are due to decreased activity of sulfate transferase (Carroll and Spencer, 1965) and ATP-sulfurylase (Subba Rao et al., 1963; Levi et al., 1968). Vitamin A does not appear to be an essential part of the sulfurylase enzyme but may be involved in its stabilization (Levi and Wolf, 1969). The neurological manifestations of vitamin A deficiency appear to be due to the failure of certain bony foramina to enlarge with the resultant pressure and subsequent degeneration of nerves. (See McLean and Urist, 1968.) The first evidence of the relationship between vitamin A and bone formation was reported by Mellanby, who also is known for his comprehensive description of the pathology of rickets. (See Mellanby, 1950.)

Dissolution of cartilage matrix occurs in hypervitaminosis A, and this leads to increased plasma levels of chondroitin sulfate and increased sulfur excretion (Thomas et al., 1960). The effect on bone growth due to increased osteoclastic activity, possibly mediated through the lysosomes, has been discussed. (See Chapter 14.) For a discussion of the postulated mechanism of action of excessive vitamin A on the lysosomal system of skeletal cells, see Fell (1970).

It should be evident that the effects of nutrients on bone are much more pronounced and more readily detected in the growing organism. In the adult, the amount of calcium in the skeleton is very large, and x-ray assessment of skeletal calcium content is generally insensitive to even a 30 percent loss in bone calcium (Lachmann, 1955). It is probably for this reason that adaptation can take place and that no clinical syndrome attributable solely to dietary calcium deficiency has been defined (Hegsted, 1967). With repeated stresses and drain on calcium stores coupled with consistently low dietary intakes of calcium and/or vitamin D, bone structure may be affected to the point where abnormality is clinically detectable. Such is probably the case in osteomalacia of pregnancy. A similar set of conditions has been suggested in the etiology of osteoporosis of old age, in which the stress is chronic, representing a small but steady drain on bone calcium as a result of low dietary intakes over the better part of a lifetime (Chinn, 1981). However, the data are certainly controversial.

Conclusion

The bone cells are far from inert calcified vestiges organized to give shape and rigidity, as well as flexibility, to the mass of functioning cytoplasm that comprises the total organism. In fact, they are living, metabolizing cells. They are responsible for maintaining the calcium ion concentration of the blood and other extracellular fluids so that, as a result, intracellular concentrations of calcium are suitable for function of all body cells. The extracellular bank of bone calcium becomes available if the metabolizing bone cells provide the necessary conditions for withdrawal: carbonic anhydrase synthesis, lysosomal enzyme activity, and probably cAMP formation. Through sensitivity to hormonal signals received by the bone cells, the calcium homeostasis in the total organism is maintained.

chapter 18

muscle cells

"Muscle, as a material of inquiry, offers great advantages. Its function is motion, one of the simplest and oldest signs of life which has always been looked upon by man as the criterion of life. Motion, owing to its mechanical character, can be observed with the naked eye and registered by relatively simple means. It is accompanied by very fast and intense chemical changes and changes in energy which can be measured with greater ease and accuracy than the relatively slow functions of parenchymatous organs. All this has made muscle the classical object of biological research and up to the present century the greater half of physiology was muscle physiology."

Albert Szent-Györgyi, 1948

The interaction of actin and myosin confers contractility and movement on most, perhaps all, cells. Cell contractility reaches its most complex development in the highly specialized muscle cell, or fiber. Muscle produces movement by effectively transducing into mechanical work some of the ATP it synthesizes. The transduction is efficiently carried out because the structural organization of the fibers is closely integrated with the specialized function of unidirectional shortening or contraction.

Structural Organization

The muscle is an organ composed of many long cells or fibers which are made up of many longitudinally arrayed fibrils. The fibrils are composed of the myofil-

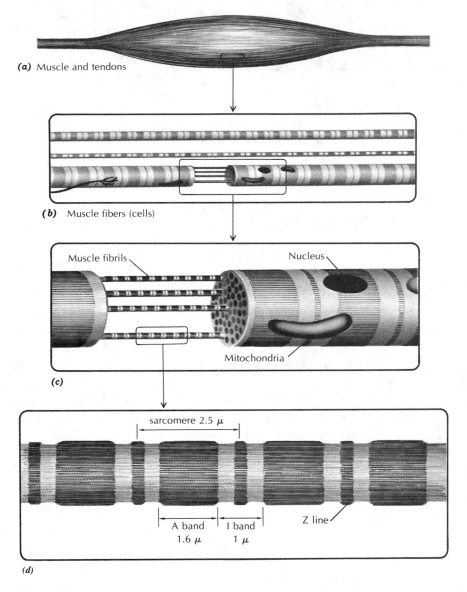

(a) Muscle and tendons

(b) Muscle fibers (cells)

Muscle fibrils

Nucleus

Mitochondria

(c)

sarcomere 2.5 μ

A band
1.6 μ

I band
1 μ

Z line

(d)

Figure 18.1
The organization of striated muscle. The muscle *(a)* is an organ composed of numerous elongated cells or fibers *(b)*. The fiber in turn is composed of numerous
contractile elements or fibrils *(c)*, which under the phase contrast microscope *(d)*
can be seen to have a striated structure of repeating units (sarcomeres) composed
of two types of bands—the A band and the I band. The latter is divided by a structure
called the Z line. In the electron microscope the band structure can be seen in far
greater detail. (From A. G. Loewy and P. Siekevitz, *Cell Structure and Function*,
2nd ed., Holt Rinehart and Winston, Inc., New York, 1969, p. 402.)

aments, myosin and actin (Fig. 18.1). Examination of the muscle fiber using a light microscope reveals its most characteristic feature, the cross striations of alternating light and dark bands. The striations are not part of the *sarcoplasm* (muscle cytoplasm) but are due to the close arrangement of myofibrils which are aligned in register with one another and give the impression that the bands cross the entire cell and are part of the fiber.

The dark bands are the *A bands* which are anisotropic under polarizing light; the lighter bands are the isotropic or *I bands*. The dark-appearing A band contains both the thicker myosin filaments and the thinner actin filaments. The lighter-appearing I band is comprised of only actin filaments. In the middle portion of the A band is a less dense portion called the *H zone,* in which there are only thick filaments. By electron microscopy, an *M band* is also seen in the center of the H band. An M-band protein links the thick myofilaments together at this central location. The myosin filament is continuous through the length of the A band. The I bands are bisected by a dark line, the *Z line.* The actin filaments begin at the Z line and are continuous through the I band, extending into the A band and terminating at the edge of the H zone. The thin filaments appear to be anchored in the Z line, a filamentous latticework consisting mainly of α-actinin.

In good preparations, projections are visible from the thick myosin filaments. The portion of the muscle fiber between the two Z lines is the *sarcomere,* a complete unit that is repeated throughout the length of the fiber and is the contractile unit or mechanism that enables the muscle to perform its specialized function of unidirectional shortening or contraction. Fig. 18.2 illustrates the detail of one sarcomere.

In addition to the precise arrangement of fibrils and myofilaments, two other characteristics of muscle structure are visible through electron microscopy: vesicles and mitochondria. There are two sets of vesicles which do not appear to

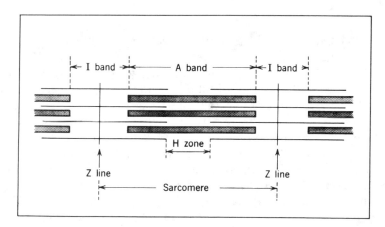

Figure 18.2
Schematic diagram of morphology of striated muscle fibers. (From L. Mandelkern, *Contractile Protiens and Muscle,* K. Laki, ed., Marcel Dekker, Inc., New York 1971, p. 499.)

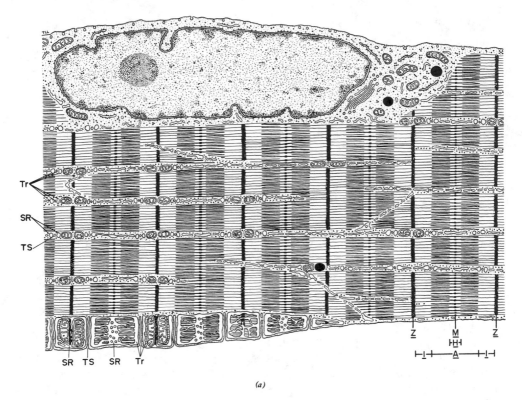

Figure 18.3a
Muscle with low metabolic activity. Tr, triad; SR, sarcoplasmic reticulum; TS, Tubular system. (From T. L. Lentz, *Cell Fine Structure*, W. B. Saunders Co., Philadelphia, 1971, p. 87.)

connect with each other and are closely associated with the myofibrils: a system of transverse tubules called the *T-system,* and the *sarcoplasmic reticulum* (Figs. 18.3 and 18.4). The T-system appears to be invaginations of the cell membrane or *sarcolemma,* and this system of tubules comes close to every sarcomere of every myofibril. The sarcoplasmic reticulum is a series of interconnected transverse and longitudinal vesicles and is the muscle version of the endoplasmic reticulum. In most mammalian muscle, three circular profiles occur near the level of the junction of the A and I bands. The two lateral and larger vesicles are the terminal dilatations of the sarcoplasmic reticulum and the central vesicle is a section through the T-system. This group is called the *triad.*

Between the myofibrils and parallel to the muscle fiber are rows of elongated mitochondria. In muscles with a low rate of activity (Fig. 18.3a), relatively few mitochondria are in the area between the myofibrils and there are also few in the area at either end of the nucleus. The mitochondria have rather sparse cristae and a matrix of low density. In muscles with a high metabolic rate (Fig. 18.3b), the mitochondria are lined up in long chains between the myofibrils, and they

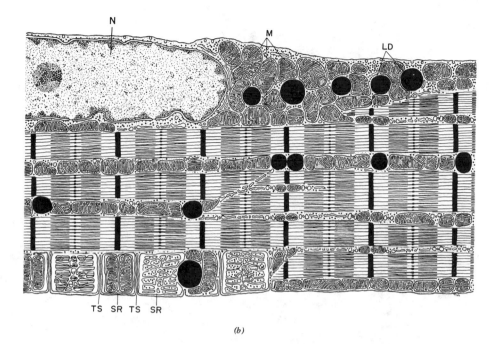

Figure 18.3*b*
Muscle with high metabolic activity. N, nucleus; M, mitochondria; LD, lipid droplets;
TS, tubular system; SR, sarcoplasmic reticulum. (From T. L. Lentz, *Cell Fine Structure,*
W. B. Saunders Co., Philadelphia, 1971, p. 89.)

are very abundant at either end of the nucleus. Each of the mitochondria has a
complex arrangement of cristae and a dense matrix. Muscle cells with a high
metabolic rate also have numerous lipid droplets close to the mitochondria and
often near the I band, whereas in muscles with a lower metabolic activity there
are few lipid droplets but abundant glycogen granules.

The nuclei in striated muscle are elongated and are located at the periphery of
the muscle fiber, just inside the sarcolemma. The fibers are multinucleate cells
and there are usually one or two nucleoli. A small Golgi complex is usually near
the end of the nucleus. There are a few ribosomes and little visible sarcoplasm
although it is present and does provide the matrix in which the myofilaments are
aligned. Its metabolic role is important to muscle function. For example, the
activity of peptidyl transferase, an integral component of ribosomes that stud the
endoplasmic reticulum, catalyzes peptide bond formation. When rats are fed low
protein diets, peptidyl transferase activity is reduced (von der Decken, 1977). In
this manner, muscle protein synthesis can be regulated within the cell.

Cardiac muscle is striated in an identical manner, but there are several specific
differences between it and skeletal muscle. The nucleus in cardiac muscle fibers
is centrally located and surrounded by an area rich in mitochondria. The mitochondria between the myofibrils are large and numerous with many cristae, and

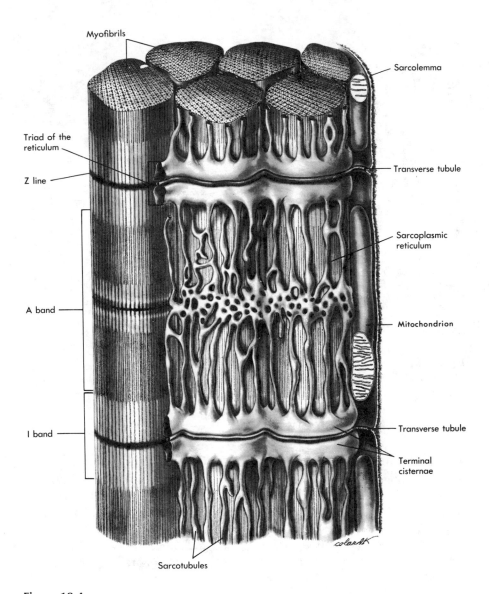

Labels on figure:
Myofibrils
Sarcolemma
Triad of the reticulum
Z line
Transverse tubule
A band
Sarcoplasmic reticulum
Mitochondrion
I band
Transverse tubule
Terminal cisternae
Sarcotubules

Figure 18.4

Schematic representation of the distribution of the sarcoplasmic reticulum around the myofibrils of skeletal muscle. The longitudinal sarcotubules are confluent with transverse elements called the terminal cisternae. A slender transverse tubule (T tubule) extending inward from the sarcolemma is flanked by two terminal cisternae to form the so-called triads of the reticulum. The location of these with respect to the cross banded pattern of the myofibrils varies from species to species. In frog muscle, depicted here, the triads are at the Z line. In mammalian muscle, there are two to each sarcomere, located at the A-I junctions. (From W. Bloom and D. W. Fawcett, *A Textbook of Histology*, 9th ed., W. B. Saunders Company, Philadelphia, 1968, p. 281.)

they are associated with lipid droplets and large numbers of glycogen granules which are also between the myofilaments. Some differences are apparent also in the tubular systems. In skeletal muscle separate cellular units are not visible, but in cardiac muscle cellular units are visibly connected with specialized arrangements of plasma membrane called *intercalated disks.* The disks do not extend across the width of the muscle fibers in a straight line but go across in a steplike manner. This arrangement is believed to provide sites of low electrical resistance to permit the spread of excitation throughout the cardiac muscle. The cardiac muscle is adapted structurally and metabolically for its sustained activity.

A three-dimensional representation of portions of several myofibrils puts into perspective all of the component structures of the muscle fiber (Fig. 18.4).

Structural Components

Skeletal muscle has been studied in greater detail than have either cardiac or smooth muscle. It is approximately 75 percent water and 20 percent protein; the remaining 5 percent includes inorganic material, the so-called organic "extractives," and glycogen and its derivatives. Of the protein, 60–70 percent of the total quantity in muscle is structural protein, the protein of the fibrils; the remaining 30–40 percent is in the sarcoplasm and various organelles. The water-soluble sarcoplasmic proteins, easily extractable with cold water, include all of the glycolytic enzymes and myoglobin. The enzyme-containing water extract is called *myogen.* The water-insoluble structural proteins are fibrous proteins and constitute almost 90 percent of the myofibril of which 54 percent is myosin, 20–25 percent actin, and 11 percent tropomyosin. The remaining 10 percent of the structural protein in the myofilaments is accounted for by troponin, α-actinin, and β-actinin.

Skeletal muscle makes up about 45 percent of the total body mass and is, by far, the largest endogenous source of amino acids. Under fasting conditions muscle can supply amino acids and fill energy requirements. Both sarcoplasmic and contractile elements contribute equally to the metabolic demands (Low and Cerauskis, 1977). Changes of lower magnitude occur in cardiac muscle.

MYOSIN

Myosin, the most abundant of muscle proteins, is the major component of the A band. It has a molecular weight of approximately 470,000 and is a long asymmetrical molecule with two identical long polypeptide chains and two short ones. The long chains each contain about 1,800 amino acids and are the longest known polypeptides. Each chain is an α-helix, and the two chains coil about each other in an α-helix. The two long chains form the tail of the molecule and part of the globular head that, in addition, contains the two small chains (Fig. 18.5). Myosin can be fragmented into two fractions: *light meromyosin,* the thin tail region, and *heavy meromyosin,* the more bulbous head region (Fig. 18.6). It is the latter region that forms the side projections on the filaments and has ATPase activity and affinity for actin. The light meromyosin has affinity for other myosin

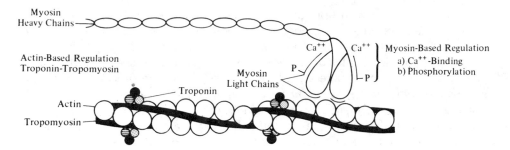

Figure 18.5
The troponin-tropomyosin-actin complex and its interaction with myosin. (From R. S. Adelstein and E. Eisenberg, *Ann. Rev. Biochem.* 49:925, 1980.)

molecules and aligns them, forming the backbone of the filaments. The structure of the myosin is closely integrated with its function.

Myosin is believed to be present as the magnesium salt, magnesium myosinate. It also binds sodium and potassium ions, and practically all of the ATP present in muscle fibers is probably bound to myosin (Szent-Györgyi, 1958). That myosin is an ATPase was first discovered by Engelhardt and Ljubimowa (1939).

ACTIN

Actin appears to be a single polypeptide chain containing about 450 amino acids. Estimates of molecular weight range from approximately 45,000 to 70,000. Actin is present in two forms. In the absence of salts, it is in the form of globular *G-actin*. Each molecule binds one calcium ion and one ATP. Binding of ATP to G-actin leads to its polymerization and the formation of *F-actin* (Fig. 18.6). F-actin is a supercoiled arrangement of two strands of G-actin (Huxley, 1963; Hanson and Lowy, 1963). For each molecule of G-actin added to the F-actin chain, one molecule of ATP is split. The ADP binds firmly to the actin and the phosphate is released. F-actin corresponds to the thin myofilaments seen in sections.

ACTOMYOSIN

When actin and myosin are mixed together *in vitro* they form actomyosin, which has high viscosity. This basic reaction was discovered by Szent-Györgyi in 1947. This interaction is the foundation of muscle contraction. It is the heavy meromyosin fragment of the myosin molecule that combines with actin. The spatial arrangement of the actin and myosin is illustrated in Figs. 18.7 and 18.8.

Actomyosin is not only a contractile protein, but it also functions as an enzyme that specifically hydrolyzes ATP and makes use of the energy of hydrolysis for muscle contraction. It is, therefore, responsible for the conversion of the chemical energy of ATP into the mechanical energy of contraction. Dissociation of actomyosin accompanies the hydrolysis and, when hydrolysis is complete, actin and myosin reaggregate.

A paradox is apparent when the dissociation of actomyosin occurs in the pres-

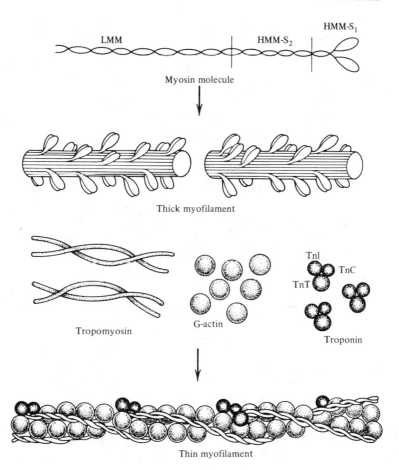

Figure 18.6
Diagram indicating the molecular structure of the thick myofilaments (top) and thin myofilaments (bottom) in the myofibril. The myosin molecule is made of two polypeptide chains 140 nm long, having at one end the S_1 head (LMM-light meromyosin; HMM-S_2, heavy meromyosin-S_2; HMM-S_1, heavy meromyosin-S_1). The thick filament results from the assembly of myosin molecules. The thin filament is the result of the association of G-actin monomers, tropomyosin, and the troponins (TnT, troponin T; TnC, troponin C; and TnI, troponin I). (From E. D. P. DeRobertis and E. M. F. DeRobertis, *Cell and Molecular Biology*, 7th ed., W. B. Saunders Co., 1980, p. 592.)

ence of ATP and Mg^{++} leading to a large and rapid decrease in viscosity *in vitro*, or a relaxed state. This reverts to rigor when there is no longer any ATP to hydrolyze, and actin and myosin reaggregate. How actomyosin requires the energy of ATP to maintain a relaxed state and also uses the energy of ATP to contract muscle is dependent on whether Ca^{++} are present. The role of Ca^{++} becomes somewhat clearer with the understanding of the roles of some of the other muscle proteins.

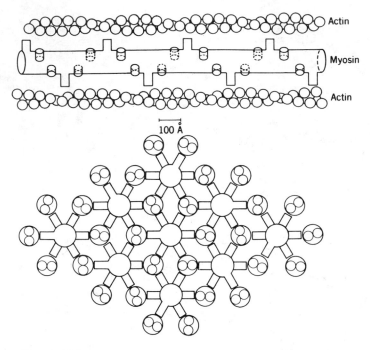

Actin

Myosin

Actin

100 Å

Figure 18.7
Spatial arrangement of myosin and actin filaments in straited muscle. (From R. E. Davies, *Nature* 199:1068, 1963.)

Actin and myosin and their interactions with ATP have been reviewed recently
(Adelstein and Eisenberg, 1980).

TROPOMYOSIN AND OTHER PROTEINS

The tropomyosin fraction of muscle protein is small. Like light meromyosin it
consists of two polypeptide chains twisted in an α-helix and coiled about each
other (Fig. 18.6). They are believed to be similar if not identical chains each
having a molecular weight of 64,000.

The tropomyosin, usually referred to as tropomyosin A, is found mostly in
invertebrate muscle such as the hinge muscle in clams (Laki, 1971c), but tropomyosin B is in the filaments of the I band (Bodwell, 1971). It is associated with
troponin, another minor protein with a major role, as part of the troponin-tropomyosin-F-actin complex (Fig. 18.6). Troponin (Tn) is a complex of three polypeptides (Fig. 18.6): TnC binds calcium, TnI binds to actin (the I-band protein),
and TnT binds to tropomyosin. The troponin complex is situated at regular intervals
along the thin filaments and regulates seven actin monomers. Ca^{++} is necessary
for the conversion of energy released by ATP into the energy of contraction. In
the absence of Ca^{++}, actomyosin requires ATP to maintain its relaxed state. Rigor
sets in if muscle can no longer generate ATP.

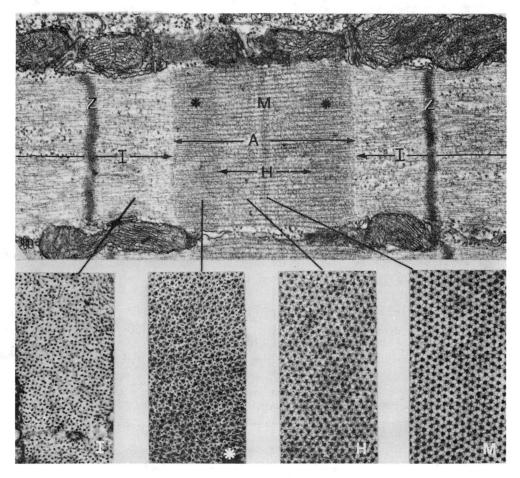

Figure 18.8

Electron micrographs illustrating the appearance of a sarcomere of striated muscle in longitudinal and transverse sections. The upper micrograph shows the Z, I, A, H, and M bands in a longitudinal section of a relaxed sarcomere.

Cross sections taken at the levels indicated are shown in the lower four micrographs (33,000×). The first of these shows thin filaments in the I bands. The second shows thin filaments interdigitating with thick filaments in the A band, forming hexagonal patterns around them; this section is cut through the region marked (*). The third shows thick filaments in the H zone. The fourth micrograph shows thick filaments at the level of the M line, where fine interconnections link them together. (From A. W. Ham and D. H. Cormack, *Histology*, 8th ed., J. B. Lippincott Co., Philadelphia, 1979, p. 545.)

Muscle Contraction

What muscles do and their characteristic appearance have been known for centuries. Within the last few years, however, ultrastructural and biochemical approaches have brought us enticingly close to understanding the exact roles of muscle proteins in the contraction process.

SLIDING FILAMENTS

The contractile material that forms the myofibrils consists of a long series of partially overlapping arrays of myosin and actin filaments which Huxley (1963) referred to as the *interdigitating filaments* (Fig. 18.8). The change in muscle length (contraction) was postulated to occur without change in filament length by the sliding of filaments over each other. The *sliding filament model* (Huxley, 1969) proposed that the change in muscle length occurs when the overlapping filaments slide past each other, with the actin (I bands) being drawn further into the myosin filaments (A bands) as the muscle shortens. The I bands move out again as the muscle relaxes or lengthens (Fig. 18.9).

The sliding of the filaments is believed to be accomplished by the alternate attachment and detachment of myosin to actin. The globular part of the myosin molecule is the part that forms the visible crossbridge. The suggestion is that flexible joints in the myosin filament permit the globular head to interact with the actin filament (Fig. 18.5). A possible mechanism for the linkage of the globular head of myosin to actin, that is, the attachment of the thick and thin filaments, is shown in Fig. 18.10. The postulated tilting of the myosin globular head group is considered to be the *power stroke of muscle contraction.*

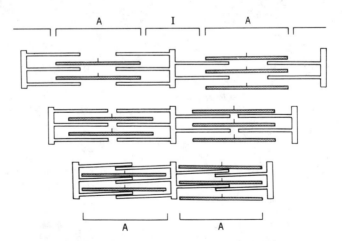

Figure 18.9
Sliding filament model of muscle contraction. (From A. L. Lehninger, *Biochemistry,* Worth Publishers Inc., New York, 1970, p. 586.)

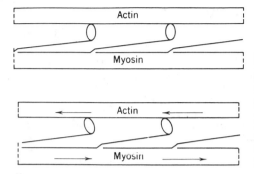

Figure 18.10
Diagram illustrating a possible mechanism for producing relative sliding movement by tilting of crossbridges. If separation of filaments is maintained by electrostatic force-balance, tilting must give rise to movement of filaments past each other. (From H. E. Huxley, *Science* 164:1356, 1969.)

The hydrolysis of ATP drives the cyclic association and dissociation of actin and myosin. ATP becomes bound to a receptor site on the myosin head which causes the myosin-ATP to be converted into a "charged" intermediate form. The charged intermediate has great affinity for the actin molecule in the thin filament, and this binding is associated with the hydrolysis of the ATP and the release of energy. The energy release causes the crossbridge to swivel to a new angle, pulling the thick filament along with respect to the thin filament thereby shortening the muscle. The detachment of the crossbridge occurs very rapidly when a new ATP binds to the actin-myosin complex causing it to revert to a low energy state. In a living cell, ATP is readily available for the recharging of the myosin head; but the absence of ATP accounts for the rigor mortis that develops in muscle after death. The low energy complexes, therefore, are called "rigor complexes"; the high energy state or the combination of actin with the charged ATP intermediates are the "active complexes." For additional discussion of the reaction cycle see Stryer (1981, pp. 821–825) and Adelstein and Eisenberg (1980).

A muscle can shorten as much as 43 percent. One ATP is required each time a myosin crossbridge interacts with actin. Each interaction results in shortening of about 10 nm.

ROLE OF CALCIUM IONS

Regulation of muscle contraction depends on the presence of Ca^{++} which is stored in sacs in the sarcoplasmic reticulum. The muscle fiber at rest is electrically polarized with the outside of the membrane positive with respect to the inside. Contraction is initiated when the nerve signal reaches the muscle cell, travels along the sarcolemma of the muscle fiber, and reaches the terminal dilatation of the triad. This induces a reversal of polarization and the release of Ca^{++} from the reticulum sacs into the fluid surrounding the filaments. The Ca^{++}, by binding to troponin, is directly responsible for activating the contractile mechanism by releasing the restraint the troponin exerted as part of the troponin-tropomyosin-F-actin complex thus permitting the crossbridges to attach and contraction to occur.

Calcium is quickly removed and returned to the storage vesicles in the membranes of the sarcoplasmic reticulum and the muscle relaxes. Calcium surrounding the filaments is lowered to 10^{-6} M or less whereas the level inside the sarcoplasmic reticulum rises to 10^{-3} M or more. This is accomplished through the action of ATP in the operation of a calcium pump (Ebashi and Lipmann, 1962). A Ca^{++}-activated ATPase localized in the outer surface of the sarcoplasmic reticulum is coupled to Ca^{++} uptake (Hasselbach and Elfvin, 1967). The protein calsequestrin, within the sarcoplasmic reticulum, can bind 40 Ca^{++} per molecule. Interference with the operation of the Ca^{++} pump interferes with muscle relaxation, and the ATP-deprived muscle will go into a state of rigor. Both the initial release of the Ca^{++} and the return to the storage sac is extremely rapid, usually requiring only a fraction of a second.

Calcium can accumulate in the transverse tubules, which is, in effect, an extracellular site. When this happens, muscle fatigue is believed to occur (Bianchi and Narayan, 1982).

Both external and membrane concentrations of magnesium are important in muscle contraction and are believed to control Ca^{++} interactions with the muscle protein (Altura, 1981; Potter et al., 1981).

Taurine is another substance that may modulate cation fluxes, particularly in the heart (Huxtable, 1980). It comprises over 60 percent of the free amino acids in many tissues. Tissue levels of this amino acid are maintained at relatively constant amounts even during prolonged starvation or when dietary taurine is varied considerably.

According to Maruyama (1971), "The most exciting prospect in the field of regulatory proteins is the elucidation of how the binding of calcium to troponin changes its conformation and how the changes are transmitted to F-actin through tropomyosin so as to permit the interaction between myosin and actin." Fortunately, we can continue to flex our muscles as we await the answer.

SOURCE OF ENERGY FOR CONTRACTION

Glycolysis can provide the energy for muscle contraction and so can respiratory activity. The muscles of all vertebrates do both. In addition, β-oxidation of free fatty acids also provides energy. The close integration of lipid utilization with the citric acid cycle has been discussed by Hochachka et al. (1977). The immediate source of energy for muscle contraction is ATP, but the amounts of ATP in muscle are extremely small compared to the chemical energy required to support muscle work. The myosin as ATPase is responsible for the hydrolysis of ATP to ADP and inorganic phosphate. However, analysis of ATP in muscle before and after single contractions shows no decrease in ATP nor any increase in ADP, indicating another source of ATP. (See Lehninger, 1970, p. 596.) The high energy compound, creatine phosphate (phosphocreatine), is that source. The prompt resynthesis of ATP from ADP is achieved through the action of creatine kinase, which transfers a high energy phosphate from creatine phosphate to the ADP. The creatine phosphate is regenerated by the transfer of high energy phosphate from ATP to creatine through aerobic metabolism using stored glucose for energy.

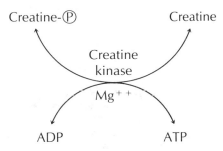

Creatine is highly mobile due to its small size. It is present in 10–1,000-fold greater amounts than ADP. The ATP and creatine phosphate are energy sources that can be used rapidly but the recharging of ATP by oxidative phosphorylation requires more time and occurs during the recovery period. At moderate rates of exercise, a sufficient amount of ATP can be synthesized from stored glycogen. However, this cannot be maintained during rapid or prolonged strenuous exercise. Under such conditions, muscle contraction is carried on anaerobically, and large amounts of lactic acid accumulate leading to "muscle fatigue." Lactic acid disappears when fatigued muscle is exposed to oxygen, and the muscle's ability to contract is regained. After muscular exercise, any lactic acid that accumulates is reconverted into glycogen. (See Chapter 11.)

There are three phases in the operation of muscle in strenuous exercise. The first phase, involving prompt resynthesis of ATP through the action of creatine phosphate, lasts only a few seconds. The second phase is the arrival of oxygen through increased respiration for resynthesis of creatine phosphate. Oxygen diffusion through the sarcoplasm is enhanced by its attachment to myoglobin. Only half the creatine phosphate is split during the peak period of activity, and all of this can be resynthesized in a brief recovery period. The third energy contribution, glycogenolysis followed by glycolysis, comes about only after oxidation can no longer keep up with the need of muscle. The quantity of available glycogen depends on the nutritional state of the muscle. Both glycogenolysis and glycogen synthesis proceed in a precisely regulated fashion. Cohen (1980) and his colleagues have provided a stimulus for a resurgence of interest in this area. Of central importance in the coordinated control mechanism is the enzyme phosphorylase kinase. This enzyme is completely dependent on Ca^{++}. Ca^{++} binds to calmodulin, a recently discovered subunit of phosphorylase kinase. This binding leads to the activation of the kinase. One action of phosphorylase kinase is to phosphorylate a single serine residue of glycogen phosphorylase, converting it to the active a form (Titani et al., 1975). Glycogen phosphorylase a then breaks down glycogen into the phosphorylated monomer, glucose-1-phosphate. Phosphorylase kinase also catalyzes phosphorylation of glycogen synthetase causing inactivation of the latter enzyme. Through the interaction of Ca^{++} with the calmodulin subunit of phosphorylase kinase on the one hand and the thin-filament subunit, troponin C, on the other, glycogen metabolism and muscle contraction are thought to be under synchronous control (Cheung, 1982b). The information flow is as follows:

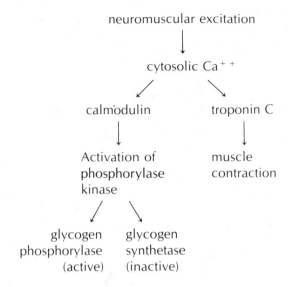

neuromuscular excitation

↓

cytosolic Ca^{++}

calmodulin   troponin C

↓   ↓

Activation of   muscle
phosphorylase   contraction
kinase

glycogen   glycogen
phosphorylase   synthetase
(active)   (inactive)

Muscle phosphorylase constitutes approximately 5 percent of the soluble protein in muscle (Fischer et al., 1971). Since phosphorylase contains stoichiometric amounts of pyridoxal phosphate, and since levels of the enzyme vary with dietary intake of vitamin B$_6$, muscle phosphorylase has been postulated to serve as a repository for vitamin B$_6$ (Black et al., 1977). The payment of the oxygen debt after strenuous exercise is a slow process and may take more than an hour after the conclusion of the exercise. In studies designed to determine how energy for the most efficient muscular work can be provided, Margaria (1972) showed that short periods of strenuous muscle work interspersed with periods of rest could permit up to 30 times more work for the energy expended.

A picture of the energy flow in muscle is shown in Fig. 18.11. The muscle fiber operates as an energy converter of the chemical energy of ATP into mechanical work. The ATP is generated in the muscle through four separate systems: the mitochondria; from creatine phosphate; from ADP and myokinase; and from the anaerobic glycolysis of glycogen to lactic acid. The energy conversion is accomplished by exploiting certain cellular capabilities and certain potentialities of molecular structure. It is a beautiful example of the integration of structure and function which, when efficiently used, can become more efficient with use.

The human skeletal muscle does not require the speed and efficiency of the hummingbird's wing, but cardiac muscle must be equipped for nonstop activity. Metabolic adaptations in heart muscle and a high content of myoglobin permit the utilization of free fatty acids, ketones, and lactate as energy sources. Under basal conditions, 35 percent of the caloric needs of the heart are provided by carbohydrate, 60 percent by fat, mostly as circulating free fatty acids, and the remainder by ketones and amino acids. As activity is increased, the nutrients used in the metabolic adaptations of heart muscle will depend, in part, on the nutritional status of the individual. As a result of exercise, marked changes have been observed in the lipid composition of the plasma membrane of myocardial cells

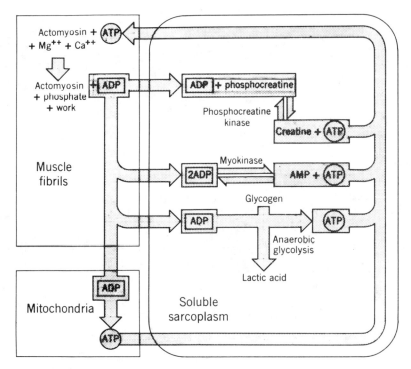

Figure 18.11
Energy flow in muscle. The muscle is seen here as a mechanochemical transducer using energy from ATP to produce work. The ATP is generated locally by four separate systems: (1) by the mitochondria, (2) from phosphocreatine, (3) from ADP and myokinase, and (4) from the anaerobic glycolysis of glycogen to lactic acid. (Redrawn from Siekevitz, 1959.) (From A. G. Loewy and P. Siekevitz, *Cell Structure and Function,* 2nd ed., Holt Rinehart and Winston, Inc., New York, 1969, p. 423.)

(Tibbits et al., 1981). The increased levels of total phospholipid and phosphatidylserine that occur are likely to influence electrical coupling in a manner that improves contractility.

Goldberg (1972) reported that skeletal muscle catabolizes certain amino acids at a rapid rate and appears to be the major site in the body for the catabolism of leucine, isoleucine, and valine. Accompanying food deprivation, catabolism of leucine, isoleucine, and valine increased the rates in normal rats three to five times. The increased ability of muscle to catabolize branched chain amino acids in food-deprived rats coincides with the increased concentrations of these amino acids in the blood. A similar situation with respect to these branched chain amino acids appears to prevail in physiological situations where muscle growth is decreased, such as in diabetes or following hypophysectomy. Goldberg's (1972) studies have also indicated that six amino acids are preferentially catabolized by muscle: leucine, isoleucine, valine, alanine, aspartic acid, and glutamic acid;

whereas other tissues catabolize the amino acids not degraded by muscle. Addition of other energy sources had little or no effect on this preferential catabolism by muscle. It is not known whether the catabolism of certain amino acids by muscle plays a role in the control of muscle protein synthesis and degradation.

During food deprivation, another metabolic adaptation occurs: the tendency to utilize glucose is reduced. It appears that glucose metabolism in muscle during starvation is inhibited at the level of pyruvate oxidation (Ruderman et al., 1977).

Conclusion

Perhaps at times the explorations through these various specialized cells have seemed to probe rather deeply into the hows and whys but, as Szent-Györgyi (1948) explained, "I cannot take the girl in my right arm and her smile in my left hand and study the two independently. Similarly, we cannot separate life from matter and what we can only study is matter and its reactions. But if we study this matter and its reactions, we study life itself." If we study nutrients and their reactions, we study living.

chapter 19

nerve cells

"The night before Easter Sunday of that year (1920) I awoke, turned on the light, and jotted down a few notes on a tiny slip of thin paper. Then I fell asleep again. It occurred to me at six o'clock in the morning that during the night I had written down something most important, but I was unable to decipher the scrawl. The next night, at three o'clock, the idea returned. It was the design of an experiment to determine whether or not the hypothesis of chemical transmission that I had uttered seventeen years ago was correct. I got up immediately, went to the laboratory, and performed a simple experiment on a frog heart according to the nocturnal design . . . its results became the foundation of the theory of chemical transmission of the nervous impulse."

Otto Loewi, 1960

The structure of the neuron creates certain logistical problems particularly in relation to nutrient supply. How does the center of synthetic activity located in the nucleus and other cell body organelles relate to the activity of the distant terminals? How do nutrients and metabolites enter and traverse the length of an axon, particularly one well insulated with a sheath of myelin? How are the nutrient needs and product requirements of the terminals monitored by the metabolic center in the cell body? These are only a few of the questions that are beginning to be asked and answered through the combined efforts of scientists from a variety of related and unrelated disciplines. In the sections to follow, certain aspects of specialized function peculiar to nerve cells, and significant to nutritionists, will be presented.

Neurons and Related Cells

The *neurons* are the cells specialized to carry on the rapid communications required for coordinated function both within the organism and between the organism and its environment. The exploitation of two characteristics of protoplasm—irritability and conductivity—permit these cells to react to various stimuli in a fraction of a second and to transmit the excitation to another location. In addition, some nerve cells possess a secretory capability that enables integration of function through localized and selective effects.

During embryological development certain cells derived from neural epithelium do not develop as neurons but as cells that occupy space between neurons. These cells have been called *neuroglia* or *glial cells* from the suggestion that they were the neural glue that held the neuron population together. The glial cells outnumber neurons by 10 to 1. They are generally divided into the macroglia and microglia. There are two types of macroglia cells: the *oligodendrocytes* and the *astrocytes*. In addition to macroglia and microglia, there are *ependymal cells* that line the cavities of the central nervous system much like an epithelial layer. These cells often have cilia and microvilli that extend into the ventricle lumens and spinal canal. Generally, the glial cells appear to act as the metabolic stabilizers of the neurons (Hyden, 1967); specifically, their functions are only beginning to be understood since early work centered on the neuron, and the glial cells were considered merely supporting connective tissue. Research should advance more rapidly since it is now possible to physically separate neurons, astrocytes, and oligodendrocytes (Farooq and Norton, 1978; Snyder et al., 1980).

The oligodendrocytes are the metabolic appendices of the neuron (Hyden, 1967) and both metabolic and functional collaboration exists between the two cell types. They may function in the provision of nutrients to the neurons they enclose. In the central nervous system these cells are thought to provide the myelin sheath much as the related Schwann cells do for the peripheral nerve fibers. (See below.) The astrocytes, interposed between capillaries and neurons, are believed to mediate ion transport and monitor the materials that pass into the neurons. In this way, they may function as part of the blood-brain barrier (ibid).

The microglia are smaller than the other glial cells. Their fine structure resembles that of macrophages, and they are believed to have a phagocytic function and to be active primarily in damaged nervous tissue.

Neuroglia that form myelin are sensitive to a variety of diseases involving the myelin sheath, the so-called demyelinating diseases, of which multiple sclerosis is one.

For detailed discussion of the fine structure of the glial cells, see Peters et al. (1970).

Each neuron and its immediate surrounding glial cells, mostly oligodendrocytes, form a biochemical and functional unit with a specificity that is the result of their relationship to other neurons in the nervous system (Peters et al., 1970). Most neurons are extremely elongated and bipolar so that one end normally receives information and the other pole transmits that information to other nerve cells or to muscle or gland cells. Information is received at points of contact on the *perikaryon* or *cell body* and on extensions from the cell body called *dendrites* (Fig. 19.1). The *axon,* or conducting portion of the nerve cell, arises from a cone-shaped region of the perikaryon called the *axon hillock.* The axon is a cylindrical structure that can vary in length from microns to meters, and it may have collateral branches along its course. It is capable of propagating an impulse at speeds up to 100 meters per second (Bodian, 1967), a rate of more than 3 miles per minute or 180 miles per hour! Axons surrounded by a single fold of a sheath cell are the unmyelinated fibers and are usually of extremely fine caliber. Axons enclosed in concentric wrappings of sheath cell membranes are myelinated axons. The *myelin sheath* is composed of layers of lipid and protein and is, in fact, a concentric lamellar specialization of the membrane of the Schwann cells (Fig 19.2).

The myelin sheath is interrupted at regular intervals designated as the *nodes of Ranvier.* The distance from one node to another is proportional to the thickness of the fiber: the thicker the fiber, the longer its internodes. Each internode is formed by and surrounded by one Schwann cell.

The functional contact between neurons is the *synapse,* the site of transmission of impulses. Contact may occur between the axon and cell body, axo-somatic; between the axon terminals of one neuron and the dendrites of another, axo-dendritic; or more rarely, between axon and axon, axo-axionic. The term synapse

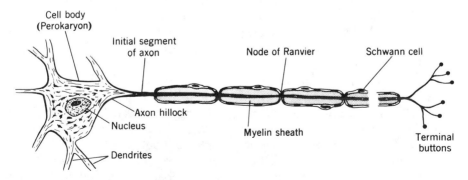

Figure 19.1
Motor neuron with myelinated axon.

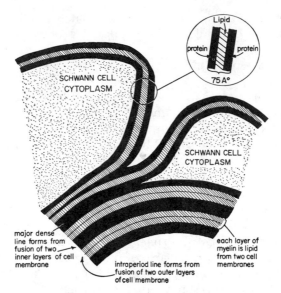

Figure 19.2
Diagram illustrating the fine structure of cell membranes and how cell membranes of Schwann cells become myelin sheaths. (From A. W. Ham and D. H. Cormack, *Histology*, 8th ed., J. B. Lippincott Company, Philadelphia, 1979, p. 526.)

includes the entire neurochemical mechanism and involves transmitter and receptor substances, synthetic and hydrolytic enzymes, and the membrane structures on each side of the contact. Details of the synapse will be presented in a later section. The cytoplasm of the two neurons is not continuous at a synapse; but the nerve impulse that has traveled down the axon of one neuron arrives at the terminals and sets off an impulse in the neuron with which it connects. This point of contact is dynamically polarized, that is, it transmits an impulse in one direction only. The number of synapses on a neuron varies from just a few to several hundred thousand.

The degree of differentiation that enables the neuron to perform its highly specialized function occurs at the expense of other cellular capabilities. After embryonic and early postnatal life, neurons are no longer capable of division and the number of neurons is not increased although changes in volume and in the complexity of the neuron processes and functional contacts can take place. The neuron is, in fact, one of the most active biosynthesizing cells in the body and such high rates of protein synthesis are often incompatible with cell division. The high rate of protein synthesis and turnover is probably related to the continuous passage of protein from the perikaryon down the axon to the nerve endings for use there or for export. For a discussion of brain cell development during pre- and postnatal life, see Chapter 21.

It is estimated that there are 14–30 billion nerve cells in man and, since no cell renewal takes place, the loss of each brain cell is a loss of capital. The contemplation of such downhill development is enough to make anyone nervous. Additional reading may be found in Kuffler and Nichols (1976) and Aidley (1978).

Neuron Structure

In common with all other cells, the surface of neurons is covered with a plasma membrane. However, there is both structural diversity and chemical heterogeneity among membranes in general and even among the membranes of nerve cells. (See Johnston and Roots, 1972.) Neuronal plasma membranes and those of glial cells and subcellular organelles differ from the myelin sheath structurally and in composition. The study of the morphology and biochemistry of all membranes, and especially nerve membranes, is a relatively new field of investigation and on its development rests our understanding of the specialized functions of the diverse membranes in the cells of the nervous system.

PERIKARYON AND AXON

The perikaryon, or cell body, is usually angular or polygonal with slight concavity of the surface between the points at which its dendrites and axon arise. Both size and shape of the cell body varies with different kinds of neurons. The cytoplasmic matrix, *neuroplasm*, is filled with organelles that appear to be in concentric formation around the nucleus. The neuroplasm that extends into the axon is called the *axoplasm*. The dendrites are extensions of the perikaryon and contain the same organelles, but these organelles are not present in the axon. The distribution of organelles within the neuron and its relationship with supporting glial cells and capillaries are shown in Fig. 19.3.

The nucleus is usually in a central position in the cell and is large and spherical. Chromatin granules are fine and dispersed evenly in the nucleoplasm and the single nucleolus is prominent. The nuclear envelope is perforated by many pores which appear to be covered with diaphragms.

The rough endoplasmic reticulum is abundant in the perikaryon, arranged as parallel aggregations of cisternae. The ribosomes stud the outer surface of the membranes and, in addition, are arranged on the membranes in loops, spirals, and rows. Free ribosomes also are abundant and appear as polysomes in rosettes or clusters in the neuroplasm and extend into the dendrites; however, they are absent where the axon originates and in the axon itself. Before examination by electron microscopy, chromophilic material in the perikaryon was designated as *Nissl bodies* which were shown to be principally ribonucleoprotein. Examination of the fine structure indicated that the Nissl bodies are, in fact, arrays of rough endoplasmic reticulum and clusters of free ribosomes. The abundance of free

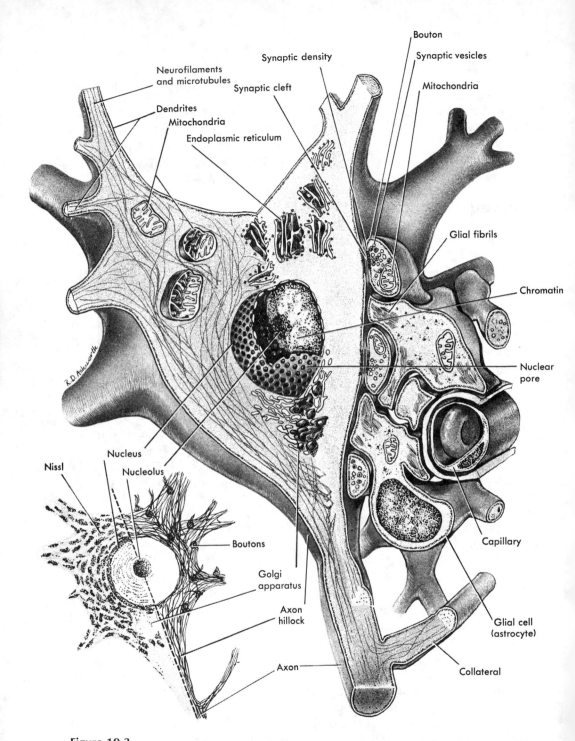

Figure 19.3

Diagram of a neuron and supporting glial cells, capillary and synaptic ending (bouton). Structures seen by low power electron microscopy are represented. The drawing at the lower left shows the perikaryon as it would appear in the light microscope stained with the Nissl stain (left of dotted line) and with metal stains (right of dotted line) which reveal neurotubules and neurofilaments. (From W. D. Willis and R. G. Grossman, *Medical Neurobiology*, 3rd ed., C. V. Mosby, St. Louis, 1981).

ribosomes in the neuron is associated with the high rate of protein synthesis required to replenish that metabolized by the cell. According to the axonal flow theory (Weiss and Hiscoe, 1948), new protein is more or less continuously synthesized in the cell body and flows from there down to the end of the axon. The rate of migration of labeled protein was shown to be approximately 1.5 mm per day (Droz and Leblond, 1963). This *slow stream* movement is thought to be necessary for axon growth and maintenance. *Fast stream* movement also occurs at a rate of 5–10 mm per hour. Both fast and intermediate stream movement are associated with movement of organelles and substances that support synaptic function, such as glycoproteins, phospholipids, neurosecretory granules, mitochondria, and the neurotransmitter synthesizing enzymes. Having arrived at the nerve endings, proteins may have half-lives of merely 12 hours or as long as 50–100 days (Cuénod and Shonbach, 1971).

The Golgi complex is well developed and often arranged as an arc halfway between the nuclear envelope and the perikaryon membrane; but sometimes the Golgi complex completely encircles the nucleus. It consists of short stacks of flat cisternae with clusters of small vesicles nearby. Areas of the Golgi are connected with smooth endoplasmic reticulum which, in turn, are connected with cisternae of rough endoplasmic reticulum, but there are no sharp divisions in the sequence.

Mitochondria are small and numerous and are scattered throughout the perikaryon and down through the axon to its endings where they appear to be particularly numerous. They have few cristae and these sometimes run parallel to the long axis of the organelle. Neuron mitochondria have been shown to contain DNA (Lehninger, 1967) and may be involved in protein synthesis.

Neurotubules (250 Å average diameter) were first observed by De Robertis and Franchi (1953) in extruded axoplasm from myelinated nerves. They course through the perikaryon, into the dendrites, and down the axon running parallel to the long axis. They are unbranched, uniform in size, and straight, running without interruption from the cell body to the terminal synapses. They appear to be formed of 13 parallel filaments arranged to form the tubes, and closely resemble the microtubules in cilia and flagella (Stephens, 1968). Neurotubules can be considered the microtubules of nerve cells. They consist of a single well-defined protein, *tubulin,* a globular protein that contains the nucleotide guanosine-5'-diphosphate and can be resolved into two slightly different subunits each with a molecular weight of about 55,000 (Bray, 1974).

Neurotubules appear to function as mechanical support and in transport down the axon to nerve endings of transmitter substances synthesized in the perikaryon (Smith et al., 1970). It has been suggested also that they function in the continual transport through the axon of protein synthesized in the cell (Droz and Leblond, 1963). Dense cores in the neurotubules observed in electron micrographs are thought to be products in transit. Methods now available for isolating and preserving neurotubules should permit both ultrastructural and biochemical analysis and further insight into function.

Neurofilaments (100 Å average diameter) and *glial filaments* (80 Å average diameter) fall into the class called intermediate filaments. Their biochemical characteristics, which have been fairly extensively studied, show them to be distinct from each other and from neurotubules. They are present in all parts of the cytoplasm of the cell body and run down the axon in remarkably straight, parallel arrays without interruption from cell body to the terminal synapses. Neurofilaments appear to be linked to each other and to neurotubules through side-arm appendages. They are believed to function as a three-dimensional lattice that provides tensile strength to the axons. The function of glial filaments remains unknown. Intermediate filaments have been reviewed recently by Lazarides (1982).

Microfilaments (70 Å average diameter) have been observed in neurons as randomly dispersed structures that occur in parallel bundles close to the membrane surface or as a loose meshwork of filaments in actively moving regions of cells in culture (Bray, 1974). Microfilaments appear to consist of actin and are associated with endocytosis. (See Chapter 9.)

The *axon terminals* at the synapse are swollen to form different shapes called end-bulbs, end-feet or boutons, cups, and so forth. Each of these swollen terminals contains many mitochondria and numerous tiny vesicles, *synaptic vesicles,* which aggregate close to the terminal membrane. The membrane itself appears to be somewhat thicker as does the opposing membrane of the postsynaptic surface. Between the two membranes is the *synaptic cleft,* a separation approximately 200 Å in width (Fig. 19.4). The manner in which these structures function in the transmission of nerve impulses will be discussed in a later section.

MYELIN SHEATH

The myelin sheath became the model for ultrastructural investigation of membranes after its layered structure was first suggested by Schmitt and his coworkers (1935) and then verified by electron microscopy (Fernández-Moran, 1950; 1952). Perhaps this was because (1) it was the only membrane that could be obtained with any degree of purity and integrity and (2) it was so accessible. The formation of this interesting structure was shown to be the result of the spiral wrapping of the Schwann cell membrane around the axon (Geren and Schmitt, 1954) which produces a concentric tightly packed membrane of uniform thickness. In the formation of the myelin sheath, the axon lies in a trough formed by the cytoplasm of the Schwann cell which surrounds the axon. The cell rotates around the axon and produces the myelin spiral. According to Robertson (1955) the Schwann cells along an axon operate individually rather than in concert since the direction of the spiral is not consistent. A diagram illustrating how the Schwann cell membranes come together and fuse to form the spiral is shown in Fig. 19.5. For detailed molecular models based on x-ray diffraction and high resolution electron microscopy, see Vandenheuvel (1963), Fernández-Moran (1967), Kirschner and Caspar (1972), and Worthington (1972). Interference with the general supply of nutrients to the cells producing the myelin sheaths during early development can result in inadequate myelinization and impaired brain formation. (See Chapter

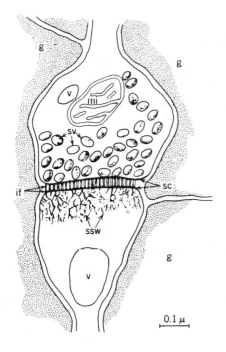

Figure 19.4

A common form of synapse in the mammalian brain. The axonal (presynaptic) side above; the dendritic (postsynaptic) side below; g, glia; if, intersynaptic filaments; mi, mitochondria; sc, synaptic cleft; ssw, subsynaptic web; sv, synaptic vesicles; v, vesiculate body. (From E. D. P. DeRobertis et al., *Cell Biology*, 5th ed., W. B. Saunders Company, Philadelphia, 1970, p. 514.)

21.) During starvation, appreciable loss of neural components is not a problem in adults. (See Morell and Norton, 1980.)

Periodic interruptions occur in the myelin sheath that are designated the nodes of Ranvier. These nodes occur where two adjacent Schwann cells meet one another. Although no myelin is present at these areas of contact, there are villi and projections of the two Schwann cells that interdigitate (Fig. 19.6). As the myelin approaches the node, the lamellae of the membrane separate from the compact myelin, and each splits into its component plasma membranes which are continuous with a membrane from the adjacent layer. The interruptions in the myelin sheath at the nodes play a role in the speed of nerve conduction and will be discussed under function.

Myelin contains lipids, proteins, polysaccharides, salts, and water. Its unusual degree of metabolic inertness was demonstrated in early studies. Brain cholesterol of adult rats given deuterium did not become labeled whereas considerable amounts of deuterium were taken up by brain cholesterol in young rats (Waelsch et al., 1940a; 1940b; 1941). This suggested that the adult brain does not synthesize cholesterol. Studies indicated that the other major lipids in myelin—cerebroside, cephalins, and sphingomyelin—also underwent little metabolic turnover (Davison et al., 1959; Davison and Dobbing, 1960). It was concluded, therefore, that myelin was one of the more permanent tissues in the body although the reasons for the inertness were not clear.

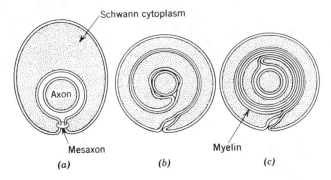

Figure 19.5
Diagram of the development of nerve myelin. (a) Axon
enveloped by a relatively large Schwann cell. (b) Intermediate stage. (c) Later stage showing formation of a few
layers of compact myelin. (Adapted from J. D. Robertson,
Prog. Biophys. 10:344, 1960.)

The lipid composition of myelin in human brains from ages 10 months to 55
years was studied by O'Brien (1965). No differences in total lipid content of
myelin were found related to age. Lipid constituted between 78 and 81 percent
of the dry weight, the highest lipid content for any tissue of the body with the
exception of adipose tissue. There was more than twice as much cholesterol as
any of the other lipids in myelin. Only 1 in 17 fatty acids was polyunsaturated,
and 1 in 5 fatty acids had a chain longer than 18 carbon atoms. The stability of
myelin is attributed to both the small proportion of lipids containing polyunsaturated fatty acids and the presence of very long chain fatty acids (O'Brien, 1965).
Data on erythrocyte membranes had provided evidence that an increase in the
proportion of lipids containing unsaturated fatty acids led to a less stable membrane (Kogl et al., 1960). Myelin has been shown to have a low proportion of
polyunsaturated fatty acids and, therefore, should be expected to have greater
stability. (For a discussion of the relation of chain saturation to lipid packing, see
Chapter 9).

Sphingolipids containing fatty acids with chain lengths of 19–26 carbon atoms
are proportionately 10 times greater in myelin than in any other membrane analyzed. In certain genetic disorders, for example, Niemann-Pick disease, there is
a seven- to tenfold deficiency of sphingolipids containing these long chain fatty
acids (O'Brien, 1964). Similar deficiencies in sphingolipids containing long chain
fatty acids have been reported for multiple sclerosis (Gerstl et al., 1963). O'Brien
(1965) concluded that deficiency of long chain sphingolipid molecules results in
either cessation of myelin formation or production of unstable myelin. Since
myelin formed in the baby is "chemically mature," O'Brien (1965) suggested that

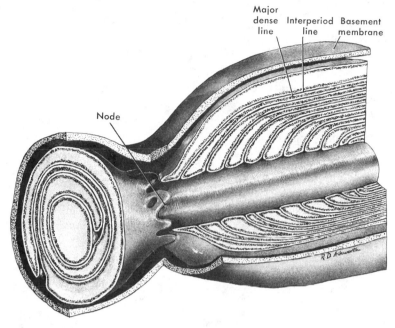

Figure 19.6
Diagram of a node of Ranvier showing myelin sheath formed by two adjacent Schwann cells with unmyelinated gap between. (From W. D. Willis and R. G. Grossman, *Medical Neurobiology*, 3rd ed., C. V. Mosby, St. Louis, 1981.)

myelination begins only when a specific chemical composition is reached; that is, when saturated glycerophosphatides and long chain sphingolipids are present in high proportions.

The proteins of the myelin sheath are distinct from those of other cells in that (1) they are present in low amount and (2) fewer types of protein are present than in most cell membranes. Among the missing proteins are those that act as ion transporters. Benjamins and Morell (1978) have discussed the proteins of myelin and their metabolism.

A detailed account of myelin has been provided by Morell and Norton (1980).

Neuron Function

The primary function of a neuron is to receive information in the form of an impulse and to carry that information along its axon to its terminals. These two facets of nerve function, *excitation* and *conduction*, depend on electrical activity.

Excitation refers to the series of events that lead to a change in membrane potential when the impulse is received, and conduction to the propagation of that change in potential away from the point of excitation. Once started, conduction is a self-propagating process and depends on expenditure of energy by the nerve cell. Neurons function in sequence and in parallel, activity from one being transmitted to another (Grundfest, 1967). Neurons also transmit information to effectors such as secretory cells and muscle fibers and the message may be excitatory or inhibitory. A diagram of a motor end plate for transmission from nerve to striated muscle is shown in Fig. 19.7.

MEMBRANE POTENTIAL

The specialized function of the neuron depends on the exploitation of a characteristic of the plasma membrane: the maintenance of a difference in composition between the intra- and extracellular fluids thereby establishing an electrical potential across the membrane; in other words, nerve cells are electrogenic. A *resting*

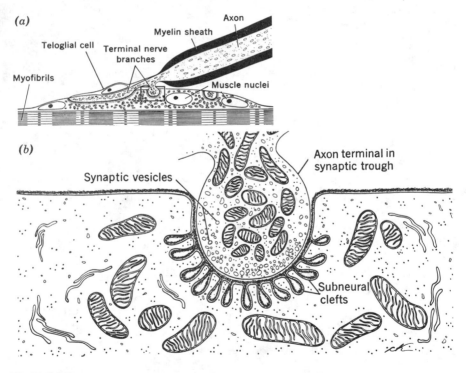

Figure 19.7
Diagram of a motor endplate for neuromuscular transmission in striated muscle. *(a)* Based on appearance under light microscope. *(b)* Based on an electron micrograph of an area comparable to rectangle on *(a)*. (From W. Bloom and D. W. Fawcett, *A Textbook of Histology*, 9th ed., W. B. Saunders Company, Philadelphia, 1968, p. 287.)

membrane potential is present in all cells, with the interior of the cell negative to the exterior; but the magnitude of the potential varies with the type of cell. In most polarized cells, the resting membrane potential is kept within narrow limits; however, in nerve (and muscle) cells a decrease in membrane potential changes the characteristics of the membrane and permits a sudden increase in permeability to Na^+. It is this unique difference that permits the generation of self-propagating impulses described below.

The neuron, like all other cells, maintains a higher concentration of K^+ in its intracellular fluid than is present in the extracellular environment. Extracellular fluid has a higher concentration of Na^+. The plasma membrane of the neuron forms the boundary between these two fluids. In the resting condition, the plasma membrane is highly permeable to K^+ but only slightly permeable to Na^+ (Fig. 19.8a). As a result of this and its gradient, K^+ tends to leak out of the axon at a fairly high rate. This results in an excess of negative charges inside the cell due to the negative charges of the macromolecular proteins. The differential concentrations of Na^+ and K^+ are maintained by the metabolic activity of the neuron involving the sodium pump and the electrical gradient across the membrane. (See Chapter 9.) Na^+ that leaks into the neuron is pumped back out, and the K^+ that

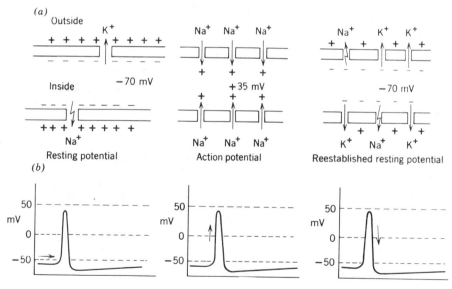

Figure 19.8
(a) Movement of sodium and potassium ions during action potential. In resting condition, membrane is highly permeable to K^+ but only slightly to Na^+. Na^+ ions are pumped out and the leaked K^+ ions pumped back in. When stimulated, membrane becomes very permeable to Na^+ ions leading to depolarization and to peak of action potential. Reversal in polarity occurs when membrane again becomes essentially impermeable to Na^+ ions and more permeable to K^+ ions. (b) Action potential spike showing rapid reversal in polarity from -70 mV to $+35$ mV and back again.

diffuses out is pumped back in. As a result, there is a concentration of K^+ within the cell at least 10 times higher than outside, and a concentration of Na^+ that is 10 times lower. The interior of the cell is about -70 mV in relation to the extracellular fluid. This is the *resting potential* of the nerve cell.

When the nerve is stimulated, an alteration of the membrane's permeability to ions occurs. The membrane becomes very permeable to Na^+ that enters at a rate faster than it can be pumped out and depolarization is initiated. The initial depolarization event is caused by the energy of the stimulus itself, for example, a touch of the skin or a sound. Immediately following the movement of Na^+ into the cell, K^+ diffuses out. After an initial decrease of 15 mV, the *firing level,* the rate of depolarization increases and the membrane potential drops to zero. This depolarization lasts for only a few milliseconds and reaches a peak at about $+35$ mV. The increased voltage difference from the resting potential to this peak is the *action potential*. A sudden reversal occurs, and the potential falls rapidly at first toward the resting level, becoming slower after repolarization is about two-thirds complete. The rapid reversal in polarity from -70 mV to $+35$ mV and back again is called the *spike* (Fig. 19.8b). This reversal is brought about when the "Na^+ gate" closes and the membrane once again becomes essentially impermeable to Na^+ and more permeable to K^+, thus permitting repolarization and reestablishment of the resting potential.

Only an extremely small fraction, on the order of one millionth, of the cell's Na^+ and K^+ cross the plasma membrane during an impulse. Thus, generation of an action potential is a highly efficient means of transmitting a signal over great distances.

The Na^+ gate or channel is a protein that has been partially purified and characterized (Barchi et al., 1980). It appears to have two important features: (1) charged groups that act as a voltage-sensing unit and cause opening or closing of the channel and (2) a highly selective pore that permits entry of ions on the basis of size and charge. Sodium and lithium are the only inorganic cations that can pass through the channel. The K^+ channel is less well understood. For further information on the ion channels of nerve cells, see Keynes (1979).

The action potential has two characteristics that are important in nerve stimulation: (1) After reaching a certain threshold of activation, regardless of the intensity of the stimulation, the height of the spike remains the same. This is referred to as an *all-or-none* response, which occurs at the point where and the moment when the impulse arises. (2) The impulse is *nondecremental,* that is, the amplitude of the spike remains the same as it is propagated along the course of the fiber. This characteristic is particularly important for conduction of impulses over long distances.

PROPAGATION OF THE NERVE IMPULSE

The architecture of the neuron is particularly well adapted to its function of transmitting information over relatively long distances. The propagation of the nerve impulse depends on the elongated conductile portion, the axon, that both separates and connects the areas of information reception and output. The characteristics of the axon enable it to generate signals that can be propagated rapidly along the cell with as little distortion as possible despite its length. This is achieved by the interaction of the intracellular fluid of the axon, the extracellular fluid surrounding the axon, and the membrane that separates these two compartments (Baker, 1966). The electrical system established is capable of generating spikes that can propagate themselves along the conductile membrane to the end of the axon. The manner in which this occurs intracellularly differs between myelinated and unmyelinated nerves. The *local circuit theory* describes conduction in unmyelinated nerves. Conduction in myelinated nerves is referred to as *saltatory conduction*. Intercellular conduction, or the transfer of information from one neuron to the others or to effector cells, is referred to as *synaptic transmission*. Each of these will be discussed separately.

Local Circuit Theory

When a receptor is stimulated, a nerve impulse, or spike, is induced. This is an all-or-none response and is propagated along the axon without decrement. Each spike is followed by a short period of complete refractoriness during which it cannot react to another stimulus. This ensures that each spike is separated from the next. This type of propagation is restricted almost exclusively to axons and operates in the following manner: the point of stimulation becomes depolarized, or positive on the inside and negative on the outside. The next adjacent region still has a normal resting potential, and this causes a current to flow from the stimulated or depolarized area to the adjacent polarized area causing it to become depolarized. The area toward which the current flows is referred to as a sink. The area from which the current flows is returned to its normal state of polarization. Repetition of this series of events causes the impulse to be propagated: each depolarized area setting up a flow of current that depolarizes the adjacent area causing the action potential to travel along the membrane as a chain reaction (Fig. 19.9). The wave of depolarization is followed by such a rapid wave of repolarization that only a very short section of the axon is depolarized at one time.

The energy required for the specialized activity of the neuron involves the operation of the sodium pump which depends on the generation of a supply of ATP. It is suggested that the active ion transport involved in impulse propagation may be the major energy-consuming process of the neuron, and it has been correlated with the presence of a Na^+- and K^+-stimulated ATPase in the membrane. There is reason to believe that an electrogenic sodium pump is present in nerve cells; that is, a pump that generates a potential because the Na^+ pumped out is not balanced by the K^+ coming in. (See Kerkut and York, 1971.) It is suggested that an electrogenic pump might provide a mechanism for metabolism to control the critical level of the membrane potential of the cell. However, both the electrogenic and the coupled Na^+-K^+ pumps have identical properties, and it is suggested that the efflux of Na^+ may occur through both mechanisms. There is still much to be learned about how important a role, if any, an electrogenic

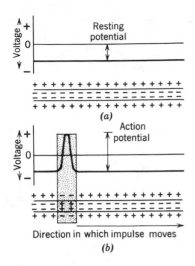
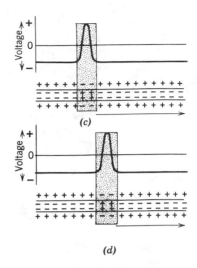

Figure 19.9
Conduction of nerve impulse in nonmyelinated nerve. The curves represent electrical changes, and the cylinders represent an axon and the electrical charges inside and outside its membrane. *(a)* In a resting nerve cell (one that is not conducting an impulse), the inside of the cell is negative to the outside. Thus a voltage difference exists which is referred to as the resting potential (electrical potential = voltage). *(b)* When the axon is stimulated, the inside becomes positive or depolarizes at the point of stimulation. This increased voltage difference is called the action potential. Although the excited region quickly recovers its original negativity or repolarizes the impulse does not disappear. *(c)* Instead, it moves forward along the axon. At the same time that the original excited region repolarizes, the region in front of it depolarizes. *(d)* These events are repeated down the length of the axon, which in this way conducts an impulse. (From J. D. Ebert et al., *Biology*, Holt, Rinehart and Winston, Inc., New York, 1973, p. 406.)

pump may have in the activity and control of the neuron. However, whether the pump is electrogenic or a coupled Na^+-K^+ pump, the energy required to drive it appears to be generated by the mitochondria present in the axoplasm and released by the ATPase in the membrane.

Saltatory Conduction

A pattern of current flow similar to that described by the Local Circuit Theory occurs in myelinated axons but, since the myelin sheath is a relatively effective insulator, little current can flow through it. Instead, the depolarization of the myelinated axon leaps from one node of Ranvier to the next. This is called saltatory conduction (after the Latin, *salta*, a leap or jump). The internodes act as passive conductors and the depolarization leaps from node to node (Fig. 19.10). At each node the action potential is boosted to the same height by the ionic mechanism.

The amount of Na+ and K+ that is exchanged is much reduced, and much less work is required for saltatory propagation. Since the myelin sheath improves the efficiency of the axon, the rate of conduction is 50 times faster in myelinated than in nonmyelinated axons. Furthermore, the thicker the myelin and the longer the internodes, the faster the conduction of the action potential. A fiber of 15 microns has an internode distance of about 2.5 mm. Fibers vary in diameter from about 1–20 microns.

Synaptic Transmission
Synaptic transmission involves the transfer of the information or impulse carried by a neuron to either another neuron or to effector sites. In most instances the transfer must be accomplished across a gap between membranes, the *synaptic cleft,* and this is accomplished through the aegis of a chemical waiting to be released for the performance of this particular mission, the *transmitter substance.*

The Synapse.   The term *synapse* was coined by Sherrington in 1897 from the Greek meaning "to fasten together," and was meant to designate a site where the axon terminal of one neuron made functional contact with another neuron. The term has been expanded to include not only the axon to dendrite contact but also functional contacts between neurons and effector cells such as muscle and gland cells. The synapse then becomes the most important structure of the nerve cell, one that enables it to perform its primary function, the transmission

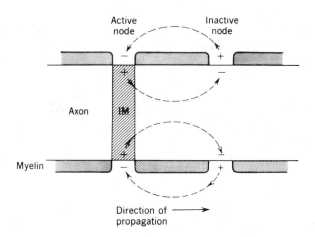

Figure 19.10
Saltatory conduction. Local current flow around an impulse in a myelinated nerve. IM = Impulse. (From W. F. Ganong, *Review of Medical Physiology,* 5th ed., Lange Medical Publications, Los Altos, California, 1971, p. 25.)

of impulses. However, the synapse is not a site of cytoplasmic contact. It is an interface at which two neurons or neurons and effector cells are functionally related. (See Fig. 19.4 and 19.7.)

The *presynaptic membrane* is the plasma membrane of the axon; the *postsynaptic membrane* is the plasma membrane of the dendrite cell body, axon, or effector site of an adjoining cell. A salient functional characteristic of the synapse is that it has directionality. An impulse is transmitted across the synaptic cleft only from the presynaptic to the postsynaptic membrane. The transmission is mediated by means of a chemical released from the presynaptic ending. Such a synapse is referred to as a chemical synapse.

Through synaptic transmission the integrative function of the nervous system operates, permitting the action potential of an axon to exert its influence across the synaptic cleft. This is effected by the release of specific neurotransmitter substances at the nerve terminal which, in turn, affect the excitability of the postsynaptic membrane.

Synaptic Vesicles.   Neurotransmitters accumulate in synaptic vesicles clustered against the presynaptic membrane (Hubbard and Kwanbunbumpen, 1968; Jones and Kwanbunbumpen, 1968). There is considerable evidence that the neurotransmitter in some vesicles is acetylcholine (Whittaker and Sheridan, 1965) and, in others, may be serotonin (5-hydroxytryptamine, 5-HT), γ-aminobutyric acid, and three catecholamines: epinephrine, norepinephrine, and dopamine (Rude et al., 1969; Tranzer et al., 1969). The vesicles containing the various transmitter substances are found within the presynaptic bouton at the axon ending along with numerous mitochondria. The mitochondria may be concerned with the need to provide energy for the energy-consuming processes involved in the synthesis of transmitter substances, the formation of the vesicles, and the storage of the neurotransmitters.

Synaptic vesicles are a constant and specific component of practically all synapses (Palay, 1967). De Robertis and Bennett (1954) showed, by use of the electron microscope, that vesicles are related to the secretion of the acetylcholine demonstrated at nerve endings by Fatt and Katz (1952). Later work has shown that the synaptic vesicles are the basic structural unit for the storage and quantal release of transmitter substance.

Receptor Sites.   The involvement and release of transmitter substance presupposes that there are receptor sites on the postsynaptic membrane. De Robertis (1971) has shown that the receptor sites undergo conformational changes when the transmitter binds to the receptor on the outer surface of the membrane. This produces the conformational change that permits translocation of ions through the membrane during synaptic transmission. There is evidence also that the isolated receptor sites show group specificity for various bivalent amines.

Postsynaptic Potentials.   When the action potential reaches the presynaptic membrane, instead of crossing the membrane, it causes the release of discrete units of constant size, or quanta, of transmitter substance from the synaptic vesicles (Fatt and Katz, 1952). The release of the soluble constituents of the granules from the vesicles appears to be by a process of reverse pinocytosis, also called exocytosis (Axelrod, 1974). The neurotransmitter crosses the gap in a few microseconds and attaches to specific receptor sites on the postsynaptic membrane. In the case of *excitatory synapses,* the attachment of the transmitter to the receptor sites causes fine channels in the membrane to open permitting Na^+ and K^+ to flow through the membrane. This produces an intense ionic flux that depolarizes the membrane. When a critical level of about -60 mV is reached the neuron discharges an impulse, the *excitatory post-synaptic potential* (EPSP). This may last for only a millisecond and by then the transmitter has either diffused out into surrounding areas or has become degraded by enzymes. For example, the enzyme acetylcholinesterase is known to destroy the neurotransmitter acetylcholine, which is released from some synaptic vesicles (De Robertis, 1967).

Structurally the *inhibitory synapse* appears very similar to the excitatory one when examined with an electron microscope, but its stimulation produces an inhibitory effect by driving the internal voltage of a nerve cell in a negative direction. If the resting potential of the cell is -70 mV, and inhibitory impulses drive it down to -75 or -80 mV, the result is an increase in membrane potential and depression of neuronal excitatory impulses. The transient increase in membrane potential is the *inhibitory postsynaptic potential* (IPSP).

The action of both inhibitory and excitatory synapses is due to changing the permeability of the synaptic membrane to the flow of ions. In the case of inhibitory synapses, Eccles (1965) has shown that it is the outward flow of K^+ through the membrane that increases the negative potential within the cell. It appears that hydrated ions, to which the membrane is permeable under the influence of inhibitory transmitter substances, are smaller than the hydrated ions to which the membrane is impermeable. The hydrated Na^+ is larger than the hydrated K^+. The difference between excitatory and inhibitory synaptic transmission is that the membrane is freely permeable to Na^+ in excitatory transmission and blocks its passage in inhibitory synaptic transmission. It appears likely that the channels through which the ions flow are selectively opened by transmitter substance; the excitatory neurotransmitter opening the larger channels to permit flow of Na^+, and the inhibitory neurotransmitter opening the smaller channels to permit flow of K^+ (Fig. 19.11).

Mechanism of Action.   It is now well established that extracellular Ca^{++} is essential for release of acetylcholine. Although some details remain to be unraveled, it appears that when the synaptic membrane becomes depolarized, Ca^{++} channels are opened. Once inside the presynaptic terminus, Ca^{++} is presumed to bind with an activator or fusion-promoting factor. Transmitter-containing synaptic vesicles can then fuse with the presynaptic membrane. At myoneural junc-

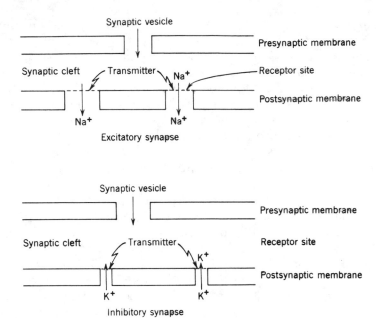

Figure 19.11
Diagram showing excitatory transmission with inward flow of Na$^+$ ions and inhibitory transmission with outward flow of K$^+$ ions.

tions the amount of transmitter released varies directly with the Ca^{++} concentration and inversely with the Mg^{++} concentration at the terminal membrane. A recent account of the roles of calcium in synaptic transmission has been provided by Llinás (1982).

An actomyosinlike protein, *neurostenin*, has been isolated from mammalian brain (Puszkin et al., 1968). It is comprised of a neurotubular protein, *neurin*, which has actinlike properties (Puszkin and Berl, 1970), and *stenin*, which has myosinlike properties. Berl et al. (1973) postulate that these proteins may be the means by which transmitter release takes place. Drawing an analogy to actomyosin, these investigators suggest that neurin may be associated with the membrane and stenin with the vesicles. Like actomyosin, neurostenin is a Mg^{++}- and Ca^{++}-activated ATPase. A model of transmitter substance release involving neurostenin at synaptic junctions is shown in Fig. 19.12. Synaptic vesicles in contact with the presynaptic membrane come under the influence of Ca^{++} either released from binding sites in the membrane or entering the synaptic ending following depolarization that follows electrical stimulation. The Ca^{++} triggers interaction between neurin and stenin, which is associated with conformational change in the membranes. Transmitter is then released into the synaptic cleft. The action is terminated by the efflux of Ca^{++}, and the vesicle then separates from the mem-

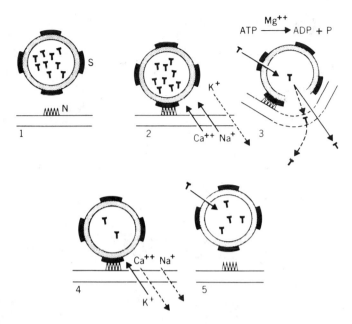

Figure 19.12
Schematic diagram to explain release of transmitter material
as a result of interaction between neurin (N) associated with
synaptic membranes and stenin (S) associated with vesicle
membranes. Stage 1, synaptic vesicle close to the presynaptic
membrane. Stage 2, synaptic vesicle in intimate contact with
the presynaptic membrane and the influx of Ca^{++} in response
to stimulation. Stage 3, the Ca^{++} triggers interaction between
neurin and stenin. Conformational changes in the membranes
result in opening of the membranes. Transmitter (T) is released
into the synaptic cleft or replaces transmitter in the membrane.
Stage 4, the action is terminated by efflux of Ca^{++}. Stage 5,
the vesicle separates from the membrane. (From S. Berl et al.,
Science 179:441, 1973.)

brane. This model suggests that transmitter release is similar to many other secretory processes in its dependence on Ca^{++}.

In summary, synaptic transmission is a process whereby a chemical substance
acts to reinitiate and modify the electrical signal. This occurs between the presynaptic and postsynaptic membranes. The chemical transmitter reacts with specific receptor sites on the postsynaptic membrane which leads to a change in
ionic permeability of the postsynaptic membrane. Whether the change in ionic
permeability leads to depolarization or hyperpolarization of the membrane determines whether the stimulus is excitatory or inhibitory. An outline summarizing

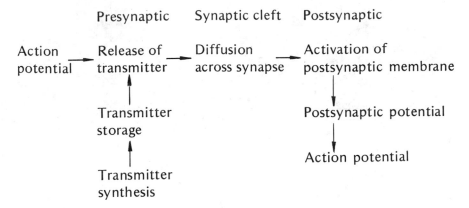

Figure 19.13
Outline of processes involved in storage and release of chemical transmitter. (From *Best and Taylor's Physiological Basis of Medical Practice,* 9th ed., J. R. Brobeck, ed., Williams and Wilkins Company, Baltimore, 1973, p. 1–58.)

the processes involved leading to synaptic transmission of an action potential is presented in Fig. 19.13. The neurotransmitter substances and their receptors are a current subject of intense investigation. Synapses and the molecular basis of synaptic transmission have been reviewed by Cottrel and Usherwood (1977) and Adams (1978).

Transmitter Substances

The transmitter substances are relatively simple compounds and, except for acetylcholine, are derived from simple amino acid precursors: the three catecholamines, norepinephrine, epinephrine, and dopamine from tyrosine; γ-aminobutyric acid from glutamic acid; and serotonin from tryptophan. The precursors of acetylcholine are equally ubiquitous, choline and acetyl CoA. It is generally accepted that these are the neurotransmitters released from nerve endings. A number of amino acids also serve as transmitters, including glycine, glutamic acid, and histamine. See Coyle (1980) for a discussion of excitatory amino acids and their receptors. It is also accepted that transmitter substance is synthesized within the neuron, packaged and stored in vesicles, and released through the presynaptic membrane into the synaptic cleft where it exercises its function as a transmitter and then is either metabolized or removed from the site. It appears quite clear that the cells from which the transmitters are released are responsible for their synthesis. Snyder et al. (1973) propose that the nerve terminals that utilize certain amino acids as transmitters have high affinity selective transport systems for the accumulation of those particular amino acids.

THE CATECHOLAMINES: NOREPINEPHRINE, EPINEPHRINE, AND DOPAMINE

The synthesis of catecholamines was assumed at first to take place in the cell body, and von Euler (1958) suggested that the storage granules were transported down the axon to the endings by axoplasmic flow. There is evidence also (Dahlström and Häggendahl, 1966) that synthesis occurs all along the axon and that storage particles are filled with transmitter both during passage and in the axon terminals. The process leading to catecholamine formation according to Axelrod (1974) starts with synthesis of the four required enzymes in the cell body and their passage down the axon to the nerve endings where the catecholamine synthesis takes place. Dopamine-β-hydroxylase is packaged in the vesicles along with norepinephrine and is released with it. This appears to be important in relation to a number of disorders which will be mentioned in a subsequent section.

The pathway for synthesis of all three catecholamines was established by Udenfriend's laboratory (Nagatsu et al., 1964). Synthesis proceeds through tyrosine to norepinephrine in three enzymatically catalyzed sequential steps (Fig. 19.14). The hydroxylation of tyrosine to dopa is the first and the rate-limiting step in norepinephrine synthesis and occurs through the action of tyrosine hydroxylase, an enzyme that is confined to neurons and to cells in the adrenal medulla where norepinephrine is synthesized (Udenfriend, 1966). Tyrosine hydroxylase can also catalyze the prior hydroxylation of phenylalanine to tyrosine (Nagatsu et al., 1964). It appears to be a soluble enzyme present in the axoplasm of the neuron (Wurzberger and Musacchio, 1971). A reduced pteridine factor and oxygen are required for its activity (Brenneman and Kaufman, 1964), and iron is an essential cofactor for the enzyme action (Petrack et al., 1968).

Decarboxylation of dopa to dopamine is catalyzed by the L-aromatic amino acid decarboxylase, dopa decarboxylase (Lovenberg et al., 1962), which is relatively nonspecific and requires pyridoxal phosphate for activity (Sourkes, 1966; 1972). This enzyme has been located in the cytosol.

The last step in synthesis requires the action of dopamine-β-hydroxylase to catalyze the formation of norepinephrine from dopamine. This is a copper-containing enzyme synthesized only in neurons and the adrenal medulla (Kaufman, 1966). The reaction requires oxygen, ascorbic acid, and fumarate. The ascorbic acid serves as a reducing agent for the Cu^{++} and acts as a cosubstrate. Fumarate apparently speeds up the reoxidation of the Cu^{++}. Catalase is also necessary to destroy peroxides formed by the auto-oxidation of ascorbate and dopamine (Axelrod, 1972). This reaction takes place in the vesicle where the product is stored (Geffen and Livett, 1971). Dopamine-β-hydroxylase has been located both in cell bodies and at the terminals (Mollinoff et al., 1970). At the terminal, it is present both in the membrane of the granule and in the soluble contents of the vesicle (Viveros et al., 1968).

Dopamine, a precursor of norepinephrine, has also been located in abundance in certain nerve terminals. In patients with Parkinson's disease there is depletion of dopamine in brain ganglia apparently due to low activity of dopamine-β-

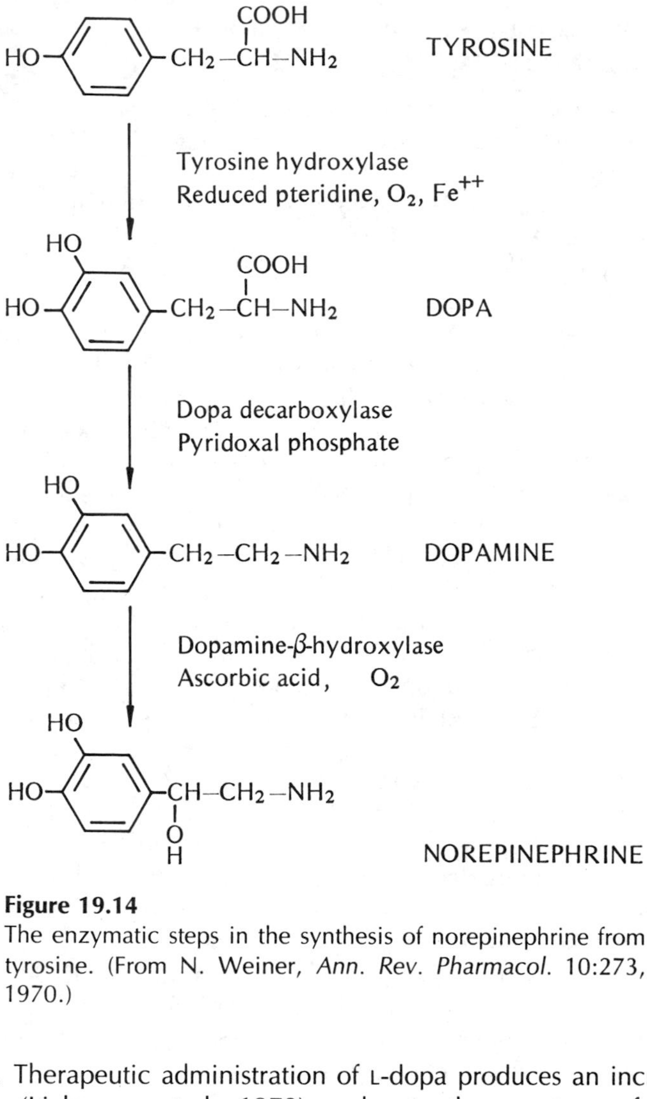

Figure 19.14
The enzymatic steps in the synthesis of norepinephrine from tyrosine. (From N. Weiner, *Ann. Rev. Pharmacol.* 10:273, 1970.)

hydroxylase. Therapeutic administration of L-dopa produces an increase in enzyme activity (Lieberman et al., 1972), and eases the symptoms of the disease. This apparent paradox is due to decreased decarboxylation of L-dopa peripherally, which apparently makes more dopa available for entry into the brain where it may be decarboxylated to dopamine (Dairman et al., 1972).

Lower than normal dopamine-β-hydroxylase activity has also been noted in the brains of schizophrenic patients and, in addition, both tryptophan and methionine administration have been found to exacerbate the symptoms of this disorder. One clue appears to be related to the relative quantities of the N-methylated and O-methylated products that are produced by the amine-methylating enzymes in the brain which use 5-methyltetrahydrofolic acid as the methyl donor (Snyder et al., 1974).

Axelrod (1974) found that the concentration of dopamine-β-hydroxylase released into the blood was low in a variety of other disease states including Down's syndrome, a neurological disease involving muscle spasticity (torsion dystonia), a cancer of nervous tissue (neuroblastoma), and in certain forms of hypertension. These findings suggested to him that functional abnormalities in the autonomic nervous system are associated with low levels of dopamine-β-hydroxylase in the blood.

The conversion of norepinephrine to epinephrine occurs almost exclusively in the adrenal medulla (Axelrod, 1972) and is catalyzed by the enzyme phenylethanolamine-N-methyl-transferase (PNMT). This enzyme is the only one unique to epinephrine production. The methyl group for the methylation was found to come from methionine. For discussion of epinephrine synthesis and secretion, see Fuller (1973).

Both norepinephrine and epinephrine are in constant flux, continuously being released, metabolized, synthesized, and reaccumulated; yet the level in the tissues is maintained remarkably constant (Axelrod, 1971). Biosynthesis is under precise control. One factor affecting rate of synthesis was shown to be its release from synaptic vesicles (Weiner and Alousi, 1967); another, the rapid feedback inhibition which appears to control tyrosine hydroxylase activity (Sedvall and Kopin, 1967). The suggestion is that concentration of free neuronal norepinephrine is reduced following transmitter release, and this cuts off the feedback inhibition thus stimulating the activity of tyrosine hydroxylase (Weiner et al., 1972). The activity and amounts of tyrosine hydroxylase, dopamine-β-hydroxylase, and PNMT transferase appear to be regulated physiologically. The activity of the enzymes may be influenced by endogenous inhibitors. The amount of the enzymes is subject to neuronal and hormonal influences such as glucocorticoids from the adrenal cortex (Fuller, 1973).

The storage of catecholamines is in the form of granules in synaptic vesicles at nerve endings and also in the adrenal medulla. The granules also contain ATP in the ratio of 1 mole of ATP to 4 moles of the catecholamine; a specific protein with a molecular weight of about 40,000; and Mg^{++} (Potter, 1966). The storage vesicles for norepinephrine have been observed by electron microscopy as dense-core vesicles at the nerve endings. Only the bound amines in the vesicles and not those in the soluble fraction are released by stimulation of the nerve (Kopin, 1967).

The release of the catecholamine from the synaptic vesicle involves the presence of Ca^{++} and takes place along with the release of adenine and AMP. The AMP is in the same ratio as in the granules. Protein is also released (Kirshner et al., 1966), and the ratio of protein to the amine is the same as in the granule. This suggested that the whole granule complex was released but there is evidence that uptake of transmitter occurs concomitantly with release and is greatly enhanced by ATP (von Euler, 1971).

After release, norepinephrine may be taken up by the blood, O-methylated by the enzyme catechol-O-methyl-transferase (COMT), or returned to the nerve terminals (Axelrod, 1971). It is generally concluded that reuptake by nerve terminals is the major mechanism for terminating neurotransmitter action (Rosell et al., 1963; Iversen, 1967; Axelrod, 1974). The uptake process requires ATP and Mg^{++} (Weiner et al., 1972). A schematic drawing of a nerve terminal that synthesizes norepinephrine, releases it, reaccumulates or inactivates it, is shown in Fig. 19.15. The pathways for norepinephrine metabolism are shown in Fig. 19.16.

Riboflavin deficiency has been associated with decreased tissue concentrations of norepinephrine and epinephrine, particularly in the liver. This has been attributed to decreased hepatic levels of monoamine oxidase (MAO) in riboflavin-deficient rats (Sourkes, 1972), and interference in catecholamine uptake from the

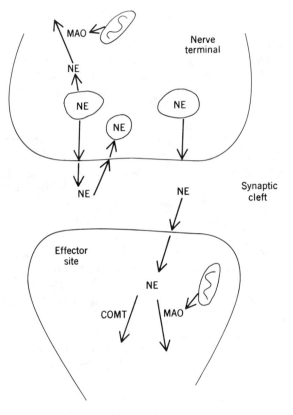

Figure 19.15
Schematic drawing of fate of norepinephrine (NE) released from nerve terminal into synaptic cleft. NE binds to effector site to elicit response. Its activity is terminated either through action of catecholamine-O-methyl-transferase (COMT) or monoamine oxidase (MAO), which is released by mitochondrion. A major mechanism for terminating activity is reuptake and storage by the nerve terminal.

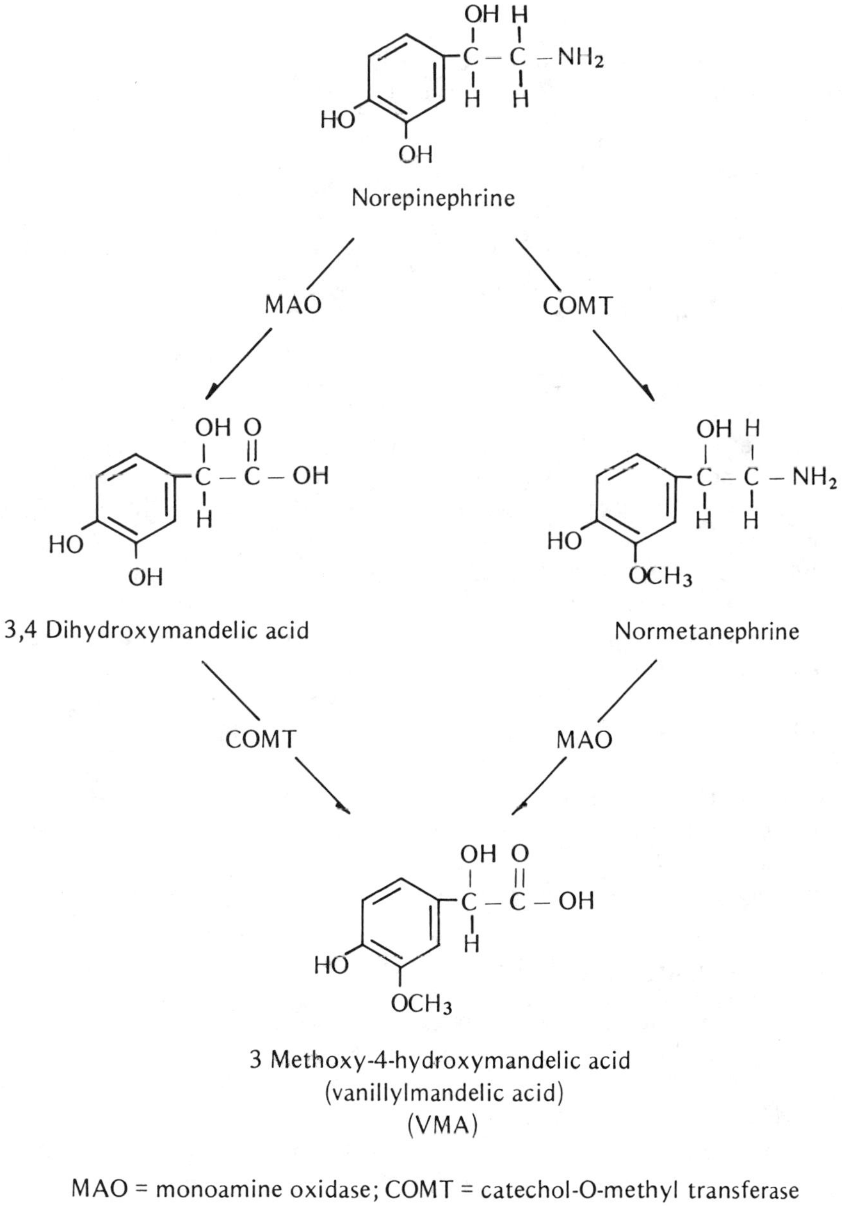
OH H
C C NH2
H H
HO
OH
Norepinephrine
MAO
COMT
OH O
C C OH
H
HO
OH
3,4 Dihydroxymandelic acid
OH H
C C NH2
H H
HO
OCH3
Normetanephrine
COMT
MAO
OH O
C C OH
H
HO
OCH3
3 Methoxy-4-hydroxymandelic acid
(vanillylmandelic acid)
(VMA)
MAO = monoamine oxidase; COMT = catechol-O-methyl transferase

Figure 19.16
Pathways of norepinephrine metabolism. (From I. J. Kopin, *The Neurosciences,* G. C. Quarton et al., eds., The Rockefeller University Press, New York, 1967, p. 431.)

blood for conversion to vanillylmandelic acid. Sourkes (ibid.) has shown that MAO contains covalently bound FAD and that activity can be restored gradually in riboflavin-deficient rats when the vitamin is added to a deficient diet.

ACETYLCHOLINE

Acetylcholine is synthesized in nerve fibers and retained in an inactive form in synaptic vesicles (Ritchie and Goldberg, 1970). These vesicles also contain the enzyme choline acetylase, which promotes the synthesis of acetylcholine from choline and acetyl CoA. For optimal activity, this enzyme requires Mg^{++}, K^+, and Ca^{++}. Ca^{++} is required for the release of acetylcholine from the vesicles into the synaptic cleft. The receptor site has been purified and some of its properties characterized (Heidmann and Changeaux, 1978).

Synthesis and release of acetylcholine appear to be closely regulated. In studies of acetylcholine release from ganglia, Birks and MacIntosh (1961) could show a total amount released that was five times the amount of acetylcholine originally present, suggesting that synthesis and release kept pace with each other.

Acetylcholine is hydrolyzed almost immediately after its release by acetylcholinesterase, which is present at the nerve terminals. The released choline is partially returned into the presynaptic neuron terminal where it can be reused for acetylcholine synthesis (MacIntosh, 1959). The uptake depends on Na^+ (Birks, 1963) and appears as though it may be part of an active transport system utilizing the Na^+ gradient to transport choline into the cell. The fate of the acetate is not clear.

A reduction in the number of functional acetylcholine receptor sites appears to be responsible for the symptoms of myasthenia gravis, a neuromuscular disorder (Fambrough et al., 1973; Fulpius et al., 1980).

A summary of the synaptic chemistry of acetylcholine is presented in Fig. 19.17.

GAMMA AMINOBUTYRIC ACID (GABA)

Gamma aminobutyric acid and the enzyme that synthesizes it (glutamate decarboxylase) are exclusively localized in the central nervous system (Wingo and Awapara, 1950). The pathway may be viewed as a shunt around the oxidative decarboxylation of α-ketoglutarate to succinate via succinyl-S-CoA (Fig. 19.18). It has been estimated that up to 40 percent of the metabolism of α-ketoglutarate is through this pathway (McKhann et al., 1960). Since transamination restores glutamate that has been decarboxylated, there is no net change in the glutamate level of the cell.

For many years GABA has been known to serve as an inhibitory substance in lobster. It has now emerged as an important inhibitory transmitter in the mammalian central nervous system, but many questions remain unanswered, particularly with regard to pathways (McGeer et al., 1982). Perhaps this sequence of events was influenced by certain gustatory advantages of selecting the lobster as a research animal.

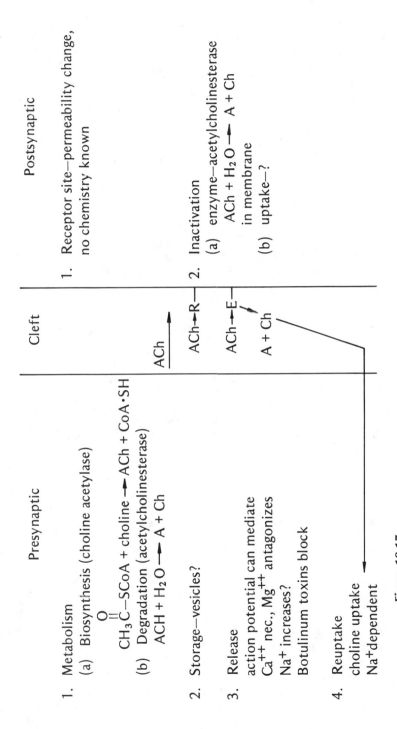

Figure 19.17
Synaptic chemistry of acetylcholine. (From E. A. Kravitz, *The Neurosciences*, G. C. Quarton et al., eds., The Rockefeller University Press, New York, 1967, p. 439.)

Presynaptic

1. Metabolism
   (a) Biosynthesis (choline acetylase)

$$CH_3\overset{\displaystyle O}{\overset{\|}{C}}-SCoA + choline \longrightarrow ACh + CoA\cdot SH$$

   (b) Degradation (acetylcholinesterase)
   $$ACH + H_2O \longrightarrow A + Ch$$

2. Storage—vesicles?

3. Release
   action potential can mediate
   Ca^{++} nec., Mg^{++} antagonizes
   Na^+ increases?
   Botulinum toxins block

4. Reuptake
   choline uptake
   Na^+ dependent

Cleft

$$ACh \longrightarrow$$

$$ACh \rightarrow R$$

$$ACh \rightarrow E$$
$$A + Ch$$

Postsynaptic

1. Receptor site—permeability change, no chemistry known

2. Inactivation
   (a) enzyme—acetylcholinesterase
   $$ACh + H_2O \longrightarrow A + Ch$$
   in membrane
   (b) uptake—?

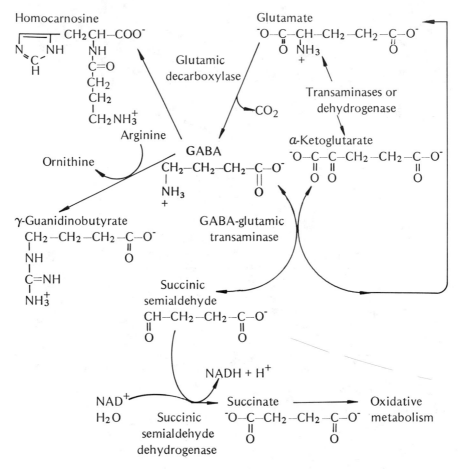

Figure 19.18
Sequence of reactions for the synthesis and destruction of GABA. (From E. A. Kravitz, *The Neurosciences*, G. C. Quarton et al., eds., The Rockefeller University Press, New York, 1967, p. 441.)

The key synthetic enzyme of GABA, glutamate decarboxylase, is distributed fairly evenly throughout the brain. Uptake studies utilizing radioactively labeled GABA indicate that 25–45 percent of nerve endings in the brain contain GABA (Iverson and Schon, 1973).

SEROTONIN

Serotonin, 5-hydroxytryptamine (5-HT), is associated with nerve terminals, especially in the brain. Its function, in a manner similar to acetylcholine in lower animals, led to the belief that 5-HT functions as a transmitter substance in mammals (Page, 1969). Subsequently, the storage of 5-HT coexisting with storage of norepinephrine was demonstrated in large granular vesicles in pineal nerve terminals through electron microscopy (Jaim-Etcheverry and Zieher, 1971). Selective depletion of the vesicles at pineal nerve endings was produced by an inhibitor of 5-HT synthesis at the hydroxylation step (Koe and Weissman, 1966). Through electron microscopic autoradiography, Bloom and Costa (1971) observed certain synapses in the brain that are specific 5-HT synapses.

The oxidation of tryptophan to the hydroxy derivative is analogous to the conversion of phenylalanine to tyrosine and can be catalyzed by the same enzyme, phenylalanine hydroxylase (Fig. 19.19). The subsequent decarboxylation of 5-

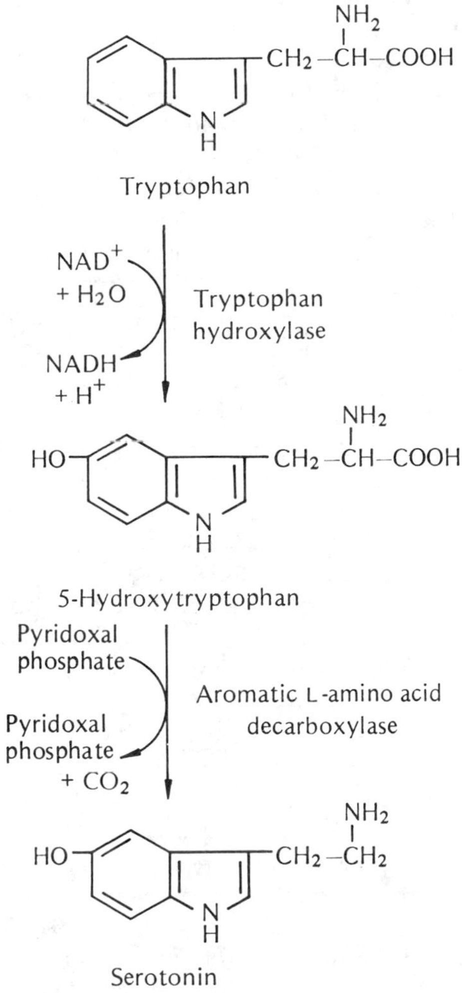

Tryptophan

NAD^+ + H_2O / Tryptophan hydroxylase

$NADH$ + H^+

5-Hydroxytryptophan

Pyridoxal phosphate / Aromatic L-amino acid decarboxylase

Pyridoxal phosphate + CO_2

Serotonin

Figure 19.19
Biosynthesis of serotonin.

hydroxytryptophan is carried out by 5-hydroxytryptophan decarboxylase (Clark et al., 1954) to yield 5-hydroxytryptamine, or serotonin. The latter reaction can also be catalyzed by aromatic L-amino acid decarboxylase that also catalyzes the decarboxylation of dopa to dopamine (Lovenberg et al., 1962). Pyridoxine depletion affects the decarboxylase enzymes more than the transaminases (Scriver and Hutchinson, 1963). The personality changes reported in subjects placed on a pyridoxine-deficient diet, as well as the abnormal electroencephalograms observed, could well be related to interference with the decarboxylation involved in production of the catecholamines, serotonin, and GABA (Sauberlich et al., 1970).

The synthesis of serotonin, like the synthesis of the catecholamines, occurs in the tissues where it is found. In the case of serotonin, the major loci are the brain and gastrointestinal tract.

Further metabolism of serotonin is by way of oxidative deamination to form 5-hydroxyindoleacetic acid (5-HIAA) and this reaction is catalyzed by MAO (Fig. 19.20). The urinary excretion of 5-HIAA amounts to 2–8 mg per day.

Several investigators have reported diurnal peaks of serotonin concentration (Dixit and Buckley, 1967; Sheving et al., 1968). There is evidence to suggest that this variation is related to diurnal fluctuations of plasma and brain tryptophan concentration. The functional meaning of the changes in concentration of serotonin are not clear (Bloom and Costa, 1971), but some findings provide for interesting speculation especially for nutritionists. Fernstrom and Wurtman (1974) found that following the ingestion of a meal high in carbohydrate there is an increase in the rate at which the brain synthesizes the neurotransmitter serotonin. This response occurs in rats within an hour after eating and is preceded by a change in the concentration of amino acids in the plasma. The concentration of most amino acids decreases, but the concentration of tryptophan increases in the plasma, and there is a proportional increase in the uptake by the brain. The rate of serotonin synthesis also increases in the serotonergic neurons. This increase in the availability of tryptophan for serotonin synthesis takes on added interest when it is realized that tryptophan is the least abundant amino acid in protein, and tryptophan hydroxylase is a low affinity enzyme. Therefore, only when the tryptophan concentration is higher than normal can the enzyme function at the maximum rate. When the available tryptophan was increased by injection, brain tryptophan and brain serotonin increased, and the diurnal variations in plasma were paralleled by changes in brain serotonin.

Since insulin lowers the amino acid concentration of plasma, plasma tryptophan levels were determined following insulin injection. Contrary to expectation, plasma tryptophan, and brain tryptophan and serotonin, were increased. Never before had there been evidence of neurotransmitter synthesis in the brain being increased by a hormone.

Further work indicated that plasma tryptophan was increased by protein intake but that neither brain tryptophan nor serotonin was elevated. It soon became apparent that brain tryptophan and serotonin were more a reflection of the ratio of tryptophan to other neutral amino acids than of the plasma level of tryptophan

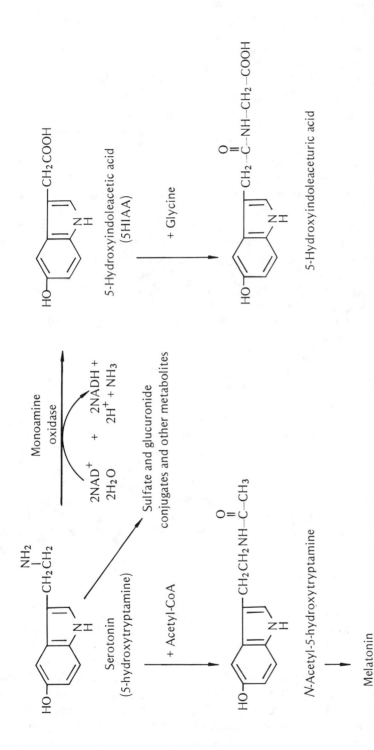

Figure 19.20

Catabolism of serotonin. In oxidative deaminations catalyzed by monoamine oxidase, an aldehyde is formed first and then oxidized to the corresponding acid. Some of the aldehyde is also reduced to the corresponding alcohol. The heavy arrow indicates the major metabolic pathway. (From W. F. Ganong, *Review of Medical Physiology*, 5th ed. Lange Medical Publications, Los Altos, California, 1971, p. 182.)

alone. A high protein diet would elevate all amino acids and thereby lower the ratio of tryptophan to other amino acids; but a high carbohydrate diet would, through stimulation of insulin secretion, increase the ratio. It then became apparent that the reason plasma tryptophan did not decrease following insulin administration was that it, like fatty acids, was carried by plasma albumin and, under usual circumstances, it competed with the other neutral amino acids for the transport system into the brain. Insulin not only released fatty acids from the albumin carrier and pulled them from the plasma, it also pulled amino acids from the plasma; that is, all the amino acids with exception of tryptophan which immediately became attached to the albumin that the fatty acids had freed. As a result, tryptophan content of the plasma remained high, and the tryptophan was protected from the action of insulin. Fernstrom and Wurtman (1974) postulate that the sensitivity of brain serotonin concentration to dietary change suggests that the serotoninergic neurons release more serotonin into synapses with a high carbohydrate diet, thereby transmitting specific signals through the neurons and conveying the message of "carbohydrate-richness" to other parts of the brain or to neuroendocrine mechanisms, to bring about some metabolic consequence. It also has been suggested that brain serotonin level in rats can influence both motor activity and food consumption.

Other nutrients that modify brain function, choline and tyrosine, have also been identified. Wurtman (1982) describes the recent progress that has been made. What other nutrient-modifiers of brain function remain to be discovered? The possibilities for speculation are enticing. Lát (1967; Lát et al., 1973) showed that associative and discriminatory types of learning are closely correlated with "nonspecific excitability level" or "tonus" of the central nervous system. He also showed that rats with an inherited high excitability level self-selected a high carbohydrate diet. If such rats were fed a high protein diet their excitability levels decreased. Similarly, rats with a low excitability level self-selected high protein diets and their excitability levels increased when fed high carbohydrate. Could it be that such dietary responses are related to plasma-borne messages to the brain which are translated into behavior by neurotransmitters? An interesting thought.

Conclusion

Understanding of the mechanisms involved in nerve cell function and the roles played by electrolytes in conduction and transmission of nerve impulses should make it apparent that any disturbance in the maintenance of electrolyte concentrations in the intra- and intercellular environment could interfere with function. Since the single neuron is ineffective unless its message can be passed along to other neurons or to effector cells, the synthesis of transmitter substances becomes a key factor in the coordination attained by the nerve cells. These simple transmitter chemicals which, except for acetylcholine, are derived from amino acids or are amino acids themselves, may be closely associated with nutrient intake or dependent on specific nutrients for their synthesis. The well-known associations of electrolytes such as Ca^{++}, Mg^{++}, K^+ and Na^+ to nerve function, and of vitamins such as thiamin, pyridoxine, nicotinic acid, ascorbic acid, and vitamin B_{12}, make abundantly clear that an intimate relationship exists between these nutrients and nerve function. The prominence of nerve function derangement in disorders of amino acid metabolism can be understood both in relationship to the high rate of protein synthesis in the neuron and the need for substrate for the synthesis of transmitter substance. This definitely becomes a case of matter over mind.

chapter 20

adipocytes

"If one attempts to summarize the results of the isotope work on fats, one is compelled to conclude that the normal animal's body fats, despite their qualitative and quantitative constancy, are in a state of rapid flux. It can readily be understood why the classical methods of metabolism, which were mainly limited to the measurement of changes in amount or relative composition, failed to detect this dynamic state."

Rudolf Schoenheimer, 1949

Adipocytes, or fat cells, are normally present in loose connective tissue either singly or in small groups. When large numbers of these cells are organized, the resulting lobules constitute adipose tissue. The specialized capability of fat cells is the storage of a fuel reserve, which may vary in extent from an approximate 40-day reserve in the average person to one sufficient for a year or more in some obese individuals. At first, fat cells were thought to be placid repositories of excess fuel which, when organized into subcutaneous layers, served as insulating material to prevent loss of body heat. Another recognized function of adipose tissue was its ability to cushion and support abdominal organs. However, the highly specialized role of fat cells in the homeostasis of the organism was established by Schoenheimer and Rittenberg (1935), who demonstrated that even when the quantity of depot fat remained constant, it was continually being degraded and synthesized.

In most mammals there are two distinct types of fat cells which differ considerably in size, number, distribuion, and metabolic activity. The bulk of the fat cells are the *white adipose cells* organized as adipose tissue in the subcutaneous layers, the mesenteries and omentum, the retroperitoneal regions, and as isolated fat cells in loose connective tissue. White adipose tissue may actually appear yellow because it contains carotene. *Brown adipose cells are much less abundant* and occur only in restricted areas. Although present in humans and other primates to a limited extent, brown adipose cells are abundant in hibernating animals and their specialized role will be discussed in a later section. Unless otherwise indicated, the material that follows refers to white or ordinary adipose cells.

White Fat Cell

STRUCTURE

The number, dimensions, and composition of fat cells varies with individuals, with subcutaneous site sampled, and with nutritional state. The fat cell number in human subjects calculated by dividing the total body fat by the average fat cell content ranges from approximately $21-43 \times 10^9$ (Salans et al., 1971). It is generally believed that the number of adipose cells reaches a maximum during adolescence or early adult life and tends to remain fixed after that (Hirsch and Knittle, 1970). However, it is granted that years of excessive calorie intake in adult humans could lead to hyperplasia as well as hypertrophy of existing cells (Salans et al., 1971). Bray and Gallagher (1970) reported a marked increase in cell number in an adult who became obese after the development of a hypothalamic tumor.

Overfeeding in infancy results in an increase in the number of fat cells. This appears to play an important role in adult obesity since there are more cells available waiting to be filled (Knittle and Hirsch, 1967). Moderate overfeeding of an adult leads only to larger cells, with no increase in number (Hirsch et al., 1966; Björstein and Sjöström, 1971). A difference in fat cell size and in the appearance of the cells in the adipose tissue in a 2-day-old and an 8-week-old rat is pictured in Fig. 20.1.

Undernutrition during gestation results in lower body weight at birth and decreased adiposity of offspring. Recent evidence indicates, however, that the body weights are not lowered permanently and that the sex of the offspring as well as the timing and duration of the maternal nutritional deprivation influence the fetal outcome. Jones and Friedman (1982) report hyperphagia and obesity in male rats born of underfed mothers; female littermates were not affected, although all pups showed an increase in fat cell size.

The prominent and distinguishing feature of the adipocyte is the large central lipid droplet that dwarfs and dislocates the other cellular contents. The lipid, surrounded by a thin rim of cytoplasm, appears homogeneously opaque in elec-

2 days

8 weeks

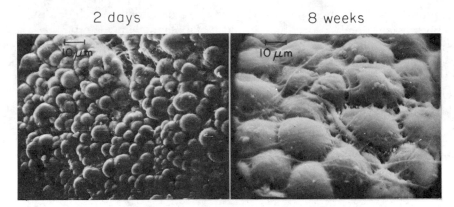

Figure 20.1
Adipose tissue taken from a 2-day-old and an 8-week-old rat showing difference
in size of fat cell. Scanning electron micrograph of epididymal adipose tissue.
Magnification 1000. (Courtesy of Dr. Jerry Regunburg.)

tron micrographs (Fig. 20.2). The nucleus, distorted to a crescent shape, lies
between the lipid and the plasma membrane. In histological preparations the lipid
is dissolved out, and the fat cell in cross section often looks like a signet ring. All
the cell organelles are distributed in the rim of cytoplasm between the lipid and
the plasma membrane. The mitochondria tend to be spherical and contain a dense
matrix. The cristae extend across the entire organelle. In addition, there is a small
Golgi complex, a few short cisternae of rough endoplasmic reticulum, and some
free ribosomes. The plasma membrane often has pinocytotic invaginations.

The conspicuous lipid droplet does not appear to be surrounded by a typical
lipoprotein membrane, although a dense interface between the lipid and the
cytoplasm is apparent in some sections. Ham and Cormack (1979, p. 240) indicate
that the droplets are frequently covered by an orderly array of fine filaments. Even
though electron micrographs do not reveal a typical membrane surrounding the
lipid in the adipose cell, during cell fractionation the cell lipases are extracted
with the lipid. It is assumed that a close structural relationship must exist between
the lipid and the lipases. Galton (1971) has suggested that the presence of a
membrane would provide for both the stabilization and attachment of the enzymes. Despite the ready-made function waiting to be assigned, no membrane
has as yet been identified.

FUNCTION

The constant turnover of the lipid content of the adipocyte requires the controlled
transport of glucose and fatty acids into the cell where they are converted to
triacylglycerol during lipogenesis, and the transport of fatty acids and glycerol
out of the cell after they have been released during lipolysis.

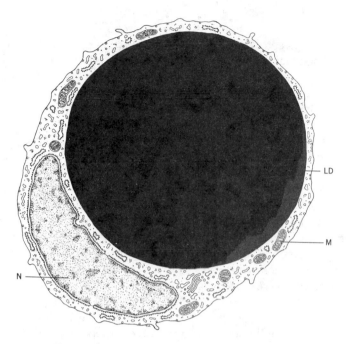

Figure 20.2
White adipose cell. N, nucleus; M, mitochodrion; LD, lipid
droplet (From T. L. Lentz, *Cell Fine Structure*, W. B. Saunders
Co., Philadelphia, 1971, p. 71.)

Lipogenesis

The liver is recognized as the primary site of fatty acid synthesis in humans (Shrago et al., 1966) and in pigeons (Goodridge and Ball, 1966). Even in the rat whose fat cells have a much higher capability for fatty acid synthesis, the major portion of fat that is eventually stored in adipose tissue cells is derived from hepatic synthesis (Markscheid and Shafrir, 1965; Zurier et al., 1967; Hollenberg, 1967). The liver exports fatty acids to the circulation as lipoproteins. In addition to the fatty acids synthesized in the liver from acetyl CoA, fatty acids are taken up from the circulating free fatty acids, incorporated into triacylglycerols in the liver and exported to the plasma. Another source of plasma triacylglycerols are those arriving via the lymphatic system after intestinal absorption and incorporation into chylomicra and lipoproteins. (See Chapter 6.)

Fatty Acid Transport.   Neither lipoproteins nor chylomicra can leave the plasma by penetrating the endothelial wall of the capillaries. The enzyme *lipoprotein lipase,* also known as the *clearing factor* or *clearing factor lipase,* has been found in human adipose tissue (Marshall, 1965) and a number of other tissues (Nilsson-Ehle et al., 1980). It appears to be synthesized locally by parenchymal cells, particularly in adipose tissue. It then appears to be secreted, becoming bound to local capillary endothelial surfaces (Brown et al., 1981) probably through an ionic interaction with the plasma membrane (Olivecrona et al., 1977). The enzyme liberates the triacylglycerol from the molecules (Harlan et al., 1967) and also may be involved in the uptake of the triacylglycerol and fatty acids by the tissue (Nestel et al., 1969).

Also present in loose connective tissue, and particularly numerous along the small blood vessel walls, are the *mast cells* which are distinguished in stained preparations by large quantities of dense granules. These granules contain two substances: histamine and the sulfated mucopolysaccharide, heparin. Heparin, secreted by the mast cell into the intercellular substance of loose connective tissue, participates in the action of lipoprotein lipase (Patten and Hollenberg, 1967). The mechanism of its participation is not clear. It apparently causes lipoprotein lipase to be released from capillary endothelium to the blood. Heparin appears to act by stabilizing the enzyme rather than by activating it, although the precise mechanism is not known (Brown et al., 1981). In any case, heparin is essential for the effect of lipoprotein lipase in "clearing" the plasma; that is, dissipating the chylomicra which give plasma a milky appearance.

Plasma lipoprotein lipase, then, is responsible for clearing the blood of chylomicra. Membrane-bound lipoprotein lipase in capillaries assists the flow of lipids into the various tissues according to need. Where there is little need, blood is shunted around the capillaries. The amount of lipoprotein lipase in different regions of the vascular tissue is regulated by local synthesis and by secretion of the enzyme by parenchymal cells coupled with rapid clearance from the blood (Olivecrona and Bengtsson, 1981).

Nilsson-Ehle and colleagues (1980) have reviewed plasma lipoprotein metabolism. They indicate that the roles and regulation of lipolytic enzymes should soon be understood at the molecular level.

Much of the free fatty acid penetrates the endothelium and then associates with the membrane of the fat cell (Vaughan et al., 1964; Knittle and Hirsch, 1965; Donabedian and Karmen, 1967). The mechanism controlling subsequent passage of the free fatty acids through the plasma membrane has not been clarified. It is assumed to be an active process (Shapiro et al., 1957; Galton et al., 1971), and could be similar to fatty acid transport through mitochondrial membranes. The free fatty acid remaining in the plasma and the glycerol released are circulated back to the liver or to other tissues.

Lipoprotein lipase activity is integrated into the total metabolic scheme. It has high activity in the fed state when lipogenesis is required, and low activity during fasting or starvation when fat must be mobilized from fat cells (Hollenberg, 1959). An inverse correlation has been observed in man between lipoprotein lipase activity of adipose tissue and the levels of serum triacylglycerols (Persson et al., 1966). Insulin, which promotes lipogenesis, appears to increase the activity of lipoprotein lipase, but whether this is a primary or secondary function of insulin is not clear (Avruch et al., 1972).

Glucose Transport.   Insulin is of particular importance in the transport of glucose into the fat cell. In addition to the insulin requirement, the process is an active one that is Na^+-dependent (Letarte and Renold, 1969; Morgan and Neely, 1972).

The mechanism by which insulin facilitates glucose entry is the subject of intensive study.

Cuatrecasas (1973a) demonstrated that insulin receptors are located on the outer surface of the fat cell membrane and that approximately 10,000 molecules of insulin can be bound per fat cell (Cuatrecasas, 1971a). The binding of insulin to the membrane is a saturable, time- and temperature-dependent reaction. The binding is highly specific for insulin, the binding of proinsulin being 20 times less (Cuatrecasas, 1971b). New affinity-labeling and affinity-purification techniques have made it possible to identify the insulin receptor and to deduce its subunit composition and stoichiometry (Massague et al., 1980).

The mechanism by which insulin acts to permit the entry of glucose into the fat cell is not completely clear. A promising hypothesis to explain insulin action on the fat cell is that the insulin molecule combines with the plasma membrane at a site near the glucose carrier. Galton (1971) reported that an alteration in membrane structure takes place. He postulated an enhancement of carrier activity. Recently, Wardzala and his associates (1978) have found that the number of glucose transporters in adipocyte plasma membranes increases in response to insulin stimulation. This is accomplished by displacing glucose from the receptor with cytochalasin B. The reaction was made specific by blocking the binding of cytochalasin B to nonreceptor sites with cytochalasin E, which does not bind to the transporter. The transporters which appear in the fat cell membrane after insulin stimulation are supplied from a cytoplasmic pool (Cushman and Wardzala, 1980). The mechanism by which insulin causes the repositioning of glucose transporters is unknown.

The glucose transporter has been isolated from the erythrocyte membrane. It is a glycoprotein which spans the membrane with the carbohydrate moiety positioned on the outside of the cell. The glucose transporter in adipocytes and muscle cells is believed to be similar to that of the erythrocyte. A recent review has been provided by Baldwin and Lienhard (1981).

It is interesting that only about 5 percent of the insulin receptors need to be filled to cause maximal activation of glucose transport (Kono and Barham, 1971). The effect of insulin on adipocytes is greater than on liver cells. This may be related to the fact that adipocyte insulin receptors occur in groups of two or more, whereas in hepatocyte receptors they are single units (Jarett et al., 1980). The roles proposed for cGMP and cAMP as the major intracellular signals for insulin action (Goldberg et al., 1973) is now subject to question, although it is possible that both cyclic nucleotides have limited, indirect roles. These concepts have been reviewed by Czech (1977).

The responsiveness of the adipocyte to insulin was reported to be related to the size of the cell: the larger the mean cell size, the less responsive it was to insulin (Salans et al., 1968). Adipose cells of obese individuals which are larger and filled with lipid displayed a diminished response to insulin, but after weight loss and reduction of adipose cell size, the response to insulin returned to normal. One explanation offered was that the overfilled cell might have distorted membrane receptor sites (Jungas, 1966) which returned to normal after weight loss. However, some investigators were unable to find differences in the sensitivity to insulin in adipose cells from obese and nonobese individuals (Davidson, 1972), and others (Bray, 1969) suggested that the state of nutrition as well as cell size affected insulin-stimulated glucose metabolism in the fat cell.

Salans et al. (1974) suggested that the disparity in results attributed to insulin in human adipose tissue reflects the composition of the diet ingested prior to tissue sampling as well as cell size, and that the dietary and morphologic effect could be dissociated. Adipose cells examined under conditions of similar nutrition and growth showed no difference in insulin response according to size.

Upon entry into the adipose cell, glucose may proceed through the glycolytic pathway to the cleavage of fructose-1,6-diphosphate to the trioses, dihydroxyacetone phosphate, and phosphoglyceraldehyde. Oxidative breakdown of dihydroxyacetone phosphate can continue, or it can be reduced to glycerol phosphate. The reaction is catalyzed by an NAD-linked glycerol phosphate dehydrogenase and provides the link between glycolysis and lipogenesis (Fig. 20.3). The glycerol phosphate is a major acceptor for long chain fatty acids in the synthesis of neutral lipid.

Fatty Acid Synthesis.   The conversion of glucose into lipid occurs readily. In mouse adipose cells, 90 percent of ^{14}C-glucose appears in glyceride fatty acids (Jansen et al., 1966a; 1966b). In human fat cells, only 16 percent or less is found in the fatty acid moiety and 80 percent in the glyceride-glycerol. Human adipose tissue does not appear to be an important site for synthesis of fatty acids based on ^{14}C recovery (Bjorntorp et al., 1968) and on studies of key enzyme levels (Shrago et al., 1966). However, data supporting fatty acid synthesis in human adipose cells have been presented by Jacob (1963) and by Goldrick et al. (1969).

The enzymes involved in fatty acid synthesis in the fat cell show an adaptive response to changes in diet and in hormonal balance. These changes are referred to as long-term changes and take two to four days to come into effect (Lowenstein, 1972). These responses in the fat cell have been ascribed to the rate of glucose utilization, which is controlled by insulin. However, there is no evidence that insulin exerts a direct effect on the enzyme levels for fatty acid synthesis.

If the fatty acids are not synthesized in the human fat cell, they are transported there by lipoprotein triacylglycerols and phospholipids after hepatic synthesis. For further details of fatty acid synthesis, see Chapters 11 and 13.

Triacylglycerol Synthesis.   Glucose can be used by adipose tissue to form the entire triacylglycerol molecule (Farvarger, 1965). Long chain fatty acids synthesized in the fat cell from glucose or transported there following hepatic synthesis react with L-α-glycerophosphate leading to the formation of diacylglycerols and then triacylglycerols. Unsaturated fatty acids are elongated by enzyme systems in the endoplasmic reticulum. (See Chapter 11.) Because mammals lack enzymes to introduce double bonds after the ninth carbon, linoleate and linolenate are dietary requirements. (See Chapter 2.) The metabolic sequence shown in Fig. 20.4 has been demonstrated in mitochondria from rat adipose tissue (Shapiro et al., 1960; Steinberg et al., 1961; Roncari and Hollenberg, 1967).

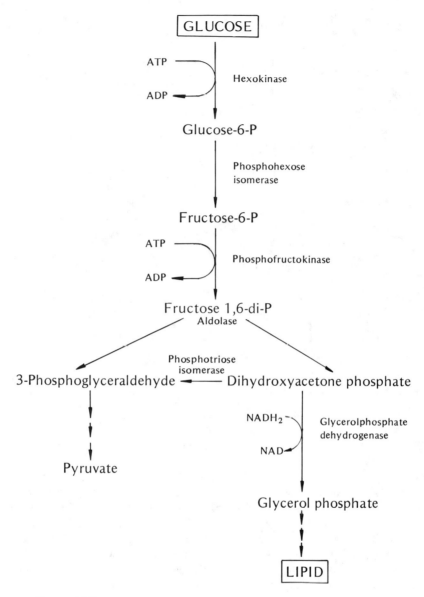

Figure 20.3
Glycolytic sequence leading to the formation of glycerol phosphate.

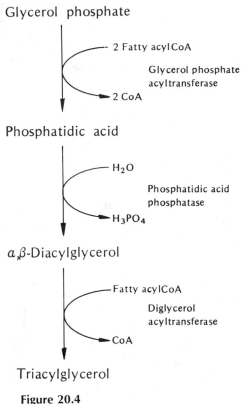

Glycerol phosphate

2 Fatty acylCoA

Glycerol phosphate
acyltransferase

2 CoA

Phosphatidic acid

H_2O

Phosphatidic acid
phosphatase

H_3PO_4

a,β-Diacylglycerol

Fatty acylCoA

Diglycerol
acyltransferase

CoA

Triacylglycerol

Figure 20.4
Steps in the synthesis of triacylglycerol.

Lipolysis

The hydrolysis of fat prior to its release from the adipocyte is a tightly controlled series of reactions—so tightly controlled in some individuals that one wonders if it occurs at all. All of the steps in the pathway leading from stored lipid in the fat cell to fatty acids and glycerol available for transport are separate from the pathways leading to lipogenesis. This separation of power increases the complexity of metabolic activity in the fat cell but also provides for finer control.

Since a specific function of the adipocyte is to store fuel in periods of plenty and to release it during periods of deprivation, it is particularly important that the reactions leading to storage and release of fat be integrated with the needs of the total organism. *Hormone-sensitive lipase,* the enzyme that catalyzes triacylglycerol hydrolysis in adipose tissue (Vaughan et al., 1964), is much more active in fat cells of fasted than of fed animals (Hollenberg, 1965). Increased activity of the enzyme occurs also after brief exposure of fat cells to at least 12 hormones including epinephrine, norepinephrine, glucagon, and ACTH (Vaughan, 1966; Butcher and Sutherland, 1967). Activity of the enzyme is decreased after fat cells are exposed to insulin or prostaglandin E_1 (Butcher and Baird, 1968; Manganiello et al., 1971). Since hormone-sensitive lipase is the rate-determining enzyme in lipolysis, its activity controls the overall rate of lipolysis (Hollett and Auditore, 1967).

Changes in hormone-sensitive lipase activity induced by hormones are associated with changes in the intracellular content of cAMP (Manganiello et al., 1971). The model shown in Fig. 20.5 incorporates the second messenger concept of cAMP action (Sutherland, 1972), the theory of allosteric regulation suggested by Monod et al. (1965), and the concept of enzymatic interconversion as postulated by Segal (1973) or by Rodbell (1973). The hormone that initiates lipolysis binds to the regulatory site of adenyl cyclase on the outer surface of the plasma membrane of the fat cell. (See Chapter 9.) An allosteric effect exposes the catalytic component on the inner surface of the membrane, which converts ATP to cAMP in the cell. The activation of protein kinase is effected by binding of cAMP, which causes dissociation of a receptor unit-catalytic unit complex thereby liberating the free catalytic unit. (See Chapter 11.) The protein kinase then transforms the inactive hormone-sensitive triacylglycerol lipase to the active form. It is this hormone that controls the rate of lipolysis. Hormone stimulation of lipolysis in human adipose tissue appears to be effected by a mechanism basically similar to that in rat adipose tissue (Khoo et al., 1974). The di- and monoacylglycerol lipase activities are not correlated with the level of the hormone (Vaughan, 1967), but their activities follow sequentially after the rate-controlling lipase is activated.

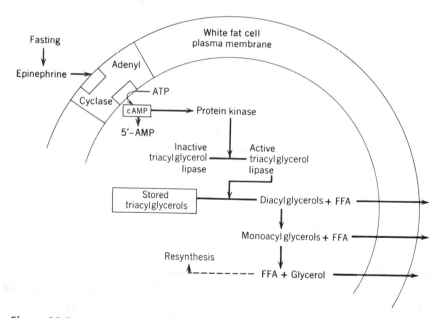

Figure 20.5
Model of lipolysis in white fat cell. Adipose cell of rat responds to glucagon and ACTH; human adipose cell does not. Level of cAMP is the major controlling factor in lipolysis.

Vitamin C deficiency, in addition to its well-known impairment of connective tissue synthesis, affects lipid metabolism. Hypovitaminosis C leads to both hypercholesterolemia and raised plasma triglyceride levels. Marginal vitamin C deficiency has been proposed as a risk factor in the pathogenesis of atherosclerosis (Ginter, 1978). If vitamin C is thus involved it may be related to changes in lipolytic enzyme activities.

Fatty Acid Acceptors.   The fatty acids released by hydrolysis in the fat cell are made water-soluble for transport by the plasma through the formation of an albumin-FFA complex. Lipolysis in the fat cell, therefore, is influenced by the plasma albumin available for the removal of the fatty acids from the cell. Increase in the amount of albumin available for transport is effected not by increasing albumin synthesis but simply by the expedient of increasing the blood flow to the adipose tissue. This has been shown to occur when fat mobilization is increased by norepinephrine, glucagon, or fasting in humans (Nielsen et al., 1968) and in rats (Mayerle and Havel, 1969). Although the concentration of fatty acids in the plasma is low, a significant amount can be transported to other tissues because of its rapid turnover. For discussion of the importance of fatty acids in the total fuel economy, see Chapter 23.

Fate of Liberated Glycerol.   For want of an enzyme, glycerol is lost. Lost, that is, as far as the metabolic machinery of the adipocyte is concerned. Almost all of the glycerol liberated by hydrolysis of triacylglycerol diffuses into the plasma because the fat cell lacks glycerokinase thereby preventing the reuse of the glycerol in the esterification of acyl CoA. Glycerokinase has been found in rat adipose tissue (Robinson and Newsholme, 1967), but its activity does not appear to have any significance. The glycerol liberated by hydrolysis is carried by the plasma to tissues, such as the liver and kidney, that can provide the enzyme required for its phosphorylation.

For a brief review of adipose cell metabolism, see Galton and Wallis (1982).

Brown Fat Cell

Brown fat, a specialized form of adipose tissue, is much less widely distributed than white fat. However, at birth brown fat is usually more abundant than the common white variety. It is found in newborn animals and in adult cold-adapted animals where it forms what is sometimes called the hibernating gland. Brown fat develops during embryonic life in certain specific sites: the interscapular region, back of the neck, and the axillae in rodents and humans; also, in humans, around the neck, kidneys, adrenals, and in the abdomen (Dawkins and Hull, 1965; Aherne and Hull, 1966; Dyer, 1968). No new areas develop after birth except in animals subjected to prolonged cold (Smith and Horwitz, 1969). Although the fat content in brown adipose tissue usually decreases with age, some masses are present even in old individuals. Total depletion of brown fat has been reported for both children and adults dying of cold exposure.

STRUCTURE

Brown fat cells are not only smaller than the white cells but contain more cytoplasm in relation to the lipid, and the lipid is in many smaller droplets (Fig. 20.6). The nucleus, usually with two nucleoli, is not generally in a central position but it does not have a distorted shape. There are many large mitochondria with abundant cristae and relatively dense matrices. However, the subunits usually observed on the inner membrane of the cristae have not been demonstrated. This finding suggests that oxidative phosphorylation, a key function of mitochondria, probably does not take place and this is consistent with the thermogenic function of the tissue. (See below.) There are few cisternae of either smooth or rough endoplasmic reticulum. Some free ribosomes and glycogen granules can be observed in the cytoplasm as well as a small Golgi apparatus. Pinocytotic vesicles

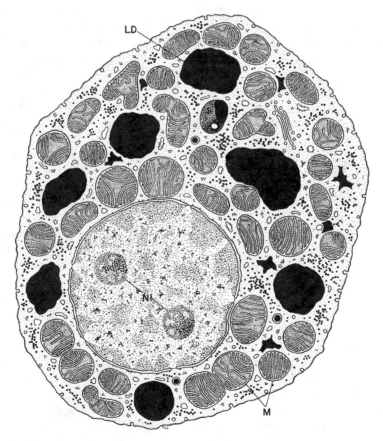

Figure 20.6
Brown adipose cell. LD, lipid droplet; M, mitochondrion; NI, nucleoli. (From T. L. Lentz, *Cell Fine Structure*, W. B. Saunders Co., Philadelphia, 1971, p. 73.)

appear at frequent intervals in the plasma membrane (Napolitano, 1965). A rich blood supply comes to brown adipose tissue and is in part responsible for its color. Color is due also to the high content of iron-containing cytochromes in the mitochondrial membranes.

FUNCTION

The functions of brown fat in newborn mammals and adult hibernating animals remained a mystery until the early 1960s. Smith (1961) observed the high heat-producing potential of brown fat and suggested that production of heat was its specific function. The high concentrations of cytochromes in the numerous mitochondria and the ample quantities of fat for substrate suggested a high capacity for oxidative metabolism. It was soon found that the oxygen consumption of these cells, when expressed on a lipid-free dry weight basis, was higher than that of any other body cells (Joel, 1965). In a series of experiments on newborn rabbits, Dawkins and Hull (1965) clearly demonstrated that brown fat cells are the main site of heat production in response to cold. The rich blood supply in the tissue rapidly removes the heat to other parts of the body, thereby protecting the bare-skinned newborn rabbit. The explanation of how exposure to cold in most mammalian neonates including humans leads to increased heat production without shivering becomes apparent. Mammals must shiver for extra heat production when their brown fat storage is gradually replaced by white fat, since white fat plays no part in nonshivering thermogenesis. A clear demonstration of the specialization of brown fat cells for this purpose was presented by Hull and Segall (1966), who showed that the cells of brown fat became depleted when newborn rabbits were exposed to cold for 48 hours but there was little change in the white fat cells. In contrast, starving newborn rabbits in a warm environment depleted white fat cells, but the brown fat cells were unchanged. Hittleman et al. (1969) also demonstrated that the stimulus to lipolysis in brown fat of rabbits was cold; in white fat it was lack of calories. Pigs are presumed to contain no brown fat and so were thought to lack cold- or dietary-induced thermogenesis. Recently, however, they have been found to exhibit dietary-induced thermogenesis (Gurr et al., 1980). The assumption that pigs lack brown adipose tissue thus may be incorrect.

Only recently was brown fat identified in humans (Heaton, 1972). Both the structure and function of brown fat in humans and animals appears similar. Silverman et al. (1964) reported that skin temperature was maintained best at the interscapular region in infants exposed to cold. Cold exposure was also related to increased plasma glycerol levels indicating lipolysis (Dawkins and Scopes, 1965).

There is a considerable body of evidence indicating that the oxidative metabolism of brown fat is mediated by norepinephrine (Hull and Segall, 1965a; Schiff et al., 1966). This apparently occurs through local secretion at sympathetic nerve endings (Hull and Segall, 1965b) since the response to cold is very rapid. Furthermore, electrical stimulation leads to heat production and cutting the sympathetic nerves supplying the tissue abolishes this response. When brown fat is removed from newborn rabbits the oxygen consumption following injection of norepinephrine is greatly reduced (Hull and Segall, 1965b).

The metabolic specialization of the brown fat cell is its capacity to shift to oxidation of fatty acids for the production of heat. The shift is initiated by temperature receptors in the skin which stimulate the temperature regulating center in the brain. Impulses are relayed through the sympathetic nerves to brown fat tissue leading to norepinephrine release at the nerve endings. A suggested model of the sequence that follows is presented in Fig. 20.7. Norepinephrine at the brown fat cell membrane interacts with adenyl cyclase and stimulates the production of cAMP. The ensuing events leading to triacylglycerol hydrolysis are probably similar to those postulated for the white fat cell: cAMP binds to the receptor unit-catalytic unit complex and liberates the free catalytic unit which activates the protein kinase. The protein kinase converts the hormone-sensitive lipase to the active state leading to hydrolysis of stored triacylglycerol into glycerol and FFA. However, the presence of glycerokinase in the brown fat cell (Treble and Ball, 1963) permits reutilization of some of the free glycerol. The increased concentration of FFA has been shown by Prusiner et al. (1968) to uncouple oxidation and phosphorylation in brown fat cells. Myant (1971) suggests that reversible uncoupling of mitochondria, combined with the increased supply of oxidizable substrate, may be the explanation for the increased oxygen consump-

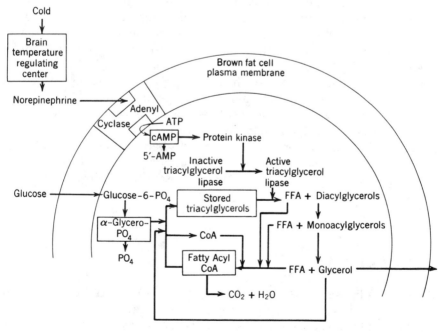

Figure 20.7
Model of lipolysis in brown fat cell.

tion in brown fat cells of cold-stressed newborn animals. There is evidence also that coupling of oxidative phosphorylation can be restored to brown fat tissue by the removal of endogenously produced fatty acids (Bulychev et al., 1972). This finding is of particular interest when considered along with a report on the presence of a fatty acid binding protein (FABP) in the cytosol in many tissues including adipose tissue (Ockner et al., 1972). The FABP appears to be a regulator of cellular fatty acid concentration. These two lines of evidence point to the possibility that the FABP, through control of the concentration of the liberated fatty acids in the brown fat cells, can shift mitochondrial metabolism so that oxidation and phosphorylation become uncoupled and thermogenesis is possible.

In order for catecholamine-induced thermogenesis to operate maximally, the Na^+-K^+ membrane pump must be functional. When the pump is inhibited by ouabain, norepinephrine-stimulated adipocyte respiration is reduced by 53 percent (Horwitz, 1979). The role of the Na^+-K^+ pump in the response of brown adipose cells to neural stimulation is not understood.

Although in most species born with brown fat the tissue is converted to white fat by adulthood, in some animals it is retained and can increase; for example, in laboratory rats kept in a cold environment. The blood supply from the brown adipose tissue conducts the heat produced to warm the body without shivering much as the water pipes in a hot water home heating system provide a similar service. In animals that hibernate, a large quantity of brown fat remains throughout life. The importance of the brown fat is not so much in providing comfort during the long sleep but rather in providing the source of heat for awakening and emergence from the hibernating state. The stimulus for increased heat production in brown fat is the release of the norepinephrine at nerve endings as the animal begins to arouse. This initiates the lipolytic reesterification cycle that produces the heat carried by the blood to warm the rest of the body. The heat generated by brown fat in a bat arousing from hibernation has been visually demonstrated by thermography. A scan of the temperature-dependent intensity of infrared radiation from the body surface was registered on a photographic plate. A sharply delineated hot area corresponded to the location of the interscapular fat (Hayward and Ball, 1966). Skin temperature measurements between the shoulder blades of newborn babies have indicated the presence of brown fat which has been identified morphologically as well (Dyer, 1968; Mrosovsky and Rowlatt, 1968).

For a review of thermogenesis in brown adipost tissue, see Himms-Hagen (1983).

Conclusion

In the white adipose tissue cell there is a continual cycle of hydrolysis of triacylglycerols to glycerol and fatty acids followed by triacylglycerol resynthesis. The α-glycerophosphate for resynthesis is derived from glycolysis in the cell. Some of the fatty acids released are reincorporated into triacylglycerol; some are synthesized in the cell; and some are derived from the triacylglycerols of the lipoproteins and chylomicra delivered by the plasma. Free fatty acids are continually released into the plasma where a small quantity circulates free and the rest are picked up by albumin. The quantity of free fatty acids released by the fat cell and circulated to supply fuel needs is determined by the relative rates of lipolysis and lipogenesis which are under hormonal control and closely integrated into the total body need for endogenous lipid as an energy source.

The continual cycle of hydrolysis in the brown fat cell differs from that in the white fat cell in that the major portion of fatty acids are not released to the circulation for an energy source but are oxidized by the mitochondria of the brown fat cell for the purpose of producing heat, rather than ATP. Triggered by the stimulus of cold, the cutaneous nerve endings elicit the series of events leading to nonshivering thermogenesis in neonates. Although the original stimulus to norepinephrine release may differ in arousal from hibernation, the mechanisms of thermogenesis appear to be the same.

part five

the complex organism

"Man is, first of all, a nutritive process. He consists of a ceaseless motion of chemical substances. One can compare him to the flame of a candle, or to the fountains playing in the gardens of Versailles. Those beings, made of burning gases or of water, are both permanent and transitory. Their existence depends on a stream of gas or of liquid. Like ourselves, they change according to the quality and the quantity of the substances which animate them. As a large river coming from the external world and returning to it, matter perpetually flows through all the cells of the body. During its passing, it yields to tissues the energy they need, and also the chemicals which build the temporary and fragile structures of our organs and humors. The corporeal substratum of all human activities originates from the inanimate world and, sooner or later, goes back to it. Our organism is made from the same elements as lifeless things. Therefore, we should not be surprised, as some modern physiologists still are, to find at work within our own self the usual laws of physics and of chemistry as they exist in the cosmic world. Since we are parts of the material universe, the absence of those laws is unthinkable."

Alexis Carrel, 1935

chapter 21

cellular growth

"I wish you wouldn't squeeze so," said the Dormouse, who was sitting next to her. "I can hardly breathe."

"I can't help it," said Alice very meekly: "I'm growing."

"You've no right to grow here," said the Dormouse.

"Don't talk nonsense," said Alice more boldly; "you know you're growing too."

"Yes, but I grow at a reasonable pace," said the Dormouse; "not in that ridiculous fashion." And he got up very sulkily and crossed over to the other side of the court.

Lewis Carroll, *Alice's Adventures in Wonderland*

To paraphrase the Dormouse, "growth does not occur in a ridiculous fashion." Growth of the total organism is a series of highly regulated processes that begins with the fertilization of the ovum and terminates with maturity; maturity being defined as the attainment of the body size, conformation, and physiological capabilities characteristic of the species, and of the hereditary material with which the organism is endowed. Growth is represented by an increase in size and weight, the acquisition of active protoplasmic mass, and the accumulation of adipose tissue.

The changes in body composition accompanying normal growth will be discussed in the following chapter. This chapter will deal with the phenomenon of growth at the cellular level and the effect of nutrition on the course of cellular growth.

The Stages of Development

The life span of all living organisms can be divided into two discrete phases: prenatal life that culminates with birth, and postnatal life that ends with death. These phases are divided into several periods each of which is characterized by discrete morphological, physiological, and biochemical features. The rate of change and the timing of these events differ among various species, but the pattern is common to all.

The stages of development from conception to maturity in the human are described in Table 21.1. The human differs from most mammalian species in one major respect: the relative length of the periods of childhood and adolescence. No other animal can boast of enjoying so long a period between birth and maturity. Indeed, a period comparable with adolescence in the human is virtually nonexistent in other species. Brody (1945) observed that growth curves of many animals are superimposed on each other when growth is expressed in terms of weight as a percentage of mature weight (Fig. 21.1). The curve for the human, however, shows a long, slow period of growth unmatched by any other species and one that does not conform to the pattern of other mammals until midadolescence.

Different species are born at different levels of maturity, as determined by body composition and physiological function. Birth is not a mark of equal development. However, certain physiological events tend to occur sequentially in many species. There are exceptions, of course, and the time intervals vary, but for the most part mammalian species tend to grow and develop in a recognizable pattern. Extrapolations then can be made from one species to another if they are made with care; consideration must be given to the variation in time at which a specific event occurs. The latter point is especially important in extrapolating from one species to another in terms of cellular growth and the effects of over- and undernutrition during critical periods of growth. The critical period varies from one species to another. For a specific organ or tissue, it may be prenatal in one species and postnatal in another. Since humans have such a long developmental period, the detrimental effects of environmental factors may be less than in some other species. In addition, there may be more than one critical period of cellular growth in some human tissues.

TABLE 21.1
Age Periods of Life before Maturity

Name of Period	Ages Represented (approximate)	Some Characterizing Features
Embryonic	First trimester of prenatal life	Rapid differentiation Establishment of systems and organs
Early fetal	Second trimester of prenatal life	Accelerated growth Elaboration of structures Early functional activities
Late fetal	Third trimester of prenatal life	Rapid increase in body mass Completion of preparation for postnatal experience
Parturient	Period of labor and delivery	Risk of trauma and anoxia Cessation of placental function
Neonatal and early infancy	First month of postnatal life	Postnatal adjustments in circulation Initiation of respiration and other functions
Middle infancy	1 month to 1 year	Rapid growth and maturation Maturation of functions, especially of nervous system
Late infancy	1–2 years	Decelerating growth Progress in walking and other voluntary motor activities and in control of excretory functions
Childhood Preschool	2–6 years	Slow growth Increased physical activity Further coordination of functions and motor mechanisms Rapid learning
School	Girls: 6–10 years Boys: 6–12 years	Steady growth Developing skills and intellectual processes

Adolescent
  Prepubertal
  (late school or early adolescent)
	Girls: 10–12 years
	Boys: 12–14 years
		Accelerating growth
		Rapid weight gain
		Early adolescent endocrine and sex organ changes

Pubertal (adolescence proper)	Girls: 12–14 years Boys: 14–16 years	Secondary sex character maturation Maximum postnatal growth increase

TABLE 21.1 (continued)

Name of Period	Ages Represented (approximate)	Some Characterizing Features
Postpubertal	Girls: 14–18 years Boys: 16–20 years	Decelerating and terminal growth Rapid muscle growth and increased skills Rapid growth and maturing functions of sex organs Need for self-reliance and independence

Source: From P. S. Timiras, *Developmental Physiology and Aging,* The MacMillan Co., New York, 1972, p. 4.

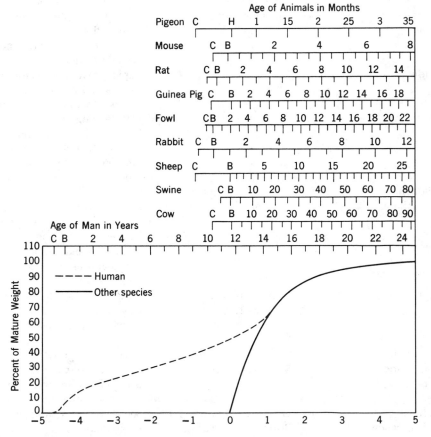

Figure 21.1
Weight-growth equivalence of farm animals, laboratory animals, and man. (From S. Brody, *Bioenergetics and Growth,* Reinhold Publishing Co., New York, 1945, p. 492.)

Determination of Cell Number and Size

In early studies growth was assessed by the change in whole body weight or the weight of specific organs and tissues (Donaldson, 1924; Dunn et al., 1947). Later, the number and size of cells were determined from the amount of DNA in an organ or tissue. DNA is located almost entirely in the nucleus and, for a given species, the amount of DNA per diploid nucleus is a constant (Boivin et al., 1948; Mirsky and Ris, 1949; Thomson et al., 1953). For the rat this amount has been shown to be 6.2 micromicrograms (Enesco and Leblond, 1962). The number of cells can be calculated from the following formula:

$$\text{Number of nuclei (millions)} = \frac{\text{total organ DNA (mg)} \times 10^3}{6.2}$$

The size of the cell thus can be calculated by dividing organ weight by the number of cells as shown below.

$$\text{Weight/nucleus (ng)} = \frac{\text{total organ weight (gm)} \times 10^3}{\text{number of nuclei (millions)}}$$

This formula can be used also to calculate protein, RNA, or any other cell constituent by dividing the total organ content of the substance by the number of nuclei.

These calculations are valid only for cells containing a diploid nucleus. The parenchymal cells of liver, however, are polyploid and, in addition, contain different quantities of DNA. Measurement of DNA in liver, therefore, does not give an accurate assessment of cell number. Total DNA, however, is closely associated with total liver mass (Campbell and Kosterlitz, 1950).

Although adipocytes have a diploid nucleus, difficulties arise in determining cell number in adipose tissue. Rodbell (1964) reported that only 20 percent of

TABLE 21.2
Total DNA in Fat Cells in Epididymal Fat Pad of Male Sprague-Dawley Rats from 12–182 Days of Age

Age	Total DNA in Fat Cells (%)
12	4.13
15	4.34
18	7.79
21	14.78
28	12.28
35	21.72
56	19.23
70	18.13
182	15.27

Source: From M. P. Cleary, M. R. C. Greenwood, and J. A. Brasel, *J. Nutr.* 107:1969 (1977).

the cells in a fat depot in young adult rats were lipid-filled fat cells. The remaining cells were termed the stromal-vascular cells and included fibroblasts. Cleary et al. (1977) reported that the ratio of the number of fat cells to total fat pad DNA varies with age (Table 21.2). Thus, total DNA is not an adequate measure of the fat-storing capacity of a fat depot. Various techniques have been developed to measure only the lipid-filled cells in a fat depot. For example, fixation of adipose tissues with osmium tetroxide separates adipocytes from other cell types (Hirsch and Gallian, 1968), and osmium-fixed cells can then be counted electronically. Fat cells can be isolated also by collagenase treatment (Rodbell, 1964), and DNA of the isolated cells can then be determined. Other methods involve indirect determination of fat cell number following measurement of fat cell size (di Girolamo et al., 1971; Sjöstrom et al., 1971). Fat cell size can be expressed as lipid/cell or by cell diameter or volume.

Phases of Cell Growth

Using some of the techniques described above, Enesco and Leblond (1962) and Winick and Nobel (1965) studied cell growth in the prenatal and postnatal rat. Growth was shown to occur in three stages. Initially, growth proceeds by cell division (hyperplasia) alone, as indicated by increasing amounts of DNA. Growth then proceeds by simultaneous cell division and cell enlargement (hyperplasia and hypertrophy), as indicated by increase in weight or protein per nucleus. Finally, cell division ceases and growth occurs only by cell enlargement (hypertrophy), that is, DNA content of the organ then remains relatively constant (Fig. 21.2).

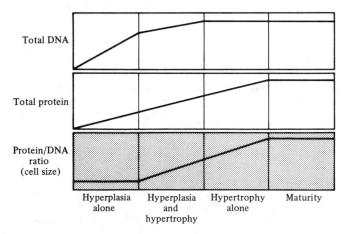

Figure 21.2
Periods of cellular growth. Plotted are the relationships between DNA and protein during the three phases of organ growth. (From M. Winick, *Hosp. Pract.* 5:37, 1970.)

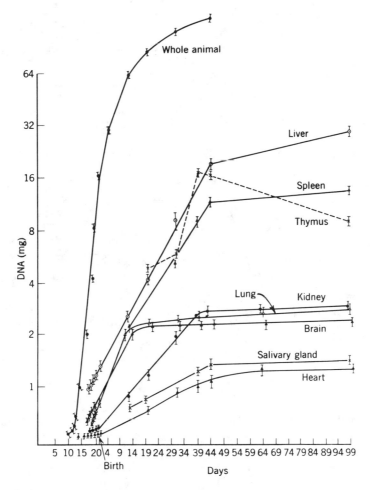

Figure 21.3
DNA (mg) during normal growth in the rat. Points represent mean
values for at least 10 animals or organs. I represents range. (From
M. Winick and A. Noble, *Develop. Biol.* 12:451, 1965.)

Cell division is very rapid in prenatal life, as demonstrated by the steep slope
of the lines representing tissue DNA content for the rat (Fig. 21.3). Following
birth, cell division continues for varying periods of time in different organs, lev-
eling off first in brain and lung at about 13 days of age and continuing in other
organs until about 44–65 days of age. Total DNA is decreased in thymus after
the thirty-ninth day, an indication of the loss of cells associated with atrophy of
the gland.

The total protein content of organs, like organ weight, increases until maturity
(Fig. 21.4). During early prenatal life, cellular protein and DNA increase proportionately indicating that growth is due to cell division alone. In the late prenatal

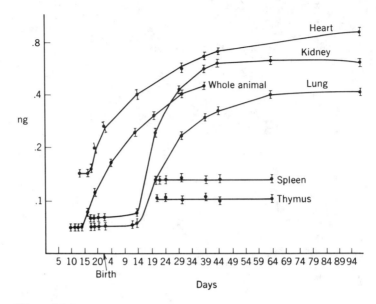

Figure 21.4
Protein per nucleus during normal growth in the rat. Symbols the
same as for Fig. 3. (From M. Winick and A. Noble, *Develop. Biol.*
12:451, 1966.)

period and thereafter, protein increases more rapidly than DNA because cell
growth is largely due to increase in cell size. When protein synthesis and degradation come into equilibrium, growth ceases. This situation is reflected in the
change from a positive nitrogen balance as seen in growing animals, and nitrogen
equilibrium as observed in the adult.

Protein content per nucleus remains static in spleen and thymus indicating that
growth in these organs occurs chiefly by cell proliferation.

A comparison of DNA, total protein, and protein per nucleus is shown in Fig.
21.5 for the whole animal body, and for lung, heart, and kidney, and emphasizes
the differences in patterns of growth for various organs. It will be noted that the
increase in number of cells is very rapid in early life and gradually tapers off as
protein increases. Enesco and Leblond (1962) estimate that the number of cells
for the whole rat body increases from 52×10^6 cells at 10 days before birth to
$3,000 \times 10^6$ at birth and then to $67,000 \times 10^6$ at 95 days of age. When the
rate of cell division decreases, total protein continues to increase at the same
rate; this results in a marked increase in protein per cell.

Total organ RNA increases during growth and, with the exception of liver, the
increase is proportional to that of DNA. Thus RNA/DNA ratio is constant for each
organ. Tissues that are most actively involved in protein synthesis such as liver,
heart, and skeletal muscle have high RNA/DNA ratios. The patterns of RNA/DNA

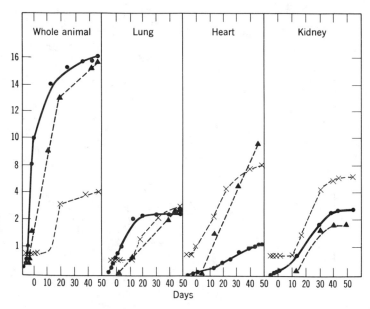

Figure 21.5
Comparison between DNA content, total protein content, and protein per nucleus in various organs during normal growth of the rat. ●– –● DNA (mg); ▲ – – – ▲ total protein (mg × 10^{-2}); X– – –X protein per nucleus. (From M. Winick and A. Noble, *Develop. Biol.* 12:451, 1966.)

ratio and protein/DNA ratio are similar, but the RNA/DNA ratio reaches its highest level earlier in development.

Similar data are difficult to obtain from humans; however, some information is available for fetal material. The DNA content of various organs in the normal human fetus is shown in Table 21.3. Total cell number increases in all organs from 13 weeks of gestation until term. Cell size as indicated by weight/DNA remains unchanged throughout gestation in heart, kidney, spleen, thyroid, thymus, esophagus, stomach, large and small intestines, and tongue. In brain, lungs, liver, adrenal gland, and diaphragm, an increase in cell size starts slowly, beginning at the 7th month of gestation.

Cell Growth of Specific Tissues

PLACENTA

Growth of the placenta follows the same three-stage pattern described for other tissues (Winick and Noble, 1966). In the rat, placental DNA increases until the seventeenth day of gestation, that is, 4 days before term. Placental weight, protein,

TABLE 21.3
DNA Content of Various Organs in Normal Human Fetuses (milligrams)

Weeks of gestation	13	17	23	25	27	31	33	34	49	40
Fetal weight (gm)	31.7	163	320	580	610	1080	1525	1720	3300	4040
Brain	25	85	134	251	240	285	385	—	620	685
Heart	0.51	2.8	8.1	15.4	17.3	18.2	38.6	40.2	54.7	55.6
Liver	16.5	50	53.9	97.3	105.1	175	203	247	328	329
Kidney	0.72	6.8	—	38.7	59.6	—	73	79	107	128
Spleen	0.41	1.2	2.5	7.7	9.8	15.3	—	64.4	84.6	90.9
Thyroid	0.02	0.10	—	0.84	0.97	2.7	—	4.5	5.8	6.9
Adrenal	0.24	0.71	1.31	1.87	2.14	5.84	6.97	8.04	10.2	12.6
Right lung	3.0	23.6	50.9	64	—	66.4	68.5	—	148.7	166.8
Left lung	2.5	18.7	37.5	41.8	—	55.6	59.4	—	126	132
Thymus	0.39	3.99	10.96	21.8	26.5	47.3	105.4	160.6	249	303
Esophagus	0.17	0.60	0.64	0.78	0.80	1.38	3.69	4.21	6.1	6.9
Stomach	0.53	2.3	3.6	5.0	5.7	6.8	22.3	26.8	32.7	40.7
Small intestine	3.8	6.1	16.2	26.3	32.8	48.7	157	179	512	529
Large intestine	0.37	2.97	5.8	10.0	11.2	26.3	47.2	525	129.6	137.2
Diaphragm	0.38	2.1	5.2	6.8	7.2	18.7	24.7	31.7	385	45.3
Tongue	0.39	1.21	2.4	3.5	3.7	4.9	—	—	—	—

Source: From M. Winick et al., *Nutrition and Development,* John Wiley, New York, 1972, p. 88.

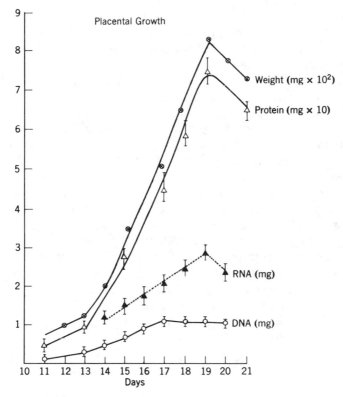

Figure 21.6
Total weight, protein, DNA, and RNA during development of
rat placenta. Each point represents the average of at least 15
separate determinations. The bars on the figure represent the
range. (From M. Winick and A. Noble, *Nature* 212:34, 1966.)

and RNA increase until day 19 (Fig. 21.6). Until day 16, cell number increases
with no increase in cell size as indicated by proportional increases in DNA and
protein. From day 16 through 18 hyperplasia and hypertrophy occur simultaneously; thereafter, placental cell growth is by hypertrophy alone.

Human placenta follows the same pattern of growth. Cell division ceases at
about 34–36 weeks of pregnancy; weight, protein, and RNA increase until near
term (Winick et al., 1967). RNA/DNA ratio of human placenta, however, is only
half that of the rat. The reason for this difference is not known.

BRAIN

When cellular growth of the total rat brain is measured by determining DNA
content, cell synthesis appears to cease at about 20 days of age (Winick and
Noble, 1965). Increases in protein and weight continue for several months. How-

ever, different regions of the brain exhibit different patterns of growth (Fish and Winick, 1969). In the rat, cell division in the cerebellum ceases at 17 days postnatally, in cerebral cortex at 21 days, and in brainstem as early as 14 days. There is a well defined increase in DNA in the hippocampus between the fourteenth and seventeenth days, which is probably due to migration of neurons into this area. Total protein content of cerebellum is not reached until nearly 100 days of age. Net protein synthesis decreases in cerebrum, and cerebral cells decrease in size with aging. In contrast, the protein/DNA ratio increases in brainstem cells due not only to an increase in cell size but also to myelination and extension of neuronal processes from other brain regions into the brainstem.

Less is known of cell growth in human brain. Analysis of brain tissue obtained from therapeutic abortions and autopsy of healthy infants who died from accidents suggests that DNA synthesis is nearly linear prenatally, begins to decline after birth, and reaches a maximum at 8–12 months of age (Winick, 1970). In more detailed studies, Dobbing and Sands (1970) described two peaks of DNA synthesis in human brain, one occurring at about 26 weeks of gestation and the second around the time of birth. These peaks were interpreted as a reflection of the peak rates of neuronal division and of glial division respectively.

Studies of postnatal changes in normal human brain are limited. Increases in lipid content (i.e., cholesterol and phospholipid) continue for several years (Rosso et al., 1970).

MUSCLE

Enesco and Leblond (1962) examined gastrocnemius muscle in rats at 17, 34, and 80–95 days of age. They noted a steady increase in number of nuclei from 17–34 days of age along with a rapid increase in weight/nucleus. From 34–56 days there was a less rapid gain in number of nuclei and in weight/nucleus. Histological study indicated a progressive hypertrophy of muscle fibers. Gordon et al. (1966) reported that hyperplasia of muscle fiber ceases at about 90 days of age in the rat, but hypertrophy continues to approximately 140 days.

Cheek et al. (1968) also have reported on changes in muscle cell population from analysis of DNA in the noncollagen protein in carcass (eviscerated animal minus skin) for male and female rats up to 14 weeks of age. As shown in Fig. 21.7, male rats have considerably more muscle cells than females. Following castration, however, muscle cell number in males approaches that of females, suggesting an androgen effect on muscular growth.

Sex differences in muscle cell number and size in humans have been observed. In boys, the increase in muscle cell number from 2 months to 16 years of age is fourteenfold (Cheek, 1968). There is a marked increase in muscle cell number at 10.5 years of age so that when number of cells is plotted against age there is a steep slope from age 10.5 to age 16 (Fig. 21.8). On the other hand, muscle cell number increases linearly for girls and after age 11 is well below the levels reported for males.

Cheek (1968) also has compared cell size as determined by protein/DNA ratio with body size (indicated by total body water) in boys and girls (Fig. 21.9). Muscle

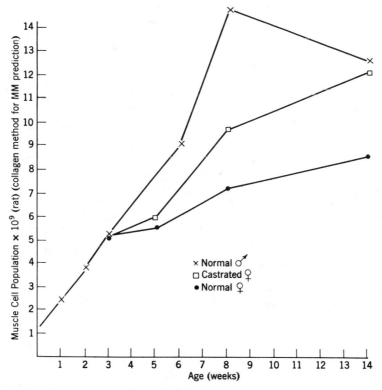

Figure 21.7
The increase in the muscle cell population of female rats is compared
with that of the male. Note the lesser number of muscle cells in the
female. Castrated female rats show muscle cell growth resembling more
that of the male. The value for the number of muscle nuclei for males
at 8 weeks equals 15.09 ± 1.38 and at 14 weeks the value is 12.52
± 1.56 (p < 0.02). At 22 weeks the value is 12.30 ± 1.33. Possibly
the peak for the muscle nuclei at 8 weeks is due to enhanced mitoses.
(From D. B. Cheek, ed., *Human Growth,* Lea and Febiger, Philadelphia,
1968, p. 311).

cell size tends to increase linearly in boys. In girls, muscle cell size is higher than
that for boys throughout childhood and early adolescence. Thereafter muscle cell
size increases in male and surpasses that of females.

ADIPOSE TISSUE

Some of the technical difficulties in the assessment of cellular growth in adipose
tissue were alluded to earlier. Early work using total fat depot DNA indicated that
DNA content continues to increase well into adulthood in rats (Enesco and Leblond, 1962). However, the osmium-fixation method used by Hirsch and Han

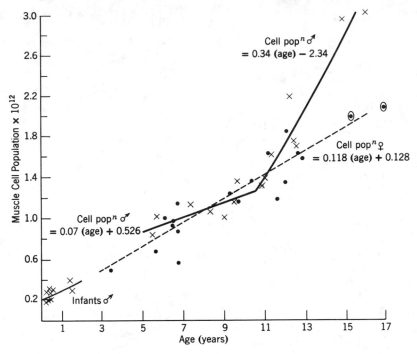

Figure 21.8
Muscle cell population against age is shown for male infants, for boys, and for girls. Note the sex difference and the breaking line relationship (or quadratic relationship) for boys. The intersection of the two lines for boys occurs at $10\frac{1}{2}$ years. The points with a circle represent sexually mature girls. (From D. B. Cheek, ed., *Human Growth,* Lea and Febiger, Philadelphia, 1968, p. 345).

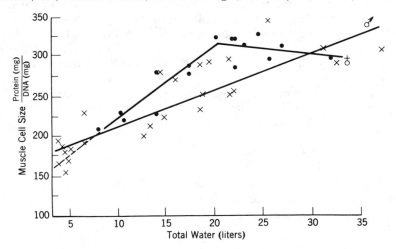

Figure 21.9
The changes in muscle cell size with growth are shown for male infants, boys, and girls. Note that the increase in cell size for girls outstrips that for boys but eventually boys overtake girls and finally have bigger muscle cells. (From D. B. Cheek, ed., *Human Growth,* Lea and Febiger, Philadelphia, 1968, p. 345).

(1969) indicated that fat cell number increases until 10–14 weeks of age and fat cell size increases until at least 26 weeks of age (Fig. 21.10). A later study in which ^{3}H-thymidine was incorporated into adipocytes indicated that fat cells developed as much as 2–3 months earlier than would be detected by the osmium-fixation method (Greenwood and Hirsch, 1974). Most of the fat cells in the rat developed by 5 weeks of age but contained no lipid. These results were supported

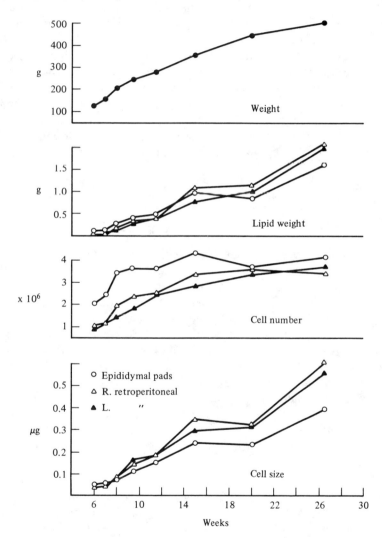

Figure 21.10
Observations of adipose cellularity at eight different times during growth and development of Sprague-Dawley rats. The large increase in fat accumulation between 19 and 26.5 weeks is clearly related to change in cell size rather than to an increase in cell number. In earlier intervals, both processes are involved in the growth of the depot. (From J. Hirsch and P. Han, *J. Lipid Res.* 10:77, 1969.)

by measurements of thymidine kinase and DNA polymerase activity. The activity of these enzymes was virtually nonexistent after 35 days of age (Cleary et al., 1979). In addition, the proportion of lipid-filled fat cells varies with age as a percent of total DNA. Cell size in adipose as in other tissues changes little in the early postnatal period but increases thereafter (Hirsch and Han, 1969; Cleary et al., 1977).

Reports on the integrated changes in fat cell size and number during normal development in humans are conflicting and may be attributed to the different techniques used and to small sample size. Hirsch and Knittle (1970) reported a threefold increase in fat cell number during the first year of life followed by a slower gradual increase until adolescence. Final cell number was attained after age 13. Fat cell size increased rapidly during the first two years of life followed by little change up to age 13. Adult fat cell size was reached at a later time. Additional work by Knittle et al. (1977) appeared to confirm these findings for children over 2 years of age. In contrast, Hager et al. (1977) found little change in fat cell number during the first year of life but a large increase in fat cell size.

Effect of Diet on Cellular Growth

Until recently, the emphasis on dietary interaction with cellular growth focused on undernutrition, and techniques were developed to induce undernutrition in animals. Early studies suggested that malnutrition in young animals and children can result in permanent growth retardation and that the likelihood of permanent damage is greater the earlier the period of undernutrition (Dunn et al., 1947). Systematic studies of the effects of undernutrition at various periods in the life of rats were carried out by McCance and Widdowson. (See Widdowson, 1964; McCance and Widdowson, 1974.) Malnutrition was produced in rats during the suckling period (the first 3 weeks of life) by increasing the size of the litter suckled by one dam to 17–20 young. These young were unable to obtain enough milk from the lactating female and therefore grew poorly. Other rats were suckled in small groups of 3 rats; these animals grew rapidly and were moderately over-nourished. At weaning, all animals were given unlimited access to food. The undernourished rats grew rapidly for a few weeks, then weight gain slackened and at 100 weeks of age they were considerably smaller than the initially well nourished rats (Fig. 21.11).

When well nourished rats were restricted in food intake from the third to sixth week and then allowed to refeed, they also grew rapidly at the outset of refeeding but never attained the full body size of rats well nourished for the entire period (Fig. 21.12). However, final body weight was much greater than that of animals subjected to malnutrition during the first three weeks of life.

When food restriction occurred as late as the ninth to twelfth week of life no permanent effect on growth resulted (Fig. 21.13). Animals rapidly attained normal weight and even slightly surpassed their continually well nourished counterparts.

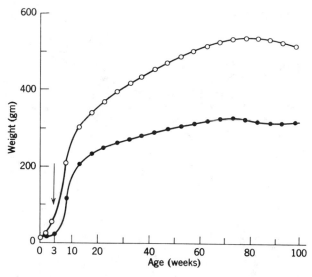

Figure 21.11
Body weight of rats suckled in small (○) and large (●) litters. Arrow shows weaning. (From R. A. McCance and E. M. Widdowson, *Proc. R. Soc. London B,* 156:326, 1962.)

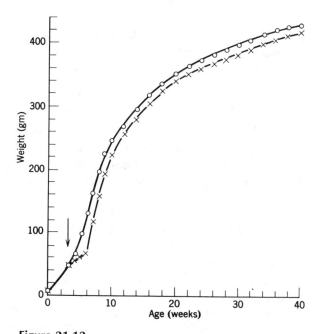

Figure 21.12
The effect of undernutrition from the 3rd to the 6th week of life on the growth in weight of rats suckled in small groups. ○, unlimited food after weaning; x, unlimited food after the 6th week. Arrow shows weaning. (From E. M. Widdowson and R. A. McCance, *Proc. R. Soc. London B,* 158:329, 1963.)

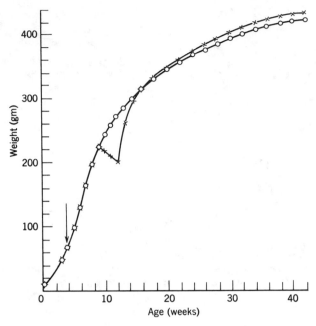

Figure 21.13

The effect of undernutrition from the 9th to the 12th week on the growth in weight of rats suckled in small groups. o, unlimited food after weaning; x, unlimited food except from the 9th to the 12th week. Arrow shows weaning. (From E. M. Widdowson and R. A. McCance, *Proc. Roy. Soc. B,* 158:329, 1963.)

These studies clearly demonstrate that undernutrition in very early life in the rat results in permanent growth stunting and, further, that beyond a certain period of life transient undernutrition has no long-term effect on growth.

Cellular Basis for Permanent Growth Retardation

In a classic study, Winick and Noble (1966) tested a hypothesis to establish the cellular basis for permanent growth retardation in animals subjected to malnutrition in early life. They reasoned that if malnutrition occurred during the period of cell division, permanent damage would result; but if malnutrition occurred when cell size only was affected then the animal likely would recover. Since the timing of periods of cellular growth of different organs was known to be different it was expected that the critical period would vary from organ to organ.

In order to test this hypothesis, three groups of animals were subjected to food deprivation during one of three periods: birth to 21 days of age, 21–42 days, and 65–82 days. Following the period of food restriction, animals were allowed access to unlimited food until they reached 133 days of age when the experiment was terminated. Analyses for DNA, RNA, and protein were made on organs from groups of animals at the end of the restriction period and at the end of the recovery period. *Ad libitum*-fed animals of the same age served as controls. Weight and DNA content of some organs following food restriction are shown in Table 21.4 and the same data following refeeding are shown in Table 21.5. In general, RNA and protein content of the animal body and organs followed the pattern for weight.

Food restriction resulted in reduced weight, total protein, and RNA in all animals regardless of the timing of the period of malnutrition. DNA, however, was lowered only in those organs in which cell division was occurring at the time of food deprivation. When food intake was restricted from birth to 21 days of age (when cell division is most rapid in all organs), animals failed to recover body or organ size because of the permanent decrease in cell number. In animals who were restricted from 21–42 days of age, all organs were permanently reduced in cell number and size except brain and lung (cell division had ceased in these organs prior to the period of food deprivation). In animals 65–82 days of age at the time of food restriction, cell number was reduced only in the lymphoid organs (thymus and spleen) although cell size was reduced to varying degrees in all organs, as indicated by decreased organ weight without reduction in DNA content. At the end of refeeding, recovery was complete for all organs except thymus.

With this simple but elegant study, Winick and Noble (1966) defined the events occurring at the cellular level which clarified the significance of timing of nutri-

TABLE 21.4

Weight and DNA Content of Animal and Organs after Food Restriction

| | Period of Restriction | | | | | |
| | Birth–21 days | | 21–42 days | | 65–82 days | |
	Weight gm	DNA mg	Weight gm	DNA mg	Weight gm	DNA mg
Whole animal: control	59	97.8	119	—	267	—
restricted	29	42.2	62	—	188	—
Brain: control	1.49	2.18	1.59	2.94	1.80	3.28
restricted	1.23	1.48	1.40	2.81	1.67	3.39
Lung: control	0.39	1.96	1.11	3.17	1.50	3.56
restricted	0.14	1.06	0.64	3.48	1.16	3.61
Heart: control	0.36	0.622	0.65	0.798	1.01	1.39
restricted	0.19	0.377	0.55	0.698	0.75	1.33
Thymus: control	0.33	2.74	0.38	10.3	0.75	1.06
restricted	0.07	0.99	0.15	2.85	0.43	0.76
Spleen: control	0.29	2.30	0.48	5.29	0.77	10.62
control	0.06	0.76	0.17	2.07	0.30	2.67

Source: Adapted from M. Winick and A. Noble. *J. Nutr.* 89: 300 (1966).

TABLE 21.5
Weight and DNA Content of Animal and Organs after Refeeding

	Period of Restriction					
	Birth-21 days		21–42 days		65–82 days	
	Weight gm	DNA mg	Weight gm	DNA mg	Weight gm	DNA mg
Whole animal: control	376	—	382	—	374	—
restricted	297	—	314	—	379	—
Brain: control	1.88	3.10	1.92	2.97	1.87	3.02
restricted	1.60	2.42	1.88	2.92	1.91	3.13
Lung: control	2.21	3.34	2.19	3.28	2.16	3.18
restricted	1.87	1.82	2.20	3.20	2.10	3.22
Heart: control	1.42	1.43	1.31	1.40	1.28	1.47
restricted	0.94	1.12	1.01	1.09	1.34	1.45
Thymus: control	0.72	1.47	0.65	1.30	0.65	1.32
restricted	0.40	0.82	0.29	0.96	0.33	1.07
Spleen: control	0.56	0.68	0.60	10.58	0.58	10.06
restricted	0.37	6.94	0.48	7.63	0.59	9.94

Source: Adapted from M. Winick and A. Noble, *J. Nutr.* 89: 300 (1966).

tional insult on later development of the animal. Cell division is time dependent. Thus, reduction in cell number as a result of undernutrition results in permanent stunting of growth.

The effects of increased energy intake during critical periods of cell proliferation have received little attention. The assumption is that overnutrition would lead to increases in cell number. Rats raised in small litters (3–4) are larger than rats raised in normal or large litters. (See Widdowson, 1964; McCance and Widdowson, 1974.) The overnourished rats have increased amounts of DNA in various organs, but cell sizes, assessed by protein/DNA and RNA/DNA, are not affected. However, overnutrition in rats raised in small litters does appear to increase both number and size of fat cells compared with pups raised in either normal or large litters (Knittle and Hirsch, 1968; Johnson et al., 1973; Faust et al., 1980).

Malnutrition and Cellular Growth of Specific Tissues

PLACENTA

Malnutrition during gestation markedly reduces placental weight (Winick, 1968; Zamenhof et al., 1971) essentially because of a decrease in cell number. Cell size remains normal. Winick (ibid) reported that rats fed a severely deficient protein diet (5 percent casein) from day 5 of gestation had small placentas con-

TABLE 21.6
Effect of Maternal Malnutrition on Rat Placenta

Parameter	Mg/Placenta	
	Control	Experimental
Weight	0.405	0.320
Protein	23.0	21.7
RNA	1.00	1.80
DNA	1.06	0.82
RNA/DNA	0.99	2.10
Protein/DNA	27.0	28.2

Source: From M. Winick, *Diagnosis and Treatment of Fetal Disorders,* Springer Verlag, New York, 1969.

taining reduced amounts of DNA and protein but elevated levels of RNA (Table 21.6). As a result, RNA/DNA ratio is about twice that for normal placental tissue. The significance of this finding is not known. High RNA/DNA ratios are found in tissues requiring protein synthesis. The increase in RNA/DNA may represent an attempt by the organ to promote protein synthesis by a compensatory increase in RNA synthesis per cell.

Reduction in cell number in placental tissue apparently also occurs in human undernutrition. Examination of placentas from a population in which undernutrition was common indicated a reduction in cell number as compared with placentas obtained from well nourished women (Winick et al., 1972). Incidence of low birth weight infants was also high in this undernourished population and may reflect intrauterine growth retardation resulting from maternal malnutrition.

BRAIN

More attention has been given to the effect of malnutrition on cell growth in brain than in any other body tissue. The studies of Winick and Noble (1966) indicated that brain weight and cell number were decreased when rats were subjected to undernutrition during the first 3 weeks of life and that these changes could not be reversed by subsequent adequate feeding. Undernutrition later in life produced a reduction in cell size only, which was readily reversed in the nutritionally rehabilitated animal. This work was rapidly confirmed and extended by a number of investigators. Guthrie and Brown (1968) subjected rats to malnutrition for 3, 5, 7, and 9 weeks after birth. Depression of brain weight and DNA was no greater in the nutritionally rehabilitated rats that had been undernourished for 5–9 weeks than for those that had been undernourished for only 3 weeks. These data indicate that undernutrition beyond the critical period in postnatal brain development is of no further detriment to the animal.

Decrease in brain cell number as a result of undernutrition in postnatal life is due almost entirely to reduction in cells of the cerebellum. According to Chase et al. (1969), cells of the cerebrum are not affected. When fetal growth retardation

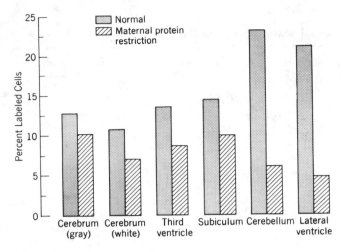

Figure 21.14
Effect of maternal protein restriction on regional DNA content
of fetal brain. (From M. Winick, *Fed. Proc.* 29:1510, 1970.)

occurs as a result of maternal dietary restriction, the number of cells of the cerebral region also is reduced although not nearly to the extent of those of cerebellar (Fig. 21.14). Other areas of the brain also are markedly affected. Malnutrition during either prenatal or postnatal life results in a reduction of brain cells to about 85 percent of normal. The combined effects of nutritional insult in both prenatal and postnatal life result in a reduction of cell number to 40 percent of normal brain (Winick, 1980).

Undernutrition during the first 3 weeks of life also was shown to interfere with the synthesis of lipids in rat brain. This results in substantially reduced quantities of cholesterol (Dobbing, 1964), cerebroside (Culley and Mertz, 1965), and slightly reduced amounts of phospholipid (Culley and Mertz, ibid.) It was found that the incorporation of sulfatide into myelin of rat brain is reduced both *in vivo* and *in vitro* and that the activity of galactocerebroside sulfokinase, the enzyme catalyzing the incorporation of sulfatide, also is reduced (Chase et al., 1969). Myelination is retarded when undernutrition occurs early in life (Fishman et al., 1971), but is relatively unaffected in the later phase of myelination even under the condition of severe undernutrition (Fishman et al., 1972).

In children, malnutrition during the first year of life results in a reduction in the number of brain cells. Brain tissue of children who died of malnutrition before age one was found to contain fewer cells than normal. Children who died of protein-energy malnutrition at an older age and who presumably were reasonably well nourished during the first year of life had brains of normal cell number but somewhat lower in cell size (Winick, 1970). Thus the protein/DNA ratio was reduced. These data are similar to observations in rats and confirm that, in the human, malnutrition during the first year of life interferes with cell division.

Malnutrition beyond 1 year interferes with cell size only. In the latter case, recovery should have been possible had the children lived.

MUSCLE

Muscle tissue is markedly affected by malnutrition during both prenatal and postnatal life. Widdowson (1970) reported that the quadriceps muscle of guinea pigs born of poorly nourished mothers weighed about half as much as muscle from young of well nourished mothers. Protein content was reduced about half; DNA was reduced by about one-quarter. Muscle fiber size was normal, but the number of muscle fibers was markedly reduced. Undernutrition during the period of hyperplastic growth in rats also results in a decrease in muscle DNA (Winick and Noble, 1965; Cheek, 1968; Graystone and Cheek, 1969; Howarth, 1972; Srivasta et al., 1974; Millward et al., 1975).

Food restriction in the postnatal rat results in proportionate decreases in DNA and protein in gastrocnemius muscle so that cell number is reduced but cell size remains essentially normal (Winick and Noble, 1966). In rats above the age of 65 days, only cell size is affected and complete recovery from the effects of undernutrition is attained when the animals are allowed an adequate diet. Similarly, Graystone and Cheek (1969) found muscle cell size to be normal or large in young rats fed a diet restricted in calories but adequate in protein and other nutrients. However, cell division was decreased as was total muscle mass.

Protein intake may have a greater effect on rat muscle growth than energy intake. For example, a reduction in both DNA content and protein/DNA ratio was observed in muscles of young rats fed diets low in both protein and energy (Hill et al., 1970). Diets adequate in protein but restricted in energy produced a less severe response on muscle growth. For reviews of studies in rats, see Trenkle (1974) and Young (1974).

In contrast, marked reductions in muscle cell size occurred in infants suffering from malnutrition during the first year of life (Cheek and Hill, 1970). After rehabilitation, the number of muscle nuclei increased to normal for the body size of the child, but cells did not attain normal size. Cheek and Hill (ibid) suggest that these differences are due to differences in the type of food restriction imposed. In protein-energy restriction small muscle fibers are found, but with low calorie intake (as in their animal studies) muscle size is normal or increased. These results suggest that the nature of the nutritional insult as well as the timing of the insult may affect the cellular response to undernutrition.

ADIPOSE TISSUE

Until recently it was assumed that fat cell number was determined during some early critical phase of development. It now appears that this may not be the case. Examination of older animals has shown increases in fat cell number in some depots (Bertrand et al., 1980). This increase is prevented in normal rats by chronic food restriction (ibid). Genetically obese rats have increases in both fat cell size and number (Johnson et al., 1971). In these animals fat depots continue to develop even when food is restricted during the suckling period (Johnson et al., 1973), postweaning (Zucker, 1967; Martin and Gahagan, 1977), or both pre- and post-weaning (Cleary et al., 1980). The development of the hyperplastic obesity occurs at the expense of lean body mass (Cleary et al., ibid) and normal muscle growth (Shapira et al., 1980; Cleary and Vasselli, 1981).

A high fat diet may increase body weight and fat cell number in susceptible strains of rats (Schemmel et al., 1970; Faust et al., 1978; Obst et al., 1981). When these fat cells have developed, weight loss does not decrease fat cell number (Faust et al., ibid).

Most studies on abnormal human adipose tissue development have focused on overnutrition and its contribution to obesity. Unfortunately, few of these studies

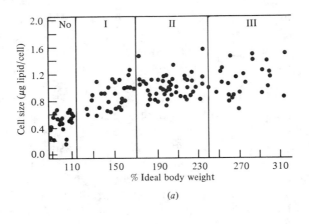

(a)

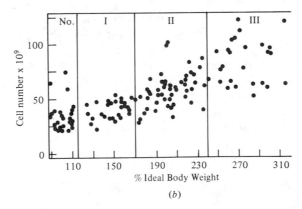

(b)

Figure. 21.15
(a) Fat cell size in comparison to % ideal body weight. (b) Fat cell number in comparison to % ideal body weight. (From J. Hirsch and B. Batchelor, *Clin. Endocrinol. Metabolism* 5:299, 1976.)

include data on fat cell number. Knittle et al. (1977; 1979) reported no statistical difference in body weight or fat cell size and number during the first year of life in children who subsequently developed hyperplastic obesity and those who did not. No food intake data were reported for these children. It is clear that children who develop obesity during childhood have greatly increased fat cell numbers, but the contribution of overeating has been difficult to assess.

Dietary restriction to prevent or treat obesity in children can halt the increase in fat cell number if energy restriction is severe (Knittle, 1974). However, in a study of severely obese 8 to 10-year-old girls who were treated by both diet and exercise over a period of 18 months, there was a significant increase in fat cell number when compared with a control population (Hager et al., 1978). In the human, as in the rat, once fat cells have developed, they are there to stay.

Two primary types of obesity have been correlated with the age of onset of obesity in both humans and animals. Hyperplastic-hypertrophic obesity, characterized by increases in both fat cell number and size, has been associated with an early or juvenile onset. Hypertrophic obesity, in which there is an increase in fat cell size only, has been associated with adult onset. This classification was derived from both human and animal studies. However, the recent reports of increases in fat cell number in adult rats fed high fat diets and hyperplastic obesity in adult humans have brought this classification under scrutiny. Data from a large number of subjects indicate that the amount of body fat correlates best with fat cell number (Fig. 21.15) and, according to Hirsch and Batchelor (1976), classification according to age of onset is valid in most cases.

Malnutrition, Mental Development, and Behavior

Few recent developments in the area of nutritional science have attracted as much public attention as the possible effect of early malnutrition on later mental development and behavior. The observation that children suffering from protein-energy malnutrition were apathetic, listless, and unresponsive to environmental stimuli suggested that there may have been an impairment in learning behavior that persisted during and following nutritional rehabilitation. Detailed observations on children who had recovered from protein-energy malnutrition suggested that there was some impairment in learning ability as compared with other children living in the same social environment (Cravioto and Robles, 1965; Cravioto et al., 1966). It was not clear, however, if the apparent retardation was a reflection of lowered intelligence or a retardation in the development of learning behavior as a result of loss of learning time. Cravioto et al. (1966) suggested that malnutrition could act in two ways: one deriving from a direct interference with the development of the central nervous system (as indicated from studies with experimental animals), and a second from a series of indirect effects including interference with learning during a critical period of development and changes in motivation and personality. Learning progresses in stages. By failing to respond to learning stimulation during the period of malnutrition, the child would become less able to benefit from later experiences. As a result the child would fail to learn because there was no foundation for the next developmental stage.

Most of the early animal experiments were designed to test the hypothesis that early malnutrition produced irreversible damage to the central nervous system which would be reflected in "animal intelligence" and could be measured by problem-solving tests. As an example, Barnes et al. (1966) used a Y-shaped water maze to evaluate the learning of visual discrimination. Subsequent studies in a number of laboratories tended to show that the *behavioral* responses of previously malnourished animals were perhaps more significant than scores on tests of "learning" (Barnes, 1967; Levitsky and Barnes, 1970). Studies of animal behavior have shown a lack of exploratory behavior as evidenced by limited activity when given free access to an "open field" (Frankova and Barnes, 1968a; Guthrie, 1968; Simonson et al., 1971; Hsueh et al., 1973), by increased excitability, and heightened emotional activity (Frankova and Barnes, 1968b; Guthrie, 1968; Simonson et al., 1971). The most characteristic change in adult behavior according to Levitsky and Barnes (1970) is in emotional responsiveness.

Early social or environmental isolation have been shown to result in an increase in emotional responsiveness in the adult rat whereas various forms of environmental stimulation (such as daily handling) have been shown to decrease emotionality. Levitsky and Barnes (1972) therefore studied the interactions between early malnutrition and environmental conditions on various aspects of adult behavior. Environmental stimulation was provided by handling the rats for three minutes once a day and providing a 1-hour "play" period five days a week with five other animals in a box containing toys. The results of the experiment indicated that the behavioral effects of early malnutrition were completely eliminated by environmental stimulation early in life although these animals were severely retarded in body weight (and presumably in brain weight and brain cell number). Thus, it would seem that the structural and biochemical deficits of brain resulting from early malnutrition cannot account entirely for learning and behavioral problems in later life.

The protective effect of early stimulation is not well understood but possibly could be due to a true physiological effect on brain tissue. Bennett et al. (1969) demonstrated that brain weight of malnourished rats allowed access to toys and other environmental stimuli were comparable with those of normal controls. The effect of stimulation also could be entirely behavioral in nature. Thus, as Cravioto et al. (1966) suggested earlier, the effect of malnutrition on development as reflected in intellectual performance may be due to the behavioral responses resulting from malnutrition. Monckeberg et al. (1972) also have stressed the significance of the interaction of malnutrition and environment on mental development in the human.

It is clear from animal studies that malnutrition in early life is associated both with defects in development of the central nervous system and with impaired behavioral response. Observations on malnourished children (Cravioto and Robles, 1965; Cravioto et al., 1966; Winick, 1970; Hertzig, 1972) suggest that similar effects occur in the human. Although extrapolations from animal studies to humans must be made with caution, as Dobbing (1973) has warned, the beneficial effects of environmental stimulation on subsequent behavioral development of malnourished animals may apply to the malnourished human as well. Indeed, a number of studies have shown that environmental enrichment of deprived populations can improve development (Campbell and Stanley, 1966; Caldwell, 1967; Schaeffer and Aaronson, 1972; Winick et al., 1975). Winick et al. (ibid) studied the effects of previous undernutrition on subsequent development of Korean children adopted into American families prior to age two. Some of the children had been severely undernourished prior to adoption. Subsequent examinations between the ages of 7–16 showed no effect of previous undernutrition on body weight (using Korean standards), nor was there a significant difference in I.Q. between previously undernourished and adequately nourished children. For a more extensive review of malnutrition and mental development, see Winick (1979).

The effect of specific nutrients on brain function was discussed in Chapter 19.

Conclusion

Cellular growth is a carefully regulated process that proceeds in three stages: hyperplasia, hyperplasia with simultaneous hypertrophy, and hypertrophy alone. Hyperplasia represents the critical stage in development and occurs in different organs for varying periods of time. Undernutrition during the period of cell division results in permanent growth retardation. Undernutrition at any time following the period of cell division results in reduction of cell size from which the system can recover with adequate feeding. The effect of overnutrition, particularly in adipose tissue during different stages of development, is less well defined and is an area for future studies.

chapter 22

body composition

Primitive man believed that by consuming the flesh of an animal he would acquire the characteristics of that animal: that eating the lion's heart would make a person brave, but a jackal's heart would make him timid; the deer's flesh would make him swift, but the bear's, clumsy. One might interpret such statements as evidence that humans, from earliest times, suspected that the food they ate became part of their substance and contributed specific characteristics. Such interpretation, perhaps, attributes unwarranted prescience to our forebears, but, despite the mask of Greek mythology, drinking the water in which a steel sword rusted could lead to the acquisition of strength if the individual happened to be anemic, and such practices and rites could indeed influence the composition of the body.

The Arabic scientist, Al-Biruni, who lived in the first half of the eleventh century stated in his Book of Drugs: *". . . the body in equilibrium has the power to transform nutriment into its own substance by complete digestion and by assimilation, thus replacing what part of the diet has been lost by disassimilation. That is the reason why the body must act* on food before it can derive any benefit from it." (See Taton, 1963.) And in Hamlet, Shakespeare said, "A man may fish with the worm that hath eat of a king, and eat of the fish that hath fed of that worm." A vivid illustration of the cycle of Nature and the continuity of matter; yet this predates by 200 years Lavoisier's experimental establishment of the Law of Conservation of Mass! Indeed, we could idly speculate about elements in our body constituents that at one time might have contributed to Pepys' dyspepsia or Solomon's sagacity.

What started as magic and progressed through myth and into the arena of science has come within the purview of the physical anthropologist, the physicist, the radiologist, the physician, as well as the various "sects" in human biology. Perhaps of greatest concern to the nutritionist are the compositional changes associated with the entire life cycle from the developing embryo to the extremes of aging. If we can assume that compositional changes determine nutrient needs, then knowledge of changing body composition constitutes the matériel for nutritionists.

Except for a few isolated studies, all the reported work investigating human body composition has appeared within the last 45 years and was inaugurated by the first of a series of papers from Behnke's laboratory (1941–42). Although the literature has become extensive and the methodology expanded, it is still easy to agree with Brozek (1961), who suggested that "the field is in the state of late adolescence rather than full-blown maturity."

Methods

During the last few decades, the interest centered on the estimation of the chemical composition of the human body has led to the development of nondisruptive methods, some of which give some insight into the dynamic state of metabolism. Final tests of their validity would be a comparison with data from chemical analysis. The purpose of this section is not to delve deeply into the specifics of each method but to understand the rationale behind them and the parameters they measure.

CHEMICAL ANALYSIS

Ways of estimating chemical composition of the human appear at first to be both obvious and impossible: obvious because the gross chemical composition of most

680   THE COMPLEX ORGANISM

TABLE 22.1
Percentage of Water and Fat in Five Adult Bodies

Subject	2	3	4	5	7
Age	46	60	48	25	42
Weight as percentage of standard	84	110	95	100	70
Percentage of fat in body	19.4	27.0	4.3	14.9	23.6
Percentage of water in body	55.1	51.4	70.8	61.8	56.0

Source: From E. M. Widdowson, *Human Body Composition,* J. Brozek, ed., Pergamon Press, Oxford, 1965, p. 35.

biological materials can be determined by analytical laboratory procedures; impossible because chemical dissection of humans today is frowned on just slightly less than anatomical dissection was in Leonardo da Vinci's day. However, despite mores and the tedious unpleasantness of the work, several nineteenth-century investigators reported on chemical analyses of human cadavers. (See McCance and Widdowson, 1951.) Not until the middle of the twentieth century were the results of detailed chemical analyses of adults published in the United States by Mitchell et al. (1945) and by Forbes et al. (1953; 1956), and in England by Widdowson and her coworkers (1951). A compilation by Widdowson (1965) of the data from these original studies which utilized dissimilar laboratory techniques revealed that the most variable body constituent was fat and this, of course, was no real surprise (Table 22.1). However, when calculations were made on the basis of fat-free tissue, the largest constituent, water, was shown to be remarkably

TABLE 22.2
Composition of the Fat-Free Body Tissue of Five Adults

Subject	2	3	4	5	7	Mean
Water, %	69.4	70.4	73.0	72.5	73.2	71.7
Total N, g/kg	37.5	38.1	33.0	31.1	31.0	34
Na, meq/kg	82.6	78.2	—	92	97	80[a]
K, meq/kg	66.5	66.6	—	71.5	73	69
Cl, meq/kg	43.9	55.5	—	—	—	50
Ca, g/kg	24.0	21.5	20.7	21.3	24.8	22.4
P, g/kg	11.6	11.3	11.1	14.0	12.9	12.0
Mg, g/kg	—	0.49	0.47	0.48	0.43	0.47
Fe, mg/kg	—	—	—	87.5	60.0	74
Cu, mg/kg	—	—	—	1.6	1.8	1.7
Zn, mg/kg	—	—	—	33.3	22.0	28
B, mg/kg	0.30	0.36	0.45	—	—	0.37
Co, mg/kg	0.022	0.024	0.018	—	—	0.021

Source: From E. M. Widdowson, *Human Body Composition,* J. Brozek, ed., Pergamon Press, Oxford, 1965, p. 37.

[a]Mean of subjects 2 and 3 only.

consistent, as were the electrolytes associated with body water (Table 22.2). The greatest range in these studies was apparent in the quantities of iron reflecting obvious differences in intakes coupled with limited capacity of the body to excrete this mineral. The data are expressed on a fat-free basis in order to compensate for the most variable component, the adipose stores. Essential lipid, which is part of every cell, is not included in the fat-free body in Table 22.2.

The disadvantages of direct analysis, both apparent and real, coupled with the importance of studying living organisms, led to the exploration of various indirect approaches to the problem of body composition.

NUTRITIONAL ANTHROPOMETRY

Even to the unpracticed eye, body measurements are a fair indication of the stores of fat, and thus of relative body composition. Certainly body weight has been used (and misused) as such a measure and often can give a fair indication of the magnitude of adipose stores in an individual. However, if body measurements are to be used for assessing human nutriture, it is apparent that selection and standardization of measurements are essential. A Committee on Nutritional Anthropometry, established by the Food and Nutrition Board of the National Research Council, employed the combined talents of physical anthropologists and nutritionists. The report of the Committee (Brozek, 1956) lists the minimum number of measurements that would indicate skeletal build and the thickness of subcutaneous fat: height, weight, and skinfold thickness.

Although height-weight relationships are the most readily attained parameters for comparison and are simple to use, they are neither definitive nor instructive by themselves. Gross departures from norms become evident but probably would be so by visual appraisal. One danger inherent in the use of such tables is the attempt to evaluate population groups of unlike genetic and nutritional backgrounds with norms for the United States. However, comparison within groups can be informative (Mitchell, 1963).

Various simple indices for estimating adiposity have been utilized that are based on weight (W) and height (H). These include W/H, W/H^2 (Quetelet index or body mass index (BMI)), $W^{1/3}/H$ (Ponderal index), $H/W^{1/3}$ (Sheldon index), H^3/W (Nicholson and Zilvas leanness index), W/H^3 (Rohrer index). An analysis of these indices for estimating obesity was made by Watson et al. (1979) who found that W/H and W/H^2 were the best indication of body fat.

In general, the BMI seems to be most useful. For example, Rolland-Cachera et al. (1982) provided BMI charts and graphs based on age and sex that permit estimation of adiposity in any child. Keys (1980) used the BMI in an analysis of the relationship of obesity to the probability of death from coronary heart disease. Why an expression that relates W/H^2 (BMI), and has the dimensions of mass per unit area, has predictive value in terms of obesity or adiposity remains an interesting question.

Attempts at relating anthropometric measurements to age of children in some parts of the world is difficult when birth dates cannot be verified, and Jelliffe (1969) stressed the need for measurements that are independent of age. So-called age-independent measurements are based on the ratio of a nutritionally labile tissue, such as muscle mass or subcutaneous fat, to a measurement likely to be less affected by acute short-term malnutrition such as height, head circumference, or the length of a single bone. (See Chapter 26.) A suggested measurement of weight for height has the disadvantage of possibly masking a general growth failure with a body weight that is relatively proportional to height (Downs, 1964). Jelliffe and Jelliffe (1971) suggest that in areas where malnutrition is prevalent in childhood, anthropometric tests of nutritional status may have to take into consideration the age incidence of malnutrition in that locale. They suggest the development of composite anthropometric indices including weight, height or possibly arm length, midarm muscle, and fat measurements that might be used to indicate mass, linear growth, and protein and calorie reserves, respectively.

The ease and rapidity of obtaining anthropometric measurements with tape measure and calipers make them extremely attractive for estimating body fat, body muscle, and the weight of the lean body mass. Behnke (1963) presented the formulas used and the data obtained on groups of individuals to support the value of specific body measurements in screening procedures.

The prediction of lean body weight (LBW) through anthropometric assessment, based on equations developed by Behnke, was tested by Wilmore and Behnke (1968) among college-age men. The highest correlation coefficients were achieved when at least five body diameters and four joint thicknesses were measured. The equation employed was

$$LBW = D^2 \times h$$

where D represents the mean of the respective measurements, and h is height in decimeters. The respective diameters in cm were biocromial, bideltoid, chest, bi-iliac, bitrochanteric, knee, ankle, elbow, and wrist. The joint measurements were the sum of the right and left side. Comparisons with lean body weight calculated from body density using different equations yielded correlation coefficients between 0.906 and 0.924. The conclusion was that LBW can be predicted rather accurately from body diameters at least in the relatively normal young adult population. In order to simplify the calculation, Wilmore and Behnke (ibid) recommended that the biocromial, bitrochanteric, wrist, and ankle diameters provide the basis for acceptable prediction; these sites are readily accessible and have well-defined marks.

SKINFOLD THICKNESS

Since the subcutaneous adipose tissue constitutes approximately 50 percent of the adipose tissue stores, skinfold measurements can serve a useful purpose in judging the total body fat of individuals. In addition, they are simple, rapid, easily interpreted, and can be used in the clinic or in the field. Keys and Brozek (1953) have reviewed the literature on skinfold measurements with respect to standardization, sites, and consistency of measurements. Data on young American soldiers were included in the report of the 1956 conference (Newman, 1956; Pascale et al., 1956). At subsequent conferences, data were presented on middle-aged men (Brozek et al., 1963), older women (Young et al., 1963a; Wessel et al., 1963), adolescent boys and girls in different cultures (Young, 1965), and trained and untrained athletes (Pařízková, 1965). A summary of various studies was prepared by Lohman (1981) who compared the accuracy of predicting body density from skinfold measurements. On the average, such predictions of body density are reasonably accurate; inconsistencies may be due to both biological and technical errors.

Standardization of skinfold measurements involves both site of measurement and the pressure exerted by the calipers on the double fold. Specially designed calipers (Fig. 22.1) exert a pressure of 10 gm/mm^2 on a contact surface of 20–40 mm^2. A trained technician using standard calipers on the triceps (Fig. 22.2) or subscapular skinfold can obtain a rapid estimation of total body fatness. Several investigators using only the triceps, which is easiest to measure, have obtained extensive data which permit determination of the normal variation in the American population (Brozek et al., 1963; Seltzer and Mayer, 1965; Seltzer et al., 1965).

A report published by the Department of Health, Education and Welfare (1973a) presents data on the distribution of skinfold measurements, at three anatomical

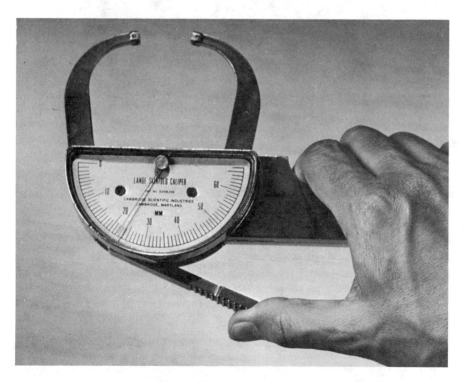

Figure 22.1
A standard skinfold caliper.

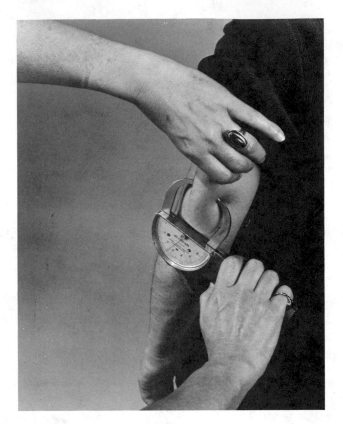

Figure 22.2
Skinfold caliper measuring a relatively thick triceps skinfold
in a young woman.

sites, on children aged 6 through 11 years in the United States. Data on over
7,000 children are discussed as related to age, sex, race, and geographic regions.
This report is one of a continuing series of publications on body dimensions and
composition. A report on height and weight of youths 12 through 17 (DHEW,
1973b) presents an analysis of the adolescent growth spurt.

Garn et al. (1971) studied the relative values of subscapular and triceps fat fold
measurements made under actual field conditions. They found that correlations
of the two measurements were high and that the subscapular fold systematically
had higher correlations with weight than the triceps fat fold. They were able to
demonstrate also that summing the two fat fold measurements did not offer any
advantage. Based on their analysis of the data from the Michigan phase of the
Ten-State Nutrition Survey, they concluded that fat fold measurements effectively
provide indications of fatness under field conditions in a mass scale nutrition
survey. Lohman (1981) found that among young adults the best two skinfolds for

prediction of body density are the abdomen and triceps. The next best sites are the subscapular and thigh.

The triceps fat fold measurement can be used to ascertain the arm muscle circumference through the use of a nomogram. The arm muscle circumference is read where a line joining the fat fold measurement and the arm circumference crosses. Figures are given also for determining the equivalent muscle area, arm area, and fat area (Gurney and Jelliffe, 1973).

A high correlation was shown between pinch-caliper and x-ray measurements of skin and subcutaneous fat (Garn, 1956) and, since the fat-plus-skin thickness at the midaxillary line at the level of the lowest rib can be measured on full-size or miniature chest plates, Garn (1957) suggests that mass radiography as used in tuberculosis detection could be extended to the assessment of obesity. Young et al. (1963b) reported good correlation between skinfold thickness and x-ray measurements of fat-pad thickness made at lower thorax and suprailiac locations in young women. Theoretically, the skinfold measurements should be twice the x-ray measurement since the calipers measure a double thickness; however, a correction has to be made for compression even though standard calipers are used, and Young et al. (1963b) point out that compression varies with location.

Lohman (1981), after a careful review of the use of skinfolds for the calculation of body density (D_B), and hence body fatness, suggests the development of a generalized approach involving:

1. A need for standard measurement procedures.
2. Random sampling and use of large samples with reporting of frequency distributions for body density in order to characterize the peculiarities of the specific sample.
3. Attention to the precise identification of each skinfold site and the technique used in measurement. The abdominal, triceps, and subscapular sites should be included in any series of skinfold measurements.
4. Use of body density as the criterion variable.
5. Recognition of the curvilinear relation between body density and skinfolds.
6. Cross validation of any developed equation on another sample of subjects to test the validity of the equation.

Equations that Lohman (1981) believes have general validity are those of Sloan (1967), Durnin and Womersley (1974), Jackson and Pollock (1978) and Jackson et al. (1980). In addition, Lohman presents the following equation based on the data of Sloan (1967), Sinning (1974), Lohman et al. (1978) and Boileau et al. (1981).

$$D_B = 1.0982 - 0.000815x + 0.0000084x^2$$

where x = the sum of triceps, abdomen, and subscapular skinfolds. The respective equations were developed from measurements of fairly large samples and the approach employed conformed to the suggested recommendations.

Both biological variation and measurement error contribute to the uncertainty of calculation of body density and fatness from skinfold measurements. Biological variation in fatness is associated with age, maturation, sex, and fat distribution. Measurement error is associated with inappropriate selection of skinfold calipers, failure to calibrate the calipers properly, site selection and identification, and intra- and interexaminer error. Lohman (1981) calculated the biological plus technical error to be about 3.3 percent.

A common equation for the calculation of body fatness (f) from body density (D_B) is that proposed by Brozek et al. (1963).

$$f = \frac{4.570}{D_B} - 4.142$$

Another is the equation proposed by Siri (1961)

$$f = \frac{4.95}{D_B} - 4.50$$

Within densities of 1.10–1.03, the two equations yield results within 1 percent. For subjects with more than 30 percent fat, the Siri equation gives higher values than the equation of Brozek et al.

The skinfold method is useful in the appraisal of nutritional status because it is inexpensive, fast, noninvasive, easy to learn, and requires no elaborate technology.

Other procedures that have been used to assess subcutaneous fatness include computed tomography (Borkan et al., 1982) and ultrasound (Bullen et al., 1965; Haymes et al., 1976; Borkan et al., 1982), and electrical conductivity (Booth et al., 1966). These procedures, with the possible exception of the ultrasound technique, are useful for research purposes but are not widely applicable for assessment of body fatness.

BODY DENSITY

Early studies by Behnke et al. (1942) and Welham and Behnke (1942) on Navy personnel, some of whom were overweight according to height-weight standards but obviously not overfat, led to the use of body density for estimating the variable quantity of body fat. From this emerged the concept of *lean body mass*, which they defined as the whole body minus nonessential or excess lipids. The lean body mass was conceived as relatively constant in gross chemical composition, with fat acting as a diluent (Behnke, 1941–1942). The concept was quantitatively expressed by Pace and Rathbun (1945) on the basis of an average water content of 73.2 percent of the lean body mass. On this basis, they developed the equation:

$$\% \text{ body fat} = 100 - \frac{\% \text{ body water}}{0.732}$$

This concept of lean body mass differs from the fat-free body in that essential structural lipids are included. Behnke's group first estimated essential lipids as constituting 10 percent of the total mass, but later this was revised to 2 percent.

Although the concept is different, the discrepancy between the fat-free body and the lean body mass that contains 2 percent essential lipid is negligible.

The rationale of Behnke's group for using body density as an estimate of body composition was based on the concept of a relatively constant lean body mass coupled with a variable fat mass. Since the density of fat is less than that of other body components, as the percentage of body fat increases, the body density decreases. In practice, specific gravity is substituted for density and calculated as weight divided by volume:

$$\text{Sp. gr.} = \frac{W}{V}$$

The essential measurement, body volume, may be obtained by employing Archimedes' principle of water displacement. Body volume therefore is calculated by subtracting the weight under water from the weight in air:

$$V = \text{wt in air} - \text{wt under water}$$

Several methods have been devised for obtaining weight under water, one of which is shown in Fig. 22.3. Corrections must be made for residual air in the lungs.

On the basis of chemical analyses and specific gravity determinations on shaved, eviscerated guinea pigs, Rathbun and Pace (1945) derived an equation for the conversion of specific gravity to percent body fat. The values presented in Table 22.3 are based on the following equation, which was corrected for the density of human fat:

$$\% \text{ body fat} = 100 \left(\frac{5.548}{\text{sp. gr.}} - 5.004 \right)$$

Using this formula and the formula by which percent body fat is derived (shown previously), Pace and Rathbun (1945) derived the equation to predict from specific gravity both the fat content and water content of the whole body:

$$\% \text{ body water} = 100 \left(4.24 - \frac{4.061}{\text{sp. gr.}} \right)$$

Since the estimation of specific gravity involves the use of expensive equipment and an extremely cooperative subject, it cannot be used in the clinic to estimate body fatness. Equations for predicting specific gravity from skinfold thickness measurements of men were presented by Brozek and Keys (1951), and Young et al. (1962) presented a formula for predicting specific gravity of young women from one skinfold measurement and the percentage of "standard weight." The predicted specific gravity then can be converted to percent fat using the Rathbun-Pace formula. Based on such calculations, Young et al. (1962) presented data on the Cornell (University) reference young woman of normal weight (Table 22.4).

The difficulties and restrictions encountered in measuring body density by hydrometry led to the development of methods for measuring body volume by helium

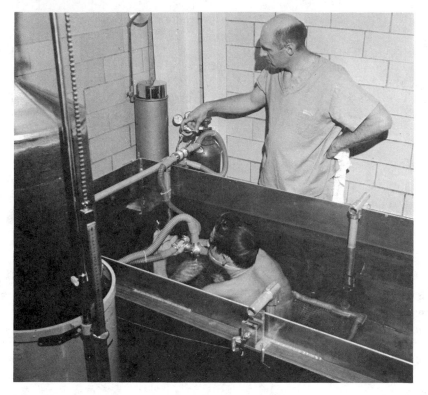

Figure 22.3
Subject in position for obtaining underwater weight which is measured using a suspended metal mesh cot. The outputs from four transducers placed at each corner of the cot frame are balanced and integrated into one voltage that is recorded on a strip chart. The subject bends forward so that his head goes underwater and his weight is recorded. He exhales as he submerges and continues to exhale until he reaches voluntary end-expiration. At this point his breathing circuit is switched to a small demand spirometer and he breathes pure oxygen for seven minutes. The volume of air in his lungs at the time the subject is weighed is determined by the quantity of nitrogen he expires in seven minutes (nitrogen wash-out method for determining the residual volume of the lungs). (Courtesy of Dr. E. R. Buskirk.)

displacement (Siri, 1953; Fomon et al., 1963), by air displacement (Falkner, 1963; Gnaedinger et al., 1963; Gundlach et al., 1980), and by a combination of water (body) and air (head) displacement (Irsigler et al., 1975), each of which obviates the necessity for correcting for residual air in the lungs. However, each of these methods and the chambers they require for use are of value as research tools but do not provide quick and easy means for determining body volume.

TABLE 22.3
Conversion of Values for Body Specific Gravity of Humans to Fat Content on Basis of Equation, Percent Fat = 100 [5.548/(Specific Gravity) Minus 5.044]

Body Sp. Gr.	Percent Fat of Body Weight	Body Sp. Gr.	Percent Fat of Body Weight
1.002	49.3	1.052	23.0
1.004	48.2	1.054	22.0
1.006	47.1	1.056	21.0
1.008	46.0	1.058	20.0
1.010	44.9	1.060	19.0
1.012	43.8	1.062	18.0
1.014	42.7	1.064	17.0
1.016	41.7	1.066	16.1
1.018	40.6	1.068	15.1
1.020	39.5	1.070	14.1
1.022	38.5	1.072	13.1
1.024	37.4	1.074	12.2
1.026	36.3	1.076	11.2
1.028	35.3	1.078	10.3
1.030	34.2	1.080	9.3
1.032	33.2	1.082	8.4
1.034	32.2	1.084	7.4
1.036	31.1	1.086	6.5
1.038	30.1	1.088	5.5
1.040	29.1	1.090	4.6
1.042	28.0	1.092	3.7
1.044	27.0	1.094	2.7
1.046	26.0	1.096	1.8
1.048	25.0	1.098	0.9
1.050	24.0	1.100	0.0

Source: From E. N. Rathbun and N. Pace, *J. Biol. Chem.* 158: 667, 1945.

TABLE 22.4
Cornell Reference Young Woman

	Percent	Percent
Fat	29	0[a]
Water	52	73
Cell solids	14	20
Bone mineral	5	7

Source: From C. M. Young et al., *J. Amer. Diet. Ass.* 40: 102, 1962.
[a]Calculated on fat-free basis.

DILUTION TECHNIQUES

Dilution techniques freed the investigator from the limitations imposed by either chemical analysis of a cadaver or the indirect and somewhat imprecise methods of anthropometry and densitometry for estimation of body composition *in vivo*. The more illusive compartmentalization of body components could now be studied. Dilution methodology is based on the concept that certain substances distribute themselves evenly within a specific body water compartment and that the dilution of a known amount of substance introduced into an unknown volume permits calculation of that unknown volume.

Total Body Water

A comparatively safe and valid approach to measuring total body water as a component of body composition is deuterium oxide dilution (D_2O) or tritium dilution. The latter is a β-emitter and the former a stable isotope. Because deuterium is a stable isotope, it has been used extensively to measure total body water. Orally ingested D_2O is readily absorbed in the gastrointestinal tract and equilibrates with the body water in a few hours. The equilibrium concentration can be determined in blood, urine, or saliva. About 2 percent of D_2 exchanges with H^+ in the body, but this slight correction is easy to make. Apparently D_2O is not selectively excreted by the kidneys and is nontoxic in tracer amounts. A variety of analytical techniques have been used to measure D_2O concentration including infrared absorption, falling drop, freezing point elevation, mass spectrometry, and gas chromatography. All involve elaborate sample preparation by prior distillation or lyophilization. A newer method should provide superior D_2O analysis because it does not require elaborate sample preparation. The raw sample containing D_2O is exposed to gamma ray irradiation with subsequent measurement of neutron emission. In addition, D_2O doses as low as 10–20 gm can be used (Stansell and Hyder, 1976). The combination of total body water and body density measurements improves the accuracy for calculation of body fatness, because body water is one of the largest body compartments.

Simultaneous Multiple Isotope Dilution

D_2O and tritium distribute evenly throughout the total body water and therefore can be used for the determination of total body water. Thiocyanate and inulin distribute themselves within the extracellular fluid but do not penetrate the plasma membrane. The use of simultaneous measurement of total body water and extracellular water permits the calculation of intracellular water by difference.

The most detailed and extensive compilation of data employing the multiple isotope dilution method comes from the laboratories of Moore and his associates at Harvard and the Peter Bent Brigham Hospital in Boston. Table 22.5 indicates the direct measurements that were made employing the multiple isotope dilution technique and those that could then be derived. From this listing, it is readily apparent that research in body composition has attained a certain degree of sophistication. For the methods, both biochemical and statistical, and the detailed

TABLE 22.5
Compositional Ratios and Derivations

Ratio or Derivation	Abbreviation	Dimensions	Normal Range[a]
Total body fat	TBF	kg or % B.Wt.[b]	12–20 % B.Wt.
Total body solids	TBS	kg or % B.Wt.	40–60 % B.Wt.
Fat-free solids	FFS	kg or % B.Wt.	25–40 % B.Wt.
Intracellular water	ICW	L. or % B.Wt.	30–40 B.Wt.
Residual sodium	Res Na	mEq or % Na_e	8–15 % Na_e
Average intracellular potassium concentration	Av. ICK conc.	mEq/liter	140–160 mEq/liter
Ratio of whole body hematocrit to large vessel hematocrit	WBH/LVH	%/%	0.85–0.91
Ratio of total exchangeable sodium to total exchangeable potassium	Na_e/K_e	mEq/mEq	0.85–1.00
Ratio of sum of total exchangeable sodium plus total exchangeable potassium to body weight	$\dfrac{Na_e + K_e}{B.Wt.}$	mEq/kg	70–90 mEq/kg
Concentration of total exchangeable cation (sodium plus potassium) in total body water	$\dfrac{Na_e + K_e}{TBW}$	mEq/liter	150–160 mEq/liter
Body cell mass	BCM	kg or % B.Wt.	35–45 % B.Wt.
Ratio of intracellular water to total body water; relative predominance of the cell	ICW/TBW	liter/liter × 100	50–55%
Ratio of red cell volume to total exchangeable potassium	RV/K_e	ml/mEq	0.50–0.55 ml/mEq
Ratio of total exchangeable potassium to dry body weight	K_e/DBW	mEq/kg	90–110 mEq/kg
Ratio of total exchangeable potassium to fat-free solids	K_e/FFS	mEq/kg	200–250 mEq/kg
Ratio of red cell volume to plasma volume	RV/PV	ml/ml	0.70–0.80
Ratio of plasma volume to total exchangeable sodium	PV/Na_e	ml/mEq	0.95–1.10 ml/mEq
Dry fat-free, marrow-free whole bone (matrix plus mineral)	B	kg or % B.Wt.	6–8 % B.Wt. (10.3 % FFB)
Ratio of total exchangeable potassium to resting 24-hour creatinine excretion	K_e/creatinine	mEq/mg	1.75–2.25 mEq/mg

Source: From F. D. Moore et al., *The Body Cell Mass and Its Supporting Environment*, W. B. Saunders Co., Philadelphia, 1963, p. 20.

[a]Broad range only.

[b]The term "B.Wt." is used for body weight throughout.

data from clinical studies, the reader is referred to the published monograph (Moore et al., 1963). Only a few of the pertinent concepts will be discussed here.

Since total body water (*TBW*) can be determined directly, the formula of Pace and Rathbun (1945) can be employed to calculate the percent of body fat, and from that the simple calculations for total body fat (*TBF*), total body solids (*TBS*), and fat-free solids (*FFS*):

$$(1) \ \% \ fat = 100 - \frac{\% \ water}{0.732}$$

$$(2) \ TBF \ (kg) = \% \ fat \times \frac{B.Wt. \ (kg)}{100}$$

$$(3) \ TBS \ (kg) = B.Wt. \ (kg) - TBW$$

$$(4) \ FFS = TBS - TBF$$

A nomogram illustrating the relationship between the water phase and the fat-free solid phase of the body is shown in Fig. 22.4. The theoretical aspects of the relationship between body water and fat-free solids permit evaluation of both normal and abnormal conditions of hydration on the basis that water content of fat-free tissue normally ranges from 69–74 percent.

From the direct determination of total exchangeable potassium (K_e) by isotope dilution using ^{42}K, another important concept has evolved, that of *body cell mass*. The body cell mass as defined by Moore et al. (1963) is the "chemically homogeneous mass of tissue in the body that contains all the cellular elements concerned with respiration, physical and chemical work, and mitotic activity." It is comprised of all the cells of the body capable of converting or using the chemical energy of food. It does not include the fluids bathing the cells nor any solids outside the cell membrane. The body cell mass is the composite of oxygen-requiring, carbon dioxide-producing, glucose-metabolizing cells of the body and constitutes from 35–45 percent of the body weight in the normal adult male and from 30–40 percent in the adult female. The body cell mass differs from both the *fat-free body* of chemical analysis and the concept of *lean body mass* set forth by Behnke. Each of the latter designations is heterogeneous both in its chemistry and energy exchange and includes not only the metabolizing cells but also skeletal and cartilaginous material, collagen, and other noncellular, nonfat portions which are not actively metabolizing nor even constant in mass.

In contrast, the body cell mass is comprised essentially of two large groups of tissues: muscle, both skeletal and smooth; and parenchyma (heart, brain, liver, kidneys, diaphragm, and endocrine glands). These two moieties differ in that the muscle functions intermittently, resting between contractions, whereas the parenchymal cells are unceasingly involved in the oxidative and synthetic processes basic to all cell life. In terms of total body energy expenditure, the muscle is concerned primarily with "activity" (including gastrointestinal activity) and the parenchyma with the basal metabolic rate.

All cells in the normal body contain potassium at a concentration of approximately 150 mEq/kg cell water (Moore and Boyden, 1963). Potassium is not present

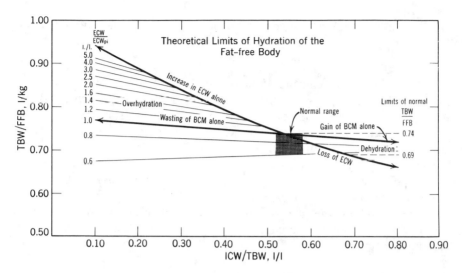

Figure 22.4

Theoretical limits of hydration of the fat-free body. The hydration coefficient of the fat-free body (the ratio TBW/FFB shown on the vertical coordinates) in the normal adult is usually assumed to be 0.732. It is variously estimated by dissection in animals and in humans as varying from 0.67–0.74. These limits of normal (TBW/FFB) are shown to the right, as well as in the shaded area identified as "normal range" and coordinated with an ICW/TBW ratio (horizontal coordinates of 0.51–0.58). This ratio, ICW/TBW, indicates the relative predominance of the cell mass in the aqueous phase of body composition. One other ratio is needed to express relative hydration. This is the ratio of the observed extracellular water to the extracellular water before illness, ECW/ECW_{pi}, shown as an added coordinate to the left. If the body wastes by a loss of body cell mass alone, the average hydration of the fat-free body increases slightly because the average water content of the body cell mass is lower than that of the extracellular fluid within which this wasting occurs. If body composition changes by an increase in extracellular water alone, then average hydration of the fat-free body increases sharply, and this describes the upper limit of body hydration. The overhydration commonly observed in a wide variety of pathological states lies somewhere between these two limits. Its exact position can be estimated by the ratio of extracellular water as observed to that predicted from regression relations, before illness. Given the observed ICW/TBW ratio and the calculated ratio ECW/ECW_{pi}, this diagram can be used as a nomogram to read off the TBW/FFB ratio. From this, in turn, body fat may be calculated with greater accuracy than that resulting from the use of a fixed coefficient such as 0.732. The much rarer dehydration states are described by similar limits and are shown to the right of the normal range. (From F. D. Moore et al., *The Body Cell Mass and Its Supporting Environment*, W. B. Saunders Co., Philadelphia, 1963, p. 16.)

to any extent in the extracellular compartment. Thus the total amount of potassium in the body is a linear function of the body cell mass:

$$BCM \text{ (gm)} = K_e \times 8.33$$

where K_e is the total exchangeable potassium in mEq and 8.33 is the coefficient applied to yield the wet weight of the body cell mass in grams. Moore and Boyden (1963) point out that the coefficient is not precise but lies somewhere between 7.0 and 10.0. Thus the measurement of exchangeable potassium can be converted into body cell mass in grams.

Since the muscle mass may vary widely among individuals or even in the same person, depending on use and state of health, a partition of the K_e into these two components can provide important information. Creatinine excretion is a linear function of the skeletal muscle mass and remains relatively constant in the normal individual. Determination of creatinine excretion permits the calculation of the K_e/creatinine ratio:

$$\text{Muscle mass} = \frac{K_e}{\text{creatinine}}$$

The K_e/creatinine ratio reported for normal subjects in the Moore monograph ranged around 2.0 mEq/mg. Distortions in the ratio are indicative of changes in the relationship between the creatinine-producing and the noncreatinine-producing moieties comprising the body cell mass. As the athlete builds up skeletal muscle, the ratio falls; however, in wasting disease, the ratio rises.

Creatinine excretion alone can be used as a predictor of the mass of muscle tissue since a highly significant linear relationship exists between creatinine excretion during growth and muscle mass. A factor of 20 was derived by Cheek (1968, p. 191) indicating 1 gm of urinary creatinine per day as equivalent to 20 kg of muscle mass, and he presented equations suggesting that this factor could be used with a high degree of confidence. Nevertheless, there is considerable individual variability in urinary creatinine excretion complicated by a diurinal pattern of excretion. Muscular exercise, dietary creatine and creatinine from meat and fish, dietary restriction or fasting, and other factors modify creatinine excretion so that the coefficient of variation has been found to range between 2 and 30 percent (Boileau et al., 1972).

A recent analysis suggests that total plasma creatinine (i.e., the plasma volume multiplied by the plasma creatinine concentration) may provide a more reliable estimate of striated muscle mass. Schutte et al. (1981) found that each milligram of total plasma creatinine represented 0.88 kg of striated muscle. The authors suggested that future studies are necessary to verify their observation and emphasize control of the following: normal hydration following an overnight fast, no recent strenuous exercise, and use of no subject with a disease or medical treatment likely to alter either plasma volume or plasma creatinine concentration.

[40]K ANALYSIS

Isotropic dilution using [42]K involves the intravenous injection of the radioisotope into the subject, a waiting time for equilibration, and the subsequent withdrawal of samples for analysis of dilution, whereas measuring the naturally occurring ^{40}K involves only counting the gamma rays emitted from the body. Since ^{40}K comprises 0.012 percent of naturally occurring potassium, the quantity in the body can be measured by a low level scintillation counter and, from the count, the total body potassium can be calculated.

A schematic representation of a whole body scintillation counter is shown in Fig. 22.5. The counter is 6 feet in length with an inner diameter of 20 inches for the subject. The motor-driven canvas sling on which the subject lies is moved into the well of the counter which is surrounded by a layer of liquid scintillator solution about 6 inches in thickness. The scintillator converts the photon energies of the gamma rays into light impulses or scintillations which are detected, amplified, and counted. For additional details, see Reba et al. (1968). The rapid procedure (3-30 minutes depending on the instrument) is without risk or discomfort to the subject. These advantages tend to offset the high cost and complexity of the instrument. The results obtained are highly reproducible permitting comparisons between laboratories. Data showing the relationship of total body potassium to body weight from different laboratories are shown in Fig. 22.6.

Methods for the measurement of total potassium content of the human by means of ^{40}K were first reported by Anderson and Langham (1959). In 1,590 individuals ranging in age from 1–79 years, sex differences and age trends were observed in the ratio of muscle mass to the other body constituents which contain little or no potassium. The use of whole body ^{40}K counting for the estimation of body fat was conceived by Forbes et al. (1961), who reported on 50 subjects, both males and females, ranging in age from 7–44 years. From the ^{40}K count, total body potassium was calculated, based on a potassium content of 68.1 mEq/kg:

$$LBW \text{ (kg)} = \frac{\text{measured total K (mEq)}}{68.1}$$

Schematic drawing of whole body counter

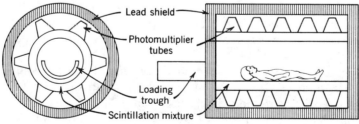

Figure 22.5
Schematic representation of 4-pi whole body liquid scintillation counter. (From R. C. Reba et al., *Human Growth*, D. B. Cheek, ed., Lea and Febiger, Philadelphia, 1968, p. 675.)

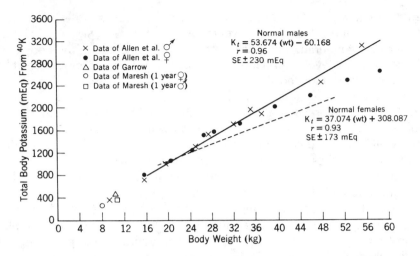

Figure 22.6
Relationship of total body potassium to body weight. Values obtained from the literature relating total K to weights outside the range of those reported in the present study are added. The solid lines are the calculated regression relationships obtained in the present study. A sex difference becomes apparent after body weight exceeds 21 kg. (From R. C. Reba et al., *Human Growth*, D. B. Cheek, ed., Lea and Febiger, Philadelphia, 1968, p. 679.

Fat content was then calculated as the difference between total body weight and lean body weight. The authors were able to show good correlations with skinfold thickness and W/H ratio indices of fatness.

In subsequent studies, Forbes and Hursh (1963) and Barter and Forbes (1963) indicate their awareness of the variation in potassium content of individual body tissues and of how contributions from bone and viscera could lead to error in the calculation of lean body mass. Therefore, Forbes (1972) included correction figures for both the influence of adiposity and for the calibration of their instrument in estimating LBM by ^{40}K counting. These data were compared with estimates obtained from body density and total body water measurements. The data derived through these three methods are comparable when height differences are taken into account and when only narrow age groupings are compared, indicating that a properly calibrated whole body counter can provide valid estimates of LBM (Krzywicki et al., 1974; Ward et al., 1975).

Uncertainties in the accurate determination of total body potassium from ^{40}K occur because of errors due to counting statistics, instability of counter performance, instability of background or high background, differences in body geometry, and variations of counting sensitivity (Smith et al., 1979). The oral administration of ^{42}K, using a technique attributed to Burkinshaw, enabled Smith et al. (ibid) to establish individual calibrations for 40 subjects who varied widely in body composition. The ^{42}K calibration technique for the ^{40}K measurements is comparable to the use of an internal standard as frequently employed in radioactive isotope counting procedures.

NEUTRON ACTIVATION ANALYSIS

In vivo neutron activation analysis is the only technique currently available for the simultaneous detection of elemental composition of the living organism. The accidental exposure of workers to radiation led to the discovery that fast neutrons are captured by target elements in the body to produce unstable isotopes of these elements. These isotopic atoms, by the emission of one or more gamma rays, revert to a stable condition. Thus, the body remains temporarily radioactive and, if placed in a whole body counting system, the emitted radiation can be recorded. The following stable elements can be measured because of the induced nuclides: oxygen (^{16}O), hydrogen (^{2}H), nitrogen (^{13}N), calcium (^{49}Ca), phosphorus (^{32}P), sodium (^{24}Na), chlorine (^{38}Cl), and magnesium (^{27}Mg). The sensitivity of the technique is dependent on the neutron energy, the target amount, and the ability of the element to capture neutrons as well as the sensitivity of the whole body counting system. Low radiation doses of 0.28–2.0 rem are possible (Cohn et al., 1974).

The neutron activation technique has been used to validate other body composition procedures. For example, Hill et al. (1978) used the procedure to show that there is a high correlation coefficient between fat-free body weight, determined from skinfolds using the Durnin and Womersley (1974) equation, and total body nitrogen (TBN) (r = 0.89–0.95) depending on the group studied. The following regression equation was calculated:

$$TBN(g) = 28.8 \; FFWt \; (kg) + 228$$

The ratio TBN/FFWt was 33.8 gm/kg, a value very close to the 34 gm/kg found by Widdowson (1965) from chemical analysis of the adult body.

McNeill et al. (1979) found that the mean percentage of nitrogen in normal men was 2.5 percent or 1.75 kg in a 70 kg man. N/K ratios ranged from 7.5–20 gm/gm which indicated that K cannot be used as a predictor of N. Body protein can be calculated from TBN using the standard conversion factor of 1 gm N = 6.25 gm protein.

Cohn et al. (1980) have documented the loss of muscle mass and body protein content with advanced age and suggested that nonmuscle lean mass remains relatively constant, but that skeletal muscle is particularly susceptible to the aging process. TBN decreased progressively from 2.06 kg in the 3rd decade to 1.78 kg in the 8th decade among 73 men studied.

Burkinshaw et al. (1981) compared TBN, TBK, and fat-free weight in 91 healthy subjects, 62 men and 29 women. The error in calculating TBN was determined to be approximately 76 gm, indicating that the measurement of fat-free weight from skinfolds and body weight is reasonably valid because the error in calculating TBN from these measurements (156 gm) was about that of the direct determination. They concluded that the elaborate technique of neutron activation analysis may be most useful in special patient populations with abnormal hydration or obesity, that is, in patients with skinfolds that are difficult to measure.

URINARY 3-METHYLHISTIDINE

Urinary creatinine excretion was discussed in a previous section in relation to fat-free body weight and skeletal muscle mass. More recently, investigations of a unique natural marker of skeletal muscle metabolism have been conducted. The major site of 3-methylhistidine (3-Mehis) production is the actin of all muscle fibers and the myosin of white fibers. Methylation of histidine residues takes place following incorporation into the chains of myofibrillar proteins. When these proteins are catabolized, the released 3-Mehis is neither metabolized nor reused for protein synthesis, but is excreted in the urine. Assuming muscle protein synthesis and catabolism are in balance, 3-Mehis excretion should be proportional to muscle mass. By placing subjects on a meat-free diet for several days to eliminate exogenous sources of 3-Mehis, it was determined that the urinary excretion of 3-Mehis averaged 225 μmol/day. Urinary 3-Mehis excretion was more highly correlated to fat-free body weight ($r = 0.89$) than was urinary creatinine excretion ($r = 0.67$). The results suggested that endogenous urinary 3-Mehis may well be related to muscle weight, a major component of fat-free weight (Lukaski and Mendez, 1980). In additional work with 3-Mehis, Lukaski et al. (1981a; 1981b) found that measurements of TBN and TBK confirmed the validity of the 3-Mehis estimation of muscle mass. The equations of Burkinshaw et al. (1978) were used to estimate the muscle and nonmuscle components of the fat-free weight. The approach utilized measurements of TBN and TBK on the premise that the K/N ratio is different in muscle and nonmuscle tissue.

Although dietary restrictions and complete urine collections make routine use of 3-Mehis analysis impractical for routine appraisal of body composition, the method is useful for continued experimental appraisal of muscle mass. Problems associated with augmented muscle catabolism such as occur with hard or extended exercise, nutritional deficiencies, hormonal imbalance, aging, injury or other trauma and disease all need to be explored.

ELECTROMAGNETIC ANALYSIS

An electromagnetic device that was used initially for estimating the amount of lean tissue in live animals has been adapted for human use (Harrison and Van Itallie, 1982). The operating principle involves the differences in electrical conductivity and the dielectric properties of lean tissue and fat. Lean tissue contains electrolytes whereas fat does not. The procedure is simple and involves placing the subject on a stretcher within a large uniform solenoidal coil. An electrical current is induced. The field need only be activated for about one-half second to obtain the mass conductivity of the body. Mass conductivity divided by body weight (specific conductivity) is proportional to the lean fraction of the body. Multiple measurements can be made in a few seconds. Fluid or electrolyte disorders complicate the measurement, and correction procedures for variations in body size and configuration may be necessary. Nevertheless, the procedure may have wide applicability in clinical metabolic facilities. Work on animals indicates agreement among electromagnetic, ^{40}K, and chemical carcass analyses.

DUAL-PHOTON ABSORPTIOMETRY

Skeletal mass or total bone mineral is difficult to assess. However, an estimate now can be provided by the technique of *dual-photon absorptiometry*. In a whole body scanning procedure, Peppler and Mazess (1981) used ^{153}Gd (an isotope of gadolinium) as the dual energy source which was coupled to a scintillation detector. Although the scan time was about 70 minutes, the absorbed radiation dose was minimal. The precision of estimating total bone mass *in vivo* was calculated as about ± 4 percent for normal subjects with a standard error of estimate of 36 gm or about 13 gm of calcium. The precision of measurement was checked by scans of two skeletons. In another study, measurement of total bone mineral (TBM) by dual-photon absorptiometry was compared with total calcium (TCa), measured with neutron activation analysis. The two procedures provided similar values for skeletal mass. The radiation dose was much smaller with the dual-photon procedure. Interestingly, the bone mineral in the radius shaft was highly correlated with both TBM (r = 0.97) and TCa (r = 0.98) and could be used to estimate these variables with standard errors of estimate of 9 and 6 percent, respectively (Mazess et al., 1981). The dual-photon absorption technique shows considerable promise in refining the calculations for body composition since reasonable assumptions about bone mass and density have been difficult when body fatness is calculated from total body density equations.

Compositional Changes During the Life Cycle

Pioneer studies of the effects of age and species on body composition were carried out over a century ago by von Bezold (1857), who reported that every individual animal possessed a normal water, organic matter, and salt content that was typical of its species and age and that was approximately constant in higher vertebrates. The classic analytical studies of Moulton (1923) on the changes during development of several different mammalian species, which he compared with data he assembled for humans, led to his concept of *chemical maturity*. Moulton defined chemical maturity as the point at which the concentration of water, proteins, and salts becomes comparatively constant in the fat-free body. He showed that there was a rapid decrease in the water content of fat-free mammalian tissue and an increase in protein and ash content from conception to the time of chemical maturity, when the change suddenly became less and a practically constant concentration was reached. The data he assembled for humans are shown in Table 22.6. There is a striking inverse relationship of water to both nitrogen and ash

TABLE 22.6
Percentage Composition of Humans on a Fat-free Basis

Age	Investigator	No. of Individuals	Water (%)	Nitrogen (%)	Ash (%)
FETUS					
35 days	Fehling[a]	1	97.54	0.39	0.001
2.5 months	Michel[b]	1	93.82	0.69	
3 months	Fehling[a]	2	91.84	0.81	1.005
3–4 months	Michel[b]	1	89.95	1.1	1.73
4 months	Fehling[a]	2	92.46	0.92	1.23
4.5 months	Fehling[a]	5	90.38	1.11	1.62
5 months	Fehling[a]	3	87.43	1.26	2.40
5 months	Michel[b]	1	87.81	1.32	1.95
5 months	Michel[b]	1	86.73	1.39	2.49
6 months	Michel[b]	1	85.03	1.64	2.51
6 months	Fehling[a]	4	86.00	1.78	2.72
7 months	Fehling[a]	1	84.97	1.71	2.89
7 months	Michel[b]	1	84.74	1.56	2.49
Full term	Fehling[a]	1	81.52	2.08	2.81
EXTRAUTERINE					
Newborn	Camerer and Söldner[c]	6	81.87	2.13	3.08
Newborn	Klose[d]	1	80.2	2.32	3.52
3 months	Sommerfeld	1	80.73	2.61	3.14
4 months	Steinitz and Weigert[e]	1	77.75	2.97	3.94
33 yr	Moleschott[f]	1	69.33	3.3	9.44?

Source: From C. R. Moulton, *J. Biol. Chem.* 57: 79, 1923.

[a]H. Fehling, *Arch. Gynäk.*, 1877, xi, 523.

[b]C. Michel, *Compt. rend. Soc. biol.*, 1899, li, 422.

[c]W. Camerer, *Z. Biol.*, 1900, xxxix, 173; xl, 529; 1902, xliii, l. Söldner, *Z. Biol.*, 1903, xliv, 61.

[d]E. Klose, *Jahrb. Kinderh.*, 1900, xxx, 253.

[e]F. Steinitz and R. Weigert, *Beitr. chem. Physiol. u. Path.*, 1905, vi, 206.

[f]J. Moleschott, *Physiologie der Nahrungsmittel*, Giessen, 2nd ed., 1859, 224.

(Fig. 22.7). Comparable data on cattle are shown in Fig. 22.8. Curves for swine, guinea pigs, dogs, cats, rabbits, rats, and mice show similar slopes.

Moulton related the variation in mammalian composition at birth to relative maturity: animals born with a high water content were less mature, and those with a relatively low water content more mature. He also related chemical development to the degree of physical development at birth: animals with relatively great development, such as guinea pigs and cattle, quickly get on their feet at birth and are well developed physically, whereas rats and mice, which are very immature at birth, have the highest water content and greater part of their chemical

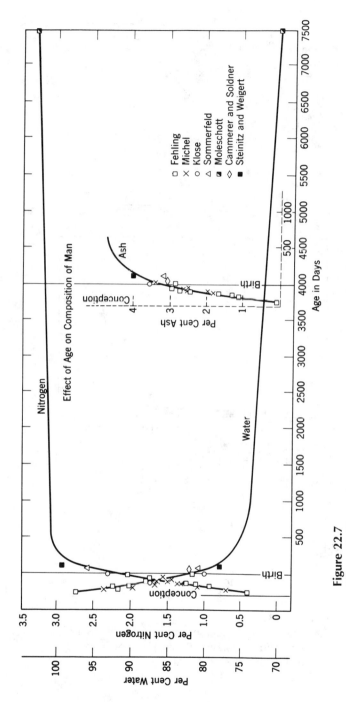

Figure 22.7

Effect of age on the composition of man. (From C. R. Moulton, *J. Biol. Chem.* 57:79, 1923.)

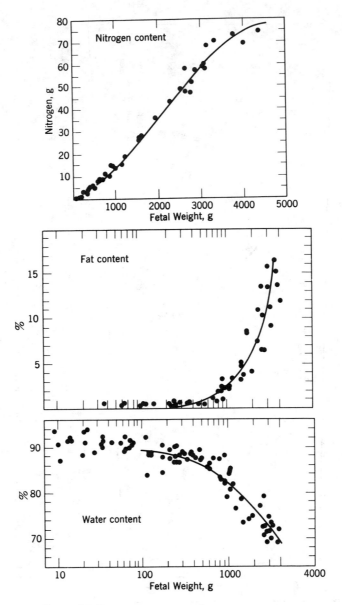

Figure 22.8
Effect of age on the composition of cattle. Data of
Moulton and coworkers. (From C. R. Moulton, *J.
Biol. Chem.* 57:79, 1923.)

development occurs after birth. Humans, pigs, dogs, and cats are in an inter-mediate group.

Decades later, confirmation of Moulton's suggestion relating chemical devel-opment to physiological development was presented by Widdowson and Dick-erson (1964). Table 22.7 presents data on the chemical composition of newborn for eight mammalian species. The guinea pig contains the highest concentration of nitrogen, calcium, magnesium, and phosphorus, making it the most highly developed chemically. It is also the most highly developed functionally. In con-trast, rats, rabbits, and mice are least developed both chemically and functionally.

HUMAN FETAL DEVELOPMENT

Investigation of the human fetus presents problems not encountered in animal studies, and establishing criteria for normality of the fetus in an interrupted preg-nancy may be difficult. Despite the vastness of the problem and the enormity of the difficulties encountered, Hytten and Leitch (1971) have amassed and presented data on chemical changes during fetal development and the associated changes in the human maternal organism from their own studies at Aberdeen and from selected sources in the literature. Figure 22.9 presents the weight gain of the human fetus during the gestation period. As the fetus grows and develops, total body water, which is the largest contributor to weight, falls from approximately 92 percent to 70 or 72 percent at term. This change is accompanied by an increase in protein and, particularly during the last two months of gestation, by an increase in fat content. The relative amounts of nitrogen, fat, and water in the developing fetus are shown in Fig. 22.10. Deposition of protein far exceeds that of fat until the last 2 months of gestation when relatively large amounts of fat are accumulated. The premature human infant whose body weight may be half that of a full-term baby may have only 10 percent of the fat; this, in itself, is enough to explain the scrawny appearance of prematures and the need to protect them against body heat loss.

The concentration of calcium in the fetus increases progressively from under 2 gm/kg for the smallest fetuses to over 8 gm/kg at term, or approximately 28 gm. Sodium content also rises progressively to 6–7 gm at term and, when calculated on the basis of concentration per 100 gm of fat-free tissue, it remains almost constant at 230–240 mg during fetal development. About 30 percent of the sodium in the skeleton is nonexchangeable and therefore not measured by dilution tech-niques. Potassium rises to about 6 gm at term and, on the basis of 100 gm of fat-free tissue, the values increase from approximately 165 mg in the smallest fetuses to about 205 mg at term. The potassium is primarily in the intracellular water and hence is related to cell mass. Great variation is observed in the iron content of fetuses and the analyses of Widdowson and Spray (see Hytten and Leitch, 1971, p. 376) show a range of from 200 mg in smaller to approximately 375 mg in full-term fetuses.

Body composition changes in 41 fetuses of malnourished Indian mothers were reported to be more closely related to body weight than to gestational age (Apte and Lyengar, 1972). Although the calcium, phosphorus, and magnesium contents

TABLE 22.7
Chemical Composition of Newborn Mammals

Constituent	Man	Pig	Dog	Cat	Rabbit	Guinea Pig	Rat	Mouse
Body weight (gm)	3,560	1,260	328	118	54	80	5.9	1.6
Composition[a]								
Water (gm)	82.3	82.0	84.5	82.2	86.5	77.5	86.2	85.0
Total N (gm)	2.3	1.8	2.1	2.4	1.8	2.9	1.6	2.1
Ca (gm)	1.0	1.0	0.5	0.7	0.5	1.2	0.3	0.3
P (gm)	0.6	0.6	0.4	0.4	0.4	0.8	0.4	0.3
Mg (gm)	0.03	0.03	0.02	0.03	0.02	0.05	0.03	0.03
Fe (mg)	9.4	2.9	—	5.5	13.5	6.7	5.9	6.7
Cu (mg)	0.5	0.3	—	0.3	0.4	0.7	0.4	0.7
Zn (mg)	1.9	1.0	—	2.9	2.3	3.5	2.4	4.6

Source: From E. M. Widdowson and J. W. T. Dickerson, *Mineral Metabolism*, Vol. II, Part A, C. L. Comar and F. Bronner, eds., Academic Press, New York, 1964, p. 40.

[a]Data expressed per 100 gm fat-free body tissue.

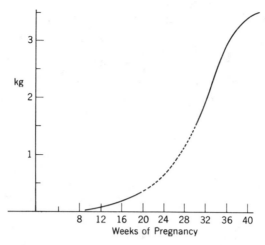

Figure 22.9
The average curve of fetal growth. The curve up
to 20 weeks is based on unpublished data of Dr.
T. Lind; from 32 weeks to term on data of Thomson et al. (1968). The intermediate dotted line
has been fitted arbitrarily. (From F. E. Hytten and
I. Leitch, *The Physiology of Human Pregnancy,*
2nd ed., Blackwell Scientific Publications, Oxford, 1971, p. 292.)

of the body per unit of fat-free weight increased progressively with gestational
age, the values were considerably lower than those reported in the literature.
Body iron was almost 30 percent lower than reported values. This study emphasizes that the chemical composition of nutrient stores in the developing fetus can
be considerably influenced by the state of maternal nutrition.

Susceptibility to modification of body composition in the premature infant may
be comparable to that of the fetus. Kagan et al. (1972) found that even minor
changes in the diet during the first month affected the body composition of prematures. The differences in body composition, which were apparent in total body
water and the distribution of body water into the intra- and extracellular compartments, were influenced primarily by the amount of the electrolytes in the
milks offered and the ratio of electrolytes, particularly potassium, to protein. The
data presented make it clear that the metabolism of the young premature infant
is modified by the composition of the diet.

The fetus is but one of three products of conception, albeit the most important
with respect to size and consequence. The comparative increments during development of protein, fat, and calcium in fetus, placenta, and amniotic fluid are
shown in Table 22.8. There are insufficient data on iron, but it is estimated that
the fetus and placenta together contain approximately 450 mg.

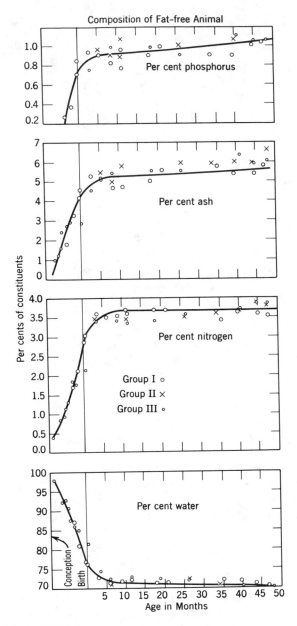

Figure 22.10
Nitrogen, fat, and water content of human fetus. (From F. E. Hytten and I. Leitch, *The Physiology of Human Pregnancy*, 2nd ed., Blackwell Scientific Publications, Oxford, 1971, pp. 371, 373.)

TABLE 22.8
Protein, Fat, and Calcium in the Products of Conception

	Weeks of Pregnancy			
	10	**20**	**30**	**40**
		Protein		
Fetus	0.3	27	160	440
Placenta	2	16	60	100
Amniotic fluid	0.08	0.5	2	3
Total	2	44	222	543
		Fat		
Fetus	2	2	80	440
Placenta		1	3	4
Amniotic fluid		0.1	0.4	0.5
Total	2	3	83	445
		Calcium		
Fetus	Negligible	1.5	10	28
Placenta	Negligible	0.05	0.13	0.65
Amniotic fluid	Negligible	Negligible	Negligible	Negligible
Total	Negligible	1.5	10	29

Source: From F. E. Hytten and I. Leitch, *The Physiology of Human Pregnancy*, 2nd ed., Blackwell Scientific Publications, Oxford, 1971, p. 382–383.

MATERNAL WEIGHT GAIN

Distribution

In addition to the nutrients incorporated into the products of conception, significant additions occur in the maternal body. However, in order to evaluate the composition of the weight gain, it is important to know whether any interference with the normal physiological adjustment was imposed through dietary restriction. Regulation of weight gain during pregnancy has long been the subject of debate and, until relatively recently, many obstetricians have tried to manipulate weight gain. Fortunately this practice is falling into disrepute, and evidence is accumulating that restriction of weight gain during pregnancy may significantly affect the incidence of prematurity, low birth weight, and the attendant mortality and morbidity (Singer et al., 1968). Weight gain in a healthy young woman who eats to appetite during pregnancy is estimated to be approximately 27.5 lb (12.5 kg) at term. The estimated weight gain at 10 weeks is 1.5 lb (0.65 kg); at 20 weeks, 9 lb (4 kg); at 30 weeks, 19 lb (8.5 kg); with the remainder during the last 10 weeks of pregnancy (Fig. 22.11). The distribution of this weight gain among the products of conception during the course of pregnancy and the more difficult estimations of the weight of the uterus, breasts, and blood volume, each of which add considerably to the total, is summarized in Table 22.9. In this analysis of

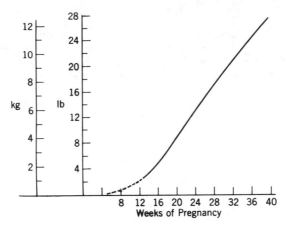

Figure 22.11
Mean weight gain in pregnancy of 2,868 normo-
tensive primigravidae (Thomson and Billewicz,
1957). (From F. E. Hytten and I. Leitch, *The Physiology of Human Pregnancy,* 2nd ed., Blackwell
Scientific Publications, Oxford, 1971, p. 280.)

weight gain there is approximately 3.5 kg not accounted for and assumed to be
fat (Hytten and Leitch, 1971, p. 357). A weight gain of about 25 lb was recommended by the Committee on Maternal Nutrition (1970).

Composition

Measurement of changes of body composition during pregnancy are a summation
of the changes in the maternal tissue and the products of conception. Estimates
of body composition rely primarily on measurements of body water employing
the usual dilution and tracer techniques and/or body density. From these measurements body fat and lean body mass can be calculated according to the formulas presented previously. However, the validity must be questioned for pregnancy since the constant proportions of water to lean body mass cannot be fixed
at 73 percent as for the nonpregnant. Some of the nonfat weight added during
pregnancy has a water content of 90 percent. Whether or not the ratio between
protein and mineral of the lean mass is unchanged during pregnancy will determine whether body fat can be estimated using both body water and body density
measurements. There have been few studies in which these methods have been
applied during pregnancy (McCartney et al., 1959).

Lean body mass was determined by whole body ^{40}K counting in pregnant
teenagers (King et al., 1973) at the beginning and end of a 100-day study period.
The increase in potassium deposition amounted to twice the estimate of Hytten
and Leitch and was supported by nitrogen retention data from the same subjects,
which also were twice the accepted estimates of daily deposition during the third
trimester of pregnancy. The observed nitrogen retentions of women during pregnancy compared to the theoretical gain, according to Hytten and Leitch, is shown

TABLE 22.9
Analysis of Weight Gain

Tissues and Fluids Accounted For and Total Weight Gained (gm)	Increase in Weight Up to:			
	10 weeks	**20 weeks**	**30 weeks**	**40 weeks**
Fetus	5	300	1,500	3,400
Placenta	20	170	430	650
Amniotic fluid	30	350	750	800
Uterus	140	320	600	970
Mammary gland	45	180	360	405
Blood	100	600	1,300	1,250
Extracellular extravascular fluid	0	30	80	1,680
1. No edema or leg edema				
2. Generalized edema	0	500	1,526	4,897
Total				
1. No edema or leg edema	340	1,950	5,020	9,155
2. Generalized edema	340	2,420	6,466	12,372
Total weight gained				
1. No edema or leg edema	650	4,000	8,500	12,500
2. Generalized edema	650	4,500	10,000	14,500
Weight not accounted for				
1. No edema or leg edema	310	2,050	3,480	3,345
2. Generalized edema	310	2,080	3,534	2,128

Source: From F. E. Hytten and I. Leitch, *The Physiology of Human Pregnancy,* 2nd ed., Blackwell Scientific Publications, Oxford, 1971, p. 356.

in Fig. 22.12. The interesting and important point brought out by King et al. (1973) is that the retention appears to be similar during the three trimesters and is considerably greater than the theoretical gain. This study emphasizes that women stored more nitrogen on higher intakes and this was accumulated as maternal lean body mass.

Estimations of total body water have been the subject of major interest to obstetricians because of their concern with the development of edema. This concern has probably led to widespread but fortunately, in most cases, mild iatrogenic disorders brought about by the use of diuretic agents. The change in body water observed during the course of pregnancy (Fig. 22.13) indicates that at term there is an excess of approximately 2.5 liters of water over what can be accounted for in the maternal tissue and the products of conception. In some cases this excess was observable as edema although in most cases the edema was clinically slight. This water has been a source of worry to obstetricians who assumed it to be indicative of some derangement in metabolism when, instead, it appears to be of physiological rather than pathological significance.

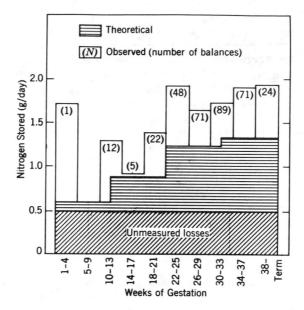

Figure 22.12
Observed nitrogen retention of women during gestation. The theoretical values are from Hytten and Leitch. (From D. H. Calloway, *Nutrition and Fetal Development,* Vol. 2, M. Winick, ed., John Wiley, New York 1974, p. 79.)

If there is an accumulation of approximately 2.5 liters of water and, in most cases, this is not visible as edema, the question of where the water is located becomes intriguing. Hytten and Leitch (1971, p. 353) point to a neglected paper (Fekete, 1954) that reported increased uptake of water in the connective tissue which was marked in pregnant women and particularly so when edema was present. They suggested that the water accumulated during pregnancy was in the mucopolysaccharide basement membranes of connective tissue and was associated with the softening of the tissue. They suggested also that this might be associated with increased diffusibility of solutes and facilitation of the nutrition of the cells. Such a normal accumulation of fluid is called physiological edema and usually is associated with better reproductive performance and fewer low birth weight and premature infants. The presence of such edema and the changes in the skin during pregnancy have been corroborated by Robertson (1971). Clarification of the changes in connective tissue water content and the extent of these changes in normal pregnancy could resolve the question of whether the edema of pregnancy is indeed a normal physiological adjustment.

That part of the maternal weight gain that cannot be accounted for in the products of conception or maternal tissue is assumed to be fat (Hytten and Leitch, 1971, p. 357) and amounts to approximately 3.5 kg. Calloway (1974) questions whether some of this unaccounted weight gain should not be attributed instead

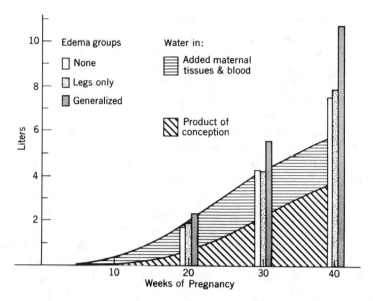

Figure 22.13
The measured gain in body water during pregnancy in three edema groups compared to the calculated water accumulation in the product of conception and added maternal blood and tissues. (From F. E. Hytten and Leitch, *The Physiology of Human Pregnancy,* 2nd ed., Blackwell Scientific Publications, Oxford, 1971, p. 349.)

to increase in lean body mass accumulated when the nitrogen and energy intakes during pregnancy are sufficiently high. In an animal model (Naismith, 1971), fat stored during pregnancy was used as a source of energy during lactation. Carcass analyses in lactating rats on days 2 and 16 postpartum showed that when the protein intake was high (25 percent), 70 percent of the fat stored during pregnancy was lost during lactation with no loss of body protein; whereas, on low protein intakes (11 percent), 10 percent of body protein in addition to the calories from fat were used for the synthesis of a reduced volume of milk. Such a study supports the suggestion that stored fat during pregnancy may indeed be a source of energy for lactation and serves to protect lean body mass.

NUTRITIONAL REQUIREMENTS DURING PREGNANCY

Meeting both fetal and maternal requirements and hence setting up nutrient allowances for pregnancy has, for the most part, been based on the suggested allowances for the nonpregnant woman with the superimposed additional requirements for pregnancy. Such an additive approximation of need has been questioned by Beaton (1961), who points out that physiological and nutritional adaptations occur that permit pregnancy to proceed if the minimal nutrient requirements are met. When the minima are not met, harm results to the mother or fetus; above the minimal levels, the pregnant woman can adapt to wide ranges of intakes. This also appears to be evident in the data presented by Thomson (1958; 1959a; 1959b) and by Oldham and Sheft (1951).

Metabolic alterations promoting the retention of essential nutrients probably are dependent on adjustments in hormonal regulation. Animal studies suggest that growth hormone acts to decrease protein catabolism during pregnancy, thereby promoting retention (Beaton et al., 1955; Beaton, 1957). The increased demand for oxygen, by stimulation of erythropoietin secretion, and the consequent stimulation of hematopoiesis lead to increased oxygen-carrying power in the form of more erythrocytes carrying hemoglobin. Increased hemoglobin synthesis coupled with the higher plasma transferrin levels that are present during pregnancy undoubtedly are associated with increased iron absorption. The need for sodium to maintain the increased body water compartments is accomplished by stimulation of aldosterone secretion, which promotes sodium reabsorption by the kidney tubules. Physiological adaptation in pregnant rats to levels of sodium intake adequate for nonpregnant animals is observed in the histological evidence of increased renin secretion which, in turn, triggers increased secretion of aldosterone (Pike et al., 1966). As long as the required increase in hormone production can be maintained, the requisite increase in retention will occur. A fundamental question arises about the degree of stress to which the pregnant body should be subjected in order to meet its nutritional requirements and to maintain body composition. From studies of rats on restricted sodium intake, physiological adjustment leading to increased stimulation of aldosterone secretion takes place to the point of disruption in the fine structure of aldosterone-secreting cells (Smiciklas et al., 1971a; 1971b) and in loss of aldosterone-secreting capacity (Khokhar and Pike, 1973). Maternal weight gain was reduced, the young were smaller and lighter, and there were significant reductions in tissue sodium and plasma volume. What starts as a physiological adjustment can be extended until it attains pathological proportions.

The bases for recommended allowances set up by various national and supranational organizations vary. (See Chapter 25.) The ranges suggested for various nutrients for pregnancy are shown in Table 22.10.

COMPOSITIONAL CHANGES BETWEEN BIRTH AND MATURITY

Only one study giving chemical analysis of a child has appeared in the literature (see Widdowson and Dickerson, 1964), and it is presented in Table 22.11 along with data on a full-term baby and an adult. Although it had been suggested that some dehydration may have taken place before death, the water, nitrogen, and potassium contents appear to have attained a composition similar to that of the adult. Values lower than the adult for calcium, phosphorus, and magnesium indicate that the bones were not chemically mature. Copper and zinc concentrations were not yet at the adult level and the low iron apparently was indicative of anemia. Fig. 22.14 shows how the composition of the newborn changes when the body weight doubles at 5 months and triples at one year.

TABLE 22.10
Daily Recommended Allowances for Nonpregnant and Pregnant Women Doing Light Work

	United Nations		United States		United Kingdom	
	Nonpregnant	Pregnant	Nonpregnant	Pregnant	Nonpregnant	Pregnant
Weight, kg	55		55		55	
Weight gain, kg		10 ± 2		11		12.5
Energy, kcal	2,200	2,550	2,000	2,300	2,200	2,400
Protein, gm	29	38	44	74	55	60
Calcium, gm	0.4–0.5	1.0–1.2	0.8	1.2	0.5	1.2
Iron, mg	14–28	14–28[a]	18	18[b]	12	15
Vitamin A, RE, mg	750	1500	800	1000	2,500	2,500
Vitamin D, mg	2.5	12.5	5	10	100	400
Thiamin, mg	0.9	1.0	1.0	1.4	0.9	1.0
Riboflavin, mg	1.3	1.5	1.2	1.5	1.3	1.6
Nicotinic acid, mg equiv.	14.5	16.8	13	15	15	18
Vitamin B_6, mg	—	—	2.0	2.6	—	—
Folate, µg	200	400	400	800	—	—
Vitamin B_{12}, µg	2.0	3.0	3.0	4.0	—	—
Ascorbic acid, mg	30	50	60	80	30	60

Sources: FAO, 1974; National Research Council, 1980; Department of Health and Social Security, 1969.

[a]Assuming previous iron intake has been satisfactory.
Lower level is the recommendation where over 25 percent of calories are from animals foods.
Upper level is the recommendation where under 10 percent of calories are from animal foods.

[b]Supplement of 30–60 mg

713

TABLE 22.11
Composition of the Whole Body of a 4½-year-old Boy Compared with that of a Full-Term Baby and an Adult

	Full-Term Baby	Boy 4½ Years	Adult
Body weight (kg)	3.5	14.0	65
Composition[a]			
Water (gm)	823	695	720
Total N (gm)	22.6	38.2	34.0
Na (mEq)	82	—	80
K (mEq)	53	65	69
Cl (mEq)	55	—	50
Ca (gm)	9.6	21.1	22.4
P (gm)	5.6	10.5	12.0
Mg (gm)	0.26	0.36	0.47
Fe (mg)	93.9	64.2	74
Cu (mg)	4.7	3.3	1.7
Zn (mg)	19.2	22.3	28

Source: From E. M. Widdowson and J. W. T. Dickerson, *Mineral Metabolism,* C. L. Comar and F. Bronner, eds., Vol. II, Part A, Academic Press, New York, 1964, p. 17.

[a]Results expressed per kg of fat-free body tissue.

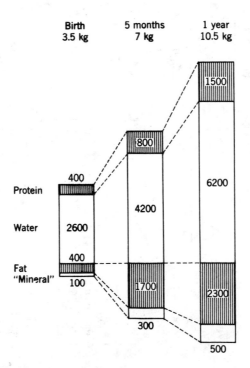

Figure 22.14
Body composition in a normal newborn infant and at 5 and 12 months of age. (From B. Friis-Hansen, *Ped.* 47:264, 1971.)

Garn et al. (1956) studied a group of 300 clinically healthy infants from 1 to 12 months of age to determine whether subcutaneous fat was indicative of nutritive status, and concluded that it was not. They noted that the amount of subcutaneous fat increased rapidly in all infants from 1 to 6 months of age but that thereafter some gained and others lost fat, and group differences disappeared. No relationship appeared to exist between the amount of fat deposited during the first 6 months and the subsequent rate of growth.

Fig. 22.15 shows the continuous increase observed in triceps fat fold measurements in males and females from age 1 to 18. Fat fold measurements in females is unchanged until the sharp prepubertal gain, which is followed by an equally sharp increase during the adolescent stage. Extension of the curves would reveal a short plateau lasting until approximately age 22 that is followed by the adult gain, with peak fatness occurring at about age 45. Fat loss then occurs into old age. The picture for males differs sharply from females after age 3, when there is a preschool loss that is not regained until the prepubertal gain between ages 8 and 13. This is followed by another loss during the adolescent stage, reaching a trough about age 18. Adult gain in triceps fat fold measurement peaks about age 50 and is followed by a drop associated with increased age.

A study measuring total body water throughout the life span using deuterium dilution (Edelman et al., 1952) included a group of 11 children with an average age of 4.5 years. The mean total body water was 58.9 percent of body weight,

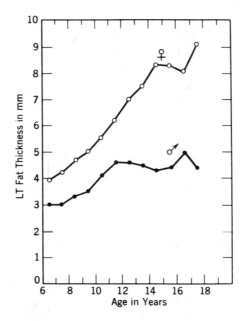

Figure 22.15
Continuous increase in lower thoracic (LT) fat in girls and parallel increase in boys, terminating at 11.5 years. By 14.5 years the adult female/male fat ratio of 180 per cent has been attained. (From S. M. Garn and J. A. Haskell, *Science* 129:1615, 1959.)

TABLE 22.12
Summary of Total Body Water Data as a Function of Age in Normal Children

No. Subjects	Age Range	Weight kg	Surface Area m²	Total Body Water liters		Total Body Water % B.Wt		Total Body Water liters/m²	
				Mean	Range	Mean	Range	Mean	Range
6	2–28 (days)	3.16	0.198	2.42	1.67–3.17	76.7	71.8–83.0	12.1	9.8–13.8
9	1–9 (months)	6.94	0.328	4.27	3.08–6.15	62.6	53.0–70.9	12.9	11.3–14.6
11	1–9 (years)	16.6	0.650	9.77	5.90–16.2	58.9	55.2–62.8	14.2	13.1–16.7

Source: From I. S. Edelman et al., *Surg. Gynec. Obstet.* 95: 1, 1952.

a figure not too different from the Widdowson data, which calculated to 53.8 percent and which the authors indicated might have been abnormally low. A summary of total body water as a function of age in normal children clearly indicated the reduction in percentage of body water from birth to 9 years of age (Table 22.12). A sex differential becomes apparent in the 10–16 age group, and the female has a lower percentage of body water associated with added increments of body fat. Fig. 22.16, which shows the absolute and relative amounts of body water as a function of age, illustrates this clearly. Similar and confirming data for total body water measured in 86 subjects ranging in age from 1 day to 15 years were obtained by Friis-Hansen (1961). Thirty-seven of these subjects received a thiosulfate injection simultaneously with the deuterium, thereby permitting estimation of both total body water and extracellular fluid volume, and calculation of intracellular fluid volume (Table 22.13).

In an attempt to determine whether a correlation exists between subcutaneous fat and total body fat in healthy children in the age groups 9–12 and 13–16, Pařizková (1961) determined body density and skinfold thickness in 123 boys and 118 girls. In both age groups and sexes high correlations were observed, suggesting that the relationship of the density and percentage of fat in children is similar to that found in adults. Nomograms were constructed for each sex in each

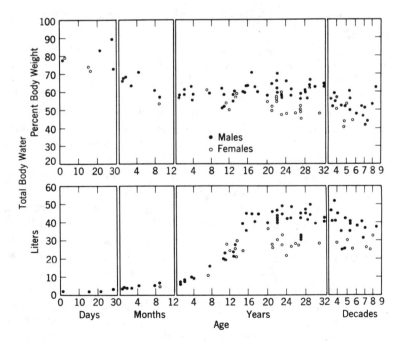

Figure 22.16
Total body water as a function of age. In the upper section, the body water is plotted as percentage of body weight (i.e., relative water volume). In the lower section the body water is plotted in liters (i.e., absolute water volume). (From I. S. Edelman et al., *Surg. Gynec. Obstet.* 95:1, 1952.)

TABLE 22.13
Mean Values of Total Body Water, Extracellular Water, and Intracellular Water[a] (Percent of Body Weight)

Age of Subjects	TBW	ECW	ICW
0–1 day	78.4	44.5	33.9
1–30 days	74.0	39.7	31.8
1–3 months	72.3	32.2	43.3
3–6 months	70.1	30.1	42.1
6–12 months	60.4	27.4	35.2
1–2 years	58.7	25.6	33.6
2–3 years	63.5	26.7	38.3
3–5 years	62.2	21.4	(45.7)
5–10 years	61.5	22.0	(42.3)
10–15 years	57.3	18.7	(46.7)

Source: From B. Friis-Hansen, *Ped.* 28: 169, 1961.

[a]TBW minus ECW is not in all cases equal to ICW because both determinations were not carried out in all subjects within each group. The figures in parentheses are based on only one or two measurements and are less significant.

age group for determining body density and hence percentage fat from two skinfold measurements.

Hunt and Giles (1956) suggested that in addition to consideration of chemical maturity as defined by Moulton, *mature hydration,* although more limited, might be useful. Mature hydration, according to their definition, is the minimal, or mature, percentage of water in the fat-free body. Hunt and Heald (1963), in a study of 55 adolescent boys, found extreme variability in the hydration of the fat-free body early in adolescence. They suggest that perhaps mature hydration occurs temporarily before adolescence but that this is followed by fattening and accumulation of enough body water to make the fat-free body as hydrated as the newborn. Later the body becomes more lean, its composition more stable, and by 18 years body composition is that of mature males.

Forbes and Hursh (1963), on the basis of ^{40}K measurements and calculation of lean body mass, found that the weight of the lean body rises rapidly in males during the midportion of the second decade, reaching a maximum by the nineteenth year, after which there is a slow fall. They also reported an increase in fat during the early "teen" years, but at a much slower rate (Fig. 22.17). An abrupt fall in fat at age 16 is followed by a slow sustained rise during middle age. It is the concomitant rapid increase in lean body mass and decrease in fat to which they attribute the "muscular" appearance of the male in late adolescence. The rise in lean body mass in females is less rapid than in males and the maximum, two-thirds that of the male, is reached at about 15 years of age. The increase in total fat is greater in females during the early years and the curve is an uninterrupted one. Plotted as ^{40}K concentrations related to age, the peak occurs at about age 9 and then falls; however, a second peak in body potassium concentration occurs in males at age 16 (Fig. 22.18). It is this second peak that corresponds to the one

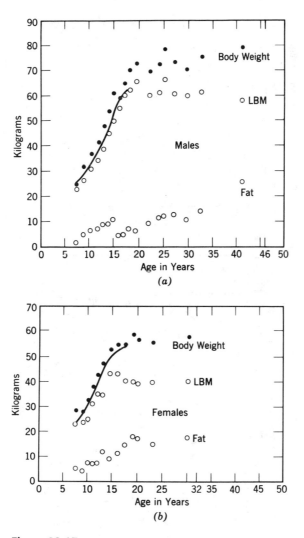

Figure 22.17
Plot of average body weight, lean body mass (LBM), and fat for males (a) and females (b). The solid lines represent the 50th percentile for body weight for normal children. (From G. B. Forbes and J. B. Hursh, *Ann. N. Y. Acad. Sci.* 110:255, 1963.)

described by Forbes and Hursh. In a study of children and young adults, Forbes et al. (1961) reported good correlations between ^{40}K measurements and both skinfold thickness and height-weight ratios, and between ^{40}K and both circumferential measurements and total fat (Barter and Forbes, 1963).

Attainment of maturity does not imply cessation of change, and alterations in relative and absolute body composition do, indeed, continue in adult life. These changes, however, proceed at a slower rate as the individual ages and are ob-

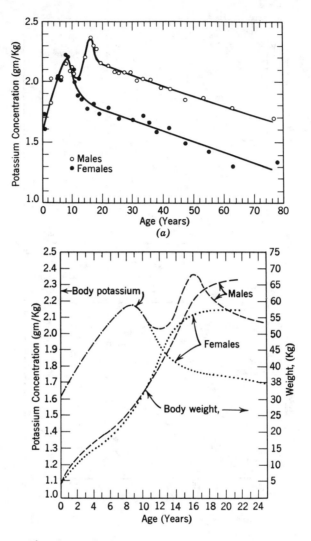

Figure 22.18
(a) Average body potassium concentrations of males and females as a function of chronologic age (grams per kilogram of gross body weight). (b) Change in male and female potassium concentrations in relation to growth (as indicated by weight gain). (From E. C. Anderson and W. H. Langham, *Science* 130:713, 1959.)

servable, often without benefit of the investigator's tools, as increases in body fat in males (Fig. 22.19) and females (Fig. 22.20). Increases in age are associated also with decreases in both body water (Fig. 22.21) and body cell mass. Table 22.14 clearly shows the concomitant and related changes in the three parameters with age at a constant body weight. The sex difference in adult body composition is readily apparent. Comparable data have been obtained by densitometry (Behnke et al., 1942; Brozek, 1952; Young et al., 1963a; 1963b), skinfold measurements (Brozek, 1952; Brozek et al., 1963), creatinine excretion (Norris et al., 1963), exchangeable potassium (Moore et al., 1963a; Olesen, 1965), ^{40}K measurements (Anderson and Langham, 1959; Forbes and Hursh, 1963; Meneeley et al., 1963), and total body water measurements (Edelman et al., 1952; Siri, 1956; Friis-Hansen, 1965). For an extensive review of the *in vivo* quantification of human fat, muscle, and bone, see Malina (1969).

COMPOSITIONAL CHANGES WITH WEIGHT CHANGE

Since the major components of body weight are water, fat, and body cell mass, changes in weight can be reflections of alterations in any one of these fractions.

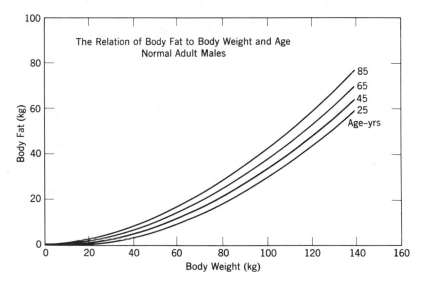

Figure 22.19
Body fat and body weight in relation to age in normal adult males of various age groups. This plot can also be used as a nomogram entered with body weight and age. Note that with progressing increase of weight the fraction of fat increases even in a population identified as "normal." (From F. D. Moore et al., *The Body Cell Mass and its Supporting Environment,* W. B. Saunders Co., Philadelphia, 1963, p. 162.)

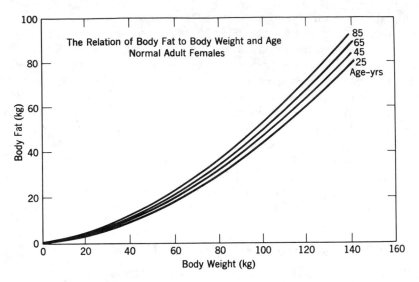

Figure 22.20
The relation of body fat and body weight to age in normal adult females of various age groups. This figure is drawn as is Fig. 22.19 for use in predicting the degree of obesity in normal adult female subjects. Both here and in the previous figure the standard hydration coefficient for the fat-free body (0.732) is used. (From F. D. Moore et al., *The Body Cell Mass and Its Supporting Environment*, W. B. Saunders Co., Philadelphia, 1963, p. 163.)

Excessive hydration, which is observed in a variety of pathological conditions, may be due to increase of extracellular water or wasting of body cell mass or both. (See Fig. 22.4.) Dehydration, which occurs more rarely, results from the reverse situation: loss of extracellular water or gain in body cell mass. These abnormal conditions are not relevant in this context. Changes in the relative proportions of fat comprising body weight may attain pathological status, but such conditions may be viewed as the extremes in the continuum from emaciation to obesity. Increases in body cell mass are the result of intensive physical activity and are observed in trained athletes.

Obesity
The effects of plethora rather than paucity of body fat is of major concern in the United States, where the combination of an abundant food supply and energy-conserving devices has made obesity a major public health problem. However, in many countries of the world where food shortages and famines are endemic, accumulation of excess body fat, though no less a health problem to the individual, may be an economic status symbol.

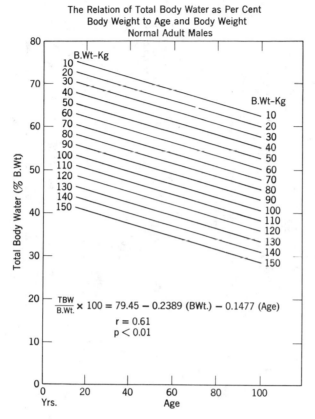

Figure 22.21

Total body water (as percent of body weight) related to
age and body weight in normal adult males of all ages.
This chart can be used as a nomogram. It is entered with
the person's age, progressing vertically upward to the
observed body weight. The vertical coordinate is then
crossed to the predicted total body water, indicated not
in liters, but in percent of body weight. The parabolic
expression on which this nomogram is based is shown
at the bottom. (From F. D. Moore et al., *The Body Cell
Mass and Its Supporting Environment,* W. B. Saunders
Co., Philadelphia, 1963, p. 159.)

Body weight gain in the adult indicates an increase in both the absolute and
relative amounts of body fat, but in spite of rather widespread misconception,
the body weight gain is not due to fat alone: it includes water, body cell mass,
and cell solids. The predicted body composition for an obese young man and
young woman shows the composition of the weight increment over a "reference"
man or woman (Table 22.15). Although the largest fraction of the increased weight

TABLE 22.14
Normal Values for Fat, Total Body Water, and Body Cell Mass Related to Body Weight and Age

Wgt. (kg)	Fat (kg)				Total Body Water (liters)				Body Cell Mass[a] (kg)			
	Age				Age				Age			
	25	45	65	85	25	45	65	85	25	45	65	85
Adult Males												
60	9.6	12.0	14.5	17.0	36.9	35.1	33.3	31.5	27.3	24.6	22.1	19.8
80	18.1	21.3	24.5	27.8	45.3	43.0	40.6	38.2	33.5	30.1	27.0	24.0
100	29.1	33.2	37.2	41.3	51.9	48.9	46.0	43.0	38.3	34.3	30.6	27.1
120	42.8	47.6	52.5	57.3	56.5	53.0	49.4	45.9	41.8	37.3	32.9	28.9
140	59.1	64.7	70.3	76.1	59.2	55.1	51.0	46.8	45.7	38.7	33.9	29.4
Adult Females												
60	17.9	19.8	21.8	23.5	30.8	29.4	28.0	26.7	21.2	19.6	18.3	16.8
80	29.5	32.0	34.6	37.1	37.0	35.1	33.2	31.4	25.6	23.4	21.7	19.8
100	44.0	47.1	50.3	53.4	41.0	38.7	36.4	34.1	28.2	25.7	23.8	21.4
120	61.3	65.1	68.9	72.6	43.0	40.2	37.4	34.7	29.6	26.8	24.5	21.8
140	81.4	85.8	90.3	94.6	42.9	39.7	36.4	33.2	29.6	26.4	23.8	20.9

Source: From F. D. Moore et al., *The Body Cell Mass and Its Supporting Environment,* W. B. Saunders Co., Philadelphia, 1963, p. 167, 168.

[a]Calculated as $K_e \times 8.33$.

TABLE 22.15

***a*. Composition of "Excess Tissue" in a 25-year-old Normal Male of 100 kg Body Weight[a]**

Compartments	Predicted Normal Body Composition		"Excess Tissue"	
			Absolute	Relative
	70 kg	100 kg	+30.0 kg	100%
Fat	13.7 kg	29.1 kg	+15.4 kg	51%
Extracellular water	17.2 liter	21.8 liter	+ 4.6 liter	15%
Body cell mass	30.6 kg	38.3 kg	+ 7.7 kg	26%
Remainder	8.5 kg	10.8 kg	+ 2.3 kg	8%

[a]A normal 25-year-old male, of 70 kg body weight is used as a "reference man".

***b*. Composition of "Excess Tissue" in a 25-year-old Normal Female of 90 kg Body Weight[a]**

Compartments	Predicted Normal Body Composition		"Excess Tissue"	
			Absolute	Relative
	60 kg	90 kg	+30.0 kg	100%
Fat	17.9 kg	36.6 kg	+18.7 kg	63%
Extracellular water	14.2 liter	18.2 liter	+ 4.0 liter	13%
Body cell mass	21.2 kg	26.7 kg	+ 5.5 kg	18%
Remainder	6.7 kg	8.5 kg	+ 1.8 kg	6%

[a]A normal 25-year-old female of 60 kg body weight is used as a "reference woman".

Source: From K. H. Olesen, *Human Body Composition,* J. Brozek, ed., Pergamon Press, Oxford, 1965, p. 185.

is due to fat, a substantial proportion is due to the increase in water, body cell mass, and cell solids. Similar findings on "obesity tissue" were obtained by densitometric (Brozek et al., 1963) and by multiple isotope dilution techniques (Moore et al., 1963).

Parizková (1972) reported that obese children are sometimes taller and have a larger lean body mass than normal children of the same age. Skeletal development also may be greater than in normal weight children, and bicristal (pelvic) width greater in obese boys but not girls (Table 22.16). The distribution of fat was described as similar to that in an old woman with the usual sexual difference in fat distribution not apparent (Fig. 22.22).

Body weight loss in the obese individual is not just loss of excess body fat but also includes loss of body water and body cell mass. A partitioning of the "obesity tissue" lost by obese young men (Brozek et al., 1963) indicates that fat constituted

TABLE 22.16
Mean Values of Anthropometric Measures and Body Composition in Normal and Obese Boys and Girls (13–14 years)

	Height (cm)	Weight (kg)	Fat (%)	LBM (kg)	Bicristal Breadth (cm)	Chest Circumference (cm)	Arm (cm)	Femur Bicondylar Breadth (cm)
Boys								
Normal	161.8	50.4	12.5	43.9	22.8	78.6	23.1	9.6
Obese	161.2	68.9	29.5	48.6	27.7	88.3	27.0	10.1
Girls								
Normal	156.9	50.4	18.1	40.7	26.8	79.2	24.3	8.6
Obese	157.5	88.9	31.9	46.7	27.4	95.1	29.6	10.0

Source: From J. Pařizková, *Nutritional Aspects of Physical Performance,* J. F. De Wijn and R. A. Binkhorst, eds., Nutricia Ltd., Zoetermeer, The Netherlands, 1972, p. 148.

64 percent; extracellular water, 4 percent; and cell residue, 32 percent. Some of the confusion that crops up in the literature concerning the composition of weight loss stems from the partition of body weight into two components: body fat and lean body weight. In this context, lean body weight includes body cell mass plus skeletal and supporting structures. As body weight decreases, the proportional weight of the skeletal and supporting tissues to total weight increases, thereby masking any decrease in body cell mass which accompanies weight loss. In addition, an increase in muscle mass during weight reduction due to physical activity obscures a decrease in body cell mass. Just such an erroneous interpretation of observed constancy in lean body weight appears in the data of Christian et al. (1963), who ascribe weight loss in obese individuals to loss of excess body

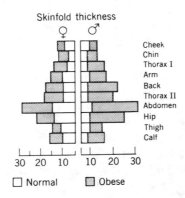

Figure 22.22
Differences in skinfold thickness at different sites in normal and obese boys and girls. (From J. Pařizková, *Physical Activity—Human Growth and Development,* G. L. Rarick, ed., Academic Press, New York, 1973, p. 114.)

fat only. In a study of weight loss in adolescent girls in which estimates of body composition were made by skinfold thickness, anthropometric measurements, and underwater determinations of specific gravity, Goldman et al. (1963) found two subjects in whom weight loss appeared to be 90–100 percent fat, and two who exceeded 100 percent! These subjects had been exercising and had undoubtedly added to their muscle mass, and the authors point to this to account for the illusion that the estimated fat loss was so high a proportion of the total weight loss.

Drenick (1975) demonstrated the importance of early water loss from the body with 30 days of fasting. Although other components also were lost by the 10 obese subjects, the average net body water loss over the 30-day period was about 11.8 liters, and a substantial portion of the water loss occurred within the first 10 days. The rate of daily water loss was highest on the first day of fasting then declined gradually to reach a relatively constant value at 12 days. (See Figure 22.23.) Intraindividual variations from day-to-day were found. Thus, the caloric equivalent for body weight loss reflects the composition of the fluid, tissue, or substrate lost. In general, the caloric equivalent tends to increase with days of

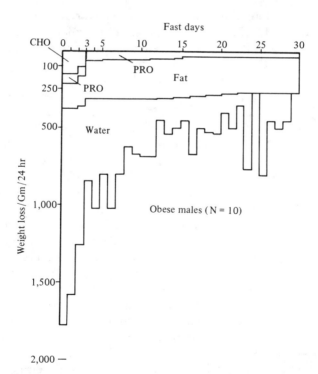

Figure 22.23
Contribution to daily weight loss of fluid and nutrients.
(From E. J. Drenick, *Obesity in Perspective, Vol. 2, Part 2*, G. A. Bray, ed, DHEW Publ. No. (NIH) 75-708, Washington, DC: U. S. Government Printing Office, 1975, p. 345.

TABLE 22.17
Mean Caloric Equivalents of Body Weight Loss in Humans[a]

Study	n	Days	kcal/kg
Undernutrition	5	4	2730
Starvation	1	4	2840
Starvation with work	6	5	2840
Semistarvation with work	6	12	4300
Semistarvation with work	13	24	5320
Reducing	12	63	6170
Prolonged semistarvation	32	168	7510
Obesity, reducing		14 or more	6000–8200

[a]n, number of subjects, days; days on experimental regimen; kcal/kg, kcal deficit/kg weight loss.

Source: From E. R. Buskirk and J. Mendez. *Human Nutrition—A Comprehensive Treatise, Vol. 3A,* R. B. Alfin-Slater and D. Kritchevsky, eds., Plenum, New York, 1980, p. 87.

fasting or semistarvation. The caloric equivalents of body weight loss in humans is summarized in Table 22.17. The data were accumulated from a variety of studies in the literature (Buskirk and Mendez, 1980). Various factors influence the caloric equivalent of the weight loss including amount of body fat, severity of the dietary restriction, degree of physical activity, magnitude of the negative caloric balance, composition of the diet, salt intake, ambient environment, fluid intake, drug therapy, and status of neurogenic and hormonal control mechanisms. Of particular concern in regard to hormonal mechanisms are those involving pituitary, thyroid, and adrenal functions.

A relatively recent development has been the focus on adipocyte number (fat cell number) in relation to obesity. In order to estimate adipocyte number, an analysis of body composition is required since calculation of the total number of adipocytes involves knowledge of total body fat and average fat content per cell. Several investigators have utilized the hypothesis that onset of obesity in early childhood is characterized by an increase in both the number (hyperplasia) and size (hypertrophy) of the adipocytes, whereas adult onset obesity involves only hypertrophy (Bjorntorp, 1974; Hirsch and Batchelor, 1976; Knittle et al., 1977). Although the hypothesis has several flaws stemming largely from the fact that adipocytes are impossible to identify unless they have a requisite amount of fat, the fact that body composition analyses are necessary to experimentally explore such hypotheses provides an additional rationale for improving techniques for body composition assessment.

The fact that obese people who participate in regular exercise may not change their body fat stores appreciably has been attributed to their apparent elevated number of adipocytes (hyperplastic obesity). In order to test this concept, Krotkiewski et al. (1979), exposed a group of obese women to a program of regular exercise of moderate intensity (3 × per week for 55 minutes per day) for 6 months. Table 22.18 shows the fatness data. There were no changes in body weight, body

TABLE 22.18
Characteristics and Body Fatness of Women Who Completed an Exercise Program Lasting Six Months

Variable	Before	at 3 Mo	at 6 Mo
Age (yr)	37.0 ± 7.5	37.3 ± 7.5	37.5 ± 7.5
Body Weight (kg)	78.8 ± 9.8	78.8 ± 10.1	80.0 ± 12.1
Fat Weight (kg)	34.1 ± 5.5	33.2 ± 5.7	34.1 ± 9.8
Fat Cell Weight (mg) (x̄ of 5 regions)	0.54 ± 0.08	0.52 ± 0.05	0.54 ± 0.07
Fat Cell Number (x 10¹⁰)	6.3 ± 1.7	6.4 ± 1.6	6.3 ± 1.8

Source: From M. K. Krotkiewski et al., *Metabolism* 28:651, 1979.

$N = 27.$

Values are means ± standard deviations.

fat, body cell mass, adiposity, or average cell size after either 3 or 6 months of exercise. Nevertheless, there appeared to be a modest relationship between adipocyte number and weight gain or loss. (See Figure 22.24.) Obese women with fewer adipocytes decreased their weight with regular exercise, whereas those with more adipocytes gained weight. Thus, the hypothesis that hyperplastic obesity blunts the effects of such interventions as exercise (and possibly diet) remains intriguing and warrants further exploration.

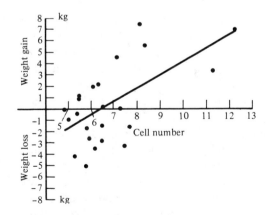

Figure 22.24
The relationship between total fat cell number ($\times$ 10¹⁰) and body weight change in obese women after 6 mo. of training. Regression coefficient r = 0.48 (p < 0.01). (From M. Krotkiewski et al., *Metabolism* 28:653, 1979.)

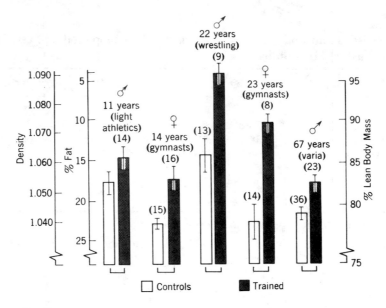

Figure 22.25
Differences between trained and untrained control subjects of different ages in body density, fat, and lean body mass proportions. (From J. Pařízková, *Physical Activity—Human Growth and Development*, G. L. Rarick, ed., Academic Press, New York, 1973, p. 100.)

Physical Activity

If comparison is made between physically active and inactive individuals of the same age, height, and weight, the physically active always have a higher body density, indicating a greater proportion of lean body mass. Pařízková (1963; 1965; 1981) has shown this for both sexes at all age levels (Fig. 22.25). In a study of gymnasts training for Olympic competition, Pařízková (1963) observed that body weight did not change during the first stage of training but that both the amount of subcutaneous and total body fat fell significantly with a concurrent development of lean body mass. After interruption of training, changes occurred in the opposite direction (Fig. 22.26). There was no difference in the response of male and female athletes. The effects of physical activity were also observed in obese children who were subjected to the combined effects of a reduction diet and intense physical training (Pařízková, 1965). At the end of a six to seven week period all the children lost weight and showed a reduction in skinfold thickness and an increase in body density (Fig. 22.27). Similar results have been reported from other laboratories (Goldman et al., 1963) for adolescent girls and boys. In a study involving obese high school boys, Christakis et al. (1966) reported that planned physical activity increased body weight loss and was accompanied by a reduction in skinfold thickness. Indeed, the effect of physical activity on body composition, observed as "overweightness" but obviously not "overfatness", in Navy personnel and in

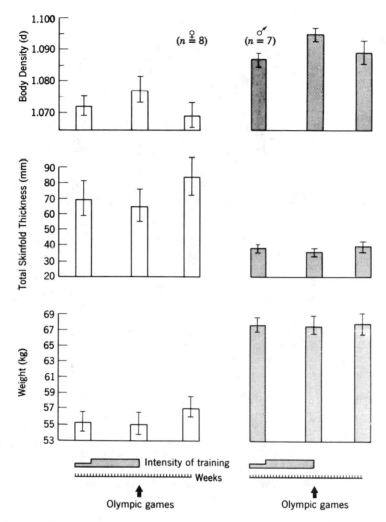

Figure 22.26
Body density, skinfold thickness, and weight changes in
gymnasts during and following Olympic training. (From
J. Pařízková, *Ann. N. Y. Acad. Sci.* 110:661, 1963.

professional football players served as the catalyst for studies on body composition
(Behnke et al., 1942; Welham and Behnke, 1942).

Profiles have been determined for athletes involved in different sports. (See
Wilmore, 1982.) That portion of the profile related to body composition for
athletes involved in four different sports is shown in Table 22.19. There are
important sex differences. Men are invariably heavier, have larger fat-free body
weights, and are leaner than women competitors in the same sport. Many of the
male competitors are quite lean indeed. Many women, particularly those who

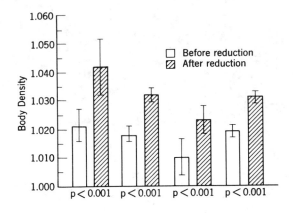

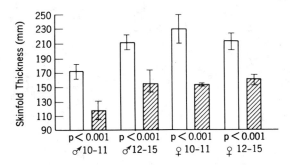

Figure 22.27
Changes in body density and skinfold thickness in obese children after program of physical activity in a summer camp. (From J. Pařízková, *Human Body Composition,* J. Brozek, ed., Pergamon Press, Oxford, 1965, p. 166.)

compete in distance events on a world-class level, are also quite lean and may average about 10 percent body fat.

Recent interest in weight training (using weights or machines) in exercise programs has stimulated investigation of the effects on body composition. In a comparison of the effects of a running program and a circuit weight training program, Gettman et al. (1978) found that weight training not only improved strength, but resulted in decreased body fatness. The running program also decreased body fatness but did not improve strength. Thus, both programs modified the body composition of the participants.

An assessment of body build that has been utilized in the analysis of musculoskeletal size is the relationship of fat-free body weight (FFW) to height (Ht). Values for comparisons among athletes are derived by relating FFW vs Ht to those established from the regression of FFW on Ht derived from nonathletes. Using this

TABLE 22.19
Physical Characteristics and Average Body Composition of Athletes Involved with Different Sports

Athletic Group	Sex	N	Age (yr)	Height (cm)	Weight (kg)	Fat (%)	Fat (kg)	Fat-free Weight (kg)	Reference
Basketball	F	21	19.1	169.1	62.6	20.8	13.0	49.6	Sinning (1973)
	M	13	25.3	197.0	90.9	9.5	8.6	82.4	Parr et al. (1978)
Runners	F	11	32.4	169.4	57.2	15.2	8.7	48.5	Wilmore & Brown (1974)
	M	20	26.2	177.0	63.1	4.7	3.0	60.0	Pollock et al. (1977)
Swimmers	F	9	19.4	168.0	63.8	26.3	16.8	47.0	Conger & McNab (1967)
	M	13	21.8	182.0	79.1	8.5	6.7	72.4	Sprynarova & Pařízková (1971)
Shotputters	F	9	21.5	167.6	78.1	28.0	21.9	56.2	Malina et al. (1971)
	M	12	27.7	187.0	108.6	16.4	17.8	90.8	Fahey et al. (1975)

Note: The procedures for measuring body fatness varied from study to study. Additional profiles for athletes appear in Wilmore (1982).

733

TABLE 22.20
Comparison of Characteristics Including the Potassium-to-Body-Weight Ratio and Total Body Calcium Between Marathon Runners and Normal Men

Group	Age (yrs)	Weight (kg)	Height (m)	K/Wt (gm/kg)	TBCa (gm)
Runners	42.0 ± 1.4	73.6 ± 1.5	1.75 ± 0.02	1.97 ± 0.04	1175.0 ± 24.3
Normals	45.0 ± 1.9	79.3 ± 2.4	1.74 ± 0.02	1.75 ± 0.05	1020.0 ± 79.8
p value	NS	< 0.2	NS	< 0.001	< 0.05

Source: From J. F. Aloia et al, *Metabolism* 27:1793, 1978.

Values are mean ± standard error of the mean.

K/Wt = potassium per body weight.

TBCa = total body calcium.

technique, large differences were found both between specific groups of athletes and between groups of athletes and nonathletes. Track runners had the least amount of FFW related to Ht among athletes and their values tended to be within 1 standard error of the regression line for nonathletes. Professional football players were 2–3 standard errors above the regression line for nonathletes. Track field-event athletes also tended to fall well above the regression line. Such an analysis for the body density of the fat-free weight may be different not only among athletes, but between athletes and nonathletes since no distinction can be made between muscle tissue and skeletal tissue or hydration of these tissues. However, women athletes had a greater FFW relative to Ht than did the men when compared to the nonathletic population (Slaughter and Lohman, 1980). The latter observation may well reflect the fact that only the more athletically gifted women are currently engaged in athletics and as this population grows, the difference in FFW/Ht between women athletes and nonathletes will become similar to that for men.

Evidence for the differences in density of the fat-free mass among athletes and others is suggested by data on body potassium from whole body counting and on calcium from neutron activation analysis in marathon runners and nonathletes (Aloia et al., 1978). When the values for total body potassium and calcium are corrected for age and body size, the marathon runners have higher values of 7 and 11 percent, respectively. (See Table 22.20.) Such differences are intriguing and should be explored among other groups of athletes and nonathletes, that is, those who vary in age, sex, fitness, and habitual activity.

Summary

Under the thicknesses of their skinfolds, all men are surprisingly alike; and for women, beauty may not be skin, but skinfold deep, the depth varying with the fashion of the times. Today's fashion, for health rather than cosmetic reasons, is leanness for both men and women since excess fat has been implicated in the etiology of many of the diseases of middle age, and actuarial tables hold dire warnings for the obese. Estimation of body composition by various analytical laboratory methods has helped to establish norms and is invaluable to the physician and surgeon in patient management. Normative data permit evaluation and calibration of simpler methods that become the tools of the investigator of large population groups or of the practitioner in office or clinic. Since it is not only what we eat, but how much and what the body does with it, that makes us what we are, the nutritionist is an integral part of the team in prophylaxis and therapeutics.

Claude Bernard said, "Every time that a new and reliable means of experimental analysis makes its appearance, we invariably see science make progress in the questions to which this means of analysis can be applied." How clearly this has been demonstrated in the investigation of body composition.

chapter 23

determination of nutrient needs: energy, protein, minerals

> Methods for assessment of nutrient needs are based on the fundamental concepts of nutrition already discussed: ingestion of food, digestion, absorption, transportation to the cells, metabolism in cells, storage, and finally excretion from the body (including expired gases, urine, feces, and sweat). Quantitatively, nutrient requirements depend on the additive needs of the individual cells, which vary according to physiological demands imposed by the life cycle: growth, reproduction, lactation. The amounts supplied by the diet, however, must be sufficient to cover the net cellular requirements plus both unabsorbed nutrients and endogenous losses. In other words, the gross dietary requirement is the sum of cellular needs plus overall body losses.
>
> It is at this point that we integrate the physiological and biochemical aspects of nutrition with the "nutritional aspects of nutrition." The additional responsibility of the nutritionist is to determine nutrient requirements and how they can be met.

The assessment of nutritional requirements, like so many complex subjects, is easier to discuss than to accomplish. At best, experiments designed to determine nutrient needs can provide only estimations of requirements. Biological systems are complex and highly variable and, in this respect, human beings are notorious. Genetic background, previous diet, environment, stress, and other factors influence to varying degrees the response to diet. Many of these factors can be controlled in carefully conducted experiments with laboratory animals of relatively short life span. Every human being, however, represents a multitude of uncontrollable variables even when maintained under the most rigid conditions.

A second complicating factor is that studies with humans rarely can be carried out for long periods of time partly because of expense of operation, but more often because few subjects will remain cooperative for more than several weeks at a time. The regimentation of eating prescribed kinds and amounts of foods and of collecting excreta require a fair degree of motivation even for a short period. The few studies that have been conducted over a period of months, however, suggest that long-term effects of diet may be quite different from effects observed in the usual periods of 6–8 weeks.

In spite of the difficulties inherent in human metabolic research, however, a large body of data has accumulated to form a working basis for evaluating the nutrient needs of humans.

Definition of Requirements

The term requirement has been loosely used and often misused. *Minimum requirement* has referred to the least amount of a nutrient that will prevent clinical symptoms of deficiency or support a well defined biochemical response such as maintenance of nitrogen equilibrium in the adult, normal hemoglobin levels, or a specified level of a metabolite in blood or urine. As will be seen later, these are very different criteria and do not necessarily measure the same state of nutrition. Therefore quantitative estimations of minimum requirement should *always* be expressed in terms of the criterion used for evaluation.

A question remains regarding *what* criterion should be used to evaluate minimum requirement. Is the minimum the lowest level that will prevent deficiency symptoms, or is it some undefined point in cellular adaptation to diminishing nutrient supply? Adaptation is a normal process in maintaining cell function, but when the adaptive shift becomes the fixed metabolic pathway, abnormalities ensue. It would seem that the true minimum requirement lies somewhere between the initial shift to alternative metabolic pathways and the final expression of adaptive failure and, in a complex organism, varies among cells according to their metabolic rates and requirements. Simply stated, the problem is that there is at present no definitive criterion for determining the point in the continuum at which adaptive mechanisms are no longer normal. The inability to define precisely minimum requirement is a valid reason for the margin of safety used in developing dietary standards. The margin of safety is, in a sense, a cushion against ignorance.

Summary of Methods for Determining Nutrient Needs

Early attempts to determine the nutrient needs of animals were based on studies of body composition on the logical assumption that substances present in the body are primarily those necessary for life. The mere presence of substances in tissues does not establish a dietary requirement; many substances are synthesized in cells from dietary components or are simply carried in the food or water as contaminants. However, the proportions of nutrients comprising the animal body suggest grossly the relative amounts needed or retained in the body and thus very early provided clues to the nutrient needs of humans.

Survey studies of nutrient intake also provide reasonable estimates of human nutrient needs. Dietary intake of a group of healthy people, for example, compared with nutrient intake of a population group in which nutritional disease is endemic, yields data that distinguish roughly between nutrient intakes that are compatible with health and those that lead to disease. Similarly, many estimates of the energy needs of children are based on energy intakes of normally growing children. The British standard for ascorbic acid (British Medical Association, 1950) also is based on the results of dietary surveys which indicated that intakes of 30 mg were compatible with apparent health in the majority of the population of Great Britain. Dietary surveys, however, cannot provide *precise* estimates of nutrient requirements; quantitative estimations of nutrient needs demand the refinement of controlled experiments.

One of the earliest recorded controlled dietary studies was the classical experiment on scurvy patients performed by James Lind about 1747. (See Todhunter, 1962.) To 12 seamen with scurvy Lind gave a basic diet and to 2 he gave daily supplements including cider, elixir of ferric sulphate, vinegar, sea water, citrus fruit, and an obscure medical treatment of the period. The result of Lind's rather crude experiment is nutrition history. The important characteristics of Lind's experiment are first, the control of dietary intake and second, the measurement of change in clinical condition as a result of dietary change alone.

Similarly, the determination of quantiative human requirements demands that dietary intake be precisely controlled in order to correlate nutrient intake with organism response. In other words, a specific response is measured against a known intake. The kinds of studies applicable to determination of human requirements are grouped arbitrarily below and will be discussed here and in Chapter 24.

1. Balance studies.
   (a) Energy balance.
   (b) Chemical balance.
2. Biochemical measurements of nutrient, nutrient metabolites or related functional and structural components.
   (a) Urinary excretions.
   (b) Blood levels.
3. Clinical evaluation and performance tests.

Other techniques such as those involving isotope tracers or tissue biopsy are essentially variations of 1 and 2. The basis of metabolic experiments is depicted in Fig. 23.1; factors most commonly measured are indicated by bold type.

Balance Studies

Balance studies are based on the principle of the conservation of energy and matter. In terms of body metabolism, as shown in Fig. 23.1, the balance method is simply a comparison of nutrient intake and output (loss from body) and thus is a measurement of body gain or loss. The technique is applicable only when a stable component is under study or when end products of metabolism are clearly recognized. For example, heat is the end product of energy metabolism and all forms of energy can be expressed as heat. Therefore the balance experiment can be used in studies of energy exchange. Protein balance is determined by measurement of its metabolically stable component, nitrogen. Mineral elements are stable substances and therefore lend themselves to the balance technique.

Vitamins, however, are not biologically stable substances; the end products of vitamin metabolism are numerous and many are as yet unidentified. Vitamins synthesized by bacteria in the gastrointestinal tract further complicate the picture. The balance technique therefore is not generally applicable to the vitamins.

In its simplest form the balance method is represented by the following equation:

$$\text{Balance} = \text{Intake} - \text{Excretion products}$$

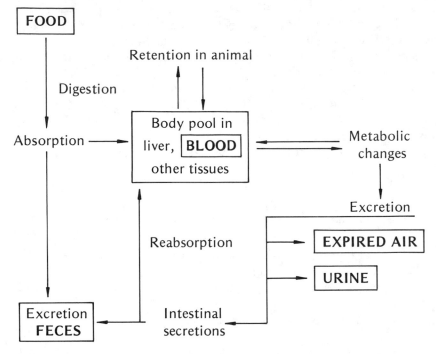

Figure 23.1
Summary of nutrient metabolism. (From P. L. Altman and D. S. Dittmer, eds., *Biology Data Book. Fed. Amer. Soc. Exp. Biol.*, Washington, D. C., 1964, p. 192.)

Excretion products are usually defined as substances excreted by way of the intestinal tract and kidneys, but in certain instances, for example energy balance, excretion via the lungs and skin is even more important. Although excretion by way of sweat need not be determined in studies of protein and mineral balance, the significance of these losses must be taken into account in the *interpretation* of data. (See Consolazio et al. 1963a; 1963b; Calloway et al., 1971.)

INTERPRETATION OF BALANCE STUDIES

The teminology used in interpretation of balance studies tends to be confusing: positive balance, negative balance, and equilibrium. A positive balance is expressed mathematically by a dietary intake greater than excretion products and indicates that the body is gaining in the nutrient under study. Positive balance is the normal response to growth or gain in body substance and therefore is expected during childhood, adolescence, late pregnancy, and repletion following dietary restriction or loss of body substance as a result of surgery, injury from burns, or other trauma.

Conversely, negative balance means that excretion of a nutrient is greater than the intake and indicates that dietary intake is too low to replace nutrients lost

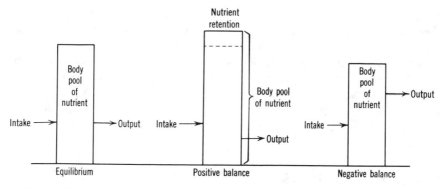

Figure 23.2
Relationship between nutrient intake and output in balance experiments.

from the body or to prevent destruction of body tissue. Loss of body weight, when corrected for body water losses, is usually indicative of a negative energy balance.

Equilibrium represents the steady state, when intake and excretion are essentially equal. The normal adult maintained on an adequate diet, therefore, should be in a state of equilibrium with respect to energy, nitrogen, and the mineral elements, assuming first that weight is maintained, and second, that the quantity of nutrient in the body remains relatively constant. The adult is, in a sense, in a dynamic steady state.

The theoretical relationship between nutrient intake and output in balance studies is shown in Fig. 23.2. The use of the terms positive balance and negative balance is unfortunate; one does not readily conceive of balance under conditions of obvious imbalance. The terms are widely accepted, however, and must be clearly understood. Returning to the balance equation and Fig. 23.2 it should be clear that, on constant dietary intake, as the body gains in a nutrient, it must excrete less; when the body loses a nutrient, it excretes more. Balance, then, must be interpreted as referring to the overall economy of the body and obviously provides no information on the dynamic exchanges within and between individual cells. (See Chapter 7.)

USES AND LIMITATIONS OF THE BALANCE TECHNIQUE

The balance technique has been used widely as a criterion of dietary adequacy of protein and the mineral elements and as a measure of the physiological utilization of these nutrients from foods. It has been used less often for the experimental study of energy balance which lends itself readily to studies of energy expenditure alone.

In the normal adult, nitrogen and mineral equilibrium can be obtained at any level above the minimum requirement. Therefore reliable data on requirements can be obtained by measuring balance at various levels of dietary intake and calculating the intake at equilibrium by regression.

Balance studies, however, reflect previous dietary intake (Hegsted et al., 1952; Kelley and Ohlson, 1954; Allison, 1957). In addition, the animal body adapts to different levels of intake, although the time required for adaptation varies among nutrients. Adaptation to varying levels of protein occurs within days (Allison, ibid), whereas adaptation to changes in calcium intake may require several months (Malm, 1958). With the proper attention given to the effect of previous intake and the power of adaptation, the balance technique is a useful and valuable tool for the study of nutrient requirements.

Energy Requirement

From an experimental standpoint, the determination of energy requirement does not necessarily involve the balance of energy intake against output. Methods for determination of energy needs are based primarily on energy expenditure alone and include the direct measurement of heat loss from the body or calculation of heat production from gaseous exchange (oxygen consumed and carbon dioxide expired). The various instruments used in determining energy exchange have been described by Swift and French (1954), Consolazio and Johnson (1971), and Buskirk and Mendez (1980). The following discussion will stress the principles underlying calorimetric methods, and scant attention will be given to details of operation.

For information on various aspects of the measurement of energy metabolism, see Ross Laboratories (1980).

PRINCIPLES OF CALORIMETRY

In studies of animal energy exchange, the use of the kilocalorie (kcal), or the kilojoule (kJ), a heat unit, must be considered a convenience rather than a primary concern. Interest in the origin of animal heat sparked the early work in calorimetry, and body heat loss has long been known to result from oxidation processes within the cell. The *primary* biological advantage, however, is not the production of heat to warm the body but the transformation of the energy bound in foodstuffs into a form of energy that can be used by the animal for internal and external work. Heat produced as an end result of cellular oxidation is beneficial to the animal in maintaining body temperature, but it is of no value as a source of external or internal work. (An exception is the brown adipose tissue that functions largely as a source of body heat.) Heat is a byproduct of metabolism. In other words, heat is a fringe benefit of animal oxidations; ATP is the net income that maintains life. (See Chapter 13.)

The animal's source of useful energy is the chemical energy supplied by food. Other forms of energy, such as solar energy utilized by the green plant for syntheses, are useful only for driving a few cellular reactions such as those occurring in the skin. Lying on a sunny beach, for example, can produce a beautiful suntan, but it is the picnic lunch that you bring along that sustains you.

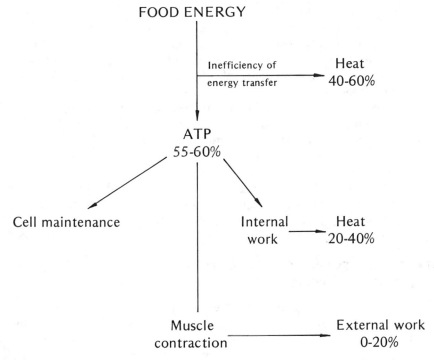

Figure 23.3
Summary of animal energy expenditure and heat loss. (From A. C. Brown and
G. Brengelmann, *Physiology and Biophysics,* T. C. Ruch and H. D. Patton, eds.,
W. B. Saunders, Philadelphia, 1965, p. 1034.)

Obviously, if an animal does not eat, the body's need for energy must be
supplied by its own substance. Glycogen from liver and muscle, fatty acids from
adipose tissues, or even structural protein all serve as substrate for cellular oxidation equally as well as the carbohydrate, fat, and protein from ham sandwiches
and deviled eggs.

The oxidation of foodstuffs provides chemical energy for cellular reactions. As
energy is transformed from one form to another (as occurs in the metabolism of
foodstuffs in the cell), the capacity of the total energy to perform work decreases.
The transformation of chemical energy (as in food) to mechanical energy (work)
is never complete. (See Fig. 23.3.) When the large molecules of carbohydrates,
fats, and proteins are broken down into progressively smaller fragments by the
enzymes of intermediary metabolism, the change is from a highly organized to
a disorganized state. The step-by-step process, however, insures the capture of
about 40 percent of the energy in the useful form of ATP. The rest is lost as heat.
(See Chapter 13.) However, when molecules are disrupted violently, as in the
oxygen-charged atmosphere of a bomb calorimeter, the state of disorganization
is such that all of the potential energy of the food is manifested as heat.

When ATP is utilized for cellular synthetic reactions and in work performance, still more energy is wasted. Lehninger (1965b) estimated that the total energy required for synthesis of phosphatidyl choline is about 17 kcal/mole of the complete molecule. The synthesis of 1 mole of phosphatidyl choline is accomplished, however, at the expense of 8 moles of ATP or a total of about 56 kcal (8×7 kcal). The efficiency of synthesis therefore is only about 34 percent.

The synthesis of a complex protein is even more expensive in terms of ATP utilization. Each peptide bond with a free energy of about 5 kcal requires an investment of at least 3 high energy phosphate bonds yielding a biosynthetic efficiency of roughly 25 percent.

Muscle contraction also is a fairly expensive process. The overall ability of the animal body to convert potential energy of food to mechanical work amounts to only 20–25 percent of the total available energy. In comparison with man-made machines, however, the efficiency of the animal body is very good.

TOTAL ENERGY EXPENDITURE: HEAT LOSS
PLUS EXTERNAL WORK PERFORMED

All of the energy transformed within the animal body can be accounted for as heat eliminated from the body and as work done by the animal on the environment. In the resting animal (that is, when no external work is being performed), essentially all of the energy transformed within the body is dissipated as heat. This state is referred to as the *resting metabolism*. Heat loss thus includes both the heat produced from inefficient transfer of the energy of oxidation and final degradation of internal work into heat. For example, the work of the heart and lungs is converted into heat by the friction of blood in the capillaries and the movement of air in and out of the body.

When external work is performed, energy expenditure is equivalent to the heat produced *plus* the work done. All forms of work, however, are not easily measured. Lifting a known weight to a known height or riding a stationary cycle ergometer are forms of work that can be calculated easily as heat energy. The heat equivalent of work energy is 1 kcal to 427 kilogram meters of work where kilogram meters = weight × distance.

If, conceivably, a gymnasium-size calorimeter could be constructed and an individual allowed (or forced) to perform all his or her usual activities within, the total amount of heat measured should be quite close to the individual's actual energy expenditure. In certain instances, such as lifting an object, a small amount of energy would reside in the object lifted; in other instances, such as freely riding a bicycle, heat is produced by friction of the wheels. Heat produced during the latter activity therefore emanates from the object, not from the individual.

In any case, the direct measurement of heat loss is expensive and complicated in operation and rarely is used now in practical human calorimetry. Lavoisier's work suggested that oxygen consumption and heat production were closely correlated in the resting animal. Atwater and Rosa (1899) proved conclusively that the *total* energy expenditure is related quantitatively to oxygen consumption. The calculation of energy expenditure in kcal from oxygen consumption is known as *indirect calorimetry*. This method is simple and relatively inexpensive in operation and offers the added advantage of measuring the total energy expenditure, that is, resting metabolism plus work performed. For these reasons, indirect calorimetry has generally replaced measurement of heat loss as a method for determining energy expenditure.

FACTORS CONTRIBUTING TO THE TOTAL ENERGY REQUIREMENT

Total metabolism and therefore total energy expenditure ultimately are determined by the internal and external work of the body and are, in effect, a result of mitochondrial activity in cells in which respiratory rate can differ widely. In the rat, for example, kidney tissue respires at a very high rate; liver, heart, brain, and diaphragm are less active than kidney but also respire at high rates. In comparison, skin, skeleton, ligaments, and blood respire at relatively low rates (Field et al., 1939).

Total energy expenditure can be viewed most conveniently as an overall expression of varying degrees of tissue (or mitochondrial) activity necessary for the internal and external work of the body. Moreover, internal and external work are inseparable when external work is performed, because it is obvious that any form of activity (or external work) affects the internal work of the body.

The determination of energy needs, therefore, requires a separation of the total energy expenditure into physiological entities that can be defined and measured. The most significant factors that affect the total energy requirements of an individual are:

1. Basal metabolism.
2. Calorigenic effect of food (specific dynamic action or specific dynamic effect).
3. Activity.

Basal Metabolism
The energy expenditure during basal metabolism has been aptly called "the cost of living" and is loosely comparable to the minimum requirement for the nutrients. It refers to the metabolic activity required to maintain life: respiration, heart beat, maintenance of body temperature, and other essential functions.

Many factors influence the internal work of the body even when at rest, for example, physiological state, environmental temperature, food intake, and such subtleties as degree of muscle tension. In order to minimize influences that would raise metabolic activity and invalidate baseline comparison among individuals, the degree of cellular metabolism or basal metabolic rate (BMR) must be determined under closely controlled and standardized conditions. The BMR therefore is determined when an individual is in the postabsorptive state (at least 12 hours after eating) and is lying down, completely relaxed, in a room of comfortable temperature.

Numerous determinations of basal metabolic rate have been made on humans and other species.[1] It is clear that metabolic rate varies with body size. For many years, however, there has been considerable discussion and disagreement in attempts to establish a constant relationship between metabolic rate and a unit of body size that would apply to large and small animals alike.

In clinical practice it is customary to express BMR in relation to surface area, that is, kcal per hour per square meter (m^2) of body surface (kcal per m^2/hr). This relationship is based on the assumption that heat loss and therefore BMR are proportional to surface area. Many formulas for calculation of body surface from weight and height have been proposed; the formula of DuBois and DuBois (1916) is one that appears to be well accepted:

$$A = W^{0.425} \times H^{0.725} \times 71.84$$

where A is surface area in m^2; W is weight in kg, and H is height in cm. Simple, easy-to-use clinical tables as shown in Table 23.1 have been substituted for the formula for most practical work.

From a comparison of data on metabolic rate of several mammalian species, however, Kleiber concluded that although metabolic rate is not proportional to body weight *per se,* there is a linear relationship between metabolic rate and the three-fourth power of body weight. (See Kleiber, 1947.) Moreover, this relationship is more precise than that of BMR and surface area and thus is applicable to all species. Originally proposed in 1932, the concept of metabolic body size defined as body weight in $kg^{3/4}$ was officially accepted at the Conference on Energy Metabolism in Tyrone, Scotland, in 1964. As a general rule covering all species, metabolic rate can be computed in kcal per day as $70 \times W^{3/4}$. More precise formulas for predicting metabolic rate of humans are:

For men: $M = 71.2 \times W^{3/4}[1 + 0.004(30 - a) + 0.010(s - 43.4)]$
For women: $M = 65.8 \times W^{3/4}[1 + 0.004(30 - a) + 0.018(s - 42.1)]$

where M = metabolic rate in kcal per day
W = body weight in kg
a = age in years (formula is based on assumption of a decrease of about 0.4 percent of the metabolic rate for each year above age 30)
s = specific stature in $cm/W^{1/3}$ (assuming each additional cm per $kg^{1/3}$ in specific stature produces an average increase of 1 percent of the metabolic rate of men and 1.8 percent of the metabolic rate of women)

A comparison of metabolic rate of the human calculated either from surface area or the three-fourth power of body weight yields comparable results. For example, daily basal energy expenditure for a 132 lb (60 kg) woman, 5 ft 6 in (167 cm) tall, 45 years old, then may be calculated from a surface area of 1.68 m^2 (Fig. 23.4). At 34.9 kcal per m^2/hr, the total expenditure would be approximately 1,409 kcal ($1.68 \times 34.9 \times 24$). Using the Kleiber formula, metabolic rate is calculated as 1,416 kcal ($1417 - 0.94 + 0.03$). It should be noted, however, that despite close agreement within species, $W^{3/4}$ yields data applicable

---

[1]See Sargent (1961; 1962) for evaluation of basal metabolic data on infants and children in the United States.

TABLE 23.1
The Mayo Foundation Normal Standards: Calories per Square Meter per Hour

Males		Females	
Age at Last Birthday	Mean	Age at Last Birthday	Mean
6	53.00	6	50.62
7	52.45	6½	50.23
8	51.78	7	49.12
8½	51.20	7½	47.84
9	50.54	8	47.00
9½	49.42	8½	46.50
10	48.50	9–10	45.90
10½	47.71	11	45.26
11	47.18	11½	44.80
12	46.75	12	44.28
13–15	46.35	12½	43.58
16	45.72	13	42.90
16½	45.30	13½	42.10
17	44.80	14	41.45
17½	44.03	14½	40.74
18	43.25	15	40.10
18½	42.70	15½	39.40
19	42.32	16	38.85
19½	42.00	16½	38.30
20–21	41.43	17	37.82
22–23	40.82	17½	37.40
24–27	40.24	18–19	36.74
28–29	39.81	20–24	36.18
30–34	39.34	25–44	35.70
35–39	38.68	45–49	34.94
40–44	38.00	50–54	33.96
45–49	37.37	55–59	33.18
50–54	36.73	60–64	32.61
55–59	36.10	65–69	32.30
60–64	35.48	a	
65–69	34.80		

[a]Obtained by extrapolation.

to all mammalian species and therefore is to be preferred for research in comparative animal calorimetry. Table 23.2 provides $W^{3/4}$ for body weights ranging from 1–100 kg.

Recently, more investigators and physicians have utilized lean body mass or fat-free body weight as the reference for BMR. The premise is that stored lipid in adipose tissue constitutes a large nonmetabolic component in the body although the adipocyte itself is metabolically active. Use of lean body mass was recom-

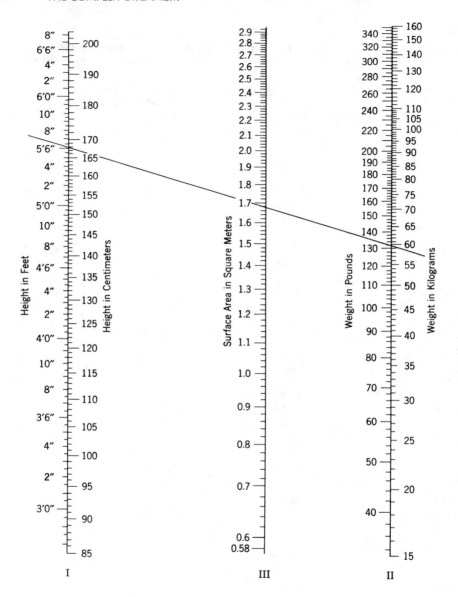

Figure 23.4
Nomogram for calculating surface area.

mended by Miller and Blyth (1952; 1953) and more recently by Tzankoff and Norris (1977; 1978), and by Cunningham (1980; 1982), among others. The latter units for BMR would be kcal per kg (fat-free)/hr.

Factors Affecting Basal Metabolism
The effect of age on basal metabolic rate is shown in Fig. 23.5. BMR is highest per square meter during the first one and one-half to two years of life, decreases

TABLE 23.2
Metabolic Body Size, $W^{3/4}$ for Body Weights from 1 to 100 kg

W, kg	$W^{3/4}$ kg$^{3/4}$	W, kg	$W^{3/4}$ kg$^{3/4}$	W, kg	$W^{3/4}$ kg$^{3/4}$	W, kg	$W^{3/4}$ kg$^{3/4}$	W, kg	$W^{3/4}$ kg$^{3/4}$
1	1.00	21	9.8	41	16.2	61	21.8	81	27.0
2	1.68	22	10.2	42	16.5	62	22.1	82	27.2
3	2.28	23	10.5	43	16.8	63	22.4	83	27.5
4	2.83	24	10.8	44	17.1	64	22.6	84	27.7
5	3.34	25	11.2	45	17.4	65	22.9	85	28.0
6	3.83	26	11.5	46	17.7	66	23.2	86	28.2
7	4.30	27	11.8	47	18.0	67	23.4	87	28.5
8	4.75	28	12.2	48	18.2	68	23.7	88	28.7
9	5.19	29	12.5	49	18.5	69	23.9	89	29.0
10	5.62	30	12.8	50	18.8	70	24.2	90	29.2
11	6.04	31	13.1	51	19.1	71	24.4	91	29.4
12	6.44	32	13.5	52	19.4	72	24.7	92	29.7
13	6.84	33	13.8	53	19.6	73	25.0	93	29.9
14	7.24	34	14.1	54	19.9	74	25.2	94	30.2
15	7.62	35	14.4	55	20.2	75	25.5	95	30.4
16	8.00	36	14.7	56	20.5	76	25.8	96	30.7
17	8.38	37	15.0	57	20.8	77	26.0	97	30.9
18	8.75	38	15.3	58	21.0	78	26.2	98	31.1
19	9.10	39	15.6	59	21.3	79	26.5	99	31.4
20	9.46	40	15.9	60	21.6	80	26.7	100	31.6

in early childhood, and increases slightly at puberty; thereafter BMR declines steadily. The reason for these age differences is not well understood. It is clear, however, that BMR is highest during periods of rapid growth and undoubtedly is associated with the increased biosynthetic activity of growth.

The sex difference noted throughout the life span often is attributed to differences in body composition between males and females. The female body generally contains more fat than the male and therefore a lower lean body mass or active protoplasmic tissue (Behnke, 1953). According to Kleiber (1961) and Mitchell (1962), the effect of the sex hormones on BMR may be more direct than their effect on body composition. Estimated basal metabolic rates for males and females over a wide range of body weight are shown in Table 23.3.

Basal heat production is increased in late pregnancy (Sandiford and Wheeler, 1924; Enright et al., 1935). Leitch (1957) attributed the increase to fetal growth and growth of maternal tissues such as mammary and uterine tissues. According to Kleiber (1961), however, the increase in BMR of pregnant rats is due mainly to increased metabolic rate of maternal tissues other than those directly involved in the reproductive process. The reason for increased BMR during pregnancy is therefore uncertain. Emerson et al. (1975) found an increase in BMR during pregnancy that was proportional to body cell mass.

Racial differences apparently do not affect basal metabolic rate and the effect

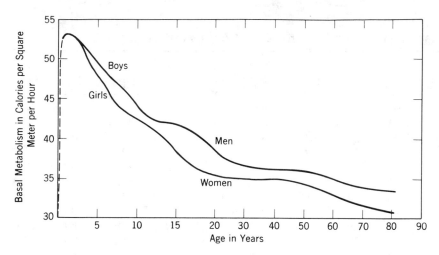

Figure 23.5
Effect of age on basal metabolism. (From H. H. Mitchell, *Comparative Nutrition of Man and Domestic Animals,* Vol. I, Academic Press, New York, 1962, p. 43.)

of environmental temperature is uncertain. Although some reports indicate that individuals living in tropical climates tend to have a basal metabolic rate lower than those living in temperate or cold climates, Consolazio et al. (1961) reported no effect of excessively hot climates on the basal metabolism.[2]

Certain pathological conditions, such as hyperthyroidism and fever, increase basal metabolism. In fever, the increase is about 7 percent for each degree (F) rise in body temperature or 13 percent for each degree (C). Both fasting and chronic undernutrition decrease the BMR to about an equal degree. Early studies by Benedict (1915) on a professional faster indicated a decrease in BMR of about 25 percent on the twentieth day of fasting; thereafter BMR remained relatively stable. Keys' studies (Keys et al., 1950) during World War II on men maintained on low calorie rations indicated a reduction of about 20 percent. The decrease in BMR as a result of undernutrition is interpreted as an adaptive mechanism of the body that conserves energy by operating at a lower level of metabolic activity; probably some of the decrease is due also to a decrease in weight and a subsequent decrease in surface area of the body.

---

[2]BMR is measured under highly standardized conditions so that, in fact, the BMR is a measure of inherent tissue metabolic rates. Resting metabolism assumes only that the individual is at rest, that is, not performing work; environmental factors are not controlled. Consequently, temperature effects are reflected in resting metabolism. The effect of environmental temperature on the resting metabolism was first shown by Lavoisier. (See Chapter 1.) An increase in metabolism occurs at either extreme of the temperature scale; in cold, the increase is accomplished by shivering: muscular contractions that result in an increase in heat production both from the inefficient transfer of the high energy of ATP and the friction of contracting muscle fibers. In severe heat, additional energy is paradoxically required to maintain body temperature; that is, the process of maintaining temperature homeostasis requires extra energy.

TABLE 23.3
Basal Metabolic Rates According to Weight and Sex

Body Weight (kg)	Kcal per 24 Hours		MJ per 24 Hours	
	Males	Females	Males	Females
3.0	150	136	0.6	0.6
4.0	210	205	0.9	0.8
5.0	270	274	1.1	1.1
6.0	330	336	1.4	1.4
7.0	390	395	1.6	1.6
8.0	445	448	1.9	1.9
9.0	495	496	2.1	2.1
10.0	545	541	2.3	2.3
11.0	590	582	2.5	2.4
12.0	625	620	2.5	2.6
13.0	665	655	2.8	2.7
14.0	700	687	2.9	2.9
15.0	725	718	3.0	3.0
16.0	750	747	3.1	3.1
17.0	780	775	3.3	3.2
18.0	810	802	3.4	3.3
19.0	840	827	3.5	3.5
20.0	870	852	3.6	3.6
22.0	910	898	3.8	3.8
24.0	980	942	4.1	3.9
26.0	1070	984	4.5	4.1
28.0	1100	1025	4.6	4.3
30.0	1140	1063	4.8	4.4
32.0	1190	1101	5.0	4.6
34.0	1230	1137	5.1	4.8
36.0	1270	1173	5.3	4.9
38.0	1305	1207	5.5	5.0
40.0	1340	1241	5.6	5.2
42.0	1370	1274	5.7	5.3
44.0	1400	1306	5.9	5.5
46.0	1430	1338	6.0	5.6
48.0	1460	1369	6.1	5.7
50.0	1485	1399	6.2	5.8
52.0	1505	1429	6.3	6.0
54.0	1555	1458	6.5	6.1
56.0	1580	1487	6.6	6.2
58.0	1600	1516	6.7	6.3
60.0	1630	1544	6.8	6.5
62.0	1660	1572	6.9	6.6
64.0	1690	1599	7.1	6.7
66.0	1725	1626	7.2	6.8
68.0	1765	1653	7.4	6.9

TABLE 23.3 (continued)

Body Weight (kg)	Kcal per 24 Hours		MJ per 24 Hours	
	Males	**Females**	**Males**	**Females**
70.0	1785	1679	7.5	7.0
72.0	1815	1705	7.6	7.1
74.0	1845	1731	7.7	7.2
76.0	1870	1756	7.8	7.3
78.0	1900	1781	7.9	7.4
80.0	—	1805	—	7.5
82.0	—	1830	—	7.7
84.0	2000	1855	8.4	7.8

Source: From FAO/WHO, "Energy Requirements and Protein Requirements," *WHO Tech. Rep. Ser.,* No. 522 (1973), pp. 107–108.

Many attempts have been made to show that BMR is higher for athletes than nonathletes due presumably to a greater mass of active protoplasmic tissue. (See Mitchell, 1962.) Slight increases have been shown in the trained athlete but differences between athletes and nonathletes generally appear to be negligible, particularly when body size and fat-free weight are taken into account.

Calorigenic Effect of Food

Determination of the basal metabolic rate requires that the subject be in the postabsorptive state, that is, without food for at least 12 hours prior to the test. The reason for withholding food is that following ingestion of food, heat production increases above the resting state. This effect was first recognized by Rubner in 1902 and was called the *specific dynamic effect* of food. The effect of food on heat production was clearly demonstrated, however, in Lavoisier's experiments. (See Chapter 1.) When foodstuffs were fed individually, the increase in heat production following ingestion of protein was observed to be considerably greater than that following carbohydrate and fat. In an ordinary mixed diet consisting of all foodstuffs, however, the calorigenic effect amounts to about 6 percent of the energy value of the dietary intake (Benedict and Carpenter, 1918). The proportions of carbohydrate, fat, and protein in the diet do not significantly influence the calorigenic effect. The use of high protein diets in weight reduction in the belief that the calorigenic effect will be increased is without scientific basis. High protein and low protein diets produce similar effects (Bradfield and Jourdan, 1973).

In passing, it might be noted that the extra heat production following ingestion of food is known also as the *specific dynamic action* (SDA) of food. We prefer the term *calorigenic effect* as a more suitable description of this confusing phenomenon.

The cause of extra heat production following ingestion of food, and particularly protein, has plagued nutritionists for many years. Numerous theories have been proposed but there is no general agreement yet. The early belief that the work of digestion caused the increase in heat production was easily disproved since even when nutrient substances were injected (thus bypassing the intestinal tract), the calorigenic effect was observed.

The calorigenic effect, then, was assumed to be related to the fate of foodstuffs after absorption. Voit proposed that when foods are ingested and transported to the cells the cellular mechanism is temporarily overwhelmed by a flood of metabolizable nutrients that, in some indefinable way, speed up the metabolic rate. The greater calorigenic effect observed for protein was attributed by Lusk (1931) to the more complicated series of reactions required for the metabolism of amino acids, that is, deamination.

Probably the most definitive early reports on this difficult and confusing subject are those of Wilhelmj et al. (1928) and Borsook and Winegarden (1931), which extended earlier work of Terroine and Bonnet (1926). The latter authors attributed the high heat increment of protein to the quantity of amino nitrogen ingested and, more specifically, to the amount of amino nitrogen deaminated, that is, urinary nitrogen. Wilhelmj et al. (1928) expressed the relationship between the calorigenic effect and ingested protein in terms of calories per millimole of deaminated amino acid (calculated from urinary nitrogen), and Borsook and Winegarden (1931) reported a positive correlation between metabolic rate and urinary nitrogen.

Passmore and Ritchie (1957) suggested that the calorigenic effect of food is a twofold process. They observed an increase in heat production in subjects within five minutes after a test meal. This finding suggests that the work of the digestive tract does indeed contribute in part to the total rise in heat production. The cellular mechanism contributing to extra heat production following the ingestion of foodstuffs remains speculative.

The most likely theory to date was proposed by Krebs (1964), who related the calorigenic effect of food to the energy requirement for synthesis of ATP. Calculating ATP yield from oxidation of triglyceride (tristearin) and carbohydrate (glucose residue from starch), he estimated that 18.1 kcal and 17.4 kcal are required to obtain 1 mole ATP when fat and carbohydrate, respectively, are oxidized, assuming complete oxidation of these foodstuffs. ATP synthesized from protein oxidation was calculated from the gross yield of ATP from each of the amino acids present in an individual protein. Calculation of ATP yield was corrected for two factors: (1) ATP required for urea synthesis and (2) incomplete oxidation of amino acids. (Much of the dietary glycine, for example, is used in the synthesis of creatine, porphyrin, or purines; some cystine and cysteine are used for synthesis of taurocholic acid; and tryptophan and, to some extent, all amino acid carbon skeletons may be incompletely oxidized.) Assuming that about 12 percent of amino acid carbon is not oxidized, and that 2 moles ATP are utilized for disposal of each gram atom of amino acid nitrogen in urea synthesis, Krebs calculated that when a protein such as ovalbumin is oxidized, at least 21.2 kcal are required to yield 1 mole ATP. Calorigenic effect is then calculated as the percentage increase in energy requirement for ATP synthesis from protein as compared with that from carbohydrate and fat, and amounts to approximately

20 percent for most proteins, varying by 1 or 2 percent according to amino acid content of the protein source.[3] Calorigenic effect thus represents the additional calories necessary for ATP formation when protein rather than carbohydrate or fat serves as oxidative substrate.

Krebs' calculations, which are based on cellular energy transformations, represented a new approach to the problem of the calorigenic effect of food. Grisolia and Kennedy (1966) criticized Krebs' calculations as being incomplete since no correction is made for ATP utilized in protein or other syntheses requiring nitrogen (purines, amino sugars, etc.). These authors do not question the basic reasoning underlying the calculation, but rather the validity of any such calculation. The problem of the calorigenic effect of food continues to be debated, and whether experimental evidence *can* be obtained that will precisely explain its metabolic basis is a moot question. The fact remains, however, that the extra heat production following ingestion of food represents a wastage of metabolizable energy and therefore is considered in establishing dietary energy requirement. In other words, the total energy intake must allow for an increase above the estimated energy expenditure. A 6 percent increase for persons consuming an ordinary varied diet is generally accepted as satisfactory.

Sims (1976) has postulated a number of mechanisms by which the calorigenic effect of food or dietary induced thermogenesis might be altered: (1) change in energy cost of fuel storage; (2) change in energy cost of fuel utilization; (3) inefficient generation of ATP; (4) uncoupling of oxidative phosphorylation; (5) inefficient utilization of ATP; (6) changes in the operation of the Na^+/K^+ ATPase pump; and (7) change in thyroid function including hormonal receptor site activity. Most of these mechanisms have an effect on protein metabolism which emphasizes the importance of the earlier discussion of protein metabolism and ATP.

Dauncey (1979) has implicated catecholamines as important in dietary-induced thermogenesis since Dauncey and Ingram (1979) found that the β-adrenergic blocker propranolol reduced the relative metabolic rate (multiple of the BMR) in pigs on a high energy intake, but not in animals on a low intake. A similar observation was reported in humans by Jung et al. (1979).

Activity

Activity is the most variable factor affecting the total energy requirement. It is the external work of the body but, clearly, external work must involve a speeding up

---

[3]Ovalbumin: kcal/mole ATP = 21.2
  Starch: kcal/mole ATP = 17.4

$$Calorigenic\ effect = \frac{\begin{bmatrix} Kcal\ required\ for\ ATP \\ synthesis\ from \\ protein\ oxidation \end{bmatrix} - \begin{bmatrix} Kcal\ required\ for\ ATP \\ synthesis\ from \\ carbohydrate\ oxidation \end{bmatrix}}{Kcal\ required\ for\ ATP\ synthesis\ from\ carbohydrate\ oxidation} \times 100$$

$$= \frac{21.2 - 17.4}{17.4} \times 100 = 21.8\ percent$$

of the internal work and therefore an increase in the metabolic rate. Moreover, as described by Benedict and Cathcart (1913) from studies of muscular work, there are essentially two components of external activity: metabolism especially involved in production of work and extraneous motion incidental to the performance of work. It is the extraneous motion that often determines the difference in energy expenditure between two individuals performing the same task.

Activity requirements also vary with body size. Obviously, more energy is required to move a large body than a small body. Energy cost of activities involving whole body movement varies too with the intensity of activity. For example, both the speed of walking and body weight influence the energy required in walking (Table 23.4).

Energy costs for various activities have been studied extensively. A large amount of the published data were compiled by Passmore and Durnin (1955). Some average data on energy expenditure for various activities are shown in Table 23.5. These figures are not representative of the cost of activity alone; they include the basal expenditure as well, and therefore they represent the total energy expenditure when activity is performed.

The total energy requirement for activity can be estimated and expressed as percent above basal expenditure; however, this is rarely done in describing the energy cost of individual activities.

Another method of grossly describing energy cost on a relative basis is to use multiples of the resting metabolic rate (Mets). One Met is equivalent to 1.1 × BMR or approximately 3.5 ml O_2 per kg/min. Assuming an exercise RQ of 0.85, the kcal equivalent of oxygen utilization would be 4.83 kcal per liter O_2.

Although not clearly established at the present time, research on animals, particularly rats, suggests that dietary thermogenesis is potentiated by exercise and that regular exercise (physical conditioning) results in greater dietary thermogenesis (Gleason et al., 1979).

The assessment of energy expenditure during pregnancy revealed 32.5 kcal per kg body/weight day ± 4 kcal during the latter half of gestation, with a small

TABLE 23.4
Relationship Between Energy Expenditure (kcal/min or kJ/min) and Speed of Walking (mph) and Gross Body Weight (lb) and (kg)

| Speed (mph) | Weight lb (kg) | | | | | | | |
| | 100 (45.5) | | 120 (54.5) | | 140 (63.6) | | 180 (81.8) | |
	kcal/min	kJ/min	kcal/min	kJ/min	kcal/min	kJ/min	kcal/min	kJ/min
2.0	2.2	9.2	2.6	10.9	2.9	12.1	3.5	14.6
2.5	2.7	11.3	3.1	13.0	3.5	14.6	4.2	17.6
3.0	3.1	13.0	3.6	15.1	4.0	16.7	4.8	20.1
3.5	3.6	15.1	4.2	17.6	4.6	19.2	5.4	22.6
4.0	4.1	17.2	4.7	19.7	5.2	21.8	6.4	26.8

Source: Adapted from R. Passmore and J.V.G.A. Durnin, Physiol. Rev. 35:801 (1955).

TABLE 23.5
Average Energy Expenditure for Various Activities[a]

Activity	kcal/minute	kJ/minute
Lying at ease	1.4–1.5	5.9–6.3
Sitting at ease	1.6	6.7
Sitting, writing	1.9–2.2	8.0–9.2
Sitting, playing cards	2.1–2.4	8.8–10.0
Sitting, playing woodwind instrument	2.0	8.4
Sitting, playing piano	2.5	10.5
Sitting, playing violin	2.7	11.3
Sitting, playing organ	3.2–3.5	13.4–14.6
Sitting, playing drums	4.0–4.2	16.7–17.6
Standing at ease	1.7–1.9	7.1–8.0
Cycling (5.5 mph)	4.5	18.8
Cycling (9.4 mph)	7.0	29.3
Cycling (13.1 mph)	11.1	46.4
Dancing, foxtrot	5.2	21.8
Dancing, rumba	7.0	29.3
Volleyball	3.5	14.7
Archery	5.2	21.8
Tennis	7.1	29.7
Football	8.9	37.2
Swimming, breaststroke (30 yd/min)	7.5	31.4
Swimming, breaststroke (40 yd/min)	10.0	42.0

Source: Adapted from R. Passmore and J.V.G.A. Durnin, *Physiol. Rev.* 35:801 (1955).

[a]Weight range 60–75 kg.

decline of about 6 percent near term. When allowance is made for the deposition of maternal and fetal tissue, the average metabolizable energy is calculated to be about 35–36 kcal per kg/day. Women who were employed or were raising small children tended to have the highest energy expenditures. These data confirm the need for considering work pace and load as well as body mass in estimating the energy requirement during pregnancy (Blackburn and Calloway, 1976b).

Other Induced Calorigenesis

Some animals can increase their heat production when exposed to cold, and they do so without shivering. This phenomenon has been labeled *nonshivering thermogenesis*. It is rare in humans, and in animals it has been associated with increased heat production in brown fat, a response mediated by the sympathetic nervous system (Himms-Hagen, 1976; also see Chapter 20). Evidence from individuals subjected to chronic cold exposure suggests that some small deposits of brown fat may be retained in "strategic" locations of the human body, such as around the neck arteries (Huttunen et al., 1981).

There is evidence also that commonly ingested items such as alcohol and caffeine as well as other methylxanthines in coffee, teas, and cola drinks induce thermogenesis. For example, Miller (1975) reported that thermogenesis was increased 2 percent following ingestion of 200 kcals of alcohol and by 14 percent following a 700 kcal breakfast, but the combined effect was a 22 percent increase in the resting metabolic rate (RMR). Similarly, 250 mg of caffeine increased the RMR by 10 percent which, together with a 700 kcal breakfast, increased the RMR 25 percent. Thus, an additive effect of food plus "drug" was noted. A similar but probably small synergistic effect was observed for food plus exercise or when psychological stress occurs with excitement, fear or anger.

CALORIMETRY

Early workers in calorimetry knew little of the details of energy transformations in the animal body. Indeed, the means by which animals utilize food and produce heat are not essential to an understanding of gross calorimetry and, in contrast to many other areas of nutrition investigation, much of the basic work in calorimetry was accomplished by 1920. Consolazio and Johnson (1971) have reviewed some of the later work.

There have been refinements in instrumentation in recent years. However, all methods of calorimetry are based on two broad principles: the measurement of heat lost from the body (direct calorimetry) or the calculation of heat production from gaseous exchange (indirect calorimetry).

Direct Calorimetry

The direct measurement of heat loss is theoretically simple but, in practice, is cumbersome and expensive. Total energy output includes sensible heat given off from the body, the latent heat of vaporized water from lungs and skin, and the heat of combustion of urine and feces.

The calorimeter is an insulated double-walled adiabatic chamber (Fig. 23.6); that is, the temperature of the two walls must be kept equal so that heat cannot flow in either direction and thus escape from the calorimeter. Heat eliminated from the subject is removed by water flowing in coils of pipe within the chamber walls. Heat loss is calculated from the difference in temperature and amount of water flowing in and out of the pipes. Heat removed by vaporization of water is calculated by measuring moisture of air leaving the calorimeter (carbon dioxide is usually absorbed in soda lime and water in sulfuric acid). For each gram of water vaporized, 0.580 kcal are required at 30°C, the temperature of the skin. In addition, corrections must be made for changes in body temperature and for any food or drink introduced into the chamber.

The data in Table 23.6 were taken in part from experiments on adult men published by Benedict and Carpenter in 1910 and indicate the magnitude of heat eliminated from the body by various avenues. Note that losses in urine and feces are minor and that a major loss in either the resting state or while performing work is by radiation and conduction from the body. Note also the differences in water vaporization between the resting and active states.

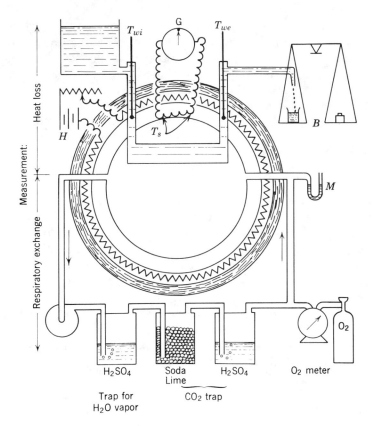

Figure 23.6
Schematic diagram showing principle of Atwater-Rosa respiration
calorimeter. The subject is surrounded by two concentric walls.
The outer wall is kept at the same temperature T_s as in the inner
wall by means of a heat source H and controlling galvanometer
G. The heat produced by the subject is carried away by water
that flows into the chamber at the temperature T_{wi} and leaves the
chamber at the temperature T_{we}. The rate of flow is measured by
the balance B. Maintenance of constant pressure is monitored by
means of the manometer M. (From M. Kleiber, *Biophysical Research Methods*, F. M. Uber, ed., Wiley-Interscience, New York,
1950.

Direct calorimetry measures the total rate of the respective heat losses by the
body as represented by the following equation:

$$\dot{M} = \dot{S} + (\dot{R} + \dot{C} + \dot{K} + \dot{E}) + \dot{W}$$

where $\dot{M}$ is the rate of free energy production
$\dot{S}$ is the rate of storage of body heat
$\dot{R}$ is the rate of radiant heat exchange
$\dot{C}$ is the rate of convective heat transfer

$\dot{K}$ is the rate of conductive heat transfer
$\dot{E}$ is the rate of evaporative heat transfer
$\dot{W}$ is the rate of work done against external forces in the environment

When employing direct calorimetry, convective and conductive heat transfer are commonly combined through the use of a common heat transfer coefficient. A ventilatory circuit is required to measure $\dot{E}$. At least two calorimeters built in more recent years have been used to measure heat loss employing gradient layers and Fourier's equation where

$$\dot{Q} = A \, (\lambda/D) \, (T_1 - T_2)$$

where $\dot{Q}$ is the rate of heat flow through the layer
A is the area of the layer
λ is the specific thermal conductivity of the layer
and T_1 and T_2 are the temperatures of the inner and outer surfaces.

The electrical circuitry of the inner and outer surfaces of the gradient layer forms a part of a Wheatstone bridge circuit so that the voltage measured is proportional to total heat flow or $\dot{Q}$.

Long-term studies cannot be undertaken easily with gradient-layer calorimetry due to limitations in size; the larger the wall area, the lower the rate of heat flow per unit surface, and the weaker the electrical signal. Thus, accuracy decreases rapidly with an increase in size. The instrument built by Benzinger and Kitzinger (1949) was coffin-size, whereas that built by Spinnler et al. (1973) and described by Jequier (1980), although somewhat larger, has a volume of only 1.56 m³. The instrument described by Poppendiek and Hody (1972) is of similar size. Despite their limitations, studies of heat loss are useful, because the efficiency of energy

TABLE 23.6
Heat Loss from Adult Men in the Resting and Active State

Subject	Number of Days on Experiment	Average Kcal per Day				Total
		By Radiation and Conduction	In Urine and Feces	In Water Vaporized	Heat Equivalent of External Work	
H. F. (resting)	3	1471	8	425	—	1904
A. L. (resting)	2	2157	22	510	—	2689
A. L. (at work)	3	2391	13	1958	459	4821

Source: From F. G. Benedict and T. M. Carpenter, "The Metabolism and Energy Transformations of Healthy Men During Rest," Carnegie Inst., Washington, 1910.

turnover can be calculated when both direct and indirect calorimetric procedures are employed. Dauncey (1980) found that the mean difference in heat loss and energy turnover measured by indirect calorimetry was only $1.2° \pm 0.14$ (SEM)% in 24-hour experiments on eight adult subjects. The 24-hour heat production increased significantly by 10 percent on a high caloric intake and decreased 6 percent on a low intake.

A unique, direct calorimeter is the suit calorimeter designed and constructed by Webb and his colleagues (1972; 1980). (See Fig. 23.7.) The subject wears a

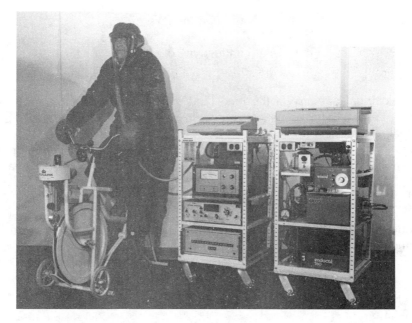

Figure 23.7
Photograph of a subject clothed in the insulated garment assembly used for direct calorimetry, and wearing a clear plastic facemask for indirect calorimetry (metabolic rate from respiratory gas exchange). The clothing assembly contains an elastic mesh undergarment which holds a network of small plastic tubes on the skin. Water circulates through them, and heat is removed directly from the body surface. Water is recirculated from the equipment cart on the right, where a pump is located along with a cooler and heater. Temperature change in water across the subject times water flow rate gives heat loss in kcal·min^{-1}. The facemask is ventilated by drawing room air through it, thence down to the left-hand cart, where it is sampled for oxygen and carbon dioxide. From O_2 and CO_2 concentrations in the diluted exhaled air, and from the flow rate of the air, oxygen consumption and carbon dioxide production are calculated. A dedicated laboratory computer, located on top of the left-hand cart, gathers the data, performs calculations, and stores results. It also drives an X-Y plotter, on the right-hand cart, to produce graphic records of heat loss to metabolism, body temperatures, and critical operating data.

union suit of elastic mesh that incorporates a network of small plastic tubing distributed over the body except for the face, hands, and soles of the feet. Water is circulated through the tubing and by measuring the rate of flow and the change in temperature of the water between that entering and leaving, body heat loss to the water is calculated. In order to prevent heat loss to the environment, an insulating overgarment is worn. Evaporative heat loss is calculated from body weight loss and garment weight gain with a correction for the difference between the masses for oxygen consumed and carbon dioxide expired. A face mask is utilized to obtain oxygen consumption measurements by indirect calorimetry. The small convective heat loss from the face is determined from the air temperature change and the rate of air flow through the mask. Using the suit calorimeter, the subject can perform relatively normal activity within the limits set by the length of tubing connecting the subject to the stationary water reservoir and other instrumentation. Exercise on a cycle ergometer or treadmill poses no problem other than that provided by the slight hobbling effect of the suit.

Indirect Calorimetry

Indirect calorimetry refers to calculation of heat production from measurement of gaseous exchange: oxygen consumed and carbon dioxide expired or both. The respiration calorimeter, a chamber somewhat similar to that used in direct calorimetry, was the first instrument to be used for the measurement of respiratory exchange. More recently, mobile lightweight and more versatile instruments have been devised; these instruments consist of masks with attachments that can be strapped to the subject for collection of gas and permit easy movement of the subject in performing various activities. (See Fig. 23.8.) Nevertheless, large facilities with hood type respiratory flow systems continue to have important uses such as in a burn and trauma unit (Kinney, 1980). An illustration of the system appears in Fig. 23.9.

The heat equivalent of respiratory exchange is not only calculated from oxygen consumed and carbon dioxide expired but also is dependent on the ratio of the moles of carbon dioxide produced to the moles of oxygen consumed, or the *respiratory quotient* (R.Q.):

$$R.Q. = \frac{\text{moles } CO_2}{\text{moles } O_2}$$

The R.Q. varies when carbohydrate, fat, and protein are oxidized because of differences in composition of the foodstuffs that determine the amount of oxygen required for complete oxidation and, consequently, the volume of carbon dioxide that is given off. For carbohydrate, the R.Q. is 1.0 since in combustion of carbohydrate, the amount of molecular oxygen required for oxidation is equal to the carbon dioxide produced. The oxidation of glucose, for example, is shown below:

$$C_6H_{12}O_6 + 6 O_2 \rightarrow 6 CO_2 + 6 H_2O$$

Fats require more oxygen that carbohydrates for combustion because the fat molecule contains a low ratio of oxygen to carbon and hydrogen. Thus for a fat such as tristearin, the R.Q. may be represented as:

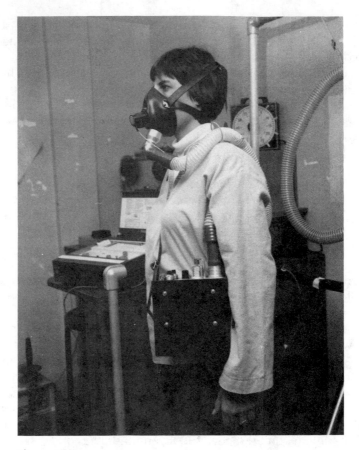

Figure 23.8
A newer portable instrument for the measurement of oxygen consumption, the OXYLOG, is comparable to the IMP (the instrument described in the first edition of this book, but no longer available), but relies on the assessment of pulmonary ventilation volume (expiratory) and the difference in partial pressure of oxygen in the inspired-expired airstreams. (From S. J. E. Humphrey and H. S. Wolff, *J. Physiol.* 267:12, 1977). The signals from the sensing elements are multiplied to provide a metered measurement of oxygen consumption. A permanent record can be made by attaching a small recorder that samples the meter every minute. The OXYLOG can be used in conjunction with other transducers, e.g., heart rate and temperature to provide a simultaneous recording of these variables.

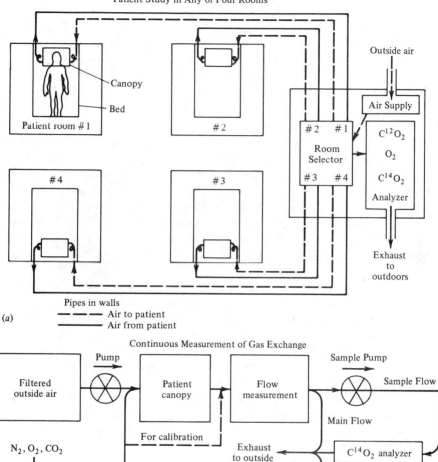

Continuous Gas Exchange
Patient Study in Any of Four Rooms

Canopy

Bed

Patient room #1

#2

Outside air

Air Supply

#2   #1

Room
Selector

#3   #4

$C^{12}O_2$

O_2

$C^{14}O_2$

Analyzer

#4

#3

Exhaust
to
outdoors

Pipes in walls
– – – – Air to patient
———— Air from patient

(a)

Continuous Measurement of Gas Exchange

Filtered
outside air

Pump

Patient
canopy

Flow
measurement

Sample Pump

Sample Flow

Main Flow

N_2, O_2, CO_2

For calibration

Exhaust
to outside

$C^{14}O_2$ analyzer

CO_2 analyzer

Flow measuring
gasistors

O_2 analyzer

Recorders, card punch

(b)

Figure 23.9
(a) Diagram of a gas-flow system with a head canopy to be used in any one of four rooms of a hospital unit. The air ventilating the canopy is returned to gas analyzer in an adjacent room for continuous analysis. (b) Steps in the airflow system. Reproduced with permission of J. M. Kinney and Ross Laboratories.

$$2\ C_{57}H_{110}O_6 + 163\ O_2 \rightarrow 114\ CO_2 + 110\ H_2O$$

$$\frac{CO_2}{O_2} = \frac{114}{163} = 0.70$$

Calculation of the R.Q. for protein is more complicated than that for fat or carbohydrate because protein is not completely oxidized and both carbon and oxygen are excreted in the urine chiefly as urea. When adjustment is made for urinary excretion, the ratio of carbon dioxide produced to oxygen consumed is approximately 1:1.2 and thus is equivalent to an R.Q. of 0.80.

The R.Q.s for individual carbohydrates, fats, and proteins differ slightly, but the average figures of 1.0, 0.7, and 0.8 respectively are accepted as representative of the foodstuffs. The R.Q. for an ordinary mixed diet consisting of the three foodstuffs is approximately 0.85. Obviously, it is impossible to make assumptions about the relative amounts of foodstuffs undergoing oxidation except at extremes of the R.Q. range. For example, if the R.Q. is nearly 1.0, one may safely assume that the foodstuff is largely carbohydrate. Similarly, an R.Q. of about 0.7 indicates a predominantly fatty acid metabolism. At intermediate levels of R.Q., no safe assumption can be made.

Since the nature of the foodstuff consumed in cellular respiratory processes determines both oxygen consumption and carbon dioxide formation (that is, the R.Q.), the caloric equivalent for a given volume of oxygen or carbon dioxide also will vary with the R.Q. Caloric equivalents of oxygen and carbon dioxide for R.Q. values between 0.7 and 1.0 are shown in Table 23.7. It is apparent from the table that when fat is oxidized, heat production represented by 1 liter of oxygen consumed is only 0.3 kcal less than when carbohydrate is oxidized, a difference of about 6 percent. The variation in caloric equivalent for carbon dioxide, however, is on the order of 30 percent. These figures apply only to mixtures of carbohydrate and fat and therefore represent what is referred to as the nonprotein R.Q.

For work requiring great accuracy, the extent of protein oxidation can be calculated from urinary nitrogen, and the nonprotein R.Q. then can be estimated. In practice, the error incurred by ignoring protein metabolism is relatively small and, particularly in short term studies, no correction is made for the effect of protein metabolism on R.Q. Calculation of heat production is made as if only fat and carbohydrate were oxidized.

Calculation of Heat Production from R.Q.   Calculation of heat production from gaseous exchange is relatively easy. Oxygen consumed and carbon dioxide produced over a known period of time are corrected to standard conditions (760 mm mercury, dry, 0°C). The R.Q. is calculated and the appropriate caloric equivalent is used to determine the total heat production. For example, consider the following hypothetical data:

Vol. O_2 consumed (standard conditions) = 14.4 liters per hour

Vol. CO_2 produced (standard conditions) = 12.0 liters per hour

TABLE 23.7
Caloric Values for Oxygen and Carbon Dioxide for Nonprotein R.Q.

Nonprotein Respiratory Quotient	Caloric Value of 1 Liter of O_2	Caloric Value of 1 Liter of CO_2	Percentage of Total O_2 Consumed by Fat	Percentage of Total Heat Produced by Fat
0.707	4.686	6.629	100.0	100.0
0.71	4.690	6.606	99.0	98.5
0.72	4.702	6.531	95.6	95.2
0.73	4.714	6.458	92.2	91.6
0.74	4.727	6.388	88.7	88.0
0.75	4.739	6.319	85.3	84.4
0.76	4.751	6.253	81.9	80.8
0.77	4.764	6.187	78.5	77.2
0.78	4.776	6.123	75.1	73.7
0.79	4.788	6.062	71.7	70.1
0.80	4.801	6.001	68.3	66.6
0.81	4.813	5.942	64.8	63.1
0.82	4.825	5.884	61.4	59.7
0.83	4.838	5.829	58.0	56.2
0.84	4.850	5.774	54.6	52.8
0.85	4.862	5.721	51.2	49.3
0.86	4.875	5.669	47.8	45.9
0.87	4.887	5.617	44.4	42.5
0.88	4.899	5.568	41.0	39.2
0.89	4.911	5.519	37.5	35.8
0.90	4.924	5.471	34.1	32.5
0.91	4.936	5.424	30.7	29.2
0.92	4.948	5.378	27.3	25.9
0.93	4.961	5.333	23.9	22.6
0.94	4.973	5.290	20.5	19.3
0.95	4.985	5.247	17.1	16.0
0.96	4.998	5.205	13.7	12.8
0.97	5.010	5.165	10.2	9.51
0.98	5.022	5.124	6.83	6.37
0.99	5.035	5.085	3.41	3.18
1.00	5.047	5.047	0	0

Source: From N. Zuntz and M. Schumberg, with modifications by G. Lusk, E. P. Cathcart and D. P. Cuthbertson, *J. Physiol* (*London*), 72:349 (1931).

$$R.Q. = \frac{12.0}{14.4} = 0.83$$

From Table 23.7, the caloric equivalent for an R.Q. of 0.83 is 4.383 for 1 liter of O_2 and 5.829 for 1 liter of CO_2.

$$\text{Heat production} = 14.4 \times 4.838 = 69.7 \text{ kcal per hour}$$
$$\text{or} = 12.0 \times 5.829 = 69.9 \text{ kcal per hour}$$

The agreement in caloric values obtained by calculation from either oxygen consumption or carbon dioxide production is quite good. However, because variation in caloric equivalents is less for oxygen than carbon dioxide over the full range of R.Q. values, measurement of oxygen consumption is preferred for most experimental work.

Calculation of Heat Production from Oxygen Consumption Alone. When only oxygen consumption is determined, an *average* caloric equivalent of 4.83 may be used to calculate total heat production. The average caloric equivalent of 1 liter of oxygen yields final computations that vary little from those obtained by first detemining R.Q., since the entire range of caloric equivalents of oxygen varies by only 6 percent. The accuracy of an average computation is heightened by the fact that rarely in practice does one encounter an R.Q. at either extreme of the range. For the most part, human beings oxidize a mixture of foodstuffs that yield R.Q. values near the middle of the range.

For example, if only oxygen consumption had been determined in the illustration cited above, heat production calculated from an average caloric equivalent of 4.83 is 69.6 kcal/hour (4.83 × 14.4) compared with 69.7 kcal/hour calculated from R.Q. Therefore, for many forms of work this simplified method is quite acceptable.

Newer Methods for Assessing Energy Turnover. A variety of methods have been tried over the years to measure indirectly physical activity, energy expenditure, or metabolic rate. For example, a radar system, based on the Doppler effect, has been described for use on a subject residing in a respiration chamber (Schutz et al., 1982). Spontaneous activity within the chamber is expressed as a percentage of time spent in activity. Percent activity is significantly correlated ($r = 0.89$) to the rate of oxygen consumption ($\dot{V}_{O_2}$) measured simultaneously. The advantages of the Doppler system were cited as (1) the capability for continuous and inconspicuous monitoring of physical activity, and (2) the possibility of utilizing activity index versus $\dot{V}_{O_2}$ relationships on an individual basis so that the energy associated with subsequent activity can be estimated from the Doppler measurements alone. Such an approach has been used by several investigators for heart rate versus $\dot{V}_{O_2}$ relationships in studying weight reduction in obese women (Warnold et al. (1978) and the energy expenditure of children (Spady, 1980).

A relatively noninvasive and nonrestrictive method for the measurement of energy expenditure using doubly labeled water ($^2H_2^{18}O$) was developed by Lifson et al. (1955). The method has been used with several species of animals, but has only recently been used with humans (Schoeller et al., 1980). The disappearance rates from body water are determined following oral administration of a known amount of the doubly labeled water. Both energy expenditure and water output over several days or weeks can be calculated. The fractional turnover rate of the labeled oxygen is dependent on both the rates of carbon dioxide (CO_2) production and water output; whereas, the fractional rate of the labeled hydrogen is dependent on the rate of water output alone. The difference is the rate of CO_2 production. Oxygen consumption and energy expenditure can be calculated from CO_2 production using indirect calorimetric equations and an estimate of the respiratory quotient (Lifson and McClintock, 1966). This method probably will be used more widely in the future, particularly if the doubly labeled water becomes less expensive.

ENERGY BALANCE

Data from calorimetric studies as just described are the basis for the establishment of energy requirements. (See Chapter 25.) These data also provide reasonable guides for the prediction of energy requirements of individuals; however, as in all determinations of nutrient requirements, studies of energy expenditure are less accurately applied to individuals than to groups. For example, differences in body size significantly affect the energy cost of the basal metabolism and activities involving whole body movement. Caloric adjustments for body size are relatively accurate for estimation of basal energy expenditure but are apt to be less accurate when applied to expenditure for activity.

Other factors also contribute to the variance among individuals. Efficiency in the performance of tasks is an obvious factor. Anyone who has seen a seasoned performer and a novice working side by side is aware of the difference.

Differences in muscle tone alone could account for the variations in energy need between two individuals apparently similar in body build and activity pattern. Relaxation of muscles during restful sleep may reduce the BMR by as much as 10 percent. Conceivably, and indeed very likely, the act of sitting quietly could require much more energy for the "high-tone" individual than for the "low-tone" individual.

One method of estimating energy expenditure requires the subject to keep an accurate record of daily activities over a period of time, usually about one week. The data shown in Table 23.8, for example, illustrate the compilation of a weekly activity record and calculation of energy expenditure for a relatively inactive man employed as a clerk (Passmore and Durnin, 1955). A similar approach was used by Widdowson et al. (1954) to estimate the energy expenditure of a group of cadets in active training. Data on energy costs for many occupational activities were compiled in the review of Passmore and Durnin (1955). On the basis of these and similar data, occupations have been classified arbitrarily as "sedentary," "light activity," and so forth. Although no system of arbitrary classification is infallible, most certainly this kind of estimation is valuable in planning group feeding programs and in roughly evaluating individual energy needs.

In this connection, it is worth mentioning that energy expenditure for certain individual activities may tend to be overestimated. Pollack et al. (1958) cite football and tennis as activities requiring a large energy expenditure when the body is in motion, but which, in fact, require only intermittent motion. In such cases, energy expended over the total period of play must be calculated separately

TABLE 23.8
Energy Output and Intake over a One-Week Period of a Clerk, age 29; ht, 66 in. (167.6 cm); wt, 66 kg (145.2 lb)

Activity	Total Time Spent Hr	Min	kcal/min	kJ/min	Kcal for Activity	MJ for Activity	Total kcal	Total MJ
In bed	54	4	1.13	4.73	3670	15.4		
Daytime dozing	1	43	1.37	5.73	140	0.59	3,810	16.0
Recreational and off work								
Light sedentary activities	31	14	1.48	6.19	2810	11.8		
Washing, shaving, dressing	3	18	3.0	12.6	590	2.47		
Playing with child		30	3.2	13.4	100	0.42		
Light domestic work	7	14	3.0	12.6	1300	5.44		
Walking	8	35	6.6	27.6	3,400	14.2		
Gardening	2	48	4.8	20.1	810	3.40		
Standing activities	6	45	1.56	6.52	630	2.64		
Watching football	2	10	2.0	8.37	260	1.09		
Total recreational and off work							9,800	41.0
Working								
Sitting activities	22	22	1.65	6.90	2,210	9.25		
Standing activities	25	57	1.90	7.95	2,960	12.4		
Walking	1	22	6.6	27.6	540	22.6		
Total working							5,710	24.0
Grand total							19,320	80.8
Daily average							2,760	11.5
Food intake (daily average determined by diet survey)							2,620	11.0

Source: Adapted from R. Passmore and J.V. G. A. Durnin, *Physiol. Rev.* 35:801 (1955).

for the periods of active play (to which figures of energy expenditure apply) *and* for periods of relative inactivity which require no greater energy expenditure of the player than that of the spectator standing on the sidelines. A careful discussion of the essential features of appropriate procedures employable in any accurate study of energy turnover has been prepared by Durnin (1978). For those contemplating similar investigations, careful reading of his suggested cautions would be helpful.

The maintenance of energy balance is so obvious that it barely merits explanation. Positive balance is indicated by an energy intake greater than expenditure and leads to weight gain which, in the adult, is largely evidenced by sagging jowls and a thickening waistline, or worse. Negative balance is synonymous with weight loss and indicates that fewer calories are taken in than are expended. The ideal for the adult, of course, is equilibrium, when energy intake and energy expenditure are nicely balanced.

Many persons are able to maintain a favorable balance of energy with little effort; appetite, thus food intake, is geared to energy expenditure. The work of Edholm et al. (1955) indicates that energy expenditure tends to regulate food intake but that the effect is delayed. This conclusion was based on the observation that caloric intake of their subjects reflected the energy expenditure of two days earlier. Clearly, the balance of energy is not a day-to-day phenomenon but is governed over a period of time. The increasing rate of obesity in the United States and other affluent countries, however, is generally accepted to be the result of reduced energy output rather than a marked increase in food intake.

ENERGY VALUE OF FOODS

The energy value of foods usually is expressed in terms of the kilocalorie. In some countries energy is expressed as kilojoules (1 kcal = 4.184 kJ); however, this practice has not yet been adopted in the United States. For a discussion of the kcal as a unit of energy, see the review by Moore (1977).

Since Lavoisier's classic experiments on the origin of animal heat, it has been known that foods burned outside the body produce the same amount of heat as foods oxidized by the slow processes of intermediary metabolism. If, then, foods are burned and heat produced is measured, the quantity of heat expressed in kilocalories represents the *gross energy value* or *heat of combustion* of the food. The instrument used to determine heat of combustion is known to all students of nutrition as the bomb calorimeter (Fig. 23.10). In effect, it consists of a bomb or small chamber immersed in a container of water. The bomb is filled with oxygen and the food contained therein is ignited by means of an electric spark. As the food burns, heat produced leads to a rise in temperature of the surrounding fluid. Thus heat production can be measured accurately. A bomb calorimeter was described by Atwater and Snell (1903). Present models, though more sleek, are technically similar to instruments used 80-odd years ago. The appearance of the ballistic bomb calorimeter speeds analyses but is no more accurate than the older instruments.

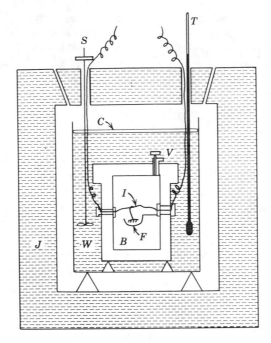

Figure 23.10
Cross section of a bomb calorimeter. J = water jacket; W = weighed amount water; S = stirrer; T = thermometer; F = platinum sample dish; B = bomb chamber; I = ignition wire. (From M. Kleiber, *Biophysical Research Methods*, F. M. Uber, ed., Wiley-Interscience, New York, 1950, p. 194.)

The heats of combustion for individual carbohydrates, proteins, and fats differ somewhat. The gross energy yield of sucrose, for example, was determined by Atwater to be 3.96 kcal/gm, whereas starch yielded 4.23 kcal/gm. Energy yield of butterfat was found to be 9.21 kcal/gm and that of lard, 9.48 kcal/gm (Atwater and Bryant, 1899). For practical use, individual figures were averaged to apply to the major foodstuffs as groups. These average (and familiar) figures are shown below:

Foodstuff	Gross Energy Value	
	kcal/g	kJ/g
Carbohydrate	4.15	17.36
Fat	9.4	39.33
Protein	5.65	23.64

The gross energy value of foodstuffs, however, does not represent the energy available to body cells, since no potentially oxidizable substrate can be considered available until it is presented to the cell for oxidation. None of the foodstuffs is completely absorbed; some potential energy, therefore, never enters the body and is excreted in the feces. Digestibility of the major foodstuffs, however, is high; on the average, 97 percent of ingested carbohydrates, 95 percent of fats, and 92 percent of proteins are absorbed from the intestinal lumen.

In addition, although carbohydrates and fats are oxidized completely to carbon dioxide and water in the processes of cellular metabolism as in the calorimeter, the cell is less efficient in oxidizing protein than is the calorimeter. In biological systems, urea, uric acid, creatinine, and other nitrogenous compounds derived from protein are excreted in the urine. Determination of both the heat of combustion and nitrogen content of urine indicates that approximately 7.9 kcal/gm of urine nitrogen is equivalent to 1.25 kcal/gm of protein (7.9/6.25). This energy represents metabolic loss and must be subtracted from the "digestible" energy of protein.

When heat of combustion is corrected for losses in digestion and for unmetabolized urinary substances, energy value of foods is designated *available energy* or *physiological fuel value*. Available energy of the major foodstuffs is shown in Fig. 23.11. The terms digestible energy and metabolizable energy are more accurately designated *apparent digestible energy* and *apparent metabolizable energy*. Fecal matter always contains some bacterial debris and materials of metabolic or body origin, sloughed-off mucosal cells, and secretions. These substances contribute to energy value of feces and, therefore, digestibility figures must represent apparent rather than true digestibility of individual foods.

Both malic and citric acid occur in varying amounts in some fruits and vegetables. These acids are absorbed and thus contribute to the tricarboxylic acid pool to yield energy. On the average, these organic acids yield approximately 2.45 kcal/gm of acid; 2.47 kcal/gm for citric acid and 2.42 kcal/gm for malic (FAO, 1974).

The contribution of organic acids to total energy value is fairly low for some vegetables and fruits. For example, cabbage, carrots, Brussels sprouts, head lettuce, and pineapple contain only 2–4 percent of organic acids as compared to total available carbohydrate. Higher amounts occur in prunes, plums, oranges, cranberries, and grapefruit. Lemon juice, however, contains a substantial amount of acids, 62.5 percent of total carbohydrate. Current food tables include organic acids as a part of total available energy.

Traditionally, tables of food composition in the United States have included data on energy, proximate composition, and the minerals and vitamins for which there are recommended dietary allowances (with the exception of vitamin D). Data for phosphorus content of foods also has been included. The trend toward more detailed identification of nutrients present in foods became evident in the previous revision of *Handbook 8* (Watt and Merrill, 1963) which, in addition to usual data, included figures on sodium and potassium of foods, and limited tables on fatty acids, cholesterol, and magnesium. The United States Department of

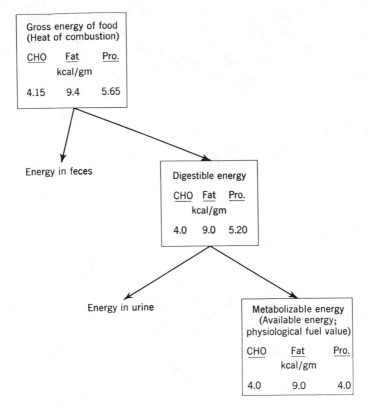

Figure 23.11
Energy value of food.

Agriculture now is updating *Handbook 8* in sections according to food categories, and currently is providing detailed nutrient data including amino acid and fatty acid content of foods.

Protein Requirements

It is convenient to speak of the protein requirement of humans because protein is the source of nitrogen in the human diet, but the true requirement is not for protein as such, but rather for specific amounts and proportions of the essential amino acids and of nonessential amino acid nitrogen. The amino acids must adequately provide for cellular synthesis of both proteins and nonprotein nitrogenous compounds. The latter requirement can be met by simple nitrogen-containing compounds such as diammonium citrate or urea (Rose et al., 1949) as well as by the naturally occurring or synthetic amino acids.

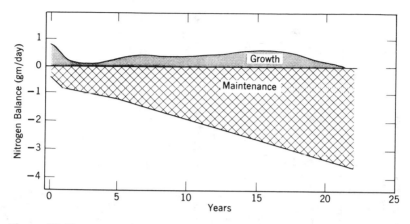

Figure 23.12
Minimum nitrogen for maintenance and growth. (From J. B. Allison, 5th Int. Cong. on Nutrition, 1960.)

The dependence of nutrient needs on physiological state was discussed in Chapter 22, and little need be added here. Obviously, both growth and body size must affect nitrogen requirements, and, as shown in Fig. 23.12, both factors also affect the nature of the requirement. Thus the need for nitrogen shifts from a high-growth, low-maintenance requirement in early infancy to a high-maintenance, low-growth requirement in adulthood. The growth requirement of the adult (adult growth), defined by Mitchell (1949) as syntheses necessary for growth of hair and nails and replacement of epidermal cells, obviously is only a fraction of the maintenance requirement of the adult body.

Maintenance requirement can be estimated from nitrogen losses from the body when subjects are maintained on a diet free or nearly free of nitrogen. These losses include endogenous urinary loss, metabolic fecal loss, losses in sweat, and from sloughing of dermal tissues. Other miscellaneous sources of loss have been quantitatively defined (Calloway et al., 1971).

A number of different procedures have been used to determine human protein requirements. The major techniques are tabulated in Table 23.9 along with the principles underlying their use and some limitations of the methods. These procedures are considered in more detail in the sections that follow.

NITROGEN BALANCE

A generally accepted method for the evaluation of human amino acid and nitrogen requirements is the nitrogen balance technique. Interpretation of nitrogen balance data is based on the premise that equilibrium in the adult is attained when the supplies of essential amino acids and total nitrogen are adequate for replacement of endogenous losses that occur through the kidney, intestinal secretions, sweat,

TABLE 23.9
Some of the Major Procedures Used for Estimation of Protein and Amino Acid Requirements in Humans

Nitrogen balance	Difference between nitrogen (N) intake and nitrogen loss. Miscellaneous losses must be accounted for.	1. Does not reveal within body distribution. 2. Difficult to measure all N losses and compensation between various routes may occur. 3. Errors are larger when N intake is large. 4. Affected by many other factors than N intake.
Nitrogen balance response curve	Nitrogen balance performed at several levels of intake around requirement level.	All the above apply, but they are minimized to some degree by using several levels of intake.
Factorial	Summation of obligatory N losses plus allowances for growth and special needs such as pregnancy and lactation.	Cannot be used for amino acid needs. Correction factor needed because even high quality proteins are not used with 100% efficiency. Factor may vary with age.
Plasma amino acids	Response of plasma amino acids to varied intakes of amino acids.	Many factors affect plasma amino acid concentrations and not all amino acids behave in the same way.
Growth	Level of amino acids or protein required to produce optimal growth when all other dietary constituents are present.	Limited to children during rapid growth.
Stable isotope infusion	Infusion of graded levels of N- or C-labeled essential amino acids and levels of stable isotope in breath, urine, or plasma are monitored.	Suitable for amino acid requirements only. As yet, the procedures are insufficiently validated.

and desquamation of epithelial cells, and for synthesis of such tissues as hair and nails. Theoretically the balance of nitrogen is expressed as:

$$B = I - (U + F + S)$$

where B is nitrogen balance, I is nitrogen intake, U is urinary nitrogen, F is fecal nitrogen, and S is loss of nitrogen through the skin. The last factor most often is overlooked in the interpretation of nitrogen balance data, and the failure to take these skin losses into account was cited by Mitchell (1949) as a source of error that may lead to underestimation of nitrogen requirement. On the basis of a wide range of reported losses, an FAO/WHO committee recently recommended a value of 8 mg N per kg/day for these miscellaneous losses (FAO/WHO, 1983). Under conditions of heavy sweating, losses could be much higher (Consolazio et al., 1963a).

Wallace (1959) suggested that errors in nitrogen balance experiments arise through the manipulations involved in feeding and in collecting excreta and that these errors are more likely to lead to overestimation rather than underestimation of nitrogen requirements. A small quantity of the food intake is apt to be lost in feeding, and a small portion of the excreta invariably cannot be recovered. These "unavoidable" losses have been estimated by Calloway et al. (1971) to be of the order of 115 mg N/day.

Clearly, there are other limitations to balance methodology. The balance of nitrogen intake against output is the sum of total body gains and losses. It is possible therefore, in a state of nitrogen equilibrium and possibly nitrogen retention, for some body tissues to be in positive balance while others are losing nitrogen. Shifting of amino acids within the total metabolic pool and possible deprivation of individual cells cannot be ascertained by the gross evaluation of nitrogen balance. This factor is probably the most significant limitation to balance methodology.

Hegsted (1976) reviewed a large number of balance studies and plotted nitrogen balance against nitrogen intake. Excessive positive balances occurred in all studies and the slope of the line implied a retention of 2 gm N/day on intakes of 14 gm N/day. These results suggest weight gains of 25 kg/year which obviously are unlikely, yet in no study was there evidence of nitrogen balance reaching a plateau as intake increased. As a result, Hegsted (ibid) suggested that balance methods be viewed with caution and skepticism.

Young and Scrimshaw (1978) are less dismissive of nitrogen balance procedures. Nonetheless they emphasize that there are limitations to such studies: (1) Body nitrogen equilibrium does not necessarily reflect a steady state of organ metabolism or nutritional state, because it fails to reveal alterations in tissue metabolism and distribution of protein within the body. (2) It is difficult to measure quantitatively all the routes of nitrogen loss from the body, and loss of nitrogen from one route may be compensated for by changes in the losses of nitrogen from another route. (3) Errors in nitrogen balance are larger when dietary intake of nitrogen is high. (4) Such factors as energy intake, diet composition, and prior nutritional status affect the sensitivity of nitrogen balance and must be considered in the evaluation of results. Nitrogen balance, and thus the interpretation of nitrogen balance data, represents the interaction of several factors. The most important of these are physiological state, body protein reserves, energy value of the diet, and the essential amino acids and nonessential amino acid nitrogen provided by the diet.

Effect of Physiological State and Body Protein Reserves

Strong positive balances are characteristic of the growing child or the woman in late pregnancy when growth of fetal tissue is most rapid. (See Calloway, 1974.) Adults depleted of labile protein respond to nitrogen feeding in the same way, that is, nitrogen retention and positive balance (Whipple, 1948). Furthermore, the extent of positive balance will reflect quantitatively the extent of protein depletion, and as protein reserves are replenished, the subject approaches equilibrium. (See Allison, 1957.)

Even when there is no marked depletion of body protein, nitrogen balance initially will reflect the previous intake. An initial negative balance in a subject placed on an experimental diet thus clearly indicates that previous dietary intake of nitrogen was higher than that of the experimental regimen, but it does not necessarily indicate that the experimental diet is inadequate. In the human, adjustment to changes in dietary protein occurs within a few days, as indicated by a relatively constant excretion of urinary nitrogen. The length of the adjustment period, however, often varies from one study to another. Forbes (1973) suggested that the period of time required for adjustment is likely longer than generally allowed and cites this possibility as a source of error in metabolic balance studies.

Effect of Energy Intake

The effect of energy intake on nitrogen balance has been widely studied (Benditt et al., 1948; Rosenthal and Allison, 1951; Oldham and Sheft, 1951; see Calloway, 1974). If dietary energy is reduced below a critical level, then energy rather than nitrogen becomes the limiting factor in nitrogen balance. Adequate energy intake, as evidenced by maintenance of body weight, is essential to prevent loss of tissue protein. When energy intake is low, increased excretion of nitrogen in the urine reflects the inadequacy of energy rather than a lack of dietary nitrogen.

Energy excess also influences nitrogen balance apparently by enhancing protein synthesis and reducing amino acid oxidation. Young (1981b) cites six human experiments in which nitrogen balance response averaged between 1–3 mg N per added kcal. It is not unlikely that some nitrogen balance studies may have underestimated requirements of protein and individual amino acids as a consequence of high energy intakes (Garza et al., 1976; 1977; Young and Scrimshaw, 1978).

Effect of Essential Amino Acid and Total Nitrogen Intake

Assuming that energy and nutrient intakes are adequate, nitrogen balance is dependent primarily on (1) the amounts and proportions of essential amino acids provided by the diet and (2) the total nitrogen intake. The minimum protein requirement therefore is a variable estimate which is affected both by the level of essential amino acids and of nonessential amino acid nitrogen in the diet. The interrelationship between amino acid composition of the diet and total nitrogen intake, for example, was illustrated in early studies by Sherman (1920), who showed that replacement of 10 percent of the protein content of a cereal diet by milk resulted in a decrease by almost 10 gm in the estimated protein requirement to maintain nitrogen equilibrium.

Because the protein requirement is a variable estimate depending on the composition of protein fed, the ultimate problem in protein nutrition is the requirement for the essential amino acids and, further, the determination of minimum levels of nonessential amino acid nitrogen required at minimum intakes of the essential amino acids. Studies on amino acid requirements necessitate the use of partially purified diets in which synthetic amino acids are incorporated. When any one of the essential amino acids is excluded from the diet, subjects immediately go into negative nitrogen balance. The missing amino acid is then fed at graded levels until the criterion of adequacy is reached.

For a comprehensive review of studies related to protein requirements, see Irwin and Hegsted (1971).

Amino acid requirements have been reported for infants (Holt and Snyderman, 1967; Fomon and Filer, 1967) and for children (Nakagawa et al., 1964). Some values are compiled in Table 23.10. Estimates for the amino acid requirements

TABLE 23.10
Protein and Amino Requirements of Children

	Mg Per Kg Per Day		
	Infants[a]	2-Year-Old Children[b]	10 to 12-Year-Old Children[a]
Histidine	28	—	—
Isoleucine	70	31	30
Leucine	161	73	45
Lysine	103	64	60
Methionine + cystine	58	27	27
Phenylalanine + tyrosine	125	69	27
Threonine	87	37	35
Tryptophan	17	13	4
Valine	93	38	33
Protein	1,800	1,390	950

Source: [a]FAO/WHO (1973).

[b]O. B. Pineda et al. *Protein Quality in Humans: Assessment and in vitro estimation,* AVI Publishing, Westport, Connecticut, 1981.

TABLE 23.11
Minimum Adult Requirements for Essential Amino Acids

Amino Acid	Amino Acid Requirements	
	Women[a]	Men[b]
	gm/day	gm/day
Isoleucine	0.45	0.70
Leucine	0.62	1.10
Lysine	0.50	0.80
Methionine + Cystine	0.55	1.10
Phenylalanine + Tyrosine	1.12	1.10
Threonine	0.31	0.50
Tryptophan	0.16	0.25
Valine	0.65	0.80

Source: [a]R. M. Leverton, *Protein and Amino Acid Nutrition,* Academic Press, New York, 1959.
[b]W. C. Rose et al., *J. Biol. Chem.* 217:987 (1955).

of adults are based primarily on studies by Rose et al. (1955), Swendseid et al. (1956a; 1956b), and Leverton (1959) and are shown in Table 23.11. Requirements reported for men are, in general, larger than those obtained from studies with women; this finding may be due in part to the larger body size of men. However, differences in interpretation of minimum requirement from the studies on men and women suggest an alternative explanation for the higher levels reported for men. Rose (ibid) defined minimum requirement as the smallest amount of an amino acid that would support a distinctly positive nitrogen balance and selected the value obtained from the subject with the highest requirement in the group studied as the proper figure to report. On the other hand, both Leverton and Swendseid defined minimum requirement as the amount of the amino acid that would keep a subject in nitrogen equilibrium or in a state in which the difference between intake and output is no more than ±5 percent. Results reported from these two studies are similar. Young (1981a; 1981b) questions the validity of these early studies on the basis of more recent data using the stable isotope infusion technique. This procedure will be discussed in a later section.

Kopple and Swendseid (1973) provided evidence that histidine may be an essential amino acid for the human adult. Subjects maintained on 40 gm of protein were in negative balance after 25 days on a diet deficient in histidine. When histidine was added subjects went into positive balance and remained so for at least 25 days. The experimental period in this study was longer than that often used in nitrogen balance studies and may account for the results obtained. These results are interesting because histidine has been thought to be nonessential for the human adult and particularly in view of the unique role that histidine plays in the maintenance of intracellular pH (see Chapter 7).

The importance of nonessential amino acid nitrogen and other forms of nitrogen (nonspecific nitrogen) on the adequacy of dietary protein and on essential amino acid requirements also must be recognized. (See Kies, 1974.) Snyderman et al. (1962) found that when milk protein was reduced until weight gain and nitrogen retention in infants were adversely affected, both weight gain and nitrogen retention could be restored to normal by administration of nonessential nitrogen in the form of glycine or urea, that is, a nonessential amino acid or a nonprotein source of nitrogen. Scrimshaw et al. (1966) studied the effect of varying levels of egg protein diluted to a constant nitrogen intake with glycine and diammonium citrate. According to their results, the minimum ratio of grams of essential amino acids per gram of total nitrogen (E/T_N) for diets approximating the amino acid pattern in whole egg apparently lies between 1.85 and 2.16; at this level, essential amino acids account for 21–25 percent of the total dietary nitrogen. These findings suggest that the relative proportions of essential and nonessential amino acids in the diet are more important than had been supposed.

FACTORIAL APPROACH

The factorial approach was used by the FAO/WHO committees on protein requirements in both 1965 and 1973 and is outlined in Table 23.12. The method is based on a major assumption (for which there is no physiological basis) that losses of nitrogen associated with a protein-free intake can be used to predict nitrogen losses that occur when nitrogen intake meets the physiological need for high quality, highly digestible protein. These total obligatory losses appear to average 50 mg N/kg or 2 mg N/basal kcal for the adult male (Smuts, 1935). For the child or the pregnant or lactating female, further allowances must be made for body nitrogen gain, the nitrogen content of the fetus, and material tissues and the milk protein output.

Certain assumptions are necessary before these minimum values can be adjusted to recommended allowances. It has been demonstrated repeatedly that nitrogen retention in children or nitrogen balance in adults cannot be achieved by feeding high quality protein at these calculated minimum levels based on obligatory losses. In other words, even high quality protein cannot be utilized with 100 percent efficiency. A 30 percent increase in nitrogen intake above total obligatory nitrogen losses was advocated by FAO/WHO (1973) to allow for inefficient utilization, but more recent data indicate that a 45 percent increase may be more accurate (Young and Scrimshaw, 1978; Beaton et al., 1979). It is not clear, however, that any one correction figure is applicable to all age groups. This possible discrepancy may explain why the FAO/WHO (1973) allowance of 0.57 gm egg protein per kg/day was found to be inadequate for many experimental subjects (Garza et al., 1976; 1977).

A further correction of 30 percent is made for individual variability. The resulting figure is termed the safe practical allowance (SPA). A final adjustment is made to allow for protein quality which includes amino acid content and protein digestibility expressed as a fraction.

Examples of these calculations for children and adults are shown in Table 23.13.

TABLE 23.12
Factorial Approach for Human Protein Requirements: FAO/WHO (1973)

A. Estimate obligatory N losses (O_N): from the sum of urinary, fecal, skin, and miscellaneous losses. These data are obtained from measurements made when subjects are consuming nonprotein diets.

B. Estimate N requirements for growth (G_N), pregnancy (P_N), and lactation (L_N) from N content and amount of new tissue in growth, and in fetal and maternal tissues in pregnancy. For lactation, N content of milk is multiplied by average milk volume.

C. Thus minimum nitrogen requirement for growth = $O_N + G_N$. *NOTE:* G_N will be zero for an adult and will vary with age for a child.

D. Adjust for efficiency of N utilization: add 30% (not to be confused with protein quality, see "G" below).

$$\text{Requirement} = (O_N + G_N) \times 1.3$$

E. Adjust for individual variability (an additional 30%).

$$\text{Safe Practical Allowance (SPA)} + [(O_N + G_N) \times 1.3] \times 1.3$$

F. Additional allowance for pregnancy (A_P) or lactation (A_L)

$$A_p = (P_N \times 1.3) \times 1.3 \quad \text{or} \quad A_L = (L_N \times 1.3) \times 1.3$$

Adjustments made both for efficiency of nitrogen utilization (+ 30%) and for individual variability (+ 30%).

G. Values for nitrogen as computed above are converted to protein (N × 6.25). These values are in terms of proteins of high quality such as egg or milk proteins and further adjustments are necessary to increase allowances when average protein quality value is less than 100%.

$$\text{Thus: Recommended Protein Allowance} = \frac{\text{SPA}}{\text{Protein Quality}}$$
$$\text{(adjusted for quality)}$$

Source: Courtesy of Dr. P. L. Pellett,

NITROGEN BALANCE RESPONSE CURVES

A diagrammatic representation of this procedure is shown in Fig. 23.13 in which nitrogen balance response is plotted against graded intakes of protein. Requirement is judged to be at the point at which the line crosses zero balance (R) or a point representing a small positive balance for growth (R_c). The slope is steeper for high quality protein than for poor quality protein; thus, requirement is lower when protein quality is high.

In theory, this procedure is the most direct way of estimating protein requirement, and no assumptions are necessary concerning the degree of utilization of

TABLE 23.13
Calculation of Protein Requirements by Factorial Approach: FAO/WHO 1973

Age Group	Weight (kg)	Obligatory Loss	Growth	Total	Inefficient Utilization +30%	Individual Variability +30%	Safe Level Of Protein Per Day Protein = N × 6.25		Safe Level Adjusted for Protein Quality NPU = 0.75 Assumed gm/day
							gm/kg	gm/day	
		mg N per kg/day							
Child 2 years	13.4	104	16	120	156	203	1.27	17	23
Child 10 years (♂)	36.9	72	6	78	101	132	0.82	30	40
Adult (♀)	55.0	49	0	49	64	83	0.52	29	39
				mg per day					
Pregnancy (extra)	—	—	—	860	1,120	1,450	—	9	12
Lactation (extra)	—	—	—	1,600	2,080	2,700	—	17	23

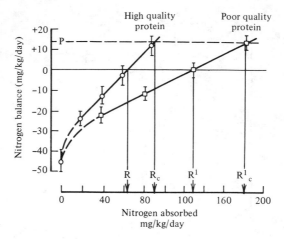

Figure 23.13
Diagrammatic representation of nitrogen balance response curves for determination of protein requirements. R and R¹ are adult N requirements for good and poor protein respectively. R_c and R^1_c are corresponding values for a child using the intersect with a small positive balance (P) rather than with the zero balance line. The slope of lines are measures of protein quality and should be compared with the slope-ratio procedures for protein quality.

high quality protein such as those required for the factorial approach. Although the nitrogen balance response curve is subject to all the limitations inherent in nitrogen balance, it is considered the means currently available for evaluating the factorial approach and for determining the relationships between obligatory losses and minimum requirements. Relatively few studies of this kind have been carried out; however, these data are used by FAO/WHO as the basis for estimation of adult protein needs (Torun et al., 1981; FAO/WHO, 1983).

PLASMA AMINO ACIDS

The levels of amino acids in the circulating plasma are controlled homeostatically, but the mechanisms of control remain unknown. Many factors affect regulation of amino acid concentrations in the circulation (Cahill, 1981). Nevertheless, plasma amino acid levels have been used in determination of nutritional status, in estimation of amino acid requirements, and in the evaluation of protein quality.

The levels of plasma amino acids and in particular the ratio of essential to nonessential amino acids were used as a means of evaluating response to low protein or low essential amino acid diets. Swendseid et al. (1963) reported that essential amino acids in plasma decreased in subjects maintained on a low protein diet, whereas the amount of nonessential amino acids was not affected. Whitehead and Dean (1964), among others, utilized the ratio of plasma nonessential to essential amino acids as a means of evaluating response to treatment of children suffering from protein-energy malnutrition. In protein-energy malnutrition the ratio is high (usually above 2) and gradually decreases as the clinical condition of the child improves under dietary treatment. The decreased ratio is due primarily to an increase in essential amino acid levels; nonessential amino acids remain unchanged. Similar changes in plasma amino acid levels were reported by Scrimshaw et al. (1966) when experimental subjects were fed diets containing decreasing levels of egg protein.

The level of amino acids in plasma has been used as a means for determining dietary amino acid requirements. Studies in rats (McLaughlan and Illman, 1967) and pigs (Mitchell et al., 1968) indicated that the limiting amino acid accumulated in plasma only when the dietary requirement had been exceeded. Results obtained by this method were in good agreement with those obtained from the growth method in young animals. In adult human males, Young et al. (1971) found the tryptophan requirement to be 3 mg/kg of body weight using the plasma tryptophan level as criterion as compared with 2–2.6 mg/kg of body weight by the nitrogen balance technique. Requirements determined by this technique are assumed to be at the sharp breakpoints in curves relating tryptophan intakes to tryptophan plasma levels. This method has been used for determining requirements for valine and lysine in young men (Young et al., 1972) and for threonine in young men and elderly women (Tontisirin et al., 1974).

Although plasma amino acids may provide estimates of amino acid requirements independent of nitrogen balance, Young and Scrimshaw (1978) caution that there is a need for qualitative and quantitative investigations of all factors and mechanisms associated with control of plasma amino acid levels before the approach can be adequately evaluated.

Plasma amino acids have been used for protein quality evaluation and identification of limiting amino acids in diets. The work in this area was reviewed by Jansen (1981).

GROWTH

Body weight gain in young infants is a measure of dietary adequacy and thus can be used to estimate both total protein requirements and requirements for individual amino acids. Two of the best known studies of essential amino acid requirements of infants used adequate growth as the criterion for meeting the need of an essential amino acid (Holt and Snyderman, 1967; Fomon and Filer, 1967).

Growth is a sensitive indicator of protein and amino acid adequacy only when growth rate is high. However, even when nitrogen balance is used for estimation of amino acid requirements of older infants (1½–2½ years of age), maintenance of adequate growth is used as the criterion of long-term dietary adequacy (Pineda et al., 1981).

STABLE ISOTOPE INFUSION TECHNIQUES

The use of continuous infusion of stable isotopes for the study of amino acid requirements is one of the more innovative techniques currently in use. Isotopic procedures for the study of amino acid metabolism have been in use for many years (Schoenheimer, 1942) and were used by Waterlow and his colleagues in investigations of children suffering from protein-energy malnutrition. (See Alleyne et al., 1972.)

Radioactive isotopes (^{3}H and ^{14}C) were used extensively in the past, but ethical considerations now preclude their use in humans. Nonradioactive tracers such as ^{2}H, ^{13}C, ^{15}N, and ^{18}C pose no such ethical problems. These tracers are now readily available, and current analytical techniques for determining isotope distribution are highly sensitive. Preferred methods are density, optical emission spectrometry, nuclear magnetic resonance, activation analysis, and mass spectrometry. (See Bier, 1982.)

The constant isotope infusion model developed by Young (1981b) is shown in Fig. 23.14. Body nitrogen metabolism is viewed as a metabolic pool from which amino acids leave either by protein synthesis or by protein breakdown. The labeled essential amino acid is administered by continuous infusion. Label dilution is measured in plasma free amino acids or in urinary urea or expired $^{13}CO_2$.

Young (1981a; 1981b) demonstrated that when the intake of a specific amino acid is very low, the oxidation of that acid is markedly reduced. Thus, a breakpoint is reached at some point in the oxidation rate as intake is reduced. Young (ibid) believes that this "breakpoint" may be at or about the requirement level. If this conclusion is correct, the estimated requirement for leucine and lysine may be in the order of 35–40 mg amino acid per kilogram body weight per day. These

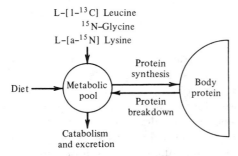

Figure 23.14
General model of whole body amino acid metabolism as studied by the application of a continuous, stable isotope infusion approach.

levels are considerably above the generally accepted leucine and lysine requirements of 11 and 9 mg respectively. Thus, essential amino acid requirements of the adult may be threefold higher than currently accepted levels.

The possible underestimation of amino acid requirements appears to apply only to adults. In children there is generally good agreement between experiments involving specific manipulation of the level of test amino acid in purified L-amino acid diets and studies of nitrogen balance and growth obtained with varying intakes of high quality protein. This difference is probably due to the sensitivity of body weight gain or nitrogen balance as criteria of dietary amino acid adequacy in the rapidly growing organism, whereas short-term nitrogen balance is a poor index of dietary amino acid adequacy for protein maintenance in the healthy adult.

Evaluation of Protein Quality

The quality of a protein is dependent on its amino acid composition and digestibility. Biological evaluation is the preferred method for determination of protein quality since it is the ability of a protein to support growth and maintenance, that is, cellular synthesis, that determines its ultimate value. Methods for evaluation of protein quality are based therefore on the retention of nitrogen in the body. Some methods, for example those utilizing nitrogen balance or growth as criteria of nitrogen retention, can be applied to studies with human subjects. The large majority of reports in the literature, however, are of studies performed with experimental animals and that sometimes utilize techniques, such as carcass analysis, that obviously are not suitable for studies with humans.

AMINO ACID SCORE (CHEMICAL SCORE)

A simple nonbiological device for estimating protein quality is called the amino acid score or chemical score. This method involves a comparison of the amino acid composition of a test food with that of a high quality protein such as egg or milk or to an amino acid reference pattern (FAO/WHO, 1973). The score is calculated from the following equation:

$$\text{Amino acid score} = \frac{\text{mg of amino acid in 1 gm of test protein}}{\text{mg of amino acid in 1 gm of reference pattern}} \times 100$$

The lowest score for any of the essential amino acids designates the "limiting amino acid" and gives a rough estimate of the protein quality of the food. In practice, only scores for lysine, methionine + cystine, and tryptophan need be calculated since one of these amino acids is usually limiting in most common foods. Although a rather crude instrument for evaluating protein quality, the amino acid score often agrees well with the results of biological evaluation.

Some amino acid reference scoring patterns that have been used to calculate amino acid scores are shown in Table 23.14.

TABLE 23.14
Some Reference Scoring Patterns

Essential Amino Acid	Whole Egg	FAO (1957)	FAO/WHO (1973)
	mg/gm Nitrogen		
Isoleucine	340	270	250
Leucine	540	306	440
Lysine	440	270	340
Total sulfur amino acids	355	270	220
Total aromatic amino acids	580	360	380
Threonine	294	180	250
Tryptophan	106	90	60
Valine	410	270	310
Total Essential Amino Acids	3,060	2,015	2,215

PROTEIN EFFICIENCY RATIO (PER)

Protein efficiency ratio is a measure of weight gain of a growing animal divided by protein intake:

$$PER = \frac{\text{weight gain (gm)}}{\text{protein intake (gm)}}$$

The PER was used as early as 1917 by Osborne and Mendel in their studies establishing differences in protein quality (Osborne et al., 1919). It has been applied most often to studies on laboratory rats, but it is also applicable to studies with human infants. It is the simplest method for evaluating protein quality since it requires only an accurate measure of dietary intake and weight gain. However, the method requires strict adherence to certain conditions: the energy intake must be adequate and the protein must be fed at an adequate but not excessive level since at high levels of dietary protein, weight gain does not increase proportionately with protein intake.

A major source of error in the PER method lies in the use of weight gain *per se* as sole criterion of protein value. In addition, PER does not account for protein needs for maintenance. Methods that precisely define protein retention therefore are likely to yield more consistently accurate results. In terms of speed of operation and expense, however, the PER method is advantageous.

NET PROTEIN RATIO (NPR)

The PER can be improved by including a group of animals consuming a protein-free diet. When modified in this way, the procedure is called *net protein ratio* (NPR). This method thus accounts for protein needs for maintenance. Pellett and

Young (1980) recommended a further modification termed *relative* NPR (RNPR). In this procedure, results of NPR are expressed on a percentage basis in relation to weight gain of animals fed a diet containing 8 percent lactalbumin.

BIOLOGICAL VALUE (BV)

Biological value is a measure of nitrogen retained for growth or maintenance and is expressed as nitrogen retained divided by nitrogen absorbed (Mitchell, 1923). It is determined by nitrogen balance and is applicable to humans as well as laboratory animals. In a quantitative sense, BV may be expressed more explicitly as:

$$BV = \frac{I - (F - F_0) - (U - U_0)}{I - (F - F_0)}$$

where I is nitrogen intake, U is urinary nitrogen, F is fecal nitrogen, and U_0 and F_0 are urinary and fecal nitrogen excreted when subjects are maintained on a nitrogen-free or nearly nitrogen-free diet. BV calculated from this equation accounts for metabolic (or endogenous) nitrogen losses. If the correction is not made, that is, if U_0 and F_0 are not in the equation, BV obtained is designated *apparent biological value*. The practice of ignoring metabolic nitrogen is not uncommon, so many values for BV represent apparent biological value of protein.

NITROGEN BALANCE INDEX

Nitrogen balance index is essentially the same as biological value (Allison, 1955). It can be determined from the slope of the line when nitrogen balance is plotted against absorbed nitrogen. More simply, nitrogen balance index can be calculated from the following equation:

$$\text{Nitrogen balance index} = \frac{B - B_0}{A}$$

where B is nitrogen balance, B_0 is nitrogen balance when nitrogen intake is zero, and A is absorbed nitrogen. Since B_0 represents metabolic nitrogen, the nitrogen balance index is a measure of dietary nitrogen retained. This method is not used as often as are some other measures of protein quality.

NET PROTEIN UTILIZATION (NPU)

Quantitatively, NPU is represented by a simple formula: N retained/N intake. The NPU thus is equivalent to biological value × digestibility and is a measure both of the digestibility of food protein and the biological value of the amino acid mixture absorbed from food.

NPU represents the proportion of *food* nitrogen retained, whereas both BV and nitrogen balance index represent the proportion of *absorbed* nitrogen retained. NPU therefore is related directly to dietary intake of nitrogen. Nitrogen retention can be measured by nitrogen balance studies (Bender and Miller, 1953) or by direct analysis of the animal body (Miller and Bender, 1955). The latter method is preferred. In any case, the method requires two groups of experimental animals equivalent in weight and age. One group is fed the test protein and the other is fed a protein-free diet. At the end of the feeding period, carcasses are analyzed for water from which nitrogen content can be calculated. (See Chapter 22.) The formula for calculating NPU is as follows:

$$NPU = \frac{\text{Body N of test group} - \text{body N of nonprotein group} + \text{N consumed by nonprotein group}}{\text{N consumed by test group}}$$

Other terms may be used to define NPU. NPU standardized (NPU_{st}) refers to determinations of NPU when proteins are fed at minimum requirement or below. NPU operative (NPU_{op}) refers to NPU determined under any other conditions. The net dietary protein value (NDpV) is a measure of utilizable protein proposed by Platt and Miller (1959) and is determined by multiplying dietary protein concentration by NPU obtained.

When NPU is determined in human subjects, the nitrogen balance technique is used. Considerable care is required because a number of factors can influence the procedure. Some such factors are psychological stress, minor infection, pattern of activity, and overall composition of the diet. Pellett and Young (1980) and Bodwell et al. (1981) described the precautions necessary for accuracy in nitrogen balance procedures in determination of protein quality in humans.

NET DIETARY PROTEIN CALORIES PERCENT (NDpCal %)

NDpCal % relates protein quality to energy intake (Platt et al., 1961). This method appears to be especially useful in evaluation of human diets in which the relation of protein to total calories may vary markedly. Thus dietary protein is expressed as percent of total calories rather than as percent of total weight.

Quantitatively, NDpCal % is obtained by the following formula:

$$NDpCal \% = \frac{\text{protein calories}}{\text{total caloric intake}} \times 100 \times NPU_{op}$$

According to calculated values from protein of highest quality, either whole egg or human milk, a diet that provides less than 5 percent of calories in the form of available protein will not meet protein needs of the human adult. For children, at least 8 percent is required. (See FAO, Protein Requirements, 1965.)

SLOPE-RATIO ASSAY

The slope-ratio assay has been used to determine protein quality in growing rats (Hegsted and Chang, 1965a; 1965b) and has been applied to adult rats (Said and

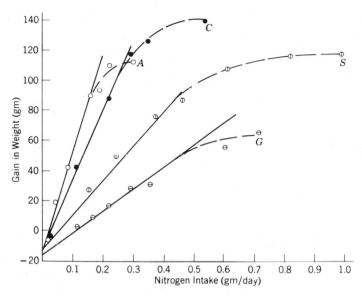

Figure 23.15
Relationship between weight gain and nitrogen intake. Broken lines drawn by inspection. Solid lines are the regression lines calculated through the points that appear to be in the linear range. A = albumin; C = casein; S = soy protein; G = gluten. (From D. M. Hegsted and Y. Chang, *J. Nutr.* 85:159, 1965.)

Hegsted, 1969). The method is essentially an application of standard bioassay procedure and involves feeding proteins at varying levels of intake including a protein-free diet. Weight, body water, or body nitrogen may be used as measures of response to dietary protein. Dietary protein levels must be selected with care because a straight line response occurs over a relatively small range of intake. At high levels of intake more protein is deaminated and used for energy. At low levels, amino acids are used more efficiently due to adaptive responses. Relative potency of the test protein is determined by comparison of its slope with that of a high quality standard protein such as albumin or lactalbumin, which is assigned a potency of 100. (See Fig. 23.15.)

OTHER TECHNIQUES

Attempts have been made to simulate the action of the mammalian digestive system using *in vitro* enzymic digestion. Satterlee et al. (1981) described a rapid technique in which a multienzyme mixture is added to a protein suspension at a specific pH and change in pH is measured after 10 minutes. This method shows good agreement with digestibility measured in rats and thus provides an indication of the availability of the protein.

When proteins are heated, chemical reactions can occur between the ϵ-amino group of lysine and certain reactive carbohydrate or lipid groupings. The absorption and the retention of lysine may be reduced, and proteins so affected show lower values when assayed by bioassy techniques. Thus, an amino acid detected by chemical analysis may be biologically unavailable. Because the ϵ-amino group of lysine is the key to the reaction, Carpenter (1973; 1981) developed a chemical assay procedure to test whether the ϵ-amino group is free or bound.

Microbiological procedures also can be used as a measure of protein availability (Ford, 1981). For example, *tetrahymena pyriformis*, first used for protein quality evaluation many years ago, was reintroduced by Dryden et al. (1977). This assay, in conjunction with a rapid procedure for digestibility (Satterlee et al., 1979) gives a quick prediction of PER.

Calcium Requirements

The greatest loss of dietary calcium occurs through the feces rather than urine and represents calcium that is not absorbed from the intestinal lumen and calcium that enters the lumen in intestinal secretions. Calcium absorption varies from roughly 15 percent to 35 percent or more. Outhouse et al. (1941) reported an average absorption of 24 percent for seven adults maintained on intakes ranging from 231–575 mg/day. A similar average absorption, 21 percent, was reported by Bricker et al. (1949b) for adult subjects on diets containing 206–752 mg calcium. Steggerda and Mitchell (1946) estimated average absorption to be about 30 percent.

Absorption of calcium and ability to maintain equilibrium on low calcium intakes varies with the previous intake of the experimental subject and the length of the experimental period. For example, Hegsted et al. (1952) found that 9 of 10 men required less than 400 mg to maintain calcium equilibrium; the subjects were inmates in a Peruvian prison and presumably had consumed a diet low in calcium for many years. Similarly, Malm (1958), in a study of men in Oslo, found the calcium requirement for equilibrium to be less than 500 mg for 21 of 26 subjects. Subjects maintained for several months on approximately 450 mg/day after consuming about 950 mg for several months absorbed about 45 percent of the intake, compared with 25 percent on the higher intake. With the increase in percentage absorption, however, the total amount of calcium absorbed was approximately the same for both levels of intake.

It is significant that some subjects in the Malm study never adjusted to low intakes of calcium over a period of several months. Other studies also indicate that in addition to the problem of adaptation to calcium intake, individual variation in calcium balance is great. The wide range of calcium intakes reported to maintain equilibrium is evident from reviews of the early literature summarized by Sherman (1920), Mitchell and Curzon (1939), Leitch and Aitken (1959), and the more recent review of Irwin and Kienholz (1973).

It would seem that calcium balance data from studies with children would be simpler to interpret since the need for calcium to support normal skeletal development is obviously high and should result in calcium retention. However, retention of dietary calcium varies considerably in children without demonstrable differences in either growth response or skeletal development. The infant fed cow's milk formula, for example, retains about 50 percent more calcium than the breast-fed infant but shows no advantage for having done so. Leitch and Aitken (1959) estimated retention of calcium necessary for skeletal growth to be between 75 and 150 mg/day between the first and tenth years of life and about 400 mg/day during the maximal pubertal growth spurt; these retentions could be effected with intakes ranging from 600 mg–1,000 mg or more.

Calcium retention is markedly affected by the level of protein in the diet (Johnson et al., 1970; Walker and Linkswiler, 1972; Anand and Linkswiler, 1974). This effect is observed even when the source of nitrogen is pure L-amino acids (Margen et al., 1974). In the studies by Linkswiler and associates, adult males maintained on a low protein diet (47 gm) retained calcium when the diet contained as little as 500 mg of calcium whereas those fed 97 gm of protein retained calcium only when dietary calcium was 800 mg or more (Fig. 23.16). On a diet containing 142 gm of protein only 3 out of 15 subjects retained calcium on levels of 1,400 mg of calcium; none were in balance at lower levels of calcium intake. Calcium absorption was increased somewhat at higher protein intakes, but this advantage

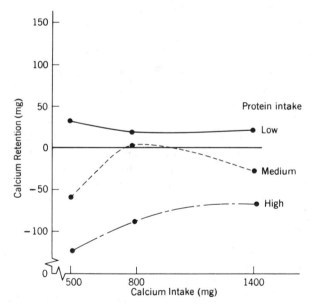

Figure 23.16
Calcium retention at three levels of calcium and three levels of protein intake; ——— = low protein; ---- = medium protein and •—•—• = high protein. (From H. M. Linkswiler, *Trans. N. Y. Acad. Sci.* (Series II), 36:333, 1974.)

was offset by markedly increased excretion of calcium in the urine. In contrast, Spencer et al. (1978) found little effect on calcium excretion when subjects were fed a high protein diet containing meat. It was postulated that the high phosphorus content of the meat diet may have influenced calcium excretion. Subsequent studies demonsrated conclusively that when both protein and phosphorus intakes are increased, urinary calcium excretion is not affected (Hegsted et al., 1981; Zemel and Linkswiler, 1981).

The influence of dietary protein and phosphorus on calcium retention could account, in part, for variations in estimated requirement from various studies. The problem of calcium requirements, however, is complicated by the lack of clinical evidence of calcium deficiency. There is no conclusive evidence that low calcium intakes significantly reduce growth rate or result in altered structure or composition of bone (Walker, 1954; Walker and Arvidsson, 1954; A.M.A. Council on Foods and Nutrition, 1963). In adults, low calcium intakes have been implicated in the etiology of senile osteoporosis (Whedon, 1959; Nordin, 1961; 1962). Other investigators (Garn et al., 1967; Newton-John and Morgan, 1968) view osteoporosis as a physiological consequence of aging. It seems likely that neither view is entirely accurate. Genetic and hormonal factors as well as degree of physical activity appear to affect skeletal integrity, and there is no clear-cut relationship between calcium intake and bone mass. However, on the basis of calcium balance studies, Heaney (1978) estimated that an average daily intake of 990 mg calcium was required to achieve balance in postmenopausal women treated with estrogen as compared with 1,500 mg for untreated women. Chinn (1981) also suggested that elderly women might benefit from high calcium intakes or calcium supplementation. In addition, treatment of osteoporosis with various forms of vitamin D has shown promising results (Gallagher et al., 1982). Whether the problem of osteoporosis is related directly to calcium intake thus remains questionable. (See Chapter 17.)

Until more precise techniques are devised for determining calcium requirements, and until the significance and limitation of physiological adaptation are fully evaluated, the problem of calcium requirements will continue to be debated as it is presently, on the basis of point of view rather than on meaningful experimental evidence.

Iron Requirements

As discussed in Chapter 6, iron is poorly absorbed from the intestinal lumen, but once absorbed very little is excreted. The inability of the intestinal mucosa to absorb more than 10–20 percent of the total dietary intake places the dietary requirement for iron far above the metabolic requirement. However, the ability of the body to conserve iron tenaciously by reusing iron from hemoglobin degradation results in a much lower dietary requirement than would be possible if iron so released were excreted in the urine. Urinary loss of iron is almost negligible (Dubach et al., 1955).

The amount of iron lost in sweat is variable and ill-defined and includes iron in sloughed off epithelial cells (Mitchell and Edman, 1962). Fecal loss includes iron contained in desquamated intestinal mucosal cells and minute amounts in intestinal secretions as well as the dietary iron that never enters the mucosal cell. The former are true losses from the body but obviously are difficult to differentiate from unabsorbed iron by the usual balance technique. Radioisotope studies indicate that the total body turnover of iron, including losses through the gastrointestinal and urinary tracts and skin, amount to approximately 14 μg/kg of body weight per day (Finch, 1959; Green et al., 1968). This loss amounts to a physiological requirement of about 0.9 mg/day for a 69 kg man and 0.8 mg/day for a nonmenstruating woman weighing 55 kg.

In women of child-bearing age, further losses occur in the menses. Menstrual blood losses vary considerably. In a study on a small group of women, Frenchman and Johnston (1949) reported losses that amounted to from 0.8–2.6 mg/day when averaged for a monthly period. In a study with a larger number of women, Hallberg et al. (1966) found menstrual losses to be less than 1.4 mg/day for all but 10 percent of normal women and less than 2.0 mg/day for all but 5 percent.

In pregnant women, additional iron is required for expansion of the red cell mass, for deposition in the fetus and placenta, and to cover the blood loss at delivery. These needs are compensated in part by the cessation of menstruation. In an early study by Coons (1932), an average positive balance of 3.2 mg was observed in 9 pregnant women who, on the average, were consuming of 14.7 mg of iron daily. These data were later confirmed by radioisotope studies (Hahn et al., 1951) and shown to be caused by increased absorption in late pregnancy as well as conservation of iron normally lost through the menses. Further confirmation of the increased absorptive capacity during pregnancy was provided by the studies of Apte and Lyengar (1969).

Therapeutic doses of iron are absorbed less efficiently than physiological doses. Despite relatively poor absorption, however, the absolute amount of iron absorbed from a therapeutic dose is higher than that from a lower intake (Smith and Pannacciulli, 1958).

The chemical balance method measures the overall retention or loss of iron from the body and has been useful in determining absorption from various foods (Schlaphoff and Johnston, 1949). The use of radioactive isotopes of iron, however, has replaced the older technique in studies of iron metabolism. (See Hallberg, 1981; also see Chapter 6.) It is surprising that the chemical balance technique and radioisotope technique have yielded similar estimates of the average dietary requirement for iron. For example, Leverton and Marsh (1942), in early balance studies, found an average of 15.9 mg of iron to be necessary for equilibrium in young women; 12.9 mg was adequate for 87 percent of their subjects. This figure is not markedly different than that obtained from estimated losses of iron from the body and radioisotope studies on availability of iron (Layrisse et al., 1968; Cook et al., 1972; see Chapter 6).

In practical terms, the dietary requirement for iron depends largely on the ability to absorb iron, which depends on the character of the diet. The establishment of a recommendation for a population group, therefore, will be influenced by usual diets consumed. (See Chapter 6 and Chapter 25.) Because of wide individual variability, dietary allowances must be established with the view of reducing the risk of deficiency in vulnerable groups. (See Beaton, 1972.)

Conclusion

Many of the techniques for determining nutrient requirements have not changed for many years. The limitations of these methods are now more readily recognized and, indeed, new interpretations have on occasion been applied to old data. As new and more refined techniques emerge, knowledge of human requirements will be refined both in terms of the individual nutrient and the effect of nutrient interrelationships on dietary requirements. The use of stable isotopes, for example, will provide much needed information on bioavailability of mineral elements (Janghorbani and Young, 1980; Janghorbani et al., 1980; 1982; see Bier, 1982). Data on human nutrient requirements are necessary to establish rational allowances for normal population groups.

chapter 24

determination of nutrient needs: vitamins

Methods for determination of vitamin requirements are of necessity different from those applicable to energy, protein, and minerals. Techniques for determining vitamin needs also have changed more over the years than those for the other nutrients and continue to change. Yet many of the classic studies conducted more than 30 years ago remain valid and indeed form the basis for the recommended dietary allowances and other standards. Confirmation of early data by new techniques, however, has increased confidence in our knowledge of human vitamin requirements and removed some of the "guess work" from the margin of safety allowed in most dietary standards. Perhaps more important, new techniques have permitted the early and accurate detection of vitamin deficiency states.

The vitamins are different chemically, and they behave differently in the metabolism of living organisms. Consequently, no single method for the assessment of vitamin requirements is equally satisfactory for all vitamins. In general, techniques that have been used to evaluate response to controlled dietary intake may be grouped into five categories:

1. Clinical evaluation.
2. Urinary excretion of the vitamin or its metabolites.
3. Blood level of the vitamin or its derivatives.
4. Urinary excretion and blood level following a test dose of the vitamin (load tests).
5. Enzyme activity and/or other biochemical or histochemical tests related to vitamin function.

In addition to differences in response among the vitamins, these techniques do not necessarily yield comparable data for any one vitamin, because, in effect, they measure different states of vitamin nutriture. Assuming that a well-nourished, healthy person is placed on a diet deficient in a single vitamin, the sequence of the developing deficiency is:

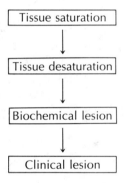

Theoretically, the five general methods for assessment of vitamin requirements should correlate with each level of vitamin status represented in the diagram; life would be simpler for the experimental nutritionist if this were so. In practice, as will be seen later, there is considerable variability and overlapping. In other words, some techniques for assessing vitamin requirements are more sensitive measurements for some vitamins than for others. Moreover, there is great variability among the rates that different vitamins become depleted from specific tissues and that different tissues are depleted of specific vitamins. In order to be useful in determining vitamin requirements, a method should be sensitive in two ways: (1) it should be *nutritionally* sensitive, that is, detectable early in deficiency, and (2) it should be *analytically* sensitive, that is, there must be an assay method that will measure small changes in level or function.

Tissue saturation applies to an optimal state of nutrition when a significant increase in tissue concentration of vitamin cannot be accomplished by an increase in dietary intake. The term is meaningful when applied to the water-soluble vitamins, but has little significance in relation to the fat-soluble vitamins. Water-soluble vitamins are excreted in the urine and, with the exception of vitamin B_{12}, do not accumulate in the body to any great degree. Although the upper limit varies, for example, 100 mg or less for thiamin and 4–5 gm for ascorbic acid, there is general agreement that beyond a certain point further loading of the body with water-soluble vitamins enriches the urine but not the body. Under this condition, the tissues are said to be saturated.

It is possible to attain small transient increases in blood ascorbic acid levels by further loading with the vitamin. When the blood level surpasses the renal excretion threshold of 1.4 mg/dl plasma, increasingly larger doses of the vitamin are required to elicit small increases in plasma ascorbic acid levels, and urinary excretion remains high (Friedman et al., 1940). Thus, for practical purposes, the body is indeed saturated.

In contrast, fat-soluble vitamins are not readily excreted in the urine and apparently can be stored to an unlimited degree in certain tissues. Since there is no apparent upper limit of accretion for these vitamins, there is no reasonable level that could be described as tissue saturation. Depletion of the body through inadequate intake of fat-soluble vitamins therefore is a long-term process; the length of time required for depletion depends primarily on the extent of tissue stores. Determination of dietary requirements for the fat-soluble vitamins thus is considerably more difficult than for the water-soluble vitamins and is limited to methods 1, 3, and 5 listed above. In addition, blood levels of fat-soluble vitamins are more difficult to interpret; a high level may merely represent mobilization from tissue stores as a result of transient inadequate dietary intake. Low levels may not be reached for months on an apparently low dietary level of vitamin when tissue stores initially are high.

Statements of minimum requirements therefore require definition of the criterion used for evaluation. The minimum requirement to prevent deficiency disease often is well below the requirement to support blood levels and/or urinary excretion. If we theorize that tissue saturation represents what is often called an optimal state of nutrition, the pathway leading to frank clinical lesions requires first that the tissues become depleted of their vitamin supply. As depletion proceeds, aberrations in cellular function result since vitamins are required chiefly as coenzymes for the biochemical reactions of cell metabolism. The appearance of clinical lesions is the final manifestation of diminishing cellular supply of a needed nutrient but does not imply that all cells are uniformly depleted. The real challenge to the experimental nutritionist is to ascertain the *order of cellular depletion*, for herein may lie the answer to the truly puzzling question, "What is minimum requirement?"

The nutritive state between tissue saturation and appearance of deficiency symptoms is an ambiguous area and is perhaps the most difficult state to evaluate. Clearly, a rather wide range of dietary intakes will support apparent health, yet they will not allow for tissue saturation or maintain comparable enzyme activities. Measurement of urinary excretion and blood levels of vitamins or related metabolites in subjects maintained on varying vitamin intakes are attempts to evaluate better this gray area of nutrition. The so-called fitness tests also have been used occasionally to determine the ability of human subjects to function properly as a *total organism;* these include such criteria as endurance, reflex action, and psychological response.

Clinical Evaluation

The chief significance of clinical evaluation is to establish the clinical course of vitamin deficiency in subjects maintained on carefully controlled vitamin intakes and thus to determine dietary levels that will prevent physical deterioration. Such studies properly should be carried on over a period of several months, since intakes that appear adequate for a short period may result in deficiency symptoms over longer periods of time as tissue supplies of a vitamin are gradually depleted. Especially significant is the identification of early symptoms of deficiency that appear before the onset of the frank disease syndrome. These early physical or mental changes correlated with analyses of blood or urine provide the basis for biochemical evaluation of nutritional status.

Table 24.1 indicates some symptoms that have been observed in vitamin deficiency states. Known minimum dietary levels that will prevent clinical symptoms also are listed. In the case of vitamin B_6 and vitamin E where requirement depends on intake of protein and polyunsaturated fatty acids (PUFA) respectively, the minimum listed is that obtained at low levels of the interrelated nutrient.

Some of the reported symptoms are highly subjective, particularly those associated with thiamin deficiency. Apprehension, anxiety, and other mental changes are difficult to evaluate. Brozek (1957) used the Minnesota Multiphasic Personality Test for the evaluation of psychological changes in his subjects, but he was not certain that the changes observed were due entirely to effects of the deficiency or possibly to negative response to the experimental regimen. Daum et al. (1949) found work output, as measured by both performance on a stationary bicycle and a standardized measure of reflex action, to be more sensitive determinants of thiamin status than the appearance of symptoms, which in early thiamin deficiency are almost always of a subjective nature.

Kinsman and Hood (1971) reported behavioral changes in experimental ascorbic acid deficiency as determined by a battery of personality and psychomotor tests including the Minnesota Multiphasic Personality Test. Subjects deprived of ascorbic acid scored high in the areas of hypochondriasis, depression, and hysteria, the so-called "neurotic triad." The results are similar to those reported in thiamin deficiency and in semistarvation (Keys et al., 1950). Because high and low levels of the vitamin were fed at different times within the study period, and psychological changes were noted only during periods of low ascorbic acid intake, these workers were able to eliminate reaction to the monotony of the experimental diet as a contributing factor. In the ascorbic acid-deficient subjects, personality changes preceded impaired function in tests of physical fitness; the latter appeared to be due to muscular and joint pains resulting from lack of the vitamin. Because psychological changes and physical performance defects may have multiple nutritional causes as well as nonnutritional etiologies, these indices are useful only in indicating that something is wrong and that the cause could be nutritional. Additional evidence is necessary to establish a cause and effect relationship between particular symptoms and a possible nutritional cause. Unfortunately, this area is extremely susceptible to nutritional misinterpretation and fraud.

TABLE 24.1
Some Clinical Evidences of Deficiency of Certain Vitamins

Vitamin	Symptoms	References
Thiamin (below 0.2–0.3 mg/1,000 kcal)	Anorexia Nausea with vomiting Constipation Calf muscle tenderness Weakness Irritability Depression Lowered blood pressure	Williams et al. (1942) Elsom et al. (1942) Najjar and Holt (1943) Foltz (1944) Brozek (1957) Horwitt et al. (1948)
Riboflavin (below 0.6 mg/day)	Cheilosis Angular stomatitis Seborrheic dermatitis (particularly nasolabial)	Horwitt et al. (1948) Hills et al. (1951)
Nicotinic acid (below 4.4 mg/ 1,000 kcal)	Dermatitis Glossitis Stomatitis Diarrhea Proctitis and vaginitis Mental depression, anxiety	Goldsmith (1956)
Ascorbic acid (below 10 mg/day)	Hyperkeratotic papules Petechiae Perifolliculosis Swollen, spongy gums Poor wound healing Fatigue Coiled hair Muscular aches Swollen joints Edema	Crandon et al. (1940) Peters et al. (1948) Hodges et al. (1971)
Vitamin B_6 (below 1.25 mg/day)	Seborrheic dermatitis Glossitis, stomatitis, cheilosis Depression Confusion Abnormal electroencephalogram Convulsions	Mueller and Vilter (1950) Coursin (1954) Baker et al. (1964)
Folacin (below 50 μg/day)	Weakness, tiredness Dyspnea Sore tongue Irritability and forgetfulness Diarrhea Headache Palpitation	Herbert (1968)

(continued)

TABLE 24.1 (continued)

Vitamin	Symptoms	References
Vitamin B$_{12}$ (below 0.5 µg/day)	Weakness, tiredness Sore tongue Paresthesia Constipation Headache Palpitation Macrocytic anemia Neurological damage	Herbert (1968)
Vitamin A (below 23–40 IU/kg)	Poor dark adaptation White papules Abnormal electroretinogram Acne Follicular hyperkeratosis Abnormalities of balance, taste, and smell	Booher et al. (1939) Hume and Krebs (1949) Hodges and Kolder (1971)
Vitamin E (below 3 mg/day)	Edema (infants) Anemia Increased erythrocyte hemolysis	Ritchie et al. (1968) Horwitt et al. (1963)

For some vitamins, the minimum requirement has been determined from the amount of the vitamin necessary to cure deficiency symptoms. Such is the case for folacin and vitamin B$_{12}$. A minimum of 50 µg/day of crystalline pteroylglutamic acid was shown to bring about a complete remission of hematological symptoms in patients with uncomplicated folacin deficiency (Herbert, 1968a). Similarly, as little as 0.1 µg/day of vitamin B$_{12}$ given intramuscularly to patients with pernicious anemia produced a reticulocyte and red cell response and a gradual return of serum vitamin B$_{12}$ levels to normal. At least 0.5 µg/day, however, was required for complete remission of hematological and neurological symptoms (ibid).

Curative doses of retinol for symptoms of vitamin A deficiency have been reported (Hodges and Kolder, 1971) and are of especial interest because so little work has been done on the requirement for vitamin A. As can be seen in Table 24.2, the curative dose varies considerably according to the deficiency symptom, from as little as 75 µg of retinol for correcting impaired dark adaption to 600 µg for curing cutaneous lesions including follicular hyperkeratosis and acne. Extrapolating on the basis of pure retinol, these levels are equivalent to 250–1998 IU. In terms of human dietaries containing both preformed vitamin A and carotene, the amounts are approximately 375–3000 IU. See Chapter 25 for further discussion of retinol equivalents and IU.

TABLE 24.2
Approximate Daily Dose of Retinol or Beta-carotene Required to Correct Clinical Defects

	Clinical Defect	Dose in Micrograms	
I	Impaired dark adaptation	$<$ 75	Retinol
		$\geq$ 150	Beta-carotene
II	Abnormal ERG	$\geq$ 150	Retinol
		$\geq$ 300	Beta-carotene
III	Abnormalities of balance, taste, smell	$\geq$ 300	Retinol
		$\geq$ 600	Beta-carotene
IV	Cutaneous lesions Follicular hyperkeratosis Acne	$\geq$ 600	Retinol
		$\geq$1200	Beta-carotene

Source: From R. E. Hodges and H. Kolder, *Summary of Proceedings, Workshop on Biochemical and Clinical Criteria for Determining Human Vitamin A Nutriture,* Food and Nutrition Board, National Academy of Sciences, Washington, D.C., 1971, p. 14.

Urinary Excretion

Although clinical evaluation provides an estimate of minimum requirements to prevent deficiency symptoms, biochemical lesions clearly must precede physical manifestation of deficiency. Measurement of urinary excretion of vitamins is a commonly used method for determination of vitamin status. Carefully controlled studies in which dietary intake was correlated with urinary excretion and appearance or absence of deficiency symptoms have formed the basis for evaluation of dietary intakes compatible with a "desirable" state of nutrition.

Urinary excretion levels may be interpreted as rough estimates of cellular function. Theoretically, as intake decreases, excretion in the urine decreases; therefore at high levels of intake, increasingly larger amounts of vitamin should be excreted in the urine. Both the absolute amount of vitamin excreted in the urine and the percentage of the intake excreted increase as the dietary intakes increase. For most water-soluble vitamins the relationship between intake and excretion is fairly linear over certain ranges of intake but when plasma levels reach the renal threshold, the proportion of intake excreted may increase dramatically. For example, the data in Table 24.3, taken from the classic report by Horwitt et al. (1950), demonstrate the effect of varying levels of riboflavin intake on excretion of the vitamin.

Symptoms of ariboflavinosis, angular stomatitis and seborrheic-type dermal lesions, appeared in subjects maintained on 0.55 mg riboflavin/day before the fourth month of experiment, but only one of the subjects receiving 0.75 and 0.85 mg/day for as long as two years showed any outward signs of deficiency. By this criterion, the riboflavin requirement would appear to be about 0.75–0.85 mg/day

TABLE 24.3
Effect of Riboflavin Intake on Urinary Excretion

No. of Subjects	Riboflavin Intake (mg)	Riboflavin Excretion in 24 Hours	
		Amount (μg)	Intake (%)
15	0.55	37	6.7
11	0.75	73	9.7
12	0.85	76	8.9
28	1.1	97	8.8
39	1.6	434	26.5
12	2.15	714	33.2
13	2.55	849	33.3
13	3.55	1714	48.3

Source: From M. K. Horwitt et al., *J. Nutr.* 41: 247, 1950.

for most people. Since riboflavin excretion increased markedly when intake was 1.6 mg as compared with 1.1 mg, Horwitt et al. (1950) concluded that tissue saturation could be reached at some point between 1.1 and 1.6 mg/day.

It would be fallacious to assume that urinary excretions of all water-soluble vitamins correlate in the same manner with dietary intake or reflect dietary changes within comparable periods of time. However, certain similarities exist. Thiamin excretion correlates with dietary intake between intakes of 0.5 and 2.0 mg/day but does not correlate well at extremely low intakes (Oldham et al., 1946; Mickelsen et al., 1947). Excretions of about 100 μg thiamin/day were reported to be compatible with adequate nutrition (Williams et al., 1942; Hathaway and Strom, 1946), but lower levels of excretion, between 50 and 100 μg, also have been judged adequate when correlated with other tests (Keys et al., 1945; Meyer et al., 1955).

According to studies of Ziporin et al. (1965), thiamin excretion approaches zero after three weeks on a diet containing less than 0.2 mg thiamin/1,000 kcal, but thiamin metabolites, pyrimidine and thiazole, remain at high levels. These workers propose that the level of metabolite output represents a measure of the rate at which body stores of thiamin are being depleted. On the basis of this assumption, minimum requirement is estimated as the amount that would replace the vitamin used for metabolic needs. Minimum requirement as estimated on this basis amounts to 0.27–0.33 mg/1,000 kcal.

Nicotinic acid metabolism is measured by the presence of its metabolites, N^1-methylnicotinamide or the 2- and 6-pyridone of N^1-methylnicotinamide, in urine. Evaluation of nicotinic acid intake must take into account the tryptophan content of the diet. Horwitt et al. (1956) and Goldsmith et al. (1961) used excretion of nicotinic acid metabolites as the basis for experiments designed to determine the extent of tryptophan conversion to nicotinic acid in the human. (See Chapter 3.)

Adjustment of urinary excretion of ascorbic acid to changes in dietary intake

TABLE 24.4
The 4-Pyridoxic Acid Excretion as Affected by Level of Vitamin B$_6$ Intake and Protein Intake

No. of Days on Specified Vitamin B$_6$ Intake	Vitamin B$_6$ Intake (mg/day)	4-Pyridoxic Acid Excretion (mg/day)
	Low Protein Diet	
6	1.66	1.01 ± 0.32[a]
2	0.16	0.67 ± 0.30
5	0.16	0.18 ± 0.18
20	0.16	0.11 ± 0.08
40	0.16	0.05 ± 0.08
7	0.76	0.12 ± 0.05
	High Protein Diet	
8	1.66	0.88 ± 0.11
2	0.16	0.46 ± 0.04
5	0.16	0.25 ± 0.13
17	0.16	0.25 ± 0.02
13	0.76	0.25 ± 0.02
2	50.16	26.20 ± 3.42

Source: From J. Kelsay et al., *J. Nutr.* 94, 490, 1968.
[a] S. D.

occurs fairly rapidly, within 10–15 days (Dodds et al., 1950). On intakes of between 50 and 60 mg of reduced ascorbic acid, subjects excrete an average of 11 mg (ibid.), but some subjects excrete half this amount. Moderate to high levels of ascorbic acid intake are reflected closely in urinary excretion (Ritchey, 1965). However, when dietary intake is below 10 mg, urinary excretions approach zero long before clinical evidence of ascorbic acid deficiency becomes apparent (Crandon, 1940).

The three forms of vitamin B$_6$ and of the metabolite, 4-pyridoxic acid, also decrease rapidly in response to a low vitamin B$_6$ intake (Table 24.4; Fig. 24.1). Other tests to be described in a later section appear to be more significant in describing changes in vitamin B$_6$ nutrition (Baker et al., 1964; Cinnamon and Beaton, 1970).

In general, urinary excretion is a useful although imprecise tool for evaluation of response to dietary intake of many water-soluble vitamins. Urinary excretions of thiamin, riboflavin, pyridoxine and, to a lesser extent, ascorbic acid respond sensitively to intake. However, urinary excretions of folacin and vitamin B$_{12}$ are not sensitive indicators of the requirements for these vitamins. In all cases, there is difficulty in determining the precise relationship between excretion rate and excretory thresholds to functional requirement of the nutrient. At low intakes, other tests appear to provide more definitive criteria.

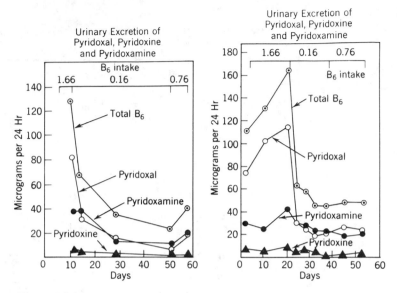

Figure 24.1
Effect of the level of intake of vitamin B_6 on the urinary excretion of pyridoxal, pyridoxamine, and pyridoxine by subjects fed a 54 gm protein diet and a 150 gm protein diet. (From J. Kelsay et al., *J. Nutr.* 94:490, 1968.)

Blood Levels

Tissue levels of vitamins are good indicators of the state of nutrition. When laboratory animals are studied, autopsies can be performed on them and various organs can be removed for analysis of tissues or subcellular particles to determine the amount and distribution of vitamins within the body. The human subject obviously is not a suitable candidate for such studies. Except for recent work on liver, skin, muscle, and adipose tissue obtained by biopsy, tissue analyses of humans are generally restricted to the most accessible tissue: blood.

Both the liquid (plasma or serum) and cell fractions of blood have been analyzed. Correlation with dietary intake depends not only on the distribution pattern peculiar to the vitamin but also on the sensitivity of analytical procedures used for determination of vitamin level. In general, blood cells contain larger amounts of vitamins than plasma, since it is within the cell that metabolic reactions that require vitamins take place. Vitamins contained in plasma, however, tend to represent the nutrient available to *all* body cells. For some vitamins, plasma level is more sensitively related to dietary intake than is the content of blood cells. In other instances, the reverse is true.

Measurement of plasma levels of thiamin and riboflavin have not been used frequently in experimental studies. An adaptation of the fluorometric method for thiamin was shown to correlate roughly with dietary intake, but there was considerable overlapping at different dietary levels (Burch et al., 1950; Dube et al., 1952). Measurement of riboflavin in red cells was shown to reflect dietary intake rather accurately (Bessey et al., 1956). The microbiological methods described by Baker and Frank (1968) are likely the most accurate methods presently available for plasma thiamin and riboflavin and have been used in a number of clinical and nutrition survey studies. However, measurements of the activity of thiamin- and riboflavin-dependent enzymes are considered to be more nutritionally sensitive. These tests will be discussed in a later section.

Blood levels of ascorbic acid are closely related to dietary intake. At comparable levels of intake, blood levels of the vitamin are higher among females than males. Dodds (1969) compiled published data on ascorbic acid blood levels of 2,130 males and 2,865 females of different ages who were maintained on known intakes of the vitamin. Below the age of puberty, no difference was found between blood values for males and females (Fig. 24.2). Above the age of puberty, however, females maintain blood levels well above those of males. The sex difference is most apparent in adults above the age of 20. These data were interpreted as evidence of hormonal regulation of ascorbic acid metabolism. The implications of this finding in terms of ascorbic acid requirements is not clear.

In studies of ascorbic acid deficiency, Hodges et al. (1971) reported that plasma ascorbic acid levels fell rapidly during the first month and then were maintained

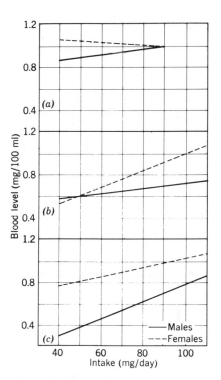

Figure 24.2
Regressions of ascorbic acid blood levels with ascorbic acid intake, males and females (a) 4–12 years of age, (b) 13–20 years, and (c) 20 years and over. (From M. L. Dodds, J. Am. Diet. Ass. 54:32, 1969.)

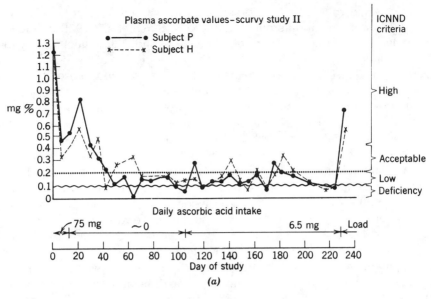

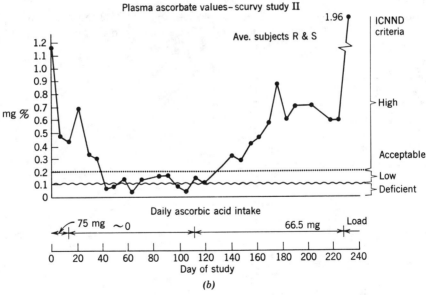

Figure 24.3a
Plasma ascorbic acid levels of 2 men during depletion and repletion with 6.5 mg
of ascorbic acid.

Figure 24.3b
Average plasma ascorbic acid levels of 2 men during depletion and repletion
with 66.5 mg of ascorbic acid. (From R. E. Hodges et al., *Am. J. Clin. Nutr.*
24:432, 1971.)

at low but measurable levels as symptoms of scurvy developed. In contrast, urinary excretion of the vitamin was essentially nil after one month. As little as 6.5 mg of ascorbic acid was sufficient to relieve clinical symptoms of deficiency with no effect on ascorbic acid blood levels (Fig. 24.3a). Subjects given 66.5 mg of ascorbic acid, however, responded with an immediate increase in plasma levels and prompt remission of clinical symptoms (Fig. 24.3 b).

Hodges and his associates (ibid) further noted that, in the presence of frank scurvy, plasma levels often were as high as 0.2 mg/dl. This finding is of particular interest since this level is above the range that was classified as a "low" level (0.1–0.19 mg/dl) of serum ascorbic acid in the Ten State National Nutrition Survey. (See Chapter 26.)

Measurement of blood vitamin A levels is of little value as an experimental tool. Individuals in a good state of vitamin A nutrition can tolerate a vitamin A-deficient diet for one to nearly two years without showing a significant decrease in the vitamin A of serum (Hume and Krebs, 1949; Hodges and Kolder, 1971). Circulating levels of this vitamin tend to be maintained as long as liver stores are available. When liver stores are depleted, blood levels fall precipitously. There is, however, considerable individual variation between serum levels of retinol and the time that symptoms appear. The data for three subjects in the study by Hodges and Kolder (1971) are shown in Table 24.5. Although a failure of dark adaptation was thought to be an early symptom of vitamin A deficiency, it was a relatively late symptom in these subjects. One subject showed symptoms of

TABLE 24.5
Serum Retinol Levels at Time of Onset of Clinical Signs and Symptoms

Subject	Time on Deficient Diet (days)	Clinical Signs and Symptoms	Serum Retinol µg/dl
1	260	White papules, anterior and shoulders	22
	321	Impaired dark adaptation	11
	449	Follicular hyperkeratosis, thighs and back	11
3	185	White papules, chest, back, and shoulders	25
	282	Follicular hyperkeratosis	25
	414	Severe acne	14
	420	Impaired dark adaptation	12
8	372	Follicular hyperkeratosis, thighs	35
	621	Impaired dark adaptation	27

Source: From R. E. Hodges and H. Kolder, *Summary of Proceedings, Workshop on Biochemical and Clinical Criteria for Determining Human Vitamin A Nutriture,* Food and Nutrition Board, National Academy of Sciences, Washington, D. C., 1971, p. 11.

follicular hyperkeratosis and impaired dark adaptation with only a small reduction in serum retinol. These results, obtained under highly controlled conditions, clearly demonstrate the almost terrifying reality of biological variation.

No experiments on vitamin A deficiency with children have been attempted. It is well known that children respond to low dietary intakes more quickly than adults, perhaps within a few months. The relative vulnerability presumably is due to the demands of growth and possibly to smaller liver stores than in adults. Underwood (1970) showed, however, that the concentration of vitamin A is higher in livers of children than of adults, although the total liver storage most likely is less than adults due to smaller liver size.

Levels of carotene in serum reflect changes in dietary intake of the provitamin (Moore, 1957), but they are of little value in determining the state of nutrition with respect to vitamin A. Attempts to determine minimum vitamin A requirement by measurement of blood levels admittedly have been discouraging.

Tocopherol blood levels also respond slowly when subjects are fed a diet deficient in the vitamin. Following depletion, however, a steady high level in plasma is reached after only one month of tocopherol feeding (Horwitt et al., 1956). Other tests, such as erythrocyte hemolysis (see following section), are more meaningful in evaluating dietary intakes of this vitamin.

Urinary Excretion and Blood Levels Following a Test Dose of Vitamin

The degree of tissue saturation can be estimated by feeding a fairly large dose of the vitamin to subjects and measuring excretion over a specific period of time, usually four hours. Such tests, sometimes called *load tests,* have been used in numerous experimental studies, and appear to be helpful in the interpretation of 24-hour excretion data.

The term *test dose return* refers to the percentage of the test dose excreted in urine samples collected during the period immediately following administration of the vitamin. Interpretation of the test dose return is based on the assumption that subjects in a state of saturation will excrete a large proportion of the administered vitamin within a relatively short period. A low percentage return indicates that body tissues are avidly retaining the needed nutrient.

The response of blood levels to a test dose of vitamin also may be used as a means for evaluating tissue levels. A combination of the two measurements, urinary excretion and various blood levels, often may provide more easily interpreted data than either alone.

Sometimes the load is not the vitamin being tested but rather is a substance that requires the vitamin for metabolism. For example, a tryptophan load test can be used to evaluate vitamin B_6 status and requirement. The excretion of xanthurenic acid is greatly increased following a load test of tryptophan when the diet does not contain pyridoxine, and this appears to be a highly sensitive test of vitamin B_6 deprivation (Baker et al., 1964). The test is based on the requirement for pyridoxal phosphate in the conversion of the tryptophan metabolite 3-hydroxykynurenine to 3-hydroxyanthranilic acid. In the absence of pyridoxine, 3-hydroxykynurenine is converted to xanthurenic acid. (See Chapter 3.) Administration of the vitamin, however, returns xanthurenic acid excretion to normal within 24 hours (Cinnamon and Beaton, 1970). This finding suggests that although xanthurenic acid excretion is a valid test for vitamin B_6 deprivation under controlled conditions, there may be little validity in results obtained randomly (as in a clinical or survey situation). A small dose of the vitamin prior to testing conceivably could obscure a long term deficiency of the vitamin. Increase in xanthurenic acid excretion following a tryptophan load also occurs in women taking oral contraceptives and who, presumably, have normal intakes of vitamin B_6 (Rose, 1978).

A strict comparison of studies reported in the literature is difficult because of differences in the amount of vitamin administered and the method of administration (orally or parenterally). Methods of test dose administration and evaluation of data were reviewed by Unglaub and Goldsmith (1954). The method remains unchanged although this test has not been used frequently in recent years.

Enzyme Activity and Other Related Tests

One of the long-term objectives of nutrition research has been to uncover sensitive tests to evaluate human response to diet. It is clearly not enough to know that a certain level of nutrient will prevent clinical deficiency; what we need to know is the level that will support normal cellular metabolism, since it seems likely that clinical lesions result only when cellular adaptive mechanisms no longer are able to cope with a diminishing supply of nutrient. Such tests are based on known metabolic functions of the vitamins and effectively combine knowledge of cellular biochemical reactions with response of the whole organism. More specifically, the best tests of this type are those utilizing an enzyme that requires a coenzyme form of the vitamin, responds early in nutritional depletion, responds only to one vitamin or its coenzyme form, occurs in blood cells or plasma, and has good analytical sensitivity. The search for such enzymes or enzyme systems has been an important part of the research in clinical and experimental nutrition in the last two decades.

The first real success in this search occurred with thiamin (Brin, 1962). The enzyme transketolase is active in erythrocytes and is depleted relatively early in thiamin deficiency. Transketolase is a thiamin pyrophosphate (TPP)-requiring enzyme which catalyzes the following two reactions in the pentose phosphate pathway. (See Chapter 11 for details):

1. xylulose-5-phosphate   sedoheptulose-7-phosphate
        +   ←   +
     ribose-5-phosphate   glyceraldehyde-3-phosphate

2. xylulose-5-phosphate   fructose-6-phosphate

$$\text{+} \quad \longleftrightarrow \quad \text{+}$$

erythrose-4-phosphate   glyceraldehyde-3-phosphate

This enzyme system appears to be highly responsive to dietary thiamin intake. When rats are placed on a thiamin-deficient diet, for example, the enzyme activity decreases even before growth rate is affected. In humans, transketolase activity is measured in red cell hemolysates.

The erythrocyte transketolase activity assay involves measurement of pentose phosphate utilization or production of heptose or hexose phosphate in hemolysates divided into two equal samples. TPP is added to one sample. Following incubation, the disappearance of pentose or the increase in heptose or hexose is measured. The degree of stimulation by TPP reflects the need for thiamin and is termed the "TPP effect." It is calculated by dividing the value obtained in the sample with TPP by that of the sample with no TPP ($\times$ 100) to obtain a percentage. In people with adequate thiamin reserves, there should be little or no stimulation by added TPP; in those with low reserves, a high percentage effect is observed.

The method is analytically and nutritionally sensitive. A major problem, however, is that most individuals show some TPP effect (Sauberlich et al., 1974). Nonetheless, it has been possible to develop standards indicating risk of thiamin deficiency on the basis of TPP effect (Table 24.6). Such standards are used in evaluation of nutrition status of individuals. (See Chapter 26.)

The levels of riboflavin and niacin coenzymes in blood have been studied and were shown to be imprecise measures of vitamin nutriture. Flavin mononucleotide (FMN) levels of plasma were found to decrease in subjects maintained on a deficient diet, but the relationship between coenzyme level and dietary intake was highly variable (Bessey et al., 1956). Flavin adenine dinucleotide (FAD) is very little affected by variations in riboflavin intake. The measurement of the activity of the enzyme glutathione reductase, however, appears to reflect riboflavin status accurately (Tillotson and Baker, 1972). This enzyme catalyzes the reduction

TABLE 24.6
Relationship of Thiamin Deficiency Risk and TPP Effect on Erythrocyte Transketolase

Risk Level	TPP Effect
ICNND Classification	
Acceptable (low risk)	0–15%
Low (medium risk)	16–20%
Deficient (high risk)	> 20%
Brin's Classification	
Normal (adequate)	0–14%
Marginally deficient (marginal)	15–24%
Severely deficient (deficient)	> 24%

Source: From H. E. Sauberlich et al., in *Laboratory Tests for the Assessment of Nutritional Status.* CRC Press, Cleveland, 1974, p.25.

of glutathione as follows:

$$GSSG + NADPH + H^+ \xrightarrow{\text{FAD}} 2\ GSH + NADP^+$$

The glutathione reductase reaction is assayed by measuring the oxidation of NADPH spectrophotometrically. The principle of the assay is similar to that of the erythrocyte transketolase test; that is, it is based on the stimulation produced by adding FAD to one sample but not to the other. Riboflavin status is evaluated on the basis of an FAD activity coefficient (rather than percentage stimulation) which is calculated by dividing values obtained with added FAD by those obtained without FAD. Guidelines for the interpretation of the activity coefficients for glutathione reductase are shown in Table 24.7.

The niacin coenzyme NAD has been determined for whole blood, serum, and red blood cells of well nourished adults (Burch et al., 1955), but the coenzyme is not a sensitive measurement at low intakes of nicotinic acid (Goldsmith, 1959). Apparently these coenzymes are maintained in blood even with extreme dietary deprivation and may not be reduced significantly even when clinical lesions are present. As yet, no enzyme test that reflects niacin nutritional status has been identified.

The activities of serum transaminases also have been evaluated in terms of vitamin B_6 nutriture. It is generally agreed that serum glutamic-pyruvate transaminase (GPT) is more closely related to dietary intake than serum glutamic-oxaloacetic transaminase (GOT) (Babcock et al., 1960; Brin et al., 1960; Cinnamon and Beaton, 1970). In vitamin B_6-depleted subjects, serum transaminases return to normal only after three to four weeks of vitamin B_6 feeding (Cinnamon and Beaton, 1970). Raica and Sauberlich (1964) suggested that the *in vitro* stimulation of serum GOT activity with pyridoxal phosphate (PLP) would provide a more definitive answer to the question of vitamin B_6 involvement in decreased serum GOT activity.

The erythrocyte hemolysis test is a test for vitamin E deficiency and is based on the effect of the vitamin in stabilization of cell membranes. The test measures the *in vitro* resistance of the erythrocyte membrane to hemolysis by hydrogen peroxide. As shown in Table 24.8, dietary supplementation of subjects depleted of vitamin E resulted in increased plasma tocopherol levels within one month, but hemolysis of red blood cells did not decrease significantly until after nine

TABLE 24.7
Riboflavin Status and FAD Activity Coefficients for Erythrocyte Glutathione Reductase

Risk Level	Coefficient
Acceptable (low risk)	<1.20
Low (medium risk)	1.2–1.4
Deficient (high risk)	>1.40

Source: From H. E. Sauberlich et al., in *Laboratory Tests for the Assessment of Nutritional Status.* CRC Press, Cleveland, 1974, p. 34.

TABLE 24.8
Effect of Supplementation of Depleted Subject with Tocopherol (15 mg/day)

Months	Plasma Tocopherol (mg/dl)	Hemolysis (%)
0	0.48	61
1	0.95	46
3	0.70	52
8	0.85	40
9	0.90	12
10	0.95	10

Source: From M. K. Horwitt, *Amer. J. Clin. Nutr.,* 8: 408, 1960.

months. This test, rather than tocopherol plasma levels, was the basis for the determination of vitamin E requirement in relation to polyunsaturated fatty acid content of the diet (Horwitt, 1960).

Conclusion

Most of the studies on which human requirements and dietary standards of the major vitamins are based were done during a 20-year period, roughly between 1940 and 1960. More highly refined tests are needed not only for establishing definitive criteria for the determination of human requirements but also for the accurate diagnosis of nutritional lesions that are amenable to dietary treatment. In addition, such tests are needed to identify cellular metabolic aberrations resulting from genetic, infectious, and degenerative diseases and from the drugs used in treatment.

Prophetically, Goldsmith (1959) stated:

> *Nutritional diagnosis implies evaluation of the biochemical milieu within and outside of the cells, as well as detection of abnormalities of function and structure of the organs and tissues of the body. Recent studies of the role of mitochondria and other cellular units in oxidative metabolism link cytology and biochemistry closely together and may lead to better correlation between pathologic anatomical changes and biochemical abnormalities of body tissues and fluids.*

New approaches to the problems of cellular metabolic disturbances will continue to be initiated primarily through studies with experimental animals followed by carefully conducted observations on humans. The measurement of enzyme activity and other functional tests appears to be superior to measurement of the vitamin itself as techniques for the determination of vitamin requirements. Nutrition research, therefore, is focusing more and more on identification of primary biochemical lesions that relate cellular function to human health. More of these lesions will become apparent as vitamin participation in cellular structure and function is better understood.

chapter 25

dietary standards

Dietary standards are derived from compilations of data from experimental studies designed to determine the nutrient requirements of humans. Quantitatively, standards are not requirements but rather are estimates of reasonable levels of nutrient intakes that should support normal function in most healthy people. Standards were originally intended as a basis for planning and evaluating diets of groups of people. They are, in fact, now used for many other purposes than originally intended.

Nutrient standards developed in different countries (and internationally) differ to varying degrees for individual nutrients, partly because populations, environmental conditions, and available food supplies differ. More often, however, these differences reflect lack of agreement on such basic issues as the appropriate criterion for defining requirement, the safety margin required to assure adequate intake, and in some few cases whether nutrient standards represent intakes of food as consumed or as purchased. Theoretically, standards are considered valid only for the group for which they were formulated. Yet, if the underlying scientific questions could be agreed on, nutrient standards for different countries would be more alike than they are different.

The first organized attempt at developing a dietary standard came as a result of food shortages during World War I when it became necessary for the United States government to devise a rational basis for shipments of food from this country to its allies in Europe. With the limited knowledge at that time of nutrition in general and of human nutrient needs in particular, recommendations could be made only for energy and, with reservations, for protein. In 1933, the British Medical Association proposed a limited set of standards, and in the same year the United States Department of Agriculture (Stiebeling, 1933) made more extensive proposals including recommendations for energy value, protein, calcium, iron, phosphorus, vitamin A, and ascorbic acid. Both sets of proposals were based primarily on results of dietary surveys from which could be calculated average nutrient intakes of presumably healthy population groups. In the mid-1930s, the vitamin era was at its peak but very few data had accumulated on the metabolic needs of the human.

The greatest impetus to the development of dietary standards (and consequently to the encouragement of laboratory research directed toward the establishment of human nutrient requirements) came as a result of the work of the League of Nations Technical Commission on Nutrition (Burnet and Aykroyd, 1935). The Commission focused international attention on the significance of diet in preventive medicine and as a means of improving the public health. Dietary standards were proposed for energy and protein expressed as an average requirement on the basis of age, sex, and activity. In retrospect, however, the proposal of standards was a minor accomplishment of the Commission. Rather, as a result of the Commission's efforts, a number of the League member governments formed nutrition councils geared specifically to the improvement of health through nutrition, and it was the lack of experimental data available to the councils that helped to stimulate research on human nutrient requirements.

More extensive recommended dietary allowances (to be discussed later) were developed in the United States by the Committee on Food and Nutrition of the National Research Council. These standards, too, were based on limited data and served to divert some attention of nutrition science from the prevailing emphasis on animal feed production to human nutrient needs.

A more detailed discussion of the development of dietary standards can be found in the review by Leitch (1942); the subject also was reviewed briefly by Young (1964).

Requirements and Allowances

Dietary standards are not dietary requirements. The term *minimum requirement* as defined in Chapter 23 represents basic physiological need and is compatible with the smallest amount of a nutrient that will prevent deficiency symptoms or support a well-defined physiological or biochemical response. The term *average requirement* is often used to denote the amount of a nutrient that will support health in most persons of a given population group and implies that the true requirement for individuals may be either above or below the average for the group. The two terms are ambiguous; the meanings tend to overlap and thus are confusing. Both, however, refer to quantitative estimates that are based on data of uncertain precision obtained from a limited number of subjects. The perfect tool for determining human requirements has not yet been devised, nor has the perfect criterion of physiological response yet been ascertained. Even if such perfection could be attained, the results would be accurate only for the individual tested at the particular time tested. An average requirement based on a broad sample still would be subject to the errors inherent in any average.

It is for this reason that the term *requirements* is usually avoided in dietary standards. *Allowances* is a more accurate description and implies the addition of an amount above the estimated requirement to cover both the variation among individuals and the lack of precision inherent in the estimated requirement. This additional amount is a safety factor referred to as a *margin of safety or allowance for safety*. The differences among dietary standards are due largely to the amount of the safety factor added, an amount determined by the philosophical goals of those who help to set the standard.

A basic problem in interpreting dietary standards results from the lack of consensus about the definition of the profusion of terms used to describe nutrient needs: "minimum requirement," "average requirement," "desirable intake," "optimal intake," "normal individuals," "substantially all healthy persons." The confusion surrounding these commonly used (but less commonly understood) terms was discussed nearly 30 years ago by Pett (1955). It is ironic that nutritional scientists have not yet been able to define precisely what is meant by such well-meaning but scientifically undefined terms. Until there is more universal agreement, groups responsible for developing dietary standards might well follow the example of the Committee for the Revision of the Dietary Standard for Canada (1983). In its report, the Committee clearly defines the terms of reference used in developing the Recommended Nutrient Intakes for Canadians (ibid) thus establishing a common understanding for use in interpreting these recommendations.

Uses of Dietary Standards

If it is recognized that dietary standards represent, in effect, value judgments based on the kinds of experimental data described in Chapters 23 and 24, and are subject to the limitations of human metabolic studies and the vagaries of human individuality, it should be clear that there are also limitations in the use of dietary standards.

An obvious and practical use of the dietary standard is in the development of *food plans* (food guides) that, loosely described, are a translation of human nutrient needs into foods or food groups that may be used conveniently by nonprofessionals in planning diets. Quantitative expressions of nutrients (in terms of milligrams, grams, etc.) have meaning for the nutritionist or dietitian, but they are of little value to the layman. Nearly all countries have developed some type of food plan based on the dietary standards adopted and the food habits and food supply of the population The *Basic Four* used in nutrition education in the United States is an example of a food plan constructed to meet nutrient needs, with the exception of calories, and is specifically adapted to common dietary practices of the American population (Page and Phipard, 1957). It is not applicable, however, to other cultures in which food habits and thus food sources of nutrients are likely to differ markedly from those of the United States. For discussions of food plans, see Hertzler and Anderson (1974), Guthrie and Scheer (1981), and Light and Cronin (1981). For derivations of the Basic Four, see King et al. (1978) and Pennington (1981).

Dietary standards commonly are used in interpreting dietary intake data collected from population surveys. The assessment of such data, however, is difficult. (See Chapter 26.) Apart from the errors inherent in the collection and calculation of food intake data, there is no clear way of determining if intakes below the dietary standard represent a hazard to health. It is generally assumed that if nutrient intakes of a large proportion of individuals are below the standard, the *risk* of deficiency is increased. However, the use of a dietary standard that includes a generous margin of safety as a basis for evaluating dietary intake can result in an overestimation of the degree of risk within a population. For this reason, some nutrition scientists suggest that a separate standard be developed for the purpose of evaluating dietary intake data. Such a standard is currently in use in Sweden (Swedish National Food Administration, 1981).

Dietary standards are used for a number of other purposes. They serve as guides for planning and procuring food for institutions and for food service programs, as for example the school lunch program. In the food industry, dietary standards may be used as the basis for formulating new products such as meal replacements. For formulated foods that replace traditional foods, the nutrient composition of the food to be replaced is likely a more appropriate guide for fortification than a dietary standard or a proportion of a standard (Food and Nutrition Board, 1980).

More recently, dietary standards have been used as a basis for the *nutrient density* concept, that is, nutrient recommendations per 1,000 kcal (Wretlind, 1977; Hansen et al., 1978; Hansen and Wyse, 1980). Expression of nutrient needs in terms of energy requirements is useful in planning diets for heterogenous groups of people and, when correctly applied, should meet the nutritional requirements of individuals with the lowest energy needs. Conversely, individuals with high energy requirements may receive a surfeit of some nutrients but it is unlikely that a modest oversupply would be disadvantageous. The nutrient density concept may have some validity in evaluating dietary intakes because, in effect, it describes the *quality* of a diet. However, for individuals with extremely low energy intakes, the diet may meet the required nutrient density but absolute intake may well be too low to meet nutrient needs.

Recommended Dietary Allowances for Americans

The dietary standards used in the United States are the Recommended Dietary Allowances (RDA) which were developed by the Food and Nutrition Board of the National Research Council, National Academy of Sciences. Every student of nutrition should be familiar with the RDA and with the basis for their formulation.

The first allowances were published in 1943 as the result of nearly two years of deliberation and study of the available literature. (See Roberts, 1958.) In presenting the first set of allowances, the following points were emphasized:

1. "That they were recommended allowances, not standards (i.e., requirements). They were goals, not necessarily absolute requirements.
2. "That they were based on the best knowledge available at the time they were formulated.
3. "That they were subject to change as soon as more evidence became available."

Consequently, the RDA were revised in 1945, again in 1948, and approximately every five years since (1953, 1958, 1963, 1968, 1974, 1980). The latest revision is shown in Table 25.1. The allowances are described as "the levels of intake of essential nutrients considered, in the judgment of the Committee on Dietary Allowances of the Food and Nutrition Board on the basis of available scientific knowledge, to be adequate to meet the known nutritional needs of practically all healthy persons."

The recommendations of the Food and Nutrition Board are discussed in detail in the report on the 1980 RDA (Food and Nutrition Board, 1980), and a general background of the basis for the new recommendations was reviewed by Harper (1980).

Contrary to previous RDA, allowances for energy are included in a separate table and are presented both as an average and as a range for each age group (Table 25.2). Recommendations for energy intake also are presented for individuals ages 51–75 and over age 76. The decreased energy intakes recommended for older adults is based on the known decline in metabolic rate of about 2 percent per decade in adults (Durnin and Passmore, 1967). The inability to estimate the degree of physical activity in the elderly is reflected in the lower figure of the range of energy recommendations which for females over 76 years of age may be as little as 1,200 kcal.

The 1980 RDA also introduced the concept of nutrient interrelationships in a more compelling manner than had been done previously. Thus, it is imperative that users of the RDA read the text in order to understand the qualifications and limitations of some figures in the table. Most significant is the extensive discussion on the effect of heme iron and ascorbic acid on total iron absorption. As shown in Table 25.3, based on the work of Monsen et al. (1978), heme iron is well absorbed (23%), and the absorption of nonheme iron can be increased from approximately 3 percent to 8 percent by the presence of ascorbic acid in a meal. (See Chapter 6.) Although this finding is probably of little significance for meat-eaters, it could be of considerable significance for vegetarians.

A third innovation in the 1980 RDA is the inclusion of a table of provisional recommendations entitled "Estimated Safe and Adequate Daily Dietary Intakes of Selected Vitamins and Minerals" (Table 25.4). These recommendations are for a number of nutrients known to be essential for humans but for which the data base is too weak to warrant inclusion in the RDA table for all age groups. Included are vitamins K, biotin, and pantothenic acid; the trace elements copper, man-

TABLE 25.1
Food and Nutrition Board, National Academy of Sciences—National Research

Age (years)	Weight (kg)	Weight (lb)	Height (cm)	Height (in)	Protein (g)	Fat-Soluble Vitamins			Vitamin C (mg)	Thiamin (mg)
						Vitamin A (μg RE)[b]	Vitamin D (μg)[c]	Vitamin E (mg α-TE)[d]		
Infants										
0.0–0.5	6	13	60	24	kg × 2.2	420	10	3	35	0.3
0.5–1.0	9	20	71	28	kg × 2.0	400	10	4	35	0.5
Children										
1–3	13	29	90	35	23	400	10	5	45	0.7
4–6	20	44	112	44	30	500	10	6	45	0.9
7–10	28	62	132	52	34	700	10	7	45	1.2
Males										
11–14	45	99	157	62	45	1000	10	8	50	1.4
15–18	66	145	176	69	56	1000	10	10	60	1.4
19–22	70	154	177	70	56	1000	7.5	10	60	1.5
23–50	70	154	178	70	56	1000	5	10	60	1.4
51+	70	154	178	70	56	1000	5	10	60	1.2
Females										
11–14	46	101	157	62	46	800	10	8	50	1.1
15–18	55	120	163	64	46	800	10	8	60	1.1
19–22	55	120	163	64	44	800	7.5	8	60	1.1
23–50	55	120	163	64	44	800	5	8	60	1.0
51+	55	120	163	64	44	800	5	8	60	1.0
Pregnant						+30	+200	+5	+2	+20	+0.4
Lactating						+20	+400	+5	+3	+40	+0.5

[a]The allowances are intended to provide for individual variations among most normal persons as they live in the United States under usual environmental stresses. Diets should be based on a variety of common foods in order to provide other nutrients for which human requirements have been less well defined. See text for detailed discussion of allowances and of nutrients not tabulated. See table 25.2 for suggested average energy intakes for mean weights and heights by individual year of age.

[b]Retinol equivalents. 1 retinol equivalent = 1 μg retinol or 6 μg β carotene. See text for calculation of vitamin A activity of diets as retinol equivalents.

[c]As cholecalciferol. 10 μg cholecalciferol = 400 IU of vitamin D.

[d]α-tocopherol equivalents. 1 mg d-α-tocopherol = 1 α-TE. See text for variation in allowances and calculation of vitamin E activity of the diet as α-tocopherol equivalents.

[e]1 NE (niacin equivalent) is equal to 1 mg of niacin or 60 mg of dietary tryptophan.

ganese, fluoride, chromium, selenium, and molybdenum; and the electrolytes sodium, potassium, and chloride. The fact that these recommendations are expressed as a range and include only seven age groupings emphasizes the provisional nature of the data.

Recommended Nutrient Intakes for Canadians

The Committee for the Revision of the Dietary Standard for Canada (1983) chose to use the term "recommended nutrient intakes" (RNI) in order to distinguish

Council–Recommended Daily Dietary Allowances,[a] Revised 1980

Water-Soluble Vitamins					Minerals					
Riboflavin (mg)	Niacin (mg NE)[e]	Vitamin B-6 (mg)	Folacin[f] (µg)	Vitamin B-12 (µg)	Calcium (mg)	Phosphorus (mg)	Magnesium (mg)	Iron (mg)	Zinc (mg)	Iodine (µg)
0.4	6	0.3	30	0.5[g]	360	240	50	10	3	40
0.6	8	0.6	45	1.5	540	360	70	15	5	50
0.8	9	0.9	100	2.0	800	800	150	15	10	70
1.0	11	1.3	200	2.5	800	800	200	10	10	90
1.4	16	1.6	300	3.0	800	800	250	10	10	120
1.6	18	1.8	400	3.0	1200	1200	350	18	15	150
1.7	18	2.0	400	3.0	1200	1200	400	18	15	150
1.7	19	2.2	400	3.0	800	800	350	10	15	150
1.6	18	2.2	400	3.0	800	800	350	10	15	150
1.4	16	2.2	400	3.0	800	800	350	10	15	150
1.3	15	1.8	400	3.0	1200	1200	300	18	15	150
1.3	14	2.0	400	3.0	1200	1200	300	18	15	150
1.3	14	2.0	400	3.0	800	800	300	18	15	150
1.2	13	2.0	400	3.0	800	800	300	18	15	150
1.2	13	2.0	400	3.0	800	800	300	10	15	150
+0.3	+2	+0.6	+400	+1.0	+400	+400	+150	h	+5	+25
+0.5	+5	+0.5	+100	+1.0	+400	+400	+150	h	+10	+50

[f]The folacin allowances refer to dietary sources as determined by *Lactobacillus casei* assay after treatment with enzymes (conjugases) to make polyglutamyl forms of the vitamin available to the test organism.

[g]The recommended dietary allowance for vitamin B-12 in infants is based on average concentration of the vitamin in human milk. The allowances after weaning are based on energy intake (as recommended by the American Academy of Pediatrics) and consideration of other factors, such as intestinal absorption; see text.

[h]The increased requirement during pregnancy cannot be met by the iron content of habitual American diets nor by the existing iron stores of many women; therefore the use of 30–60 mg of supplemental iron is recommended. Iron needs during lactation are not substantially different from those of non-pregnant women, but continued supplementation of the mother for 2-3 months after parturition is advisable in order to replenish stores depleted by pregnancy.

nutrient requirements from the various dietary guides that describe patterns of food use. (Dietary guides will be discussed later in this chapter.) The RNI are somewhat different from the RDA in quantitative recommendations (Table 25.5). The purposes of the standards are very similar (see Campbell, 1974), and clearly the differences in nutrient standards are the result of differences in philosophy concerning the means to presumably the same end. The RDA are "to be adequate to meet the known nutrition needs of practically all healthy persons." The RNI is defined as "that level of dietary intake thought to be sufficiently high to meet the requirements of almost all individuals in a group with specified characteristics (age, sex, body size, physical activity, type of diet)." As do the RDA, the RNI

TABLE 25.2
Mean Heights and Weights and Recommended Energy Intake[a]

Category	Age (years)	Weight (kg)	Weight (lb)	Height (cm)	Height (in.)	Energy Needs (kcal with range)		Energy Needs (MJ)
Infants	0.0–0.5	6	13	60	24	kg × 115	(95–145)	kg × 0.48
	0.5–1.0	9	20	71	28	kg × 105	(80–135)	kg × 0.44
Children	1–3	13	29	90	35	1300	(900–1800)	5.5
	4–6	20	44	112	44	1700	(1300–2300)	7.1
	7–10	28	62	132	52	2400	(1650–3300)	10.1
Males	11–14	45	99	157	62	2700	(2000–3700)	11.3
	15–18	66	145	176	69	2800	(2100–3900)	11.8
	19–22	70	154	177	70	2900	(2500–3300)	12.2
	23–50	70	154	178	70	2700	(2300–3100)	11.3
	51–75	70	154	178	70	2400	(2000–2800)	10.1
	76+	70	154	178	70	2050	(1650–2450)	8.6

	Age	(kg)	(lb)	(cm)	(in)	Energy (kcal)		
Females	11–14	46	101	157	62	2200	(1500–3000)	9.2
	15–18	55	120	163	64	2100	(1200–3000)	8.8
	19–22	55	120	163	64	2100	(1700–2500)	8.8
	23–50	55	120	163	64	2000	(1600–2400)	8.4
	51–75	55	120	163	64	1800	(1400–2200)	7.6
	76+	55	120	163	64	1600	(1200–2000)	6.7
Pregnancy						+300		
Lactation						+500		

Source: From *Recommended Dietary Allowances,* Food and Nutrition Board, National Academy of Sciences-National Research Council, Washington, D.C., revised 1980, p. 23.

[a]The data in this table have been assembled from the observed median heights and weights of children together with desirable weights for adults for the mean heights of men (70 in.) and women (64 in.) between the ages of 18 and 34 years as surveyed in the U.S. population (HEW/NCHS data).

The energy allowances for the young adults are for men and women doing light work. The allowances for the two older age groups represent mean energy needs over these age spans allowing for a 2-percent decrease in basal (resting) metabolic rate per decade and a reduction in activity of 200 kcal/day for men and women between 51 and 75 years, 500 kcal for men over 75 years, and 400 kcal for women over 75 years (see text). The customary range of daily energy output is shown in parentheses for adults and is based on a variation in energy needs of ± 400 kcal at any one age (see text and Garrow, 1978), emphasizing the wide range of energy intakes appropriate for any group of people.

Energy allowances for children through age 18 are based on median energy intakes of children of these ages followed in longitudinal growth studies. The values in parentheses are 10th and 90th percentiles of energy intake, to indicate the range of energy consumption among children of these ages (see text).

TABLE 25.3
Availability of Iron in Different Meals

Type of Meal	Absorption of Iron Present in Meal (%)	
	Nonheme Iron	Heme Iron
Low-availability meal <30 gm meat, poultry, fish <25 mg ascorbic acid	3	23

Medium-availability meal
  30–90 gm meat, poultry, fish
  or 25–75 mg ascorbic acid
	5	23

High-availability meal
  >90 gm meat, poultry, fish
  or > 75 ascorbic acid,
  or 30–90 gm meat, poultry, fish
  plus 25–75 mg ascorbic acid
	8	23

Source: From Monsen et al., *Am. J. Clin. Nutr.* 31:135, 1978

take into account individual variability and exceed the requirement of almost all individuals. It is noteworthy that RNI for infants under one year of age are established for four age groups: 0-2 months, 3-5 months, 6-8 months, and 9-11 months. It is noteworthy also that recommendations are estimated for each trimester of pregnancy and for individuals 75 years of age and older.

Users of the RNI are cautioned to read the text of the report carefully and to note the qualifications about the interpretation of the recommendations. For some nutrients, suggestions are made about how the RNI may be adjusted for particular situations.

FAO/WHO Standards

The Food and Agriculture Organization (FAO) and World Health Organization (WHO) of the United Nations have established standards for energy, protein, calcium, iron, and several vitamins (vitamins A, D, and B-12, and thiamin, riboflavin, niacin, folic acid, and ascorbic acid). These standards are intended for international use and, therefore, for many varied population groups. The standards with the exception of those for protein and energy, are defined as "recommended intakes" (Table 25.6), that is, "amounts considered sufficient for the maintenance of health in nearly all people" (FAO/WHO, 1974). The committee responsible for developing protein standards preferred the expression "safe level of intake," which is defined as "the amount of protein considered necessary to meet the physiological needs and maintain the health of nearly all persons in a specified group" (FAO/WHO, 1974). It seems that "safe level of intake" and "recom-

Table 25.4
Estimated Safe and Adequate Daily Dietary Intakes of Selected Vitamins and Minerals[a]

		Vitamins		
	Age (years)	Vitamin K (μg)	Biotin (μg)	Pantothenic Acid (mg)
Infants	0–0.5	12	35	2
	0.5–1	10–20	50	3
Children	1–3	15–30	65	3
and	4–6	20–40	85	3–4
Adolescents	7–10	30–60	120	4–5
	11+	50–100	100–200	4–7
Adults		70–140	100–200	4–7

				Trace Element[b]			
	Age (years)	Copper (mg)	Manganese (mg)	Fluoride (mg)	Chromium (mg)	Selenium (mg)	Molybdenum (mg)
Infants	0–0.5	0.5–0.7	0.5–0.7	0.1–0.5	0.01–0.04	0.01–0.04	0.03–0.06
	0.5–1	0.7–1.0	0.7–1.0	0.2–1.0	0.02–0.06	0.02–0.06	0.04–0.08
Children	1–3	1.0–1.5	1.0–1.5	0.5–1.5	0.02–0.08	0.02–0.08	0.05–0.1
and	4–6	1.5–2.0	1.5–2.0	1.0–2.5	0.03–0.12	0.03–0.12	0.06–0.15
Adolescents	7–10	2.0–2.5	2.0–3.0	1.5–2.5	0.05–0.2	0.05–0.2	0.10–0.3
	11+	2.0–3.0	2.5–5.0	1.5–2.5	0.05–0.2	0.05–0.2	0.15–0.5
Adults		2.0–3.0	2.5–5.0	1.5–4.0	0.05–0.2	0.05–0.2	0.15–0.5

		Electrolytes		
	Age (years)	Sodium (mg)	Potassium (mg)	Chloride (mg)
Infants	0–0.5	115–350	350–925	275–700
	0.5–1	250–750	425–1275	400–1200
Children	1–3	325–975	550–1650	500–1500
and	4–6	450–1350	775–2325	700–2100
Adolescents	7–10	600–1800	1000–3000	925–2775
	11+	900–2700	1525–4575	1400–4200
Adults		1100–3300	1875–5625	1700–5100

Source: From *Recommended Dietary Allowances,* Food and Nutrition Board, National Academy of Sciences-National Research Council, Washington, D.C., revised 1980, p. 178.

[a]Because there is less information on which to base allowances, these figures are not given in the main table of RDA and are provided here in the form of ranges of recommended intakes.

[b]Since the toxic levels for many trace elements may be only several times usual intakes, the upper levels for the trace elements given in this table should not be habitually exceeded.

TABLE 25.5
Summary Examples of Recommended Nutrient Intakes for Canadians[a,b], 1983

Age	Sex	Weight (kg)	Protein (gm/day)	Fat-Soluble Vitamins			Water-Soluble Vitamins			Minerals				
				Vitamin A (RE/day)[c]	Vitamin D (µg/day)[e]	Vitamin E (mg/day)[f]	Vitamin C (mg/day)	Folacin (µg/day)[g]	Vitamin B_{12} (µg/day)	Calcium (mg/day)	Magnesium (mg/day)	Iron (mg/day)	Iodine (µg/day)	Zinc (mg/day)
Months														
0–2	Both	4.5	11[h]	400	10	3	20	50	0.3	350	30	0.4[i]	25	2[j]
3–5	Both	7.0	14[h]	400	10	3	20	50	0.3	350	40	5	35	3
6–8	Both	8.5	16[h]	400	10	3	20	50	0.3	400	45	7	40	3
9–11	Both	9.5	18	400	10	3	20	55	0.3	400	50	7	45	3
Years														
1	Both	11	18	400	10	3	20	65	0.3	500	55	6	55	4
2–3	Both	14	20	400	5	4	20	80	0.4	500	65	6	65	4
4–6	Both	18	25	500	5	5	25	90	0.5	600	90	6	85	5
7–9	M	25	31	700	2.5	7	35	125	0.8	700	110	7	110	6
	F	25	29	700	2.5	6	30	125	0.8	700	110	7	95	6
10–12	M	34	38	800	2.5	8	40	170	1.0	900	150	10	125	7
	F	36	39	800	2.5	7	40	170	1.0	1000	160	10	110	7
13–15	M	50	49	900	2.5	9	50	160	1.5	1100	220	12	160	9
	F	48	43	800	2.5	7	45	160	1.5	800	190	13	160	8
16–18	M	62	54	1000	2.5	10	55	190	1.9	900	240	10	160	9
	F	53	47	800	2.5	7	45	160	1.9	700	220	14	160	8
19–24	M	71	57	1000	2.5	10	60	210	2.0	800	240	8	160	9
	F	58	41	800	2.5	7	45	165	2.0	700	190	14	160	8
25–49	M	74	57	1000	2.5	9	60	210	2.0	800	240	8	160	9
	F	59	41	800	2.5	6	45	165	2.0	700	190	14[k]	160	8
50–74	M	73	57	1000	2.5	7	60	210	2.0	800	240	8	160	9
	F	63	41	800	2.5	6	45	165	2.0	800	190	7	160	8
75+	M	69	57	1000	2.5	6	60	210	2.0	800	240	8	160	9
	F	64	41	800	2.5	5	45	165	2.0	800	190	7	160	8

Pregnancy (additional)											
1st trimester	15	100	2.5	2	0	305	1.0	500	15	6	25	0
2nd trimester	20	100	2.5	2	20	305	1.0	500	20	6	25	1
3rd trimester	25	100	2.5	2	20	305	1.0	500	25	6	25	2
Lactation (additional)	20	400	2.5	3	30	120	0.5	500	80	0	50	6

[a] Recommended intakes of energy and of certain nutrients are not listed in this table because of the nature of the variables on which they are based. The figures for energy are estimates of average requirements for expected patterns of activity. For nutrients not shown, the following amounts are recommended: thiamin, 0.4 mg/1000 kcal (0.48 mg/5000 kJ); riboflavin, 0.5 mg/1000 kcal (0.6 mg/5000 kJ); niacin 7.2NE/1000 kcal (8.6NE/5000 kJ); vitamin B_6, 15 μg, as pyridoxine/gm of protein; phosphorus, same as calcium.

[b] Recommended intakes during periods of growth are taken as appropriate for individuals representative of the mid-point in each age group. All recommended intakes are designed to cover individual variations in essentially all of a healthy population subsisting on a variety of common foods available in Canada.

[c] The primary units are gm/kg of body weight. The figures shown here are only examples.

[d] One retinol equivalent (RE) corresponds to the biological activity of 1 μg of retinol, 6 μg of β-carotene or 12 μg of other carotenes.

[e] Expressed as cholecalciferol or ergocalciferol.

[f] Expressed as d-α-tocopherol equivalents, relative to which β- and γ-tocopherol and α-tocotrienol have activities of 0.5, 0.1, and 0.3. respectively.

[g] Expressed as total folate.

[h] Assumption that the protein is from breast milk or is of the same biological value as that of breast milk and that between 3 and 9 months adjustment for the quality of the protein is made.

[i] It is assumed that breast milk is the source of iron up to 2 months of age.

[j] Based on the assumption that breast milk is the source of zinc for the first 2 months.

[k] After the menopause the recommended intake is 7 mg/day.

Source: Department of National Health and Welfare. *Recommended Nutrient Intakes for Canadians.* Compiled by the Committee for the Revisions of the Dietary Standard for Canada, Bureau of Nutritional Sciences, Food Directorate, Health Protection Branch, Ottawa, 1983, pp. 179–180.

Table 25.6
Recommended Intakes of Nutrients, FAO/WHO

Age	Body Weight (kg)	Energy (kcal)	Energy (MJ)	Protein (gm)	Vitamin A (µg)	Vitamin D (µg)	Thiamin (mg)	Riboflavin (mg)	Niacin (mg)	Folic Acid (µg)	Vitamin B_{12} (µg)	Ascorbic Acid (mg)	Calcium[a] (gm)	Iron[a] (mg)
Children														
<1	7.3	820	3.4	14	300	10.0	0.3	0.5	5.4	60	0.3	20	0.5–0.6	5–10
1–3	13.4	1360	5.7	16	250	10.0	0.5	0.8	9.0	100	0.9	20	0.4–0.5	5–10
4–6	20.2	1830	7.6	20	300	10.0	0.7	1.1	12.1	100	1.5	20	0.4–0.5	5–10
7–9	28.1	2190	9.2	25	400	2.5	0.9	1.3	14.5	100	1.5	20	0.4–0.5	5–10
Male adolescents														
10–12	36.9	2600	10.9	30	575	2.5	1.0	1.6	17.2	100	2.0	20	0.6–0.7	5–10
13–15	51.3	2900	12.1	37	725	2.5	1.2	1.7	19.1	200	2.0	30	0.6–0.7	9–18
16–19	62.9	3070	12.8	38	750	2.5	1.2	1.8	20.3	200	2.0	30	0.5–0.6	5–9
Female adolescents														
10–12	38.0	2350	9.8	29	575	2.5	0.9	1.4	15.5	100	2.0	20	0.6–0.7	5–10
13–15	49.9	2490	10.4	31	725	2.5	1.0	1.5	16.4	200	2.0	30	0.6–0.7	12–24
16–19	54.4	2310	9.7	30	750	2.5	0.9	1.4	15.2	200	2.0	30	0.5–0.6	14–28
Adult man (moderately active)	65.0	3000	12.6	37	750	2.5	1.2	1.8	19.8	200	2.0	30	0.4–0.5	5–9
Adult woman (moderately active)	55.0	2200	9.2	29	750	2.5	0.9	1.3	14.5	200	2.0	30	0.4–0.5	14–28
Pregnancy (later half)		+350	+1.5	38	750	10.0	+0.1	+0.2	+2.3	400	3.0	50	1.0–1.2	(9)
Lactation (first 6 months)		+550	+2.3	46	1200	10.0	+0.2	+0.4	+3.7	300	2.5	50	1.0–1.2	(9)

[a]On each line the lower value applies when over 25 percent of calories in the diet come from animal foods, and the higher value when animal foods represent less than 10 percent of calories. For women whose iron intake throughout life has been at the level recommended in this table, the daily intake of iron during pregnancy and lactation should be the same as that recommended for nonpregnant, nonlactating women of childbearing age. For women whose iron status is not satisfactory at the beginning of pregnancy, the requirement is increased and in the extreme situation of women with no iron stores, the requirement can probably not be met without supplementation.

Source: FAO/WHO, *Handbook of Human Nutritional Requirements.* FAO Nutritional Studies No. 28, Rome, 1974.

mended intake" are similar in concept and for practical purposes may be considered as different terms for essentially the same standard.

In a somewhat different vein, characteristic of most dietary standards, *energy requirement* is defined as "the energy intake that is considered adequate to meet the energy needs of the average healthy person in a specified category." Thus, some persons will need less and others more than the average requirement. Because energy expenditure for work activities in developing countries may vary from those of industralized nations, activity levels as defined by FAO/WHO are shown in Table 25.7. Accordingly, recommendations for energy requirements as indicated by body weight and occupation are shown in Table 25.8.

Other Dietary Standards

Dietary standards have been established by many other countries including Australia, South Africa, Philippines, Japan, Central America and Panama, Colombia, Guatemala, India, and most of the European countries.

A number of dietary standards were presented at the Second European Nutrition Conference (1977). The number of nutrients included in the tables of recommended allowances varies. West Germany, for example, includes 28 nutrients; other countries vary from 8 to 18 nutrients. (See Wretlind, 1982.) Although most

TABLE 25.7
Activity Levels as Defined by FAO/WHO

Light activity
   Men: office workers, most professional men (such as lawyers, doctors, accountants, teachers, architects, etc.), shop workers, unemployed men
   Women: office workers, housewives in houses with mechanical household appliances, teachers, and most other professional women
Moderately active
   Men: most men in light industry, students, building workers (excluding heavy laborers), many farm workers, soldiers not on active service, fishermen
   Women: light industry, housewives without mechanical household appliances, students, department store workers
Very active
   Men: some agricultural workers, unskilled laborers, forestry workers, army recruits and soldiers on active service, mine workers, steel workers
   Women: some farm workers (especially peasant agriculture), dancers, athletes
Exceptionally active
   Men: lumberjacks, blacksmiths, rickshaw-pullers
   Women: construction workers

Source: From FAO/WHO, *Energy and Protein Requirements,* WHO Tech. Rep. Ser., No. 522, 1973, p. 25.

TABLE 25.8
The Effects of Body Weight and Occupation on Energy Requirements

| | Men | | | | | | | |
| | Light Activity | | Moderately Active | | Very Active | | Exceptionally Active | |
Body Weight (kg)	(kcal)	(MJ)	(kcal)	(MJ)	(kcal)	(MJ)	(kcal)	(MJ)
50	2100	8.8	2300	9.6	2700	11.3	3100	13.0
55	2310	9.7	2530	10.6	2970	12.4	3410	14.3
60	2520	10.5	2760	11.5	3240	13.6	3720	15.6
65	2700	11.3	3000	12.5	3500	14.6	4000	16.7
70	2940	12.3	3220	13.5	3780	15.8	4340	18.2
75	3150	13.2	3450	14.4	4050	16.9	4650	19.5
80	3360	14.1	3680	15.4	4320	18.1	4960	20.8

| | Women | | | | | | | |
| | Light Activity | | Moderately Active | | Very Active | | Exceptionally Active | |
Body Weight (kg)	(kcal)	(MJ)	(kcal)	(MJ)	(kcal)	(MJ)	(kcal)	(MJ)
40	1440	6.0	1600	6.7	1880	7.9	2200	9.2
45	1620	6.8	1800	7.5	2120	8.9	2480	10.4
50	1800	7.5	2000	8.4	2350	9.8	2750	11.5
55	2000	8.4	2200	9.2	2600	10.9	3000	12.6
60	2160	9.0	2400	10.0	2820	11.8	3300	13.8
65	2340	9.8	2600	10.9	3055	12.8	3575	15.0
70	2520	10.5	2800	11.7	3290	13.8	3850	16.1

Source: From FAO/WHO, *Energy and Protein Requirements,* WHO Tech. Rep. Ser, No. 522, 1973, p. 31.

recommendations represent food as consumed, those of West Germany refer to food as purchased and, therefore, are higher than those of other countries. A thorough examination of dietary standards around the world should emphasize the limitations of present knowledge concerning human nutrient requirements and the divergence of opinion as to the interpretation of experimental data and how these data should be applied in improving the nutrition of population groups.

Dietary Guidelines

For many years the *Basic Four* food groups established by the U.S. Department of Agriculture (Page and Phipard, 1957) and based on the RDA served as the basis for dietary planning and nutrition education. This plan has since been replaced by a five-group plan which includes an additional "negative" group consisting of fats, sugar, and alcohol (U.S. Department of Agriculture, 1980). It was suggested that foods contributing to energy intake but containing few nutrients should be consumed sparingly. This modification of the Basic Four reflects a gradual change in public and scientific interest from the prevention of nutrient deficiencies (and hence establishment of human nutrient requirements) to prevention of chronic degenerative disease by modification of dietary intakes of food components (macronutrients), many of which are not considered "essential" by traditional definition.

Over the past two decades a number of dietary recommendations have been proposed as a means of preventing or delaying chronic disease, particularly cardiovascular disease. Among these recommendations there are some areas of consensus. However, there is greater disagreement concerning desirable levels of dietary fat, kind of fat, and cholesterol. Some of these recommendations were summarized by FAO (Dietary Fats and Oils, Table 6, 1980) and by McNutt (1980). The more recent recommendations made in the 1970s and 80s began with the "Seven Countries" study of Keys (1970). These and other epidemiological studies formed the basis for recommendations by a Commission formed to fulfill the requirements of Section 907 of Public Law 89-239 which established the Regional Medical Programs in 1965 (Report of the Inter-Society Commission for Heart Disease Resources, 1970). This report, the eighth in a series on the Prevention of Cardiovascular Diseases, studied risk factors in coronary heart disease (CHD) and evidence with regard to the possibility of preventing CHD and other atherosclerotic diseases by dietary modification.

The Commission recommended that (1) caloric intake be adjusted to achieve and maintain optimal weight, (2) dietary cholesterol be reduced to less than 300 mg per day, (3) dietary saturated fats be reduced to less than 10 percent of total calories, and (4) dietary total fat be reduced to 35 percent or less. Several recommendations were made regarding the implementation of the recommendations. They were followed in 1977, after extensive hearings, by the "Dietary Goals" of the Select Committee on Nutrition and Human Needs of the U.S. Senate. The major dietary changes dealt with intake of fat: (1) reduce overall fat consumption from approximately 40 to about 30 percent of energy intake, (2) reduce saturated fat consumption to account for about 10 percent of total energy intake, and increase polyunsaturated and monounsaturated fats to account for about 10 percent of energy intake each, and (3) reduce cholesterol consumption to about 300 mg per day. Changes in food selection and preparation were suggested to implement the goals.

The next major recommendations came in 1980 from a joint effort by the U.S. Department of Agriculture and the U.S. Department of Health, Education and Welfare (now Health and Human Services). These more general recommendations—Dietary Guidelines for Americans— were made for fat intake: avoid too much fat, saturated fat, and cholesterol (Guideline 3). The guidelines suggested that "for the U.S. population as a whole, reduction in our current intake of total fat, saturated fat, and cholesterol is sensible. This suggestion is especially appropriate for people who have high blood pressure or who smoke."

In 1972 the Food and Nutrition Board and the Council on Food and Nutrition issued a joint statement advising a lowered intake of fat and cholesterol and an increased P/S ratio in the diets of persons falling into "risk categories." "At risk" individuals included those with elevated levels of plasma lipids or whose family history includes early death from CHD. The Food and Nutrition Board more recently reviewed the evidence and published "Toward Healthful Diets" (National Research Council, 1980) which qualified the previous recommendations of the Board. The report stated: "It appears, therefore,that although high serum cholesterol and LDL levels are positive risk factors for coronary heart disease, it has not been proven that lowering these levels by dietary intervention will consistently affect the rate of new coronary events. In the light of these observations, the Board recommends that the fat content be adjusted to a level appropriate for the caloric requirements of the individual. Infants, adolescent boys, pregnant teenage girls, as well as adults performing heavy manual labor, probably have no need to reduce the fat level of their diets below 40 percent of calories. On the other hand, sedentary persons attempting to achieve weight control may be well advised to reduce the caloric density of their diets by reduction of dietary fat. It does not seem prudent at this time to recommend an increase in the dietary P/S ratio except for individuals in high risk categories."

These recommendations drew wide criticism from advocates of low-fat low-cholesterol diets. When the various positions are critically analyzed, however, the major area of disagreement is related to whether dietary recommendations for the prevention of heart disease should be made for the entire population or only for those individuals who have been diagnosed "at risk." There is basic agreement on several recommendations: (1) eat more fruits and vegetables, (2) eat a variety of foods, (3) consume all foods in moderation.

The Nutrition Committee of the American Heart Association (AHA) (Grundy, 1982) recently reviewed all of its past recommendations with the view of "updating on the basis of the best currently available evidence." Their recommendations date back to 1957 and were released on several occasions thereafter in 1961, 1965, 1968, 1973, and 1978. The 1982 statement is similar to previous ones: (1) reduction in saturated fatty acids to less than 10 percent of total calories, (2) substitution of unsaturated fats with polyunsaturates (not to exceed 10 percent of total calories) and complex carbohydrate, (3) increase in carbohydrates (preferably complex), (4) substantial reduction in dietary cholesterol, and (5) caloric intake adjusted to achieve and maintain desirable weight. The AHA has not recommended the intake of large quantities of polyunsaturated fats for various reasons, among which is the fact that "no large population has consumed large quantities of polyunsaturated fats for many years with demonstrated safety." Thus it may be prudent for the U.S. public to avoid very large amounts of polyunsaturated fats at present.

In view of the increasing concern over obesity as a major health problem in the United States, a reduction in dietary fat (and thus in caloric density) might well serve a dual purpose for many persons. This appears to be one area of general agreement.

Summary

Dietary standards are necessary and useful tools and are a means through which the science of nutrition can be applied for the improvement of human health. Standards serve as guides in planning dietaries, in evaluating food consumption of population groups, and in devising rational plans for maintaining an adequate food supply. They are never static but are assessed periodically and revised as new data become available. Standards differ among nations and reflect, in part, the needs of the population group for which they are intended and, in part, the philosophy of those who establish the standards.

It is likely that public and professional interest in dietary intake patterns in relation to chronic diseases will continue. Given that degenerative diseases have multiple causes, the role of diet in preventing or delaying these conditions is difficult to assess. However, it seems reasonable that, like the RDA, scientific evidence relating diet to health and disease should be reviewed critically and periodically, and such judgments as can be agreed upon should be made available to the public.

chapter 26

nutrition surveys

A nutrition survey is similar to any other community survey in that its goal is to define a population in terms of specific factors. It is epidemiological in nature and, in this respect, it is designed to identify the extent and distribution of malnutrition. The survey is the chief but not the only means of providing information necessary for the planning of realistic nutrition programs consistent with the needs and habits of a community and for evaluating the effect of nutrition programs already existing within a community. There are other less direct means for obtaining a fair concept of the nutritional status of population groups, but the survey as usually conducted has the advantage of providing the kind of quantitative data necessary to convince legislators (and the public) to support and encourage direct action programs for the benefit of the public health.

The classic methods for the determination of nutritional status yield four kinds of evaluative data: dietary, biochemical, clinical, and anthropometric. The four methods measure different states of nutriture and, therefore, do not necessarily correlate with each other. It is generally agreed that dietary surveys evaluate current food intake, biochemical data reflect recent nutritional status, and clinical and anthropometric examinations evaluate more long-term nutritional history.

Any one or combination of the four methods may be used in survey studies, but there is no question that interpretation of results becomes more difficult as the number of evaluative criteria increase. Perhaps surveys, more than any other kind of nutritional studies, help to remind investigators of the limitations of the procedures currently available for the evaluation of human nutritional status and of the variability inherent within the human race. In spite of the limitations, however, useful data can be obtained that grossly define the nutritional status of groups of people and lend themselves to comparison among different groups.

Contributory Information

Certain kinds of accessory information provide indications of nutritional status and should be investigated prior to or at the same time as a population survey. These factors were summarized in a WHO publication (1963a) along with the usual components of nutrition surveys and are presented in Table 26.1. The interaction of these factors with the classic methods for determining dietary and nutritional status is depicted in Fig. 26.1.

AGRICULTURAL DATA. FOOD BALANCE SHEETS

The FAO has developed food balance sheets for many countries that relate agricultural production and import and export data to arrive at a presumptive figure grossly approximating the amount of food available to a population. Similarly, the astute nutritionist or medical worker can learn much of the general nutritional situation of a population by studying available agricultural records. Such data can be valuable in roughly estimating the presence or absence of widespread food shortages, but they obviously provide no information on the distribution of available food within the different segments of the population.

VITAL AND HEALTH STATISTICS

Mortality and morbidity ratios are affected by many factors including environmental conditions of sanitation and the extent of immunization and medical care. Infants are especially vulnerable to environmental stresses and neglect. There is evidence suggesting that the high mortality rate observed among children one to four years of age in many areas of the world is the result of the interaction between malnutrition and infectious disease. Scrimshaw and Behar (1956) reported that deaths that had been attributed to diarrhea or parasitic infection among children under five years of age in a Central American community were, in fact, caused by or associated with malnutrition. It is generally accepted that the mortality rate in the preschool age range of one to four years may serve as a rough index of malnutrition in a community (Wills and Waterlow, 1958).

The occurrence of high mortality rates in a community therefore suggests that for each child who dies in early life, many others live who are being handicapped

TABLE 26.1
Information Needed for Assessment of Nutritional Status

Sources of Information	Nature of Information Obtained	Nutritional Implications
1. Agricultural data Food balance sheets	Gross estimates of agricultural production Agricultural methods Soil fertility Predominance of cash crops Overproduction of staples Food imports and exports	Approximate availability of food supplies to a population
2. Socioeconomic data Information on marketing, distribution, and storage	Purchasing power Distribution and storage of foodstuffs	Unequal distribution of available foods between the socioeconomic groups in the community and within the family
3. Food consumption patterns Cultural-anthropological data	Lack of knowledge, erroneous beliefs, prejudices, and indifference	
4. Dietary surveys	Food consumption	Low, excessive, or unbalanced nutrient intake
5. Special studies on foods	Biological value of diets Presence of interfering factors (e.g., goitrogens) Effects of food processing	Special problems related to nutrient utilization
6. Vital and health statistics	Morbidity and mortality data	Extent of risk to community Identification of high-risk groups
7. Anthropometric studies	Physical development	Effect of nutrition on physical development
8. Clinical nutritional surveys	Physical signs	Deviation from health due to malnutrition
9. Biochemical studies	Levels of nutrients, metabolites, and other components of body tissues and fluids	Nutrient supplies in the body Impairment of biochemical function
10. Additional medical information	Prevalent disease patterns, including infections and infestations	Interrelationships of state of nutrition and disease

Source: From WHO Report of Expert Committee on Medical Assessment of Nutritional Status, *Tech. Rpt. Series No. 258,* 1963a.

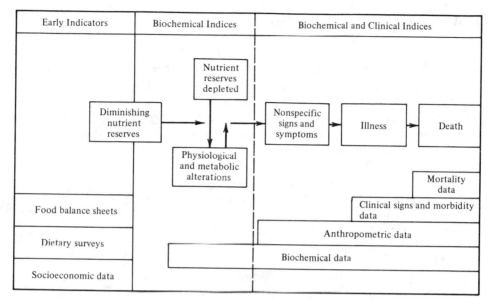

Early Indicators	Biochemical Indices	Biochemical and Clinical Indices

Figure 26.1
Continuum in evaluating dietary and nutritional status of population groups. (From M. Behar, *Nutrition in Preventive Medicine*, G. H. Beaton and J. M. Bengoa, Eds., WHO Monograph Series No. 62, WHO, Geneva, 1976, p. 556.).

by incipient malnutrition. (See Chapter 21.) Unfortunately, accurate health and vital statistics are not available in all countries, and even when statistics are available, the investigator can estimate only that a nutritional problem exists. The identification of the problem requires more specific evaluation.

Dietary Surveys

Just as the first organized attempts to develop dietary standards came as a result of the work of the League of Nations Technical Commission on Nutrition, so did the first organized efforts to evaluate the nutritional status of population groups. Bigwood's *Guiding Principles for Studies on the Nutrition of Populations* (1939) is a classic in the area of nutrition surveys, and although many of the details of procedure and methodology have been extended, improved, or replaced, the basic approach and philosophy are essentially the same today as they were 45 years ago.

Dietary surveys can be planned to determine food consumption of families or of individuals. Family food consumption or household consumption, as it is more appropriately called, is an estimate of the total amount of food used by an entire household for a fixed period of time, usually one week. The most commonly used methods are the food account, food list, and food record.

HOUSEHOLD FOOD CONSUMPTION

Food Account
The food account is a record of all food purchased or produced for family consumption over a period of several weeks. The length of time depends on the complexity of the diet since no record is made of food already in the household or of that remaining at the end of the study period. When the diet is relatively monotonous or few food supplies are routinely stored in the home, a period of two weeks is often satisfactory since under these conditions food purchases tend to represent food consumed within a brief period of time. A family that relies on a well-stocked freezer to provide a large portion of the weekly food intake is not well suited to this type of study. For this reason, the method is almost never used in the United States and has been used chiefly in areas where the diet is less complex than that of the average American family.

Food List
The food list is essentially a recall method. The homemaker is asked to estimate by weight, retail unit, or household measure, the quantity of food used by the entire household during the previous week. The method requires a well-trained interviewer who can help the homemaker recall by daily menu or purchases all food used by the household. The food list is advantageous in that only one visit to the household is necessary; because it requires little time and effort on the part of the homemaker, cooperation usually is good.

   The food list method is used for many of the food consumption surveys conducted by the United States Department of Agriculture and most often is the basis for the per capita food consumption data published by the Department. Accuracy of the food list is judged to be satisfactory for this purpose; errors tend to be due to omission of food items or incorrect estimation of amounts of food used.

Food Record
This method involves a weighed inventory of foods at the beginning and close of the study period, usually one week, together with a day-by-day record by weight of food brought into the home during the week. Records of plate and kitchen wastes are sometimes, but not always, included. The method is time consuming and therefore more expensive than the food list. At least two visits to the home are required of the interviewer and considerably more time is demanded of the homemaker. Accuracy of the method is relatively high although it is generally believed that the food list is an equally satisfactory and much less expensive means for obtaining household food consumption data.

Weighed Household Consumption
In some cases it is both feasible and advisable to obtain household food consumption by daily weighing of food prepared and served in the home. This method usually requires that an investigator be present in the home at the time that food is prepared. The method has the advantage of providing more precise information

than can be obtained by recall or record. It is perhaps the best approach to use in rural or small village situations where much food is obtained from home gardens or local barter and where retail measures or weights are uncertain. However, the method requires a greater investment in time and personnel than other techniques and is seldom used unless it is certain that data of comparable validity cannot be obtained by other means.

Summary

Surveys of household food consumption are designed to yield essentially two kinds of data: economic consumption, that is, the monetary value of food entering the home or food available for consumption; and/or physiological consumption, food actually eaten by the family. In any case, certain kinds of accessory information must be obtained, such as the number of individuals usually fed from the family food supply, the number of meals eaten away from home, and the number of guests entertained during the study period. The accuracy of the calculation of per capita intake depends on these factors as well as on the composition of the family unit. Formulas taking into consideration family composition by age and the number of meals eaten in and out of the home have been proposed (Francois, 1970; Cresta, 1970).

If wastes from purchased and prepared foods are ignored, food use data represent economic but not physiological consumption. For this reason, economic food consumption, such as the per capita food supply data, tends to be higher than physiological consumption. (See Call, 1965.) In either case, data on family food use yield no information on the distribution of food within the family.

Details of these methods can be found in several publications (Norris, 1949; NRC, 1949; Reh, 1962; FAO, 1964).

INDIVIDUAL FOOD CONSUMPTION

Evaluation of individual nutritional status leading to identification of vulnerable groups within a population group requires study of food consumed by a given individual. Four methods are commonly used to determine individual food consumption: estimation by recall, food record, dietary history, and weighed intake.

Estimation by Recall

Recall of food intake is almost always for a 24-hour period only, and for this reason it is generally designated the 24-hour recall. The subject is asked to recall all food consumed during the previous day and to estimate quantities in ordinary measures or servings. In order to increase accuracy of quantities of food consumed, the subject may be provided with measuring cups or other devices to aid in estimation. Information obtained by this method is not necessarily representative of usual intake of an individual. The method, therefore, is most useful when relatively large numbers of subjects are involved and provides a qualitative and a quantitative description of group dietary patterns. The 24-hour recall can serve as a basis for educational programs or gross evaluation of dietary intake of large groups. It is not valid as an accurate measure of food intake of one individual. When large numbers of subjects are involved, the method is considered to be indicative of the dietary pattern characteristic of the group. Because of ease of obtaining data, the 24-hour recall has gained in usage. Recently, the use of periodic 24-hour recalls by the same individual was described as a means of continuous monitoring of food consumption patterns (National Research Council, 1981).

Food Record

This method requires that the subject keep a record of food eaten for varying lengths of time, usually three to seven days. Quantities of food are estimated in common household measures. Accuracy of the method depends largely on the diligence and integrity of the subject and on the subject's ability to estimate quantities of food. The method appears to be a fairly accurate estimate of individual food consumption over a specific period of time.

Weighed Intake

A very accurate record of food consumption can be obtained by having a subject or a trained person weigh all food consumed during a given period of time. This method of obtaining food consumption data is obviously expensive and time consuming and consequently is rarely used in nutrition surveys. In spite of the accuracy of data obtained on quantities of food consumed, the method is limited in other ways. Because of the tediousness of the procedure, subjects are prone to try to find shortcuts and thus to change from their usual eating patterns.

The weighed food intake, however, is standard procedure in a laboratory-controlled metabolic study and, although a few surveys have involved weighed data, this method most often is limited to research studies. Under these circumstances, it is the researcher rather than the subject who bears the burden of tedium.

Diet History

The diet history is designed to discover the *usual* food intake pattern over a relatively long period of time and is most often obtained by interview. A series of food records kept at intervals over a period of months or years yields data comparable to the diet history but obviously is a more expensive procedure both in terms of time and personnel. The diet history often is used for studies of food habits or in clinics or hospital dietetics. Burke (1947), however, devised a method for calculation of diet histories and for their use as research tools.

The research dietary history has the disadvantage of requiring highly skilled interviewers in order to obtain useful data. Quantitative significance of the data, however, has been questioned, and in unskilled hands, the history may yield erroneous information (Maynard, 1950). When properly conducted, it has an advantage over other methods in that it relates food intake over a relatively long period of time. The method measures frequency of intake of a large number of foods or groups of foods and thus balances out possible seasonal variations in food intake.

As originally devised by Burke, the diet history method is rather time consuming. A modification of the history applicable to epidemiological studies involving thousands of subjects was described by Stefanick and Trulson (1962). The method requires less time than the diet history and is regarded as a qualitative estimation of frequency of food intake. Mann et al. (1962) described a similar modification of the Burke dietary history in which the procedure was restricted to a selection of nutrients pertinent to the problem under study.

Summary
Since all known methods for obtaining dietary data have certain advantages as well as limitations, the choice of method should depend on the population sample to be surveyed and the specific use for which the data are intended. Flores (1962), for example, pointed out some differences in collection of dietary information in nonmodernized societies as compared to modernized communities. For further discussion of the advantages and disadvantages of methods for obtaining individual food consumption, see Young et al. (1952), Chalmers et al. (1952), Trulson and McCann (1959), Adelson (1960), Cellier and Hankin (1963), Pekkarinen (1970), Balogh et al. (1971), Marr (1971), Burk and Pao (1976), and Young (1981). Alternative methods of collecting food consumption data (such as telephone interview) are discussed by Schucker (1982).

In addition to the choice of method, the investigator must decide how the collected data will be handled. It may be necessary to know only the general pattern of food intake or the range of nutrient intake for a population and the specific food groups from which nutrients are obtained. In certain epidemiological studies, the pattern of eating throughout the day can be as important as total nutrient intake. Furthermore, the consumption of food in commercial establishments and the use of highly processed convenience foods in the home have increased. It is becoming more and more important to assess the contribution of food consumed from these sources and their effects on total nutrient intake.

CALCULATION AND INTERPRETATION OF DIETARY INTAKE

The laborious computation of nutrient intake from food records is familiar to every student of nutrition. Calculation of dietaries, however, has been greatly simplified by the use of computers. Tullis et al. (1965), Hankins et al. (1965), and Mo et al. (1971) discussed computer calculations for a number of purposes: surveys, hospital and clinic records, and institution dietaries. All foods listed in Handbook 8 are provided with code numbers for use in computer calculations, and methods for coding and preparing coded data for analysis were described in an early publication of the United States Department of Agriculture (USDA) (Davenport, 1964). The USDA nutrient data bank has since been updated (Hepburn, 1982), and a number of other data banks have been developed and are currently used by various investigators. (See Samonds, 1982.)

When the diet is complex and consists of many mixed food dishes, accurate calculation is difficult and depends on having a detailed description of the food and, if possible, the recipe used in preparation. Merrill et al. (1966) described methods for calculating mixed dishes from home-prepared foods; methods also were described by the Interdepartmental Committee on Nutrition for National Defense (1963).

Several short methods for the calculation of dietary intake have been described by Leichsenring and Wilson (1951), Clark and Cofer (1962), and more recently by Pennington (1982). Foods similar in nutritive content are grouped together, and average values are used to calculate nutritive content of foods included in each group. Results obtained by these shortened procedures tend to agree rather well with the more detailed dietary calculations when large samples are involved. A short procedure described by Mann et al. (1962) was designed for the Framingham epidemiological study relating environmental and other factors to incidence of heart disease. This was aimed at identifying dietary intake as high, medium, or low with regard to specific nutrients. The accuracy of the procedure appeared to be high since even after a lapse of two years, dietary intake obtained from a second dietary history almost always fell into the same general category (Dawber et al., 1962). This type of procedure appears to have special merit for epidemiological studies in which interest is centered both on specific dietary components and the relation of diet over a long period of time to a specific health problem. The gross identification of dietary intake as high, medium, or low appears to be a reasonable approach to interpretation of data from nutritional status studies as well. Even the most precise mathematical manipulations cannot remove the sources of error inherent both in the methods for collecting data and in the food tables from which these data are calculated; therefore the use of numerical values in describing food intakes often implies a degree of accuracy that does not exist.

Currently there is no general consensus concerning the interpretation of dietary intake data. The USDA has generally used the current RDA or a fraction thereof as a baseline for judging dietary adequacy for specific nutrients. (See Pao and Mickle, 1981.) Many independent investigators conducting limited surveys have arbitrarily chosen two-thirds of the RDA as a means of estimating the probable risk of dietary inadequacy.

The Ten State Nutrition Survey conducted in 1968 by the Nutrition Section of the DHEW (now the U. S. Department of Health and Human Services) developed standards for evaluation of dietary intake data based on both the 1968 RDA and FAO/WHO standards. (See Chapter 25.) This information is shown in Table 26.2. The standards developed for energy, protein, and iron were approximately the same as the RDA; energy and protein, however, were expressed in terms of body weight for all age groups. Calcium, vitamin A, and ascorbic acid standards were lower than the RDA and were similar to the FAO/WHO standards which were considered to be more realistic for evaluation of dietary data. Thiamin, riboflavin,

TABLE 26.2
Guide to Interpretation of Nutrient Intake Data

Kcal Standards		Protein Standards	
Age	**Kcal/kg Body Weight**	**Age**	**Gm Protein/kg Body Weight**
0–1 ⎫	120	0–11 ⎫	2.2
2–5 ⎪	110	12–23 ⎪ months	1.9
6–11 ⎬ months	100	24–47 ⎬	1.7
12–23 ⎪	90	48–71 ⎭	1.5
24–47 ⎪	86	6–9 ⎫	1.3
48–71 ⎭	82	10–16 ⎬ years	1.2
6–7 ⎫	82	17–19 ⎪	1.1
8–9 ⎪	82	20 and over ⎭	1.0

For 2nd and 3rd trimesters of pregnancy, increase basic standard 20 gm.

For lactating, increase basic standard 25 gm.

Kcal Standards	
Age	**Kcal/kg Body Weight**
10–12	
Male	68
Female	64
13–16	
Male	60
Female	48
17–19	
Male	44
Female	35
20–29	
Male	40
Female ⎬ years	35
30–39	
Male	38
Female	33
40–49	
Male	37
Female	31
50–59	
Male	36
Female	30
60–69	
Male	34
Female	29
>70	
Male	34
Female	29

Calcium Standards

Age	Mg/Day
0–11 ⎫ months	550
12–71 ⎭	450
6–9 ⎫	450
10–12 ⎪	650
13–16 ⎬ years	650
17–19 ⎪	550
20 and over ⎭	400

For 2nd and 3rd trimesters of pregnancy, increase basic standard 200 kcal.

For lactating, increase basic standard 1,000 kcal.

For 3rd trimester of pregnancy, increase standard 400 mg.

For lactating, increase standard 500 mg.

(continued)

TABLE 26.2 (continued)

Vitamin B Standards

Age	Thiamin	Riboflavin	Niacin
For all age groups including adults	0.4 mg/ 1000 kcal	0.55 mg/ 1000 kcal	6.6 mg/ 1000 kcal

Iron Standards

Age		Mg/Day
0–11	months	10
12–47		15
48–71		10
6–9	years	10
10–12		
Male		10
Female		18
13–19		
Male		18
Female		18
20 and over		
Male		10
Female (to 55)		18
Female (55 on)		10

Vitamin A Standards

Age	International Units
0–1 (months)	1,500
2–5	1,500
6–11	1,500
12–23	2,000
24–47	2,000
48–71	2,000
6–7 (years)	2,500
8–9	2,500
10–12	2,500
>12	3,500

For lactating, increase standard 1,000 I.U.

Vitamin C Standards (ascorbic acid)

All age groups	30 mg/day

Source: From U. S. Department of Health, Education and Welfare, Publication No. (HSM) 72-8133 (N.D.)

and niacin were expressed in relation to energy intake as were those of FAO/WHO; absolute values, however, were similar to those of the RDA. Standards for pregnant and lactating women were adapted from the RDA.

The National Health and Nutrition Examination Survey (NHANES), which followed the Ten State Survey in 1971–1974, used similar dietary standards with minor modifications. The calcium standard for adult women was raised to 600 mg (rather than 400 mg) and the vitamin A standard for pregnant women was increased by 1,000 I.U. (similar to lactating women). The vitamin C standard was changed from 30 mg to 40 mg for children up to age 12 years, to 50 mg for ages 13–16 years, to 55 mg for males 17–19 years, and to 55 mg for adult females. These standards correspond to the 1968 RDA. (See U. S. Department of Health, Education, and Welfare, 1977a.)

Data from the second NHANES (1976–1980) are reported in percentiles which indicate the distribution of nutrient intakes in the population studied. Thus, the raw data are available, and interpretation of these data may vary according to the purpose for which they are used. For information on the two major food consumption surveys conducted in the United States, see Swan (1983). For a compilation of nutritional status and dietary evaluation studies conducted in the United States between 1957 and 1967, see Kelsay (1969).

SUMMARY

Proper interpretation of dietary data requires a sound knowledge of dietary requirements and an appreciation of the errors inherent in the methods for collecting and analyzing the data. One cannot depreciate the value of survey data as an *indication* of nutritional status, but there is little virtue in assigning to such data an accuracy that cannot possibly pertain. The human being is a highly variable creature, and the human living in an uncontrolled community setting is even more variable. There are many pitfalls in the study of population groups, and they should be recognized.

Biochemical Evaluation of Nutritional Status

Data accumulated on human response to diet under controlled conditions, that is, metabolic studies, have been used to establish standards for evaluation of the nutritional status of population groups. Biochemical tests for appraisal of nutritional status, however, usually have been selected on the basis of simplicity of the analytical procedure. Sensitivity of the method has, perhaps, too often been of secondary concern. When the study sample is large and the objective of the study is to identify nutritional problems of possible public health significance, emphasis is on the group rather than the individual. Under these circumstances, the approach is to select the most practical method that will yield useful data.

Methods applicable to the biochemical appraisal of nutritional status have been reviewed by Lowry (1952), Pearson (1962), Sauberlich et al. (1973), among others. Analytical procedures also are described in the ICNND manual (1963). Micromethods that require only a few drops of blood obtained by finger prick were developed over 30 years ago by Lowry and Bessey (1945); these methods are suitable for the study of some nutrients. Sensitive microbiological methods also have been developed (Baker and Frank, 1968) and have been applied in survey studies (Baker et al., 1967; Christakis et al., 1968). For details of methods currently used in nationwide surveys (NHANES), see Gunter et al. (1981).

Just as biochemical analyses are limited primarily to blood and excreta in human metabolic studies, so are analyses for surveys usually limited to blood and urine. Collection of urine samples obviously presents more problems than blood. A 24-hour sample rarely can be obtained and investigators are fortunate if they can obtain a timed sample over a period of four or six hours. Most often a single voided sample is analyzed and may be a fasting sample collected in the morning before any food is eaten, or a random sample taken at any time during the day. Excretion data from single samples are expressed in relation to creatinine content of the same sample on the assumption that creatinine excretion is relatively constant and thus can serve as a basis for equating excretion data from different individuals. This method is generally accepted for practical purposes but is acknowledged to be limited by vagaries of creatinine and nutrient excretions (Edwards et al., 1969; Pollack, 1970). The variability of creatinine excretion is particularly high in children aged 2–10 years (Lewis et al., 1975).

The technique most commonly used in surveys are measurements of thiamin, riboflavin, and N^1-methylnicotinamide in urine; and hemoglobin, vitamin A, carotene, and ascorbic acid in blood. (See ICNND, 1963.) The reliability of these tests appears to be relatively high in terms of identifying nutritional problems within a population. Iodine in urine also was determined in the National Nutrition Survey and in the National Health and Nutrition Examination Survey in order to correlate these data with clinical evidence of goiter in the American population. Serum proteins and serum albumin often are determined, the latter being a more sensitive indicator of protein nutriture.

The 1976–1980 NHANES included determinations of hemoglobin concentration, hematocrit, red blood cell and white blood cell counts, mean corpuscular volume, erythrocyte protoporphyrin, serum iron and total iron-binding capacity, transferrin saturation, and serum zinc, copper, vitamin C, albumin, and vitamin A (McDowell et al., 1981).

Guides for interpretation of data on urinary excretion of riboflavin, thiamin, N^1-methylnicotinamide, and iodine, and for blood hematocrit, hemoglobin, iron transferrin saturation, serum proteins, serum vitamin A, carotene, ascorbic acid, and folic acid are shown in Table 26.3. (See O'Neal et al., 1970.) The rationale behind these standards was discussed by Plough and Bridgforth (1960), Pearson (1962; 1967), and Wilson et al (1964). In the NHANES evaluations, similar guidelines were used with slightly different age groups for the hematological cutoff points (U.S. Dept. HEW, 1974). Hematological and other biochemical data from the 1976–1980 NHANES, however, are expressed in percentile distributions of the survey population. (See Fulwood et al., 1982.)

Special problems in the biochemical assessment of nutritional status during pregnancy evolved from the Vanderbilt study of pregnant women (Darby et al., 1948; Dawson et al., 1969), and it is clear that standards for pregnant and nonpregnant women differ (NRC, 1978). More data are needed on the biochemical evaluation of nutritional status of young children and the elderly.

Clinical Evaluation of Nutritional Status

The physical examination of subjects was the earliest means of evaluating nutritional status since knowledge of the nutrients evolved from the observation of deficiency symptoms. Clinical evaluation, however, is by far the most subjective area in the determination of nutritional status, and for this reason it is recommended that all clinical evaluations be conducted by one physician trained in recognition of deficiency symptoms. When the number of subjects is so large that

TABLE 26.3
Guidelines for Classification and Interpretation of Group Blood and Urine Data Collected as Part of the Ten State Nutrition Survey

Determination	Classification Category		
	Less than Acceptable		
	Deficient	Low	Acceptable[a]
Hemoglobin, gm/dl			
6–23 months	< 9.0	9.0–9.9	≥10.0
2–5 yr	<10	10.0–10.9	≥11.0
6–12 yr	<10	10.0–11.4	≥11.5
13–16 yr, male	<12	12.0–12.9	≥13.0
13–16 yr, female	<10	10.0–11.4	≥11.5
>16 yr, male	<12	12.0–13.9	≥14.0
>16 yr, female	<10	10.0–11.9	≥12.0
Pregnant, 2nd trimester	< 9.5	9.5–10.9	≥11.0
Pregnant, 3rd trimester	< 9.0	9.0–10.4	≥10.5
Hematocrit, %			
6–23 months	<28	28–30	≥31
2–5 yr	<30	30–33	≥34
6–12 yr	<30	30–35	≥36
13–16 yr, male	<37	37–39	≥40
13–16 yr, female	<31	31–35	≥36
>16 yr, male	<37	37–43	≥44
>16 yr, female	<31	31–37	≥38
Pregnant, 2nd trimester	<30	30–34	≥35
Pregnant, 3rd trimester	<30	30–32	≥33
Hemoglobin conc. MCHC g/dl RBC			
All ages	—	30	≥30
Serum iron, μg/dl			
0–5 months	—		—
6–23 months		<30	≥30
2–5 yr		<40	≥40
6–12 yr		<50	≥50
>12 yr, male		<60	≥60
>12 yr, female		<40	≥40
Transferrin saturation, %			
0–5 months		—	—
6–23 months		<15	≥15
2–12 yr		<20	≥20
>12 yr, male		<20	≥20
>12 yr, female		<15	≥15
Red cell folacin, ng/ml			
All ages	<140	140–159	≥160–650
Serum folacin, ng/ml	3.0	3.0–5.9	≥6.0
Serum protein, gm/dl			
0–11 months		<5.0	≥5.0
1–5 yr		<5.5	≥5.5
6–17 yr		<6.0	≥6.0

(continued)

TABLE 26.3 (continued)

Determination	Classification Category		Acceptable[a]
	Less than Acceptable		
	Deficient	**Low**	**Acceptable[a]**
Adult	<6.0	6.0–6.4	≧6.5
Pregnant, 2nd and 3rd trimester	<5.5	5.5–5.9	≧6.0
Serum albumin, gm/dl			
0–11 months		<2.5	≧2.5
1–5 yr		<3.0	≧3.0
6–17 yr		<3.5	≧3.5
Adult	<2.8	2.8–3.4	≧3.5
Pregnant, 1st trimester	<3.0	3.0–3.9	≧4.0
Pregnant, 2nd and 3rd trimester	<3.0	3.0–3.4	≧3.5
Serum vitamin C, mg/dl			
0–11 months	—	—	—
>1 yr	<0.1	0.1–0.19	≧0.2
Plasma carotene, μg/dl			
0–5 months		<10	≧ 10
6–11 months		<30	≧ 30
1–17 yr		<40	≧ 40
Adult	<20[b]	20–39	≧ 40
Pregnant, 2nd trimester		30–79	≧ 80
Pregnant, 3rd trimester		40–79	≧ 80
Plasma vitamin A, μg/dl			
0–5 months	< 10	10–19	≧ 20
0.5–17 yr	< 20	20–29	≧ 30
Adult	< 10	10–19	≧ 20
Urinary thiamin, μg/g creatinine			
1–3 yr	<120	120–175	≧176
4–6 yr	< 85	85–120	≧121
7–9 yr	< 70	70–180	≧181
10–12 yr	< 60	60–180	≧181
13–15 yr	< 50	50–150	≧151
Adult	< 27	27–65	≧ 66
Pregnant, 2nd trimester	< 23	23–54	≧ 55
Pregnant, 3rd trimester	< 21	21–49	≧ 50
Urinary riboflavin, μg/gm creatinine			
1–3 yr	<150	150–499	≧500
4–6 yr	<100	100–299	≧300
7–9 yr	< 85	85–269	≧270
10–15 yr	< 70	70–199	≧200
Adult	< 27	27–79	≧ 80
Pregnant, 2nd trimester	< 39	39–119	≧120
Pregnant, 3rd trimester	< 30	30–89	≧ 90
Urinary iodine, μg/gm creatinine	< 25	25–49	≧ 50

Source: From O'Neal et al., *Pediat. Res.* 4:103, 1970.

[a]Excessively high levels may indicate abnormal clinical status or toxicity.

[b]May indicate unusual diet or malabsorption.

more than one examining physician is needed, best results are obtained if physicians are trained in a group and interobserver variability is determined through repeated examinations of the same subjects by all examining physicians. In this way the reliability of the clinical data is enhanced.

Whereas the dietary survey is indicative of current food intake and biochemical analysis of relatively recent food intake, the clinical examination is more likely to reflect the result of long-term nutritional status. Scars of early skin lesions and mild skeletal deformities, for example, provide evidence of earlier deprivation even when the present diet appears adequate.

Clinical lesions, moreover, may be influenced by other factors, such as intestinal parasites or infection, which may influence absorption and metabolism of nutrients independent of dietary intake. A carefully taken medical history can help reveal significant factors contributing to nutritional status.

Symptoms and signs have been classified by WHO (1963a) and are shown in the Guide for Interpretation of Clinical Signs (Table 26.4). These symptoms and signs are listed under the nutrient-deficiency or excess with which they are usually associated. They vary in sensitivity and specificity for individual nutrients. Frank clinical lesions are generally easily recognized and evaluated, particularly in areas of the world where malnutrition is still endemic (Africa, S.E. Asia, and Latin America). In the highly developed industrialized countries, however, serious malnutrition is rarely seen except in very ill, hospitalized patients. Marginal malnutrition is not infrequently found, but it is much more difficult to define and to evaluate. It occurs usually in older people and may be due to such underlying conditions as heart disease or diabetes. ICNND (1963) published a guide for the interpretation of clinical signs of nutritional inadequacy similar to the WHO guide. Excellent discussions of the clinical examination as a means of determining nutritional status were given by the NRC (1949) and by Goldsmith (1959).

Anthropometric Assessment of Nutritional Status

Growth, as represented by height and weight for age, is believed to be one of the most definitive indications of nutritional status of young children. On the basis of data collected on children 6 to 11 years of age, Ferro-Luzzi (1966) suggested that these simple anthropometric measurements, in addition to clinical examination, provide more information at low cost than other more extensive and expensive methods of survey. When the age of the child is not accurately known, as often occurs in some primitive societies, weight/height ratio for very young children may be a useful criterion of nutritional status. Dugdale (1971) showed that the weight/height ratio for children one to five years of age is independent of age but correlates with nutritional status. Normal weight for height has been observed, however, in young children with height below the norms for their ages (Downs, 1964). These children apparently suffered from malnutrition in early life which resulted in lowered height for age; that is, although weight was proportional to height, both were similar to that observed in younger children. This phenom-

TABLE 26.4
Suggested Guide for Interpretation of Clinical Signs

Dietary Obesity
Excessive weight in relation to height or other skeletal indices
Excessive skinfolds
Excessive abdominal girth in relation to chest girth

Undernutrition
Lethargy, mental and physical (starvation)
Low weight in relation to height or other skeletal indices
Diminished skinfolds
Exaggerated skeletal prominences
Loss of elasticity of skin

Protein-Calorie Deficiency Diseases
Edema
Muscle wasting
Low body weight
Psychomotor change
Dyspigmentation of the hair
Easy pluckability of the hair
Thin, sparse hair
Moon face
Flaky paint dermatosis
Diffuse depigmentation of the skin

Vitamin A Deficiency
Xerosis of skin
Follicular hyperkeratosis, type 1
Xerosis conjunctivae
Keratomalacia
Bitot's spots

Riboflavin Deficiency
Angular stomatitis; angular scars
Cheilosis
Magenta tongue
Central atrophy of lingual papillae
Naso-labial dyssebacea
Angular palpebritis
Scrotal and vulval dermatosis
Corneal vascularization

Thiamin Deficiency
Loss of ankle jerks
Loss of knee jerks
Sensory loss and motor weakness
Calf-muscle tenderness
Cardiovascular dysfunction
Edema

TABLE 26.4 (continued)

Niacin Deficiency
Pellagrous dermatosis
Scarlet and raw tongue
Tongue fissuring
Atrophic lingual papillae
Malar and supraorbital pigmentation

Vitamin C Deficiency
Spongy and bleeding gums
Follicular hyperkeratosis, type 2
Petechiae
Ecchymoses
Intramuscular or subperiosteal hematoma
Epiphyseal enlargement (painful)

Vitamin D Deficiency
(1) *Active rickets* (in children)
Epiphyseal enlargement (over 6 months of age), painless
Beading of ribs
Craniotabes (under 1 year of age)
Muscular hypotonia

(2) *Healed rickets* (in children or adults)
Frontal and parietal bossing
Knock-knees or bowlegs
Deformities of thorax

(3) *Osteomalacia* (in adults)
Local or generalized skeletal deformities

Iron Deficiency
Pallor of mucous membranes
Koilonychia
Atrophic lingual papillae

Iodine Deficiency
Enlargement of thyroid

Excess of Fluorine (Fluorosis)
Mottled dental enamel, difficult to distinguish in early stages from enamel hypoplasia.

Source: From WHO Report of Expert Committee on Medical Assessment of Nutritional Status, Tech. Rept. Series no. 258 (1963a), pp. 59–61.

enon has been called nutritional dwarfing by Downs (ibid) and is quite common in many developing countries.

The Stuart-Meredith standards based on measurements of children in Boston in the early 1940s and of Iowa City children and adolescents in the 1930s (see Nelson, 1946) have been used frequently as standards for the evaluation of height/weight data in surveys throughout the world. They have now been superseded by more recent data collected between 1965 and 1974 by the National Center for Health Statistics in three surveys (U.S. Dept. HEW, 1977b). These data are certainly more representative of the United States population as a whole than the previously used data. In addition, longitudinal data from the growth study of the Fels Research Institute for ages 6–20 years also are included. The growth charts constructed from these data were accepted by WHO as international standards and are now generally used in both growth studies and surveys in many countries. Despite objections of applying North American standards to various racial groups, children of various racial backgrounds who come from homes of high economic status tend to fall within the standards (Edozien, 1965; Bohdal and Simmons, 1969). These findings suggest that nutritional status may be a more significant factor in promoting growth than genetic makeup, but the controversy of "nurture" versus "nature" is far from solved. In both the Ten State Nutrition Survey and the NHANES, differences were found between white and black children before puberty with the former usually being heavier and the latter slightly taller. During puberty, this changed inasmuch as black girls were heavier than white girls of the same height; black boys were slightly taller but lighter than white boys of the same age. Clearly, what is needed are longitudinal studies of children of different racial groups but similar socio-economic background in order to find answers to the "nurture" versus "nature" effect on growth.

Correlation of Dietary, Biochemical, and Clinical Data

The degree of correlation that can be expected among dietary, biochemical, and clinical data is limited by the nature of the data. Dietary data usually are derived from one day diet records whereas biochemical measurements reflect intake over weeks or months and clinical lesions usually take several months to develop. In spite of these limitations, significant correlations have been found between dietary and biochemical data (U.S. Department of Health, Education, and Welfare, N.D.; Kerr et al. 1982) as well as between dietary and clinical findings (Lowenstein, 1978), and between biochemical and clinical findings, particularly in older age groups (Wenger et al., 1979). One might expect that serum ascorbic acid would reflect dietary intake fairly well, and results of surveys tend to bear this out. Clinical evidence of ascorbic acid deficiency, such as spongy or bleeding gums, also tends to correlate rather well with a low intake of the vitamin and low or negligible levels in serum (Plough and Bridgforth, 1960).

Urinary excretions of thiamin, riboflavin, and N^1-methylnicotinamide roughly parallel dietary intake, but data generally do not agree well enough to predict either parameter from a measurement of the other.

The cost of surveys with their complex methodology often makes them prohibitive, particularly for smaller administrative units such as states or counties. Recently efforts have been made to use a few key tests and measurements that provide as much essential information as the more extensive studies now provide (Guthrie et al., 1973). Functional appraisals, as for example immune response, reproductive capability, productivity, and social competence have been suggested as indices of nutritional status. (See Solomons and Allen, 1983.) However, such research is only beginning and remains to be evaluated.

Summary

Surveys as currently conducted are valuable in grossly defining nutritional status. The investigator of population nutritional status always runs the risk of gathering data that cannot be adequately interpreted. Because the survey is limited both by current methodology and by the variability of population groups, interpretation of survey data should be made with recognition of the limitations of the procedures. Clearly there is a need for improved methodology for assessing nutritional status of population groups and for standardization of methods of evaluating survey data.

bibliography

Aasenden, R. and T. C. Peebles. Effects of fluoride supplementation from birth on human deciduous and permanent teeth. *Arch. Oral Biol.* 19:321–326 (1974).

Abdul-Nour, B. and G. C. Webster. Biological activity of reconstituted ribosomes. *Exp. Cell Res.* 20:226–227 (1960).

Abels, J. and R. F. Schilling. Protection of intrinsic factor by vitamin B_{12}. *J. Lab. Clin. Med.* 64:375–384 (1964).

Abels, J., J. J. M. Vegter, M. G. Woldring, J. H. Jans, and H. O. Nieweg. The physiologic mechanism of vitamin B_{12} absorption. *Acta Med. Scand.* 165:105–113 (1959).

Abraham, E. P. Experiments relating to the constitution of alloxazine-adenine-dinucleotide. *Biochem. J.* 33:543–548 (1939).

Ackers, G. K. Molecular sieve methods of analysis. In *The Proteins,* Vol. 1, pp. 1–94, H. Neurath and R. L. Hill, Eds., Academic Press, New York (1975).

Adams, C. *Nutritive Value of American Foods.* Agriculture Handbook No. 456, Agricultural Research Service, U.S. Department of Agriculture, Washington, D.C. (1975).

Adams, P. R. Molecular basis of synaptic transmission. *Trends Neurosci.* 1:14–17 (1978).

Addison, J. M., D. Burston, and D. M. Matthews. Evidence for active transport of the dipeptide glycylsarcosine by hamster jejunum *in vitro*. *Clin. Sci.* 43:907–911 (1972).

Adelson, S. Some problems in collecting dietary data from individuals. *J. Am. Diet. Assoc.* 36:453–461 (1960).

Adelstein, R. S. and E. Eisenberg. Regulation and kinetics of the actin-myosin-ATP interaction. *Ann. Rev. Biochem.* 49:921–956 (1980).

Adibi, S. A. Intestinal transport of dipeptides in man: relative importance of hydrolysis and intact absorption. *J. Clin. Invest.* 50:2266–2275 (1971).

Abidi, S. A. and S. J. Gray. Intestinal absorption of essential amino acids in man. *Gastroenterol.* 52:837–845 (1967).

Adibi, S. A. and Y. S. Kim. Peptide absorption and hydrolysis. In *Physiology of the Gastrointestinal Tract,* Vol. 2, pp. 1073–1095, Raven Press, New York (1981).

Adibi, S. A. and D. W. Mercer. Protein digestion in the human intestine as reflected in luminal, mucosal and plasma amino acid concentrations after meals. *J. Clin. Invest.* 52:1586–1594 (1973).

Adibi, S. A. and E. L. Morse. The number of glycine residues which limits intact absorption of glycine oligopeptides in human jejunum. *J. Clin. Invest.* 60:1008–1016 (1977).

Adibi, S. A., E. L. Morse, S. S. Masilamani, and P. M. Amin. Evidence for two different modes of tripeptide disappearance in human intestine. *J. Clin. Invest.* 56:1355–1363 (1975).

Adibi, S. A. and E. Phillips. Evidence for greater absorption of amino acids from peptide than from free form in human intestine. *Clin. Res.* 16:446. (1968).

Afzelius, B. A. The ultrastructure of the nuclear membrane of the sea urchin oocyte as studied with the electron microscope. *Exp. Cell Res.* 8:147–158 (1955).

Afzelius, B. A. The occurrence and structure of microbodies. A comparative study. *J. Cell Biol.* 26:835–843 (1965).

Aherne, W. and D. Hull. Brown adipose tissue and heat production in the new-born infant. *J. Pathol. Bacteriol.* 91:223–234 (1966).

Ahrens, E. H. Dietary fats and coronary heart disease: unfinished business. *Lancet* 2:1345–1348 (1979).

Ahrens, E. H., Jr., and W. E. Connor. Report of the task force on the evidence relating six dietary factors to the nation's health. (Symposium). *Am. J. Clin. Nutr.* 32:(Suppl)2621–2748 (1979).

Ahrens, H. and W. Korytnyk. Pyridoxine chemistry. XXI. Thin-layer chromatography and thin-layer electrophoresis of compounds in the vitamin B_6 group. *Anal. Biochem.* 30:413–420 (1969).

Aidley, D. J. *The Physiology of Excitable Cells,* 2nd ed., Liverpool University Press (1978).

Aikawa, J. *Magnesium: It's Biological Significance,* CRC Press, Boca Raton, Fla. (1981).

Aisen, P. The transferrins. In *Iron in Biochemistry and Medicine,* II, pp. 87–129, A. Jacobs and M. Worwood, Eds., Academic Press, London (1980).

Aisen, P. and E. Brown. The iron-binding function of transferrin in iron metabolism. *Semin. Hematol.* 14:31–53 (1977).

Akeson, W. R. and Stahman, M. A. A pepsin pancreatin digest index of protein quality evaluation. *J. Nutr.* 83:257–261 (1964).

Alam, S. Q. Inositols. IX. Biochemical systems. In *The Vitamins,* Vol. 3, pp. 380–394, W. H. Sebrell, Jr., and R. S. Harris, Eds., Academic Press, New York (1971).

Albright, F. and E. C. Reifenstein. *The Parathyroid Glands and Metabolic Bone Disease: Selected Studies,* Williams & Wilkins, Baltimore (1948).

Allen, D. W. and J. H. Jandl. Kinetics of intracellular iron in rabbit reticulocytes. *Blood* 15:71–81 (1960).

Allen, L. H. Calcium bioavailability and absorption: a review. *Am. J. Clin. Nutr.* 35:783–808 (1982).

Allen, T. M., E. C. Anderson, and W. H. Langham. Total body potassium and gross body composition. *J. Gerontol.* 15:348–357 (1960).

Alleyne, G. A. O., H. Flores, D. I. M. Picou, and J. C. Waterlow. Metabolic changes in children with protein-calorie malnutrtion. In *Nutrition and Development,* pp. 201–238, M. Winick, Ed., John Wiley & Sons, New York (1972).

Allfrey, V. G. Biosynthetic reactions in the cell nucleus. In *Aspects of Protein Biosynthesis,* Part A, pp. 247–365, C. B. Anfinsen, Jr., Ed., Academic Press, New York (1970).

Allfrey, V. G., V. C. Littau, and A. E. Mirsky. On the role of histones in regulating ribonucleic acid synthesis in the cell nucleus. *Proc. Nat. Acad. Sci.* 49:414–421 (1963).

Allgood, J. W. and E. B. Brown. The relationship between duodenal mucosal iron concentration and iron absorption in human subjects. *Scand. J. Haematol.* 4:217–229 (1967).

Allison, A. Lysosomes and disease. *Sci. Am.* 217(5):62–72 (1967).

Allison, J. B. Biological evaluation of protein. *Physiol. Rev.* 35:664–700 (1955).

Allison, J. B. Interpretation of nitrogen balance data. *Fed. Proc.* 10:676–683 (1957).

Allison, J. B. and J. A. Anderson. The relation between absorbed nitrogen, nitrogen balance and biological value of proteins in adult dogs. *J. Nutr.* 29:413–442 (1945).

Allison, J. B., R. W. Wannemacher, Jr., and W. L. Banks, Jr. Influence of dietary proteins on protein biosynthesis in various tissues. *Fed. Proc.* 22:1126–1130 (1963).

Aloia, J. F., S. H. Cohn, T. Babu, C. Abesamis, N. Kalici, and K. Ellis. Skeletal mass and body composition in marathon runners. *Metabolism* 27:1793–1796 (1978).

Altman, P. L. and D. S. Dittmer, Eds., *Biology Data Book,* Federation of American Societies for Experimental Biology, Washington, D.C. (1964).

Altman, P. L. and D. D. Katz, Eds., *Cell Biology Handbook,* Federation of American Societies for Experimental Biology, Bethesda, Md. (1976).

Altura, B. M. Role of magnesium ions in regulation of muscle contraction (Symposium). *Fed. Proc.* 40:2645–2679 (1981).

Alvarado, F. and R. K. Crane. Phlorizin as a competitive inhibitor of the active transport of sugars by hamster small intestine *in vitro. Biochim. Biophys. Acta* 56:170–172 (1962).

American Academy of Pediatrics Committee on Nutrition. The prophylactic requirement and the toxicity of vitamin D. *Pediatr.* 31:512–513 (1963).

American Academy of Pediatrics Committee on Nutrition. Vitamin D intake and the hypercalcemic syndrome. *Pediatr.* 35:1022–1023 (1965).

American Health Foundation. E. L. Wynder, Conf. Chairman. *Plasma Lipids: Optimal Levels for Health,* Academic Press, New York (1980).

American Medical Association Council on Foods and Nutrition. Symposium on human calcium requirements. *JAMA* 185:588–593 (1963).

Ames, S. R. Factors affecting absorption, transport and storage of vitamin A. *Am. J. Clin. Nutr.* 22:934–935 (1969).

Amos, W. H., Jr., and R. A. Neal. Isolation and identification of 3-(2′-methyl-4′-5′-pyrimidylmethyl)-4-methylthiazole-5-acetic acid (thiamine acetic acid) and 2-methyl-4-amino-5-formylaminomethylpyrimidine as metabolites of thiamine in the rat. *J. Biol. Chem.* 245:5643–5648 (1970).

Anand, B. S., S. T. Callender, and J. Skinner. A study of mucosal ferritin and transferrin. *Br. J. Haematol.* 33:609 (1976).

Anderson, E. C. and W. H. Langham. Average potassium concentration of the human body as a function of age. *Science* 130:713–714 (1959).

Anderson, J. W. Dietary fiber and diabetes. In *Medical Aspects of Dietary Fiber*, pp. 193–221, G. A. Spiller and R. M. Kay, Eds., Plenum, New York (1980).

Anderson, R. E., H. Schraer, and C. V. Gay. Ultrastructural immunocytochemical localization of carbonic anhydrase in normal and calcitonin-treated chick osteoclasts. *Anat. Rec.* 204:9–20 (1982).

Anderson, T. W., D. B. W. Reid, and G. H. Beaton. Vitamin C and the common cold: a double-blind trial. *Can. Med. Assoc. J.* 107:503–508 (1972).

Anderssen, B. Thirst and brain control of water balance. *Am. Sci.* 59:408–415 (1971).

Anderssen, B., M. F. Dallman, and K. Olsson. Observations on central control of drinking and of the release of antidiuretic hormone (ADH). *Life Sci.* 8:425–432 (1969).

Anderssen, B., L. G. Leksell, and M. Rundgren. Regulation of water intake. *Ann. Rev. Nutr.* 2:73–89 (1982).

Anderssen, B., K. Olsson, and R. G. Warner. Dissimilarities between the central control of thirst and the release of antidiuretic hormone (ADH). *Acta Physiol. Scand.* 71:57–64 (1967).

Anderssen, S. Gastric and duodenal mechanisms inhibiting gastric secretion of acid. In *Handbook of Physiology*, Section 6: Alimentary Canal, Vol. 2, pp. 865–877, C. F. Code, Ed., American Physiological Society, Washington, D.C. (1967).

Andre, J. and V. Marinozzi. Presence dans les mitochondries de particules ressemblant aux ribosomes. *J. Microscopie* 4:615–626 (1965).

Anfinsen, C. B. and H. Scheraga. Experimental and theoretical aspects of protein folding. *Adv. Protein Chem.* 29:205–316 (1975).

Angier, R. B., J. H. Boothe, B. L. Hutchings, J. H. Mowat, J. Semb, E. L. R. Stokstad, Y. SubbaRow, C. W. Waller, D. B. Consulich, M. J. Fahrenback, M. E. Hultquist, E. Kuh, E. H. Northey, D. R. Seeger, J. P. Sickels, and J. M. Smith, Jr. The structure and synthesis of the liver L. casei factor. *Science* 103:667–669 (1946).

Anning, S. T., J. Dawson, D. E. Dolby, and J. T. Ingram. The toxic effects of calciferol. *Q. J. Med.* 17:203–228 (1948).

Antonson, D. L., A. J. Barak, and J. A. Vanderhoof. Determination of the site of zinc absorption in rat small intestine. *J. Nutr.* 109:142–147 (1979).

Antony, A. C., C. Utley, K. C. Van Horne, and J. F. Kolhouse. Isolation and characterization of a folate receptor from human placenta. *J. Biol. Chem.* 256:9684–9692 (1981).

Apte, S. V. and L. Lyengar. Absorption of dietary iron in pregnancy. *Am. J. Clin. Nutr.* 23:73–77 (1969).

Apte, S. V. and L. Lyengar. Composition of the human foetus. *Br. J. Nutr.* 27:305–312 (1972).

Archer, M. C. Hazards of nitrate, nitrite, and N-nitroso compounds in human nutrition. In *Nutritional Toxicology,* Vol. 1, pp. 328–381 J. N. Hathcock, Ed., Academic Press, New York, 1982.

Arens, J. F. and D. A. van Dorp. Synthesis of some compounds possessing vitamin A activity. *Nature* 157:190–191 (1946).

Ariaey-Nejad, M. R., M. Balaghi, E. M. Baker, and II. E. Sauberlich. Thiamin metabolism in man. *Am. J. Clin. Nutr.* 23:764–778 (1970).

Arnesjo, B., A. Nilsson, J. Barrowman, and B. Borgström. Intestinal digestion and absorption of cholesterol and lecithin in the human. *Scand. J. Gastroenterol.* 4:653–665 (1969).

Arora, R. B. and C. N. Mathur. Relationship between structure and anticoagulant activity of coumarin derivatives. *Br. J. Pharmacol.* 20:29–35 (1963).

Arroyave, G. The estimation of relative nutrient intake and nutritional status by biochemical methods: proteins. *Am. J. Clin. Nutr.* 11:447–461 (1962).

Arroyave, G. Comparative sensitivity of specific amino acid ratios versus "essential to nonessential" amino acid ratio. *Am. J. Clin. Nutr.* 23:703–706 (1970).

Arroyave, G., F. Viteri, M. Béhar, and N. S. Scrimshaw. Impairment of intestinal absorption of vitamin A palmitate in severe protein malnutrition (kwashiorkor). *Am. J. Clin. Nutr.* 7:185–190 (1959).

Asatoor, A. M., A. K. Chadha, I. M. P. Dawson, M. D. Milne, and D. I. Prosser. The effect of pyridoxine deficiency on intestinal absorption of amino acids and peptides in the rat. *Br. J. Nutr.* 28:417–423 (1972).

Asatoor, A. M., B. Cheng, K. D. G. Edwards, A. F. Lant, D. M. Matthews, M. D. Milne, F. Navab, and A. J. Richards. Intestinal absorption of two dipeptides in Hartnup disease. *Gut* 11:380–389 (1970).

Asatoor, A. M., M. R. Crouchman, A. R. Harrison, F. W. Light, L. W. Loughridge, M. D. Milne, and A. J. Richards. Intestinal absorption of oligopeptides in cystinuria. *Clin. Sci.* 41:23–33 (1971).

Asatoor, A. M., B. W. Lacey, D. R. London, and M. D. Milne. Aminoacid metabolism in cystinuria. *Clin. Sci.* 23:285–304 (1962).

Aspin, N. and A. Sass-Kortsak. Copper. In *Disorders of Mineral Metabolism,* Vol

1, pp. 60–92, F. Bronner and J. Coburn, Eds., Academic Press, New York (1981).

Asquith, R. E., Ed., *Chemistry of natural protein fibers,* Plenum, New York and London (1977).

Association of Official Agricultural Chemists. *Official Methods of Analysis,* Collegiate Press, George Banta Co., Inc., Menasha, Wis. (1960).

Association of Official Analytical Chemists. *Official Methods of Analysis,* AOAC, Arlington, Va. (1980).

Association of Vitamin Chemists, Inc. *Methods of Vitamin Assay,* 3rd ed., Interscience Pub., Inc., New York (1966).

Ast, D. B., D. J. Smith, B. Wachs, and K. T. Cantwell. Newburgh-Kingston caries fluorine study. XIV. Combined clinical and roentgenographic dental findings after ten years of fluoride experience. *J. Am. Dent. Assoc.* 52:290–325 (1956).

Astaldi, G., G. Meardi, and T. Libino. The iron content of jejunal mucosa obtained by Crosby's biopsy in hemochromatosis and hemosiderosis. *Blood* 28:70–82 (1966).

Atwater, W. O. and F. G. Benedict. *Off. Exp. Stns. Bull.* No. 109, U.S. Department of Agriculture, Washington, D.C. (1902).

Atwater, W. O. and A. P. Bryant. The availability and fuel value of food materials. *Storrs Agr. Ext. Sta. Ann. Rept.,* pp. 73–110 (1899).

Atwater, W. O. and E. B. Rosa. Description of new respiration calorimeter and experiments on the conservation of energy in the human body. *Off. Exp. Sta. Bull.* No. 63, U.S. Department of Agriculture, Washington, D.C. (1899).

Atwater, W. O. and J. F. Snell. Description of a bomb calorimeter and method of its use. *J. Am. Chem. Soc.* 25:659–699 (1903).

Auerbach, C. The chemical production of mutations. *Science* 158:1141–1147 (1967).

Aukland, K. and G. Nicolaysen. Interstitial fluid volume: local regulatory mechanisms. *Physiol. Rev.* 61:556–643 (1981).

Aurbach, G. D. and L. R. Chase. Cyclic 3', 5'-adenylic acid in bone and the mechanism of action of parathyroid hormone. *Fed. Proc.* 29:1179–1182 (1970).

Aurbach, G. D., R. Marcus, J. Heersche, and S. Marx. Hormones and other factors regulating calcium metabolism. *Ann. N. Y. Acad. Sci.* 185:386–394 (1971).

Aurbach, G. D., S. J. Marx, and A. M. Spiegel. Parathyroid hormone, calcitonin, and the calciferols. In *Textbook of Endocrinology,* pp. 922–1031, R. H. Williams, Ed., W. B. Saunders Co., 6th ed., Philadelphia and London (1981).

Avioli, L. V. Current concepts of vitamin D_3 metabolism in man. In *The Fat-Soluble Vitamins,* pp. 159–172, H. F. DeLuca and J. W. Suttie, Eds., University of Wisconsin Press, Madison (1970).

Avioli, L. V. Major minerals. In *Modern Nutrition in Health and Disease,* 6th ed., pp. 294–309, R. Goodhart and M. Shils, Eds., Lea & Febiger, Philadelphia (1980).

Avruch, J., J. R. Carter, and D. B. Martin. The effect of insulin on the metabolism of adipose tissue. In *Handbook of Physiology*, Section 7, Vol. 1, pp. 545–562, R. O. Greep and E. B. Astwood, Eds., American Physiological Society, Washington, D.C. (1972).

Axelrod, J. Noradrenaline: rate and control of its biosynthesis. *Science* 173:598–606 (1971).

Axelrod, J. Dopamine-β-hydroxylase: regulation of its synthesis and release from nerve terminals. *Pharmacol. Rev.* 24:233–243 (1972).

Axelrod, J. Neurotransmitters. *Sci. Am.* 230(6):58–71 (1974).

Babcock, M. J., M. Brush, and E. Sostman. Evaluation of vitamin B_6 nutrition. *J. Nutr.* 70:369–376 (1960).

Bach, A. C. and V. I. Babayan. Medium-chain triglycerides: an update. *Am. J. Clin. Nutr.* 36:950–962 (1982).

Bai, P., M. Bennion, and C. J. Gubler. Biochemical factors involved in the anorexia of thiamin deficiency in rats. *J. Nutr.* 101:731–738 (1971).

Bailey, A. J. and D. J. Etherington. Metablism of collagen and elastin. In *Comprehensive Biochemistry*, pp. 299–460, M. Florkin, Ed., Elsevier Scientific Publishing Co., Amsterdam and New York (1980).

Baker, E. M., III, D. C. Hammer, S. C. March, B. M. Tolbert, and J. E. Canham. Ascorbate sulfate: a urinary metabolite of ascorbic acid in man. *Science* 173:826–827 (1971a).

Baker, E. M., R. E. Hodges, J. Hood, H. E. Sauberlich, S. March, and J. E. Canham. Metabolism of ^{14}C- and ^3H-labeled L-ascorbic acid in human scurvy. *Am. J. Clin. Nutr.* 24:444–454 (1971b).

Baker, E. M., J. C. Saari, and B. M. Tolbert. Ascorbic acid metabolism in man. *Am. J. Clin. Nutr.* 19:371–378 (1966).

Baker, H. and O. Frank. *Clinical Vitaminology*, Interscience Pub., Inc., New York (1968).

Baker, H., O. Frank, S. Feingold, G. Christakis, and H. Ziffer. Vitamins, total cholesterol, and triglycerides in 642 New York City school children. *Am. J. Clin. Nutr.* 20:850–857 (1967).

Baker, H., O. Frank, J. J. Fennelly, and C. M. Leevy. A method for assaying thiamine status in man and animals. *Am. J. Clin. Nutr.* 14:197–201 (1964).

Baker, H., O. Frank, V. B. Matovitch, I. Pasher, S. Aaronson, S. H. Hunter, and H. Sobotka. A new assay method for biotin in blood, serum, urine, and tissues. *Anal. Biochem.* 3:31–39 (1962).

Baker, H., H. Ziffer, I. Pasher, and H. Sobotka. A comparison of maternal foetal folic acid and vitamin B_{12} at parturition. *Br. Med. J.* 1:978–979 (1958).

Baker, P. E. The nerve axon. *Sci. Am.* 214(3):74–82 (1966).

Baker, R. D. and G. W. Searle. Bile salt absorption at various levels of rat small intestine. *Proc. Soc. Exp. Biol. Med.* 105:512–521 (1960).

Balaghi, M. and W. N. Pearson. Metabolism of physiological doses of thiazole-2-^{14}C-labeled thiamine by the rat. *J. Nutr.* 89:265–270 (1966).

Balazs, E. A. *Chemistry and Molecular Biology of the Intercellular Matrix*, Vol. 2, *Glycosaminoglycans and proteoglycans*, Academic Press, New York (1970).

Balcerzak, S. P. and N. J. Greenberger. Iron content of isolated intestinal epithelial cells in relation to iron absorption. *Nature* 220:270–271 (1968).

Baldwin, S. A. and G. E. Lienhard. Glucose transport across plasma membranes: facilitated diffusion systems: *Trends Biochem. Sci.* 6:208–211 (1981).

Ballard, F. J. and J. M. Gunn. Nutritional and hormonal effects on intracellular protein catabolism. *Nutr. Rev.* 40:33–42 (1982).

Balnave, D. Clinical symptoms of biotin deficiency in animals. *Am. J. Clin. Nutr.* 30:1408–1413 (1977).

Balogh, M., H. A. Kahn, and J. H. Medalie. Random repeat 24-hour dietary recalls. *Am. J. Clin. Nutr.* 24:304–310 (1971).

Barchi, R. L., S. A. Cohen, and L. E. Murphy. Purification from rat sarcolemma of the saxitoxin-binding component of the excitable membrane sodium channel. *Proc. Nat. Acad. Sci. U. S.* 77:1306–1310 (1980).

Barclay, L. L., B. E. Gibson, and J. P. Blass. Cholinergic therapy of abnormal open-field behavior in thiamin-deficient rats. *J. Nutr.* 112:1906–1913 (1982).

Bard, H. Postnatal fetal and adult hemoglobin synthesis in early preterm newborn infants. *J. Clin. Invest.* 52:1789–1795 (1973).

Barer, R., S. Joseph, and G. A. Meek. The origin of the nuclear membrane. *Exp. Cell Res.* 18:179–182 (1959).

Barker, H. A., H. Weissbach, and R. D. Smyth. A coenzyme containing pseudo-vitamin B_{12}. *Proc. Nat. Acad. Sci. U. S.* 44:1093–1097 (1958).

Barnes, M. J. Ascorbic acid and the biosynthesis of collagen and elastin. *Bibl. Nutr. Dieta* 13:86–98 (1969).

Barnes, M. J. Function of ascorbic acid in collagen metabolism. *Ann. N. Y. Acad. Sci.* 258:264–277 (1975).

Barnes, R. H. Experimental animal approaches to the study of early malnutrition and mental development. *Fed. Proc.* 26:144–147 (1967).

Barnes, R. H., S. R. Cunnold, R. R. Zimmerman, H. Simmons, R. B. McLeon, and L. Krook. Influence of nutritional deprivations in early life on learning behavior of rats as measured by performance in a water maze. *J. Nutr.* 89:399–410 (1966).

Barnes, R. H., G. Fiala, and E. Kwong. Decreased growth rate resulting from prevention of coprophagy. *Fed. Proc.* 22:125–128 (1963).

Barnett, W. E. and D. H. Brown. Mitochondrial transfer ribonucleic acids. *Proc. Nat. Acad. Sci. U. S.* 57:452–458 (1967).

Barnett, W. E., D. H. Brown, and J. Epler. Mitochondrial-specific amino-acyl-RNA synthetases. *Proc. Nat. Acad. Sci. U. S.* 57:1775–1781 (1967).

Barnett, W. E. and J. L. Epler. Fractionation and specificities of two aspartyl-ribonucleic acid and two phenylalanyl-ribonucleic acid synthetases. *Proc. Nat. Acad. Sci. U. S.* 55:184–189 (1966).

Barondes, S. H. and M. W. Nirenberg. Fate of a synthetic polynucleotide directing cell-free protein synthesis. II. Association with ribosomes. *Science* 138:813–817 (1962).

Barter, J. and G. B. Forbes. Correlation of potassium-40 data with anthropometric measurements. *Ann. N. Y. Acad. Sci.* 110:264–270 (1963).

Baudhuin, P., H. Beaufay, and C. DeDuve. Combined biochemical and morphological study of particulate fractions from rat liver. *J. Cell Biol.* 26:219–243 (1965).

Bauer, G. C. H., A. Carlsson, and B. Lindquist. Metabolism and homeostatic function of bone. In *Mineral Metabolism,* Vol. 1, Part B, pp. 609–676, C. L. Comar and F. Bronner, Eds., Academic Press, New York (1961).

Baugh, C. M. and C. L. Krumdieck. Naturally occurring folates. *Ann. N. Y. Acad. Sci.* 186:7–28 (1971).

Baugh, C. M., C. L. Krumdieck, H. J. Baker, and C. E. Butterworth, Jr. Studies on the absorption and metabolism of folic acid. I. Folate absorption in the dog after exposure of isolated intestinal segments to synthetic pteroylpolyglutamates of various chain lengths. *J. Clin. Invest.* 50:2009–2021 (1971).

Baugh, C. M., J. H. Malone, and C. E. Butterworth, Jr. Human biotin deficiency. A case history of biotin deficiency induced by raw egg consumption in a cirrhotic patient. *Am. J. Clin. Nutr.* 21:173–182 (1968).

Baxter, J. H. Origins and characteristics of endogenous lipid in thoracic duct lymph in rat. *J. Lipid Res.* 7:158–166 (1966).

Baxter, R. Origin and continuity of mitochondria. In *Origin and Continuity of Cell Organelles,* pp. 46–64, J. Reinert and H. Ursprung, Eds., Springer-Verlag, New York (1971).

Bayless, T. M. and N. S. Rosensweig. A racial difference in incidence of lactase deficiency. *JAMA* 197:968–972 (1966).

Bayless, W. M. and E. H. Starling. The mechanism of pancreatic secretion. *J. Physiol.* (London) 28:325–353 (1902).

Beams, H. W. and R. G. Kessel. The Golgi apparatus: structure and function. *Int. Rev. Cytol.* 23:209–276 (1968).

Bean, W. B. Some aspects of pharmacologic use and abuse of water-soluble vitamins. In *Nutrition and Drug Interrelations,* pp. 667–685, J. N. Hathcock and J. Coon, Eds., Academic Press, New York (1978).

Bean, W. B. and R. E. Hodges. Pantothenic acid deficiency induced in human subjects. *Proc. Soc. Exp. Biol. Med.* 86:693–698 (1954).

Beare-Rogers, J. L. Time sequence of liver phospholipid alterations during deprivation of dietary choline. *Can. J. Physiol. Pharmacol.* 49:171–177 (1971).

Beaton, G. H. Urea formation in the pregnant rat. *Arch. Biochem. Biophys.* 67:1–9 (1957).

Beaton, G. H. Nutritional and physiological adaptations in pregnancy. *Fed. Proc.* 20: (Part 3, Suppl. No. 7)196–201 (1961).

Beaton, G. H. The use of nutritional requirements and allowances. In *Proceedings Western Hemisphere Nutrition Congress 3*, pp. 356–363, Futura Publishing Co., Mount Kisco, N.Y. (1971).

Beaton, G. H., D. H. Calloway, and J. Waterlow. Protein and energy requirements: a joint FAO/WHO memorandum. *Bull. WHO.* 57:65–79 (1979).

Beaton, G. H. and N. A. Fernandez. The use of nutritional requirements and allowances. In *Proceedings Western Hemisphere Nutrition Congress 2*, pp. 356–363, Futura Publishing Co., Mount Kisco, N.Y. (1972).

Beaton, G. H., M. H. Ryu, and E. W. McHenry. Studies on the role of growth hormone in pregnancy. *Endocrinology* 57:748–754 (1955).

Beattie, D. S. The synthesis of mitochondrial proteins. *Subcell. Biochem.* 1:1–23 (1971).

Beck, F. and J. B. Lloyd. Histochemistry and electron microscopy of lysosomes. In *Lysosomes in Biology and Pathology*, Vol. 2, pp. 567–599, J. T. Dingle and H. B. Fell, Eds., Wiley-Interscience, New York (1969).

Beck, W. S. Deoxyribonucleotide synthesis and the role of vitamin B_{12} in erythropoiesis. *Vitam. Horm.* 26:413–442 (1968).

Bédard, Y. C., P. H. Pinkerton, and G. T. Simon. Radioautographic observations on iron absorption by the normal mouse duodenum. *Blood* 38:232–245 (1971).

Beermann, W. and U. Clever. Chromosome puffs. *Sci. Am.* 210(4):50–58 (1964).

Beg, Z. H., J. A. Stonik, and H. B. Brewer, Jr. 3-Hydroxy-3-methyl-glutaryl coenzyme A reductase. Regulation of enzymatic activity by phosphorylation and dephosphorylation. *Proc. Nat. Acad. Sci. U. S.* 75:3678–3682 (1978).

Behar, M. Appraisal of the nutritional status of population groups. In *Nutrition in Preventive Medicine*, pp. 556–575, G. H. Beaton and J. M. Bengoa, Eds., WHO Monograph Series No. 62 (1976).

Behar, M., F. Viteri, R. Bressani, G. Arroyave, R. L. Squibb, and N. S. Scrimshaw. Principles of treatment and prevention of severe protein malnutrition in children (kwashiorkor). *Ann. N. Y. Acad. Sci.* 69:954–968 (1959).

Behnke, A. R. Fat content and composition of the body. *Harvey Lect.* 37:198–226 (1941–42).

Behnke, A. R. The relation of lean body weight to metabolism and some consequent systematizations. *Ann. N. Y. Acad. Sci.* 56:1095–1142 (1953).

Behnke, A. R. Anthropometric evaluation of body composition throughout life. *Ann. N. Y. Acad. Sci.* 110:450–464 (1963).

Behnke, A. R., B. G. Feen, and W. C. Welham. The specific gravity of healthy men. *JAMA* 118:495–498 (1942).

Beiler, J. M., J. N. Moss, and G. J. Martin. Formation of a competitive antagonist of vitamin B_{12} by oxidation. *Science* 114:122–123 (1951).

Bell, P. H., W. F. Barg, Jr., D. F. Colucci, M. C. Davies, C. Dziobkowski, M. E. Englert, E. Heyder, R. Paul, and E. H. Snedeker. Purification and structure of porcine calcitonin-1. *J. Am. Chem. Soc.* 90:2704–2706 (1968).

Bell, R. R., H. H. Draper, and J. G. Bergan. Sucrose, lactose, and glucose tolerance in northern Alaskan Eskimos. *Am. J. Clin. Nutr.* 26:1185–1190 (1973).

Bemis, J. A., G. M. Bryant, J. C. Arcos, and M. I. Argus. Swelling and contraction of mitochondrial particles: a reexamination of the existence of a contractile protein extractable with 0.6 M-potassium chloride. *J. Mol. Biol.* 33:299–307 (1968).

Bender, A. E. Determination of nutritive value of proteins by chemical analysis. In *Progress in meeting protein needs of infants and preschool children,* National Academy of Sciences, Pub. 843, pp. 407–424, L. Voris, Ed., National Research Council, Washington, D.C. (1961).

Bender, A. E. and B. H. Doell. Note on the determination of net protein utilization by carcass analysis. *Br. J. Nutr.* 11:138–143 (1957).

Bender, A. E. and D. S. Miller. A new brief method of estimating net protein value. *Biochem. J.* 53:vii (1953).

Benditt, E. P., E. M. Humphreys, R. W. Wissler, C. H. Steffee, L. E. Frazier, and P. R. Cannon. The dynamics of protein metabolism. I. The interrelationship between protein and caloric intakes and their influence upon the utilization of ingested protein for tissue synthesis by the adult protein-depleted rat. *J. Lab. Clin. Med.* 33:257–268 (1948).

Benedict, F. G. *A study of prolonged fasting.* Carnegie Institute of Washington Pub. No. 203 (1915).

Benedict, F. G. and T. M. Carpenter. *The metabolism and energy transformations of healthy men during rest.* Carnegie Institute of Washington Pub. No. 126 (1910).

Benedict, F. G. and T. M. Carpenter. *Food ingestion and energy transformations with special reference to the stimulating effect of nutrients.* Carnegie Institute of Washington Pub. No. 261 (1918).

Benedict, F. G. and E. P. Cathcart. *Muscular work. (A metabolic study with special reference to the efficiency of the human body as a machine.)* Carnegie Institute of Washington Pub. No. 187 (1913).

Benjamin, H. R., H. H. Gordon, and E. Marples. Calcium and phosphorus requirements of premature infants *Am. J. Dis. Child.* 65:412–425 (1943).

Benjamins, J. A. and P. Morell. Proteins of myelin and their metabolism. *Neurochem. Res.* 3:137–174 (1978).

Bennett, E. L., M. R. Rosenzweig, and M. C. Diamond. Rat brain: effects of environment enrichment on wet and dry weights. *Science* 163:825–826 (1969).

Bennett, G. Migration of glycoprotein from Golgi apparatus to cell coat in the columnar cells of the duodenal epithelium. *J. Cell Biol.* 45:668–673 (1970).

Bennett, G. and C. P. Leblond. Formation of cell coat material for the whole surface of columnar cells in the rat small intestine, as visualized by radioautography with L-fucose-^{3}H. *J. Cell Biol.* 46:409–416 (1970).

Benson, A. A. On the orientation of lipids in chloroplast and cell membranes. *J. Am. Oil Chem. Soc.* 43:265–270 (1966).

Benzinger, T. H. and C. Kitzinger. Direct calorimetry by means of the gradient principle. *Rev. Sci. Instrum.* 20:849–860 (1949).

Benzonana, G., B. Entressangles, G. Marchis-Mouren, L. Pasero, L. Sarda, and P. Desnuelle. Further studies on pig pancreatic lipase. In *Metabolism and Physiological Significance of Lipids,* pp. 141–154, R. M. C. Dawson and D. N. Rhodes, Eds., John Wiley & Sons, New York (1964).

Berendes, H. D. Factors involved in the expression of gene activity in polytene chromosomes. *Chromosoma* 24:418–437 (1968).

Beresford, C. H., R. J. Neale, and O. G. Brooks. Iron absorption and pyrexia. *Lancet* 1:568–575 (1971).

Berg, P. and E. J. Ofengand. An enzymatic mechanism for linking amino acids to RNA. *Proc. Nat. Acad. Sci. U. S.* 44:78–86 (1958).

Berger, E. Y. Intestinal absorption and excretion. In *Mineral Metabolism,* Vol. 1, Part A, pp. 249–286, C. L. Comar and F. Bronner, Eds., Academic Press, New York (1960).

Bergström, S., H. Danielsson, and B. Samuelsson. The enzymatic formation of prostaglandin E_2 from arachidonic acid. Prostaglandins and related factors 32. *Biochim. Biophys. Acta* 90:207–210 (1964).

Bergström, S., R. Ryhage, B. Samuelsson, and J. Sjövall. The structure of prostaglandin E, F, and F_2. *Acta Chem. Scand.* 16:501–502 (1962).

Berk, P. D., R. B. Howe, J. R. Bloomer, and N. I. Berlin. The life span of the red cell as determined with labeled bilirubin. In *Formation and Destruction of Blood Cells,* pp. 91–107, T. J. Greenwalt and G. A. Jamieson, Eds., J. B. Lippincott, Philadelphia (1970).

Berl, S., S. Puszkin, and W. J. Nicklas. Actomyosin-like protein in the brain. *Science* 179:441–446 (1973).

Berlin, J. D. The localization of acid mucopolysaccharides in the Golgi complex of intestinal goblet cells. *J. Cell Biol.* 32:760–766 (1967).

Bernard, C. (1878a), *Leçons sur les phénomènes de la vie communs aux animaux et aux végétaux,* p. 121, Bailliere, Paris. Cited by H. Rahn in *Claude Bernard and the Internal Environment,* p. 179, E. D. Robin, Ed., Marcel Dekker Inc., New York (1979).

Bernard, C. (1878b). In *Selected Readings in the History of Physiology,* 2nd ed., p. 326, J. F. Fulton, Ed., Charles C. Thomas, Springfield, Ill., (1966).

Bernard, R. A. and B. P. Halpern. Taste changes in vitamin A deficiency. *J. Gen. Physiol.* 52:444–464 (1968).

Bernhard, W. and N. Granboulan. Electron microscopy of the nucleolus in vertebrate cells. In *The Nucleus,* Vol. 3, *Ultrastructure in Biological Systems,* pp. 81–149, A. J. Dalton and C. Haguenau, Eds., Academic Press, New York (1968).

Bernstein, D. S., N. Sadowsky, D. M. Hegsted, C. D. Guri, and F. J. Stare. Prevalence of osteoporosis in high- and low-fluoride areas in North Dakota. *JAMA* 198:499–504 (1966).

Bernstein, L. H., S. Gutstein, S. Weiner, and G. Efron. The absorption and mal-absorption of folic acid and its polyglutamates. *Am. J. Med.* 48:570–579 (1970).

Berry, H. K. Hereditary disorders of amino acid metabolism associated with mental deficiency. *Ann. N. Y. Acad. Sci.* 66–73 (1969).

Bertles, J. F. The occurrence and significance of fetal hemoglobins. In *Regulation of Hematopoiesis*, Vol. 1, pp. 731–765, A. S. Gordon, Ed., Appleton-Century-Crofts, New York (1970).

Bertrand, H. A., T. T. Lynd, E. J. Masoro, and B. P. Yu. Changes in adipose mass and cellularity through the adult life of rats fed ad libitum or a life-promoting restricted diet. *J. Gerontol.* 35:835–872 (1980).

Bessey, O. A., M. K. Horwitt, and R. H. Love. Dietary deprivation of riboflavin and blood riboflavin levels in man. *J. Nutr.* 58:367–383 (1956).

Bessis, M. The blood cells and their formation. In *The Cell*, Vol. 5, pp. 163–217, J. Brachet and A. E. Mirsky, Eds., Academic Press, New York (1961).

Best, C. H. and M. E. Huntsman. The effects of the components of lecithine upon deposition of fat in the liver. *J. Physiol.* (London) 75:405–412 (1932).

Bhatnagar, R. S., S. S. R. Rapaka, T. Z. Liu, and S. M. Wolfe. Hydralazine-induced disturbances in collagen biosynthesis. *Biochim. Biophys. Acta* 271:125–132 (1972).

Bhattacharyya, M. H. and H. F. DeLuca. The regulation of rat liver calciferol-25-hydroxylase. *J. Biol. Chem.* 218:2969–2973 (1973).

Bhattathiry, E. P. M. and M. D. Siperstein. Feedback control of cholesterol synthesis in man. *J. Clin. Invest.* 42:1613–1618 (1963).

Bianchi, C. P. and S. Narayan. Muscle fatigue and the role of transverse tubules. *Science* 215:295–296 (1982).

Bidder, F. and C. Schmidt. *Die Verdauungssaefte und der Stoffwechsel.* pp. 333–339, Mitau, Leipzig (1852).

Bie, P. Osmoreceptors, vasopressin, and control of renal water excretion. *Physiol. Rev.* 60:961–1048 (1980).

Biehl, J. P. and R. W. Vilter. Effects of isoniazid on pyridoxine metabolism. *JAMA* 156:1549–1552 (1954).

Bier, D. M. Stable isotope methods for nutritional diagnosis and research. *Nutr. Rev.* 40:129–134 (1982).

Bieri, J. G. Chromatography of tocopherols. In *Lipid Chromatographic Analysis*, Vol. 2, pp. 459–478, G. V. Marinetti, Ed., Marcel Dekker Inc., New York (1969).

Bieri, J. G. Biological activity and metabolism of N-substituted tocopheramines: implications on vitamin E function. In *The Fat-Soluble Vitamins*, pp. 307–316, H. F. DeLuca and J. W. Suttie, Eds., University of Wisconsin Press, Madison (1970).

Bieri, J. G. and P. M. Farrell. Vitamin E. *Vitam. Horm.* 34:31–75 (1976).

Bieri, J. G., E. G. McDaniel, and W. E. Rogers, Jr. Survival of germfree rats without vitamin A. *Science* 163:574–575 (1969).

Bieri, J. G. and M. C. McKenna. Expressing dietary values for fat-soluble vitamins: changes in concepts and terminology. *Am. J. Clin. Nutr.* 34:289–295 (1981).

Bieri, J. G., T. J. Tolliver, and G. L. Catignanl. Simultaneous determination of α-tocopherol and retinol in plasma or red cells by high pressure liquid chromatography. *Am. J. Clin. Nutr.* 32:2143–2149 (1979).

Bigler, W. N. and D. M. Kelly. Liquid chromatographic analysis of ascorbate and ascorbate-2-sulfate. *Ann. N. Y. Acad. Sci.* 258:70–71 (1975).

Bigwood, E. J. *Guiding principles for studies on the nutrition of populations.* League of Nations Health Organization, Geneva (March 1939).

Bihler, I. and R. K. Crane. Studies on the mechanism of intestinal absorption of sugars. V. The influence of several cations and anions on the active transport of sugars, *in vitro,* by various preparations of hamster small intestine. *Biochim. Biophys. Acta* 59:78–93 (1962).

Bikle, D. B., R. L. Morrissey, and D. T. Zolock. The mechanism of action of vitamin D in the intestine. *Am. J. Clin. Nutr.* 32:2322–2338 (1979).

Binder, H. J., D. C. Herting, V. Hurst, S. C. Finch, and H. M. Spiro. Tocopherol deficiency in man. *N. Eng. J. Med.* 273:1289–1297 (1965).

Bird, O. D., E. L. Wittle, R. Q. Thompson, and V. M. McGlohon. Pantothenic acid antagonists. *Am. J. Clin. Nutr.* 3:298–304 (1955).

Birge, S. J., W. A. Peck, M. Berman, and G. P. Whedon. Study of calcium absorption in man. A kinetic analysis and physiologic model. *J. Clin. Invest.* 48:1705–1713 (1969).

Birks, R. I. The role of sodium ions in the metabolism of acetylcholine. *Can. J. Biochem. Physiol.* 41:2573–2597 (1963).

Birks, R. and F. C. MacIntosh. Acetylcholine metabolism of a sympathetic ganglion. *Can. J. Biochem. Physiol.* 39:787–827 (1961).

Birnstiel, M. L., M. I. H. Chipchase, and W. G. Flamm. On the chemistry and organization of nucleolar proteins. *Biochim. Biophys. Acta* 87:111–122 (1964).

Bischoff, T. L. W. and C. Voit. *Die Gesetze der Ernährung des Fleischfressers,* Winter, Leipzig (1860).

Bisswanger, H. and E. Schmincke-Ott, Eds., *Multifunctional proteins,* Wiley-Interscience, New York (1980).

Bito, L. Z. Blood-brain barrier: evidence for active cation transport between blood and the extracellular fluid of brain. *Science* 165:81–83 (1969).

Bizzi, A., E. Veneroni, S. Garattini, L. Puglisi, and R. Paoletti. Hypersensitivity to lipid mobilizing agents in essential fatty acid (EFA) deficient rats. *Eur. J. Pharmacol.* 2:48–52 (1967).

Björn-Rasmussen, E. Iron absorption from wheat bread. *Nutr. Metab.* 16:101–110 (1974).

Björn-Rasmussen, E., L. Hallberg, B. Isaksson, and B. Arvidsson. Food iron absorption in man: application of the two-pool extrinsic tag method to measure heme and nonheme iron absorption from the whole diet. *J. Clin. Invest.* 53:247–253 (1974).

Björn-Rasmussen, E., L. Hallberg, and R. B. Walker. Food iron absorption in man. I. Isotopic exchange between food iron and inorganic iron salt added to food: studies on maize, wheat, and eggs. *Am. J. Clin. Nutr.* 25:317–323 (1972).

Björnstein, I. and L. Sjöström. Number and size of adipose tissue fat cells in relation to metabolism in human obesity. *Metabolism* 20:703–715 (1971).

Björntorp, P. Effects of age, sex, and clinical conditions on adipose tissue cellularity in man. *Metabolism* 23:1091–1102 (1974).

Björntorp, P., T. Schersten, and A. Gottfries. Effects of glucose infusions on adipose tissue lipogenesis in man. *Acta Med. Scand.* 183:565–571 (1968).

Black, A. L., B. M. Guirard, and E. E. Snell. Increased muscle phosphorylase in rats fed high levels of vitamin B_6. *J. Nutr.* 107:1962–1968 (1977).

Black, R., M. Tripp, P. Whanger, and P. Weswig. Selenium proteins in ovine tissues: III. Distribution of selenium and glutathione peroxidases in tissue cytosols. *Bioinorg. Chem.* 8:161–172 (1978).

Blackburn, M. W. and D. H. Calloway. Basal metabolic rate and work energy expenditure of mature pregnant women. *J. Am. Diet. Assoc.* 69:24–28 (1976).

Blair, J. A. Isolation of *iso*xanthopterin from human urine. *Biochem. J.* 68:385–387 (1958).

Blair, J. A., I. T. Johnson, and A. J. Matty. Aspects of intestinal folate transport in the rat. *J. Physiol.* (London) 256:197–208 (1976).

Blake, C. C. F., M. J. Geisow, S. J. Oatley, B. Rérat, and C. Rérat. Structure of prealbumin: secondary, tertiary, and quaternary interactions determined by Fourier refinement at 1.8 Å. *J. Mol. Biol.* 121:339–356 (1978).

Bland, J. H. *Clinical Metabolism of Body Water and Electrolytes*, W. B. Saunders Co., Philadelphia (1963).

Blankenhorn, D. H., J. Hirsh, and E. H. Ahrens, Jr. Transintestinal intubation: technique for measurement of gut length and physiological sampling at known loci. *Proc. Soc. Exp. Biol. Med.* 88:356–362 (1955).

Blayney, L., R. Bailey-Wood, A. Jacobs, A. Henderson, and J. Muir. The effects of iron deficiency on the respiratory function and cytochrome content of rat heart mitochondria. *Circ. Res.* 39:744–748 (1976).

Blobel, G. Synthesis and segregation of secretory proteins: the signal hypothesis. In *International Cell Biology*, pp. 318-325, B. R. Brinkley and K. R. Porter, Eds., Rockefeller University Press, New York (1977).

Block, R. J. and Mitchell, H. H. The correlation of the amino-acid composition of proteins with their nutritive value. *Nutr. Abst. Rev.* 16:249 (1946).

Blomhoff, R., P. Helgerud, M. Rasmussen, T. Berg, and K. R. Norum. *In vivo* uptake of chylomicron ^3H retinyl ester by rat liver: evidence for retinol transfer from parenchymal to nonparenchymal cells. *Proc. Nat. Acad. Sci. U. S.* 79:7326–7330 (1982).

Blomstrand, R. and E. H. Ahrens, Jr. Absorption of fats studied in a patient with chyluria. *J. Biol. Chem.* 233:327–330 (1958).

Blomstrand, R. and L. Forsgren. Intestinal absorption and esterification of vitamin D_3-1,2-^{3}H in man. *Acta Chem. Scand.* 21:1662–1663 (1967).

Blomstrand, R. and L. Forsgren. Vitamin K_1-^{3}H in man: its intestinal absorption and transport in the thoracic duct lymph. *Int. Z. Vitaminforsch* 38:45–64 (1968).

Bloom, F. E. and E. Costa. The effects of drugs on serotonergic nerve terminals. *Adv. Cytopharmacol.* 1:379–395 (1971).

Bloom, S. R. *Gut Hormones,* Churchill Livingstone, New York (1978).

Bloom, S. R. Control of glucagon secretion: an overview. In *Glucagon: Physiology, Pathophysiology, and Morphology of the Pancreatic A-Cells,* pp. 100–113, R. H. Unger and L. Orci, Eds., Elsevier, New York (1981).

Bloom, W. and D. W. Fawcett. *A Textbook of Histology,* 9th ed., W. B. Saunders Co., Philadelphia (1968).

Blunt, J. W., Y. Tanaka, and H. F. DeLuca. 25-Hydroxycholecalciferol: a biologically active metabolite of vitamin D_3. *Biochemistry* 8:671–675 (1969).

Boass, A. and T. H. Wilson. Intestinal absorption of intrinsic factor and B_{12}-intrinsic factor complex. *Am. J. Physiol.* 207:27–32 (1964).

Bockaert, J., C. Roy, R. Rajerison, and S. Jard. Specific binding of (^{3}H)-lysine-vasopressin to pig kidney plasma membranes. *J. Biol. Chem.* 248:5922–5931 (1973).

Bodian, D. Neurons, circuits, and neuroglia. In *The Neurosciences,* pp. 6–24, G. C. Quarton, T. Melnechuk, and F. O. Schmitt, Eds., Rockefeller University Press, New York (1967).

Bodwell, C. E. Tropomyosin B. In *Contractile Proteins and Muscle,* pp. 155–177, K. Laki, Ed., Marcel Dekker Inc., New York (1971).

Bodwell, C. E., J. S. Adkins, and D. T. Hopkins, Eds., *Protein quality in humans: assessment and in vitro estimation,* AVI Publishing Co., Westport, Conn. (1981).

Bohdal, M. and W. K. Simmons. A comparison of the nutritional indices in health: African, Asian, and European children. *Bull. WHO* 40:166–174 (1969).

Boileau, R. A., D. H. Horstman, E. R. Buskirk, and J. Mendez. The usefulness of urinary creatinine excretion in estimating body composition. *Med. Sci. Sports* 4:85–90 (1972).

Boileau, R. A., J. H. Wilmore, T. G. Lohman, M. H. Slaughter, and W. F. Riner. Estimation of body density from skinfold thicknesses, body circumferences, and skeletal widths in boys aged 8 to 11 years: comparison of two samples. *Hum. Biol.* 53:575–592 (1981).

Boivin, A., R. Vendrely, and C. Vendrely. L'acide desoxyribonucleique du noyau cellulaire, dépositaire des caractères hère ditaires: arguments d'ordre analytique. *C. R. Acad. Sci., Paris,* 226:1061–1063 (1948).

Bolin, T. D. The effect of diet on lactase activity in the rat. *Gastroenterol.* 60:432–437 (1971).

Bolin, T. D., R. C. Pirola, and A. E. Davis. Adaptation of intestinal lactase in the rat. *Gastroenterol.* 57:406–409 (1969).

Bonjour, J. P. Biotin in man's nutrition and therapy. *Int. J. Vitam. Nutr. Res.* 47:107–118 (1977).

Bonjour, J. P. and R. L. Malvin. Stimulation of ADH release by the renin-angiotensin system. *Am. J. Physiol.* 218:1555–1559 (1970).

Booher, L. E., E. C. Callison, and E. M. Hewston. An experimental determination of the minimum vitamin A requirements of normal adults. *J. Nutr.* 17:317–331 (1939).

Booth, C. C. Effect of location along the small intestine on absorption of nutrients. In *Handbook of Physiology,* Section 6: Alimentary Canal, Vol. 3, pp. 1513–1527, C. F. Code, Ed., American Physiological Society, Washington, D.C. (1968).

Booth, C. C. and M. C. Brain. The absorption of tritium-labelled pyridoxine hydrochloride in the rat. *J. Physiol.* 164:282–294 (1962).

Booth, C. C. and D. L. Mollin. The site of absorption of vitamin B_{12} in man. *Lancet* 1:18–21 (1959).

Booth, R. A. D., B. A. Goddard, and A. Paton. Measurement of fat thickness in man: a comparison of ultrasound, calipers and electrical conductivity. *Br. J. Nutr.* 20:719–727 (1966).

Border, P. M. and G. A. J. Pitt. Spermatogenesis in rats after administration of 3-dehydroretinol (vitamin A-2), p. 41, *Abstracts 12th International Congress of Nutrition* (1981).

Borgström, B. Digestion and absorption of fat. *Gastroenterol.* 43:216–219 (1962).

Borgström, B. Fat digestion and absorption. In *Intestinal Absorption, Biomembranes,* Vol. 4B, pp. 555–626, D. H. Smyth, Ed., Plenum, London (1974).

Borkan, G. A., S. G. Gerzof, A. H. Robbins, D. E. Hults, C. K. Silbert, and J. E Silbert. Assessment of abdominal fat content by computed tomography. *Am. J. Clin. Nutr.* 36:172–177 (1982).

Borle, A. B. Calcium metabolism at the cellular level. *Fed. Proc.* 32:1944–1950 (1973).

Bornstein, P., H. P. Ehrlich, and A. W. Wyke. Procollagen: conversion of the precursor to collagen by a neutral protease. *Science* 175:544–546 (1972).

Bornstein, P. and W. Traub. The chemistry and biology of collagen. In *The Proteins,* Vol. 4, pp. 412–632, H. Neurath and R. L. Hill, Eds., Academic Press, New York (1979).

Borsook, H. and G. Keighley. The energy of urea synthesis. I and II. *Proc. Nat. Acad. Sci. U. S.* 19:626–631; 720–725 (1933).

Borsook, H. and H. M. Winegarden. The work of the kidney in the production of urine. *Proc. Nat. Acad. Sci. U. S.* 17:13–28 (1931).

Bouillon, R., H. Van Baelen, W. Rombauts, and P. De Moor. The purification and characterization of the human serum binding protein for the 25-hydroxycholecalciferol (transcalciferin). Identity with group-specific component. *Eur. J. Biochem.* 66:285–291 (1976).

Bowen, R. H. The Golgi apparatus—its structure and functional significance. *Anat. Rec.* 32:151–193 (1926).

Bowers, W. E. Lysosomes in lymphoid tissues: spleen, thymus, and lymph nodes. In *Lysosomes in Biology and Pathology,* Vol. 1, pp. 167–191, J. T. Dingle and H. B. Fell, Eds., Wiley-Interscience, New York (1969).

Boyd, W. C. Applications of biochemistry to problems of variation and heredity. *Ann. N. Y. Acad. Sci.* 134:858–863 (1966).

Boyle, I. T., R. W. Gray, and H. F. DeLuca. Regulation by calcium of *in vivo* synthesis of 1,25-dihydroxycholecalciferol and 21,25-dihydroxycholecalciferol. *Proc. Nat. Acad. Sci. U. S.* 68:2131–2134 (1971).

Brace, R. A. Progress toward resolving the controversy of positive vs negative interstitial fluid pressure. *Circ. Res.* 49:281–297 (1981).

Bradfield, R. B. A rapid tissue technique for the field assessment of protein-calorie malnutrition. *Am. J. Clin. Nutr.* 25:720–729 (1972).

Bradfield, R. B. and M. H. Jourdan. Relative importance of specific dynamic action in weight-reduction diets. *Lancet* 2:640–643 (1973).

Brain, M. C. and C. C. Booth. The absorption of tritium-labelled pyridoxine HCl in control subjects and in patients with intestinal malabsorption. *Gut* 5:241–247 (1964).

Brandt, P. W. and A. R. Freeman. Plasma membrane: substructural changes correlated with electrical resistance and pinocytosis. *Science* 155:582–585 (1967).

Branton, D. and D. W. Deamer. *Membrane Structure,* Springer-Verlag, Vienna and New York (1972).

Brätter, P. and P. Schramel. *Trace Element Analytical Chemistry in Medicine and Biology.* deGruyter, Berlin (1980).

Bray, D. The fibrillar proteins of nerve cells. *Endeavour* 33:131–136 (1974).

Bray, G. A. Effect of diet and triiodothyronine on the activity of *sn*-glycerol-3-phosphate dehydrogenase and on the metabolism of glucose and pyruvate by adipose tissue of obese patients. *J. Clin. Invest.* 48:1413–1422 (1969).

Bray, G. A. and T. F. Gallagher, Jr. Regulatory obesity in man. *Clin. Res.* 18:537A (1970).

Breeze, B. B. and A. B. McCoord. Vitamin A absorption in celiac disease. *J. Pediatr.* 15:183–196 (1939).

Bremner, I., W. G. Hoekstra, N. T. Davies, and B. W. Young. Effect of zinc status of rats on the synthesis and degradation of copper-induced metallothioneins. *Biochem. J.* 174:883–892 (1978).

Brenneman, A. R. and S. Kaufman. The role of tetrahydropteridines in the enzymatic conversion of tyrosine to 3,4-dihydroxyphenylalanine. *Biochem. Biophys. Res. Commun.* 17:177–183 (1964).

Bretscher, M. S. Membrane structure: some general principles. *Science* 181:622–629 (1973).

Brewer, H. B., Jr., T. Farwell, R. Ronan, G. W. Sizemore, and C. D. Arnaud. Human parathyroid hormone: amino acid sequence of the amino-terminal residues 1-34. *Proc. Nat. Acad. Sci. U. S.* 69:3585–3588 (1972).

Brewer, H. B., Jr., and R. Ronan. Bovine parathyroid hormone: amino acid sequence. *Proc. Nat. Acad. Sci. U. S.* 67:1862–1869 (1970).

Bricker, M. L., J. M. Smith, T. S. Hamilton, and H. H. Mitchell. The effect of cocoa upon calcium utilization and requirements, nitrogen retention and fecal composition. *J. Nutr.* 39:455–461 (1949).

Brin, M. Erythrocyte transketolase in early thiamine deficiency. *Ann. N. Y. Acad. Sci.* 98:528–541 (1962).

Brin, M. The antithiamine effects of amprolium in rats on tissue transketolase activity. *Toxicol. Appl. Pharmacol.* 6:454–458 (1964).

Brin, M. Functional evaluation of nutritional status: thiamin. In *Newer Methods in Nutritional Biochemistry,* Vol. 3, pp. 407–445, A. A. Albanese, Ed., Academic Press, New York (1967).

Brin, M. A simplified Toepfer-Lehmann assay for the three vitamin B_6 vitamers. In *Methods in Enzymology,* Vol. 18, Part A, pp. 519–523, D. B. McCormick and L. D. Wright, Eds., Academic Press, New York (1970).

Brin, M., M. Tai, A. S. Ostashever, and H. Kalinsky. The relative effects of pyridoxine deficiency on two plasma transaminases in the growing and in the adult rat. *J. Nutr.* 71:416–420 (1960).

Brindley, D. N. The intracellular phase of fat absorption. In *Intestinal Absorption, Biomembranes,* Vol. 4B, pp. 621–671, D. H. Smyth, Ed., Plenum, London (1974).

Brindley, D. N. and G. Hubscher. The effect of chain length on the activation and subsequent incorporation of fatty acids into glycerides by the small intestinal mucosa. *Biochim. Biophys. Acta* 125:92–105 (1966).

Brine, C. L. and F. A. Johnston. Endogenous calcium in the feces of adult man and the amount of calcium absorbed from food. *Am. J. Clin. Nutr.* 3:418–420 (1955).

Brinkhous, K. M. Plasma prothrombin: vitamin K. *Medicine* 19:329–416 (1940).

Brinkley, B. R. The cytoskeleton: a perspective. In *Methods in Cell Biology,* Vol. 24, Part A, pp. 2–8, L. Wilson, Ed., Academic Press, New York (1982).

Brittin, G. M. and D. Raval. Duodenal ferritin synthesis during iron absorption in the iron-deficient rat. *J. Lab. Clin. Med.* 75:811–817 (1970).

Brobeck, J. R., Ed., *Best and Taylor's Physiological Basis of Medical Practice,* 9th ed., Williams & Wilkins, Baltimore (1973).

Brody, S. *Bioenergetics and Growth.* Reinhold Publishing Co., New York (1945).

Brody, T., J. E. Watson, and E. L. R. Stokstad. Folate pentaglutamate and folate hexaglutamate mediated one-carbon metabolism. *Biochemistry* 21:276–282 (1982).

Bronner, F. Dynamics and function of calcium. In *Mineral Metabolism,* Vol. 2, Part A, pp. 341–444, C. L. Comar and F. Bronner, Eds., Academic Press, New York (1964).

Bronner, F. Intestinal calcium absorption and transport. In *Membrane Transport of Calcium,* pp. 237–262, E. Carafoli, Ed., Academic Press, New York (1982).

Bronner, F. and R. S. Harris. Absorption and metabolism of calcium in human beings, studied with calcium[45]. *Ann. N. Y. Acad. Sci.* 64:314–325 (1956).

Bronner, F., J. Lipton, D. Pansu, M. Buckley, R. Singh, and A. Miller. III. Molecular and transport effects of 1,25-dihydroxyvitamin D_3 in rat duodenum. *Fed. Proc.* 41:61–65 (1982).

Brooks, V. L. and R. L. Malvin. An intercerebral, physiological role for angiotensin: effects of central blockade. *Fed. Proc.* 38:2272–2275 (1979).

Broquist, H. P., E. L. R. Stokstad, and T. H. Jukes. Biochemical studies with the "citrovorum factor." *J. Lab. Clin. Med.* 38:95–100 (1951).

Brown, A. C. and G. Brengelmann. Energy metabolism. In *Physiology and Biophysics,* pp. 1030–1049, T. C. Ruch and H. D. Patton, Eds., W. B. Saunders Co., Philadelphia (1965).

Brown, E. B. Evidence supporting the concept of heterogeneity of iron atoms bound to transferrin in the rat. In *Proteins of Iron Storage and Transport in Biochemistry and Medicine,* pp. 97–106, R. R. Crichton, Ed., North-Holland Publishing Company, Amsterdam (1975).

Brown, E. B., P. Aisen, J. Fielding, and R. R. Crichton, Eds., *Proteins of Iron Metabolism.* Grune & Stratton, New York (1977).

Brown, E. G. Evidence for the involvement of ferrous iron in the biosynthesis of δ-aminolaevulinic acid by chicken erythrocyte preparations. *Nature* (London) 182:313–315 (1958).

Brown, F. and J. F. Danielli. The cell surface and cell physiology. In *Cytology and Cell Physiology,* pp. 239–310, G. H. Bourne, Ed., Academic Press, New York (1964).

Brown, J. H. and S. H. Pollack. Stabilization of hepatic lysosomes of rats by vitamin E and selenium *in vivo* as indicated by thermal labilization of isolated lysosomes. *J. Nutr.* 102:1413–1419 (1972).

Brown, M. S., P. T. Kovanen, J. L. Goldstein. Regulation of plasma cholesterol by lipoprotein receptors. *Science* 212:628–635 (1981).

Brown, R. G., E. M. Button, and J. T. Smith. Effect of vitamin E deficiency on collagen metabolism in the rat's skin. *J. Nutr.* 91:99–106 (1967).

Brown, R. R. Normal and pathological conditions which may alter the human requirement for vitamin B_6. *Agric. Food Chem.* 20:498–505 (1972).

Brown, R. R., D. P. Rose, J. M. Price, and H. Wolf. Tryptophan metabolism as affected by anovulatory agents. *Ann. N. Y. Acad. Sci.* 146:44–56 (1969).

Brown, W. V., P. Wang-Iverson, and J. R. Paterniti. Heparin, lipoproteins and lipoprotein lipase. In *Chemistry and Biology of Heparin,* pp. 175–185, R. L.

Lundblad, W. V. Brown, K. G. Mann, and H. R. Roberts, Eds., Elsevier-North Holland, New York (1981).

Brownlee, M., Ed., *Handbook of Diabetes Mellitus,* Garland STPM Press, New York (1981).

Brozek, J. Changes of body composition in man during maturity and their nutritional implications. *Fed. Proc.* 11:784–793 (1952).

Brozek, J., Ed., *Body Measurements and Human Nutrition,* National Research Council Committee on Nutritional Anthropometry, Wayne University Press, Detroit (1956).

Brozek, J. (with technical assistance of H. Guetzkow). Psychologic effects of thiamine restriction and deprivation in normal young men. *Am. J. Clin. Nutr.* 5:109–120 (1957).

Brozek, J. Body composition. *Science* 134:920–930 (1961).

Brozek, J., F. Grande, J. T. Anderson, and A. Keys. Densitometric analysis of body composition: revision of some quantitative assumptions. *Ann. N. Y. Acad. Sci.* 110:113–140 (1963).

Brozek, J. and A. Keys. Evaluation of leanness-fatness in man: norms and interrelationships. *Br. J. Nutr.* 5:194–206 (1951).

Brozek, J., J. K. Kihlberg, H. L. Taylor, and A. Keys. Skinfold distributions in middle-aged American men: a contribution to norms of leanness-fatness. *Ann. N. Y. Acad. Sci.* 110:492–502 (1963).

Brozović, B. Absorption of iron. In *Intestinal Absorption in Man,* pp. 263–314, I. McColl and G. E. Sladen, Eds., Academic Press, London (1975).

Bruce, A. A critical evaluation of the RDA and suggestions on how they can be improved. *Voding* 41:288–292 (1980).

Brutlag, D. and A. Kornberg. Enzymatic synthesis of deoxyribonucleic acid. XXXVI. A proofreading function for the $3' \rightarrow 5'$ exonuclease activity in deoxyribonucleic acid polymerases. *J. Biol. Chem.* 247:241–248 (1972).

Buell, G. C. and R. Reiser. Glyceride-glycerol precursors in the intestinal mucosa. *J. Biol. Chem.* 234:217–219 (1959).

Bullen, B. F., A. Quaade, E. Olsen, and S. A. Lund. Ultrasonic reflections used for measuring subcutaneous fat in humans. *Hum. Biol.* 37:377–384 (1965).

Bulychev, A., R. Kramar, Z. Drahata, and O. Lindberg. Role of a specific endogenous fatty acid fraction in the coupling-uncoupling mechanism of oxidative phosphorylation of brown adipose tissue. *Exp. Cell Res.* 72:169–187 (1972).

Bunn, H. F., B. G. Forget, and H. M. Ranney, Eds., *Human Hemoglobins,* W. B. Saunders Co., Philadelphia (1977).

Burch, H. B., T. Salcedo, Jr., E. O. Carrasco, R. L. Intengan, and A. B. Caldwell. Nutrition survey and tests in Bataan, Philippines. *J. Nutr.* 42:9–30 (1950).

Burch, H. B., C. A. Storvick, R. L. Bicknell, H. C. Kung, L. G. Alejo, W. A.

Everhart, O. H. Lowry, C. G. King, and O. Bessey. Metabolic studies of precursors of pyridine nucleotides. *J. Biol. Chem.* 212:897–907 (1955).

Burchenal, J. J. Folic acid antagonists. *Am. J. Clin. Nutr.* 3:311–320 (1955).

Burgess, D. R. and B. E. Prum. Reevaluation of brush border motility: calcium induces core filament solation and microvillar vesiculation. *J. Cell Biol.* 94:97–107 (1982).

Burk, M. C. and E. M. Pao. *Methods for large scale surveys of household and individual diets.* Home Economics Research Report No. 40. U.S. Government Printing Office. Washington, D.C. (1976).

Burk, R. F. Biological activity of selenium. *Ann. Rev. Nutr.* 3:53–70 (1983).

Burke, B. The dietary history as a tool in research. *J. Am. Diet Assoc.* 23:1044–1046 (1947).

Burkinshaw, L., G. L. Hill, and D. B. Morgan. Assessment of the distribution of protein in the human body by *in vivo* neutron activation analysis. In *International Symposium on Nuclear Activation Techniques in the Life Sciences*, pp. 787–798 (IAEA-SM-227/39). Vienna: IAEA (1978).

Burkinshaw, L., D. B. Morgan, N. P. Silverton, and R. D. Thomas. Total body nitrogen and its relation to body potassium and fat-free mass in healthy subjects. *Clin. Sci.* 61:457–462 (1981).

Burnet, E. and W. D. Aykroyd. Nutrition and public health. *League of Nations Quart. Bull.* IV, No. 2 (1935).

Burr, G. W. and M. M. Burr. A new deficiency disease produced by the rigid exclusion of fat from the diet. *J. Biol. Chem.* 82:345–367 (1929).

Burr, I. M., H. P. Taft, W. Stauffacher, and A. E. Renold. On the role of cyclic AMP in insulin release: II. Dynamic aspects and relations to adrenergic receptors in the perfused pancreas of adult rats. *Ann. N. Y. Acad. Sci.* 185:245–262 (1971).

Buskirk, E. R. and J. Mendez. Energy: caloric requirements. In *Human Nutrition: A Comprehensive Treatise, 3A, Nutrition and the Adult Macronutrients*, pp. 49–95, R. B. Alfin-Slater and D. Kritchevsky, Eds., Plenum, New York (1980).

Butcher, R. W. and C. E. Baird. Effects of prostaglandins on adenosine 3',5'-monophosphate levels in fat and other tissues. *J. Biol. Chem.* 243:1713–1717 (1968).

Butcher, R. W., C. E. Baird, and E. W. Sutherland. Effects of lipolytic and antilipolytic substances on adenosine 3',5'-monophosphate levels in isolated fat cells. *J. Biol. Chem.* 243:1705–1712 (1968).

Butcher, R. W. and E. W. Sutherland. The effects of the catecholamines, adrenergic blocking agents, prostaglandins E_1, and insulin on cyclic AMP levels in the rat epididymal fat pad *in vitro*. *Ann. N. Y. Acad. Sci.* 139:849–859 (1967).

Butow, R. A., W. F. Bennett, D. B. Finkelstein, and R. E. Kellems. Nuclear-cytoplasmic interactions in the biogenesis of mitochondria in yeast. In *Mem-*

brane *Biogenesis: Mitochondria, Chloroplasts, and Bacteria,* pp. 155–199, A. Tzagoloff, Ed., Plenum, New York (1975).

Butterworth, C. E., Jr., C. M. Baugh, and C. L. Krumdieck. A study of folate absorption and metabolism in man utilizing carbon-14-labeled polyglutamates synthesized by the solid phase method. *J. Clin. Invest.* 48:1131–1142 (1969).

Buzina, R., A. Brodarec, M. Jusic, N. Milanovic, K. Bernhard, G. Brubacher, S. Christeller, and J. P. Vuilleumier. The assessment of dietary vitamin intake of 24 Istrian farmers. I. Laboratory analysis versus food tables. *Int. J. Vitam. Nutr. Res.* 41:129–140 (1971).

Caasi, P. I., J. W. Hauswirth, and P. P. Nair. Biosynthesis of heme in vitamin E deficiency. *Ann. N. Y. Acad. Sci.* 203:93–102 (1972).

Caddell, J. L. Magnesium deficiency in protein-calorie malnutrition: a follow-up study. *Ann. N. Y. Acad. Sci.* 162:874–890 (1969).

Cahill, G. F., Jr., T. T. Aoki, and R. J. Smith. Amino acid cycles in man. In *Biological Cycles,* Vol. 18, *Current Topics in Cellular Regulation,* pp. 389–400, R. W. Estabrook and P. Srere, Eds., Academic Press, New York (1981).

Caldwell, B. M. Descriptive evaluations of child development and of developmental settings. *Pediatr.* 40:46–54 (1967).

Call, D. L. An examination of caloric availability and consumption in the United States, 1909–1963. *Am. J. Clin. Nutr.* 16:374–379 (1965).

Callahan, J. W. and J. A. Lowden, Eds. *Lysosomes and Lysosomal Storage Diseases,* Raven Press, New York (1981).

Callender, S. T., B. J. Mallett, and M. D. Smith. Absorption of hemoglobin iron. *Br. J. Haematol.* 3:186–192 (1957).

Callender, S. T., S. R. Marney, and G. T. Warner. Eggs and iron absorption. *Br. J. Haematol.* 19:657–665 (1970).

Callender, S. T. and G. T. Warner. Iron absorption from bread. *Am. J. Clin. Nutr.* 21:1170–1174 (1968).

Callow, R. R., E. Kodicek, and G. A. Thompson. Metabolism of tritiated vitamin D. *Proc. R. Soc. Lond. (Biol.)* 164:1–20 (1966).

Calloway, D. H. Nitrogen balance during pregnancy. In *Nutrition and Fetal Development,* Vol. 2, pp. 79–94, M. Winick, Ed., John Wiley & Sons, New York (1974).

Calloway, D. H. and S. Margen. Variation in endogenous nitrogen excretion and dietary nitrogen utilization as determinants of human protein requirement. *J. Nutr.* 101:205–216 (1971).

Calloway, D. H., E. L. Murphy, and D. Bauer. Determination of lactose intolerance by breath analysis. *Am. J. Dig. Dis.* 14:811–815 (1969).

Calloway, D. H., A. C. F. Odell, and S. Margen. Sweat and miscellaneous nitrogen losses in human balance studies. *J. Nutr.* 101:775–786 (1971).

Campbell, D. T. and J. C. Stanley. In *Experimental and Quasi-Experimental Designs for Research,* p. 84, Rand McNally & Co., Chicago (1966).

Campbell, H. A. and K. P. Link. Studies on the hemorrhagic sweet clover disease. IV. The isolation and crystallization of the hemorrhagic agent. *J. Biol. Chem.* 138:21–33 (1941).

Campbell, J. A. Approaches in revising dietary standards. *J. Am. Diet. Assoc.* 64:175–178 (1974).

Campbell, R. M. and H. W. Kosterlitz. The effects of growth and sex in the composition of the liver cells in the rat. *J. Endocrinol.* 6:308–318 (1950).

Canadian Council on Nutrition. Dietary standard for Canada. *Can. Bull. Nutr.* 6:1–76 (1964), Suppl. (1968).

Canadian Pediatric Society. The use and abuse of vitamin A. *Can. Med. Assoc. J.* 104:521–522 (1971).

Canas, F., J. S. Brand, W. F. Neuman, and A. R. Terepka. Some effects of vitamin D_3 on collagen synthesis in rachitic chick cortical bone. *Am. J. Physiol.* 216:1092–1096 (1969).

Canham, J. E., E. M. Baker, R. S. Harding, H. E. Sauberlich, and I. C. Plough. Dietary protein—its relationship to vitamin B_6 requirements and function, *Ann. N. Y. Acad. Sci.* 166:16–29 (1969).

Cannigia, A., C. Gennari, L. Cesari, and S. Romano. Intestinal absorption of ^{45}Ca in adult and old human subjects. *Gerontologia* 10:193–198 (1964).

Cannon, W. B. Organization for physiological homeostasis. *Physiol. Rev.* 9:399–431 (1929).

Capaldi, R. A. A dynamic model of cell membranes. *Sci. Am.* 230(3):26–34 (1974).

Carafoli, E. Ca^{2+} pumping systems in the plasma membrane. In *Calcium and Phosphate Transport Across Biomembranes,* pp. 9–14, F. Bronner and M. Peterlik, Eds., Academic Press, New York (1981a).

Carafoli, E. The uptake and release of calcium from mitochondria. In *Mitochondria and Microsomes,* pp. 357–374, C. P. Lees, G. Shatz, and G. Dallner, Eds., Addison-Wesley Publishing Co., London (1981b).

Carafoli, E. The regulation of the cellular functions of Ca^{2+}. In *Disorders of Mineral Metabolism,* Vol. 2, *Calcium Physiology,* pp. 1–42, F. Bronner and J. W. Coburn, Eds., Academic Press, New York (1982).

Carafoli, E. and M. Crompton. The regulation of intracellular calcium. *Curr. Top. Membr. Transp.* 10:151–216 (1978).

Carafoli, E., P. Gazzotti, F. D. Vasington, G. L. Sottocasa, G. Sandri, E. Panfil, and B. deBernard. Soluble Ca^{2+} binding factors isolated from mitochondria. In *Biochemistry and Biophysics of Mitochondrial Membranes,* pp. 623–640, G. F. Azzone, E. Carafoli, A. L. Lehninger, E. Quagliariello, and N. Siliprandi, Eds., Academic Press, New York (1972).

Carafoli, E., P. Patriarca, and C. S. Rossi. A comparative study of the role of mitochondria and the sarcoplasmic reticulum in the uptake and release of Ca^{++} by the rat diaphragm. *J. Cell. Physiol.* 74:17–30 (1969).

Carafoli, E. and C. S. Rossi. Calcium transport in mitochondria. *Adv. Cytophar-macol.* 1:209–227 (1971).

Care, A. D., R. F. L. Bates, and H. J. Gitelman. Evidence for a role of cyclic AMP in the release of calcitonin. *Ann. N. Y. Acad. Sci.* 185:317–326 (1971).

Carey, M. C., D. M. Small, and C. M. Bliss. Lipid digestion and absorption. *Ann. Rev. Physiol.* 45:651–677 (1983).

Carlisle, E. M. Silicon as an essential element. *Fed. Proc.* 33:1758–1766 (1974).

Carlisle, E. M. The nutritional essentiality of silicon. *Nutr. Rev.* 40:193–198 (1982).

Carlsson, A. and B. Lindquist. Comparison of intestinal and skeletal effects of vitamin D in relation to dosage. *Acta Physiol. Scand.* 35:53–55 (1955).

Carnes, W. H. Role of copper in connective tissue metabolism. *Fed. Proc.* 30:995–1000 (1971).

Caro, L. G. and G. E. Palade. Protein synthesis, storage and discharge in the pancreatic exocrine cell. An autoradiographic study. *J. Cell Biol.* 20:473–495 (1964).

Carpenter, K. J. Damage to lysine in food processing: its measurement and its significance. *Nutr. Abst. Revs.* 43:423–451 (1973).

Carpenter, K. J. Effects of different methods of processing maize on its pellagra-genic activity. *Fed. Proc.* 40:1531–1535 (1981).

Carpenter, K. J. Individual amino acid levels and bioavailability. In *Protein quality in humans: Assessment and in vitro estimation*, pp. 239–259, C. E. Bodwell, J. S. Adkins and D. T. Hopkins, Eds., AVI Publishing Co., Westport, Conn. (1981).

Carr, F. H. and E. A. Price. Colour reactions attributed to vitamin A. *Biochem. J.* 20:497–501 (1926).

Carrel, Alexis. *Man the Unknown*, Harper & Bros., New York (1935).

Carroll, J. and B. Spencer. Vitamin A and sulphotransferases in foetal rat liver. *Biochem. J.* 96:79P (1965).

Carter, E. G. A. Quantitation of urinary niacin metabolites by reversed-phase liquid chromatography. *Am. J. Clin. Nutr.* 36:926–930 (1982).

Carter, E. G. A. and K. J. Carpenter. The bioavailability for humans of bound niacin from wheat bran. *Am. J. Clin. Nutr.* 36:855–861 (1982).

Casey, C. E., P. A. Walravens, and K. M. Hambidge. Availability of zinc: loading test with human milk, cow's milk and infant formulas. *Pediatr.* 68:394–396 (1981).

Caspary, W. F. and R. K. Crane. Active transport of myo-inositol and its relation to the sugar transport system in hamster small intestine. *Biochim. Biophys. Acta* 203:308–316 (1970).

Castelli, W. P., T. Gordon, M. C. Hjortland, A. Kagan, J. T. Doyle, C. G. Hames, S. B. Hulley, and W. J. Zukel. Alcohol and blood lipids. *Lancet* 2:153–155 (1977).

Castle, W. B. Gastric intrinsic factor and vitamin B_{12} absorption. In *Handbook of Physiology*, Section 6, Vol. 3, pp. 1529–1552, C. F. Code, Ed., American Physiological Society, Washington, D.C. (1968).

Cellier, K. M. and M. E. Hankin. Studies of nutrition in pregnancy. I. Some considerations in collecting dietary information. *Am. J. Clin. Nutr.* 13:55–62 (1963).

Center for Disease Control. *Ten state nutrition survey in the United States, 1968–1970. V. Dietary.* (DHEW Publication No. [HSM] 72-8133). Health Services and Mental Health Administration, Altanta (1972).

Century, T. J., I. R. Fenichel, and S. B. Horowitz. The concentrations of water, sodium and potassium in the nucleus and cytoplasm of amphibian oocytes. *J. Cell Sci.* 7:5–13 (1970).

Cerecedo, L. R. Thiamine antagonists. *Am. J. Clin. Nutr.* 3:273–281 (1955).

Chalmers, F., M. Clayton, L. Gates, R. Tucker, A. Wertz, C. Young, and W. Foster. The dietary record—how many and which days? *J. Am. Diet Assoc.* 28:711–717 (1952).

Chambers, T. J. and C. T. Magnus. Calcitonin alters behaviour of isolated osteoclasts. *J. Pathol.* 136:27–39 (1982).

Chanarin, I. and J. Perry. Evidence for reduction and methylation of folate in the intestine during normal absorption. *Lancet* 2:776–778 (1969).

Chandra, R. K., B. Au, G. Woodford, and P. Hyam. Iron status, immune response and susceptibility to infection. In *Iron Metabolism*, pp. 249–268, (Ciba Foundation Symposium 51 [new ser.]), Elsevier North-Holland, New York (1977).

Chaney, S. G. Principles of Nutrition II: Micronutrients. In *Textbook of Biochemistry with Clinical Correlations*, pp. 1197–1239, T. M. Devlin, Ed., John Wiley & Sons, New York (1982).

Chao, F. C. Dissociation of macromolecular ribonucleoprotein of yeast. *Arch. Biochem. Biophys.* 70:426–431 (1957).

Chapman, D. Recent physical studies of phospholipids and natural membranes. In *Biological membranes*, D. Chapman, Ed., Academic Press, London (1968).

Chapman, D. and R. B. Leslie. Structure and function of phospholipids in membranes. In *Membranes of Mitochondria and Chloroplasts*, pp. 91–126, E. Racker, Ed., Van Nostrand Reinhold Co., New York (1970).

Charley, P. J., C. Stitt, E. Shore, and P. Saltman. Studies in the regulation of intestinal iron absorption. *J. Lab. Clin. Med.* 61:397–410 (1963).

Charlton, R. W. and T. H. Bothwell. Iron absorption. *Ann. Rev. Med.* 34:55–68 (1983).

Chase, H. P. and J. Dupont. Abnormal levels of prostaglandins and fatty acids in blood of children with cystic fibrosis. *Lancet* 2:236–238 (1978).

Chase, H. P., W. F. B. Lindsley, Jr., and D. O'Brien. Undernutrition and cerebellar development. *Nature* 221:554–555 (1969).

Chase, L. R. and G. D. Aurbach. Renal adenyl cyclase: anatomically separate sites for parathyroid hormone and vasopressin. *Science* 159:545–547 (1968).

Chatterjee, I. B. Biosynthesis of L-ascorbate in animals. In *Methods in Enzymology,* Vol. 18, Part A, pp. 28–34, D. B. McCormick and L. D. Wright, Eds., Academic Press, New York (1970).

Chatterjee, I. B., A. K. Majumder, B. K. Nandi, and N. Bubramanian. Synthesis and some major functions of vitamin C in animals. *Ann. N. Y. Acad. Sci.* 258:24–47 (1975).

Chaudhuri, C. R. and I. B. Chatterjee. L-Ascorbic acid synthesis in birds: phylogenetic trend. *Science* 164:435–436 (1969).

Chavez, J. F. and P. L. Pellett. Protein quality of some representative Latin American diets by rat bioassay. *J. Nutr.* 106:792–801 (1976).

Chaykin, G. Nicotinamide coenzymes. *Ann. Rev. Biochem.* 36:149–170 (1967).

Cheek, D. B., Ed. *Human Growth,* Lea & Febiger, Philadelphia (1968).

Cheek, D. B. Muscle cell growth in normal children. In *Human Growth,* pp. 337–351, D. B. Cheek, Ed., Lea & Febiger, Philadelphia (1968).

Cheek, D. B., J. A. Brasel, and J. E. Graystone. Muscle cell growth in rodents: sex differences and the role of hormones. In *Human Growth,* pp. 306–325, D. B. Cheek, Ed., Lea & Febiger, Philadelphia (1968).

Cheek, D. B. and D. E. Hill. Muscle and liver cell growth: role of hormones and nutritional factors. *Fed. Proc.* 29:1510–1515 (1970).

Chen, P. S. and H. B. Bosmann. Effect of vitamins D_2 and D_3 on serum calcium and phosphorous in rachitic chicks. *J. Nutr.* 83:133–139 (1964).

Chesters, J. Biochemical functions of zinc in animals. *World Rev. Nutr. Diet.* 32:135–164 (1978).

Cheung, W. Y. Adenosine 3′,5′-monophosphate: on the mechanism of action. *Perspect. Biol. Med.* 15:221–235 (1972).

Cheung, W. Y. Calmodulin plays a pivotal role in cellular regulation. *Science* 207:19–27 (1980).

Cheung, W. Y. Calmodulin: an overview. *Fed. Proc.* 41:2253–2257 (1982a).

Cheung, W. Y. Calmodulin. *Sci. Am.* 246(6):62–70 (1982b).

Chinn, H. I. *Effects of dietary factors in skeletal integrity in adults: calcium, phosphorous, vitamin D and protein,* Life Sciences Research Office, FASEB, Bethesda, Md. (1981).

Chisolm, J. J., Jr. Lead Poisoning. *Sci. Am.* 224(2):15–23 (1971).

Chole, R. A. and C. A. Quick. Experimental temporal bone histopathology in rats deprived of dietary retinol and maintained with supplemental retinoic acid. *J. Nutr.* 108:1008–1016 (1978).

Chong, Y. H. Erythrocyte transketolase activity. *Am. J. Clin. Nutr.* 23:261–266 (1970).

Chopra, I. J. Triiodothyronines in health and disease. *Monogr. Endocrinol.*, Vol. 18. F. Gross, M. Grumbach, A. Labhart, M. B. Lipsett, T. Mann, L. T. Samuels, and J. Zander, Eds., Springer-Verlag, Berlin (1981).

Chow, C. K. Nutritional influence on cellular antioxidant defense systems. *Am. J. Clin. Nutr.* 32:1066–1081 (1979).

Christakis, G., A. Miridjanian, L. Nath, H. S. Khurana, C. Cowell, M. Archer, O. Frank, H. Ziffer, H. Baker, and G. James. A nutritional epidemiologic investigation of 642 New York City children. *Am. J. Clin. Nutr.* 21:107–126 (1968).

Christakis, G., S. Sajecki, R. W. Hillman, E. Miller, S. Blumenthal, and M. Archer. Effect of a combined nutrition education and physical fitness program on the weight status of obese high school boys. *Fed. Proc.* 25:15–19 (1966).

Christensen, H. N. *Biological Transport*, W. A. Benjamin, New York (1962).

Christensen, H. N. Membrane domination of biological energy exchanges: a message of the 1978 Nobel Award in chemistry. *Perspect. Biol. Med.* 24:358–373 (1981).

Christian, J. E., L. W. Combs, and W. V. Kessler. Body composition: relative *in vivo* determinations from potassium-40 measurements. *Science* 140:489–490 (1963).

Chung, Y. C., Y. S. Kim, A. Shadchehr, A. Garrido, I. L. MacGregor, and M. H. Sleisenger. Protein digestion and absorption in human small intestine. *Gastroenterol.* 76:1415–1421 (1979).

Chvapil, M., J. N. Ryan, and C. F. Zukoski. The effect of zinc and other metals on the stability of lysosomes. *Proc. Soc. Exper. Biol. Med.* 140:642–646 (1972).

Cinnamon, A. D. and J. R. Beaton. Biochemical assessment of vitamin B_6 status in man. *Am. J. Clin. Nutr.* 23:696–702 (1970).

Clark, B. and G. Hubscher. Glycerokinase in mucosa of the small intestine of the cat. *Nature* 195:599–600 (1962).

Clark, B. F. and K. A. Marcker. How proteins start. *Sci. Am.* 218(1):36–42 (1968).

Clark, C. T., H. Weissbach, and S. Udenfriend. 5-Hydroxytryptophan decarboxylase: preparation and properties. *J. Biol. Chem.* 210:139–148 (1954).

Clark, F. and E. Cofer. A short method for calculating nutritive value of food issues. *J. Am. Diet. Assoc.* 40:301–307 (1962).

Clark, S. L., Jr. The ingestion of proteins and colloidal materials by columnar absorptive cells of the small intestine in suckling rats and mice. *J. Biophys. Biochem. Cytol.* 5:41–50 (1959).

Cleary, M. P., M. R. C. Greenwood, and J. A. Brasel. A multifactor analysis of growth in the rat epididymal fat pad. *J. Nutr.* 107:1969–1974 (1977).

Cleary, M. P., B. E. Klein, J. A. Brasel, and M. R. C. Greenwood. Thymidine kinase and DNA polymerase activity during postnatal growth of the epididymal fat pad. *J. Nutr.* 109:48–54 (1979).

Cleary, M. P. and J. R. Vasselli. Reduced organ growth when hyperphagia is prevented in genetically obese (fa/fa) Zucker rats. *Proc. Soc. Exp. Biol. Med.* 167:616–623 (1981).

Cleary, M. P., J. R. Vasselli, and M. R. C. Greenwood. Development of obesity in Zucker obese (fa/fa) rat in absence of hyperphagia. *Am. J. Physiol.* 238:284–292 (1980).

Cleaver, J. E. Defective repair replication of DNA in xeroderma pigmentosum. *Nature* 218:652–656 (1968).

Clifton, G., S. R. Bryant, and C. G. Skinner. N^1-(substituted) pantothenamides, antimetabolites of pantothenic acid. *Arch. Biochem. Biophys.* 137:523–528 (1970).

Cohen, A. C. Pyridoxine in the prevention and treatment of convulsions and neurotoxicity due to cycloserine. *Ann. N. Y. Acad. Sci.* 166:346–349 (1969).

Cohen, N., A. Gelb, and H. Sobotka. Intestinal absorption of folic acid *in vitro*. *Clin. Res.* 12:206A (1964).

Cohen, P. The role of calmodulin and troponin in the regulation of phosphorylase kinase from mammalian skeletal muscle. In *Calcium and Cell Function*, Vol. 1, pp. 183–199, W. Y. Cheung, Ed., Academic Press, New York (1980).

Cohenour, S. H. and D. H. Calloway. Blood, urine and dietary pantothenic acid levels of pregnant teenagers. *Am. J. Clin. Nutr.* 25:512–517 (1972).

Cohlan, S. Q. Excessive intake of vitamin A as a cause of congenital anomalies in the rat. *Science* 117:535–536 (1953).

Cohn, S. H., K. J. Ellis, and S. Wallach. *In vivo* neutron activation analysis—clinical potential in body composition studies. *Am. J. Med.* 57:683–686 (1974).

Cohn, S. H., D. Vartsky, S. Yasumura, A. Sawitsky, I. Zanzi, A. Vaswani, and K. J. Ellis. Compartmental body composition based on total body nitrogen, potassium, and calcium. *Am. J. Physiol.* 239:E524-E530 (1980).

Cohn, Z. A. and B. Benson. The *in vitro* differentiation of mononuclear phagocytes. II. The influence of serum on granule formation, hydrolase production, and pinocytosis. *J. Exper. Med.* 121:835–848 (1965).

Collins, F. D., A. J. Sinclair, J. P. Royle, P. A. Coats, A. T. Maynard, and R. F. Lenard. Plasma lipids in human linoleic acid deficiency. *Nutr. Metab.* 13:150–167 (1971).

Collip, J. B., L. I. Pugsley, H. Selye, and D. L. Thomson. Observations concerning the mechanism of parathyroid hormone action. *Br. J. Exp. Pathol.* 15:335–336 (1934).

Combs, J. F., Jr. and G. M. Pesti. Influence of ascorbic acid on selenium nutrition in the chick. *J. Nutr.* 106:958–966 (1976).

Committee for the Revision of the Dietary Standard for Canada. *Recommended Nutrient Intakes for Canadians,* Bureau of Nutritional Sciences, Food Directorate, Health Protection Branch, Department of National Health and Welfare, Ottawa (1983).

Committee on Maternal Nutrition. *Maternal Nutrition and the Course of Pregnancy.* National Research Council, National Academy of Sciences, Washington, D.C. (1970).

Committee on Nutrition of the American Academy of Pediatrics. The practical significance of lactose intolerance in children. *Pediatr.* 62:240–245 (1978).

Committee on Nutritional Misinformation, Food and Nutrition Board. Supplementation of human diets with vitamin E. *Nutr. Rev.* 31:327–328 (1973).

Condon, J. R., J. R. Nassim, J. C. Millard, A. Hilbe, and E. M. Stainthorpe. Calcium and phosphorus metabolism in relation to lactose intolerance. *Lancet* 1:1027–1029 (1970).

Conger, P. R. and R. B. J. Macnab. Strength, body composition and work capacity of participants and nonparticipants in women's intercollegiate sports. *Res. Q.* 38:184–192 (1967).

Conn, E. E. and P. K. Stumpf. *Outlines of Biochemistry,* 3rd ed., p. 71, John Wiley & Sons, New York (1972).

Connell, A. M. Dietary fiber. In *Physiology of the Gastrointestinal Tract,* Vol. 2, pp. 1291–1299, L. R. Johnson, Ed., Raven Press, New York (1981).

Conover, T. E. and M. Bárány. The absence of a myosin-like protein in liver mitochondria. *Biochem. Biophys. Acta* 127:235–238 (1966).

Conrad, M. E. and W. H. Crosby. The natural history of iron deficiency induced by phlebotomy. *Blood* 20:173–185 (1962).

Conrad, M. E. and W. H. Crosby. Intestinal mucosal mechanisms controlling iron absorption. *Blood* 22:406–415 (1963).

Consolazio, C. F. and H. L. Johnson. Measurement of energy cost in humans. *Fed. Proc.* 30:1444–1453 (1971).

Consolazio, C. F., R. E. Johnson, and E. Marek. *Metabolic Methods. Clinical Procedure in the Study of Metabolic Functions.* C. V. Mosby, St. Louis (1951).

Consolazio, C. F., L. O. Matoush, R. A. Nelson, R. S. Harding, and J. E. Canham. Excretions of sodium, potassium, magnesium and iron in human sweat and the relation of each to balance requirements. *J. Nutr.* 79:407–415 (1963b).

Consolazio, C. F., R. A. Nelson, L. O. Matoush, R. S. Harding, and J. E. Canham. Nitrogen excretion in sweat and its relation to nitrogen balance requirements. *J. Nutr.* 79:399–406 (1963a).

Consolazio, C. F., R. Shapiro, J. E. Masterson, and P. S. L. McKinzie. Energy requirements of men in extreme heat. *J. Nutr.* 73:126–134 (1961).

Contractor, S. D. and B. Shane. 4-Pyridoxic acid-5'-phosphate: metabolite of pyridoxol in the rat. *Biochem. Biophys. Res. Commun.* 39:1175–1181 (1970).

Cook, J. D. Absorption of food iron. *Fed Proc.* 36:2028–2032 (1977).

Cook, J. D., M. Layrisse, C. Martinez-Torres, R. Walker, E. Monsen, and C. A. Finch. Food iron absorption measured by an extrinsic tag. *J. Clin. Invest.* 51:805–815 (1972).

Cook, J. D., V. Minnich, C. V. Moore, A. Rasmussen, W. B. Bradley, and C. A. Finch. Absorption of fortification iron in bread. *Am. J. Clin. Nutr.* 26:861–872 (1973).

Cook, J. D. and E. R. Monsen. Food iron absorption. I. Use of a semisynthetic diet to study absorption of nonheme iron. *Am. J. Clin. Nutr.* 28:1289–1295 (1975).

Cook, J. D. and E. R. Monsen. Food iron absorption. III. Comparison of the effects of animal proteins on non-heme iron. *Am. J. Clin. Nutr.* 29:859–867 (1976).

Cook, J. D. and E. R. Monsen. Vitamin C, the common cold and iron absorption. *Am. J. Clin. Nutr.* 30:235–241 (1977).

Cooke, N. E., J. Walgate, and J. G. Haddad, Jr. Human serum binding protein for vitamin D and its metabolites. II. Specific, high affinity association with a protein in nucleated tissue. *J. Biol. Chem.* 254:5965–5971 (1979).

Coombs, R. R. A. and H. B. Fell. Lysosomes in tissue damage mediated by allergic reactions. In *Lysosomes in Biology and Pathology*, Vol. 2, pp. 3–18, J. T. Dingle and H. B. Fell, Eds., Wiley-Interscience, New York (1969).

Coon, M. J. Oxygen activation in the metabolism of lipids, drugs and carcinogens. *Nutr. Rev.* 36:319–338 (1978).

Coons, C. M. Iron retention by women during pregnancy. *J. Biol. Chem.* 97:215–226 (1932).

Cooper, C. W., W. H. Schwesinger, A. M. Mahgoub, and D. A. Ontjes. Thyrocalcitonin: stimulation of secretion by pentagastrin. *Science* 172:1238–1240 (1971).

Cooper, J. R. The role of ascorbic acid in the oxidation of tryptophan to 5-hydroxytryptophan. *Ann. N. Y. Acad. Sci.* 92:208–211 (1961).

Cooper, T. G. *The Tools of Biochemistry*, John Wiley & Sons, New York (1977).

Cooperman, J. Microbiological assay of folic acid activity in serum and whole blood. In *Methods in Enzymology*, Vol. 18, Part B. D. B. McCormick and L. D. Wright, Eds., Academic Press, New York (1971).

Copenhaver, J. S. and W. B. Bell. The production of bovine hyperkeratosis (X disease) with an experimentally-made pellet feed. *Vet. Med.* 49:96–101 (1954).

Copp, D. H. Parathyroids and homeostasis of blood calcium. In *Bone as a Tissue*, pp. 289–299, K. Rodahl, J. T. Nicholson, and E. M. Brown, Jr., Eds., McGraw-Hill, New York (1960).

Copp, D. H., E. C. Cameron, B. A. Cheney, A. G. F. Davidson, and E. G. Henze. Evidence for calcitonin—a new hormone from the parathyroid that lowers blood calcium. *Endocrinology* 70:638–649 (1962).

Copping, A. M. Inhibitors of pantothenic acid. In *Antivitamins,* pp. 169–177, J. C. Somogyi, Ed., *Bibl. Nutr. Dieta,* Vol. 8, S. Karger, Basel, Switz. (1966).

Cori, C. F. The fate of sugar in the animal body. I. The rate of absorption of hexoses and pentoses from the intestinal tract. *J. Biol. Chem.* 66:691–715 (1925).

Cori, C. F. Mammalian carbohydrate metabolism. *Physiol. Rev.* 11:143–275 (1931).

Cori, C. F. and B. Illingworth. The prosthetic group of phosphorylase. *Proc. Nat. Acad. Sci. U. S.* 43:547–552 (1957).

Correy, E. L. Growth and glycogen content of the fetal liver and placenta. *Am. J. Physiol.* 112:263–267 (1935).

Corrigan, J. J. and F. I. Marcus. Coagulopathy associated with vitamin E ingestion. *JAMA* 230:1300–1301 (1974).

Cottrel, G. A. and P. Usherwood, Eds. *Synapses.,* Blackie & Sons, London (1977).

Cousins, R. J. Regulation of zinc absorption: role of intracellular ligands. *Am. J. Clin. Nutr.* 32:339–345 (1979).

Cousins, R. J. Regulatory aspects of zinc metabolism in liver and intestine. Nutr. Rev. 37:97–103 (1979).

Coward, D. G., M. B. Sawyer, and R. G. Whitehead. Microtechniques for the automated analysis of serum total protein and albumin, urinary urea, creatinine, and hydroxyproline for nutrition surveys in developing countries. *Am. J. Clin. Nutr.* 24:940–946 (1971).

Cox, E. V. and A. M. White. Methylmalonic acid excretion: an index of vitamin-B_{12} deficiency. *Lancet* 2:853–856 (1962).

Cox, T. M., J. Mazurier, G. Spik, J. Montreuil, and T. J. Peters. Iron-binding proteins and influx of iron across the duodenal brush border. *Biochim. Biophys. Acta* 588:120–128 (1979).

Coyle, J. T. Excitatory amino acid receptors. In *Neurotransmitter Receptors, Part I,* pp. 3–40, S. J. Enna and H. I. Yamamura, Eds., Chapman and Hall, New York (1980).

Cramer, C. F. Quantitative studies on the absorption and excretion of calcium for Thiry-Vella intestinal loops in the dog. In *The Transfer of Calcium and Strontium Across Biologic Membranes,* pp. 75–84, R. H. Wasserman, Ed., Academic Press, New York (1963).

Crampton, R. F., M. T. Lis, and D. M. Matthews. Sites of maximal absorption and hydrolysis of two dipeptides by rat small intestine *in vivo. Clin. Sci.* 44:583–594 (1973).

Crandon, J. H., C. C. Lund, and D. B. Dill. Experimental human scurvy. *N. Eng. J. Med.* 223:353–369 (1940).

Crane, R. K. Intestinal absorption of sugars. *Physiol. Rev.* 40:789–825 (1960).

Crane, R. K. Na$^+$-dependent transport in the intestine and other animal tissues. *Fed. Proc.* 24:1000–1006 (1965).

Crane, R. K. Absorption of sugars. In *Handbook of Physiology,* Section 6: Alimentary Canal, Vol. 3, pp. 1323–1351, C. F. Code, Ed., American Physiological Society, Washington, D.C. (1968).

Crane, R. K. and P. Mandelstam. The active transport of sugars by various preparations of hamster intestine. *Biochim. Biophys. Acta* 45:460–476 (1960).

Cravioto, J., E. R. DeLicardie, and H. G. Birch. Nutrition, growth and neurointegrative development: an experimental and ecologic study. *Pediatr.* 38:319–372 (1966).

Cravioto, J. and B. Robles. Evolution of adaptive and motor behavior during rehabilitation from kwashiorkor. *Am. J. Orthopsychiatry* 35:449–464 (1965).

Cresta, M. New method of assessing food consumption by age-groups on the basis of overall family data. *Nutrition Newsletter* 8:37–49 (1970).

Crichton, R. Studies on the structure of ferritin and apoferritin from horse spleen. I. Tryptic digestion of ferritin and apoferritin. *Biochim. Biophys. Acta* 194:34–42 (1969).

Crick, F. H. C. On the genetic code. *Science* 139:461–464 (1963).

Crick, F. H. C. The genetic code—yesterday, today, and tomorrow. *Cold Spring Harbor Symp. Quant. Biol.* 31:3–9 (1966a).

Crick, F. H. C. Codon-anticodon paring: the wobble hypothesis. *J. Mol. Biol.* 19:548–555 (1966b).

Crick, F. H. C. Central dogma of molecular biology. *Nature* 227:561–563 (1970).

Crick, F. H. C., L. Barnett, S. Brenner, and R. J. Watts-Tobin. General nature of the genetic code for proteins. *Nature* 192:1227–1230 (1961).

Crokaert, R. Du dosage chimique de l'acide pantothénique. *Bull. Soc. Chim. Biol.* 31:903–907 (1949).

Csáky, T. Z. Significance of sodium ions in active intestinal transport of non-electrolytes. *Am. J. Physiol.* 201:999–1001 (1961).

Csáky, T. Z. A possible link between active transport of electrolytes and non-electrolytes. *Fed. Proc.* 22:3–7 (1963).

Csallany, A. S., H. H. Draper, and S. N. Shah. Conversion of a d-a-tocopherol-C^{14} to tocopheryl-p-quinone *in vivo. Arch. Biochem. Biophys.* 98:142–145 (1962).

Csallany, A. S. and H. H. Draper. Dimerization of a-tocopherol *in vivo. Arch. Biochem. Biophys.* 100:335–337 (1963).

Cuatrecasas, P. Insulin-receptor interactions in adipose tissue cells: direct measurement and properties. *Proc. Nat. Acad. Sci. U. S.* 68:1264–1268 (1971a).

Cuatrecasas, P. Properties of the insulin receptor of isolated fat cell membranes. *J. Biol. Chem.* 246:7265–7274 (1971b).

Cuatrecasas, P. Insulin receptor of liver and fat cell membranes. *Fed. Proc.* 32:1838–1846 (1973a).

Cuatrecasas, P., D. H. Lockwood, and J. R. Caldwell. Lactase deficiency in the adult. *Lancet* 1:14–18 (1965).

Cuénod, M. and J. Schonback. Synaptic proteins and axonal flow in the pigeon visual pathway. *J. Neurochem.* 18:809–816 (1971).

Culley, W. J. and E. T. Mertz. Effect of restricted food intake on growth and composition of preweanling rat brain. *Proc. Soc. Exp. Biol. Med.* 118:233–235 (1965).

Cummings, J. H., M. J. Hill, H. Houston, W. J. Branch, and D. J. A. Jenkins. The effect of meat protein and dietary fiber on colonic function and metabolism. I. Changes in bowel habit, bile acid excretion and calcium absorption. *Am. J. Clin. Nutr.* 32:2086–2093 (1979).

Cunningham, J. J. A reanalysis of the factors influencing basal metabolic rate in normal adults. *Am. J. Clin. Nutr.* 33:2372–2374 (1980).

Cunningham, J. J. An individualization of dietary requirements for energy in adults. *J. Am. Diet. Assoc.* 80:335–338 (1982).

Curran, P. F., J. J. Hajjar, and I. M. Glynn. The sodium-alanine interaction in rabbit ileum. Effect of alanine on sodium fluxes. *J. Gen. Physiol.* 55:297–308 (1970).

Curtis, K. J., Y. S. Kim, J. M. Perdomo, D. B. A. Silk, and J. S. Whitehead. Protein digestion and absorption in the rat. *J. Physiol.* 274:409–419 (1978).

Cushman, S. W. and L. J. Wardzala. Potential mechanism of insulin action on glucose transport in the isolated rat adipose cell. *J. Biol. Chem.* 255:4758–4762 (1980).

Czech, M. P. Molecular basis of insulin action. *Ann. Rev. Biochem.* 46:359–384 (1977).

Czech, M. P. Insulin action and the regulation of hexose transport. *Diabetes* 29:399–409 (1980).

Czech, M. P. Insulin action. *Am. J. Med.* 70:142–150 (1981).

Daems, W. Th., E. Wisse, and P. Brederoo. Electron microscopy of the vacuolar apparatus. In *Lysosomes in Biology and Pathology,* Vol. 1, pp. 64–112, J. T. Dingle and H. B. Fell, Eds., Wiley-Interscience, New York (1969).

Daft, F. S., E. G. McDaniel, L. G. Herman, M. K. Romine, and J. R. Hegner. Role of coprophagy in utilization of B vitamins synthesized by intestinal bacteria. *Fed. Proc.* 22:129–133 (1963).

Dagley, S. and D. E. Nicholson. *An Introduction to Metabolic Pathways,* John Wiley & Sons, New York (1970).

Dahlqvist, A. The intestinal disaccharidases and disaccharide intolerance (Editorial) *Gastroenterol.* 43:694–696 (1962).

Dahlqvist, A. Localization of the small-intestinal disaccharidases. *Am. J. Clin. Nutr.* 20:81–88 (1967).

Dahlqvist, A. and B. Borgström. Digestion and absorption of disaccharides in man. *Biochem. J.* 81:411–418 (1961).

Dahlström, A. and J. Häggendal. Studies on the transport and life-span of amine storage granules in a peripheral adrenergic neuron system. *Acta Physiol. Scand.* 67:278–288 (1966).

Daiger, S. P., M. S. Schanfield, and L. L. Cavalli-Sforza. Group-specific component (Gc) proteins bind vitamin D and 25-hydroxyvitamin D. *Proc. Nat. Acad. Sci. U. S.* 72:2076–2080 (1975).

Dairman, W., J. G. Christenson, and S. Udenfriend. Changes in tyrosine hydroxylase and dopa decarboxylase induced by pharmacological agents. *Pharmacol. Rev.* 24:269–289 (1972).

Dalderup, C. B. M. Vitamins. In *Side Effects of Drugs,* Vol. 6, pp. 000, L. Meyler and A. Herxheimer, Eds., Excerpta Medica Foundation, Amsterdam (1967).

Dallman, P. R. Tissue effects of iron deficiency, In *Iron in Biochemistry and Medicine,* pp. 337–375, A. Jacobs and M. Worwood, Eds., Academic Press, New York (1974).

Dalton, A. J. Golgi apparatus and secretion granules. In *The Cell,* Vol. 2, pp. 603–619, J. Brachet and A. E. Mirsky, Eds., Academic Press, New York (1961).

Dalvi, R. R., H. E. Sauberlich, and R. A. Neal. An examination of the metabolism of thiamin by rat liver alcohol dehydrogenase. *J. Nutr.* 104:1476–1483 (1974).

Dam, H. Vitamin K. *Vitam. Horm.* 6:27–53 (1948).

Dam, H. Interrelations between vitamin E and polyunsaturated fatty acids in animals. *Vitam. Horm.* 20:527–540 (1962).

Dam, H. and H. Granados. Peroxidation of body fat in vitamin E deficiency. *Acta Physiol. Scand.* 10:162–171 (1945).

Dam, H., F. Schønheyder and E. Tage-Hansen. Studies on the mode of action of vitamin K. *Biochem. J.* 30:1075–1079 (1936).

Daniel, P. M., O. E. Pratt, and E. Spargo. The metabolic homeostatic role of muscle and its function as a store of protein. *Lancet* 2:446–448 (1977).

Danielli, J. F. and H. Davson. A contribution to the theory of permeability of thin films. *J. Cell Comp. Physiol.* 5:495–508 (1935).

Daniels, A. L., M. K. Hutton, E. M. Knott, O. E. Wright, and M. Forman. Calcium and phosphorus needs of preschool children. *J. Nutr.* 10:373–388 (1935).

Darby, W. J., R. O. Cannon, and M. M. Kaser. The biochemical assessment of nutritional status during pregnancy. *Obstet. Gynecol. Surv.* 3:704–715 (1948).

Darby, W. J., N. W. McNutt, and E. N. Todhunter. Niacin. *Nutr. Rev.* 33:289–297 (1975).

Das, M. and A. N. Radhakrishnan. Glycyl-L-leucine hydrolase, a versatile "master" dipeptidase from monkey small intestine. *Biochem. J.* 135:609–615 (1973).

Daum, K., W. W. Tuttle, and M. Wilson. Thiamine requirements and their implications. *J. Am. Diet. Assoc.* 25:398–404 (1949).

Dauncey, M. J. Energy metabolism in man and the influence of diet and temperature: a review. *J. Hum. Nutr.* 33:259–269 (1979).

Dauncey, M. J. Metabolic effects of altering the 24 h energy intake in man, using direct and indirect calorimetry. *Br. J. Nutr.* 43:257–269 (1980).

Dauncey, M. J. and D. L. Ingram. Effect of dietary composition and cold exposure on non-shivering thermogenesis in young pigs and its alteration by the β-blocker propranolol. *Br. J. Nutr.* 41:361–370 (1979).

Dauncy, M. J., J. C. L. Shaw, and J. Urman. The absorption and retention of magnesium, zinc, and copper by low birth weight infants fed pasteurized human breast milk. *Pediatr. Res.* 11:1033–1038 (1977).

Davenport, E. Calculating the nutritive value of diets (ARS Pub. 62-10-1), U.S. Department of Agriculture, Washington, D.C. (1964).

Davenport, H. W. *Physiology of the Digestive Tract,* 3rd ed., Year Book Medical Publishers, Chicago (1971).

Davenport, H. W. Why the stomach does not digest itself. *Sci. Am.* 226(1): 86–94 (1972).

David, J. S. K., P. Malathi, and J. Ganguly. Role of the intestinal brush border in the absorption of cholesterol in rats. *Biochem. J.* 98:662–668 (1966).

Davidson, M. B. Effects of obesity on insulin sensitivity of human adipose tissue. *Diabetes* 21:6–12 (1972).

Davis, J. O. and R. H. Freeman. Mechanisms regulating renin release. *Physiol. Rev.* 56:1–56 (1976).

Davis, J. O. and R. H. Freeman. The other angiotensins. *Biochem. Pharmacol.* 26:93–97 (1977).

Davis, R. E. A molecular theory of muscle contraction: calcium-dependent contractions with hydrogen bond formation plus ATP-dependent extensions of part of the myosin-actin cross-bridges. *Nature* 199:1068–1074 (1963).

Davison, A. N. and J. Dobbing. Phospholipid metabolism in nervous tissue. II. Metabolic stability. *Biochem. J.* 75:565–570 (1960).

Davison, A. N., R. S. Morgan, M. Wajda, and G. P. Wright. Metabolism of myelin lipids: incorporation of [3-^{14}C] serine in brain lipids of the developing rabbit and their persistence in the central nervous system. *J. Neurochem.* 4:360–365 (1959).

Davson, H. The blood-brain barrier. *J. Physiol.* 255:1–28 (1976).

Dawber, T. R., G. Pearson, P. Anderson, G. V. Mann, W. B. Kannel, D. Shurtleff, and P. McNamara. Dietary assessment in the epidemiologic study of coronary heart disease: the Framingham Study. II. Reliability of measurement. *Am. J. Clin. Nutr.* 11:226–234 (1962).

Dawkins, M. J. R. and D. Hull. The production of heat by fat. *Sci. Am.* 213 (2):62–67 (1965).

Dawkins, M. J. R. and J. W. Scopes. Non-shivering thermogenesis and brown adipose tissue in the human newborn infant. *Nature* 206:201–202 (1965).

Dawson, E. B., R. R. Clark, and W. J. McGanity. Plasma vitamins and trace metal changes during teen-age pregnancy. *Am. J. Obstet. Gynecol.* 104:953–958 (1969).

Dawson, R. B., S. Rafal, and L. R. Weintraub. Absorption of hemoglobin iron: the role of xanthine oxidase in the intestinal heme-splitting reaction. *Blood* 35:94–103 (1970).

Dayhoff, M. O., Ed., *Atlas of protein sequence and structure 1972*, Vol. 5, Suppl. No. 3, 1978, National Biomedical Foundation (1979).

Dean, R. T. *Lysosomes,* Edward Arnold Publishers, London (1977).

Dean, R. T. and A. J. Barrett. Lysosomes. *Essays Biochem.* 12:1–40 (1976).

Dean, R. T. and J. D. Judah. Post-translational proteolytic processing of polypeptides. In *Comprehensive Biochemistry,* Vol. 19B, Part 1, pp. 233–298, M. Florkin, Ed., Elsevier Scientific Publishing Co., Amsterdam and New York (1980).

Debognie, J. C., A. D. Newcomer, D. B. McGill, and S. F. Phillips. Absorption of nutrients in lactase deficiency. *Dig. Dis. Sci.* 24:225–231 (1979).

De Duve, C. The Lysosome. *Sci. Am.* 208(5):64–72 (1963).

De Duve, C. The lysosome concept. In *Ciba Foundation Symposium on Lysosomes,* pp. 1–31, A. V. S. de Reuck and M. P. Cameron, Eds., Little, Brown & Co., Boston (1963a).

De Duve, C. Evolution of the peroxisome. *Ann. N. Y. Acad. Sci.* 168:369–381 (1969b).

De Duve, C. The lysosome in retrospect. In *Lysosomes in Biology and Pathology,* Vol. 1, pp. 3–40, J. T. Dingle and H. B. Fell, Eds., Wiley-Interscience, New York (1969a).

De Duve, C. Biochemical studies on the occurrence, biogenesis and life history of mammalian peroxisomes. *J. Histochem. Cytochem.* 21:941–948 (1973).

De Duve, C. Microbodies in the living cell. *Sci. Am.* 248(5):74–84 (1983).

De Duve, C. and P. Baudhuin. Peroxisomes (microbodies and related particles). *Physiol. Rev.* 46:323–357 (1966).

De Duve, C., A. C. Pressman, R. Gianetto, R. Wattiaux, and F. Applemans. Tissue fractionation studies. 6. Intracellular distribution patterns of enzymes in rat-liver tissue. *Biochem. J.* 60:604–617 (1955).

De Duve, C. and R. Wattiaux. Functions of lysosomes. *Ann. Rev. Physiol.* 28:435–492 (1966).

De Duve, C., R. Wattiaux, and M. Wibo. Effects of fat-soluble compounds on lysosomes *in vitro. Biochem. Pharmacol.* 9:97–116 (1962).

Deen, W. M., M. P. Bohrer, C. R. Robertson, and B. M. Brenner. Determinants of the transglomerular passage of macromolecules. *Fed. Proc.* 36:2614–2618 (1977).

DeGrazia, J. A., P. I. Vonovich, H. Fellows, and C. Rich. A double isotope method for measurement of intestinal absorption of calcium in man. *J. Lab. Clin. Med.* 66:822–831 (1965).

Dekaban, A. S., R. Aamodt, W. F. Rumble, G. S. Johnston, and S. O'Reilly. Kinky hair disease. Study of copper metabolism with use of ^{67}Cu. *Arch. Neurol.* 32:672–675 (1975).

DeLalla, O. and J. W. Gofman. Ultracentrifugal analysis of serum lipoproteins. In *Methods of Biochemical Analysis,* Vol. 1, pp. 459–478, D. Glick, Ed., Interscience Pub., Inc., New York (1954).

Delange, R. J. and E. L. Smith. Chromosomal proteins. In *The Proteins,* Vol. 4, pp. 119–243, H. Neurath and R. L. Hill, Eds., Academic Press, New York, (1979).

Della-Fera, M. A. and C. A. Baile. Cholecystokinin octapeptide: continuous picomole injections into the cerebral ventricles of sheep suppress feeding. *Science* 206:471–473 (1979).

Della-Fera, M. A. and C. A. Baile. Cholecystokinin antibody injected in cerebral ventricles stimulates feeding in sheep. *Science* 212:687–689 (1981).

DeLuca, H. F. Recent advances in the metabolism of vitamin D. *Ann. Rev. Physiol.* 43:199–209 (1981).

DeLuca, H. F. and J. W. Blunt. Vitamin D. In *Methods in Enzymology,* Vol. 18, Part C, pp. 709–733, D. B. McCormick and L. D. Wright, Eds., Academic Press, New York (1971).

DeLuca, H. F. and G. W. Engstrom. Calcium uptake by rat kidney mitochondria. *Proc. Nat. Acad. Sci. U. S.* 47:1744–1750 (1961).

DeLuca, H. F., G. W. Engstrom, and H. Rasmussen. The action of vitamin D and parathyroid hormone *in vitro* on calcium uptake and release by kidney mitochondria. *Proc. Nat. Acad. Sci. U. S.* 48:1604–1609 (1962).

DeLuca, H. F., R. T. Franceschi, B. P. Halloran, and E. R. Massaro. Molecular events involved in 1,25-dihydroxyvitamin D_3 stimulation of intestinal calcium transport. *Fed. Proc.* 41:66–71 (1982).

DeLuca, H. F. and H. K. Schnoes. Vitamin D: recent advances. *Ann. Rev. Biochem.* 52:411–439 (1983).

DeLuca, L., N. Maestri, F. Bonanni, and D. Nelson. Maintenance of epithelial cell differentiation: the mode of action of vitamin A. *Cancer* 30:1326–1331 (1972).

DeLuca, L. M. and S. S. Shapiro. Modulation of cellular interactions by vitamin A and derivatives (retinoids). *Ann. N. Y. Acad. Sci.* 359:1–430 (1981).

DeLuise, M., T. J. Martin, P. B. Greenberg, and V. Michelangeli. Metabolism of porcine, human and salmon calcitonin in the rat. *J. Endocrinol* 53:475–482 (1972).

De Meyts, P. and J. Hanoune. Plasma membrane receptors and function. In *The Liver: Biology and Pathobiology,* pp. 551–580, I. Arias, H. Popper, D. Schachter, and D. A. Shafritz, Eds., Raven Press, New York (1982).

Demopoulos, H. B. The basis of free radical pathology. *Fed. Proc.* 32:1859–1861 (1973).

Dempsey, G. P., S. Bullivant, and W. B. Watkins. Endothelial cell membranes: polarity of particles as seen by freeze-fracturing. *Science* 179:190–192 (1973).

Dennis, V. W., W. W. Stead, and J. L. Myers. Renal handling of phosphate and calcium. *Ann. Rev. Physiol.* 41:257–271 (1979).

Denton, R. M. and J. G. McCormack. Calcium ions, hormones, and mitochondrial metabolism. *Clin. Sci.* 61:135–140 (1981).

Department of Health, Education, and Welfare. *Height and Weight of Youths 12–17 Years, United States* (Vital and Health Statistics Series 11, No. 124, DHEW Publication No. [HSM] 73-1606), U.S. Government Printing Office, Washington, D. C. (1973b).

Department of Health, Education, and Welfare. *Skinfold Thickness of Children 6–11 years, United States* (Vital and Health Statistics Series 11, No. 120, DHEW Publication No. [HSM] 73-1602), U.S. Government Printing Office, Washington, D. C. (1973a).

De Pierre, J. W. and L. Ernster. Enzyme topology of intracellular membranes. *Ann. Rev. Biochem.* 46:201–262 (1977).

Deren, J. J. Development of intestinal structure and function. In *Handbook of Physiology*, Section 6: Alimentary Canal, Vol. 3, pp. 1099–1123, C. F. Code, Ed., American Physiological Society, Washington, D.C. (1968).

DeRobertis, E. Ultrastructure and cytochemistry of the synaptic region. *Science* 156:907–914 (1967).

DeRobertis, E. Molecular biology of synaptic receptors. *Science* 171:963–971 (1971).

DeRobertis, E. and H. S. Bennett. Submicroscopic vesicular component in the synapse. *Fed. Proc.* 13:35A (1954).

DeRobertis, E. and C. M. Franchi. The submicroscopic organization of axon material isolated from myelin nerve fibers. *J. Exp. Med.* 98:269–276 (1953).

DeRobertis, E. and H. Franco Ruffo. Submicroscopic organization of the mitochondrial body and other cytoplasmic structures of insect testis. *Exp. Cell Res.* 12:66–79 (1957).

DeRobertis, E. D. P. and E. M. F. DeRobertis. *Cell and Molecular Biology*, 7th ed., W. B. Saunders Co., Philadelphia (1980).

DeRobertis, E. D. P., W. W. Nowinski, and F. A. Saez. *Cell Biology*, 5th ed., p. 53, W. B. Saunders Co., Philadelphia (1970).

Desai, I. D. Assay methods. In *Vitamin E, A Comprehensive Treatise*, pp. 67–98, L. J. Machlin, Ed., Marcel Dekker Inc., New York (1980).

Deshmukh, D. S. and J. Ganguly. Demonstration of oxidation and reduction of retinal in rat intestine. *Indian J. Biochem.* 4:18–21 (1967).

Deshmukh, D. S., P. Malathi, K. Subba Rao, and J. Ganguly. Absorption of retinoic acid (vitamin A acid) in rats. *Indian J. Biochem.* 1:164–166 (1964).

Deshmukh, D. S., S. K. Murthy, S. Mahadevan, and J. Ganguly. Studies on metabolism of vitamin A: absorption of retinal (vitamin A aldehyde) in rats. *Biochem. J.* 96:377–382 (1965).

Devlin, T. M., Ed., *Textbook of Biochemistry with Clinical Correlations*, John Wiley & Sons, New York (1982).

DeVries, J. X., W. Gunthert, and R. Derig. Determination of nicotinamide in human plasma and urine by ion-pair reversed high phase high-performance liquid chromatography. *J. Chromatogr.* 221:161–165 (1980).

DeVries, W. H., W. M. Grovier, J. S. Evans, J. D. Gregory, G. D. Novelli, M. Soodak, and F. Lipmann. Purification of coenzyme A from fermentation sources and its further partial identification. *J. Am. Chem. Soc.* 72:4838. (1950).

Dickerson, R. E. The structure and history of an ancient protein. *Sci. Am.* 226(4):58–72 (1972).

Dickerson, R. E. Cytochrome c and the evolution of energy metabolism. *Sci. Am.* 242:137–153 (1980).

Dickerson, R. E. and I. Geis. *The Structure and Action of Proteins*, W. A. Benjamin, Menlo Park, Calif. (1969).

Dietrich, L. S. Regulation of nicotinamide metabolism. *Am. J. Clin. Nutr.* 24:800–804 (1971).

Dietrich, L. S., L. Martinez, and L. Franklin. Role of the liver in systemic pyridine nucleotide metabolism. Naturwissenschaften 55:231—232 (1968).

diGirolamo, M., S. Mendlinger, and J. W. Fertig. A simple method to determine fat cell size and number in four mammalian species. *Am. J. Physiol.* 221:850–858 (1971).

Dimroth, P. The role of biotin and sodium in the decarboxylation of oxaloacetate by the membrane-bound oxaloacetate decarboxylase from *Klebsiella aerogenes. Eur. J. Biochem.* 121:435–441 (1982).

Dingle, J. T. Action of vitamin A on the stability of lysosomes *in vivo* and *in vitro.* In *Ciba Foundation Symposium on Lysosomes,* pp. 384–398, A. V. S. deReuck and M. P. Cameron, Eds., Little, Brown & Co., Boston (1963).

Dingle, J. T. and J. A. Lucy. Vitamin A, carotenoids and cell function. *Biol. Rev.* 40:422–461 (1965).

Dinning, J. S. and P. L. Day. Vitamin E deficiency in the monkey I. Muscular dystrophy, hematologic changes, and the excretion of urinary nitrogenous constituents. *J. Exp. Med.* 105:395–402 (1957).

Dintzis, H. M. Assembly of the peptide chains of hemoglobin. *Proc. Nat. Acad. Sci. U. S.* 47:247–261 (1961).

Dirks, J. H., J. R. Clapp, and R. W. Berliner. The protein concentration in the proximal tubule of the dog. *J. Clin. Invest.* 43:916–921 (1964).

Disler, P. B., S. R. Lynch, R. W. Charlton, J. D. Torrance, T. H. Bothwell, R. B. Walker, and R. Mayet. The effect of tea on iron absorption. *Gut* 16:193–200 (1974).

Dixit, B. N. and J. P. Buckley. Circadian changes in brain 5-hydroxytryptamine and plasma corticosterone in the rat. *Life Sci.* 6:755–758 (1967).

Dobbing, J. The influence of early nutrition on the development and myelination of the brain. *Proc. R. Soc. Lond. Ser.* B 159:503–509 (1964).

Dobbing, J. The developing brain: a plea for more critical interspecies extrapolation. *Nutr. Rep. Int.* 7:401–406 (1973).

Dobbing, J. and J. Sands. Timing of neuroblast multiplication in developing human brain. *Nature* 226:639–640 (1970).

Dobbs, R. E. Control of glucagon secretion: nutrients, gastroenteropancreatic hormones, calcium and prostaglandins. In *Glucagon: Physiology, Pathophysiology, and Morphology of the Pancreatic A-Cells,* pp. 115–133, R. H. Unger and L. Orci, Eds., Elsevier, New York (1981).

Dobzhansky, T. *Heredity and the Nature of Man,* Harcourt, Brace and World, New York (1964).

Dodds, M. L. Sex as a factor in blood levels of ascorbic acid. *J. Am. Diet. Assoc.* 54:32–33 (1969).

Dodds, M. L., E. L. Price, and F. L. MacLeod. A study of the relation and adjustment of blood plasma level and urinary excretion of ascorbic acid to intake. *J. Nutr.* 40:255–263 (1950).

Doisy, E. A., Jr. Micronutrient controls on biosynthesis of clotting proteins and cholesterol. In *Trace Substances in Environmental Health,* Vol. 6, p. 193, D. Hemphill, Ed., University of Missouri, Columbia (1972).

Donabedian, R. K. and A. Karmen. Fatty acid transport and incorporation into human erythrocytes *in vitro. J. Clin. Invest.* 46:1017–1027 (1967).

Donaldson, H. H. In *The Rat,* 2nd ed, Wistar Institute Press, Philadelphia (1924).

Donaldson, R. M., Jr., I. L. Mackenzie, and J. S. Trier. Intrinsic factor-mediated attachment of vitamin B_{12} to brush border and microvillous membranes of hamster intestine. *J. Clin. Invest.* 46:1215–1228 (1967).

Doumeng, C. and S. Maroux. Arminotripeptidase, a cytosol enzyme from rabbit intestinal mucosa. *Biochem. J.* 177:801–808 (1979).

Dowdle, E. B., D. Schachter, and H. Schenker. Active transport of Fe^{59} by everted segments of rat duodenum. *Am. J. Physiol.* 198:609–613 (1960).

Dowling, J. E. and G. Wald. The biological function of vitamin A acid. *Proc. Nat. Acad. Sci. U. S.* 46:587–608 (1960).

Downs, E. F. Nutritional dwarfing. A syndrome of early protein-calorie malnutrition. *Am. J. Clin. Nutr.* 15:275–281 (1964).

Drake, J. R. and C. D. Fitch. Status of Vitamin E as an erythropoietic factor. *Am. J. Clin. Nutr.* 33:2386–2393 (1980).

Drapanas, T., J. S. Williams, J. C. McDonald, W. Heyden, T. Bow, and R. P. Spencer. Role of the ileum in the absorption of vitamin B_{12} and intrinsic factor (NF). *JAMA* 184:337–341 (1963).

Draper, H. H., J. G. Bergan, M. Chiu, A. S. Csallany, and A. V. Boaro. A further study of the specificity of the vitamin E requirement for reproduction. *J. Nutr.* 84:395–400 (1964).

Draper, H. H. and A. S. Csallany. Metabolism and function of vitamin E. *Fed. Proc.* 28:1690–1695 (1969).

Draper, H. H. and A. S. Csallany. Metabolism of vitamin E. In *The Fat-Soluble*

Vitamins, pp. 347–353, H. F. DeLuca and J. W. Suttie, Eds., University of Wisconsin Press, Madison (1970).

Draper, H. H., A. S. Csallany, and M. Chiu. Isolation of a trimer of a-tocopherol from mammalian liver. *Lipids* 2:47–54 (1967).

Draper, H. H. and C. A. Scythes. Calcium, phosphorus, and osteoporosis. *Fed. Proc.* 40:2434–2438 (1981).

Drenick, E. J. Weight reduction by prolonged fasting. In *Obesity in Perspective,* Vol. 2, Part 2, pp. 341–360, G. A. Bray, Ed. (DHEW Publ. No. [NIH] 75-708), U.S. Government Printing Office, Washington, D.C. (1975).

Dreyer, W. J., D. S. Papermaster, and H. Kuhn. On the absence of ubiquitous structural protein subunits in biological membranes. *Ann. N. Y. Acad. Sci.* 195:61–74 (1972).

Droz, B. and C. P. Leblond. Axonal migration of proteins in the central nervous system and peripheral nerves as shown by radioautography. *J. Comp. Neurol.* 121:325–346 (1963).

Drummond, J. C. The nomenclature of the so-called accessory food factors. *Biochem. J.* 14:660. (1920).

Dryden, J. J., J. G. Kendrick, L. D. Satterlee, L. J. Schroeder, and R. G. Block. Predicting protein digestibility and quality using an enzyme—*Tetrahymena pyriformis* W. bioassay. *J. Food Biochem.* 1:35–43 (1977).

Drysdale, J. W. and H. N. Munro. Small-scale isolation of ferritin for the assay of the incorporation of ^{14}C-labelled amino acids. *Biochem. J.* 95:851–858 (1965).

Drysdale, J. W. and H. N. Munro. Regulation of synthesis and turnover of ferritin in rat liver. *J. Biol. Chem.* 241:3630–3637 (1966).

Dubach, R. V., C. V. Moore, and S. Callender. Studies in iron transportation and metabolism. IX. Excretion of iron as measured by the isotope technique. *J. Lab. Clin. Med.* 45:599–615 (1955).

Dubé, R. B., E. C. Johnson, H. H. Yü, and C. A. Storwick, with technical assistance of S. Kosko and S. McFarland. Thiamine metabolism of women on controlled diets. II. Daily blood thiamine values. *J. Nutr.* 48:307–316 (1952).

Dubois, D. and E. F. Dubois. Clinical calorimetry. A formula to estimate the approximate surface area if height and weight be known. *Arch. Intern. Med.* 17:863–871 (1916).

Dugdale, A. E. An age-independent anthropometric index of nutritional status. *Am. J. Clin. Nutr.* 24:174–180 (1971).

Dunn, M. S., E. A. Murphy, and L. B. Rockland. Optimal growth of the rat. *Physiol. Rev.* 27:72–94 (1947).

Dupont, J. and M. M. Mathias. Bio-oxidation of linoleic acid via methylmalonyl-CoA. *Lipids* 4:478–483 (1969).

Durnin, J. V. G. A. Indirect calorimetry in man: a critique of practical problems. *Proc. Nutr. Soc.* 37:5–12 (1978).

Durnin, J. V. G. A., and R. Passmore. *Energy, work and leisure*. Heinemann Educational Books, London (1967).

Durnin, J. V. G. A. and J. Wormersley. Body fat assessed from total body density and its estimation from skinfold thickness measurements on 481 men and women aged 16 to 72 years. *Br. J. Nutr.* 32:77–97 (1974).

Dustin, P. *Microtubules,* Springer-Verlag, New York (1978).

Dyer, R. F. Morphological features of brown adipose cell maturation *in vivo* and *in vitro*. *Am. J. Anat.* 123:255–282 (1968).

Dyerberg, J. Dietary manipulation of prostaglandin synthesis: beneficial or detrimental. In *Cardiovascular Pharmacology of the Prostaglandins.* pp. 233–244, A. G. Herman, P. M. Vanhoutte, H. Denolin, and A. Goossens, Eds., Raven Press, New York (1982).

Dziewiatkowski, D. D. Vitamin A and endochondral ossification in the rat as indicated by the use of sulphur-35 and phosphorus-32. *J. Exp. Med.* 100:11–24 (1954).

Eanes, E. D. and A. H. Reddi. The effect of fluoride on bone mineral apatite. *Metab. Bone Dis. Rel. Res.* 2:3–10 (1979).

Eanes, E. D., J. D. Termine, and A. S. Posner. Amorphous calcium phosphate in skeletal tissues. *Clin. Orthop.* 53:223–235 (1967).

Ebashi, S. and F. Lipmann. Adenosine triphosphate-linked concentration of calcium ions in a particulate fraction of rabbit muscle. *J. Cell Biol.* 14:389–400 (1962).

Ebel, J. G., A. N. Taylor, and R. H. Wasserman. Vitamin D-induced calcium-binding protein of intestinal mucosa. *Am. J. Clin. Nutr.* 22:431–436 (1969).

Ebert, J. D., A. G. Loewy, R. S. Miller, and H. A. Schneiderman. *Biology,* Holt, Rinehart & Winston, New York (1973).

Eccles, J. C. The Synapse. *Sci. Am.* 212(1):56–66 (1965).

Eck, R. V. Genetic code: emergence of a symmetrical pattern. *Science* 140:477–480 (1963).

Eckhert, C. D., M. V. Sloan, J. R. Duncan, and L. S. Hurley. Zinc binding: a difference between human and bovine milk. *Science* 195:789–790 (1977).

Edelman, I. S., H. B. Haley, P. R. Schloerb, D. B. Sheldon, B. J. Friis-Hansen, G. Stoll, and F. D. Moore. Further observations on total body water. I. Normal values throughout the life span. *Surg. Gynecol. Obstet.* 95:1–12 (1952).

Edholm, O. G., J. G. Fletcher, E. M. Widdowson, and R. A. McCance. The energy expenditure and food intake of individual men. *Br. J. Nutr.* 9:286–300 (1955).

Edidin, M. Rotational and translational diffusion in membranes. *Ann. Rev. Biophys. Bioeng.* 3:179–201 (1974).

Edkins, J. S. The chemical mechanism of gastric secretion. *J. Physiol.* (London) 34:183–185 (1906).

Edozien, J. C. Establishment of a biochemical norm for the evaluation of nutritional status in West Africa. *J. West Afr. Sci. Assoc.* 10:1–21 (1965).

Edstrom, J. E. and W. Beermann. The base composition of nucleic acids in chromosomes, puffs, nucleoli, and cytoplasm of *Chirononus* salivary gland cells. *J. Cell Biol.* 14:371–379 (1962).

Edwards, O. M., R. I. S. Bayliss, and S. Millen. Urinary creatinine excretion as an index of the completeness of 24-hour urine collections. *Lancet* 2:1165–1166 (1969).

Ehret, C. F. and E. L. Powers. Macronuclear and nucleolar development in *Paramecium bursaria*. *Exp. Cell Res.* 9:241–259 (1955).

Eichholz, A. and R. K. Crane. Studies on the organization of the brush border in intestinal epithelial cells. I. Tris disruption of isolated hamster brush borders and density gradient separation of fractions. *J. Cell Biol.* 26:687–691 (1965).

Eisenberg, S. Plasma lipoprotein conversions: the origin of low density and high density lipoproteins. *Ann. N. Y. Acad. Sci.* 348:30–44 (1980).

El-Gorab, M. I. and B. A. Underwood. Solubilization of β-carotene and retinol into aqueous solutions of mixed micelles. *Biochim. Biophys. Acta* 306:58–66 (1973).

El-Gorab, M. I., B. A. Underwood, and J. D. Loerch. The roles of bile salts in the uptake of beta-carotene and retinol by rat everted gut sacs. *Biochim. Biophys. Acta* 401:265–277 (1975).

Elias, H. Three-dimensional structure identified from single sections. *Science* 174:993–1000 (1971).

Elsom, K. O'S., J. G. Reinhold, J. T. L. Nicholson, and C. Chornock. Studies of the B vitamins in the human subject. V. The normal requirement for thiamine; some factors influencing its utilization and excretion. *Am. J. Med. Sci.* 203:569–577 (1942).

Elson, D. Preparation and properties of a ribonucleoprotein isolated from *Escherichia coli*. *Biochim. Biophys. Acta* 36:362–371 (1959).

Elson, D. A ribonucleic acid particle released from ribosomes by salt. *Biochim. Biophys. Acta* 53:232–234 (1961).

Elvehjem, C. A. The relative value of inorganic and organic iron in hemoglobin formation. *JAMA* 98:1047–1050 (1932).

Elvehjem, C. A., R. J. Madden, S. M. Strong, and D. W. Wooley. The isolation and identification of the anti-black tongue factor. *J. Biol. Chem.* 123:137–149 (1938).

Elwood, P. C., D. Newton, J. D. Eakins, and D. A. Brown. Absorption of iron from bread. *Am. J. Clin. Nutr.* 21:1162–1169 (1968).

Emerson, G. A., E. Wurtz, and O. H. Johnson. The antiriboflavin effect of galactoflavin. *J. Biol. Chem.* 160:165–167 (1945).

Emerson, K., E. L. Poindexter, and M. Kothari. Changes in total body composition during normal and diabetic pregnancy. Relation to oxygen consumption. *Obstet. Gynecol.* 45:505–511 (1975).

Emerson, K., B. N. Saxena, and E. L. Poindexter. Caloric cost of normal pregnancy. *Obstet. Gynecol.* 40:786–794 (1972).

Emmett, A. D. and G. O. Luros. Water-soluble vitamines. *J. Biol. Chem.* 43:265–280 (1920).

Enesco, M. and C. P. Leblond. Increase in cell number as a factor in the growth of the organs and tissues of the young male rat. *J. Embryol. Exp. Morphol.* 10:530–562 (1962).

Engelhardt, W. A. and M. N. Ljubimowa. Myosin and adenosinetriphosphatase. *Nature* 144:668–669 (1939).

Engle, P. L., M. Irwin, R. E. Klein, C. Yarbrough, and J. W. Townsend. Nutrition and mental development in children. In *Nutrition Pre- and Postnatal Development*, pp. 291–306, M. Winick, Ed., Plenum, New York (1979).

Enns, T. Facilitation by carbonic anhydrase of carbon dioxide transport. *Science* 155:40–47 (1967).

Enochs, M. R. and L. R. Johnson. Trophic effects of gastrointestinal hormones: physiological implications. *Fed. Proc.* 36:1942–1947 (1977).

Enright, L. V., V. Cole, and F. A. Hitchcock. Basal metabolism and iodine excretion during pregnancy. *Am. J. Physiol.* 113:221–228 (1935).

Epstein, A. N., J. T. Fitzsimons, and B. J. Simons. Drinking caused by the intracranial injection of angiotensin in the rat. *J. Physiol.* 200:98–100P (1969).

Erdös, E. G. The angiotensin I converting enzyme. *Fed. Proc.* 36:1760–1765 (1977).

Ericcson, J. L. E. Mechanism of cellular autophagy. In *Lysosomes in Biology and Pathology*, Vol. 2, pp. 345–394, J. T. Dingle and H. B. Fell, Eds., Wiley-Interscience, New York (1969).

Ericsson, J. L. E. and B. F. Trump. Electron microscopic studies of the epithelium of the proximal tubule of the rat kidney. III. Microbodies, multivesicular bodies, and the Golgi apparatus. *Lab. Invest.* 15:1610–1633 (1966).

Ericsson, J. L. E., B. F. Trump, and J. Weibel. Electron microscopic studies of the proximal tubule of the rat kidney. II. Cytosegresomes and cytosomes: their relationship to each other and to the lysosome concept. *Lab. Invest.* 14:1341–1365 (1965).

Ernster, L. and B. Kuylenstierna. Outer membrane of mitochondria. In *Membranes of Mitochondria and Chloroplasts*, pp. 172–212, E. Racker, Ed., Van Nostrand Reinhold Co., New York (1970).

Erslev, A. J. Humoral regulation of red cell production. *Blood* 8:349–357 (1953).

Ertel, R., N. Brot, B. Redfield, J. E. Allende, and H. Weissbach. Binding of guanosine 5'-triphosphate by soluble factors required for polypeptide synthesis. *Proc. Nat. Acad. Sci. U. S.* 59:861–868 (1968).

Essner, E. and A. Novikoff. Cytological studies on two functional hepatomas. Interrelations of endoplasmic reticulum, Golgi apparatus, and lysosomes. *J. Cell Biol.* 15:289–312 (1962).

Evans, G. W. Transferrin function in zinc absorption and transport. *Proc. Soc. Exp. Biol. Med.* 151:775–778 (1976).

Evans, G. W. Normal and abnormal zinc absorption in man and animals: the tryptophan connection. *Nutr. Rev.* 38:137–141 (1980).

Evans, G. W., C. I. Grace and H. J. Votava. A proposed mechanism of zinc absorption in the rat. *Am. J. Physiol.* 228:501–505 (1975).

Evans, G. W. and P. E. Johnson. Zinc binding factor in acrodermatitis enteropathica. *Lancet* 2:1310. (1976).

Evans, H. M. The pioneer history of vitamin E. *Vitam. Horm.* 20:379–387 (1963).

Exton, J. H. The effects of glucagon on hepatic glycogen metabolism and gluconeogenesis. In *Glucagon: Physiology, Pathophysiology, and Morphology of the Pancreatic A-Cells,* pp. 195–219, R. H. Unger and L. Orci, Eds., Elsevier, New York (1981).

Fahey, T. D., L. Akka, and R. Rolph. Body composition and $\dot{V}_{O_2max}$ of exceptional weight-trained athletes. *J. Appl. Physiol.* 39:559–561 (1975).

Fairbanks, B. W. and H. H. Mitchell. The availability of calcium in spinach, in skim milk powder, and in calcium oxalate. *J. Nutr.* 16:79–89 (1938).

Falkner, F. An air displacement method of measuring body volume in babies: a preliminary communication. *Ann. N. Y. Acad. Sci.* 110:75–79 (1963).

Fambrough, D. M., D. B. Drachman, and S. Satyamurti. Neuromuscular junction in myasthenia gravis: decreased acetylcholine receptors. *Science* 182:293–295 (1973).

Farooq, M. and W. T. Norton. A modified procedure for isolation of astrocyte- and neuron-enriched fractions from rat brain. *J. Neurochem.* 31:887–894 (1978).

Farquhar, M. G. Lysosome function in regulating secretion: disposal of secretory granules in cells of the anterior pituitary gland. In *Lysosomes in Biology and Pathology,* Vol. 2, pp. 462–482, J. T. Dingle and H. B. Fell, Eds., Wiley-Interscience, New York (1969).

Farquhar, M. G. and G. E. Palade. Cell junctions in amphibian skin. *J. Cell Biol.* 26:263–291 (1965).

Fasella, P. Pyridoxal phosphate. *Ann. Rev. Biochem.* 36:185–210 (1967).

Fasman, G. D., Ed. Proteins. In *Handbook of Biochemistry and Molecular Biology,* 3rd ed., Vol. 1–3, CRC Press, Cleveland (1976).

Fatt, P. and B. Katz. Spontaneous subthreshold activity of motor nerve endings. *J. Physiol.* 117:109–128 (1952).

Faust, I. M., P. R. Johnson, and J. Hirsch. Long-term effects of early nutritional experience on the development of obesity in the rat. *J. Nutr.* 110:2027–2034 (1980).

Faust, I. M., P. R. Johnson, J. S. Stern, and J. Hirsch. Diet-induced adipocyte number increase in adult rats: a new model of obesity. *Am. J. Physiol.* 235:E279–286 (1978).

Favarger, P. Relative importance of different tissues in the synthesis of fatty acids. In *Handbook of Physiology,* Section 5, Adipose Tissue, pp. 19–23, A. E. Renold and G. F. Cahill, Eds., American Physiological Society, Washington, D.C. (1965).

Fawcett, D. W. Observations on the cytology and electron microscopy of hepatic cells. *J. Nat. Cancer Inst.* 15 (Suppl. 5):1475–1502 (1955).

Fawcett, D. W. Physiologically significant specializations of the cell surface. *Circulation* 26:1105–1125 (1962).

Fawcett, D. W. *The Cell. Its Organelles and Inclusions.* W. B. Saunders Co., Philadelphia (1966).

Fawcett, D. W. *The Cell,* W. B. Saunders Co., Philadelphia (1981).

Fawcett, D. W., J. A. Long, and A. L. Jones. The ultrastructure of endocrine glands. *Recent Prog. Horm. Res.* 25:315–368 (1969).

Fedorko, M. E. and J. G. Hirsch. Cytoplasmic granule formation in myelocytes. *J. Cell Biol.* 29:307–316 (1966).

Fekete, S. The significance of mucopolysaccharides in the pathogenesis of tox-aemias of pregnancy. *Acta Med. Acad. Sci. Hung.* 5:293 (1954). Cited in Hytten and Leitch, *The Physiology of Human Pregnancy,* 2nd ed., F. A. Davis Co., Philadelphia (1971).

Feldherr, C. M. Structure and function of the nuclear envelope: nucleo-cyto-plasmic exchanges. *Adv. Cytopharmacol.* 1:89–98 (1971).

Feldherr, C. M. Structure and function of the nuclear envelope. *Adv. Cell Mol. Biol.* 2:273–307 (1972).

Feldman, S. L. and R. J. Cousins. Influence of cadmium on the metabolism of 25-hydroxycholecalciferol in chicks. *Nutr. Rep. Int.* 8:25–59 (1973).

Felig, P., T. Pozefsky, E. Marliss, and G. F. Cahill, Jr. Alanine: key role in gluconeogenesis. *Science* 167:1003–1004 (1970).

Felig, P. and J. Wahren. Protein turnover and amino acid metabolism in the regulation of gluconeogenesis. *Fed. Proc.* 33:1092–1097 (1974).

Fell, H. B. The effect of vitamin A on the breakdown and synthesis of intercellular material in skeletal tissue in organ culture. *Proc. Nutr. Soc.* 24:166–170 (1965).

Fell, H. B. The direct action of vitamin A on skeletal tissue *in vitro.* In *The Fat-Soluble Vitamins,* pp. 187–202, H. F. DeLuca and J. W. Suttie, Eds., University of Wisconsin Press, Madison (1970).

Fernández-Moran, H. Sheath and axon structures in the internode portion of vertebrate myelinated nerve fibers. An electron microscope study of rat and frog sciatic nerves. *Exp. Cell Res.* 1:309–340 (1950).

Fernández-Moran, H. The submicroscopic organization of vertebrate nerve fibers. An electron microscope study of myelinated and unmyelinated nerve fibers. *Exp. Cell Res.* 3:282–359 (1952).

Fernández-Moran, H. Cell-membrane ultrastructure. *Circulation* 26:1039–1065 (1962).

Fernández-Moran, H. Membrane ultrastructure in nerve cells. In *The Neurosciences,* pp. 281–304, G. C. Quarton, T. Melnechuk, and F. O. Schmitt, Eds., Rockefeller University Press, New York (1967).

Fernstrom, J. D. and R. J. Wurtman. Nutrition and the brain. *Sci. Am.* 230(2):84–91 (1974).

Ferrari, G., U. Ventura, and G. Rindi. The Na^+-dependence of thiamine intestinal transport *in vitro. Life Sci.* 10:67–75 (1971).

Ferro-Luzzi, G. Rapid evaluation of nutritional level. *Am. J. Clin. Nutr.* 19:247–254 (1966).

Fidge, N. H. and D. S. Goodman. The enzymatic reduction of retinal to retinol in rat intestine. *J. Biol. Chem.* 243:4372–4379 (1968).

Fidge, N. H., T. Shiratori, J. Ganguly, and D. S. Goodman. Pathways of absorption of retinal and retinoic acid in the rat. *J. Lipid Res.* 9:103–109 (1968).

Field, J., H. S. Belding, and A. W. Martin. An analysis of the relation between basal metabolism and summated tissue respiration in the rat. *J. Cell Comp. Physiol.* 14:143–157 (1939).

Filer, L. J. and G. A. Martinez. Caloric and iron intake by infants in the U.S.: an evaluation of 4,000 representative six-month-olds. *Clin. Pediatr. (Phila.)* 2:470–476 (1963).

Filer, L. J., Jr., F. H. Mattson, and S. J. Fomon. Triglyceride configuration and fat absorption by the human infant. *J. Nutr.* 99:293–298 (1970).

Finch, C. A. Body iron exchange in man. *J. Clin. Invest.* 38:392–396 (1959).

Finch, C. A. Ferrokinetics and hemoglobin synthesis in man. *Vitam. Horm.* 26:515–523 (1968).

Finch, C. A. and H. Huebers. Perspectives in iron metabolism. *N. Engl. J. Med.* 306:1520–1528 (1982).

Fincke, M. L. and H. C. Sherman. The availability of calcium from some typical foods. *J. Biol. Chem.* 110:421–428 (1935).

Fischer, E. H., L. M. G. Heilmeyer, and R. H. Haschke. Phosphorylase and the control of glycogen degradation. *Curr. Top. Cell Regul.* 4:211–251 (1971).

Fischer, P. W., A. Giroux, and M. R. L'Abbe. The effect of dietary zinc on intestinal copper absorption. *Am. J. Clin. Nutr.* 34:1670–1675 (1981).

Fish, I. and M. Winick. Cellular growth in various regions of the developing rat brain. *Pediatr. Res.* 3:407–412 (1969).

Fisher, J. W. Introduction to conference on erythropoietin. *Ann. N. Y. Acad. Sci.* 149:9–11 (1968).

Fishman, M. A., P. Madyastha, and A. L. Prensky. The effects of undernutrition on the development of myelin in the rat central nervous system. *Lipids* 6:458–465 (1971).

Fishman, M. A., A. L. Prensky, M. E. Tumbleson, and B. Daftari. Relative resistance of the later phase of myelination to severe undernutrition in miniature swine. *Am. J. Clin. Nutr.* 25:7–10 (1972).

Fitch, C. D. Experimental anemia in primates due to vitamin E deficiency. *Vitam. Horm.* 26:501–514 (1968).

Fitzsimons, J. T. The role of a renal thirst factor in drinking induced by extracellular stimuli. *J. Physiol.* 201:349–368 (1969).

Fitzsimons, J. T. Angiotensin, thirst, and sodium appetite: retrospect and prospect. *Fed. Proc.* 37:2669–2675 (1978).

Fitzsimons, J. T. and B. J. Simons. The effect on drinking in the rat of intravenous infusion of angiotensin, given alone or in combination with other thirst stimuli. *J. Physiol.* 203:45–57 (1969).

Flamm, W. G. and M. L. Birnstiel. Inhibiting DNA replication and its effect on histone synthesis. *Exp. Cell Res.* 33:616–619 (1964).

Fleischer, S., G. Rouser, B. Fleischer, A. Casu, and G. Kritchevsky. Lipid composition of mitochondria from bovine heart, liver, and kidney. *J. Lipid Res.* 8:170–180 (1967).

Fleshler, B. and R. A. Nelson. Sodium dependency of L-alanine absorption in canine Thiry-Vella loops. *Gut* 11:240–244 (1970).

Fletcher, J. and E. R. Huehns. Function of transferrin. *Nature* 218:1211–1218 (1968).

Flickinger, C. J. The development of Golgi complexes and their dependence upon the nucleus in *Amebae*. *J. Cell Biol.* 43:250–262 (1969).

Flohé, I., W. A. Guenzler, and R. Ladenstein. Glutathione peroxidase. In *Glutathione*, pp. 115–138, I. M. Arias and W. B. Jacoby, Eds., Raven Press, New York (1976).

Florendo, N. T. Ribosome substructure in intact mouse liver cells. *J. Cell Biol.* 41:335–339 (1969).

Flores, M. Dietary studies for assessment of the nutritional status of populations in nonmodernized societies. *Am. J. Clin. Nutr.* 11:344–355 (1962).

Flynn, M. A., C. Gehrke, B. R. Maier, R. K. Tsutakawa, and D. J. Hentges. Effect of diet on fecal nutrients. *J. Am. Diet. Assoc.* 71:521–526 (1977).

Folin, O. A theory of protein metabolism. *Am. J. Physiol.* 13:117–138 (1905).

Foltz, E. E., C. J. Barborka, and A. C. Ivy. The level of vitamin B-complex in the diet at which detectable symptoms of deficiency occur in man. *Gastroenterol.* 2:323–344 (1944).

Fomon, S. J. and L. F. Filer. Amino acid requirements of normal growth. In *Amino Acid Metabolism and Genetic Variation*, pp. 391–400, W. L. Nyan, Ed., McGraw-Hill, New York (1967).

Fomon, S. J., R. L. Jensen, and G. M. Owen. Determination of body volume of infants by a method of helium displacement. *Ann. N. Y. Acad. Sci.* 110:80–90 (1963).

Fomon, S. J., M. K. Younoszai, and L. N. Thomas. Influence of vitamin D on linear growth of normal full-term infants. *J. Nutr.* 88:345–350 (1966).

Food and Agricultural Organization. Protein requirements. *FAO Nutr. Stud.*, No. 16. FAO, Rome (1957).

Food and Agricultural Organization. Program of food consumption surveys. FAO, Rome (1964).

Food and Agricultural Organization. Amino acid content of foods and biological data on proteins. *FAO Nutr. Stud.*, No. 24. FAO, Rome (1970).

Food and Agricultural Organziation. *Dietary Fats and Oils* (Report of an expert consultation). *FAO Food Nutr. Ser.*, No. 20. Rome (1980). (Table 6—Recommendations of 18 scientific and medical committees on dietary fats and coronary heart disease, pp. 40–41.)

Food and Agricultural Organization/World Health Organization. Protein requirements. *WHO Tech. Rep. Ser.*, No. 301, *FAO Nutr. Meet. Rep. Ser.*, No. 37. FAO, Rome and WHO, Geneva (1965).

Food and Agricultural Organization/World Health Organization. Energy and protein requirements (Report of a joint FAO/WHO ad hoc expert committee on energy and protein requirements.) *WHO Tech. Rep. Ser.*, No. 522, WHO, Geneva, *FAO Nutr. Meet. Rep. Ser.*, No. 52, FAO, Rome (1973).

Food and Agricultural Organization/World Health Organization. Handbook on human nutritional requirements (Report of R. Passmore, B. M. Nicol, M. N. Rao, G. H. Beaton and E. M. DeMayer.) *FAO Nutr Stud.*, No. 28/*WHO Monogr. Ser.*, No. 61. Rome/Geneva (1974).

Food and Agricultural Organization/World Health Organization. Energy and protein requirements. FAO, Rome (1983).

Food and Nutrition Board, National Research Council. *Recommended Dietary Allowances*, 9th ed., National Academy of Sciences, Washington, D.C. (1980).

Forbes, G. B. Growth of the lean body mass in man. *Growth* 36:325–338 (1972).

Forbes, G. B. Another source of error in the metabolic balance method. *Nutr. Rev.* 31:297–300 (1973).

Forbes, G. B. Body composition and the natural history of fatness. In *Obesity in America*, pp. 95–102, G. A. Bray, Ed. (NIH Publication No. 79-359). U.S. Department of Health, Education, and Welfare, Washington, D.C. (1979).

Forbes, G. B., J. Gallup, and J. B. Hursh. Estimation of total body fat from potassium-40 content. *Science* 133:101–102 (1961).

Forbes, G. B. and J. B. Hursh. Age and sex trends in lean body mass calculated from K^{40} measurements: with a note on the theoretical basis for the procedure. *Ann. N. Y. Acad. Sci.* 110:255–263 (1963).

Forbes, R. M. Nutritional interactions of zinc and calcium. *Fed. Proc.* 19:643–647 (1960).

Forbes, R. M., A. R. Cooper, and H. H. Mitchell. The composition of the adult human body as determined by chemical analysis. *J. Biol. Chem.* 203:359–366 (1953).

Forbes, R. M. and J. W. Erdman, Jr. Bioavailability of trace mineral elements. *Ann. Rev. Nutr.* 3:213–231 (1983).

Forbes, R. M., H. H. Mitchell, and R. A. Cooper. Further studies on the gross composition and mineral elements of the adult human body. *J. Biol. Chem.* 223:969 975 (1956).

Ford, J. E. Microbiological methods for protein quality assessment. In *Protein quality in humans: assessment and in vitro estimations,* pp. 278–300, C. E. Bodwell, J. S Adkins, and D. T. Hopkins, Eds., AVI Publishing Co., Westport, Conn. (1981).

Forsgren, L. Studies on the intestinal absorption of labelled fat-soluble vitamins (A, D, E, and K) via the thoracic-duct lymph in the absence of bile in man. *Acta Chir. Scand. (Suppl.)* 399:3–29 (1969).

Forster, J. Versuche uber die Bedeutung der Aschebestandtheile in der Nahrung. *Z. Biol.* 9:297–380 (1873).

Foster, G. V., I. MacIntyre, and A. G. E. Pearse. Calcitonin production and the mitochondrion-rich cells of the dog thyroid. *Nature* 203:1029–1030 (1964).

Fourman, P. and P. Royer. *Calcium Metabolism and the Bone.*, 2nd ed., F. A. Davis Co., Philadelphia (1968).

Fox, C. F. The structure of cell membranes. *Sci. Am.* 226(2):30–38 (1972).

Fox, H. C. and D. S. Miller. Ackee toxin: a riboflavin antimetabolite? *Nature* 186:561–562 (1960).

Foy, H. and A. Kondi. Comparison between erythroid aplasia in marasmus and kwashiorkor and the experimentally induced erythroid aplasia in baboons in riboflavin deficiency. *Vitam. Horm.* 26:653–681 (1968).

Francois, P. J. Food consumption surveys—study on a general formula for the estimation of per caput, household and group consumption. *Nutr. Newsletter* 8:10–26 (1970).

Franke, W. W. Isolated nuclear membranes. *J. Cell Biol.* 31:619–623 (1966).

Franke, W. W. Structure, biochemistry, and functions of the nuclear envelope. *Int. Rev. Cytol. (Suppl.)* 4:71–236 (1974).

Franke, W. W., B. Deumling, B. Ermen, E. D. Jarasch, and H. Kleinig. Nuclear membranes from mammalian liver. I. Isolation procedure and general characteristics. *J. Cell. Biol.* 46:379–395 (1970).

Franke, W. W. and U. Scheer. The ultrastructure of the nuclear envelope of amphibian oocytes: a reinvestigation. I. The mature oocyte. *J. Ultrastruct. Res.* 30:288–316 (1970a).

Franke, W. W. and U. Scheer. The ultrastructure of the nuclear envelope of amphibian oocytes: a reinvestigation. II. The immature oocyte and dynamic aspects. *J. Ultrastruct. Res.* 30:317–327 (1970b).

Frankova, S. and R. H. Barnes. Influence of malnutrition in early life on exploratory behavior of rats. *J. Nutr.* 96:477–484 (1968a).

Frankova, S. and R. H. Barnes. Effect of malnutrition in early life on avoidance conditioning and behavior of adult rats. *J. Nutr.* 96:485–493 (1968b).

Fransson, L. Å. Structure and metablism of the proteoglycans of dermatan sulfate. In *Chemistry and Molecular Biology of the Intracellular Matrix*, Vol. 2, pp. 823–842. E. A. Balazs, Ed., Academic Press, New York (1970).

Fraser, D., B. S. L. Kidd, S. W. Kooh, and L. Paunier. A new look at infantile hypercalcemia. *Pediatr. Clin. North Am.* 13:503–525 (1966).

Fraser, D. R. and E. Kodicek. Investigations on vitamin D esters synthesized in rats. Detection and identification. *Biochem. J.* 106: 485–490 (1968a).

Fraser, D. R. and E. Kodicek. Investigations on vitamin D esters synthesized in rats. Turnover and sites of synthesis. *Biochem. J.* 106:491–496 (1968b).

Fraser, D. R. and E. Kodicek. Enzyme studies on the esterification of vitamin D in rat tissues. *Biochem. J.* 109:457–467 (1968c).

Fraser, D. R. and E. Kodicek. Unique biosynthesis by kidney of a biologically active vitamin D metabolite. *Nature* (London) 228:764–766 (1970).

Fraser, D. R. and E. Kodicek. Regulation of 25-hydroxycholecalciferol-1-hydroxylase activity in kidney by parathyroid hormone. *Nature (New Biol.)* 241:163–166 (1973).

Frazer, A. C. Fat absorption and metabolism. *Analyst* 63:308–314 (1938).

Frederick, J. F., Ed., *Origins and Evolution of Eukaryotic Intracellular Organelles*, Vol. 361, *Ann. N. Y. Acad. Sci.* (1981).

Freedman, R. A., M. Weiser, and K. J. Isselbacher. Calcium translocation by Golgi and lateral-based membrane vesicles from rat intestine: decrease in vitamin D-dependent rats. *Proc. Nat. Acad. Sci. U. S.* 74:3612–3616 (1977).

Freeman, D., K. McCorkle, and C. B. Srikant. Effect of hyperglucagonemia on glucagon binding and biologic activity. *Diabetes* 26, (Suppl. 1) 366. (1977).

Freeman, H. J. and Y. S. Kim. Digestion and absorption of protein. *Ann. Rev. Med.* 29:99–116 (1978).

Freeman, R. H. and J. O. Davis. Physiological actions of angiotensin II on the kidney. *Fed. Proc.* 38:2276–2279 (1979).

Freeman, R. H., J. O. Davis, T. E. Lohmeier, and W. S. Spielman. [Des-Asp[1]] angiotensin II: mediator of the renin-angiotensin system? *Fed. Proc.* 36:1766–1770 (1977).

Frenchman, R. and F. A. Johnston. Relation of menstrual losses to iron requirement. *J. Am. Diet. Assoc.* 25:217–220 (1949).

Frieden, E. The ferrous to ferric cycles in iron metabolism. *Nutr. Rev.* 31:41–44 (1973).

Frieden, E. Ceruloplasmin: a multi-functional metalloprotein of vertebrate plasma. In *Metal Ions in Biological Systems*, Vol. 13, pp. 117–142, H. Sigel, Ed., Marcel Dekker Inc., New York (1981).

Friedland, N. "Normal" lactose tolerance test. *Arch. Intern. Med.* 116:886–888 (1965).

Friedman, G. J., S. Sherry, and E. P. Ralli. The mechanism of the excretion of vitamin C by the human kidney at low and normal plasma levels of ascorbic acid. *J. Clin. Invest.* 19:685–689 (1940).

Friedmann, T. Prenatal diagnosis of genetic disease. *Sci. Am.* 225 (5):34–42 (1971).

Friedrich, Von W. Antagonisten des Vitamins B_{12}. *Bibl. Nutr. Dieta* 8:178–225 (1966).

Friend, B. Nutrients in United States food supply. A review of trends, 1909–1913 to 1965. *Am. J. Clin. Nutr.* 20:907–914 (1967).

Friis-Hansen, B. Hydrometry of growth and aging. In *Human Body Composition,* pp. 191–209, J. Brozek, Ed., Pergamon Press, Oxford (1965).

Friis-Hansen, B. Body water compartments in children: changes during growth and related changes in body composition. *Pediatr.* 28:169–181 (1961).

Friis-Hansen, B. Body composition during growth. *In vivo* measurements and biochemical data correlated to differential anatomical growth. *Pediatr.* 47:264–274 (1971).

Frohman, L. A. CNS peptides and glucoregulation. *Ann. Rev. Physiol.* 45:95–107 (1983).

Frost, D. and P. Lish. Selenium in biology. *Ann. Rev. Pharmacol.* 15:259–284 (1975).

Fujimoto, D. and N. Tamiya. Incorporation of ^{18}O from air into hydroxyproline by chick embryo. *Biochem. J.* 84:333–335 (1962).

Fuller, R. W. Control of epinephrine synthesis and secretion. *Fed. Proc.* 32:1772–1781 (1973).

Fulpius, B. W., R. Miskin, and E. Reich. Antibodies from myasthenic patients that compete with cholinergic agents for binding to nicotinic receptors. *Proc. Nat. Acad. Sci. U. S.* 77:4326–4330 (1980).

Fulwood, R., C. L. Johnson, J. D. Bryner, E. W. Gunter, and C. R. McGrath. *Hematological and Nutritional Biochemistry Reference Data for Persons 6 Months–74 Years of Age: United States, 1976–80.* National Center for Health Statistics, U.S. Department of Health and Human Services, Hyattsville, Md. (1982).

Funk, C. The etiology of the deficiency diseases. *J. State Med.* 20:341–368 (1912).

Gaber, B. P. and P. Aisen. Is divalent iron bound to transferrin. *Biochim. Biophys. Acta* 221:228–233 (1970).

Gad, P. and S. L. Clark, Jr. Involution and regeneration of the thymus in mice, induced by bacterial endotoxin and studied by quantitative histology and electron microscopy. *Am. J. Anat.* 122:573–585 (1968).

Gadian, D. G. and G. K. Radda. NMR studies of tissue metabolism. *Ann. Rev. Biochem.* 50:69–83 (1981).

Gall, J. G. Octagonal nuclear pores. *J. Cell Biol.* 32:391–399 (1967).

Gallo-Torres, H. E. Obligatory role of bile for the intestinal absorption of vitamin E. *Lipids* 5:379–384 (1970a).

Gallo-Torres, H. E. Intestinal absorption and lymphatic transport of d,1-3,4-^{3}H$_2$-α-tocopheryl nicotinate in the rat. *Int. Z. Vitaminforsch.* 40:505–514 (1970b).

Galli, C., E. Agradi, A. Petroni, and A. Socini. Modulation of prostaglandin production in tissues by dietary essential fatty acids. *Acta Med. Scand. (Suppl.)* 642:171–179 (1980).

Gallup, P. M. and M. Paz. Posttranslational protein modifications with special attention to collagen and elastin. *Physiol. Rev.* 55:418–487 (1975).

Galton, D. J. *The Human Adipose Cell: A Model for Errors in Metabolic Regulation,* Appleton-Century-Crofts, New York (1971).

Galton, D. J. and S. Wallis. The regulation of adipose cell metabolism. *Proc. Nutr. Soc.* 41:167–173 (1982).

Gamow, G. Possible relation between deoxyribonucleic acid and protein structures. *Nature* 173:318. (1954).

Gamow, G. and M. Ycas. *Mr. Tompkins Inside Himself,* Viking Press, New York (1967).

Ganguly, J. Absorption of vitamin A. *Am. J. Clin. Nutr.* 22:923–933 (1969).

Ganong, W. F. *Review of Medical Physiology,* 5th ed., Lange Medical Publications, Los Altos, Calif. (1971).

Ganong, W. F. The renin-angiotensin system and the central nervous system. *Fed. Proc.* 36:1771–1775 (1977).

Garabedian, M., M. F. Holick, H. F. DeLuca, and I. T. Boyle. Control of 25-hydroxycholecalciferol metabolism by the parathyroid glands. *Proc. Nat. Acad. Sci. U. S.* 69:1673–1676 (1972).

Garabedian, M., Y. Tanaka, M. F. Holick, and H. F. DeLuca. Response of intestinal calcium transport and bone calcium mobilization to 1,25-dihydroxy-vitamin D$_3$ in thyroparathyroidectomized rats. *Endocrinol.* 94:1022–1027 (1974).

Garby, L. and W. D. Noyes. Studies on hemoglobin metabolism. II. Pathways of hemoglobin iron metabolism in normal man. *J. Clin. Invest.* 38:1484–1486 (1959).

Gardner, G., V. Edgerton, B. Senewiratne, R. Barnard, and Y. Ohira. Physical work capacity and metabolic stress in subjects with iron deficiency anemia. *Am. J. Clin. Nutr.* 30:910–917 (1977).

Garfield, R. E., S. Sims, and E. E. Daniel. Gap junctions: their presence and necessity in myometrium during parturition. *Science* 198:958–960 (1977).

Garn, S. M. Comparison of pinch-caliper and x-ray measurements of skin plus subcutaneous fat. *Science* 124:178–179 (1956).

Garn, S. M. Selection of body sites for fat measurement. *Science* 125:550–551 (1957).

Garn, S. M. The evolutionary and genetic control of variability in man. *Ann. N. Y. Acad. Sci.* 134:602–615 (1966).

Garn, S. M., G. R. Greaney, and R. W. Young. Fat thickness and growth progess during infancy. In *Body Measurements and Human Nutrition*, pp. 122–140, J. Brozek, Ed., Wayne University Press, Detroit (1956).

Garn, S. M. and J. A. Haskell. Fat changes during adolescence. *Science* 129:1615–1616 (1959a).

Garn, S. M. and J. A. Haskell. Fat and growth during childhood. *Science* 130:1711–1712 (1959b).

Garn, S. M., C. C. Rohmann, and B. Wagner. Bone loss as a general phenomenon in man. *Fed. Proc.* 26:1729–1736 (1967).

Garn, S. M., N. N. Rosen, and M. B. McCann. Relative values of different fat fold in a nutritional survey. *Am. J. Clin. Nutr.* 24:1380–1381 (1971).

Garraway, W. M., J. P. Whisnant, A. J. Furlan, L. H. Phillips, II, L. T. Kurland, and W. M. O. Fallon. The declining incidence of stroke. *N. Engl. J. Med.* 300:449–452 (1979).

Garren, L. D., G. N. Gill, and G. M. Walton. The isolation of a receptor for adenosine 3',5'-cyclic monophosphate (cAMP) from the adrenal cortex: the role of the receptor in the mechanism of action of cAMP. *Ann. N. Y. Acad. Sci.* 185:210–226 (1971).

Garrod, A. E. The incidence of alkaptonuria: a study in chemical individuality. *Lancet* 2:1616–1620 (1902).

Garza, C., N. S. Scrimshaw, and V. R. Young. Human protein requirements: the effect of variations in energy intake within the maintenance range. *Am. J. Clin. Nutr.* 29:280–287 (1976).

Garza, C., N. S. Scrimshaw, and V. R. Young. Human protein requirements: a long term metabolic nitrogen balance study in young men to evaluate the 1973 FAO/WHO safe level of egg protein intake. *J. Nutr.* 107:335–353 (1977).

Gay, C. V. and W. J. Mueller. Carbonic anhydrase and osteoclasts: localization by labeled inhibitor autoradiography. *Science* 183:432–434 (1974).

Gedalia, I. and I. Zipkin. *The Role of Fluoride in Bone Structure*, Warren H. Green Inc., St. Louis (1973).

Geffen, L. B. and G. V. Livett. Synaptic vesicles in sympathetic neurons. *Physiol. Rev.* 51:98–157 (1971).

Geiger, E. The role of the time factor in protein synthesis. *Science* 111:594–599 (1950).

Gemsa, D. Stimulation of prostaglandin E release from macrophages and possible role in the immune response. In *Lymphokines*, Vol. 4, pp. 335–375, E. O. Pick, Ed. Academic Press, New York (1981).

Geren, B. B. and F. O. Schmitt. Electron microscope studies of the Schwann cell and its constituents with particular reference to their relation to the axon. In *8th Congress of Cell Biology, Leiden*, pp. 251–260, Interscience Publishers, New York (1954).

Gershoff, S. N. Vitamin B_6. In *Present Knowledge of Nutrition*, 4th ed., pp. 149–161, Nutrition Foundation, Washington, D.C. (1976).

Gerstl, B., M. G. Tavaststjerna, R. B. Hayman, J. K. Smith, and L. F. Eng. Lipid studies of white matter and thalamus of human brains. *J. Neurochem.* 10:889–902 (1963).

Gettman, L. R., J. J. Ayres, M. L. Pollock, and A. Jackson. The effect of circuit weight training on strength, cardiorespiratory function, and body composition of adult men. *Med. Sci. Sports* 10:171–176 (1978).

Gholson, R. K. The pyridine nucleotide cycle. *Nature* 212:933–935 (1966).

Gibor, A. and S. Granick. Plastids and mitochondria: inheritable systems. *Science* 145:890–897 (1964).

Giese, A. C. *Cell Physiology*, 3rd ed., W. B. Saunders Co., Philadelphia (1968).

Giese, A. C. *Cell Physiology*, 4th ed., W. B. Saunders Co., Philadelphia (1973).

Gilat, T., S. Russo, E. Gelman-Malachi, T. A. M. Aldor. Lactase in man: a nonadaptable enzyme. *Gastroenterol.* 62:1125–1227 (1972).

Gilbert, W. and B. Müller-Hill. Isolation of the *lac* repressor. *Proc. Nat. Acad. Sci. U. S.* 56:1891–1898 (1966).

Gillham, N. W. *Organelle Heredity,* Raven Press, New York (1978).

Gillman, T., M. Hathorn, and P. A. S. Canham. Experimental dietary siderosis. *Am. J. Path.* 35:349–368 (1959).

Gilula, N. B. Gap junctions and cell communication. In *International Cell Biology* 1976–1977, pp. 61–69, B. R. Brinkley and K. R. Porter, Eds., Rockefeller University Press, New York (1977).

Ginter, E. Marginal vitamin C deficiency, lipid metabolism and atherogenesis. *Adv. Lipid Res.* 16:167–220 (1978).

Glaser, M., H. Simpkins, S. J. Singer, M. Sheetz, and S. I. Chan. On the interactions of lipids and proteins in the red blood cell membrane. *Proc. Nat. Acad. Sci. U. S.* 65:721–728 (1970).

Glaser, M. and S. J. Singer. Circular dichroism and the conformations of membrane proteins. Studies with red blood cell membranes. *Biochemistry* 10:1780–1787 (1971).

Glasinovic, J. C., M. Duval, and S. Eislinger. Hepatic cellular uptake of taurocholate in the dog. *J. Clin. Invest.* 5:419–426 (1975).

Glass, G. B. J. *Gastric Intrinsic Factor and Other Vitamin B_{12} Binders,* Georg Thieme Publishers, Stuttgart (1974).

Glass, G. B. J., Ed., *Gastrointestinal Hormones,* Raven Press, New York (1980).

Gleeson, M., J. F. Brown, and J. J. Waring. Thermogenic effects of diet and exercise. *Proc. Nutr. Soc.* 38:82A (1979).

Gnaedinger, R. H., E. P. Reineke, A. M. Pearson, W. D. Van Huss, J. A. Wessel, and H. J. Montoye. Determination of body density by air displacement, helium dilution and underwater weighing. *Ann. N. Y. Acad. Sci.* 110:96–108 (1963).

Gofman, J. W., O. DeLalla, F. Glazier, N. K. Freeman, F. T. Lingren, A. V. Nicholls, B. Strisower, and A. R. Tamplin. The plasma lipoprotein transport system in health, metabolic disorders, atherosclerosis and coronary heart disease. *Plasma* 2:413–484 (1954).

Goldberg, A. L. Mechanisms of growth and atrophy of skeletal muscle. In *Muscle Biology*, Vol. 1, pp. 89–118, R. G. Cassens, Ed., Marcel Dekker Inc. New York (1972).

Goldberg, A. L. and T. W. Chang. Regulation and significance of amino acid metabolism in skeletal muscle. *Fed. Proc.* 37:2301–2307 (1978).

Goldberg, N. D., R. F. O'Dea, and M. K. Maddox. Cyclic GMP. *Adv. Cyclic Nucleotide Res.* 3:155–223 (1973).

Goldberger, J. The transmissibility of pellagra. *Public Health R.* 31:3159–3173 (1916).

Goldberger, J. and G. A. Wheeler. Experimental pellagra in the human subject brought about by a restricted diet. *Public Health R.* 30:3336–3339 (1915).

Goldberger, J. and G. A. Wheeler. Experimental black tongue of dogs and its relation to pellagra. *Public Health R.* 43:172–217 (1928).

Goldblatt, M. W. A depressor substance in seminal fluid. *J. Soc. Chem. Ind.* (*London*) 52:1056–1057 (1933).

Goldblatt, M. W. Properties of human seminal plasma. *J. Physiol.* (*London*) 84:208–218 (1935).

Golde, D. W., J. M. Cline, D. Metcalf, and C. F. Fox, Eds., *Hemopoietic Cell Differentiation*, Academic Press, New York (1978).

Goldfischer, S. Peroxisomes in disease. *J. Histochem. Cytochem.* 27:1371–1373 (1979).

Goldman, R. F., B. Bullen, and C. Seltzer. Changes in specific gravity and body fat in overweight female adolescents as a result of weight reduction. *Ann. N. Y. Acad. Sci.* 110:913–917 (1963).

Goldrick, R. B., B. C. E. Ashley, and M. L. Lloyd. Effects of prolonged incubation and cell concentration on lipogenesis from glucose in isolated human omental fat cells. *J. Lipid Res.* 10:253–259 (1969).

Goldsmith, G. A. Experimental niacin deficiency. *J. Am. Diet. Assoc.* 32:312–316 (1956).

Goldsmith, G. A. *Nutritional Diagnosis.* Charles C. Thomas, Springfield, Ill. (1959).

Goldsmith, G. A., O. N. Miller, and W. G. Unglaub. Efficiency of tryptophan as a niacin precursor in man. *J. Nutr.* 73:172–176 (1961).

Goldstein, J. L., R. G. W. Anderson, and M. S. Brown, Coated pits, coated vesicles, and receptor-mediated endocytosis. *Nature* 279:679–685 (1979).

Goldstein, L. Nucleocytoplasmic relationship. In *Cytology and Cell Physiology*, 3rd ed., pp. 559–635, G. H. Bourne, Ed., Academic Press, New York (1964).

Goldwasser, E. Erythropoietin and the differentiation of red blood cells. *Fed. Proc.* 34:2285–2292 (1975).

Goldwasser, E. and G. Inana. Molecular aspects of the initiation of erythropoiesis.

In *Hemopoietic Cell Differentiation,* pp. 15–24, D. W. Golde, J. M. Cline, D. Metcalf, and C. F. Fox, Eds., Academic Press, New York (1978).

Gonzales, F. and M. J. Karnovsky. Electron microscopy of osteoclasts in healing fractures of rat bone. *J. Biophys. Biochem. Cytol.* 9:299–316 (1961).

Goodenough, U. W. and R. P. Levine. The genetic activity of mitochondria and chloroplasts. *Sci. Am.* 223(5):22–29 (1970).

Goodman, DeW. S. Preparation of human serum albumin free of long-chain fatty acids. *Science* 125:1296–1297 (1957).

Goodman, DeW. S. Biosynthesis of vitamin A from β-carotene. *Am. J. Clin. Nutr.* 22:963–965 (1969a).

Goodman, DeW. S. Retinol transport in human plasma. *Am. J. Clin. Nutr.* 22:911–912 (1969b).

Goodman, DeW. S. Retinol transport in human plasma. In *The Fat-Soluble Vitamins,* pp. 203–212, H. F. DeLuca and J. W. Suttie, Eds., University of Wisconsin Press, Madison (1970).

Goodman, DeW. S. Vitamin A metabolism. *Fed Proc.* 39:2716–2722 (1980).

Goodman, DeW. S., R. Blomstrand, B. Werner, H. S. Huang, and T. Shiratori. The intestinal absorption and metabolism of vitamin A and β-carotene in man. *J. Clin. Invest.* 45:1615–1623 (1966).

Goodman, DeW. S. and H. S. Huang. Biosynthesis of vitamin A with rat intestinal enzymes. *Science* 149:879–880 (1965).

Goodman, DeW. S., H. S. Huang, M. Kanai, and T. Shiratori. The enzymatic conversion of all-*trans*-β-carotene in retinal. *J. Biol. Chem.* 242:3543–3554 (1967).

Goodman, DeW. S. and R. P. Noble. Turnover of plasma cholesterol in man. *J. Clin. Invest.* 47:231–241 (1968).

Goodnight, S. H., Jr., W. S. Harris, W. E. Connor, and D. R. Illingsworth. Polyunsaturated fatty acids, hyperlipidemia, and thrombosis. *Arteriosclerosis* 2:87–113 (1982).

Goodridge, A. G. and E. G. Ball. Lipogenesis in the pigeon: *in vitro* studies. *Am. J. Physiol.* 211:803–808 (1966).

Gopalan, C., P. S. Venkatachalam, and B. Bhavani. Studies of vitamin A deficiency in children. *Am. J. Clin. Nutr.* 8:833–840 (1960).

Gordon, E. E., K. Kowalski, and M. Fritts. Muscle proteins and DNA in rat quadriceps during growth. *Am. J. Physiol.* 210:1033–1040 (1966).

Gorter, E and F. Grendel. On bimolecular layers of lipoids on the chromocytes of the blood. *J. Exp. Med.* 41:439–443 (1925).

Göthlin, G. and J. Ericsson. Fine structural localization of acid phosphomonoesterase in the brush border region of osteoclasts. *Histochemie* 28:337–344 (1972).

Gottlieb, A. A., A. Kaplan, and S. Udenfriend. Further evidence for the accumulation of a hydroxyproline-deficient, collagenase-degradable protein during collagen biosynthesis *in vitro. J. Biol. Chem.* 241:1551–1555 (1966).

Gottschalk, C. W. and W. E. Lassiter. Mechanisms of urine formation. In *Medical Physiology,* Vol 2., pp. 1165–1205, V. B. Mountcastle, Ed., C. V. Mosby, St. Louis (1980).

Graber, S. E. and S. B. Krantz. Erythropoietin and the control of red cell production. *Ann. Rev. Med.* 29:51–66 (1978).

Graham, L. A., J. J. Caesar, and A. S. V. Burgen. Gastrointestinal absorption and excretion of Mg^{28} in man. *Metabolism* 9:646–659 (1960).

Graham, R. C. and M. J. Karnovsky. The early stages of absorption of injected horseradish peroxidase in the proximal tubules of mouse kidney: ultrastructural cytochemistry by a new technique. *J. Histochem. Cytochem.* 14:291–302 (1966).

Granick, S. Ferritin. IV. Occurrence and immunological properties of ferritin. *J. Biol. Chem.* 149:157–167 (1943).

Granick, S. Iron metabolism and hemochromatosis. *Bull. N. Y. Acad. Med.* 25:403–428 (1949).

Granick, S. Structure and physiological functions of ferritins. *Physiol. Rev.* 31:489–511 (1951).

Granick, S. Iron metabolism. *Bull. N. Y. Acad. Med.* 30:81–105 (1954).

Gräsbeck, R. Intrinsic factor and the transcobalamins with reflections on the general function and evolution of soluble transport proteins. *Scand. J. Clin. Lab. Invest., Suppl.* 95:7–18 (1967).

Gräsbeck, R., K. Simons, and I. Sinkkonen. Isolation of intrinsic factors from human gastric juice. *Acta Chem. Scand.* 19:1777–1778 (1965).

Gräsbeck, R., K. Simons, and I. Sinkkonen. Isolation of intrinsic factor and its probable degradation product, as their vitamin B_{12} complexes, from human gastric juice. *Biochim. Biophys. Acta* 127:47–58 (1966).

Gray, G. M. Carbohydrate absorption and malabsorption. In *Physiology of the Gastrointestinal Tract,* Vol. 2, pp. 1063–1072, L. R. Johnson, Ed., Raven Press, New York (1981).

Gray, G. M., K. A. Conklin, and R. R. W. Townley. Sucrase-isomaltase deficiency. Absence of an inactive enzyme variant. *N. Engl. J. Med.* 294:750–753 (1976).

Gray, G. M. and H. L. Cooper. Protein digestion and absorption. *Gastroenterol.* 61:535–544 (1971).

Gray, G. M., B. C. Lally, and K. A. Conklin. Action of intestinal sucrase-isomaltase and its free monomers on an α-limit dextrin. *J. Biol. Chem.* 254:6038–6043 (1979).

Gray, R., I. Boyle, and H. F. DeLuca. Vitamin D metabolism: the role of kidney tissue. *Science* 172:1232–1234 (1972).

Gray, T. K. and P. L. Munson. Thyrocalcitonin. Evidence for physiological function. *Science* 166:512–513 (1969).

Graystone, J. E. and D. B. Cheek. The effects of reduced caloric intake and increased insulin-induced caloric intake on the cell growth of muscle, liver and cerebrum and on the skeletal collagen in the postweaning rat. *Pediatr. Res.* 3:66–76 (1969).

Greaves, J. D. and L. A. Schmidt. Relation of bile to absorption of vitamin E in the rat. *Proc. Soc. Exp. Biol. Med.* 37:40–42 (1937).

Green, C. The transport of sterol across the mucosa. In *Biochemical Problems of Lipids*, pp. 144–148, A. C. Frazer, Ed., Elsevier, Amsterdam (1963).

Green, D. E. The mitochondrion. *Sci. Am.* 210(1):63–74 (1964).

Green, D. E. Membrane proteins: a perspective. *Ann. N. Y. Acad. Sci.* 195:150–172 (1972).

Green, D. E. and Y. Hatefi. The mitochondrion and biochemical machines. *Science* 133:13–19 (1961).

Green, D. E., W. F. Loomis, and V. H. Auerbach. Studies on the cyclophorase system. I. The complete oxidation of pyruvic acid to carbon dioxide and water. *J. Biol. Chem.* 172:389–403 (1948).

Green, D. E. and A. Tzagoloff. Role of lipids in the structure and function of biological membranes. *J. Lipid Res.* 7:587–602 (1966).

Green, J. Antagonists of vitamin A. *Bibl. Nutr. Dieta* 8:33–43 (1966a).

Green, J. Antagonists of vitamin K. *Vitam. Horm.* 24:619–632 (1966b).

Green, N. M. Evidence for a genetic relationship between avidins and lysozymes. *Nature* 217:254–256 (1968).

Green, N. M. Spectrophotometric determination of avidin and biotin. In *Methods in Enzymology*, Vol. 13, Part A, pp. 418–424, D. B. McCormick and L. D. Wright, Eds., Academic Press, New York (1970).

Green, R., W. E. Carlson, and C. A. Evans. The inactivation of vitamin B_1 in diets containing whole fish. *J. Nutr.* 23:165–175 (1942).

Green, R., R. W. Charlton, H. Seftel, T. H. Bothwell, F. Mayet, E. B. Adams, C. A. Finch, and M. Layrisse. Body iron excretion in man: a collaborative study. *Am. J. Med.* 45:336–353 (1968).

Greenberg, D. M. Studies in mineral metabolism with the aid of artificial radioactive isotopes. VIII. Tracer experiments with radioactive calcium and strontium on the mechanism of vitamin D action in rachitic rats. *J. Biol. Chem.* 157:99–104 (1945).

Greenberger, N. J., S. P. Balcerzak, and G. A. Ackerman. Iron uptake by isolated intestinal brush borders: changes induced by alterations in iron stores. *J. Lab. Clin. Med.* 73:711–721 (1969).

Greenberger, N. J. and T. G. Skillman. Medium-chain triglycerides. Physiologic considerations and clinical implications. *N. Engl. J. Med.* 280:1045–1058 (1969).

Greenwald, L. and J. Gross. The prevention of tetany of parathyroidectomized dogs. II. Lactose containing diet. *J. Biol. Chem.* 34:531–544 (1929).

Greenwood, M. R. C. and J. Hirsch. Postnatal development of adipocyte cellularity in the normal rat. *J. Lipid Res.* 15:474–483 (1974).

Greer, M. A. and Y. Grimm. Changes in thyroid secretion produced by inhibition of iodotyrosine deoxidase. *Endocrinology* 83:405–410 (1968).

Gregory, J. F. and J. R. Kirk. The bioavailability of Vitamin B$_6$ in foods. *Nutr. Rev.* 39:1–8 (1981).

Gregory, J. F., III, D. B. Manley, and J. R. Kirk. Determination of vitamin B-6 in animal tissues by reverse-phase high performance liquid chromatography. *J. Agri. Food Chem.* 29:921–927 (1981).

Griffith, W. H. and J. F. Nyc. Choline X. Effects of deficiency. In *The Vitamins,* Vol. 3, pp. 81–123, W. H. Sebrell, Jr., and R. S. Harris, Eds., Academic Press, New York (1971).

Griffith, W. H. and N. J. Wade. Choline metabolism. I. The occurrence and prevention of hemorrhagic degeneration in young rats on a low choline diet. *J. Biol. Chem.* 131:567–577 (1939).

Griminger, P. Biological activity of the various vitamin K forms. *Vitam. Horm.* 24:605–618 (1966).

Grisolia, S. and J. Kennedy. On specific dynamic action, turnover and protein synthesis. *Perspect. Biol. Med.* 9: 578–585 (1966).

Grivell, L. A. Mitochondrial DNA. *Sci. Am.* 248(3):78–89 (1983).

Grobstein, C. Differentiation of vertebrate cells. In *The Cell,* Vol. 1, pp. 437–496, J. Brachet and A. E. Mirsky, Eds., Academic Press, New York (1959).

Grobstein, C. Cytodifferentiation and its controls. *Science* 143:643–650 (1964).

Gross, S. and D. K. Melhorn. Vitamin E, red cell lipids and red cell stability in prematurity. *Ann. N. Y. Acad. Sci.* 203:141–162 (1972).

Grossman, M. I. Proposal: Use the term cholecystokinin in place of cholecystokinin-pancreozymin. *Gastroenterol.* 58:128. (1970).

Grossman, M. I. Physiological effects of gastrointestinal hormones. *Fed. Proc.* 36:1930–1932 (1977).

Grossman, M. I. Chemical messengers: a view from the gut. *Fed. Proc.* 38:2341–2343 (1979).

Grossman, M. I., V. Speranza, N. Basso, and E. Lezoche, Eds. *Symposium on Gastrointestinal Hormones and Pathology of the Digestive System,* Plenum, New York, (1977).

Grossman, R. A., C. Harinasuta, and B. A. Underwood. *Nutrition and some related diseases of public health importance in the Lower Mekong Basin: a review.* (SEADAG Papers), Asia Society, New York (1973).

Grove, S. N., C. E. Bracker, and D. J. Morré. Cytomembrane differentiation in the endoplasmic reticulum-Golgi apparatus-vesicle complex. *Science* 161: 171–173 (1968).

Growdon, J. H. and R. J. Wurtman. Dietary influences on the synthesis of neurotransmitters in the brain. *Nutr. Rev.* 37:129–136 (1979).

Grundfest, H. Synaptic and ephaptic transmission. In The *Neurosciences,* pp. 353–372, G. C. Quarton, T. Melnechuk, and F. O. Schmitt, Eds., Rockefeller University Press, New York (1967).

Grundy, S., E. H. Ahrens, and J. Davignon. The interaction of cholesterol absorption and cholesterol synthesis in man. *J. Lipid Res.* 10:304–315 (1969).

Grundy, S. M., D. Bilheimer, H. Blackburn, W. V. Brown, P. O. Kwiterovich, Jr., F. Mattson, G. Schonfeld, and W. H. Weidman. Rationale of the diet-heart statement of the American Heart Association (Report of Nutrition Committee). *Circulation* 65:839A-854A (1982).

Guarnieri, M. and R. M. Johnson. The essential fatty acids. *Adv. Lipid Res.* 8:115–174 (1970).

Gubler, C. J. Enzyme studies in thiamine deficiency. *Int. Z. Vitaminforsch.* 38:287–303 (1968).

Gudmundsson, T. V. and N. J. Y. Woodhouse. Regulation of plasma calcium in man: the influence of parathyroid hormone and calcitonin. *Hormones* (Basel) 2:26–39 (1976).

Guha, A. and O. A. Roels The influence of α-tocopherol on arylsulfatases A and B in the liver of vitamin A-deficient rats. *Biochim. Biophys. Acta* 111:364–374 (1965).

Guilarte, T. R., P. A. McIntyre, and M. Tsan. Growth of the yeasts *Saccharomyces uvarum* and *Kloeckera brevis* to the free biologically active forms of vitamin B-6. *J. Nutr.* 110:954–958 (1980).

Gundlach, B. L., H. G. M. Nijkrake, and J. G. A. J. Hautvast. A rapid and simplified plethysmometric method for measuring body volume. *Hum. Biol.* 52:23–33 (1980).

Gunsalus, I. C. The chemistry and function of the pyruvate oxidation factor (lipoic acid). *J. Cell Comp. Physiol.* 41:113–136 (1953).

Gunter, E. W., W. E. Turner, J. W. Neese, and D. D. Bayse. *Laboratory procedures used by the Clinical Chemistry Division, Centers for Disease Control, for the second health and nutrition examination study (HANES II) 1976–1980.* Nutritional Biochemistry Branch, Center for Disease Control, U.S. Department of Health and Human Services, Atlanta, Ga. (1981).

Gurney, J. M. and D. B. Jelliffe. Arm anthropometry in nutritional assessment: nomogram for rapid calculation of muscle circumference and cross-sectional muscle and fat areas. *Am. J. Clin. Nutr.* 26:912–915 (1973).

Gurr, M. I. and A. T. James. *Lipid Biochemistry: An Introduction.* Cornell University Press, Ithaca, N.Y. (1971).

Gurr, M. I. and A. T. James. *Lipid Biochemistry: An Introduction,* 3rd ed, p. 51, Chapman and Hall, New York (1980).

Gurr, M. I., R. Mawson, N. Rothwell, and M. J. Stock. Effects of manipulating dietary protein and energy intake on energy balance and thermogenesis in the pig. *J. Nutr.* 110:532–542 (1980).

Guthrie, B. E., W. E. Wolf, and E. Jeillon. Background correction and related problems in the determination of chromium in urine by graphite furnace atomic absorption spectrophotometry. *Anal. Chem.* 50:1900–1902 (1978).

Guthrie, H. A. Severe undernutrition in early infancy and behavior in rehabilitated female rats. *Physiol. Behav.* 3:619–623 (1968).

Guthrie, H. A. and M. L. Brown. Effect of severe undernutrition in early growth, brain size and composition in adult rats. *J. Nutr.* 94:419–426 (1968).

Guthrie, H. A., G. M. Owen, and G. M. Guthrie. Factor analysis of measures of nutritional status of preschool children. *Am. J. Clin. Nutr.* 26:497–502 (1973).

Guthrie, H. A. and J. C. Scheer. An evaluation of the basic four food guide. *J. Nutr. Educ.* 13:46–49 (1981).

Guttmann, St., J. Pless, R. L. Huguenin, Ed. Sandrin, H. Bossert, and K. Zehnder. Synthesis of a highly potent hypocalcaemic dotriacontapeptide, having the properties of salmon calcitonin. In *Calcitonin: Proceedings of the Second International Symposium,* pp. 74–79, Springer-Verlag, New York (1970).

Guyton, A. C., R. A Brace, and B. J. Barber. Regulatory functions of the interstitium. In *Claude Bernard and the Internal Environment,* pp. 207–227, E. D. Robin, Ed., Marcel Dekker Inc. New York (1979).

Guyton, A. C., A. E. Taylor, and H. J. Granger. *Dynamics and Control of Body Fluids.* W. B. Saunders Co., Philadelphia (1975).

Gÿorgy, P. Vitamin B_2 and the pellagra-like dermatitis in rats. *Nature* 133:498–499 (1934).

Gÿorgy, P. Crystalline vitamin B_6. *J. Am. Chem. Soc.* 60:983–984 (1938).

Gÿorgy, P. The curative factor (vitamin H) for egg white injury, with particular reference to its presence in different foodstuffs and in yeast. *J. Biol. Chem.* 131:733–744 (1939).

Gÿorgy, P., Ed., *Vitamin Methods,* Vol. 1., Academic Press, New York (1950).

Gÿorgy, P. Early experiences with riboflavin—a retrospect. *Nutr. Rev.* 12:97–100 (1954).

Gÿorgy, P. Symposium on vitamin E and metabolism. *Vitam. Horm.* 20:599–601 (1962).

Gÿorgy, P. Developments leading to the metabolic role of vitamin B_6. *Am. J. Clin. Nutr.* 24:1250–1256 (1971).

Habener, J. F., F. R. Singer, L. J. Deftos, and J. T. Potts, Jr. Immunological stability of calcitonin in plasma. *Endocrinology* 90:952–960 (1972).

Hackenbrock. C. R. Ultrastructural bases for metabolically linked mechanical activity in mitochondria. I. Reversible ultrastructural changes with change in metabolic steady state in isolated liver mitochondria. *J. Cell Biol.* 30:269–297 (1966).

Hackenbrock, C. R. Ultrastructural bases for metabolically linked mechanical activity in mitochondria. II. Electron transport-linked ultrastructural transformations in mitochondria. *J. Cell Biol.* 37:345–369 (1968).

Hackenbrock, C. R. Chemical and physical fixation of isolated mitochondria in low-energy and high-energy states. *Proc. Nat. Acad. Sci. U. S.* 61:598–605 (1968).

Hackenbrock, C. R. Molecular organization and the fluid nature of the mito-chondrial energy transducing membrane. In *The Structure of Biological Membranes,* S. Abrahamsson and I. Pascher, Eds., *Nobel Symp.* 34:199–234, Plenum, New York (1977).

Hackenbrock, C. R. and K. J. Miller. The distribution of anionic sites on the surfaces of mitochondrial membranes. *J. Cell Biol.* 65:615–630 (1975).

Haddad, J. G., Jr. and J. Walgate. 25-Hydroxyvitamin D transport in human plasma. Isolation and partial characterization of calcifidiol-binding protein. *J. Biol. Chem.* 251:4803–4809 (1976).

Haddy, F. J. and J. B. Scott. Metabolically linked vasoactive chemicals in local regulation of blood flow. *Physiol. Rev.* 48:688–707 (1968).

Haessler, H. A. and K. J. Isselbacher. The metabolism of glycerol by the intestinal mucosa. *Biochim. Biophys. Acta* 73:427–436 (1963).

Hågå, P. and S. Kran. Plasma vitamin E levels and vitamin E/β-lipoprotein relationships in small preterm infants during the early anemia of prematurity. *Eur. J. Pediatr.* 136:143–147 (1981).

Hager, A., L. Sjöström, B. Arvidsson, P. Björntorp, and U. Smith. Body fat and adipose tissue cellularity in infants—a longitudinal study. *Metabolism* 26:607–613 (1977).

Hager, A., L. Sjöström, B. Arvidsson, P. Björntrop, and U. Smith. Adipose tissue cellularity in obese school girls before and after dietary treatment. *Am. J. Clin. Nutr.* 31:68–75 (1978).

Haggis, G. H., D. Michie, A. R. Muir, K. B. Roberts, and P. M. B. Walker. *Introduction to Molecular Biology,* John Wiley & Sons, New York (1964).

Hahn, P. F., W. F. Bale, E. O. Laurence, and G. H. Whipple. Radioactive iron and its metabolism in anemia. Its absorption, transportation and utilization. *J. Exp. Med.* 69:739–753 (1939).

Hahn, P. F., W. F. Bale, J. F. Ross, W. M. Balfour, and G. H. Whipple. Radioactive iron absorption by gastrointestinal tract. *J. Exp. Med.* 78:169–188 (1943).

Hahn, P. F., E. L. Carothers, W. J. Darby, M. Martin, C. W. Sheppard, R. O. Cannon, A. S. Beam, P. M. Densen, J. C. Peterson, and G. S. McClellan. Iron metabolism in human pregnancy as studied with radioactive isotopes. *Am. J. Obstet. Gynecol.* 61:477–486 (1951).

Halestrap, A. P. Stimulation of the respiratory chain of rat liver mitochondria between cytochrome c_1 and cytochrome c by glucagon treatment of rats. *Biochem. J.* 172:399–405 (1978).

Haley, F. L. and G. S. Samuelsen. Vitamin A and the detoxification of monobromobenzene. *J. Lab. Clin. Med.* 28:1079–1082 (1943).

Hall, D., R. Cammack, and K. Rao. Non-haem iron proteins. In *Iron in Bio-*

chemistry and Medicine, pp. 279–334, A. Jacobs and M. Worwood, Eds., Academic Press, New York (1974).

Hallberg, L. Bioavailable nutrient density: a new concept applied in the interpretation of food iron absorption data. *Am. J. Clin. Nutr.* 34:2242–2247 (1981a).

Hallberg, L. Bioavailability of dietary iron in man. *Ann. Rev. Nutr.* 1:123–147 (1981b).

Hallberg, L. Iron absorption and iron deficiency. *Hum. Nutr. Clin. Nutr.* 36C:259–278 (1982).

Hallberg, L., A. M. Högdahl, L. Nilsson, and G. Rybo. Menstrual blood loss— a population study. Variation at different ages and attempts to define normality. *Acta Obstet. Gynecol. Scand.* 45:320–351 (1966).

Hallberg, L. and L. Sölvell. Determination of the absorption rate of iron in man. *Acta Med. Scand.* (Suppl 358) 168:3–17 (1960a).

Hallberg, L. and L. Sölvell. Absorption of a single dose of iron in man. *Acta Med. Scand.* (Suppl. 358) 168:19–42 (1960b).

Hallberg, L. and L. Sölvell. Iron absorption during constant intragastric infusion of iron in man. *Acta Med. Scand.* (Suppl. 358) 168:43–69 (1960c).

Halsted, C. H. The small intestine in vitamin B_{12} and folate deficiency. *Nutr. Rev.* 33:33–37 (1975).

Halsted, C. H. Drugs and water-soluble vitamin absorption. In *Nutrition and Drug Interrelations,* pp. 83–112, J. N. Hathcock and J. Coon, Eds., Academic Press, New York (1978).

Halsted, C. H., A. Reisenauer, C. Back, and G. Gotterer. *In vitro* uptake and metabolism of pteroylpolyglutamate by rat small intestine. *J. Nutr.* 106:485–492 (1976).

Halver, J. E., R. R. Smith, B. M. Tolbert, and E. M. Baker. Utilization of ascorbic acid in fish. *Ann. N. Y. Acad. Sci.* 258:81–102 (1975).

Halvorsen, O. and S. Skrede. Separation of coenzyme A and its precursors by reversed phase high performance liquid chromatography. *Anal. Biochem.* 107:103–108 (1980).

Ham, A. W. Some histophysiological problems peculiar to calcified tissue. *J. Bone Joint Surg.* 34-A:701–728 (1952).

Ham, A. W. *Histology, 6th ed., J. B. Lippincott, Philadelphia (1969).*

Ham, A. W. and D. H. Cormack. *Histology,* 8th ed., J. B. Lippincott, Philadelphia (1979).

Hamberg, M., J. Svensson, and B. Samuelsson. Thromboxanes: a new group of biologically active compounds derived from prostaglandin endoperoxides. *Proc. Nat. Acad. Sci. U. S.* 72:2994–2998 (1975).

Hambidge, K. M., C. Hambidge, M. Jacobs, and J. D. Baum. Low levels of zinc in hair, anorexia, poor growth, and hypogeusia in children. *Pediatr. Res.* 6:868–874 (1972).

Hamerman, D. Views on the pathogenesis of rheumatoid arthritis. *Med. Clin. North Am.* 52:593–605 (1968).

Hamfelt, A. and T. Tuvemo. Pyridoxal phosphate and folic acid concentration in blood and erythrocyte aspartate aminotransferase during pregnancy. *Clin. Chim. Acta* 41:287–298 (1972).

Hamilton, R. L. Synthesis and secretion of plasma lipoproteins. *Adv. Exp. Med. Biol.* 26:7–24 (1972).

Hamm, M., H. Mehansho, and L. Henderson. Transport and metabolism of pyridoxamine and pyridoxamine phosphate in the small intestine of the rat. *J. Nutr.* 109:1548–1555 (1979).

Hammarström, S. Biosynthesis and biological actions of prostaglandins and thromboxanes. *Arch. Biochem. Biophys.* 214:431–445 (1982).

Hamosh, M., and R. O. Scow. Lingual lipase and its role in the digestion of dietary lipid. *J. Clin. Invest.* 52:88–95 (1973).

Hanawalt, P. C. Repair of genetic material in living cells. *Endeavour* 31 (113):83–87 (1972).

Hancock, R. Conservation of histones in chromatin during growth and mitosis *in vitro*. *J. Mol. Biol.* 40:457–466 (1969).

Handler, J. S. and J. Orloff. Antidiuretic hormone. *Ann. Rev. Physiol.* 43:611–624 (1981).

Handler, P. Nutritional diseases (Conference on beriberi, endemic goiter, and hypovitaminosis A. Part II). *Fed. Proc.* 17:31–35 (1958).

Hankins, G. J., T. J. Eccles, Jr., B. C. Judlin, and M. C. Moore. Data processing of dietary survey data. *J. Am. Diet. Assoc.* 46:387–394 (1965).

Hanni, R. and F. Bigler. Isolation and identification of the major metabolites of retinoic acid from rat feces. *Helv. Chim. Acta* 60:881–887 (1977).

Hanni, R., F. Bigler, W. Meister, and G. Englert. Isolation and identification of three urinary metabolites of retinoic acid in the rat. *Helv. Chim. Acta* 59:2221–2227 (1976).

Hansen, R. G., G. Brown, and B. W. Wyse. Nutrient needs and their expression. *Food Technol.* 25:44–53 (1978).

Hansen, R. G. and B. W. Wyse, Expression of nutrient allowances per 1000 kilocalories. *J. Am. Diet. Assoc.* 76:223–227 (1980).

Hanson, J. and J. Lowy. The structure of F-actin and of actin filaments isolated from muscle. *J. Mol. Biol.* 6:46–60 (1963).

Hardinge, M. G., J. B. Swarner, and H. Crooks. Carbohydrates in foods. *J. Am. Diet. Assoc.* 46:197–204 (1965).

Hardman, J. G., G. A. Robison, and E. W. Sutherland. Cyclic nucleotides. *Ann. Rev. Physiol.* 33:311–336 (1971).

Harlan, W. R., Jr., P. S. Winesett, and A. J. Wasserman. Tissue lipoprotein lipase in normal individuals and in individuals with exogenous hypertriglyceridemia and the relationship of this enzyme to assimilation of fat. *J. Clin. Invest.* 46:239–247 (1967).

Harmon, H. J., J. D. Hall, and F. L. Crane. Structure of mitochondrial cristae membranes. *Biochim. Biophys. Acta* 344:119–155 (1974).

Harper, A. A. and H. S. Raper. Pancreozymin, a stimulant of the secretion of pancreatic enzymes in extracts of the small intestine. *J. Physiol. (London)* 102:115–125 (1943).

Harper, A. E. Recommended dietary allowances—1980. *Nutr. Rev.* 38:290–294 (1980).

Harper, H. A. *Review of Physiological Chemistry,* Lange Medical Publishers, Los Altos, Calif. (1971).

Harris, F., R. Hoffenberg, and E. Black. Calcium kinetics in vitamin D deficiency rickets. II. Intestinal handling of calcium. *Metabolism* 14:1112–1121 (1965).

Harris, R. S. Reliability of nutrient analyses and food tables. *Am. J. Clin. Nutr.* 11:377–381 (1962).

Harris, S. A. and K. Folkers. Synthesis of vitamin B_6. *J. Am. Chem. Soc.* 61:1245–1247 (1939).

Harris, S. A., D. E. Wolf, R. Mozingo, G. E. Arth, R. C. Anderson, N. R. Easton, and K. Folkers. Biotin. V. Synthesis of dl-biotin, dl-allobiotin and dl-epi-al-lobiotin. *J. Am. Chem. Soc.* 67:2096–2100 (1945).

Harrison, G. G. and T. B. Van Itallie. Estimation of body composition: a new approach based on electromagnetic principles. *Am. J. Clin. Nutr.* 35:1176–1179 (1982).

Harrison, P. M., G. A. Clegg, and K. May. Ferritin structure and function. In *Iron in Biochemistry and Medicine,* II, pp. 131–171, A. Jacobs and M. Worwood, Eds., Academic Press, London (1980).

Harrison, P. M., R. J. Hoare, T. G. Hoy, and I. G. Macara. Ferritin and hae-mosiderin: structure and function. In *Iron in Biochemistry and Medicine,* pp. 73–114, A. Jacobs and M. Worwood, Eds., Academic Press, New York (1974).

Hart, E. B., H. Steenbock, J. Waddell, and C. A. Elvehjem. Iron in nutrition. VII. Copper as a supplement to iron for hemoglobin building in the rat. *J. Biol. Chem.* 77:797–812 (1928).

Hartsuck, J. A. and W. N. Lipscomb. Carboxypeptidase A. In *The Enzymes,* 3rd Ed., Vol. 3, pp. 1–56, P. D. Boyer, Ed., Academic Press, New York and London (1971).

Hasilik, A. Biosynthesis of lysosomal enzymes. *Trends Biochem. Sci.* 5:237–240 (1980).

Haskell, B. E. and E. E. Snell. Microbiological determination of the vitamin B_6 group. In *Methods in Enzymology,* Vol. 18, Part A, pp. 512–519, D. B. Mc-Cormick and L. D. Wright, Eds. Academic Press, New York (1970).

Haslewood, G. A. D. *The Biological Importance of Bile Salts.* North-Holland Publishing Co., Amsterdam (1978).

Hasselbach, W. and L. G. Elfvin. Structural and chemical asymmetry of the calcium-transporting membranes of the sarcotubular system as revealed by electron microscopy. *J. Ultrastruct. Res.* 17:598–622 (1967).

Hathaway, M. L. and J. E. Strom. A comparison of thiamine synthesis and excretion in human subjects on synthetic and natural diets. *J. Nutr.* 32:1–8 (1946).

Hathcock, J. N. Thiamin deficiency effects on rat leukocyte pyruvate decarboxylation rates. *Am. J. Clin. Nutr.* 31:250–252 (1978).

Haugen, R. and K. R. Norum. Coenzyme-A-dependent esterification of cholesterol in rat intestinal mucosa. *Scand. J. Gastroenterol.* 11:615–621 (1976).

Hauschka, P. V., P. A. Friedman, H. P. Traverso, and P. M. Gallop. Vitamin K-dependent α-carboxyglutamic acid formation by kidney microsomes *in vitro*. *Biochem. Biophys. Res. Commun.* 71:1207–1213 (1976).

Hauschka, P. V., J. B. Lian, and P. M. Gallop. Direct identification of the calcium-binding amino acid α-carboxyglutamate in mineralized tissues. *Proc. Nat. Acad. Sci. U. S.* 72:3925–3929 (1975).

Hausler, M. R. and T. A. McCain. Vitamin D metabolism and action. *N. Engl. J. Med.* 297:974–983; 1041–1050 (1977).

Hayaishi, O. and Y. Shizuta. Binding of pyridoxal phosphate to apoenzymes as studied by optical rotatory dispersion and circular dichroism. *Vitam. Horm.* 28:245–264 (1970).

Haymes, E. M., H. M. Lundegren, J. L. Loomis, and E. R. Buskirk. Validity of the ultrasonic technique as a method of measuring subcutaneous adipose tissue. *Ann. Hum. Biol.* 3:245–251 (1976).

Hayward, J. S. and E. G. Ball. Quantitative aspects of brown adipose tissue thermogenesis during arousal from hibernation. *Biol. Bull.* 131:94–103 (1966).

Heading, R. C., H. P. Schedl, L. D. Steginka, and D. L. Miller. Intestinal absorption of glycine and glycyl-L-proline in the rat. *Clin. Sci. Mol. Med.* 52:607–614 (1977).

Heaney, R. P., R. R. Recker, and P. D. Saville. Menopausal changes in calcium balance performance. *J. Lab. Clin. Med.* 92:953–963 (1978).

Heaney, R. P. and T. G. Skillman. Secretion and excretion of calcium by the human gastrointestinal tract. *J. Lab. Clin. Med.* 64:29–41 (1964).

Heaton, J. M. The distribution of brown adipose tissue in the human. *J. Anat.* 112:35–39 (1972).

Hegsted, D. M. Mineral intake and bone loss. *Fed. Proc.* 26:1747–1754 (1967).

Hegsted, D. M. Nutritional research on the value of amino acid fortification: experimental studies in animals. In *Amino Acid Fortification of Protein Foods*, pp. 157–, N. S. Scrimshaw and A. M. Altschul, Eds., MIT Press, Cambridge, Mass. (1971).

Hegsted, D. M. Problems in the use and interpretations of the recommended dietary allowances. *Ecol. Food Nutr.* 1:255–265 (1972).

Hegsted, D. M. Balance studies. *J. Nutr.* 106:307–311 (1976).

Hegsted, D. M. and Y. Chang. Protein utilization in growing rats at different levels of intake. *J. Nutr.* 87:19–25 (1965a).

Hegsted, D. M. and Y. Chang. Protein utilization in growing rats. I. Relative growth index as a bioassay procedure. *J. Nutr.* 85:159–168 (1965b).

Hegsted, D. M., C. A. Finch, and T. D. Kinney. The influence of diet on iron absorption. II. The interrelation of iron and phosphorus. *J. Exp. Med.* 90:147–156 (1949).

Hegsted, D. M., I. Moscoso, and C. C. Collazos. A study of the minimum calcium requirements of adult men. *J. Nutr.* 46:181–201 (1952).

Hegsted, D. M. and R. Neff. Efficiency of protein utilization in young rats at various levels of intake. *J. Nutr.* 100:1173–1179 (1970).

Hegsted, M., S. A. Schuette, M. B. Zemel, and H. M. Linkswiler. Urinary calcium and calcium balance as affected by level of protein and phosphorous intake. *J. Nutr.* 111:553–562 (1981).

Heidmann, T. and J.-P. Changeux. Structural and functional properties of the acetylcholine receptor protein in its purified and membrane-bound states. *Ann. Rev. Biochem.* 47:317–357 (1978).

Heinz, E. and P. M. Walsh. Exchange diffusion, transport, and intracellular level of amino acids in Ehrlich carcinoma cells. *J. Biol. Chem.* 233:1488–1493 (1958).

Helbock, H. J. and P. Saltman. The transport of iron by rat intestine. *Biochim. Biophys. Acta* 135:979–990 (1967).

Heller, J. Structure of visual pigments. II. Binding of retinal and conformational changes on light exposure in bovine visual pigment 500. *Biochemistry* 7:2914–2920 (1968).

Hellman, L. and J. J. Burns. Metabolism of L-ascorbic acid-l-C^{14} in man. *J. Biol. Chem.* 230:923–930 (1958).

Helminen, H. J. and J. L. E. Ericsson. Studies on mammary gland involution. II. Ultrastructural evidence for auto- and heterophagocytosis. *J. Ultrastruct. Res.* 25:214–227 (1968).

Hems, D. A. and P. D. Whitton. Control of hepatic glycogenolysis *Physiol. Rev.* 60:2–50 (1980).

Henderson, L. M. Niacin. *Ann. Rev. Nutr.* 3:289–307 (1983).

Hengen, N., V. Seiberth, and M. Hengen. High-performance liquid chromatographic determination of free nicotinic acid and its metabolite, nicotinuric acid, in plasma and urine. *Clin. Chem.* 24:1740–1743 (1978).

Henkin, R. I. Newer aspects of copper and zinc metabolism. In *Newer Trace Elements in Nutrition*, pp. 255–312, W. Mertz and W. E. Cornatzer, Eds., Marcel Dekker Inc., New York (1971).

Henkin, R. J., P. J. Schecter, R. Hoye, and C. F. T. Mattern. Idiopathic hypogeusia with dysgeusia, hyposmia, and dysosmia. *JAMA* 217:434–440 (1971).

Hentges, D. J. Does diet influence human fecal microflora composition? *Nutr. Rev.* 38:329–336 (1980).

Hepburn, F. N. The USDA national nutrient data bank. *Am. J. Clin. Nutr.* 35(5 Suppl):1297–1301 (1982).

Hepner, G. W., C. C. Booth, J. Cowan, A. V. Hoffbrand, and D. L. Mollin. Absorption of crystalline folic acid in man. *Lancet* 2:302–306 (1968).

Herbert, V. Studies of the mechanism of the effect of hog intrinsic factor concentrate on the uptake of vitamin B_{12} by rat liver slices. *J. Clin. Invest.* 37:646–650 (1958).

Herbert, V. Mechanism of intrinsic factor action in everted sacs or rat small intestine. *J. Clin. Invest.* 38:102–109 (1959).

Herbert, V. Biochemical and hematologic lesions in folic acid deficiency. *Am. J. Clin. Nutr.* 20:562–568 (1967).

Herbert, V. Folic acid deficiency in man. *Vitam. Horm.* 26:525–536 (1968a).

Herbert, V. Nutritional requirements for vitamin B_{12} and folic acid. *Am. J. Clin. Nutr.* 21:743–752 (1968b).

Herbert, V. and W. B. Castle. Intrinsic factor. *N. Engl. J. Med.* 270:1181–1185 (1964).

Herbert, V. and S. S. Shapiro. The site of absorption of folic acid in the rat *in vitro*. *Fed. Proc.* 21:250 (1962).

Herbert, V., R. R. Streiff, and L. W. Sullivan. Notes on vitamin B_{12} absorption: autoimmunity and childhood pernicious anemia; relation of intrinsic factor to blood group substance. *Medicine* 43:679–687 (1964a).

Herbert, V. and R. Zalusky. Interrelations of vitamin B_{12} and folic acid metabolism: folic acid clearance studies. *J. Clin. Invest.* 41:1263–1276 (1962).

Herman, A. G. Introductory remarks about the nomenclature of prostaglandins and their biosynthesis and metabolism. In *Cardiovascular Pharmacology of the Prostaglandins*, pp. 1–5, A. G. Herman, P. M. Vanhoutte, H. Denolin, and A. Goossens, Eds., Raven Press, New York (1982).

Herman, R. H. Mannose metabolism. *Am. J. Clin. Nutr.* 24:488–498 (1971).

Hernandez, H. H., I. L. Chaikoff, and J. Y. Kiyasu. Role of pancreatic juice in cholesterol absorption. *Am. J. Physiol.* 181:523–526 (1955).

Hers, H. G. α-Glucosidase deficiency in generalized glycogen-storage disease (Pompe's disease). *Biochem. J.* 86:11–16 (1963).

Hers, H. G. The control of glycogen metabolism in the liver. *Ann. Rev. Biochem.* 45:167–189 (1976).

Hers, H. G. and F. Van Hoof. Genetic abnormalities of lysosomes. In *Lysosomes in Biology and Pathology,* Vol. 2, pp. 19–40, J. T. Dingle and H. B. Fell, Eds., Wiley-Interscience, New York (1969).

Hertzig, E., H. G. Birch, S. A. Richardson, and J. Tizard. Intellectual levels of school children severely malnourished during the first two years of life. *Pediatr.* 49:814–824 (1972).

Hertzler, A. A. and H. L. Anderson. Food guides in the United States. *J. Am. Diet. Assoc.* 64:19–28 (1974).

Herzog, V. Pathways of endocytosis in secretory cells. *Trends Biochem. Sci.* 6:319–322 (1981).

Hess, A. F., M. Weinstock, and F. D. Helman. The antirachitic value of irradiated phytosterol and cholesterol. *J. Biol. Chem.* 63:305–308 (1925).

Hess, G. P. and J. A. Rupley. Structure and function of proteins. *Ann. Rev. Biochem.* 40:1013–1044 (1971).

Hicks, S. J., J. W. Drysdale, and H. N. Munro. Preferential synthesis of ferritin and albumin by different populations of liver polysomes. *Science* 164:584–585 (1969).

Highley, D. R., M. C. Davies, and L. Ellenbogen. Hog intrinsic factor. Some physico-chemical properties of vitamin B_{12}-binding fractions from hog pylorus. *J. Biol. Chem.* 242:1010–1015 (1967).

Hilker, D. M. and J. C. Somogyi. Antithiamins of plant origin: their chemical nature and mode of action. *Ann. N. Y. Acad. Sci.* 378:137–145 (1982).

Hill, D. E., A. B. Holt, A. Parra, and D. B. Cheek. The influence of protein calorie versus caloric restriction on the body composition and cellular growth of muscle and liver in weanling rats. *Johns Hopkins Med. J.* 127:146–163 (1970).

Hill, G. L., J. A. Bradley, J. P. Collins, I. McCarthy, C. B. Oxby, and L. Burkinshaw. Fat-free body mass from skinfold thickness: a close relationship with total body nitrogen. *Br. J. Nutr.* 39:403–405 (1978).

Hill, H. A. O., J. M. Pratt, and R. J. P. Williams. Identification and investigation of cobalamins and cobamide coenzymes by nuclear magnetic resonance and electron paramagnetic resonance spectroscopy. In *Methods in Enzymology,* Vol. 13, Part C, pp. 5–31, D. B. McCormick and L. D. Wright, Eds., Academic Press, New York (1971).

Hillman, R. S. Mechanisms underlying abnormal erythropoiesis. In *Regulation of Hematopoiesis,* Vol. 1, pp. 579–609, A. S. Gordon, Ed., Appleton-Century-Crofts, New York (1970).

Hillman, R. W. Tocopherol excess in man. Creatinuria associated with prolonged ingestion. *Am. J. Clin. Nutr.* 5:597–600 (1957).

Hills, O. W., E. Liebert, D. L. Steinberg, and M. K. Horwitt. Clinical aspects of dietary depletion of riboflavine. *AMA Arch. Intern. Med.* 87:682–693 (1951).

Hilz, H. and F. Lipmann. The enzymatic activation of sulfate. *Proc. Nat. Acad. Sci. U. S.* 41:880–890 (1955).

Himms-Hagen, J. Cellular thermogenesis. *Ann. Rev. Physiol.* 38:315–351 (1976).

Himms-Hagen, J. Brown adipose tissue thermogenesis in obese animals. *Nutr. Rev.* 41:261–267 (1983).

Hirano, S., P. Hoffman, and K. Meyer. The structure of keratosulfate of bovine cornea. *J. Org. Chem.* 26:5064–5069 (1961).

Hirsch, J. and B. Batchelor. Adipose tissue cellularity in human obesity. *Clin. Endocrinol. Metab.* 5:299–311 (1976).

Hirsch, J. and E. Gallian. Methods for the determination of adipose cell size in man and animals. *J. Lipid Res.* 9:110–119 (1968).

Hirsch, J. and P. W. Han. Cellularity of rat adipose tissue: effects of growth, starvation and obesity. *J. Lipid Res.* 10:77–82 (1969).

Hirsch, J. and J. L. Knittle. Cellularity of obese and nonobese human adipose tissue. *Fed. Proc.* 29:1516–1521 (1970).

Hirsch, J., J. L. Knittle, and L. B. Salans. Cell lipid content and cell number in obese and non-obese human adipose tissue. *J. Clin. Invest.* 45:1023A (1966).

Hirsch, P. F., G. F. Gauthier, and P. L. Munson. Thyroid hypocalcemic principle and recurrent laryngeal nerve injury as factors affecting the response to parathyroidectomy in rats. *Endocrinology* 73:244–252 (1963).

Hittleman, K. J., O. Lindberg, and B. Cannon. Oxidative phosphorylation and compartmentation of fatty acid metabolism in brown fat mitochondria. *Eur. J. Biochem.* 11:183–192 (1969).

Hoagland, M. B. An enzymatic mechanism for amino acid activation in animal tissues. *Biochim. Biophys. Acta* 16:288–289 (1955).

Hoagland, M. B., E. B. Keller, and P. C. Zamencnik. Enzymatic carboxyl activation of amino acids. *J. Biol. Chem.* 218:345–358 (1956).

Hochachka, P. W., J. R. Neely, and W. R. Driedzic. Integration of lipid utilization with Krebs cycle activity in muscle. *Fed. Proc.* 36:2009–2014 (1977).

Hochstein, P. and S. K. Jain. Association of lipid peroxidation and polymerization of membrane proteins with erythrocyte aging. *Fed. Proc.* 40:183–188 (1981).

Hodge, H. C. and F. A. Smith. Occupational fluoride exposure. *J. Occup. Med.* 19:12–39 (1977).

Hodges, R. E., J. Hood, J. E. Canham, H. E. Sauberlich, and E. M. Baker. Clinical manifestations of ascorbic acid deficiency in man. *Am. J. Clin. Nutr.* 24:432–443 (1971).

Hodges, R. E. and H. Kolder. Experimental vitamin A deficiency in human volunteers. In *Summary of Proceedings, Workshop on Biochemical and Clinical Criteria for Determining Human Vitamin A Nutriture*, pp. 10–16, J. G. Bieri, Chmn., National Academy of Sciences, Washington, D.C. (1971).

Hodgkin, D. C., J. Kamper, J. Lindsey, M. MacKay, J. Pickworth, J. H. Robertson, C. B. Shoemaker, J. G. White, R. J. Prosen, and K. N. Trueblood. The structure of vitamin B_{12}. I. An outline of the crystallographic investigation of vitamin B_{12}. *Proc. R. Soc. Lond., Ser. A* 242:228–263 (1957).

Hodgkin, D. C., J. Pickworth, J. H. Robertson, K. N. Trueblood, R. J. Prosen, and J. G. White. The crystal structure of the hexacarboxylic acid derived from B$_{12}$ and the molecular structure of the vitamin. *Nature* 176:325–328 (1955).

Hoedemaker, P. J., J. Abels, J. J. Wachters, A. Arends, and H. O. Nieweg. Investigations about the site of production of Castle's gastric intrinsic factor. *Lab. Invest.* 13:1394–1399 (1964).

Hoekstra, W. G., J. W. Suttie, H. E. Gauther, and W. Mertz. *Trace element metabolism in animals.* Vol 2, University Park Press, Baltimore (1974).

Hoffbrand, A. V. and T. J. Peters. The subcellular localization of pteroylpolyglutamate hydrolase and folate in guinea pig intestinal mucosa. *Biochim. Biophys. Acta* 192:479–485 (1969).

Hoffman, H. and G. W. Grigg. An electron microscopic study of mitochondria formation. *Exp. Cell Res.* 15:118–131 (1958).

Hoffman, N. E. The relationship between uptake *in vitro* of oleic acid and micellar solubilization. *Biochim. Biophys. Acta* 196:193–203 (1970).

Hofmann, A. and B. Borgström. Physico-chemical state of lipids in intestinal content during their digestion and absorption. *Fed. Proc.* 21:43–50 (1962).

Hofmann, A. and B. Borgström. Hydrolysis of long-chain monoglycerides in micellar solution by pancreatic lipase. *Biochem. Biophys. Acta* 70:317–331 (1963).

Hohman, W. and H. Schraer. The intracellular distribution of calcium in the mucosa of the avian shell gland. *J. Cell Biol.* 30:317–331 (1966).

Hohman, W. and H. Schraer. Low temperature ultramicroincineration of thin-sectioned tissue. *J. Cell Biol.* 55:328–354 (1972).

Hokin, C. E. Dynamic aspects of phospholipids during protein secretion. *Int. Rev. Cytol.* 23:187–208 (1968).

Holcomb, K. J. and S. A. Fusari. Liquid chromatographic determinations of folic acid in multivitamin-mineral preparations. *Anal. Chem.* 53:607–609 (1981).

Holick, M. F., M. Garabedian, and H. F. DeLuca. 1,25-Dihydroxycholecalciferol: metabolite of vitamin D$_3$ active on bone in anephric rats. *Science* 176:1146–1147 (1972a).

Holick, M. F., A. Kleiner-Bosaller, H. K. Schnoes, P. M. Kaster, I. T. Boyle, and H. F. DeLuca. 1,24,25-Trihydroxyvitamin D$_3$: a metabolite of vitamin D$_3$ effective on intestine. *J. Biol. Chem.* 248:6691–6696 (1973).

Holick, M. F., H. K. Schnoes, and H. F. DeLuca. Identification of 1,25-dihydroxycholecalciferol, a form of vitamin D$_3$ metabolically active in the intestine. *Proc. Nat. Acad. Sci. U. S.* 68:803–804 (1971a).

Holick, M. F., H. K. Schnoes, H. F. DeLuca, R. W. Gray, I. T. Boyle, and T. Suda. Isolation and identification of 24,25-dihydroxycholecalciferol: a metabolite of vitamin D$_3$ made in the kidney. *Biochemistry* 11:4251–4255 (1972b).

Holick, M. F., H. K. Schnoes, H. F. DeLuca, T. Suda, and R. J. Cousins. Isolation and identification of 1,25-dihydroxycholecalciferol: a metabolite of vitamin D active in intestine. *Biochemistry* 10:2799–2804 (1971).

Hollander, D. Vitamin K_1 absorption by everted intestinal sacs of the rat. *Am. J. Physiol.* 225:360–364 (1973).

Hollander, D., K. S. Muralidhara, and E. Rim. Colonic absorption of bacterially synthesized vitamin K_2 in the rat. *Am. J. Physiol.* 230:251–255 (1976).

Hollander, D. and E. Rim. Vitamin K_2 absorption by rat everted small intestinal sacs. *Am. J. Physiol.* 231:415–419 (1976).

Hollenberg, C. H. Effect of nutrition on activity and release of lipase from rat adipose tissue. *Am. J. Physiol.* 197:667–670 (1959).

Hollenberg, C. H. Adipose tissue lipases. II. In *Handbook of Physiology,* Section 5, Adipose Tissue, pp. 301–307, A. E. Renold and G. F. Cahill, Eds., American Physiological Society, Washington, D.C. (1965).

Hollenberg, C. H. Distribution of radioactive glycerol and fatty acids among adipose tissue triglycerides after administration of glucose-U-^{14}C. *J. Lipid Res.* 8:328–334 (1967).

Hollett, C. R. and J. V. Auditore. Localization and characterization of a lipase in rat adipose tissue. *Arch. Biochem. Biophys.* 121:423–430 (1967).

Holley, R. W., J. Apgar, G. A. Everett, J. T. Madison, M. Marquisee, S. H. Merrill, J. R. Penswick, and A. Zamir. Structure of a ribonucleic acid. *Science* 147:1462–1465 (1965).

Holloway, W. D., C. Tasman-Jones, and S. P. Lee. Digestion of certain fractions of dietary fiber in humans. *Am. J. Clin. Nutr.* 31:927–930 (1978).

Holman, C. A., E. B. Mawer, and D. J. Smith. Tissue distribution of cholecalciferol (vitamin D_3) in the rat. *Biochem. J.* 120:29P (1970).

Holoubek, V. and T. Crocker. DNA-associated acidic proteins. *Biochim. Biophys. Acta* 157:352–361 (1969).

Holst, A. and T. Frolich. Experimental studies relating to ship-beriberi and scurvy. 2. On the etiology of scurvy. *J. Hyg. (Camb.)* 7:634 (1907).

Holt, J. H. and D. Miller. The localization of phosphomonoesterase and aminopeptidase in brush borders isolated from intestinal epithelial cells. *Biochim. Biophys. Acta* 58:239–243 (1962).

Holt, L. E. and S. E. Snyderman. The amino acid requirement of children. In *Amino Acid Metabolism and Genetic Variation,* pp. 381–390, W. L. Nyan, Ed., McGraw-Hill, New York (1967).

Holter, H. Pinocytosis. In *Biological Structure and Function,* Vol. 1, pp. 157–168, T. W. Goodwin and O. Lindberg, Eds., Academic Press, London (1961).

Holzel, A., V. Schwarz, and K. W. Sutcliffe. Defective lactose absorption causing malnutrition in infancy. *Lancet* 1:1126–1128 (1959).

Holtzmann, E. Golgi apparatus, GERL, and lysosomes in secretion and protein uptake by adrenal medulla cells. *J. Cell Biol.* 35:58A (1967).

Holtzmann, E. *Lysosomes: A Survey,* Springer-Verlag, New York (1976).

Hooper, C. E. S. Cell turnover in epithelial populations. *J. Histochem. Cytochem.* 4:531–540 (1956).

Hopkins, F. G. Feeding experiments illustrating the importance of accessory factors in normal dietaries. *J. Physiol. (London)* 44:425–460 (1912).

Hoppner, K., B. Lampi, and D. E. Perrin. The free and total folate activity in foods available on the Canadian market. *Can. Inst. Food Sci. Tech. J.* 5:60–66 (1972).

Hoppner, K., B. Lampi, and D. C. Smith. Data on folacin activity in foods: availability, applications and limitations. In *Folic Acid. Biochemistry and Physiology in Relation to the Human Nutrition Requirement*, pp 69–82, National Research Council, National Academy of Sciences, Washington, D.C.

Horowitz, M. I. and W. Pigman, Eds., *The Glycoconjugates. Vol. 1 Mammalian Glycoproteins and Glycolipids.* Academic Press, New York and London (1977).

Horowitz, S. B. and I. R. Fenichel. Analysis of sodium transport in the amphibian oocyte by extractive and radioautographic techniques. *J. Cell Biol.* 47:120–131 (1970).

Horst, R. L., R. M. Shepard, N. A. Jorgensen, and H. F. DeLuca. The determination of 24,25-dehydroxyvitamin D in plasma from normal and nephrectomized man. *J. Lab. Clin. Med.* 93:277–285 (1979).

Horton, J. E., L. G. Raisz, H. A. Simmons, J. J. Oppenheim, and S. E. Mergenhagen. Bone resorbing activity in supernatant fluid from cultured human peripheral blood leukocytes. *Science* 177:793–795 (1972).

Horton, R., R. Zipser, and M. Fichman. Prostaglandins, renal function and vascular regulation. *Med. Clin. North Am.* 65:891–914 (1981).

Horwitt, M. K. Effects of limited tocopherol intake in man with relationships to erythrocyte hemolysis and lipid oxidations. *Am. J. Clin. Nutr.* 8:408–419 (1960).

Horwitt, M. K. Vitamin E and lipid metabolism in man. *Am. J. Clin. Nutr.* 8:451–461 (1960).

Horwitt, M. K. Interrelations between vitamin E and polyunsaturated fatty acids in adult men. *Vitam. Horm.* 20:541–558 (1962).

Horwitt, M. K., B. Century, and A. A. Zeman. Erythrocyte survival time and reticulocyte levels after tocopherol depletion in man. *Am. J. Clin. Nutr.* 12:99–106 (1963).

Horwitt, M. K., A. E. Harper, and L. M. Henderson. Niacin-tryptophan relationships for evaluating niacin equivalents. *Am. J. Clin. Nutr.* 34:423–427 (1981).

Horwitt, M. K., C. C. Harvey, O. W. Hills, and E. Liebert. Correlation of urinary excretion of riboflavin with dietary intake and symptoms of ariboflavinosis. *J. Nutr.* 41:247–264 (1950).

Horwitt, M. K., C. C. Harvey, W. S. Rothwell, J. L. Cutler, and D. Haffron. Tryptophan-niacin relationships in man. *J. Nutr.* 60: (Suppl. 1) 1–43 (1956).

Horwitt, M. K., E. Liebert, O. Kreisler, and P. Wittman. *Investigations of human requirements for B-complex vitamins* (National Research Council Bull. 116), National Academy of Sciences, Washington, D.C. (1948).

Horwitz, B. A. Cellular events underlying catecholamine-induced thermogenesis: cation transport in brown adipocytes. *Fed. Proc.* 38:2170–2176 (1979).

Hostmark, A. T. The effect of insulin on epinephrine and glucagon inactivated glycogen synthase I in the isolated perfused rat liver. *Acta Physiol. Scand.* 88:248–255 (1973).

Howard, L., C. Wagner, and S. Schenker. Malabsorption of thiamine in folate-deficient rats. *J. Nutr.* 104:1024–1032 (1974).

Howarth, R. E. Influence of dietary protein on rat skeletal muscle growth. *J. Nutr.* 102:37–43 (1972).

Howell, B. J., F. W. Baumgardner, K. Bondi, and H. Rahn. Acid-base balance in cold-blooded vertebrates as a function of body temperature. *Am. J. Physiol.* 218:600–606 (1970).

Howell, J. McC. and A. N. Davison. The copper content and cytochrome oxidase activity of tissues from normal and swayback lambs. *Biochem. J.* 72:365–368 (1959).

Hoyumpa, A. M., K. J. Breen, S. Schenker, and F. A. Wilson. Thiamine transport across the rat intestine. II. Effect of ethanol. *J. Lab. Clin. Med.* 86:803–816 (1975b).

Hoyumpa, A. M., Jr., H. M. Middleton, F. A. Wilson, and S. Schenker. Thiamine transport across the rat intestine. I. Normal characteristics. *Gastroenterol.* 68:1218–1227 (1975a).

Hryniuk, W. M. and J. R. Bertino. Growth rate and cell kill. *Ann. N. Y. Acad. Sci.* 186:330–342 (1971).

Hsia, D. Y-Y. The diagnosis of carrier of disease-producing genes. *Ann. N. Y. Acad. Sci.* 134:946–964 (1966).

Hsueh, A. M., M. Simonson, M. J. Kellum, and B. F. Chow. Perinatal under-nutrition and the metabolic and behavioral development of the offspring. *Nutr. Rep. Int.* 7:437–446 (1973).

Huang, R. C. and J. Bonner. Histone, a suppressor of chromosomal RNA synthesis. *Proc. Nat. Acad. Sci. U. S.* 48:1216–1222 (1962).

Huang, S. S. and T. M. Bayless. Milk and lactose intolerance in healthy orientals. *Science* 160:83–84 (1968).

Hubbard, J. I. and S. Kwanbunbumpen. Evidence for the vesicle hypothesis. *J. Physiol. (London)* 194:407–420 (1968).

Huebers, H. Identification of iron binding intermediates in intestinal mucosal tissue of rats during absorption. In *Proteins of Iron Storage and Transport in Biochemistry and Medicine,* pp. 381–388, R. R. Crichton, Ed., North-Holland Publishing Co., Amsterdam (1975).

Huebers, H., E. Huebers, W. Forth, and W. Rummel. Binding of iron to a non-ferritin protein in the mucosal cells of normal and iron-deficient rats during absorption. *Life Sci.* 10:1141–1148 (1971).

Huebers, H., E. Huebers, W. Rummel, and R. R. Crichton. Isolation and characterization of iron-binding proteins from rat intestinal mucosa. *Eur. J. Biochem.* 66:447–455 (1976).

Huehns, E. R. and G. H. Beaven. Developmental changes in human haemoglobins. In *The Biochemistry of Development,* pp. 175–203, P. F. Benson, Ed., J. B. Lippincott, Philadelphia (1971).

Huehns, E. R., N. Dance, G. H. Beaven, F. Hecht, A. G. Motulsky. Human embryonic hemoglobins. *Cold Spring Harbor Symp. Quant. Biol.* 29:327–331 (1964).

Huldshinsky, K. Heilung von Rachitis durch künstliche Höhensonne. *Deut. Med. Wochschr.* 45:712–713 (1919).

Hull, B. E. and L. A. Staehlin. The terminal web. *J. Cell Biol.* 81:67–82 (1978).

Hull, D. and M. M. Segall. The contribution of brown adipose tissue to heat production in the new-born rabbit. *J. Physiol. (London)* 181:449–457 (1965a).

Hull, D. and M. M. Segall. Sympathetic nervous control of brown adipose tissue and heat production in the new-born rabbit. *J. Physiol. (London)* 181:458–467 (1965b).

Hull, D. and M. M. Segall. Distinction of brown from white adipose tissue. *Nature* 212:469–472 (1966).

Hullar, T. L. Potential antimetabolites of pyridoxal phosphate. *Ann. N. Y. Acad. Sci.* 166:191–198 (1969).

Hume, E. M. and H. A. Krebs, Compilers. *Vitamin A requirement of human adults. An experimental study of vitamin A deprivation in man.* (Special Report Series No. 264). Medical Research Council, Great Britain, London (1949).

Humphrey, S. J. E. and H. S. Wolff. The oxylog. *J. Physiol. (London)* 267:12P (1977).

Hunt, E. E. and E. Giles. Allometric growth of body composition in man and other mammals. *Hum. Biol.* 30:253–273 (1956).

Hunt, E. E., Jr. and F. P. Heald. Physique, body composition, and sexual maturation in adolescent boys. *Ann. N. Y. Acad. Sci.* 110:532–544 (1963).

Hunt, J. A. and V. M. Ingram. A terminal peptide sequence of human haemoglobin? *Nature* 184:640–641 (1959).

Hunt, R. D., F. G. Garcia, and D. M. Hegsted. A comparison of vitamin D_2 and D_3 in new world primates. I. Production and regression of osteodystrophia fibrosa. *Lab. Anim. Care* 17:222–234 (1967).

Hutton, J. J., A. L. Tappel, and S. Udenfriend. Cofactor and substrate requirements of collagen proline hydroxylase. *Arch. Biochem. Biophys.* 118:231–240 (1967).

Huttunen, P., J. Hirvonen, and V. Kinnula. The occurrence of brown adipose tissue in outdoor workers. *Eur. J. Appl. Physiol.* 46:339–345 (1981).

Huxley, H. E. Electron microscope studies of natural and synthetic protein filaments from striated muscle. *J. Mol. Biol.* 7:281–308 (1963).

Huxley, H. E. The mechanism of muscular contraction. *Science* 164:1356–1366 (1969).

Huxtable, R. J. Does taurine have a function? *Fed. Proc.* 39:2678–2679 (1980).

Hyden, H. RNA in brain cells. In *The Neurosciences,* pp. 248–266, G. C. Quarton, T. Melnechuk, and F. O. Schmitt, Eds., Rockefeller University Press, New York (1967).

Hylander, E., K. Ladefoged, and S. Jarnum. The importance of the colon in calcium absorption following small-intestinal resection. *Scand. J. Gastroenterol.* 15:55–60 (1980).

Hytten, F. E. and I. Leitch. *The Physiology of Human Pregnancy,* 2nd ed., F. A. Davis Co., Philadelphia (1971).

Hyun, S. A., G. V. Vahouny, and C. R. Treadwell. Effect of α-ethylcaproic acid on cholesterol esterification and absorption. *Arch. Biochem. Biophys.* 104:139–145 (1964).

Iacono, J. M., R. M. Dougherty, R. Paoletti, C. Galli, A. C. A. Carvalho, A. Ferro-Luzzi, D. G. Therriault, G. J. Nelson, and A. Keys. Pilot epidemiological studies in thrombosis. In *The Thrombotic Process in Atherogenesis (Adv. Exp. Med. Biol.* Vol. 104), pp. 309–327, A. B. Chandler, K. Eurenius, G. C. McMillan, C. B. Nelson, C. J. Schwartz, and S. Wessler, Eds., Plenum, New York (1978).

Iacono, J. M., J. T. Judd, M. W. Marshall, J. J. Canary, R. M. Dougherty, J. F. Mackin, and B. T. Weinland. The role of dietary essential fatty acids and prostaglandins in reducing blood pressure. *Prog. Lipid Res.* Vol. 20:349–363 (1981).

ICNND. *Manual for Nutrition Surveys,* 2nd ed., U.S. Government Printing Office, Washington, D.C. (1963).

Imai, S. and K. Takeda. Actions of calcium and certain multivalent cations on potassium contracture of guinea pig's *taenia coli. J. Physiol. (London)* 190:155–169 (1967).

Imami, R. H., S. Reiser, and P. A. Christiansen. Effects of vitamin E and essential fatty acid deficiencies on the intestinal transport of L-valine and α-methyl-D-glucoside in the rat. *J. Nutr.* 100:101–109 (1970).

Imawari, M., Y. Akanuma, H. Itakura, Y. Muto, K. Kosaka, and D. S. Goodman. The effects of diseases of the liver on serum 25-hydroxyvitamin D and on the serum binding protein for vitamin D and its metabolites. *J. Lab. Clin. Med.* 93:171–180 (1979).

Imawari, M., K. Kida, and D. S. Goodman. The transport of vitamin D and its 25-hydroxy metabolite in human plasma. Isolation and partial characterization of vitamin D and 25-hydroxyvitamin D binding protein. *J. Clin. Invest.* 58:514–523 (1976).

Ingbar, S. H. and K. A. Woeber. The thyroid gland. In *Textbook of Endocrinology,* 6th ed., pp. 117–247, R. H. Williams, Ed., W. B. Saunders Co., Philadelphia (1981).

Ingebritsen, T. S. and P. Cohen. Protein phosphatases: properties and role in cellular regulation. *Science* 221:331–338 (1983).

Ingenbleek, Y., M. De Visscher, and Ph. De Nayer. Measurement of prealbumin as index of protein-calorie malnutrition. *Lancet* 2:106–109 (1972).

Ingram, V. M. Gene mutations in human haemoglobins: the chemical difference between normal and sickle cell haemoglobin. *Nature* 180:326–328 (1957).

Irsigler, K., H. Heitkamp, W. Schlick, and P. Schmid. Diet and energy balance in obesity (a methodological approach). In *Regulation of Energy Balance in Man*, pp. 72–83, E. Jequier, Ed., Widmer Foundation de l'Imprimerie Medicine et Hygiene, Geneva (1975).

Irving, J. T. *Calcium Metabolism,* John Wiley & Sons, New York (1957).

Irwin, M. I. and D. M. Hegsted. A conspectus of research on protein requirements of man. *J. Nutr.* 101:385–430 (1971).

Isselbacher, K. J. Metabolism and transport of lipid by intestinal mucosa. *Fed. Proc.* 24:16–22 (1965).

Isselbacher, K. J. and R. M. Glickman. On the role of protein synthesis in the intestinal absorption of fat. In *Transport Across the Intestine*, pp. 245–250, W. C. Burland and P. D. Samuel, Eds., Churchill Livingstone, Edinburgh (1972).

Ito, S. Structure and function of the glycocalyx. *Fed. Proc.* 28:12–25 (1969).

IUPAC-IUB Commission on Biochemical Nomenclature. Tentative rules. *J. Biol. Chem.* 241:2987–2994 (1966).

IUPAC-IUB Commission on Biochemical Nomenclature. Rules for the nomenclature of lipids. *Eur. J. Biochem.* 2:127–131 (1967).

IUPAC-IUB Commission on Biochemical Nomenclature. The nomenclature of lipids. Recommendations (1976). *Lipids* 12:455–468 (1977).

Iversen, L. L. *The Uptake and Storage of Noradrenaline in Sympathetic Nerves,* Cambridge University Press, London (1967).

Iversen, L. L. and Schon, F. E. The use of autoradiographic techniques for the identification and mapping of transmitter specific neurons in CNS. In *New Concepts in Neurotransmitter Mechanisms*, pp. 153–193, A. J. Mandell, Ed., Plenum, New York (1973).

Ivy, A. C. and E. Oldberg. A hormone mechanism for gallbladder contraction and evacuation. *Am. J. Physiol.* 86:599–613 (1928).

Iwasaki, K., S. Sabol, A. J. Wahba, and S. Ochoa. Translation of the genetic message. VII. Role of initiation factors in formation of the chain initiation complex with *Escherichia coli* ribosomes. *Arch. Biochem. Biophys.* 125:542–547 (1968).

Jackson, A. S. and M. L. Pollock. Generalized equations for predicting body density of men. *Br. J. Nutr.* 40:497–504 (1978).

Jackson, A. S., M. L. Pollock, and A. Ward. Generalized equations for predicting body density of women. *Med. Sci. Sports Exer.* 12:175–182 (1980).

Jacob, E., S. J. Baker, and V. Herbert. Vitamin B_{12}-binding proteins. *Physiol. Rev.* 60:918–960 (1980).

Jacob, F. and J. Monod. Genetic regulatory mechanisms in the synthesis of proteins. *J. Mol. Biol.* 3:318–356 (1961).

Jacob, M. I. Fatty acid synthesis in cell-free preparations of human adipose tissue. *Biochim. Biophys. Acta* 70:231–241 (1963).

Jacobs, A. and M. Worwood. Iron. In *Disorders of Mineral Metabolism,* Vol. 1, pp. 1–58, F. Bronner and J. W. Coburn, Eds., Academic Press, New York (1981).

Jacobson, L. O., E. Goldwasser, W. Fried, and L. Pizak. Role of the kidney in erythropoiesis. *Nature* 179:633–634 (1957).

Jacobson, W. and I. A. B. Cathie. The inactivation of folic acid antagonists by normal and leukaemic cells. *Biochem. Pharmacol.* 5:130–142 (1960).

Jagerstad, M., B. Akesson, and C. Fehling. Effect of methionine on the metabolic fate of liver folates in vitamin B_{12}-deficient rats. *Br. J. Nutr.* 44:361–369 (1980).

Jaim-Etcheverry, G. and L. M. Zieher. Ultrastructural aspects of neurotransmitter storage in adrenergic nerves. *Adv. Cytopharmacol.* 1:343–361 (1971).

James, W. P. T., W. J. Branch, and D. A. T. Southgate. Calcium binding by dietary fiber. *Lancet* 1:638–639 (1978).

James, W. P. T. and A. M. Hay. Albumin metabolism: effect of the nutritional state and the dietary protein intake. *J. Clin. Invest.* 47:1958–1972 (1968).

Jamieson, J. D. Role of the Golgi complex in the intracellular transport of secretory proteins. *Adv. Cytopharmacol.* 1:183–190 (1971).

Jamieson, J. D. and G. E. Palade. Intracellular transport of newly synthesized proteins in the exocrine process. *J. Cell Biol.* 27:47A (1965).

Jamieson, J. D. and G. E. Palade. Role of the Golgi complex in the intracellular transport of secretory proteins. *Proc. Nat. Acad. Sci. U.S.* 55:424–431 (1966).

Jamieson, J. D. and G. E. Palade. Intracellular transport of secretory proteins in the pancreatic exocrine cell. I. Role of the peripheral elements of the Golgi complex. *J. Cell Biol.* 34:577–596 (1967a).

Jamieson, J. D. and G. E. Palade. Intracellular transport of secretory proteins in the pancreatic exocrine cell. II. Transport to condensing vacuoles and zymogen granules. *J. Cell Biol.* 34:597–615 (1967b).

Jamieson, J. D. and G. E. Palade. Production of secretory proteins in animal cells. In *International Cell Biology,* pp. 308–317, B. R. Brinkley and K. R. Porter, Eds., Rockefeller University Press, New York (1977).

Jamison, R. L. The renal concentrating mechanism: micropuncture studies of the renal medulla. *Fed. Proc.* 42:2392–2397 (1983).

Janghorbani, M., M. J. Christensen, F. H. Steinke, and V. R. Young. Feasibility of intrinsic labelling of poultry meat with stable isotope of selenium (^{74}Se) for use in human metabolism studies. *J. Nutr.* 111:817–822 (1981).

Janghorbani, M., B. T. G. Ting, and V. R. Young. Accurate analysis of stable isotopes 68_{Zn}, 70_{Zn}, and 58_{Fe} in human feces with neutron activation analysis. *Clin. Chim. Acta* 108:9–24 (1980).

Janghorbani, M. and V. R. Young. Stable isotope methods for bioavailability assessment of dietary minerals in humans. In *Advances in Nutritional Research,* Vol. 3, pp. 127–155, H. H. Draper, Ed., Plenum, New York (1980).

Jansen, C. and I. Harrill. Intakes and serum levels of protein and iron for 70 elderly women. *Am. J. Clin. Nutr.* 30:1414–1422 (1977).

Jansen, G. R. Biochemical parameters and protein quality. In *Protein Quality in Humans: Assessment and in Vitro Estimation.* pp. 118–142, C. E. Bodwell, J. S. Adkins and D. T. Hopkins, Eds., AVI Publishing Co., Westport, Conn. (1981).

Jansen, G. R., C. F. Hutchison, and M. E. Zanetti. Studies on lipogenesis *in vivo. Biochem. J.* 99:323–332 (1966a).

Jansen, G. R., M. E. Zanetti, and C. F. Hutchison. Studies on lipogenesis *in vivo. Biochem. J.* 102:864–869 (1966b).

Jardetzky, O. Simple allosteric model for membrane pumps. *Nature* 211:269–270 (1966).

Jarett, L., J. B. Schweitzer, and R. M. Smith. Insulin receptors: differences in structural organization on adipocyte and liver plasma membranes. *Science* 210:1127–1128 (1980).

Jeanloz, R. W. Mucopolysaccharides of higher animals. *The Carbohydrates,* Vol. 2, pp. 589–625, W. Pigman, D. Horton, and A. Herp, Eds., Academic Press, New York (1970).

Jeans, P. C. and G. Stearns. Effect of vitamin D on linear growth in infancy: effect of intakes above 1,800 U.S.P. units daily. *J. Pediatr.* 13:730–740 (1938).

Jeejeebhoy, K. N., R. C. Chu, E. B. Marliss, G. R. Greenberg, and A. Bruce-Robertson. Chromium deficiency, glucose intolerance, and neuropathy reversed by chromium supplementation in a patient receiving long-term total parenteral nutrition. *Am. J. Clin. Nutr.* 30:531–538 (1977).

Jelliffe, D. B. Field anthropometry independent of precise age. *J. Pediatr.* 75:334–335 (1969).

Jelliffe, D. B. and E. F. P. Jelliffe. Age-independent anthropometry. *Am. J. Clin. Nutr.* 24:1377–1379 (1971).

Jequier, E. Studies with direct calorimetry in humans: thermal body insulation and thermoregulatory responses during exercise. In *Assessment of Energy Metabolism in Health and Disease,* pp. 15–20, Proceedings of the First Ross Conference on Medical Research, Ross Laboratories, Columbus, Ohio (1980).

Jewell, P. A. and E. B. Verney. An experimental attempt to determine the site of the neurohypophyseal osmoreceptors in the dog. *Philos. Trans. R. Soc. Lond. Ser. B,* 240:197–324 (1957).

Joel, C. D. The physiological role of brown adipose tissue. In *Handbook of Physiology,* Section 5, Adipose Tissue, pp. 59–85, A. E. Renold and G. F. Cahill, Eds., American Physiological Society, Washington, D.C. (1965).

Johansson, C. Gastrointestinal interactions. VII. Characteristics of the absorption pattern of sugar, fat, and protein from composite meals in man. Quantitative study. *Scand. J. Gastroenterol.* 10:33–42 (1975).

Johansson, S., S. Lindstedt, U. Register, and L. Wadström. Studies on the metabolism of labeled pyridoxine in man. *Am. J. Clin. Nutr.* 18:185–196 (1966).

Johns, D. G. and D. M. Valerino. Metabolism of folate antagonists. *Ann. N. Y. Acad. Sci.* 186:378–386 (1971).

Johnson, J. D. The regional and ethnic distribution of lactose malabsorption. Adaptive and genetic hypotheses. In *Lactose Digestion: Clinical and Nutritional Implications,* pp. 11–22, D. M. Paige and T. M. Bayless, Eds., Johns Hopkins University Press, Baltimore (1981).

Johnson, J., B. Hainline, and K. Rajagopalan. Characterization of the molybdenum cofactor of sulfite oxidase, xanthine oxidase, and nitrate reductase. *J. Biol. Chem.* 255:1783–1786 (1980a).

Johnson, J., W. Waud, K. Rajagopalan, M. Duran, F. Beemer, and S. Wadman. Inborn errors of molybdenum metabolism: combined deficiencies of sulfite oxidase and xanthine oxidase in a patient lacking the molybdenum cofactor. *Proc. Nat. Acad. Sci. U. S.* 77:3715–3719 (1980b).

Johnson, L. C. Histogenesis and mechanisms in the development of osteofluorosis. In *Fluorine Chemistry,* Vol. 4, pp. 424–441, J. H. Simons, Ed., Academic Press, New York (1965).

Johnson, N. E., E. N. Alcantara, and H. Linkswiler. Effect of level of protein intake on urinary and fecal calcium and calcium retention of young adult males. *J. Nutr.* 100:1425–1430 (1970).

Johnson, P. and W. F. R. Pover. Intestinal absorption of α-tocopherol. *Life Sci.* 4:115–117 (1962).

Johnson, P. R., J. S. Stern, M. R. C. Greenwood, L. M. Zucker, and J. Hirsch. Effect of early nutrition on adipose tissue cellularity and pancreatic insulin release in the Zucker rat. *J. Nutr.* 103:738–743 (1973).

Johnson, P. R., L. M. Zucker, J. A. F. Cruce, and J. Hirsch. Cellularity of adipose depots and the genetically obese Zucker rat. *J. Lipid Res.* 12:706–714 (1971).

Johnson, R., S. Baker, J. Fallon, E. Maynard, J. Ruskin, Z. Wen, K. Ge, and H. Cohen. An occidental case of cardiomyopathy and selenium deficiency. *N. Engl. J. Med.* 304:1210–1213 (1981).

Johnston, F. A., T. J. McMillan, and G. D. Falconer. Calcium retained by young women before and after adding spinach to the diet. *J. Am. Diet. Assoc.* 28:933–938 (1952).

Johnston, J. M. Recent developments in the mechanism of fat absorption. In *Advances in Lipid Research,* Vol. 1, pp. 105–131, R. Paoletti and D. Kritchevsky, Eds., Academic Press, New York (1963).

Johnston, J. M. Mechanism of fat absorption. In *Handbook of Physiology,* Section

6: Alimentary Canal, Vol. 3, pp. 1353–1375, C. F. Code, Ed., American Physiological Society, Washington, D.C., 1968.

Johnston, J. M. and B. Borgström. The intestinal absorption and metabolism of micellar solutions of lipids. *Biochim. Biophys. Acta* 84:412–423 (1964).

Johnston, P. V. and B. I. Roots. *Nerve Membranes. A Study of the Biological and Chemical Aspects of Neuron-Glia Relationships.* Pergamon Press, Oxford (1972).

Jones, A. P. and M. I. Friedman. Obesity and adipocyte abnormalities in offspring of rats undernourished during pregnancy. *Science* 215:1518–1519 (1982).

Jones, D., J. Scholler, and K. Folkers. The vitamin activity of coenzyme Q_7 in reproduction in the rat. *Int. J. Vitam. Nutr. Res.* 41:215–220 (1971).

Jones, S. F. and S. Kwanbunbumpen. On the role of synaptic vesicles in transmitter release. *Life Sci.* 7:1251–1255 (1968).

Jost, J-P. and H. V. Rickenberg. Cyclic AMP. *Ann. Rev. Biochem.* 40:741–774 (1971).

Jung, R. T., P. S. Shetty, and W. P. T. James. The effects of beta adrenergic blockade on basal metabolism and peripheral thyroid metabolism. *Proc. Nutr. Soc.* 38:57A (1979).

Jungas, R. L. Role of cyclic-3′,5′-AMP in the response of adipose tissue to insulin. *Proc. Nat. Acad. Sci. U. S.* 56:757–763 (1966).

Jurkowitz, B. Determination of vitamin A acid in human plasma after oral administration. *Arch. Biochem. Biophys.* 98:337–341 (1962).

Jusko, W. J. and G. Levy. Absorption, metabolism and excretion of riboflavin-5′-phosphate in man. *J. Pharm Sci.* 56:58–62 (1967).

Jusko, W. J., G. Levy, and S. J. Yaffe. Effect of age on intestinal absorption of riboflavin in humans. *J. Pharm. Sci.* 59:487–490 (1970).

Kagan, B. M., V. Stanincova, N. S. Felix, J. Hodgman, and D. Kalman. Body composition of premature infants: relation to nutrition. *Am. J. Clin. Nutr.* 25:1153–1164 (1972).

Kagawa, Y. and N. Shimazono. Catabolism of L-ascorbate in animal tissues. In *Methods in Enzymology,* Vol. 18, Part A, pp. 46–50, D. B. McCormick and L. D. Wright, Eds., Academic Press, New York (1970).

Kahn, S. B., S. Fein, S. Rigberg, and I. Brodsky. Correlation of folate metabolism and socioeconomic status in pregnancy and in patients taking oral contraceptives. *Am. J. Obstet. Gynecol.* 108:931–935 (1970).

Kanai, M., A. Raz, and D. W. Goodman. Retinol-binding protein: the transport protein for vitamin A in human plasma. *J. Clin. Invest.* 47:2025–2044 (1968).

Kanda, Y., D. S. Goodman, R. E. Canfield, and F. J. Morgan. The amino acid sequence of human plasma prealbumin. *J. Biol. Chem.* 249:6796–6805 (1974).

Kannel, W. B. and T. Gordon. Framingham study, epidemiological investigation of cardiovascular diseases. Framingham diet study, diet and regulation of serum cholesterol. DHEW Report, Section 24, Washington, D.C. (1970).

Kaplan, B. H. The control of heme synthesis. In *Regulation of Hematopoiesis,* Vol. 1, pp. 677–700, A. S. Gordon, Ed., Appleton-Century-Crofts, New York (1970).

Kaplowitz, P. B., R. D. Platz, and L. J. Kleinsmith. Nuclear phosphoproteins. III. Increase in phosphorylation during histone-phosphoprotein interaction. *Biochim. Biophys. Acta* 229:739–748 (1971).

Karlson, P. *Introduction to Modern Biochemistry,* 2nd ed., Academic Press, New York (1965).

Karlson, P. *Introduction to Modern Biochemistry,* 3rd ed., Academic Press, New York (1968).

Karmen, A., I. McCaffrey, and R. L. Bowman. A flow-through method for scintillation counting of carbon-14 and tritium in gas-liquid chromotographic effluents. *J. Lipid Res.* 3:372–377 (1962).

Karmen, A., M. Whyte, and DeW. S. Goodman. Fatty acid esterification and chylomicron formation during fat absorption. I. Triglycerides and cholesterol esters. *J. Lipid Res.* 4:312–321 (1963).

Karrer, P., R. Morf, and K. Schöpp. Zur Kenntnis des Vitamins-A aus Fischtranen. *Helv. Chim. Acta* 14:1036–1040 (1931).

Karrer, P., K. Schöpp, and F. Penz. Synthesen von Flavinen IV. *Helv. Chim. Acta* 18:426–429 (1935).

Kasparek, S. Chemistry of tocopherols and tocotrienols. In *Vitamin E: A Comprehensive Treatise,* pp. 7–65, L. J. Machlin, Ed., Marcel Dekker Inc., New York (1980).

Kasper, C. B. Biochemical distinctions between the nuclear and microsomal membranes from rat hepatocytes. *J. Biol. Chem.* 246:577–581 (1971).

Kasper, H. Fecal fat excretion, diarrhea and subjective complaints with highly dosed oral fat intake. *Digestion* 3:321–330 (1970).

Katz, J., S. Rosenfeld, and A. L. Sellers. Albumin metabolism in aminonucleoside nephrotic rats. *J. Lab. Clin. Med.* 62:910–934 (1963).

Katz, J., A. L. Sellers, and G. Bonorris. Effect of nephrectomy on plasma albumin catabolism in experimental nephrosis. *J. Lab. Clin. Med.* 63:680–693 (1964).

Katz, J. H. The delivery of iron to the immature red cells in erythropoiesis. A critical review. *Ser. Haematol.* 6:15–29 (1965).

Katz, J. H. Transferrin and its functions in the regulation of iron metabolism. In *Regulation of Hematopoiesis,* Vol. 1, pp. 539–577, A. S. Gordon, Ed., Appleton-Century-Crofts, New York (1970).

Kaufman, S. Coenzymes and hydroxylases: ascorbate and dopamine-β-hydroxylase; tetrahydropteridines and phenylalanine and tyrosine hydroxylases. *Pharmacol. Rev.* 18:61–69 (1966).

Kavenoff, R., L. C. Klotz, and B. H. Zimm. On the nature of chromosome-sized DNA molecules. *Cold Spring Harbor Symp. Quant. Biol.* 38:1–8 (1973).

Kay, R. M. Origin, functions and physiological significance of dietary fiber. *J. Lipid Res.* 23:221–242 (1982).

Kay, R. M., and S. M. Strasberg. Origin, chemistry, physiological effects and clinical importance of dietary fibre. *Clin. Invest. Med.* 1:9–24 (1978).

Kayden, H. J. and L. Bjornson. The dynamics of vitamin E transport in the human erythrocyte. *Ann. N. Y. Acad. Sci.* 203:127–140 (1972).

Keenan, T. W. and D. J. Morré. Phospholipid class and fatty acid composition of Golgi apparatus isolated from rat liver and comparison with other cell fractions. *Biochemistry* 9:19–25 (1970).

Kelley, L. and M. A. Ohlson. Experimental variables in predicting protein minima for rats. *J. Nutr.* 52:325–335 (1954).

Kelly, R. B., M. R. Atkinson, J. A. Huberman, and A. Kornberg. Excision of thymine dimers and other mismatched sequences by DNA polymerase of *Escherichia coli. Nature* 224:495–501 (1969).

Kelsay, J. L. A compendium of nutritional status studies and dietary evaluation studies conducted in the United States, 1957–1967. *J. Nutr.* 99:(Suppl. 1, Part III), 123–166 (1969).

Kelsay, J. L. Effect of diet fiber level on bowel function and trace mineral balances of human subjects. *Cereal Chem.* 58:2–5 (1981).

Kelsay, J. L. Effects of fiber on mineral and vitamin bioavailability. In *Dietary Fiber in Health and Disease*, G. V. Vahouny and D. Kritchevsky, Eds., Plenum, New York (1982).

Kelsay, J. L., A. Baysal, and H. Linkswiler. Effect of vitamin B_6 depletion on the pyridoxal, pyridoxamine and pyridoxine content of the blood and urine of men. *J. Nutr.* 94:490–494 (1968).

Kelsay, J. L., K. M. Behall, and E. S. Prather. Effect of fiber from fruits and vegetables on metabolic responses of human subjects. II. Calcium, magnesium, iron and silicon balances. *Am. J. Clin. Nutr.* 32:1876–1880 (1979).

Kennedy, E. P. and A. L. Lehninger. Oxidation of fatty acids and tricarboxylic acid cycle intermediates by isolated rat liver mitochondria. *J. Biol. Chem.* 179:957–972 (1949).

Keresztesy, J. C. and J. R. Stevens. Crystalline vitamin B_6. *Proc. Soc. Exp. Biol. Med.* 38:64–65 (1938).

Kerkut, G. A. and B. York. *The Electrogenic Sodium Pump.* Scientichnica, Ltd., Bristol, Eng. (1971).

Kerr, G. R., E. S. Lee, M-K. M. Lam, R. J. Lorimer, E. Randall, R. N. Forthofer, M. A. Davis, and S. M. Magnetti. Relationships between dietary and biochemical measures of nutritional status in HANES I data. *Am. J. Clin. Nutr.* 35:294–308 (1982).

Keshan Disease Research Group. Observations on effect of sodium selenite in prevention of Keshan disease. *Chin. Med. J. (Engl.)* 92:471–476 (1979).

Keusch, G. T. and M. Katz, Eds., Effective interventions to reduce infection in malnourished populations (Proceedings of a symposium held on June 12–16,

1977 Port-au-Prince, Haiti), *Am. J. Clin. Nutr.* 31:2031–2126; 2198–2356 (1977).

Keynes, R. D. Ion channels in the nerve-cell membrane. *Sci. Am.* 240(3):126–135 (1979).

Keys, A., Ed., Coronary heart disease in seven countries. *Circulation* 41: Suppl. I) 1–211 (1970).

Keys, A. Overweight, obesity, coronary heart disease and mortality. *Nutr. Rev.* 38:297–307 (1980).

Keys, A. and J. Brozek. Body fat in adult man. *Physiol. Rev.* 33:245–325 (1953).

Keys, A., J. Brozek, A. Henschel, O. Mickelsen, and H. L. Taylor. *The Biology of Human Starvation,* Vols. 1, 2, University of Minnesota Press, Minneapolis (1950).

Keys, A., A. Henschel, H. L. Taylor, O. Mickelsen, and J. Brozek. Experimental studies on man with restricted intake of the B vitamins. *Am. J. Physiol.* 144:5–42 (1945).

Khokhar, S. A. and R. L. Pike. Aldosterone producing capacity of adrenal glands of sodium-restricted pregnant rats. *J. Nutr.* 103:1126–1130 (1973).

Khoo, J. C., A. A. Aquino, and D. Steinberg. The mechanism of activation of hormone-sensitive lipase in human adipose tissue. *J. Clin. Invest.* 53:1124–1131 (1974).

Kies, C. Non-specific nitrogen in the nutrition of human beings. *Fed. Proc.* 31:1172–1177 (1972).

Kies, C. Comparative value of various sources of nonspecific nitrogen for the human. *J. Agri. Food Chem.* 22:190–193 (1974).

Kimberg, D. V., D. Schachter, and H. Schenker. Active transport of calcium by intestine. Effect of dietary calcium. *Am. J. Physiol.* 200:1256–1262 (1961).

Kimmich, G. A. Intestinal absorption of sugar. In *Physiology of the Gastrointestinal Tract,* Vol. 2, pp. 1035–1061, L. R. Johnson, Ed., Raven Press, New York (1981).

Kimmich, G. A. and J. Randles. Evidence for an intestinal Na^+: sugar transport coupling stoichiometry of 2.0. *Biochim. Biophys. Acta* 596:439–444 (1980).

Kimura, K. K. *The nutritional significance of dietary fiber.* Life Sciences Research Office, Federation of American Societies for Experimental Biology, Bethesda, Md. (1977).

Kimura, K. K. *The nutritional significance of dietary fiber,* Life Sciences Research Office, Federation of American Societies for Experimental Biology, Bethesda, Md. (1977).

King, J. C., D. H. Calloway, and S. Margen. Nitrogen retention, total body ^{40}K and weight gain in teenage pregnant girls. *J. Nutr.* 103:772–785 (1973).

King, J. C., S. H. Cohenour, C. G. Corruccini, and B. Schneeman. Evaluation and modification of the basic four food guide. *J. Nutr. Educ.* 10:27–29 (1978).

Kingsbury, K. J., S. Paul, A. Crossley, and D. M. Morgan. Fatty acid composition of human depot fat. *Biochem. J.* 78:541–550 (1961).

Kinney, J. M. The application of indirect calorimetry to clinical studies. In *Assessment of Energy Metabolism in Health and Disease*, pp. 42–48, Proceedings of the First Ross Conference on Medical Research, Ross Laboratories, Columbus, Ohio (1980).

Kinney, T. D., D. M. Hegsted, and C. A. Finch. The influence of diet on iron absorption. I. The pathology of iron excess. *J. Exp. Med.* 90:137–145 (1949).

Kinsella, J. E., G. Bruckner, J. Mai, and J. Shimp. Metabolism of trans fatty acids with emphasis on the effects of trans, trans-octadecadienoate on lipid composition, essential fatty acid, and prostaglandins: an overview. *Am. J. Clin. Nutr.* 34:2307–2318 (1981).

Kinsman, R. A. and J. Hood. Some behavioral effects of ascorbic acid deficiency. *Am. J. Clin. Nutr.* 24:444–454 (1971).

Kint, J. A., G. Dacremont, D. Carton, E. Orye, and C. Hooft. Mucopolysaccharidoses: secondarily induced abnormal distribution of lysosomal isoenzymes. *Science* 181:352–354 (1973).

Kirschner, D. A. and D. L. D. Caspar. Comparative diffraction studies on myelin membranes. *Ann. N. Y. Acad. Sci.* 195:309–320 (1972).

Kirshner, N., C. Halloway, W. J. Smith, and A. G. Kirshner. Uptake and storage of catecholamines. In *Mechanisms of Release of Biogenic Amines*, pp. 109–123, U. S. von Euler, S. Rosell, and B. Unvas, Eds., Pergamon Press, Oxford, (1966).

Kishimoto, Y. and N. S. Radin. Determination of brain gangliosides by determination of ganglioside stearic acid. *J. Lipid Res.* 7:141–145 (1966).

Klavins, J. V., T. D. Kinney, and N. Kaufman. The influence of dietary protein on iron absorption. *Br. J. Exp. Pathol.* 43:172–180 (1962).

Kleiber, M. Body size and metabolic rate. *Physiol. Rev.* 27:511–541 (1947).

Kleiber, M. *The Fire of Life: An Introduction to Animal Energetics*. John Wiley & Sons, New York (1961).

Kleiber, M. Joules vs. calories in nutrition. *J. Nutr.* 102:309–312 (1972).

Klein, R. L. and B. A. Afzelius. Nuclear membrane hydrolysis of adenosine triphosphate. *Nature* 212:609 (1966).

Kleinig, H. Nuclear membranes from mammalian liver. II. Lipid composition. *J. Cell Biol.* 46:396–402 (1970).

Klevay, L. M. Hair as a biopsy material. I. Assessment of zinc nutriture. *Am. J. Clin. Nutr.* 23:284–289 (1970a).

Klevay, L. M. Hair as a biopsy material. II. Assessment of copper nutriture. *Am. J. Clin. Nutr.* 23:1194–1202 (1970b).

Klingenberg, M., P. Riccio. H. Aguilla, B. B. Buchanan, and K. Grebe. Mechanism of carrier transport and ADP, ATP carriers. In *The Structural Basis of Membrane Function*, pp. 293–311, Y. Hatefi and L. Djavadi-Ohaniancie, Eds., Academic Press, New York (1976).

Klotz, I. M. and D. W. Darnall. Protein subunits: a table (2nd ed.) *Science* 166:126–127 (1969).

Knappe, J. Mechanism of biotin action. *Ann. Rev. Biochem.* 39:757–776 (1970).

Knittle, J. L. Obesity and the cellularity of the adipose depot. *Triangle* 13:57–62 (1974).

Knittle, J. L., F. Ginsberg-Fellner, and R. E. Brown. Adipose tissue development in man. *Am. J. Clin. Nutr.* 30:762–766 (1977).

Knittle, J. L. and J. Hirsch. Effect of chain length on rates of uptake of free fatty acids during *in vitro* incubations of rat adipose tissue. *J. Lipid Res.* 6:565–571 (1965).

Knittle, J. L. and J. Hirsch. Infantile nutrition as a determinant of adult adipose tissue metabolism and cellularity. *Clin. Res.* 15:323A (1967).

Knittle, J. L. and J. Hirsch. Effect of early nutrition on the development of rat epididymal fat pads. Cellularity and metabolism. *J. Clin. Invest.* 47:2091–2098 (1968).

Knittle, J. L., K. Timmers, F. Ginsberg-Fellner, R. E. Brown, and D. P. Katz. The growth of adipose tissue in children and adolescents. *J. Clin. Invest.* 63:239–246 (1979).

Knochel, J. P. The pathophysiology and clinical characteristics of severe hypophosphatemia. *Arch. Int. Med.* 137:203–220 (1977).

Knox, W. E. Antizymes, adaptation and homeostasis. *N. Engl. J. Med.* 295:784–785 (1976).

Kocian, J., I. Skala, and K. Bakos. Calcium absorption from milk and lactose-free milk in healthy subjects and patients with lactose intolerance. *Digestion* 9:311–324 (1973).

Kodicek, E. The fate of ^{14}C-labeled vitamin D_2 in rats and infants. In *Drugs Affecting Lipid Metabolism,* p. 515, S. Garattini and G. Paoletti, Eds., Elsevier, Amsterdam (1960).

Kodicek, E. Antivitamins of nicotinic acid and of biotin. In *Antivitamins,* p. 8, J. C. Somogyi, Ed., S. Karger, Basel, Switz. (1966).

Koe, B. K. and A. Weissman. *p*-Chlorophenylalanine: a specific depletor of brain serotonin. *J. Pharmacol. Exp. Ther.* 154:499–516 (1966).

Koenig, H. Lysosomes in the nervous system. In *Lysosomes in Biology and Pathology,* Vol. 2, pp. 111–162, J. T. Dingle and H. B. Fell, Eds., Wiley-Interscience, New York (1969).

Koenig, H. and A. Jibril. Acidic glycolipids and the role of ionic bonds in the structure-linked latency of lysosomal hydrolases. *Biochim. Biophys. Acta* 65:543–545 (1962).

Koeppe, R. E., II and R. M. Stroud. Mechanism of hydrolysis by serine proteases. *Biochemistry* 15(16):3450–3458 (1976).

Kögl, F., J. de Gier, I. Mulder, and L. M. Van Deenen. Metabolism and functions of phosphatides. Specific fatty acid composition of the red blood cell membranes. *Biochim. Biophys. Acta* 43:95–103 (1960).

Kögl, F. and B. Tönnis. Über das Bios-Problem. Darstellung von Krystallisiertem Biotin aus Eigelb. *Z. Physiol. Chem.* 242:43–73 (1936).

Koketsu, K. and S. Miyamoto. Release of $_{45}$Ca from frog nerves. *Nature* 189:402–403 (1961).

Kolhouse, J. F., H. Kondo, N. C. Allen, E. Podell, and R. H. Allen. Cobalamin analogues are present in human plasma and can mask cobalamin deficiency because current radioisotope dilution assays are not specific for the cobalamin. *N. Engl. J. Med.* 299:785–792 (1978).

Komai, T., K. Kawai, and H. Shindo. Active transport of thiamine from rat small intestine. *J. Nutr. Sci. Vitaminol. (Tokyo)* 20:163–177 (1974).

Kono, T. and F. W. Barham. The relationship between the insulin-binding capacity of fat cells and the cellular response to insulin. *J. Biol. Chem.* 246:6210–6216 (1971).

Kopin, I. J. The adrenergic synapse. In *The Neurosciences,* pp. 427–432, G. C. Quarton, T. Melnechuk, and F. O. Schmitt, Eds., Rockefeller University Press, New York (1967).

Kopple, J. D. and M. E. Swendseid. Evidence for a dietary histidine requirement in normal man. *Fed. Proc.* 33:671A (1973).

Korn, E. D. Structure of biological membranes. *Science* 153:1491–1498 (1966).

Korn, E. D. Current concepts of membrane structure and function. *Fed. Proc.* 28:6–11 (1969).

Kornberg, A. Biologic synthesis of deoxyribonucleic acid. *Science* 131:1503–1508 (1960).

Kornberg, A. Active center of DNA polymerase. *Science* 163:1410–1418 (1969).

Kornberg, A. *DNA Replication,* W. H. Freeman & Co., San Francisco (1980).

Körner, W. F. and J. Völlm. New aspects of the tolerance of retinol in humans. *Int. J. Vitam. Nutr. Res.* 45:363–372 (1975).

Koschara, W. von. Isolierung eines gelben Farbstoffs (Uropterin) aus Menschenharn. *Z. Phys. Chem.* 240:127–151 (1936).

Koshland, D. E., Jr., A. Goldbeter, and J. B. Stock. Amplification and adaptation in regulatory and sensory systems. *N. Engl. J. Med.* 217:220–225 (1982).

Krane, S. M., J. M. Dayer, S. R. Goldring, and D. R. Robinson. Mechanisms of cell cooperation in arthritic disease. In *Cellular Interactions,* pp. 231–239, J. T. Dingle and J. L. Gordon, Eds., Elsevier North-Holland, Amsterdam (1981).

Krantz, S. B. and E. Goldwasser. On the mechanism of erythropoietin-induced differentiation. II. The effect of RNA synthesis. *Biochim. Biophys. Acta* 103:325–332 (1965).

Kravitz, E. A. Acetylcholine, γ-aminobutyric acid, and glutamic acid: physiological and chemical studies related to their roles as neurotransmitter agents. In *The Neurosciences,* pp. 433–444, G. C. Quarton, T. Melnechuk, and F. O. Schmitt, Eds., Rockefeller University Press, New York (1967).

Krebs, H. A. The metabolic fate of amino acids. In *Mammalian Protein Metabolism,* Vol. 1, pp. 125–176, H. N. Munro and J. B. Allison, Eds., Academic Press, New York (1964).

Krebs, H. A. and K. Henseleit. Untersuchungen über die Harnstoffbildung im Tierkörper. *Z. Phys. Chem.* 210:33–66 (1932).

Krehl, W. A., L. J. Tepley, and C. A. Elvehjem. Corn as an etiological factor in the production of nicotinic acid deficiency in the rat. *Science* 101:283. (1945a).

Krehl, W. A., L. J. Tepley, P. S. Sarma, and C. A. Elvehjem. Growth retarding effect of corn in nicotinic acid low rations and its counteraction by tryptophan. *Science* 101:489–490 (1945b).

Kreil, G. Transfer of proteins across membranes. *Ann. Rev. Biochem.* 50:317–348 (1981).

Krishnamurthy, S., J. G. Bieri, and E. L. Andrews. Metabolism and biological activity of vitamin A acid in the chick. *J. Nutr.* 79:503–510 (1963).

Krishnarao, G. V. G. and H. H. Draper. Influence of dietary phosphate on bone resorption is senescent mice. *J. Nutr.* 102:1143–1145 (1972).

Kromphardt, H., H. Grobecker, K. Ring, and E. Heinz. Uber den Einfluss von Alkali-Ionen auf den Glycintransport in Ehrlich-Ascites-Tumorzellen. *Biochim. Biophys. Acta* 74:549–551 (1963).

Krotkiewski, M., K. Mandroukas, L. Sjöström, L. Sullivan, H. Wetterqvist, and P. Björntorp. Effects of long-term physical training on body fat, metabolism, and blood pressure in obesity. *Metabolism* 28:650–658 (1979).

Kruse, H., E. Orent, and E. McCollum. Studies on magnesium-deficient animals. I. Symptomology resulting from magnesium deprivation. *J. Biol. Chem.* 96:519–539 (1932).

Krzysik, B. A. and S. A. Adibi. Cytoplasmic dipeptidase activities of kidney, ileum, jejunum, liver, muscle and blood. *Am. J. Physiol.* 233:E450–E456 (1977).

Krzywicki, H. J., G. M. Ward, D. P. Rahman, R. A. Nelson, and C. F. Consolazio. A comparison of methods for estimating human body composition. *Am. J. Clin. Nutr.* 27:1380–1385 (1974).

Kuehl, F. A., Jr., and R. W. Egan. Prostaglandins, arachidonic acid and inflammation. *Science* 210:978–984 (1980).

Kuenzig, W. R., R. Avenia, and J. J. Kamm. Studies on the antiscorbutic activity of ascorbate 2-sulfate in the guinea pig. *J. Nutr.* 104:952–956 (1974).

Kuffler, S. W. and J. G. Nicholls. *From Neurons to Brain,* Sinauer, Stamford, Conn. (1976).

Kuhn, I. N., M. Layrisse, M. Roche, C. Martinez, and R. B. Walker. Observations on the mechanism of iron absorption. *Am. J. Clin. Nutr.* 21:1184–1188 (1968).

Kuhn, R., K. Reinemund, F. Weygand, and R. Ströbele. Über die Synthese des Lactoflavins (Vitamin B$_2$). *Berichte.* 68:1765–1774 (1935).

Kuksis, A. and S. Mookerjea. Choline. *Nutr. Rev.* 36:201–207 (1978a).

Kuksis, A. and S. Mookerjea. Inositol. *Nutr. Rev.* 36:233–238 (1978b).

Kuman, A., H. Yamamura, and Y. Nishizuka. Mode of action of adenosine 3′,5′-cyclic phosphate on protein kinase from rat liver. *Biochem. Biophys. Res. Commun.* 41:1290–1297 (1970).

Kummerow, F. A. Possible role of vitamin E in unsaturated fatty acid metabolism. *Fed. Proc.* 23:1053–1058 (1964).

Kurtz, A., W. Jelkmann, and C. Bauer. Mesangial cells derived from rat glomeruli produce an erythropoiesis stimulating factor in cell culture. *FEBS Lett.* 137:129–132 (1982).

Kurzrok, R. and C. C. Lieb. Biochemical studies of human semen. II. The action of semen on the human uterus. *Proc. Soc. Exp. Biol. Med.* 28:268–272 (1930).

Lachman, E. Osteoporosis: the potentialities and limitations of its roentgenologic diagnosis. *Am. J. Roentgenol.* 74:712–715 (1955).

Lack, C. H. Lysosomes in relation to arthritis. In *Lysosomes in Biology and Pathology,* Vol. 1, pp. 493–508, J. T. Dingle and H. B. Fell, Eds., North-Holland Publishing Co., Amsterdam (1969).

Laemmli, U. K., S. M. Cheng, K. W. Adolph, J. R. Paulson, J. S. Brown, and W. R. Baumbach. Metaphase chromosome structure: the role of non-histone proteins. *Cold Spring Harbor Symp Quant. Biol.* 42:351–360 (1977).

Lafontaine, J. G. and C. Allard. A light and electron microscope study of the morphological changes induced in rat liver cells by the azo dye 2-Me-DAB. *J. Cell. Biol.* 22:143–172 (1964).

Laki, K. Tropomyosin A. In *Contractile Proteins and Muscle,* pp. 273–288, K. Laki, Ed., Marcel Dekker Inc., New York (1971c).

Lambooy, J. P. Riboflavin antagonists. *Am. J. Clin. Nutr.* 3:282–290 (1955).

Lamola, A. A. and T. Yamane. Zinc protoporphyrin in the erythrocytes of patients with lead intoxication and iron deficiency anemia. *Science* 186:936–938 (1974).

Lands, W. E. M. Prostaglandin synthesis from polyunsaturated fatty acids. In *Nutritional Factors: Modulating Effects on Metabolic Processes,* pp. 489–494, R. F. Beers, Jr., and E. G. Bassett, Eds., Raven Press, New York (1981).

Lane, M. and C. P. Alfrey, Jr. The anemia of human riboflavin deficiency. *Blood* 25:432–442 (1970).

Lane, M. D. and F. Lynen. The biochemical function of biotin. VI. Chemical structure of the carboxylated active site of propionyl carboxylase. *Proc. Nat. Acad. Sci. U. S.* 49:379–385 (1963).

Langer, B. W., Jr., and P. György. Biotin. VIII. Active compounds and antagonists. In *The Vitamins,* Vol. 2, pp. 294–322, W. H. Sebrell, Jr., and R. S. Harris, Eds., Academic Press, New York (1968).

Langworthy, C. F. The value of experiments on the metabolism of matter and energy. *Exp. Sta. Rec.* 9:1003–1019 (1897–1898).

Laragh, J. H., L. Baer, H. R. Brunner, F. R. Bühler, J. E. Sealey, and E. D. Vaughan, Jr. Renin, angiotensin and aldosterone system in pathogenesis and management of hypertensive vascular disease. *Am. J. Med.* 52:837–852 (1972).

Lát, J. Self-selection of dietary components. In *Handbook of Physiology,* Section 6, Vol. 1, pp. 367–386, C. F. Code, Ed., American Physiological Society, Washington, D.C. (1967).

Lát, J., A. Pavlik, and B. Jakoubek. Interrelations between individual differences in excitability levels, habituation-rates and in the incorporation of ^{14}c-leucine into brain and nonbrain proteins in rats. *Physiol. Behav.* 11:131–137 (1973).

Latta, H., A. B. Maunsbach, and L. Osvaldo. The fine structure of renal tubules in cortex and medulla. In *Ultrastructure of the Kidney*, pp. 1–65, A. J. Dalton and F. Haguenau, Eds., Academic Press, New York (1967).

Lawson, D. E. M., D. R. Fraser, E. Kodicek, H. R. Morris, and D. H. Williams. Identification of 1,25-dihydroxycholecalciferol, a new kidney hormone controlling calcium metabolism. *Nature* 230:228–230 (1971).

Layrisse, M., C. Martinez-Torres, M. Renzy, and I. Leets. Ferritin iron absorption in man. *Blood* 45:689–698 (1975).

Layrisse, M., C. Martinez-Torres, and M. Roche. Effect of interaction of various foods on iron absorption. *Am. J. Clin. Nutr.* 21:1175–1183 (1968).

Lazarides, E. Tropomyosin antibody: the specific localization of tropomyosin in nonmuscle cells. *J. Cell Biol.* 65:549–561 (1975).

Lazarides, E. Intermediate filaments: a chemically heterogeneous, developmentally regulated class of proteins. *Ann. Rev. Biochem.* 51:219–250 (1982).

Leach, R. Role of manganese in mucopolysaccharide metabolism. *Fed. Proc.* 30:991–994 (1971).

Leach, R. and M. Lilburn. Manganese metabolism and its function. *World Rev. Nutr. Diet.* 32:123–134 (1978).

Leach, R. M., Jr. Role of manganese in the synthesis of mucopolysaccharides. *Fed. Proc.* 26:118–120 (1967).

Leach, R. M., Jr. Role of manganese in mucopolysaccharide metabolism. *Fed. Proc.* 30:991–994 (1971).

Leach, R. M., Jr. and A-M. Muenster. Studies on the role of manganese in bone formation. I. Effect upon the mucopolysaccharide content of chick bone. *J. Nutr.* 78:51–56 (1962).

Leach, R. M., Jr., A-M. Muenster, and E. Wien. Studies on the role of manganese in bone formation. II. Effect upon chondroitin sulfate synthesis in chick epiphyseal cartilage. *Arch. Biochem. Biophys.* 133:22–28 (1969).

Leblond, C. P. and G. Bennett. Role of Golgi apparatus in terminal glycosylation. In *International Cell Biology 1976–1977*, pp. 326–336, B. R. Brinkley and K. R. Porter, Eds., Rockefeller University Press, New York (1977).

Leblond, C. P. and B. Messier. Renewal of chief cells and goblet cells in the small intestine as shown by radioautography after injection of thymidine-H^3 into mice. *Anat. Rec.* 132:247–259 (1958).

Leblond, C. P. and M. Weinstock. A comparative study of dentin and bone. In *The Biochemistry and Physiology of Bone*, 2nd ed., Vol. 4, pp. 517–562, G. H. Bourne, Ed., Academic Press, New York (1976).

Lederberg, J. A view of genetics. *Science* 131:269–276 (1960).

Lee, C. Y., R. S. Shallenberger, and M. T. Vittum. Free sugars in fruits and vegetables. *N. Y. Food Life Sci. Bull. No. 1* (1970).

Lee, D. B., N. Brautbar, and C. R. Kleeman. Disorders of phosphorus metabolism. In *Disorders of Mineral Metabolism,* Vol. 3, pp. 283–421, F. Bronner and J. Coburn, Eds., Academic Press, New York (1981).

Lee, H. M., L. D. Wright, and D. B. McCormick. Metabolism of carbonyl-labeled ^{14}C-biotin in the rat. *J. Nutr.* 102:1453–1464 (1972).

Lee, W., P. Hamernyik, M. Hutchinson, V. A. Raisys, and R. F. Labbe. Ascorbic acid in lymphocytes: cell preparation and liquid-chromatographic assay. *Clin. Chem.* 28:2165–2169 (1982).

Lee, Y. C., R. K. Gholson, and N. Raica. Isolation and identification of two new nicotinamide metabolites. *J. Biol. Chem.* 244:3277–3282 (1969).

Leevy, C. M. and H. Baker. Vitamins and alcoholism. *Am. J. Clin. Nutr.* 21:1325–1328 (1968).

Lefevere, M. F., A. P. De Leenheer, and A. E. Claeys. High performance liquid chromatographic assay of vitamin K in human serum. *J. Chromatogr.* 186:749–762 (1979).

Lehman, I. R. DNA ligase: structure, mechanism, and function. *Science* 186:790–797 (1974).

Lehninger, A. L. Water uptake and extrusion by mitochondria in relation to oxidative phosphorylation. *Physiol. Rev.* 42:467–517 (1962).

Lehninger, A. L. *The mitochondrion,* W. A. Benjamin, New York (1964).

Lehninger, A. L. *Bioenergetics,* W. A. Benjamin, New York (1965b).

Lehninger, A. L. Cell organelles: the mitochondrion. In *The Neurosciences,* pp. 91–100, G. C. Quarton, T. Melnechuk, and F. O. Schmitt, Eds., Rockefeller University Press, New York (1967).

Lehninger, A. L. Acid-base changes in mitochondria and medium during energy-dependent and energy-independent binding of Ca^{++}. *Ann. N. Y. Acad. Sci.* 147:816–823 (1969).

Lehninger, A. L. *Biochemistry,* Worth Publishers, Inc., New York (1970).

Lehninger, A. L. Mitochondria and calcium ion transport. *Biochem. J.* 119:129–138 (1970).

Lehninger, A. L. The molecular organization of mitochondrial membranes. *Adv. Cytopharmacol.* 1:199–208 (1971a).

Lehninger, A. L. A soluble, heat-labile, high-affinity Ca^{2+}-binding factor extracted from rat liver mitochondria. *Biochem. Biophys. Res. Commun.* 42:312–318 (1971b).

Leichsenring, J. M., L. M. Norris, S. A. Lamison, E. D. Wilson, and M. B. Patton. The effect of level of intake on calcium and phosphorus metabolism in college women. *J. Nutr.* 45:407–418 (1951).

Leichsenring, J. M. and E. D. Wilson. Food composition table for short method of dietary analysis (2nd rev.). *J. Am. Diet. Assoc.* 27:386–389 (1951).

Leitch, I. The evolution of dietary standards. *Nutr. Abstr. Rev.* 11:509–521 (1942).

Leitch, I. Changing concepts in the nutritional physiology of human pregnancy. *Proc. Nutr. Soc.* 16:38–45 (1957).

Leitch, I. and F. C. Aitkin. Estimation of calcium requirement: re-examination. *Nutr. Abstr. Rev.* 29:393–411 (1959).

Leklem, J. E., R. R. Brown, D. P. Rose, and H. M. Linkswiler. Vitamin B$_6$ requirements of women using oral contraceptives. *Am. J. Clin. Nutr.* 28:535–541 (1975a).

Leklem, J. E., R. R. Brown, D. P. Rose, H. M. Linkswiler, and R. A. Arend. Metabolism of tryptophan and niacin in oral contraceptive users receiving controlled intakes of vitamin B$_6$. *Am. J. Clin. Nutr.* 28:146–156 (1975b).

Leklem, J. E. and R. D. Reynolds, Eds. *Methods in Vitamin B-6 Nutrition. Analysis and Status Assessment,* Plenum, New York (1980).

Lema, I. and H. H. Sandstead. Zinc deficiency, effect on collagen and glycoprotein synthesis and bone mineralization. *Fed. Proc.* 29:297A (1970).

Lenard, J. and S. J. Singer. Protein conformation in cell membrane preparations as studied by optical rotary dispersion and circular dichroism. *Proc. Nat. Acad. Sci. U. S.* 56:1828–1835 (1966).

Lengemann, F. W., R. H. Wasserman, and C. L. Comar. Studies on the enhancement of radiocalcium and radiostrontium absorption by lactose in the rat. *J. Nutr.* 68:443–456 (1959).

Lengyel, P. Biochemistry of interferons and their actions. *Ann. Rev. Biochem.* 51:251–282 (1982).

Lenhert, P. G. and D. C. Hodgkin. Structure of the 5,6-dimethylbenzimidazolylcobamide coenzyme. *Nature* 192:937–938 (1961).

Lentz, T. L. *Cell Fine Structure. An Atlas of Drawings of Whole-Cell Structure,* W. B. Saunders Co., Philadelphia (1971).

Leonard, J. V., T. C. Marrs, J. M. Addison, D. Burston, K. M. Clegg, J. K. Lloyd, D. M. Matthews, and J. W. Seakins. Intestinal absorption of amino acids and peptides in Hartnup disorder. *Pediatr. Res.* 10:246–249 (1976).

Lepkovsky, S. Crystalline factor I. *Science* 87:169–170 (1938).

Letarte, J. and A. E. Renold. Ionic effects on glucose transport and metabolism by isolated mouse fat cells incubated with or without insulin. III. Effects of replacement of Na$^+$. *Biochim. Biophys. Acta* 183:366–374 (1969).

Levander, O., B. Sutherland, V. Morris, and J. King. Selenium balance in young men during selenium depletion and repletion. *Am. J. Clin. Nutr.* 34:2662–2669 (1981).

Leveille, G. A. Modified thiochrome procedure for the determination of urinary thiamin. *Am. J. Clin. Nutr.* 25:273–274 (1972).

Levens, N. R., M. J. Peach, and R. M. Carey. Role of the intrarenal renin-angiotensin system in the control of renal function. *Circ. Res.* 48:157–167 (1981).

Levenson, S. M. and B. Tennant. Some metabolic and nutritional studies with germfree animals. *Fed. Proc.* 22:109–119 (1963).

Leventhal, B. and F. Stohlman, Jr. Regulation of erythropoiesis. XVII. Determinants of red cell size in iron deficiency states. *Pediatr.* 37:62–67 (1966).

Lever, J. D. Cytological studies on the hypophysectomized rat adrenal cortex: the alterations of its fine structure following ACTH administration and on lowering the Na/K ratio. *Endocrinol.* 58:163–180 (1956a).

Lever, J. D. Physiologically induced changes in adrenocortical mitochondria. *J. Biophys. Biochem Cytol.* 2:(Suppl. 4)313–317 (1956b).

Leverton, R. M. Amino acid requirements of young adults. In *Protein and Amino Acid Nutrition,* pp. 477 506, A. A. Albanese, Ed., Academic Press, New York (1959).

Leverton, R. M. The RDAs are not for amateurs. *J. Am. Diet. Assoc.* 66:9–11 (1975).

Leverton, R. M. and A. G. Marsh. The iron metabolism and requirement of young women. *J. Nutr.* 23:229–238 (1942).

Levey, G. S. The glucagon receptor and adenylate cyclase. *Metabolism* 24:301–310 (1975).

Levi, A. S., S. Geller, D. M. Root, and G. Wolf. The effect of vitamin A and other dietary constituents on the activity of adenosine triphosphate sulphurylase. *Biochem. J.* 109:69–74 (1968).

Levi, A. S. and G. Wolf. Purification and properties of the enzyme ATP-sulfurylase and its relation to vitamin A. *Biochim. Biophys. Acta* 178:262–282 (1969).

Levin, E. Y., B. Levenberg, and S. Kaufman. The enzymatic conversion of 3,4-dihydroxyphenylethylamine to norepinephrine. *J. Biol. Chem.* 235:2080–2086 (1960).

Levine, B. S., M. W. Walling, and J. W. Coburn. Intestinal absorption of calcium: its assessment, normal physiology, and alterations in various disease states. In *Disorders of Mineral Metabolism,* Vol. 2, pp. 103–188, F. Bronner and J. W. Coburn, Eds., Academic Press, New York (1982).

Levine, P. H., A. J. Levine, and L. R. Weintraub. The role of transferrin in the control of iron absorption. Studies on a cellular level. *J. Lab. Clin. Med.* 80:333–341 (1972).

Levitsky, D. A. and R. H. Barnes. Effect of early malnutrition on the reaction of adult rats to aversive stimuli. *Nature* 225:468–469 (1970).

Levitsky, D. A. and R. H. Barnes. Nutritional and environmental interactions in the behavioral development of the rat: long term effects. *Science* 176:68–71 (1972).

Levy, G. and W. J. Jusko. Factors affecting the absorption of riboflavin in man. *J. Pharm. Sci.* 55:285–289 (1966).

Levy, M. and M.-T. Sauner. Specificité de composition en phospholipides et en cholesterol des membranes mitochondriales. *Chem. Phys. Lipids* 2:291–295 (1968).

Levy, R. I. and J. Moskowitz. Cardiovascular research: decades of progress, a decade of promise. *Science* 217:121–129 (1982).

Lewis, J. S., M. L. Brunker, S. S. Getts, and R. Essien. Variability of creatinine excretion of normal, phenylketonuric and galactosemic children, and children treated with anticonvulsant drugs. *Am. J. Clin. Nutr.* 28:310–315 (1975).

Lieberman, A., L. S. Freedman, and M. Goldstein. Serum dopamine-β-hydroxylase activity in patients with Huntington's chorea and Parkinson's disease. *Lancet* 1:153–154 (1972).

Lifson, N., G. B. Gordon, and R. McClintock. Measurement of total carbon dioxide production by means of D_2O^{18}. *J. Appl. Physiol.* 7:704–710 (1955).

Lifson, N. and R. McClintock. Theory of use of the turnover rates of body water for measuring energy and material balance. *J. Theor. Biol.* 12:46–74 (1966).

Light, L. and F. J. Cronin. Food guidance revisited. *J. Nutr. Educ.* 13:57–62 (1981).

Lightner, D. A., A. Moscowitz, Z. J. Petryka, S. Jones, M. Weimer, E. Davis, N. A. Beach, and C. J. Watson. Mass spectrometry and ferric chloride oxidation applied to urobilinoid structures. *Arch. Biochem. Biophys.* 131:566–576 (1969).

Liljenquist, J. E., G. L. Mueller, A. D. Cherrington, U. Keller, J. L. Chiasson, J. M. Perry, W. W. Lacy, and D. Rabinowitz. Evidence for an important role of glucagon in the regulation of hepatic glucose production in normal man. *J. Clin. Invest.* 59:369–374 (1977).

Lind, James. *Treatise of the Scurvy*, printed by Sands, Murray and Cochran for A. Kincaid and A. Donaldson, Edinburgh (1753).

Lindenbaum, J. and M. J. Roman. Nutritional anemias in alcoholism. *Am. J. Clin. Nutr.* 33:2727–2735 (1980).

Linder, M. C., V. Dunn, E. Issacs, D. Jones, S. Lim, M. Van Volkom, and H. N. Munro. Ferritin and intestinal iron absorption: pancreatic enzymes and free iron. *Am. J. Physiol.* 228:196–204 (1975).

Linder, M. C. and H. N. Munro. Ferritin and free iron in iron absorption. In *Proteins of Iron Storage and Transport in Biochemistry and Medicine,* pp. 395–400, R. R. Crichton, Ed., North-Holland Publishing Co., Amsterdam (1975).

Linder, M. C. and H. N. Munro. The mechanism of iron absorption and its regulation. *Fed. Proc.* 36:2017–2023 (1977).

Lindquist, B. Effect of vitamin D on the metabolism of radiocalcium in rachitic rats. *Acta Paediatr.* 41: (Suppl. 86)1–82 (1952).

Lingren, F. T. The plasma lipoproteins: historical developments and nomenclature. *Ann. N. Y. Acad. Sci.* 348:1–15 (1980).

Linkswiler, H. M., C. L. Joyce, and C. R. Anand. Calcium retention of young adult males as affected by level of protein and of calcium intake. *Trans. N. Y. Acad. Sci. (Ser. II)* 36:333–340 (1974).

Lipkin, M. Cell proliferation in the gastrointestinal tract of man. *Fed. Proc.* 24:10–15 (1965).

Lipkin, M. Proliferation and differentiation of gastrointestinal cells in normal and disease states. In *Physiology of the Gastrointestinal Tract,* Vol. 1, pp. 145–168, L. R. Johnson, Ed., Raven Press, New York (1981).

Lipmann, F. Polypeptide chain elongation in protein synthesis. *Science* 164:1024–1031 (1969).

Lipmann, F. and N. O. Kaplan. A common factor in the enzymatic acetylation of sulfanilamide and of choline. *J. Biol. Chem.* 162:743–744 (1946).

Lippe, B., L. Hensen, G. Mendoza, M. Finerman, and M. Welch. Chronic vitamin A intoxication. *Am. J. Dis. Child.* 135:634–636 (1981).

Lipschitz, D. A., T. H. Bothwell, H. C. Seftel, A. A. Wapnick, and R. W. Charlton. The role of ascorbic acid in the metabolism of storage iron. *Br. J. Haematol.* 20:155–163 (1971).

Llinás, R. R. Calcium in synaptic transmission. *Sci. Am.* 247(4):56–65 (1982).

Lloyd, J. B. and F. Beck. Teratogenesis. In *Lysosomes in Biology and Pathology,* Vol. 1, pp. 433–449, J. T. Dingle and H. B. Fell, Eds., North-Holland Publishing Co., Amsterdam (1969).

Lo, C. and J. B. Marsh. Biosynthesis of plasma lipoproteins. Incorporation of ^{14}C-glucosamine by cells and subcellular fractions of rat liver. *J. Biol. Chem.* 245:5001–5006 (1970).

Locke, F. Towards the ideal artificial circulating fluid for the isolated frog's heart. *J. Physiol. (London).* 18:332–333 (1895).

Loewenstein, W. R. and Y. Kanno. Intercellular communication and tissue growth. I. Cancerous growth. *J. Cell Biol.* 33:225–234 (1967).

Loewi, Otto. An autobiographic sketch. *Perspect. Biol. Med.* 4:3–25 (1960).

Loewy, A. G. and P. Siekevitz. *Cell Structure and Function,* 2nd ed., Holt, Rinehart & Winston, New York (1963).

Lohman, T. G. Skinfolds and body density and their relation to body fatness: a review. *Hum. Biol.* 53:181–225 (1981).

Lohman, T. G., M. H. Slaughter, A. Selinger, and R. A. Boileau. Relationship of body composition to somatotype in college-age men. *Hum. Biol.* 5:147–157 (1978).

Lohmann, K. and P. Schuster. Untersuchungen über die Cocarboxylase. *Biochem. Z.* 294:188–214 (1937).

Lönnerdal, B., A. G. Stanislowski, and L. S. Hurley. Isolation of a low molecular weight zinc-binding ligand from milk. *J. Inorg. Biochem.* 12:71–78 (1980).

Losowsky, M. S., J. Kelleher, B. E. Walker, T. Davies, and C. L. Smith. Intake and absorption of tocopherol. *Ann. N. Y. Acad. Sci.* 203:212–222 (1972).

Lotspeich, W. D. and A. H. Wheeler. Insulin, anaerobiosis, and phlorizin in entry of D-galactose into skeletal muscle. *Am. J. Physiol.* 202:1065–1069 (1962).

Lovenberg, W., H. Weissbach, and S. Udenfriend. Aromatic L-amino acid decarboxylase. *J. Biol. Chem.* 237:89–93 (1962).

Low, R. B. and P. W. Cerauskis. Biosynthesis of muscle proteins in the fasted rat. *J. Nutr.* 107:1244–1254 (1977).

Lowell, R. T. Essentiality of vitamin C in feeds for intensively fed caged channel catfish. *J. Nutr.* 103:134–138 (1973).

Lowenstein, F. W. *A new look at dietary intake in relation to nutritional health. (Abstract) 721,* 11th International Congress of Nutrition, Rio de Janeiro, August 27-September 1, 1978.

Lowenstein, J. M. Is insulin involved in regulating the rate of fatty acid synthesis? In *Handbook of Physiology,* Section 7: Endocrinology, Vol. 1, pp. 415–424, R. O. Greep and E. B. Astwood, Eds., American Physiological Society, Washington, D.C. (1972).

Lowenstein, W. R. Permeability of the junctional membrane channel. In *International Cell Biology,* pp.70–82, B. R. Brinkley and K. R. Palmer, Eds., Rockefeller University Press, New York (1977).

Lowenthal, J. and J. A. MacFarlane. Use of a competitive vitamin K antagonist, 2-chloro-3-phytyl-*l*-,4-naphthoquinone, for the study of the mechanism of action of vitamin K and coumarin anticoagulants. *J. Pharmacol. Exp. Ther.* 157:672–680 (1967).

Lowry, O. H. Biochemical evidence of nutritional status. *Physiol. Rev.* 32:431–448 (1952).

Lowry, O. H. and O. A. Bessey. Microchemical methods for nutritional studies. *Fed. Proc.* 4:268–271 (1945).

Lubin, B. and L. J. Machlin. Vitamin E: biochemical, hematological, and clinical aspects. *Ann. N. Y. Acad. Sci.* 393:1–504 (1982).

Lucht, U. Acid phosphatase of osteoclasts demonstrated by electron microscopic histochemistry. *Histochemie* 28:103–117 (1971).

Luck, D. J. L. Genesis of mitochondria in *Neurospora crassa. Proc. Nat. Acad. Sci. U. S.* 49:233–240 (1963a).

Luck, D. J. L. Formation of mitochondria in *Neurospora crassa. J. Cell Biol.* 16:483–499 (1963b).

Luck, D. J. L. and E. Reich. DNA in mitochondria of *Neurospora crassa. Proc. Nat. Acad. Sci. U. S.* 52:931–938 (1964).

Lucy, J. A. Ultrastructure of membranes: micellar organization. *Br. Med. Bull.* 24:127–129 (1968).

Lucy, J. A. Functional and structural aspects of biological membranes: a suggested structural role for vitamin E in the control of membrane permeability and stability. *Ann. N. Y. Acad. Sci.* 203:4–11 (1972).

Lukaski, H. C. and J. Mendez. Relationship between fat-free weight and urinary 3-methylhistidine excretion in man. *Metabolism* 29:758–761 (1980).

Lukaski, H. C., J. Mendez, E. R. Buskirk, and S. H. Cohn. A comparison of methods of assessment of body composition including neutron activation analysis of total body nitrogen. *Metabolism* 30:777–782 (1981a).

Lukaski, H. C., J. Mendez, E. R. Buskirk, and S. H. Cohn. Relationship between endogenous 3-methylhistidine excretion and body composition. *Am. J. Physiol.* 240:E302–E307 (1981b).

Lukie, B. E., H. Westergaard, and J. M. Dietschy. Validation of a chamber that allows measurement of both tissue uptake rates and unstirred layer thickness in the intestine under conditions of controlled stirring. *Gastroenterol.* 67:652–661 (1974).

Lunin, N. Ueber die Bedeutung der anorganischen Salze fur die Ernahrung des Thieres (Inaugural- dissertation, Dorpat, 1880). Cited in E.V. McCollum, *A History of Nutrition,* p. 204, Houghton Mifflin, Boston (1957).

Lusk, G. *The Elements of the Science of Nutrition,* 4th ed., W. B. Saunders Co., Philadelphia (1928).

Lusk, G. The specific dynamic action (Editorial review). *J. Nutr.* 3:519–530 (1931).

Luzzati, V., H. Mustacchi, and A. Skoulios. The structure of the liquid-crystal phases of some soap + water systems. *Faraday Discuss. Chem. Soc.* 25:43–50 (1958).

Lyttleton, J. W. Nucleoproteins of white clover. *Biochem. J.* 74:82–90 (1960).

Lyttleton, J. W. Isolation of ribosomes from spinach chloroplasts. *Exp. Cell Res.* 26:312–317 (1962).

Macara, I. G., T. G. Hoy, and P. M. Harrison. Formation of ferritin from apoferritin. Kinetics and mechanism of iron uptake. *Biochem. J.* 126:151–162 (1972).

Machado, E. A., E. A. Porta, W. S. Hartroft, and F. Hamilton. Studies on dietary hepatic necrosis. II. Ultrastructural and enzymatic alterations of the hepatocytic plasma membrane. *Lab. Invest.* 24:13–20 (1971).

Machlin, L. J., E. Gabriel, and M. Brin. Biopotency of α-tocopherols as determined by curative myopathy bioassay in the rat. *J. Nutr.* 112:1437–1440 (1982).

Machlin, L. J., F. Garcia, W. Kuenzig, C. B. Richter, H. E. Spiegel, and M. Brin. Lack of antiscorbutic activity of ascorbate 2-sulfate in the rhesus monkey. *Am. J. Clin. Nutr.* 29:825–831 (1976).

MacIntosh, F. C. Formation, storage and release of acetylcholine at nerve endings. *Can. J. Biochem. Physiol.* 37:343–356 (1959).

MacIntyre, I. Human calcitonin: practical and theoretical consequences. In *Calcitonin: Proceedings of the Second International Symposium,* pp. 1–13, Springer-Verlag, New York (1970).

MacKenzie, I. L. and R. M. Donaldson. Vitamin B_{12} absorption and the intestinal cell surface. *Fed. Proc.* 28:41–45 (1969).

MacKenzie, I. L., R. M. Donaldson, Jr., W. L. Kopp, and J. S. Trier. Antibodies to intestinal microvillous membranes. II. Inhibition of intrinsic factor-mediated attachment of vitamin B_{12} to hamster brush border. *J. Exp. Med.* 128:375–386 (1968).

MacMahon, M. T. and G. Neale. The absorption of α-tocopherol in control subjects and in patients with intestinal malabsorption. *Clin Sci.* 38:197–210 (1970).

MacMahon, M. T., G. Neale, and G. R. Thompson. Lymphatic and portal venous transport of α-tocopherol and cholesterol. *Eur. J. Clin. Invest.* 1:228–294 (1971).

MacMahon, M. T. and G. R. Thompson. Comparison of the absorption of a polar lipid, oleic acid, and a non-polar lipid, α-tocopherol from mixed micellar solutions and emulsions. *Eur. J. Clin. Invest.* 1:161–166 (1970).

Madden, S. C. and G. Whipple. Plasma proteins: their source, production and utilization. *Physiol. Rev.* 20:194–217 (1940).

Magendie, F. On the nutritive value of substances which contain no nitrogen. *Ann. de Chim. et de Phys.* 3:66 (1816).

Magnusson, B., E. Björn-Rasmussen, L. Hallberg, and L. Rosander. Iron absorption in relation to iron status. Model proposed to express results of food iron absorption measurements. *Scand. J. Haematol.* 27:201–208 (1981).

Mahadevan, S. and J. Ganguly. Further studies on the absorption of vitamin A. *Biochem. J.* 81:53–58 (1961).

Mahadevan, S., P. Seshadri Sastry, and J. Ganguly. Studies on the metabolism of vitamin A. III. The mode of absorption of vitamin A esters in the living rat. *Biochem. J.* 88:531–533 (1963a).

Mahadevan, S., P. Seshadri Sastry, and J. Ganguly. Studies on the metabolism of vitamin A. IV. Studies on the mode of absorption of vitamin A by rat intestine *in vitro. Biochem. J.* 88:534–539 (1963b).

Maines, M. D. and A. Kappas. Metals as regulators of heme metabolism. *Science* 198:1215–1221 (1977).

Maitra, U. and J. Hurwitz. The role of DNA in RNA synthesis. IX. Nucleoside triphosphate termini in RNA polymerase products. *Proc. Nat. Acad. Sci. U. S.* 54:815–822 (1965).

Majaj, A. S. and K. Folkers. Hematological activity of coenzyme Q in an anemia of human malnutrition. *Int. Z. Vitaminforsch.* 38:182–195 (1968).

Malina, R. M., Quantification of fat, muscle and bone in man. *Clin. Orthoped.* 65:9–38 (1969).

Malina, R. M., A. B. Harper, H. H. Avent, and D. E. Campbell. Physique of female track and field athletes. *Med. Sci. Sports* 3:32–38 (1971).

Mallette, L. E., J. H. Exton, and C. R. Park. Effects of glucagon on amino acid transport and utilization in the perfused rat liver. *J. Biol. Chem.* 244:5724–5728 (1969).

Malm, O. J. Calcium requirements and adaptation in adult men. *Scand. J. Clin. Lab. Invest. Suppl.* 10(36):1–289 (1958).

Mandelkern, L. Muscle as a fibrous protein system. In *Contractile Proteins and Muscle,* pp. 499–568, K. Laki, Ed., Marcel Dekker, Inc., New York (1971).

Manganiello, V. C., F. Murad, and M. Vaughan. Effects of lipolytic and antilipolytic agents on cyclic 3',5'-adenosine monophosphate in fat cells. *J. Biol. Chem.* 246:2195–2202 (1971).

Manis, J. G. and D. Schachter. Active transport of iron by intestine: effects of oral iron and pregnancy. *Am. J. Physiol.* 203:81–86 (1962).

Manis, J. G. and D. Schachter. Active transport of iron by intestine: mucosal iron pools. *Am. J. Physiol.* 207:893–900 (1964).

Manis, J. and D. Schachter. Fe^{59}-amino acid complexes: are they intermediates in Fe^{59} absorption across intestinal mucosa? *Proc. Soc. Exp. Biol. Med.* 119:1185–1187 (1965).

Mann, G. V., G. Pearson, T. Gordon, and T. R. Dawber. Diet and cardiovascular disease in the Framingham study. I. Measurement of dietary intake. *Am. J. Clin. Nutr.* 11:200–225 (1962).

March, B. E., E. Wong, L. Seier, J. Sim, and J. Biely. Hypervitaminosis E in the chick. *J. Nutr.* 103:371–377 (1973).

Marchis-Mouren, G., L. Pasero, and P. Desnuelle. Further studies on amylase biosynthesis by pancreas of rats fed on a starch-rich or casein-rich diet. *Biochem. Biophys. Res. Commun.* 13:262–266 (1963).

Marcus, A. J. The role of lipids in platelet function: with particular reference to the arachidonic acid pathway. *J. Lipid Res.* 19:793–826 (1978).

Margaria, R. The sources of muscular energy. *Sci. Am.* 226(3):84–91 (1972).

Margen, S., J. Y. Chu, N. A. Kaufmann, and D. H. Calloway. Studies in calcium metabolism. I. The calciuretic effect of dietary protein. *Am. J. Clin. Nutr.* 27:584–589 (1974).

Markscheid, L. and E. Shafrir. Incorporation of lipoprotein-borne triglycerides by adipose tissue *in vitro*. *J. Lipid Res.* 6:247–257 (1965).

Marr, J. W. Individual dietary surveys: purposes and methods. *World Rev. Nutr. Diet.* 13:105–164 (1971).

Marshall, F. N. Lipoprotein lipase activity in normal human adipose tissue and its absence in human lipomas. *Experientia* 21:130–131 (1965).

Marston, H. R. and S. H. Allen. Factors affecting formiminoglutamic acid excretion in vitamin B_{12} deficiency. *Biochem. J.* 116:681–688 (1970).

Martelo, O. J., B. F. Toro, and J. Hirsch. Activation of renal erythropoietic factor by phosphorylation. *J. Lab. Clin. Med.* 87:83–88 (1976).

Martin, H. E., J. Mehl, and M. Wertman. Clinical studies of magnesium metabolism. *Med. Clin. North Am.* 36:1157–1171 (1952).

Martin, R. J. and J. Gahagan. Serum hormone levels and tissue metabolism in pair-fed and obese Zucker rats. *Horm. Metab. Res.* 9:181–186 (1977).

Mason, J. B., N. Gibson, and E. Kodicek. The chemical nature of the bound nicotinic acid of wheat bran. Studies of nicotinic acid containing macromolecules. *Br. J. Nutr.* 30:297–311 (1973).

Martinez-Torres, C. and M. Layrisse. Interest for the study of dietary absorption and iron fortification. *World Rev. Nutr. Diet.* 19:51–70 (1974).

Martinez-Torres, C., E. Romano, and M. Layrisse. Effect of cysteine on iron absorption in man. *Am. J. Clin. Nutr.* 34:322–327 (1981).

Maruyama, K. Regulatory proteins. In *Contractile Proteins and Muscle*, pp. 289–313, K. Laki, Ed., Marcel Dekker Inc., New York (1971).

Marx, S. J., C. J. Woodard, and G. D. Aurbach. Calcitonin receptors of kidney and bone. *Science* 178:999–1001 (1972).

Mason, K. E. A conspectus of research on copper metabolism and requirements of man. *J. Nutr.* 109:1979–2066 (1979).

Mason, M., J. Ford, and H. L. C. Wu. Effects of steroid and nonsteriod metabolites on enzyme conformation and pyridoxal phosphate binding. *Ann. N. Y. Acad. Sci.* 166:170–183 (1969).

Massague, J., P. F. Pilch, and M. P. Czech. Electrophoretic resolution of three major insulin receptor structures with unique subunit stoichiometries. *Proc. Nat. Acad. Sci. U. S.* 77:7137–7141 (1980).

Matschiner, J. T. Occurrence and biopotency of the various forms of vitamin K. In *The Fat-Soluble Vitamins,* pp. 377–397, H. F. DeLuca and J. W. Suttie, Eds. University of Wisconsin Press, Madison (1970).

Matseshe, J. W., S. F. Phillips, J-R. Malagelada, and J. T. McCall. Recovery of dietary iron and zinc from the proximal small intestine of healthy man: studies of different meals and supplements. *Am. J. Clin. Nutr.* 33:1946–1953 (1980).

Matsuda, T. and J. R. Cooper Thiamine as an integral component of brain synaptosomal membranes. *Proc. Nat. Acad. Sci. U. S.* 78:5886–5889 (1981).

Matthews, D. E. and D. M. Bier. *Stable isotope methods for nutrition investigation.* *Ann. Rev. Nutr.* 3:309–339 (1983).

Matthews, D. M. Absorption of water-soluble vitamins. In *Intestinal Absorption,* Vol. 4B, *Biomembranes,* pp. 847–875, D. H. Smyth Ed., Plenum, London, (1974).

Matthews, D. M. Intestinal absorption of peptides. *Physiol. Rev.* 55:537–608 (1975a).

Matthews, D. M. Intestinal transport of peptides. In *Intestinal Absorption and Malabsorption,* pp. 95–111, T. Z. Csaky, Ed., Raven Press, New York (1975b).

Matthews, D. M., J. M. Addison, and D. Burston. Evidence for active transport of the dipeptide carnosine (β-alanyl-L-histidine) by hamster jejunum *in vitro.* *Clin. Sci. Mol. Med.* 46:693–705 (1974).

Matthews, D. M. and S. A. Adibi. Peptide absorption. *Gastroenterol.* 71:151–161 (1976).

Matthews, D. M., I. L. Craft, D. M. Geddes, I. J. Wise, and C. W. Hyde. Absorption of glycine peptides from the small intestine of the rat. *Clin. Sci.* 35:415–424 (1968).

Matthews, D. M. and J. W. Payne. *Peptide transport in protein nutrition. Frontiers of Biology,* Vol. 37, North-Holland Publishing Co., Amsterdam, and Elsevier, New York (1975).

Matthews, J. L., J. H. Martin, H. W. Sampson, A. S. Kunin, and J. H. Roan. Mitochondrial granules in the normal and rachitic rat epiphysis. *Calcif. Tissue Res.* 5:91–99 (1970).

Matthews, R. G., R. Hubbard, P. K. Brown, and G. Wald. Tautomeric forms of metarhodopsin. *J. Gen. Physiol.* 47:215–240 (1964).

Maugh, T. H., II. Vitamin B_{12}: after 25 years, the first synthesis. *Science* 179:266–267 (1973).

Maunsbach, A. B. Observations on the ultrastructure and acid phosphatase activity of the cytoplasmic bodies in rat kidney proximal tubule cells. *J. Ultrastruct. Res.* 16:197–238 (1966a).

Maunsbach, A. B. Albumin absorption by renal proximal tubule cells. *Nature* 212:546–547 (1966b).

Maunsbach, A. B. Functions of lysosomes in kidney cells. In *Lysosomes in Biology and Pathology*, Vol. 1, pp. 115–154, J. T. Dingle and H. B. Fell, Eds., Wiley-Interscience, New York (1969).

Mawer, E. B., J. Backhouse, C. A. Holman, G. A. Lumb, and S. W. Stanbury. The distribution and storage of vitamin D and its metabolites in human tissues. *Clin. Sci.* 43:413–431 (1972).

Mawer, E. B., G. A. Lumb, K. Schaefer, and S. W. Stanbury. The metabolism of isotopically labelled vitamin D_3 in man: the influence of the state of vitamin D nutrition. *Clin. Sci.* 40:39–53 (1971).

Mayerle, J. A. and R. J. Havel. Nutritional effects on blood flow in adipose tissue of unanesthetized rats. *Am. J. Physiol.* 217:1694–1698 (1969).

Mazess, R. B., W. W. Peppler, C. H. Chesnut, III, W. B. Nelp, S. H. Cohn, and I. Zanzi. Total body bone mineral and lean body mass by dual-photon absorptiometry. II. Comparison with total body calcium by neutron activation analyses. *Calcif. Tissue Int.* 33:361–363 (1981).

Mazur, A. Role of ascorbic acid in the incorporation of plasma iron into ferritin. *Ann. N. Y. Acad. Sci.* 92:223–229 (1961).

Mazur, A. and A. Carleton. Relation of ferritin iron to heme synthesis in marrow and reticulocytes. *J. Biol. Chem.* 238:1817–1824 (1963).

McBride, D. E. and C. J. Wyatt. Evaluation of a modified AOAC determination for thiamin and riboflavin in foods. *J. Food Sci.* 48:748–750 (1983).

McCammon, R. W. The concept of normality. *Ann. N. Y. Acad. Sci.* 134:559–562 (1966).

McCance, R. A. and E. M. Widdowson. Absorption and excretion of iron. *Lancet* 2:680–684 (1937).

McCance, R. A. and E. M. Widdowson. Mineral metabolism of healthy adults on white and brown bread dietaries. *J. Physiol. (London)* 10:44–85 (1942).

McCance, R. A. and E. M. Widdowson. Composition of the body. *Br. Med. Bull.* 7:297–306 (1951).

McCance, R. A. and E. M. Widdowson. Nutrition and growth. *Proc. R. Soc. London (Biol.)* 156:326–337 (1962).

McCance, R. A. and E. M. Widdowson, Eds., *Calorie Deficiencies and Protein Deficiencies*, Little, Brown & Co., Boston (1968).

McCance, R. A. and E. M. Widdowson. Review lecture. The determinants of growth and form. *Proc. R. Soc. London., Ser. B* 185:1–17 (1974).

McCartney, C. P., R. E. Pottinger, and J. P. Harrod. Alterations in body composition during pregnancy. *Am. J. Obstet. Gynecol.* 77:1038–1053 (1959).

McCay, P. B. Physiological significance of lipid peroxidation. *Fed. Proc.* 40:173. (1981).

McCay, P. B., M. M. King, J. L. Poyer, and E. K. Lai. An update on antioxidant theory: spin trapping of trichloromethyl radicals *in vivo. Ann. N. Y. Acad. Sci,* 393:23–31 (1982).

McCay, P. B., P. M. Pfeifer, and W. H. Stipe. Vitamin E protection of membrane lipids during electron transport functions. *Ann. N. Y. Acad. Sci.* 203:62–73 (1972).

McClure, F. J. Cariostatic effect of phosphates. *Science* 144:1337–1338 (1964).

McCollum, E. V. *A History of Nutrition.* Houghton Mifflin, Boston (1957).

McCollum, E. V. and M. Davis. The necessity of certain lipids in the diet during growth. *J. Biol. Chem.* 15:167–175 (1913).

McCollum, E. V., N. Simmonds, J. E. Becker, and P. G. Shipley. Studies on experimental rickets. XXIII. The production of rickets in the rat by diets consisting of essentially purified food substances. *J. Biol. Chem.* 54:249–252 (1922).

McConnell, K., R. Burton, T. Kute, and P. Higgins. Selenoproteins from rat testis cytosol. *Biochim. Biophys. Acta* 588:113–119 (1979).

McCormick, A. M., J. L. Napoli, H. K. Schnoes, and H. F. DeLuca. Isolation and identification of 5,6-epoxy-retinoic acid: a biologically active metabolite of retinoic acid. *Biochem.* 17:4085–4090 (1978).

McCormick, D. B. Biotin. *Nutr. Rev.* 33:97–102 (1975).

McCormick, D. B. and J. A. Roth. Specificity, stereochemistry, and mechanism of the color reaction between *p*-dimethylominocinna maldehyde and biotin analogs. *Anal. Biochem.* 34:226–236 (1970).

McCormick, D. B. and L. D. Wright, Eds., *Methods in Enzymology,* Vol. 18, Part A, Academic Press, New York (1970).

McCormick, D. B. and L. D. Wright, Eds., *Methods in Enzymology,* Vol. 18, Part B, Academic Press, New York (1971a).

McCormick, D. B. and L. D. Wright, Eds., *Methods in Enzymology,* Vol. 18, Part C, Academic Press, New York (1971b).

McCoy, K. E. M. and P. H. Weswig. Some selenium responses in the rat not related to vitamin E. *J. Nutr.* 98:383–389 (1969).

McCoy, R. H., C. E. Meyer, and W. C. Rose. Feeding experiments with mixtures of highly purified amino acids. VIII. Isolation and identification of a new essential amino acid. *J. Biol. Chem.* 112:283–302 (1935–36).

McCulloch, E. A. Control of hematopoiesis at the cellular level. In *Regulation of Hematopoiesis,* Vol. 1, pp. 133–159, A. S. Gordon, Ed., Appleton-Century-Crofts, New York (1970).

McDonald, J. F. and S. Margen. Wine versus ethanol in human nutrition. IV. Zinc balance. *Am. J. Clin. Nutr.* 33:1096–1102 (1980).

McDowell, A., A. Engle, J. Massey, and K. Maurer. Plan and operation of the second national health and nutrition examination survey, 1976–1980 (Series

1, No. 15. DHEW Pub. [(PHS] 81-1317), Health Research Statistics and Technology). U. S. Government Printing Office, Washington D.C. (1981).

McGeer, E. G., P. L. McGeer, and S. R. Vincent. GABA enzyme and pathways. In *Neurotransmitter Interaction and Compartmentation*, pp. 299–327, H. F. Bradford, Ed., Plenum, New York (1982).

McGhee, J. D. and G. Felsenfeld. Nucleosome structure. *Ann. Rev. Biochem.* 49:1115–1156 (1980).

McGiff, J. C. Prostaglandins as regulators of blood pressure. In *Hypertension: Mechanisms, Diagnosis and Management*, pp. 189–200, J. O. Davis, J. H. Laragh, and A. Selwyn, Eds., HP Pub. Co. Inc. NY (1977).

McGiff, J. C. Prostaglandins, prostacyclin, and thromboxanes. *Ann. Rev. Pharmacol. Toxicol.* 21:479–509 (1981).

McGilvery, R. W. *Biochemistry—A functional approach*, 2nd ed., W. B. Saunders Co., Philadelphia (1979).

McGuigan, J. E. Gastrointestinal hormones. *Ann. Rev. Med.* 29:307–318 (1978).

McKhann, G. M., R. W. Albers, L. Sokoloff, O. Mickelsen, and D. B. Tower. The quantitative significance of the gamma-aminobutyric acid pathway in cerebral oxidative metabolism. In *Inhibition in the Nervous System and Gamma-aminobutyric acid*, pp. 169–181, E. Roberts, C. F. Baxter, A. Van Harreveld, C. A. G. Wiersma, W. R. Adley and K. F. Killam, Eds., Pergamon Press, New York (1960).

McKibbin, J. M. Glycolipids. In *The Carbohydrates*, Vol. 2B, pp. 711–738, W. Pigman, D. Horton, and A. Herp, Eds., Academic Press, New York (1970).

McLaren, D. S. *Nutrition and its Disorders*, 3rd ed., Churchill Livingstone, Edinburgh and New York (1981).

McLaughlan, J. M. Relationship between protein quality and plasma amino acid levels. *Fed. Proc.* 22:1122–1125 (1963).

McLaughlan, J. M. and W. I. Illman. Use of free amino acid levels for estimating amino acid requirements of the growing rat. *J. Nutr.* 93:21–24 (1967).

McLean, F. C. and A. M. Budy. Chemistry and physiology of the parathyroid hormone. *Vitam. Horm.* 19:165–187 (1961).

McLean, F. C. and M. R. Urist. *Bone. Fundamentals of the Physiology of Skeletal Tissue*, 3rd Ed., University of Chicago Press, Chicago (1968).

McMillan, J. A., S. A. Landaw, and F. A. Oski. Iron sufficiency in breast-fed infants and the availability of iron from human milk. *Pediatr.* 58:686–691 (1976).

McMillan, J. A., F. A. Oski, G. Lourie, R. M. Tomarelli, and S. A. Landaw. Iron absorption from human milk, simulated human milk and proprietary formulas. *Pediatr.* 60:896–900 (1977).

McNeill, K. G., J. R. Mernagh, K. N. Jeejeebhoy, S. L. Wolman, and J. E. Harrison. *In vivo* measurements of body protein based on the determination of nitrogen by prompt γ analysis. *Am. J. Clin. Nutr.* 32:1955–1961 (1979).

McNutt, K. Dietary advice to the public: 1957–1980. *Nutr. Rev.* 38:353–360 (1980).

McWhinnie D. L. and A. J. Mack. The interaction of wheat bran and oral iron supplements *in vivo. Hum. Nutr. Clin. Nutr.* 36C:315–318 (1982).

Mehansho, H., M. Hamm, and L. Henderson. Transport and metabolism of pyridoxal and pyridoxal phosphate in the small intestine of the rat. *J. Nutr.* 109:1538–1547 (1979).

Meister, A. Enzymology of amino acid transport. *Science* 180:33–39 (1973).

Meister, A. On the cycles of glutathione metabolism and transport. In *Current Topics in Cellular Regulation,* Vol. 18, *Biological Cycles,* pp. 21–58, R. W. Estabrook and P. Srere, Eds., Academic Press, New York and London (1981).

Meister, A. Selective modification of glutathione metabolism. *Science* 220:470–477 (1983).

Melikian, V., A. Paton, R. J. Leeming, and H. Partman-Graham. Site of reduction and methylation of folic acid in man. *Lancet* 2:955–957 (1971).

Mellanby, E. An experimental investigation on rickets. *Lancet* 1:407–412 (1919).

Mellanby, E. *A Story of Nutritional Research: The Effect of Some Dietary Factors on Bones and the Nervous System,* Williams & Wilkins, Baltimore (1950).

Mellors, A., D. Nahrwold, and R. Rose. Ascorbic acid flux across mucosal border of guinea pig and human ileum. *Am. J. Physiol.* 233:E374-E379 (1977).

Melnick, L. L. and L. Packer. Freeze-fracture faces of inner and outer membranes of mitochondria. *Biochim. Biophys. Acta* 253:503–508 (1971).

Mena, I. Manganese. In *Disorders of Mineral Metabolism,* Vol. 1, pp. 233–270, F. Bronner and J. Coburn, Eds., Academic Press, New York (1981).

Menard, M. P. and R. J. Cousins. Zinc transport by isolated brush border membrane vesicles from rat intestine. *Fed. Proc.* 41:779A (1982).

Menard, M. P., P. Oestreicher, and R. J. Cousins. Zinc transport by isolated, vascularly perfused rat intestine and intestinal brush border vesicles. In *Nutritional Bioavailability of Zinc,* pp. 233–246, G. E. Inglett, Ed. (ACS Symposium Series 210), American Chemistry Society Press, Washington, D.C. (1983).

Meneely, G. R., R. M. Heyssel, C. O. T. Ball, R. L. Weiland, A. R. Lorimer, C. Constantinides, and E. U. Meneely. Analysis of factors affecting body composition determined from potassium content in 915 normal subjects. *Ann. N. Y. Acad. Sci.* 110:271–281 (1963).

Merriam, R. W. Nuclear envelope structure during cell division in *Chaetopterus* eggs. *Exp. Cell Res.* 22:93–107 (1961).

Merrill, A. L., C. F. Adams, and L. J. Fincher. Procedures for calculating nutritive values of home-prepared foods (ARS 62-13), U.S. Department of Agriculture, Washington, D.C. (1966).

Mertz, W. Chromium occurrence and function in biological systems. *Physiol. Rev.* 49:163–239 (1969).

Mertz, W. Some aspects of nutritional trace element research. *Fed. Proc.* 29:1482–1488 (1970).

Mertz, W. Chromium—an overview. In *Chromium in Nutrition and Metabolism,* pp. 1–14, D. Sahpcott and J. Hubert, Eds., Elsevier North-Holland Biomedical Press, Amsterdam (1979).

Mertz, W. Mineral elements: new perspectives. *J. Am. Diet. Assoc.* 77:258–263 (1980).

Mertz, W. and E. E. Roginski. Chromium metabolism: the glucose tolerance factor. In *Newer Trace Elements in Nutrition,* pp. 123–153, W. Mertz and W. E. Cornatzer, Eds., Marcel Dekker Inc., New York (1971).

Mertz, W., F. W. Toepfer, E. E. Roginski, and M. M. Polansky. Present knowledge of the role of chromium. *Fed. Proc.* 33:2275–2280 (1974).

Meselson, M. and F. W. Stahl. Re replication of DNA in *E. coli. Proc. Nat. Acad. Sci. U. S.* 44:671–676 (1958).

Messer, H., W. Armstrong, and L. Singer. Essentiality and function of fluoride. In *Trace Element Metabolism in Animals,* Vol. 2, pp. 425–434, W. G. Hoekstra, J. W. Suttie, H. E. Ganther, and W. Mertz, Eds., University Park Press, Baltimore (1974).

Metcalf, D. and M. A. S. Moore. *Haemopoietic Cells,* North-Holland Publishing Co., Amsterdam (1971).

Meunier, P., R. Ferrando, J. Jouanneteau, and G. Thomas. Influence de la vitamine à sur la détoxication du benzoate de sodium par l'organisme du rat. *Compt. Rend.* 228:1254–1256 (1949).

Meyer, F. L., M. L. Brown, and M. L. Hathaway. Nutritive value of school lunches as determined by chemical analyses. *J. Am. Diet. Assoc.* 27:841–846 (1951).

Meyer, F. L., M. L. Brown, H. J. Wright, and M. L. Hathaway. A standardized diet for metabolic studies: its development and application (Technical Bulletin No. 1126), U.S. Department of Agriculture, Washington, D.C. (1955).

Meyer, J. H. and G. A. Kelly. Canine pancreatic responses to intestinally perfused proteins and protein digests. *Am. J. Physiol.* 231:682–691 (1976).

Meyer, K., E. Davidson, A. Linker, and P. Hoffman. The acid mucopolysaccharides of connective tissue. *Biochim. Biophys. Acta* 21:506–518 (1956).

Mickelsen, O., W. O. Caster, and A. Keys. A statistical evaluation of the thiamine and pyramin excretions of normal young men on controlled intakes of thiamine. *J. Biol. Chem.* 168:415–431 (1947).

Middleton, H. Uptake of pyridoxine hydrochloride by the rat jejunal mucosa *in vitro. J. Nutr.* 107:126–131 (1977).

Milhorat, A. T. Inositol. XI. Deficiency effects in human beings. In *The Vitamins,* Vol. 3, pp. 398–405, W. H. Sebrell, Jr. and R. S. Harris, Eds., Academic Press, New York (1971).

Miller, A. T. and C. S. Blyth. Estimation of lean body mass and body fat from basal oxygen consumption and creatinine excretion. *J. Appl. Physiol.* 5:73–78 (1952).

Miller, A. T. and C. S. Blyth. Lean body mass as a metabolic reference standard. *J. Appl. Physiol.* 5:311–316 (1953).

Miller, D. and R. K. Crane. The digestive function of the epithelium of the small intestine. I. An intracellular locus of disaccharide and sugar phosphate ester hydrolysis. *Biochim. Biophys. Acta* 52:281–293 (1961a).

Miller, D. and R. K. Crane. The digestive function of the epithelium of the small intestine. II. Localization of disaccharide hydrolysis in isolated brush border portion of intestinal epithelial cells. *Biochim. Biophys. Acta* 52:293–298 (1961b).

Miller, D. D., B. R. Schricker, R. R. Rasmussen, and D. VanCampen. An *in vitro* method for estimation of iron availability from meals. *Am. J. Clin. Nutr.* 34:2248–2256 (1981).

Miller, D. S. Thermogenesis in everyday life. In *Regulation of Energy Balance in Man*, pp. 209–211, I. E. Jequier, Ed., Widmer Foundation de l'Imprimerie Médecine et Hygiène, Geneva (1975).

Miller, D. S. and A. E. Bender. The determination of the net utilization of protein by a shortened method. *Br. J. Nutr.* 9:382–388 (1955).

Miller, E. J. Biochemical studies on the structure of chick bone collagen. *Fed. Proc.* 28:1839–1845 (1969).

Miller, E. J. and V. J. Matukas. Biosynthesis of collagen. The biochemist's view. *Fed. Proc.* 33:1197–1204 (1974).

Miller, F. and G. E. Palade. Lytic activities in renal protein absorption droplets. An electron microscopical cytochemical study. *J. Cell Biol.* 23:519–552 (1964).

Miller, G. J. High density lipoproteins and atherosclerosis. *Ann. Rev. Med.* 31:97–108 (1980).

Miller, L. T. and M. Edwards. Microbiological assay of vitamin B-6 in blood and urine. In *Methods in Vitamin B-6 Nutrition. Analysis and Status Assessment,* pp. 45–55, J. E. Leklem and R. D. Reynolds, Eds., Plenum, New York (1980).

Miller, O. L., Jr. The visualization of genes in action. *Sci. Am.* 228(3):34–43 (1973).

Miller, T. L. and M. J. Wolin. Fermentation by saccharolytic intestinal bacteria. *Am. J. Clin. Nutr.* 32:164–172 (1979).

Miller, W. J., J. D. Morton, W. J. Pitts, and G. M. Clifton. Effect of zinc deficiency and restricted feeding on wound healing in the bovine. *Proc. Soc. Exp. Biol. Med.* 118:427–430 (1965).

Mills, R., H. Breiter, E. Kampster, B. McKay, M. Pickens, and J. Outhouse. The influence of lactose in calcium retention in children. *J. Nutr.* 20:467–476 (1940).

Millward, D. J., P. C. Bates, J. G. Brown, S. R. Rosochacki, and M. J. Rennie. Anabolic stimulation of protein breakdown related to remodeling. In *Protein Degradation in Health and Disease*, pp. 307–329 (Ciba Foundation 75), Excerpta Medica, Amsterdam (1980).

Millward, D. J. and P. J. Garlick. The pattern of protein turnover in the whole animal and the effect of dietary variations. *Proc. Nutr. Soc.* 31:257–267 (1972).

Millward, D. J., P. J. Garlick, R. J. C. Stewart, D. O. Nanyelugo, and J. C. Waterlow. Skeletal muscle growth and protein turnover. *Biochem. J.* 150:235–243 (1975).

Millward, D. J. and J. C. Waterlow. Effect of nutrition on protein turnover in skeletal muscle. *Fed. Proc.* 37:2283–2290 (1978).

Milne, M. D. Disorders of amino acid transport. *Br. Med. J.* 1:327–336 (1964).

Milne, M. D. Genetic disorders of intestinal amino acid transport. In *Handbook of Physiology*, Section 6: Alimentary Canal, Vol. 3, pp. 1309–1321, C. F. Code, Ed., American Physiological Society, Washington, D.C. (1968).

Milne, M. D. Hereditary disorders of intestinal transport. In *Intestinal Absorption. Biomembranes*, Vol. 4B, pp. 961–1013, D. H. Smyth, Ed., Plenum, London (1974).

Milne, M. D., A. Asatoor, and L. W. Loughridge. Hartnup disease and cystinuria. *Lancet* 1:51–52 (1961).

Minot, G. R. and W. P. Murphy. Treatment of pernicious anemia by a special diet. *JAMA* 87:470–476 (1926).

Mirand, E. A., T. C. Prentice, and W. R. Slaunwhite. Current studies on the role of erythropoietin on erythropoiesis. *Ann. N. Y. Acad. Sci.* 77:677–702 (1959).

Mirsky, A. E. and H. Ris. Variable and constant components of chromosomes. *Nature* 163:666–667 (1949).

Mitchell, H. H. A method of determining the biological value of protein. *J. Biol. Chem.* 58:873–922 (1923).

Mitchell, H. H. Adult growth in man and its nutrient requirements. *Arch. Biochem.* 21:335–342 (1949).

Mitchell, H. H. *Comparative Nutrition of Man and Domestic Animals*. Academic Press, New York (1962).

Mitchell, H. H. and E. G. Curzon. The dietary requirement of calcium and its significance (Actualitiés scientifiques et industrielles No. 771, Nutrition 18), Hermann, Paris (1939).

Mitchell, H. H. and M. Edman. Nutritional significance of the dermal losses of nutrients in man, particularly of nitrogen and minerals. *Am. J. Clin. Nutr.* 10:163–172 (1962).

Mitchell, H. H., T. S. Hamilton, F. R. Steggerda, and H. W. Bean. The chemical composition of the adult human body and its bearing on the biochemistry of growth. *J. Biol. Chem.* 158:625–637 (1945).

Mitchell, H. K., E. E. Snell, and R. J. Williams. The concentration of folic acid. *J. Am. Chem. Soc.* 63:2284. (1941).

Mitchell, J. R., D. E. Becker, A. H. Jensen, B. G. Harmon, and H. W. Norton. Determination of amino acid needs of the young pig by nitrogen balance and plasma free amino acids. *J. Anim. Sci.* 27:1327–1331 (1968).

Mitchell, P. Coupling of phosphorylation to electron and hydrogen transfer by a chemiosmotic type mechanism. *Nature* 191:144–148 (1961).

Mitchell, P. Metabolic flow in the mitochondrial multiphase system: an appraisal of the chemi-osmotic theory of oxidative phosphorylation. In *Regulation of Metabolic Processes in Mitochondria,* Vol. 7, pp. 65–85, J. M. Tager, S. Papa, E. Quagliarello, and E. C. Slater, Eds., Biochimica Biophysics Acta Library, Elsevier, Amsterdam (1966).

Mitchell, P. Vectorial chemistry and the molecular mechanisms of chemiosmotic coupling: power transmission by proticity. *Trans. Biochem. Soc.* 4:399–430 (1976).

Mizrahi, A., R. D. London, and D. Bribetz. Neonatal hypocalcemia—its causes and treatment. *N. Engl. J. Med.* 278:1163–1165 (1968).

Mo, A., P. S. Peckos, and C. B. Glatkly. Computers in a dietary study. *J. Am. Diet. Assoc.* 59:111–115 (1971).

Molenaar, I., C. E. Hulstaert, and M. J. Hardonk. Role in function and ultrastructure of cellular membranes. In *Vitamin E: A comprehensive Treatise,* pp. 372–390, L. J. Machlin, Ed., Marcel Dekker Inc., New York (1980).

Molinoff, P. B., W. S. Brimijoin, R. M. Weinshilboum, and J. Axelrod. Neurally mediated increase in dopamine-β-hydroxylase activity. *Proc. Nat. Acad. Sci. U. S.* 66:453–458 (1970).

Mollenhauer, H. H. An intercisternal structure in the Golgi apparatus. *J. Cell Biol.* 24:504–511 (1965).

Moncada, S., R. J. Gryglewski, S. Bunting, and J. R. Vane. An enzyme isolated from arteries transforms prostaglandin endoperoxides to an unstable substance that inhibits platelet aggregation. *Nature* 263:663–665 (1976a).

Moncada, S., R. J. Gryglewski, S. Bunting, and J. R. Vane. A lipid peroxide inhibits the enzyme in blood vessel microsomes that generates from prostaglandin endoperoxides the substance (prostaglandin X) which prevents platelet aggregation. *Prostaglandins* 12:715–733 (1976b).

Moncada, S. and J. R. Vane. Prostacyclin in the cardiovascular system. *Adv. Prostaglandin Thromboxane Res.* 6:43–60 (1980).

Moncada, S. and J. R. Vane. Prostacyclin: its biosynthesis, actions and clinical potential. *Philos. Trans. R. Soc. Lond. (Biol.)* 294:305–329 (1981).

Monckeberg, F., S. Tisler, S. Toro, V. Guttas, and L. Vega. Malnutrition and mental development. *Am. J. Clin. Nutr.* 25:766–772 (1972).

Monod, J., J. Wyman, and J.-P. Changeux. On the nature of allosteric transitions: a plausible model. *J. Mol. Biol.* 12:88–118 (1965).

Monsen, E. R. and J. L. Balintfy. Calculating dietary iron bioavailability: refinement and computerization. *J. Am. Diet. Assoc.* 80:307–311 (1982).

Monsen, E. R., L. Hallberg, M. Layrisse, D. M. Hegsted, J. D. Cook, W. Mertz, and C. A. Finch. Estimation of available dietary iron. *Am. J. Clin. Nutr.* 31:134–141 (1978).

Montgomery, R., R. L. Dryer, T. W. Conway, and A. A. Spector. *Biochemistry. A Case-Oriented Approach,* 3d ed., C. V. Mosby, St. Louis (1980).

Mookerjea, S. Action of choline in lipoprotein metabolism. *Fed. Proc.* 30:143–150 (1971).

Moore, C. V. and R. Dubach. Observations on the absorption of iron from foods tagged with radioiron. *Trans. Assoc. Am. Physicians* 64:245–256 (1951).

Moore, C. V., R. Dubach, V. Minnich, and H. K. Roberts. Absorption of ferrous and ferric radioactive iron by human subjects and by dogs. *J. Clin. Invest.* 23:755–767 (1944).

Moore, F. D. and C. M. Boyden. Body cell mass and limits of hydration of the fat-free body: their relation to estimated skeletal weight. *Ann. N. Y. Acad. Sci.* 110:62–71 (1963).

Moore, F. D., K. H. Olesen, J. D. McMurrey, H. V. Parker, M. R. Ball, and C. M. Boyden. *The Body Cell Mass and Its Supporting Environment.* W. B. Saunders Co., Philadelphia (1963).

Moore, H. W. and K. Folkers. Vitamin B_{12}. VIII. Active compounds and antagonists. In *The Vitamins,* Vol. 2, pp. 181–184, W. H. Sebrell, Jr. and R. S. Harris, Eds., Academic Press, New York (1968).

Moore, M. A. S. and D. Metcalf. Ontogeny of the haemopoietic system: yolk sac origin of *in vivo* and *in vitro* colony forming cells in the developing mouse embryo. *Br. J. Haematol.* 18:279–296 (1970).

Moore, T. Vitamin A and carotene. *Biochem. J.* 24:692–702 (1930).

Moore, T. *Vitamin A.* Elsevier Publishing Co., Princeton, N.J. (1957).

Moore, T. The calorie as the unit of nutritional energy. *World Rev. Nutr. Diet.* 26:1–25 (1977).

Morell, P. and W. T. Norton. Myelin. *Sci. Am.* 242(5):88–118 (1980).

Morgan, E. H. Transferrin and transferrin iron. In *Iron in Biochemistry and Medicine,* pp. 29–71, A. Jacobs and M. Worwood, Eds., Academic Press, New York (1974).

Morgan, E. H., E. R. Huehns, and C. A. Finch. Iron reflux from reticulocytes and bone marrow cells *in vitro. Am. J. Physiol.* 210:579–585 (1966).

Morgan, H. E. and J. R. Neely. Insulin and membrane transport. In *Handbook of Physiology,* Section 7: Endocrinology, Vol. 1, pp. 323–331, R. O. Greep and E. B. Astwood, Eds., American Physiological Society, Washington, D.C. (1972).

Mori, S. Primary changes in eyes of rats that result from deficiency of fat-soluble A. *JAMA* 79:197–200 (1922).

Morii, H. and H. F. DeLuca. Relationship between vitamin D deficiency, thyrocalcitonin, and parathyroid hormone. *Am. J. Physiol.* 213:358–362 (1967).

Morley, C. G. D. Humoral regulation of liver regeneration and tissue growth. *Perspect. Biol. Med.* 17:411–428 (1974).

Morley, C. G. D. and H. S. Kingdon. The regulation of cell growth. I. Identification and partial characterization of a DNA synthesis stimulating factor from the serum of partially hepatectomized rats. *Biochim. Biophys. Acta* 308:260–275 (1973).

Morley, J. Role of prostaglandins secreted by macrophages in the inflammatory process. In *Lymphokines,* Vol. 4, pp. 377–394, E. O. Pick, Ed., Academic Press, New York (1981).

Morré, D. J., W. W. Franke, B. Deumling, S. E. Nyquist, and L. Ovtracht. Golgi apparatus function in membrane flow and differentiation: origin of plasma membrane from endoplasmic reticulum. In *Biomembranes,* Vol. 2, pp. 95–104, L. A. Manson, Ed., Plenum, New York (1971a).

Morré, D. J., R. L. Hamilton, H. H. Mollenhauer, R. W. Mahley, W. P. Cunningham, R. D. Cheetham, and V. S. LeQuire. Isolation of a Golgi apparatus-rich fraction from rat liver. I. Method and morphology. *J. Cell Biol.* 44:484–490 (1970).

Morré, D. J., H. H. Mollenhauer, and C. E. Bracker. Origin and continuity of Golgi apparatus. In *Origin and Continuity of Cell Organelles,* Vol. 2, pp. 82–126, J. Reinert and H. Ursprung, Eds., Springer-Verlag, New York (1971a).

Morré, D. J., T. W. Keenan, and H. H. Mollenhauer. Golgi apparatus function in membrane transformations and product compartmentalization: studies with cell fractions from rat liver. *Adv. Cytopharmacol.* 1:157–182 (1971b).

Morré, D. J. and L. Ovtracht. Dynamics of the Golgi apparatus: membrane differentiation and membrane flow. *Int. Rev. Cytol. (Suppl.)* 5:61–188 (1977).

Morrice, G., Jr., W. H. Havener, and F. Kapetansky. Vitamin A intoxication as a cause of pseudotumor cerebri. *JAMA* 173:1802–1805 (1960).

Morris, E. R. An overview of current information on bioavailability of dietary iron to humans. *Fed. Proc.* 42:1716–1720 (1983).

Morris, I. G. Gamma globulin absorption in the newborn. In *Handbook of Physiology,* Section 6: Alimentary Canal, Vol. 3, pp. 1491–1512, C. F. Code, Ed., American Physiological Society, Washington, D.C. (1968).

Morris, M. D. and I. L. Chaikoff. The origin of cholesterol in liver, small intestine, adrenal gland, and testis of the rat: dietary versus endogenous contributions. *J. Biol. Chem.* 234:1095–1097 (1959).

Morrison, A. B. and J. A. Campbell. Vitamin absorption studies. I. Factors influencing the excretion of oral test doses of thiamine and riboflavin by human subjects. *J. Nutr.* 72:435–440 (1960).

Morse, B. S. and F. Stohlman, Jr. Regulation of erythropoiesis. XVIII. The effect of vincristine and erythropoietin on bone marrow. *J. Clin. Invest.* 45:1241–1250 (1966).

Mortimore, G. E. Mechanisms of cellular protein catabolism. *Nutr. Rev.* 40:1–12 (1982).

Mortimore, G. E. and W. F. Ward. Behavior of the lysosomal system during organ perfusion. An inquiry into the mechanism of hepatic proteolysis. In *Lysosomes in Biology and Pathology,* Vol. 5, pp. 157–184, J. T. Dingle and R. T. Dean, Eds., North-Holland, London (1976).

Moses, M. J. The nucleus and chromosomes: a cytological perspective. In *Cytology and Cell Physiology*, 3rd Ed., pp. 424–558, G. H. Bourne, Ed., Academic Press, New York (1964).

Moulton, C. R. Age and chemical development in mammals. *J. Biol. Chem.* 57:79–97 (1923).

Mrsovosky, N. and U. Rowlatt. Changes in the microstructure of brown fat at birth in the human infant. *Biol. Neonate.* 13:230–252 (1968).

Mudd, S. H. Pyridoxine-responsive genetic disease. *Fed. Proc.* 30:970–976 (1971).

Mudd, S. H. and H. L. Levy. Disorders of transsulfuration. In *The Metabolic Basis of Inherited Disease*, pp. 458–503, J. B. Wyngaarden and D. S. Frederickson, Eds., McGraw-Hill, New York (1978).

Mueller, J. F. and R. W. Vilter. Pyridoxine deficiency in human beings induced with desoxypyridoxine. *J. Clin. Invest.* 29:192–201 (1950.)

Mueller, W. J., R. L. Brubaker, C. V. Gay, and J. N. Boelkins. Mechanisms of bone resorption in laying hens. *Fed. Proc.* 32:1951–1954 (1973).

Mulder, G. J. Ueber die Proteinverbindungen des Pflanzenreiches. *J. Prakt. Chem.* 16:129 (1839); 44:503–505 (1848).

Muller, D. P. R., and J. K. Lloyd. Effect of large doses of vitamin E on the neurological sequelae of patients with abetalipoproteinemia. *Ann. N. Y. Acad. Sci.* 393:133–142 (1982).

Muller, S. A., A. S. Posner, and H. E. Firschein. Effect of vitamin D deficiency on the crystal chemistry of bone mineral. *Proc. Soc. Exp. Biol. Med.* 121:844–846 (1966).

Munck, B. G. Intestinal absorption of amino acids. In *Physiology of the Gastrointestinal Tract*, Vol. 2, pp. 1097–1122, L. R. Johnson, Ed., Raven Press, New York (1981).

Munro, H. M. and J. W. Drysdale. Role of iron in the regulation of ferritin metabolism. *Fed. Proc.* 29:1469–1473 (1970).

Munson, P. L. and T. K. Gray. Function of thyrocalcitonin in normal physiology. *Fed. Proc.* 29:1206–1208 (1970).

Murakami, U. and Y. Kameyama. Malformations of the mouse fetus caused by hypervitaminosis A of the mother during pregnancy. *Arch. Environ. Health* 10:732–741 (1965).

Murata, K. Actions of two types of thiaminase on thiamin and its analogues. *Ann. N. Y. Acad. Sci.* 378:146–156 (1982).

Murphy, D. B. and G. G. Borisy. Association of high molecular weight proteins with microtubules and their role in microtubule assembly *in vitro*. *Proc. Nat. Acad. Sci. U. S.* 72:2696–2700 (1975).

Murphy, P. N. A. and S. P. Mistry. Biotin. *Prog. Food Nutr. Sci.* 2:405–455 (1977).

Muto, Y., J. E. Smith, P. O. Milch, and D. S. Goodman. Regulation of retinol-binding protein metabolism by vitamin A status in the rat. *J. Biol. Chem.* 247:2542–2550 (1972).

Myant, N. B. Developmental aspects of lipid metabolism. In *The Biochemistry of Development*, P. F. Benson, Ed. (Clinics in Developmental Medicine No. 37), J. B. Lippincott, Philadelphia (1971).

Myhre, E. Iron uptake and hemoglobin synthesis by human erythroid cell *in vitro*. *Scand. J. Clin. Lab. Invest.* 16:212–221 (1964).

Myron, D. R., T. J. Zimmerman, T. R. Shuler, L. M. Klevay, D. E. Lee, and F. H. Nielsen. Intake of nickel and vanadium by humans. A survey of selected diets. *Am. J. Clin. Nutr.* 31:527–531 (1978).

Nagatsu, T., M. Levitt, S. Udenfriend. Tyrosine hydroxylase: the initial step in norepinephrine biosynthesis. *J. Biol. Chem.* 239:2910–2917 (1964).

Nair, P. P. Vitamin E and metabolic regulation. *Ann. N. Y. Acad. Sci.* 203:53–61 (1972).

Nair, P. P., H. S. Murty, P. I. Caasi, S. K. Brooks, and J. Quartner. Vitamin E. Regulation of biosynthesis of porphyrins and heme. *J. Agric. Food Chem.* 20:476–480 (1972).

Naismith, D. J. The role of body fat accumulated during pregnancy in lactation in the rat. *Proc. Nutr. Soc.* 30:93A (1971).

Najjar, V. A. and L. E. Holt. The biosynthesis of thiamine in man and its implication in human nutrition. *JAMA* 123:683–684 (1943).

Nakagawa, I., T. Takahashi, T. Suzuki, and K. Kobayashi. Amino acid requirements of children: nitrogen balance at the minimal level of essential amino acids. *J. Nutr.* 83:115–118 (1964).

Nandi, M. A. and E. S. Parham. Milk drinking by the lactose intolerant. *J. Am. Diet. Assoc.* 61:258–261 (1972).

Naora, H., H. Naora, M. Izawa, V. G. Allfrey, and A. E. Mirsky. Some observations on differences in composition between the nucleus and cytoplasm of the frog oocyte. *Proc. Nat. Acad. Sci. U. S.* 48:853–859 (1962).

Napolitano, L. The fine structure of adipose tissues. In *Handbook of Physiology*, Section 5, Adipose Tissue, pp. 109–123, A. E. Renold and G. F. Cahill, Jr., Eds., American Physiological Society, Washington, D.C. (1965).

Narasinga Rao, B. S. Physiology of iron absorption and supplementation. *Br. Med. Bull.* 37:25–30 (1981).

Nasjletti, A. and K. U. Malik. Interrelations between prostaglandins and vasoconstrictor hormones: contribution of blood pressure regulation. *Fed. Proc.* 41:2394–2399 (1982).

Nass, M. M. K. Mitochondrial DNA. I. Intramitochondrial distribution and structural relations of single- and double-length circular DNA. *J. Mol. Biol.* 42:521–528 (1969).

Nass, M. M. K. and S. Nass. Intramitochondrial fibers with DNA characteristics. *J. Cell Biol.* 19:593–611 (1962).

Nasset, E. S. Role of the digestive system in protein metabolism. *Fed. Proc.* 24:953–958 (1965).

Nasset, E. S. and J. S. Ju. Mixture of endogenous and exogenous protein in the alimentary tract. *J. Nutr.* 74:461–465 (1961).

Nasset, E. S., P. Swartz, and H. V. Weiss. The digestion of proteins *in vivo. J. Nutr.* 56:83–94 (1955).

National Research Council. *Nutrition surveys: their techniques and value* (National Research Council Bulletin No. 117), National Academy of Sciences, Washington, D.C. (1949).

National Research Council. Committee on Nutrition of the Mother and Preschool Child, Food and Nutrition Board, *Laboratory Indices of Nutritional Status in Pregnancy*, National Academy of Sciences Press, Washington, D.C. (1978).

National Research Council. Committee on Medical and Biological Effects of Environmental Pollutants, Subcommittee on Iron. *Iron*, pp. 84–85, University Park Press, Baltimore (1979).

National Research Council. Food and Nutrition Board, *Toward Healthful Diets,* National Academy of Sciences Press, Washington, D.C. (1980).

National Research Council. *Recommended Dietary Allowances,* 9th ed., National Academy of Sciences Press, Washington, D.C. (1980).

National Research Council. Subcommittee on Mineral Toxicity in Animals, *Mineral Tolerance of Domestic Animals,* pp. 392–401, National Academy of Sciences Press, Washington, D.C. (1980).

National Research Council. Committee on Food Consumption Patterns, Food and Nutrition Board, *Assessing Changing Food Consumption Patterns*, National Academy Press, Washington, D.C. (1981).

Naughton, M. A. and H. M. Dintzis. Sequential biosynthesis of the peptide chains of hemoglobin. *Proc. Nat. Acad. Sci. U. S.* 48:1822–1830 (1962).

Navab, M., J. E. Smith, and D. S. Goodman. Rat plasma prealbumin. Metabolic studies on effects of vitamin A status and on tissue distribution. *J. Biol. Chem.* 252:5107–5114 (1977).

Neal, R. A. Isolation and identification of thiamine catabolites in mammalian urine; isolation and identification of some products of bacterial catabolism of thiamine. In *Methods in Enzymology*, Vol. 18, Part A, pp. 133–140, D. B. McCormick and A. D. Wright, Eds., Academic Press, New York (1970).

Neal, R. A. and W. N. Pearson. Studies of thiamine metabolism in the rat. I. Metabolic products found in urine. *J. Nutr.* 83:343–350 (1964).

Neame, K. D. and G. Wiseman. The transamination of glutamic and aspartic acids during absorption by the small intestine of the dog *in vivo. J. Physiol. (London)* 135:442–450 (1957).

Neame, K. D. and G. Wiseman. The alanine and oxo acid concentrations in mesenteric blood during the absorption of L-glutamic acid by the small intestine of the dog, cat and rabbit *in vivo. J. Physiol. (London)* 140:148–155 (1958).

Necheles, T. F. and L. M. Snyder. Malabsorption of folate polyglutamates associated with oral contraceptive therapy. *N. Engl. J. Med.* 282:858–859 (1970).

Needleman, S. B., Ed. *Protein Sequence Determination: A Source Book of Methods and Techniques*, 2nd ed., Springer-Verlag, New York, Heidelberg, and Berlin (1975).

Neeld, J. B., Jr., and W. N. Pearson. Macro- and micromethods for the determination of serum vitamin A using trifluoroacetic acid. *J. Nutr.* 79:454–462 (1963).

Neher, R., B. Riniker, R. Maier, P. G. H. Byfield, T. V. Gudmundsson, and I. MacIntyre. Human calcitonin. *Nature* 200:984–986 (1968).

Nelsestuen, G. L. and J. W. Suttie. The purification and properties of an abnormal prothrombin protein produced by dicoumarol-treated cows. A comparison to normal prothrombin. *J. Biol. Chem.* 247:8176–8182 (1972).

Nelson, W. E. *Textbook of Pediatrics,* W. B. Saunders Co., Philadelphia (1946).

Nestel, P. J., W. Austin, and D. Foxman. Lipoprotein lipase content and triglyceride-fatty acid uptake in adipose tissue of rats of differing body weights. *J. Lipid Res.* 10:383–387 (1969).

Neufeld, E. F. The enzymology of inherited mucopolysaccharide storage disorders. *Trends Biochem. Sci.* 2:25–26 (1977).

Neuman, W. F. The *milieu interieur* of bone: Claude Bernard revisited. *Fed. Proc.* 28:1846–1850 (1969).

Neuman, W. F. and M. W. Neuman. *The Chemical Dynamics of Bone Mineral,* University of Chicago Press, Chicago (1958).

Neupert, W., G. D. Ludwig, and A. Pfaller. Structure and biogenesis of outer and inner mitochondrial membranes of *Neurospora crassa.* In *Biochemistry and Biophysics of Mitochondrial Membranes,* pp. 559–576, G. F. Azzone, E. Carafoli, A. L. Lehninger, E. Quagliariello, and N. Silliprandi, Eds., Academic Press, New York (1972).

Neurath, H. Protein-digesting enzymes. *Sci. Am.* 211(6):68–79 (1964).

Neutra, M. and C. P. Leblond. Synthesis of the carbohydrate of mucus in the Golgi complex as shown by electron microscope radioautography of goblet cells from rats injected with glucose-H^3. *J. Cell Biol.* 30:119–136 (1966).

Neutra, M. and C. P. Leblond. The Golgi apparatus. *Sci. Am.* 220(2):100–107 (1969).

Newburgh, L. H., M. W. Johnston, and M. Falcon-Lesses. Measurement of total water exchange. *J. Clin. Invest.* 8:161–196 (1930).

Newcomer, A. D. and D. B. McGill. Lactose tolerance test in adults with normal lactase activity. *Gastroenterol.* 50:340–346 (1966).

Newman, R. W. Skinfold measurements in young American males. In *Body Measurements and Human Nutrition,* pp. 44–54, (National Research Council Committee on National Anthropometry), J. Brozek, Ed., Wayne University Press, Detroit (1956).

Newton-John, H. F. and D. B. Morgan. Osteoporosis: disease or senescence? *Lancet* 1:232–233 (1968).

Niall, H., H. Keutman, R. Sauer, M. Hogan, B. Dawson, G. D. Aurbach, and J. T. Potts, Jr. The amino acid sequence of bovine parathyroid hormone. I. *Hoppe-Seyler's Z. Physiol. Chem.* 351:1586–1588 (1970).

Nicholl, A., N. E. Miller, and B. Lewis. High density lipoprotein metabolism. *Adv. Lipid Res.* 17:53–106 (1980).

Nicholls, D. G. and M. Crompton. Mitochondrial calcium transport. *FEBS Lett.* 111:261–268 (1980).

Nicholls, L. and A. Nimalasuriya. Adaptation to a low calcium intake in reference to the calcium requirements of a tropical population. *J. Nutr.* 18:563–577 (1939).

Nicholson, F. T. L. and F. W. Chornock. Intubation studies of the human intestine. XXII. An improved technique for the study of absorption: its application to ascorbic acid. *J. Clin. Invest.* 21:505–509 (1942).

Nicolaysen, R. Studies upon the mode of action of vitamin D. III. The absorption calcium intake in reference of vitamin D on the absorption of calcium and phosphorus in the rat. *Biochem. J.* 31:122–129 (1937).

Nicolini, C., Ed. *Cell Growth,* Plenum, New York (1982).

Nielsen, F. H. Evidence of the essentiality of arsenic, nickel, and vanadium and their possible nutritional significance. In *Advances in Nutritional Research,* Vol. 3, pp. 157–172, H. H. Draper, Ed., Plenum, New York (1980).

Nielsen, F. H. and H. H. Sandstead. Are nickel, vanadium, silicon, fluorine, and tin essential for man? A review. *Am. J. Clin. Nutr.* 27:515–520 (1974).

Nielsen, F. H. and Z. Z. Ziporin. Effect of zinc deficiency on the uptake of $^{35}SO_4$- by the epiphyseal plate and primary spongiosa of the chick. *Fed. Proc.* 28:762A (1969).

Nielsen, S. L., V. Lbitsch, O. A. Larsen, H. A. Lassen, and F. Quaade. Blood flow through human adipose tissue during lipolysis. *Scand. J. Clin. Lab. Invest.* 22:124–130 (1968).

Nilsson-Ehle, P., A. S. Garfinkel, and M. C. Schotz. Lipolytic enzymes and plasma lipoprotein metabolism. *Ann. Rev. Biochem.* 49:667–693 (1980).

Nirenberg, M. The flow of information from gene to protein. In *Aspects of Protein Biosynthesis,* Part A, pp. 215–246, C. B. Anfinsen, Jr., Ed., Academic Press, New York (1970).

Nirenberg, M. W. The Genetic Code. II. *Sci. Am.* 208(3):80–94 (1963).

Nirenberg, M. W. and J. H. Matthaei. The dependence of cell-free protein synthesis in *E. coli* upon naturally-occurring or synthetic polyribonucleotides. *Proc. Nat. Acad. Sci. U. S.* 47:1588–1602 (1961).

Nirenberg, M. W., J. H. Matthaei, and O. W. Jones. An intermediate in the biosynthesis of polyphenylalanine directed by synthetic template RNA. *Proc. Nat. Acad. Sci. U. S.* 48:104–109 (1962).

Nishizawa, Y. and F. Matsuzaki. The antagonistic action of homopantothenic acid against pantothenic acid. *J. Vitaminol.* 15:8–25 (1969).

Nishizuka, Y. and O. Hayashi. Studies on the biosynthesis of nicotinamide adenine dinucleotide. I. Enzymic synthesis of niacin ribonucleotides from 3-hydroxyanthranilic acid in mammalian tissues. *J. Biol. Chem.* 238:3369–3377 (1963).

Nishizuka, Y. and F. Lipmann. Comparison of guanosine triphosphate split and polypeptide synthesis with a purified *E. Coli* system. *Proc. Nat. Acad. Sci. U. S.* 55:212–219 (1966).

Nixon, S. E. and G. E. Mawer. Digestion and absorption of protein in man. I. Site of absorption. *Br. J. Nutr.* 24:227–240 (1970a).

Nixon, S. E. and G. E. Mawer. Digestion and absorption of protein in man. II. The form in which digested protein is absorbed. *Br. J. Nutr.* 24:241–258 (1970b).

Noell, W. K. and R. Albrecht. Vitamin A deficiency effect on retina: dependence on light. *Science* 172:72–79 (1971).

Noguchi, T., A. H. Cantor, and M. L. Scott. Mode of action of selenium and vitamin E in prevention of exudative diathesis in chicks. *J. Nutr.* 103:1502–1511 (1973).

Nomura, M. Ribosomes. *Sci. Am.* 221(4):28–35 (1969).

Nomura, M. Bacterial ribosome. *Bacteriol. Rev.* 34:228–277 (1970).

Nordin, B. E. C. Pathogenesis of osteoporosis. *Lancet* 1:1011–1015 (1961).

Nordin, B. E. C. Calcium balance and calcium requirements in spinal osteoporosis. *Am. J. Clin. Nutr.* 10:384–390 (1962).

Nordin, B. E. C., A. Horsman, D. H. Marshall, M. Simpson, and G. M. Waterhouse. Calcium requirement and calcium therapy. *Clin. Orthop.* 140:216–246 (1979).

Nordin, B. E. C. and M. Peacock. The role of the kidney in serum calcium homeostasis. In *Calcitonin: Proceedings of the Second International Symposium,* pp. 472–482, Springer-Verlag, New York (1970).

Noren, O., H. Sjöström, and L. Josefsson. Studies on soluble dipeptidase from pig intestinal mucosa. I. Purification and specificity. *Biochim. Biophys. Acta* 327:446–456 (1973).

Norman, A. W. Actinomycin D and the response to vitamin D. *Science* 149:184–186 (1965).

Norman, A. W. Vitamin D metabolism and calcium absorption. *Am. J. Med.* 67:989–998 (1979).

Norman, A. W. and H. F. DeLuca. The preparation of H^3-vitamins D_2 and D_3 and their localization in the rat. *Biochem.* 2:1160–1168 (1963).

Norman, A. W., J. F. Myrtle, R. J. Midgett, H. G. Nowicki, V. Williams, and G. Popjak. 1,25-Dihydroxycholecalciferol: identification of the proposed active form of vitamin D_3 in the intestine. *Science* 173:51–54 (1971).

Norris, A. H., T. Lundy, and N. W. Shock. Trends in selected indices of body composition in men between the ages 30 and 80 years. *Ann. N. Y. Acad. Sci.* 110:623–639 (1963).

Norris, T. Dietary surveys. Their technique and interpretation. *FAO Nutr. Stud.* No. 4, Washington, D.C. (1949).

North, R. The localization by electron microscopy of acid phosphatase activity in guinea pig macrophages. *J. Ultrastruct. Res.* 16:96–108 (1966).

Northcote, D. H. The Golgi apparatus. *Endeavour* 30:26–33 (1971).

Novikoff, A. B. Mitochondria (chondriosomes). In *The Cell,* Vol. 2, pp. 299–421, J. Brachet and A. E. Mirsky, Eds., Academic Press, New York (1961a).

Novikoff, A. B. Lysosomes in the physiology and pathology of cells: contributions of staining methods. In *Ciba Foundation Symposium on Lysosomes,* pp. 36–73, A. V. S. deReuck and M. P. Cameron, Eds., Little, Brown & Co., Boston (1963).

Novikoff, A. B., H. Beaufay, and C. DeDuve. Electron microscopy of lysosome-rich fractions from rat liver. *J. Biophys. Biochem. Cytol. (Suppl.)* 2:179–184 (1956).

Novikoff, A. B., E. Essner, S. Goldfischer, and M. Heus. Nucleosidephosphatase activities of cytomembranes. In *The Interpretation of Ultrastructure,* Vol. 1, pp. 149–192, R. J. C. Harris, Ed., Academic Press, New York (1962).

Novikoff, A. B., E. Essner, and N. Quintana. Golgi apparatus and lysosomes. *Fed. Proc.* 23:1010–1022 (1964).

Noyes, W. D., T. H. Bothwell, and C. A. Finch. The role of the reticuloendothelial cell in iron metabolism. *Br. J. Haemat.* 6:43–55 (1960).

Noyes, W. D., F. Hosain, and C. A. Finch. Incorporation of radio iron into marrow heme. *J. Lab. Clin. Med.* 64:574–580 (1964).

Nyberg, W. The influence of *Diphyllobothrium latum* on the vitamin B_{12} intrinsic factor complex. II. *In vitro* studies. *Acta Med. Scand.* 167:189–192 (1960).

Nyquist, S. E., F. L. Crane, and D. J. Morré. Vitamin A: concentration in the rat liver Golgi apparatus. *Science* 173:939–941 (1971).

O'Brien, J. S. A molecular defect of myelination. *Biophys. Res. Commun.* 15:484–490 (1964).

O'Brien, J. S. Stability of the myelin membrane. *Science* 147:1099–1107 (1965).

Obst, B. E., R. A. Schemmel, D. Czajka-Narins, and R. Merkel. Adipocyte size and number in dietary obesity resistant and susceptible rats. *Am. J. Physiol.* 240:E47–E53 (1981).

Ochoa, S. Synthetic polynucleotides and the genetic code. *Fed. Proc.* 22:62–74 (1963).

Ockner, R. K., F. B. Hughes, and K. J. Isselbacher. Very low density lipoproteins in intestinal lymph: role in triglyceride and cholesterol transport during fat absorption. *J. Clin. Invest.* 48:2367–2373 (1969).

Ockner, R. K. and K. J. Isselbacher. Recent concept of intestinal fat absorption. *Rev. Physiol. Biochem. Pharmacol.* 71:107–146 (1974).

Ockner, R. K. and J. A. Manning. Fatty acid-binding protein in small intestine. Identification, isolation and evidence for its role in cellular fatty acid transport. *J. Clin. Invest.* 54:326–338 (1974).

Ockner, R. K., J. A. Manning, R. B. Poppenhausen, and W. K. L. Ho. A binding protein for fatty acids in cytosol of intestinal mucosa, liver, myocardium, and other tissues. *Science* 177:56–58 (1972).

Octave, J. N., Y.-J. Schneider, R. R. Crichton, and A. Trouet. Transferrin protein and iron uptake by isolated rat erythroblasts. *FEBS Lett.* 137:119–123 (1982).

Offenbacher, E. G. and F. X. Pi-Sunyer. Beneficial effect of chromium-rich yeast on glucose tolerance and blood lipids in elderly subjects. *Diabetes* 29:919–925 (1980).

Ohnishi, T. and T. Ohnishi. Extraction of a contractile protein from liver mitochondria. *J. Biochem.* (Tokyo) 51:380–381 (1962a).

Ohnishi, T. and T. Ohnishi. Extraction of actin- and myosin-like proteins from liver mitochondria. *J. Biochem.* (Tokyo) 52:230–231 (1962b).

Okada, Y., A. Irimajiri, and A. Inouye. Electrical properties and active solute transport in rat small intestine. II. Conductive properties of transepithelial routes. *J. Membr. Biol.* 31:221–232 (1977a).

Okada, Y., W. Tsuchiya, A. Irimajiri, and A. Inouye. Electrical properties and active solute transport in rat small intestine. I. Potential profile changes associated with sugar and amino acid transport. *J. Membr. Biol.* 31:205–219 (1977b).

Okazaki, R., T. Okazaki, K. Sakabe, K. Sugimoto, and A. Sugino. Mechanism of DNA chain growth. I. Possible discontinuity and unusual secondary structure of newly synthesized chains. *Proc. Nat. Acad. Sci. U. S.* 59:598–605 (1968).

Oldham, H., M. V. Davis, and L. J. Roberts. Thiamine excretions and blood levels of young women on diets containing varying levels of the B-vitamins with some observations on niacin and pantothenic acid. *J. Nutr.* 32:163–180 (1946).

Oldham, H., F. W. Schlutz, and M. Morse. Utilization of organic and inorganic iron by the normal infant. *Am. J. Dis. Child.* 54:252–264 (1937).

Oldham, H. and B. B. Sheft. Effect of caloric intake on nitrogen utilization during pregnancy. *J. Am. Diet. Ass.* 27:847–854 (1951).

Olesen, K. H. Body composition in normal adults. In *Human Body Composition, Approaches and Applications,* pp. 177–190, J. Brozek, Ed., Pergamon Press, Oxford, Eng. (1965).

Olinger, E. J., J. R. Bertino, and H. J. Binder. Intestinal folate absorption. II. Conversion and retention of pteroylmonoglutamate by jejunum. *J. Clin. Invest.* 52:2138–2145 (1973).

Olivecrona, T. and G. Bengtsson. Heparin and lipoprotein lipase. In *Chemistry and Biology of Heparin,* pp. 187–194, R. L. Lundblad, W. V. Brown, K. G. Mann, and H. R. Roberts, Eds., Elsevier North-Holland, New York (1981).

Olivecrona, T., G. Bengtsson, S.-E. Marklund, V. Lindahl, and M. Höök. Heparin-lipoprotein lipase interactions. *Fed. Proc.* 36:60–65 (1977).

Oliver, M. F. Serum cholesterol—the knave of hearts and the joker. *Lancet* 2:1090–1095 (1981).

Oliverio, V. T. and D. S. Zaharko. Tissue distribution of folate antagonists. *Ann. N. Y. Acad. Sci.* 186:387–399 (1971).

Olson, J. A. The alpha and omega of vitamin A metabolism. *Am. J. Clin. Nutr.* 22:953–962 (1969a).

Olson, J. A. Metabolism and function of vitamin A. *Fed. Proc.* 28:1670–1677 (1969b).

Olson, J. A. Liver vitamin A reserves of neonates, preschool children and adults dying of various causes in Salvador, Brazil. *Arch. Latinoam. Nutr.* 29:521–545 (1979).

Olson, J. A. and O. Hayaishi. The enzymatic cleavage of B-carotene into vitamin A by soluble enzymes of rat liver and intestine. *Proc. Nat. Acad. Sci. U. S.* 54:1364–1370 (1965).

Olson, J. A. and M. R. Lakshmanan. Enzymatic transformations of vitamin A, with particular emphasis on carotenoid cleavage. In *The Fat-Soluble Vitamins*, pp. 213–226, H. F. DeLuca and J. W. Suttie, Eds., University of Wisconsin Press, Madison (1970).

Olson, R. E. Vitamin E and its relation to heart disease. *Circulation* 48:179–184 (1973).

Olson, R. E., Ed., *Protein-calorie malnutrition*. Academic Press, New York and London (1975).

Omaye, S. T., J. D. Turnbull, and H. E. Sauberlich. Selected methods for the determination of ascorbic acid in animal cells, tissues, and fluids. *Methods Enzymol.* 62:3–11 (1979).

Omdahl, J. L. and H. F. DeLuca. Regulation of vitamin D metabolism and function. *Physiol. Rev.* 53:327–372 (1973).

O'Neal, R. M., O. C. Johnson, and A. E. Schaefer. Guidelines for classification and interpretation of group blood and urine data collected as part of the national nutrition survey. *Pediatr. Res.* 4:103–106 (1970).

O'Neil, R. G. Potassium secretion by the cortical collecting tubule. *Fed. Proc.* 40:2403–2407 (1981).

Onishi, T. Studies on the mechanism of decrease in the RNA content in liver cells of fasted rats. II. The mechanism of starvation-induced decrease in RNA polymerase activity in liver. *Biochim. Biophys. Acta* 217:384–393 (1970).

Oppenheimer, J. H., M. I. Surks, J. C. Smith, and R. Squef. Isolation and characterization of human thyroxine-binding prealbumin. *J. Biol. Chem.* 240:173–180 (1965).

Orci, L., M. Amherdt, F. Malaisse-Lagae, C. Rouiller, and A. E. Renold. Insulin release by emiocytosis: demonstration with freeze-etching technique. *Science* 179:82–84 (1973a).

Orci, L., F. Malaisse-Lagae, M. Ravazzola, M. Amherdt, and A. E. Renold. Exocytosis-endocytosis coupling in the pancreatic beta cell. *Science* 181:561–562 (1973b).

Orlic, D. Ultrastructural analysis of erythropoiesis. In *Regulation of Hemato-poiesis*, Vol. 1, pp. 271–296, A. S. Gordon, Ed., Appleton-Century-Crofts, New York (1970).

Orlic, D., A. S. Gordon, and J. A. G. Rhodin. An ultrastructural study of eryth-ropoietin-induced red cell formation in mouse spleen. *J. Ultrastruct. Res.* 13:516–542 (1965).

Orlic, D., A. S. Gordon, and J. A. G. Rhodin. Ultrastructural and autoradiographic studies of erythropoietin-induced red cell production. *Ann. N. Y. Acad. Sci.* 149:198–216 (1968).

Orloff, J. and J. Handler. The role of adenosine 3′, 5′-phosphate in the action of antidiuretic hormone. *Am. J. Med.* 42:757–768 (1967).

Orten, J. M. and O. W. Neuhaus. *Human Biochemistry*, 10th ed., C. V. Mosby, St. Louis (1982).

Osaki, S., D. A. Johnson, and E. Frieden. The possible significance of the ferrous oxidase activity of ceruloplasmin in normal human serum. *J. Biol. Chem.* 241:2746–2751 (1966).

Osborne, J. C., Jr. and H. B. Brewer. The plasma lipoproteins. *Adv. Protein Chem.* 31:253–337 (1977).

Osborne, T. B. *The Vegetable Proteins.* 2nd ed., Longmans, Green and Co., London (1924).

Osborne, T. B. and L. B. Mendel. *Feeding experiments with isolated food sub-stances,* Carnegie Institute of Washington Pub. No. 156, Pts. I and II (1911).

Osborne, T. B., L. B. Mendel, and E. L. Ferry. A method of expressing numerically the growth-promoting value of proteins. *J. Biol. Chem.* 37:223–229 (1919).

Oski, F. A. and S. A. Landaw. Inhibition of iron absorption from human milk by baby food. *Am. J. Dis. Child.* 134:459–460 (1980).

Outhouse, J., H. Brieter, E. Rutherford, J. Dwight, R. Mills, and W. Armstrong. The calcium requirement of man. Balance studies on seven adults. *J. Nutr.* 21:565–575 (1941).

Overton, J. A., A. Eichholz, and R. K. Crane. Studies on the organization of the brush border in intestinal cells. II. Fine structure of tris-disrupted hamster brush borders. *J. Cell. Biol.* 26:693–706 (1965).

Pace, N. and E. N. Rathbun. Studies on body composition. III. The body water and chemically combined nitrogen content in relation to fat content. *J. Biol. Chem.* 158:685–691 (1945).

Padykula, H. A. Recent functional interpretations of intestinal morphology. *Fed. Proc.* 21:873–879 (1962).

Page, I. H. The nature of arterial hypertension. *Arch. Int. Med.* 111:103–115 (1963).

Page, I. H. Serotonin and the brain. In *The Structure and Function of Nervous Tissue*, Vol. III, pp. 289–307, G. H. Bourne, Ed., Academic Press, New York, 1969.

Page, L. and E. Phipard. *Essentials of an adequate diet* (USDA Home Economics Research Report No. 3). U.S. Department of Agriculture, Washington, D.C. (1957).

Page-Thomas, D. P. Lysosomal enzymes in experimental and rheumatoid arthritis. In *Lysosomes in Biology and Pathology,* Vol. 2, pp. 87–110, J. T. Dingle and H. B. Fell, Eds., Wiley-Interscience New York, 1969.

Paige, D. M. and T. M. Bayless, Ed., *Lactose Digestion: Clinical and Nutritional Implications,* Johns Hopkins University Press, Baltimore (1981).

Paige, D. M., T. M. Bayless, S-S Huang and R. Wexler. Lactose hydrolyzed milk. *Am. J. Clin. Nutr.* 28:818–822 (1975).

Paik, W. K. and S. Kim. *Protein methylation,* Wiley-Interscience, New York (1980).

Palade, G. E. The fine structure of mitochondria. *Anat. Rec.* 114:427–451 (1952).

Palade, G. E. Intracellular aspects of the process of protein synthesis. *Science* 189:347–358 (1975).

Palay, S. L. Principles of cellular organization in the nervous system. In *The Neurosciences,* pp. 24–31, G. C. Quarton, T. Melnechuk, and F. O. Schmitt, Eds., Rockefeller University Press, New York (1967).

Palay, S. L. and L. J. Karlin. An electron microscopic study of the intestinal villus. I. The fasting animal. *J. Biophys. Biochem. Cytol.* 5:363–372 (1959b).

Palay, S. L. and L. J. Karlin. An electron microscopic study of the intestinal villus. II. The pathway of fat absorption. *J. Biophys. Biochem. Cytol.* 5:373–384 (1959a).

Palmer, J. P. and D. Porte, Jr. Control of glucagon secretion: the central nervous system. In *Glucagon: Physiology, Pathophysiology, and Morphology of the Pancreatic A-Cells,* pp. 135–159, R. H. Unger and L. Orci, Eds., Elsevier, New York (1981).

Pänkäläinen, M. and K. I. Kivirikko. Protocollagen proline hydroxylase: molecular weight, subunits and isoelectric point. *Biochim. Biophys. Acta* 221:559–565 (1970).

Pansu, D. and M. C. Chapuy. Relation, chez l'homme, entre l'action sur la calcemie de divers composes glucidiques et leur utilisation digestive. *C. R. Acad. Sci. (Paris)* 260:3103–3106 (1970).

Pao, E. M., and S. J. Mickle. Problem nutrients in the United States. *Food Technol.* 35(9):58–79 (1981).

Papavasiliou, P. S., S. T. Miller, and G. C. Cotzias. Role of liver in regulating distribution and excretion of manganese. *Am. J. Physiol.* 211:211–216 (1966).

Pappenheimer, A. M. and M. Goettsch. A cerebellar disorder in chicks, apparently of nutritional origin. *J. Exp. Med.* 53:11–16 (1931).

Pappenheimer, J. R. Passage of molecules through capillary walls. *Physiol. Rev.* 33:387–423 (1953).

Pardee, A. B. Membrane transport proteins. *Science* 162:632–637 (1968).

Pařízková, J. Total body fat and skinfold thickness in children. *Metabolism* 10:794–807 (1961).

Pařízková, J. Impact of age, diet and exercise on man's body composition. *Ann. N. Y. Acad. Sci.* 110:661–674 (1963).

Pařízková, J. Physical activity and body composition. In *Human Body Composition, Approaches and Applications, pp. 161–176,* J. Brozek, Ed., Pergamon Press, Oxford, Eng. (1965).

Pařízková, J. Obesity and physical activity. In *Nutritional Aspects of Physical Performance*, pp. 146–160, J. F. De Wijn and R. A. Binkhorst, Eds., Nutricia Ltd., Zoetermeer, The Netherlands (1972).

Pařízková, J. Body composition and exercise during growth and development. In *Physical Activity—Human Growth and Development*, pp. 97–124, G. L. Rarick, Ed., Academic Press, New York (1973).

Pařízková, J. Physical activity related to nutrition as a factor of variability of body composition. In *Food, Nutrition and Evolution—Food as an Environmental Factor in the Genesis of Human Variability*, pp. 133–141 D. N. Walcher and N. Kretchmer, Eds., Masson Publishing USA, New York, (1981).

Parr, R. B., J. H. Wilmore, R. Hoover, D. Bachman, and R. Kerlan. Professional basketball players: athletic profiles. *Physician Sportsmed.* 6:77–84 (1978).

Parsons, B. J., D. H. Smyth, and C. B. Taylor. The action of phlorizin on the intestinal transfer of glucose and water *in vitro. J. Physiol. (London)* 144:387–402 (1958).

Parsons, H. T., J. G. Lease, and E. Kelly. Interrelationship between dietary egg white and requirement for protective factor in cure of nutritional disorder due to egg white. *Biochem. J.* 31:424–432 (1937).

Parsons, H. T., A. Williamson, and M. L. Johnson. The availability of vitamins from yeasts. I. The absorption of thiamine by human subjects from various types of bakers' yeast. *J. Nutr.* 29:373–381 (1945).

Parsons, J. A. Parathyroid physiology and the skeleton. In *The Biochemistry and Physiology of Bone*, 2nd ed., Vol. 4, pp. 159–215, G. H. Bourne, Ed., Academic Press, New York (1976).

Pascale, L. R., M. I. Grossman, H. S. Sloane, and T. Frankel. Correlations between thickness of skinfolds and body density in 88 soldiers. In *Body Measurements and Human Nutrition*, pp. 55–66, J. Brozek, Ed., Wayne University Press (1956).

Passmore, R. and J. V. G. A. Durnin. Human energy expenditures. *Physiol. Rev.* 35:801–840 (1955).

Passmore, R. and F. J. Ritchie. The specific dynamic action of food and the satiety mechanism. *Br. J. Nutr.* 11:79–85 (1957).

Pastan, I. and R. L. Perlman. The role of the lac promoter locus in the regulation of β-galactosidase synthesis by cyclic 3′, 5′-adenosine monophosphate. *Proc. Nat. Acad. Sci. U. S.* 61:1336–1342 (1968).

Pastan, I. H., G. S. Johnson, and W. B. Anderson. Role of cyclic nucleotides in growth control. *Ann. Rev. Biochem.* 44:491–522 (1975).

Patriarca, P. and E. Carafoli. A study of the intracellular transport of calcium in rat heart. *J. Cell Physiol.* 72:29–38 (1968).

Patt, H. M. and H. Quastler. Radiation effects on cell renewal and related systems. *Physiol. Rev.* 43:357–396 (1963).

Patten, R. L. and C. H. Hollenberg. The mechanism of heparin stimulation of rat adipocyte lipoprotein lipase. *J. Lipid Res.* 10:374–382 (1967).

Patterson, E. I., M. H. Saltza, and E. L. R. Stokstad. The isolation and characterization of a pteridine required for the growth of *Crithidia fasciculata. J. Am. Chem. Soc.* 78:5871 5873 (1956).

Patton, J. S. Gastrointestinal lipid digestion. In *Physiology of the Gastrointestinal Tract*, Vol. 2, pp. 1123–1146, L. R. Johnson, Ed., Raven Press, New York (1981).

Patton, S. Milk. *Sci. Am.* 221(1):58–68 (1969).

Paul, A. A. and D. A. T. Southgate, Eds., McCance and Widdowson's "The Composition of Foods," 4th rev. ed., Elsevier North-Holland Biomedical Press, New York (1978).

Pauling, L. Orthomolecular psychiatry. *Science* 160:265–271 (1968).

Pauling, L. *Vitamin C and the Common Cold,* W. H. Freeman & Co., San Francisco (1970).

Pauling, L. The significance of the evidence about ascorbic acid and the common cold. *Proc. Nat. Acad. Sci. U. S.* 68:2678–2681 (1971).

Pauling L., R. B. Corey, and H. R. Branson. The structure of proteins: two hydrogen-bonded helical configurations of the polypeptide chain. *Proc. Nat. Acad. Sci. U. S.* 37:205–211 (1951).

Pauling, L., H. A. Itano, S. J. Singer, and I. C. Wells. Sickle cell anemia, a molecular disease. *Science* 110:543–548 (1949).

Pavlov, I. *The Work of the Digestive Glands.* (trans. W. H. Thompson), C. Griffin and Co., London (1910).

Payne, L. C. and C. L. Marsh. Absorption of gamma globulin by the small intestine. *Fed. Proc.* 21:909–912 (1962).

Pearson, W. N. Biochemical appraisal of the vitamin nutritional status in man. *JAMA* 180:49–55 (1962).

Pearson, W. N. Blood and urinary vitamin levels as potential indices of body stores. *Am. J. Clin Nutr.* 20:514–525 (1967).

Pearson, W. N. Thiamine. In *The Vitamins*, Vol. 7, 2nd ed., p. 53, Academic Press, New York (1967).

Pearse, B. M. F. and M. S. Bretscher. Membrane recycling by coated vesicles. *Ann. Rev. Biochem.* 50:85–101 (1981).

Peart, W. S. Renin-angiotensin system. *N. Engl. J. Med.* 292:302–306 (1975).

Pease, B. Coated vesicles. *Trends Biochem. Sci.* 5:131–134 (1980).

Pekkarinen, M. Methodology in the collection of food consumption data. *World Rev. Nutr. Diet.* 12:145–171 (1970).

Pellett, P. L. Protein quality evaluation revisited. *Food Technol.* 32(5):60–78 (1978).

Pellett, P. L. and V. R. Young, Eds., *Nutritional evaluation of protein foods.* (WHTR·3/UNUP 129), United Nations University Tokyo (1981).

Pennington, J. Considerations for a new food guide. *J. Nutr. Educ.* 13:53–55 (1981).

Pennington, J.A.T. Development of shortened food data bases. In *Proceedings of the Symposium on Dietary Data Collection, Analysis, and Significance,* pp. 65–72, V. A. Beal and M. J. Laus, Eds., Massachusetts Agr. Exp. Sta. Res. Bull. No. 675, Amherst (1982).

Peppler, W. W. and R. B. Mazess. Total body bone mineral and lean body mass by dual-photon absorptiometry. I. Theory and measurement procedure. *Calcif. Tissue Int.* 33:353–359 (1981).

Peraino, C. and A. E. Harper. Concentrations of free amino acids in blood plasma of rats force-fed L-glutamic acid, L-glutamine or L-alanine. *Arch. Biochem. Biophys.* 97:442–448 (1962).

Pereira, S. M., A. Begum, T. Isaac, and M. E. Dumm. Vitamin A therapy in children with kwashiorkor. *Am. J. Clin. Nutr.* 20:297–304 (1967).

Persson, B., P. Björntorp, and B. Hood. Lipoprotein lipase activity in human adipose tissue. I. Conditions for release and relationship to triglycerides in serum. *Metabolism* 15:730–741 (1966).

Persson, B., R. Tunell, and K. Ekengren. Chronic vitamin A intoxication during the first half year of life. *Acta Pediatr. Scand.* 54:49–60 (1965).

Peterkofsky, B. and S. Udenfriend. Enzymatic hydroxylation of proline in microsomal polypeptides leading to formation of collagen. *Proc. Nat. Acad. Sci. U. S.* 53:335–342 (1965).

Petermann, M. L. How does a ribosome translate linear genetic information? *Subcell Biochem.* 1:67–73 (1971).

Peters, A., S. L. Palay, and H. deF. Webster. *The Fine Structure of the Nervous System. The Cells and Their Processes,* Hoeber, New York (1970).

Peters, J. P., D. M. Kydd, and P. H. Lavietes. A note on the calculation of water exchange. *J. Clin. Invest.* 12:689–693 (1933).

Peters, R. A. The biochemical lesion in vitamin B deficiency. Application of modern biochemical analysis in its diagnosis. *Lancet* 1:1161–1165 (1936).

Peters, R. A., K. H. Coward, H. A. Krebs, L. W. Mapson, L. G. Parson, B. S. Platt, J. C. Spence, and J. R. P. O'Brien (Accessory Food Factors Subcommittee of the British Medical Research Council) Vitamin C requirement of human adults. *Lancet* 1:853–860 (1948).

Peters, T. The biosynthesis of rat serum albumin. *J. Biol. Chem.* 237:1181–1185 (1962).

Petith, M. and H. P. Schedl. Effects of semistarvation on large intestinal calcium transport: *in vivo* studies in the rat. *Am. J. Clin. Nutr.* 32:1006–1010 (1979).

Petith, M., H. D. Wilson, and H. P. Schedl. Vitamin D dependence of *in vivo* calcium transport and mucosal calcium binding protein in rat large intestine. *Gastroenterol.* 76:99–104 (1979).

Petrack, B., F. Sheppy, and V. Fetzer. Studies on tyrosine hydroxylase from bovine adrenal medulla. *J. Biol. Chem.* 243:743–748 (1968).

Pett, L. B. Vitamin requirements of human beings. *Vitam. Horm.* 13:213–237 (1955).

Pettijohn, D. and P. Hanawalt. Evidence for repair-replication of ultraviolet damaged DNA in bacteria. *J. Mol. Biol.* 9:395–410 (1964).

Pfaff, E. and M. Klingenberg. Adenine nucleotide translocation of mitochondria. I. Specificity and control *Eur. J. Biochem.* 6:66–79 (1968).

Pfiffner, J. J., D. G. Calkins, E. S. Bloom, and B. L. O'Dell. On the peptide nature of vitamin Bc conjugate from yeast. *J. Am. Chem. Soc.* 68:1392 (1946).

Phillips, M. I., W. E. Hoffman, and S. L. Bealer. Dehydration and fluid balance: central effects of angiotensin. *Fed. Proc.* 41:2520–2527 (1982).

Phillips, M. I., J. Weyhenmeyer, D. Felix, D. Ganten, and W. E. Hoffman. Evidence for an endogenous brain renin-angiotensin system. *Fed. Proc.* 38:2260–2266 (1979).

Phornplutkul, C., W. J. Gamble, and R. G. Monroe. Ventricular performance, coronary flow, and myocardial oxygen consumption in rats with advanced thiamin deficiency. *Am. J. Clin. Nutr.* 27:136–143 (1974).

Pierce, J. G. and T. F. Parsons. Glycoprotein hormones: structure and function. *Ann. Rev. Biochem.* 50:465–495 (1981).

Pike, R. L., J. E. Miles, and J. M. Wardlaw. Juxtaglomerular degranulation and zona glomerulosa exhaustion in pregnant rats induced by low sodium intakes and reversed by sodium load. *Am. J. Obstet. Gynecol.* 95:604–614 (1966).

Pike, R. L. and H. A. Smiciklas. A reappraisal of sodium restriction during pregnancy. *Int. J. Gynecol. Obstet.* 10:1–8 (1972).

Pimstone, B.L., M. Sheppard, B. Shapiro, S. Kronheim, A. Hudson, S. Hendricks, and K. Waligora. Localization in and release of somatostatin from brain and gut. *Fed. Proc.* 38:2330–2332 (1979).

Pincus, J. H., J. R. Cooper, J. V. Murphy, E. F. Rabe, D. Lonsdale, and H. G. Dunne. Thiamine derivatives in subacute necrotizing encephalomyelopathy. *Pediatr.* 51:716–721 (1973).

Pineda, O. B. T., F. E. Viteri, and G. Arroyave. Protein quality in relation to estimates of essential amino acids requirements, In *Protein Quality in Humans: Assessment and in Vitro Estimation,* pp. 29–42, C. E. Bodwell, J. S. Adkins, and D. T. Hopkins, Eds., AVI Publishing Co., Westport, Conn. (1981).

Pitts, G. C. and T. R. Bullard. Some interspecific aspects of body composition in mammals. In *Body Composition in Animals and Man,* pp. 45–70, (NAS Publication No. 1598), National Academy of Sciences Press, Washington, D.C. (1968)

Pitts, R. F. *Physiology of the Kidney and Body Fluids,* 2nd ed., Year Book Medical Publishers, Chicago (1968).

Platt, B. S. and D. S. Miller. The net dietary-protein value (N.D.p.v.) of mixtures of foods—its definition, determination and application. *Proc. Nutr. Soc.* 18:vii–viii (1959).

Platt, B. S., D. S. Miller, and P. R. Payne. Protein value of human foods. In *Recent Advances in Human Nutrition,* pp. 351–360, J. F. Brock, Ed., Churchhill, London (1961).

Playoust, M. R. and K. J. Isselbacher. Studies on the transport and metabolism of conjugated bile salts by intestinal mucosa. *J Clin. Invest.* 43:467–476 (1964).

Plotkin, G. R. and K. J. Isselbacher. Secondary disaccharidase deficiency in adult celiac disease (non-tropical sprue) and other malabsorption states. *N. Engl. J. Med.* 271:1033–1037 (1964).

Plough, I. C. and E. B. Bridgforth. Relation of clinical and dietary findings in nutrition surveys. *Public Health Rpt.* 75:699–706 (1960).

Polansky, M. Microbiological assay of vitamin B-6 in foods. In *Methods in Vitamin B-6 Nutrition. Analysis and Status Assessment,* pp. 21–44, J. E. Leklem and R. D. Reynolds, Eds., Plenum, New York (1980).

Polin, D., E. R. Wynosky, and C. C. Porter. Studies on the absorption of amprolium and thiamine in laying hens. *Poult. Sci.* 42:1057–1061 (1963).

Pollack, H., C. F. Consolazio, and G. J. Isaac. Metabolic demands as a factor in weight control. *JAMA* 167:216–219 (1958).

Pollack, S. and T. Campana. The relationship between mucosal iron and iron absorption in the guinea pig. *Scand. J. Haematol.* 7:208–211 (1970).

Pollack, S. and F. D. Lasky. A new iron binding protein in intestinal mucosa. In *Proteins of Iron Storage and Transport in Biochemistry and Medicine,* pp. 389–393, R. R. Crichton, Ed., North-Holland Publishing Co., Amsterdam (1975).

Pollak, P. I. Thiamine. *Encycl. Chem. Technol.* 20:173–193 (1969).

Pollock, H. Creatinine excretion as index for estimating urinary excretion of micronutrients or their metabolic end products. *Am. J. Clin. Nutr.* 23:865–867 (1970).

Pollock, M. I., A. Jackson, J. Ayres, A. Ward, A. C. Linnerud, and L. R. Gettman. Body composition of elite class distance runners. *Ann. N. Y. Acad. Sci.* 301:361–370 (1977).

Poppendiek, H. F. and G. L. Hody. Design considerations and applications of gradient layer calorimeters for use in biological heat production measurement. In *Temperature—Its Measurement and Control in Science and Industry,* Vol. 4., pp. 2079–2088, H. H. Plumb, Ed., Instrument Society of America, Pittsburgh (1972).

Pories, W. J., J. H. Henzel, C. C. Rob, and W. H. Strain. Acceleration of wound healing in man with zinc sulfate given by mouth. *Lancet* 1:121–124 (1967).

Porte, D., Jr., and J. B. Halter. The endocrine pancreas and diabetes mellitus. In

Textbook of Endocrinology, 6th ed., pp. 716–843, R. H. Williams, Ed., W. B. Saunders Co., Philadelphia (1981).

Porter, K. R. The endoplasmic reticulum: some current interpretations of its forms and functions. In *Biological Structure and Function,* Vol. 1, pp. 127–155, T. W. Goodwin and O. Lindberg, Eds., Academic Press, London (1961a).

Porter, K. R. The ground substance: observations from electron microscopy. In *The Cell,* Vol. 2, pp. 621–675, J. Brachet and A. E. Mirsky, Eds., Academic Press, New York (1961b).

Porter, K. R., A. Claude, and E. F. Fullam. A study of tissue culture cells by electron microscopy. Methods and preliminary observations. *J. Exp. Med.* 81:233–246 (1945).

Posner, A. S. Relationship between diet and bone mineral ultrastructure. *Fed. Proc.* 26:1717–1722 (1967).

Posner, A. S. Crystal chemistry of bone mineral. *Physiol. Rev.* 49:760–792 (1969).

Posner, A. S. Bone mineral on the molecular level. *Fed. Proc.* 32:1933–1937 (1973).

Poston, J. M. Cobalamin-dependent formation of leucine and β-leucine by rat and human tissue. *J. Biol. Chem.* 255:10067–10072 (1980).

Potter, J. O., S. P. Robertson, and J. D. Johnson. Magnesium and the regulation of muscle contraction. *Fed. Proc.* 40:2653–2656 (1981).

Potter, L. T. Storage of norepinephrine in sympathetic nerves. *Pharmacol. Rev.* 18:439–451 (1966).

Potts, J. T., Jr. Polypeptide hormones and calcium metabolism. *Ann. Intern. Med.* 70:1243–1265 (1969).

Potts, J. T., Jr. Recent advances in thyrocalcitonin research. *Fed. Proc.* 29:1200–1205 (1970).

Potts, J. T., Jr., H. B. Brewer, Jr., R. A. Reisfeld, P. F. Hirsch, R. Schlester, and P. L. Munson. Isolation and chemical properties of porcine thyrocalcitonin. In *Parathyroid Hormone and Thyrocalcitonin (Calcitonin),* pp. 54–67, R. V. Talmage and L. F. Belanger, Eds., Excerpta Medica Foundation, Amsterdam (1968).

Potts, J. T., Jr., H. D. Niall, H. T. Keutmann, H. B. Brewer, and L. J. Deftos. The amino acid sequence of porcine thyrocalcitonin. *Proc. Nat. Acad. Sci. U. S.* 59:1321–1328 (1968).

Prasad, A. S. Zinc in human nutrition. *CRC Crit. Rev. Clin. Lab. Sci.* 8:1–80 (1977).

Prasad, A. S., A. R. Schulert, A. Miale, Z. Farid, and H. H. Sandstead. Zinc and iron deficiencies in male subjects with dwarfism and hypogonadism but without ancylostomiasis, schistosomiasis or severe anemia. *Am. J. Clin. Nutr.* 12:437–444 (1963).

Prasad, A. S., G. J. Brewer, E. B. Schoomaker, and P. Rabbini. Hypocupremia induced by zinc therapy. JAMA 240:2166–2168 (1978).

Primosigh, J. V. and E. D. Thomas. Studies on the partition of iron in bone marrow cells. *J. Clin. Invest.* 47:1473–1482 (1968).

Prockop, D. J. Role of iron in the synthesis of collagen in connective tissue. *Fed. Proc.* 30:984–990 (1971).

Prockop, D. J. and K. Juva. Synthesis of hydroxyproline *in vitro* by the hydroxylation of proline in a precursor of collagen. *Proc. Nat. Acad. Sci. U. S.* 53:661–668 (1965).

Prockop, D. J., A. Kaplan, and S. Udenfriend. Cofactor requirements of the O-demethylating liver microsomal enzyme system. *Arch. Biochem. Biophys.* 101:494–503 (1963).

Protein Advisory Group. *Milk Intolerance—Nutritional Implications* (Report on the PAG *ad hoc* working group meeting, United Nations System, Document 1.27/9) (1972).

Prunier, J. H., A. G. Bearn, and H. Cleve. Site of formation of group-specific component and certain other serum proteins. *Proc. Soc. Exp. Biol. Med.* 115:1005–1007 (1964).

Prusiner, S. B., B. Cannon, T. M. Ching, and O. Lindberg. Oxidative metabolism in cells isolated from brown adipose tissue. II. Catecholamine regulated respiratory control. *Eur. J. Biochem.* 7:51–57 (1968).

Pryor, W. A. Free radical reactions and their importance in biochemical systems. *Fed. Proc.* 32:1862–1869 (1973).

Prystowsky, J. H., J. E. Smith, and D. S. Goodman. Retinyl palmitate hydrolase activity in normal rat liver. *J. Biol. Chem.* 256:4498–4503 (1981).

Ptashne, M. Isolation of the λ phage repressor. *Proc. Nat. Acad. Sci. U. S.* 57:306–313 (1967).

Purdy, R. H., K. A. Woeber, M. T. Holloway, and S. H. Ingbar. Preparation of crystalline thyroxine-binding prealbumin from human plasma. *Biochem.* 4:1888–1895 (1965).

Puszkin, S. and S. Berl. Actin-like properties of colchicine binding protein isolated from brain. *Nature* 225:558–559 (1970).

Puszkin, S., S. Berl, E. Puszkin, and D. D. Clarke. Actomyosin-like protein isolated from mammalian brain. *Science* 161:170–171 (1968).

Quaife, M. L. and P. L. Harris. Chemical assay of foods for vitamin E content. *Anal. Chem.* 20:1221–1224 (1948).

Quick, A. J. *Hemorrhagic Diseases,* Lea & Febiger, Philadelphia (1957).

Quill, H. and G. Wolf. Formation of α-1, 2- and α-1, 3-linked mannose disaccharides from mannosyl retinyl phosphate by rat liver membrane enzymes. *Ann. N. Y. Acad. Sci.* 359:331–344 (1981).

Rabinowitz, J. C. and E. E. Snell. The vitamin B_6 group. XIV. Distribution of pyridoxal, pyridoxamine and pyridoxine in some natural products. *J. Biol. Chem.* 176:1157–1167 (1948).

Racker, E. Resolution and reconstruction of the inner mitochondrial membrane. *Fed. Proc.* 26:1335–1340 (1967).

Racker, E. The membrane of the mitochondrion. *Sci. Am.* 218(2):32–39 (1968).

Racker, E. From Pasteur to Mitchell: a hundred years of bioenergetics. *Fed Proc.* 39:210–215 (1980).

Radda, G. K. and P. T. Seely. Recent studies on cellular metabolism by nuclear magnetic resonance. *Ann. Rev. Physiol.* 41:744–769 (1979).

Raff, R. A. and H. R. Mahler. The nonsymbiotic origin of mitochondria. *Science* 177:575–582 (1972).

Raffin. S. B., C. H. Woo, K. T. Roost, D. C. Price, and R. Schmid. Intestinal absorption of hemoglobin iron-heme cleavage by mucosal heme oxygenase. *J. Clin. Invest.* 54:1344–1352 (1974).

Rahn, H. Acid-base balance and the milieu intérieur. In *Claude Bernard and the Internal Environment,* pp. 179–190, E. D. Robin, Ed., Marcel Dekker Inc., New York (1979).

Rahn, H. and B. J. Howell. The OH^-/H^+ concept of acid-base balance. Historical development. *Respir. Physiol.* 33:91–97 (1978).

Rahn, H., R. B. Reeves, and B. J. Howell. Hydrogen ion regulation temperature, and evolution. *Am. Rev. Respir. Dis.* 112:165–172 (1975).

Raica, N., Jr., and H. E. Sauberlich. Blood cell transaminase activity in human vitamin B_6 deficiency. *Am. J. Clin. Nutr.* 15:67–72 (1964).

Rajagopalan, K. V., J. L. Johnson, and B. E. Hainline. The pterin of the molybdenum cofactor. *Fed. Proc.* 41:2608–2612 (1982).

Rambourg, A., W. Hernandez, and C. P. Leblond. Detection of complex carbohydrates in the Golgi apparatus of rat cells. *J. Cell Biol.* 40:395–414 (1969).

Rambourg, A. and C. P. Leblond. Electron microscopic observations of the carbohydrate rich cell coat present at the surface of cells in the rat. *J. Cell Biol.* 32:27–53 (1967).

Randall, H. T. Water, electrolytes, and acid-base balance. In *Modern Nutrition in Health and Disease,* 6th ed., pp. 355–394, R. S. Goodhart and M. E. Shils, Eds., Lea & Febiger, Philadelphia (1980).

Ransome-Kuti, O., N. Kretchmer, J. D. Johnson, and J. T. Gribble. A genetic study of lactose digestion in Nigerian families. *Gastroenterol.* 68:431–436 (1975).

Rasmussen, H., J. Feinblatt, N. Nagata, and M. Pechet. Effect of ions upon bone cell function. *Fed. Proc.* 29:1190–1197 (1970).

Rasmussen, H., T. Matsumoto, O. Fontaine, and D. Goodman. Role of changes in membrane lipid structure in the action of 1,25-dihydroxyvitamin D_3. *Fed. Proc.* 41:72–77 (1982).

Rasmussen, H. and N. Nagata. Renal gluconeogenesis: effects of parathyroid hormone and dibutyryl 3′,5′-AMP. *Biochim Biophys. Acta* 215:17–28 (1970).

Rasmussen, H., M. Wong, D. Bikle, and D. B. P. Goodman. Hormonal control of the renal conversion of 25-hydroxycholecalciferol to 1,25-dihydroxycholecalciferol. *J. Clin. Invest.* 51:2502–2504 (1972).

Rathbun, E. N. and N. Pace. Studies on body composition. I. The determination of total body fat by means of the body specific gravity. *J. Biol. Chem.* 158:667–676 (1945).

Raven, P. H. A multiple origin for plastids and mitochondria. *Science* 169:641–646 (1970).

Raychaudhuri, C. and I. D. Desai. Ceroid pigment formation and irreversible sterility in vitamin E deficiency. *Science* 173:1028–1029 (1971).

Reba, R. C., F. C. Leitnaker, and K. T. Woodward. In *Human Growth*, pp. 674–681, D. B. Cheek, Ed., Lea & Febiger, Philadelphia (1968).

Reddy, S. K., M. S. Reynolds, and J. M. Price. The determination of 4-pyridoxic acid in human urine. *J. Biol. Chem.* 233:691–696 (1958).

Reeves, R. B. An imidazole alphastat hypothesis for vertebrate acid-base regulation. *Respir. Physiol.* 14:219–236 (1972).

Regnault, H. W. and J. Reiset. Recherches chimiques sur la respiration des animaux des diverses classes. *Ann. Chim. Phys.* 26:(Ser. 3)299–519 (1849).

Reh, E. *Manual on household food consumption surveys* (FAO Nutritional Studies No. 18). FAO, Rome (1962).

Reid, E. W. Intestinal absorption of solutions. *J. Physiol.* (*London*) 28:241–256 (1902).

Reid, I. A. The brain renin-angiotensin system: a critical analysis. *Fed. Proc.* 38:2255–2259 (1979).

Reid, I. A., B. J. Morris, and W. F. Ganong. The renin-angiotensin system. *Ann. Rev. Physiol.* 40:377–410 (1978).

Reinhold, J. G., K. Nasr, A. Lahimgarzadeh, and H. Hedayati. Effects of purified phytate and phytate-rich bread upon metabolism of zinc, calcium, phosphorus and nitrogen in man. *Lancet* 1:283–288 (1973).

Reinhold, J. G., J. Salvador, and L. Garcia. Binding of iron by fiber of wheat and maize. *Am. J. Clin. Nutr.* 34:1384–1391 (1981).

Reisenauer, A. M., C. L. Krumdieck, and C. H. Halsted. Folate conjugase: two separate activities in human jejunum. *Science* 198:196–197 (1977).

Reiser, S. and P. A. Christiansen. Intestinal transport of amino acids studied with L-valine. *Am. J. Physiol.* 208:914–921 (1965).

Reissmann, K. R. Studies on the mechanism of erythropoietic stimulation in parabiotic rats during hypoxia. *Blood* 5:372–380 (1950).

Reizenstein, P. G. Excretion of non-labeled vitamin B_{12} in man. *Acta Med. Scand.* 165:313–320 (1959).

Rendi, R. On the occurrence of intramitochondrial RNA particles. *Exp. Cell Res.* 17:585–587 (1959).

Rennke, H. G. and M. A. Venkatachalam. Structural determinants of glomerular permselectivity. *Fed. Proc.* 36:2619–2626 (1977).

Report of Inter-Society Commission for Heart Disease Resources. *Primary Prevention of the Atherosclerotic Diseases.* XLII. Circulation A55–A94 (1970).

Reutter, F. W., R. Siebenmann, and M. Pajarola. Fluoride in osteoporosis. In *Fluoride in Medicine,* pp. 143–152, T. L. Vischer, Ed., Hans Huber, Bern (1970).

Revel, J.-P. and S. Ito. The surface components of cells. In *The Specificity of Cell Surfaces,* pp. 211–234, B. D. Davis and L. Warren, Eds., Prentice-Hall Inc., Englewood Cliffs, N.J. (1967).

Revel, M., M. Herzberg, A. Becarevic, and F. Gros. Role of protein factor in the functional binding of ribosomes to natural messenger RNA. *J. Mol. Biol.* 33:231–249 (1968).

Rhoads, R. E. and S. Udenfriend. Decarboxylation of α-ketoglutarate coupled to collagen proline hydroxylase. *Proc. Nat. Acad. Sci. U. S.* 60:1473–1478 (1968).

Riccio, P., H. Aquila, and M. Klingenberg. Purification of the carboxy-atractylate binding protein from mitochondria. *FEBS Lett.* 56:132–138 (1975).

Rich, C. and E. Feist. The action of fluoride on bone. In *Fluoride in Medicine,* pp. 70–87, T. L. Vischer, Ed., Hans Huber, Bern (1970).

Richardson, T., A. L. Tappel, and E. R. Gruger, Jr. Essential fatty acids in mitochondria. *Arch. Biochem. Biophys.* 94:1–6 (1961).

Richardson, T., A. L. Tappel, L. M. Smith, and C. R. Houle. Polyunsaturated fatty acids in mitochondria. *J. Lipid Res.* 3:344–350 (1962).

Rickes, E. L., N. G. Brink, F. R. Koniuszy, T. R. Wood, and K. Folkers. Crystalline vitamin B_{12}. *Science* 107:396–397 (1948)

Riemann, W., C. Muir, and H. C. Macgregor. Sodium and potassium in oocytes of *Triturus cristatus. J. Cell. Sci.* 4:299–304 (1969).

Riklis, E. and J. H. Quastel. Effects of cations on sugar absorption by isolated surviving guinea pig intestine. *Can. J. Biochem. Physiol.* 36:347–362 (1958).

Rindi, G., L. de Giuseppe, and G. Sciorelli. Thiamine monophosphate, a normal constituent of rat plasma. *J. Nutr.* 94:447–454 (1968).

Rindi, G., G. Ferrari, U. Ventura, and A. Trotta. Action of amprolium on the thiamine content of rat tissues. *J. Nutr.* 89:197–202 (1966).

Rindi, G., U. Ventura, L. de Guiseppe, and G. Sciorelli. The phosphorylation of thiamine in the intestinal wall during absorption *in vitro. Experientia* 22:473–474 (1966).

Ringer, S. Further observations regarding the antagonism between calcium salts and sodium, potassium and ammonium salts. *J. Physiol. (London)* 18:425–429 (1895).

Ritchey, S. J. Metabolic patterns in preadolescent children. XV. Ascorbic acid intake, urinary excretion and serum concentration. *Am. J. Clin. Nutr.* 17:57–114 (1965).

Ritchie, A. K. and A. M. Goldberg. Vesicular and synaptoplasmic synthesis of acetylcholine. *Science* 173:489–490 (1970).

Ritchie, J. H., M. B. Fish, V. M. McMasters, and M. Grossman. Edema and hemolytic anemia in premature infants: a vitamin E deficiency syndrome. *N. Engl. J. Med.* 279:1185–1190 (1968).

Rivlin, R. S. Regulation of flavoprotein enzymes in hypothyroidism and in ribo-flavin deficiency. *Adv. Enzyme Regul.* 8:239–250 (1970).

Roberts, A. B. and H. F. DeLuca. Pathways of retinol and retinoic acid metabolism in the rat. *Biochem. J.* 102:600–610 (1967).

Roberts, A. B. and C. A. Frolik. Recent advances in the *in vivo* and *in vitro* metabolism of retinoic acid. *Fed. Proc.* 38:2524–2527 (1979).

Roberts, L. J. The beginnings of the recommended dietary allowances. *J. Am. Diet. Assoc.* 34:903–908 (1958).

Robertson, E. G. The natural history of oedema during pregnancy. *J. Obstet. Gynaecol. Br. Commonw.* 78:520–529 (1971).

Robertson, J. D. The ultrastructure of adult vertebrate peripheral myelinated nerve fibers in relation to myelinogenesis. *J. Biophys. Biochem. Cytol.* 1:271–278 (1955).

Robertson, J. D. The ultrastructure of cell membranes and their derivatives. *Biochem. Soc. Symp.* 16:3–43 (1959).

Robertson, J. D. The molecular structure and contact relationships of cell mem-branes. *Progr. Biophys. Chem.* 10:343–418 (1960).

Robertson, J. D. Cell membranes and the origin of mitochondria. *Regional Neu-rochemistry, Proceedings 4th International Neurochemical Symposium,* pp. 497–534, Pergamon Press, Oxford, (1960).

Robertson, W. B. and J. Hewitt. Augmentation of collagen synthesis by ascorbic acid *in vitro. Biochem. Biophys. Acta* 49:404–406 (1961).

Robin, E. D. Relationship between temperature and plasma pH and carbon diox-ide tension in the turtle. *Nature* 195:249–251 (1962).

Robin, E. D. Claude Bernard's (extended) milieu intérieur revisited. Autoregulation of cell and subcell integrity. *Clin. Sci. Mol. Med.* 52:443–448 (1977).

Robin, E. D. Limits of the internal environment. In *Claude Bernard and the Internal Environment,* pp. 257–267, E. D. Robin, Ed., Marcel Dekker Inc., New York (1979).

Robinson, F. A. *The Vitamin Co-factors of Enzyme Systems,* pp. 638–666, Per-gamon Press, New York (1966).

Robinson, J. and E. A. Newsholme. Glycerolkinase activities in rat heart and adipose tissue. *Biochem. J.* 104:2C–4C (1967).

Robison, G. A., R. W. Butcher, and E. W. Sutherland. Cyclic AMP. *Ann. Rev. Biochem.* 37:149–174 (1968).

Robison, G. A., R. W. Butcher, and E. W. Sutherland. *Cyclic AMP.* Academic Press, New York (1971)

Robison, G. A. and E. W. Sutherland. Cyclic AMP and the function of eukaryotic cells: an introduction. *Ann. N. Y. Acad. Sci.* 185:5–9 (1971).

Rodan, G. A. and T. J. Martin. Role of osteoblasts in hormonal control of bone resorption—a hypothesis. *Calcif. Tissue Int.* 33:349–351 (1981).

Rodbell, M. Metabolism of isolated fat cells. I. Effects of hormones on glucose metabolism and lipolysis. *J. Biol. Chem.* 239:375–380 (1964).

Rodbell, M. The problem of identifying the glucagon receptor. *Fed. Proc.* 32:1854–1858 (1973).

Rodbell, M. The actions of glucagon on the adenylate cyclase system. In *Glucagon: Physiology, Pathophysiology, and Morphology of the Pancreatic A-Cells,* pp. 177–193, R. H. Unger and L. Orci, Eds., Elsevier, New York (1981).

Rodgers, G. M., J. W. Fisher, and W. J. George. Increase in hematocrit, hemoglobin and red cell mass in normal mice after treatment with cyclic AMP. *Proc. Soc. Exp. Biol. Med.* 148:380–382 (1975)

Rodgers, G. M., W. J. George, and J. W. Fisher. Increased kidney cyclic AMP levels and erythropoietin production following cobalt administration. *Proc. Soc. Exp. Biol. Med.* 140:977–981 (1972).

Rodwell, V. W., D. J. McNamara, and D. J. Shapiro. Regulation of hepatic 3-hydroxy-3-methylglutaryl coenzyme A reductase. *Adv. Enzymol.* 38:373–412 (1973).

Roe, D. A. Nutrient toxicity with excessive intake. I. Vitamins. *N. Y. State J. Med.* 66:869–873 (1966).

Roels, O. A. The influence of vitamins A and E on lysosomes. In *Lysosomes in Biology and Pathology,* Vol. 1, pp. 254–275, J. T. Dingle and H. B. Fell, Eds., North-Holland Publishing Co., Amsterdam (1969).

Roels, O. A., S. Djaeni, M. R. Trout, T. G. Lauw, A. Heath, S. H. Poey, M. S. Tarwotjo, and B. Suhadi. The effect of protein and fat supplements on vitamin A-deficient Indonesian children. *Am. J. Clin. Nutr.* 12:380–387 (1963).

Roels, O. A., M. E. Trout, and R. Dujaquier. Carotene balances on boys in Ruanda where vitamin A deficiency is prevalent. *J. Nutr.* 65:115–127 (1958).

Roels, O. A., M. Trout, and A. Guha. Vitamin A deficiency and acid hydrolases: β-glycerophosphate phosphatase in rat liver. *Biochem. J.* 93:23c–25c (1964).

Roels, O. A., M. Trout, and A. Guha. The effect of vitamin A deficiency and dietary α-tocopherol on the stability of rat-liver lysosomes. *Biochem. J.* 97:353–359 (1965).

Rogers, E. F. Thiamine antagonists. In *Methods in Enzymology,* Vol. 18, Part A, pp. 245–258, D. B. McCormick, and L. D. Wright, Eds., Academic Press, New York (1970).

Rogers, W. E., Jr. Reexamination of enzyme activities thought to show evidence of a coenzyme role for vitamin A. *Am. J. Clin. Nutr.* 22:1003–1013 (1969).

Rolland-Cachera, M. F., M. Sempe, M. Giullaud-Bataille, E. Patois, F. Pequignot-Guggenbuhl, and V. Fautrad. Adiposity indices in children. *Am. J. Clin. Nutr.* 36:178–184 (1982).

Romslo, I. Intracellular transport of iron. In *Iron in Biochemistry and Medicine, II*, pp. 325–362, A. Jacobs and M. Worwood, Eds., Academic Press, London (1980).

Roncari, D. A. K. and C. H. Hollenberg. Esterification of free fatty acids by subcellular preparations of rat adipose tissue. *Biochim. Biophys. Acta* 137:446–463 (1967).

Rose, B. O. *Clinical Physiology of Acid-base and Electrolyte Disorders.* McGraw-Hill, New York (1977).

Rose, D. P. Effects of oral contraceptives on nutrient utilization. In *Nutrition and Drug Interrelations,* pp. 151–187. J. N. Hathcock and J. Coon, Eds., Academic Press, New York (1978a).

Rose, D. P. Oral contraceptives and vitamin B_6. In *Human Vitamin B_6 Requirements,* pp. 193–201. National Academy of Sciences, Washington, D.C. (1978b).

Rose, R. Water-soluble vitamin absorption in intestine. *Ann. Rev. Physiol.* 42:157–171 (1980).

Rose, R., M. Koch, and D. Nahrwold. Folic acid transport by mammalian small intestine. *Am. J. Physiol.* 235:E678–E685 (1978).

Rose, R. C. Intestinal absorption of water-soluble vitamins. In *Physiology of the Gastrointestinal Tract,* Vol. 2, pp. 1231–1242, L. R. Johnson, Ed., Raven Press, New York (1981).

Rose, R. C. Transport and metabolism of water-soluble vitamins in intestine. *Am. J. Physiol.* 240:G97–G101 (1981).

Rose, W. C. Introductory essay. In *An Experimental Inquiry into Principles of Nutrition and the Digestive Process,* J. R. Young, 1803. University of Illinois Press, Urbana (1959).

Rose, W. C., R. L. Wixon, H. B. Lockhart, and G. F. Lambert. The amino acid requirements of man. XV. The valine requirement: summary and final observations. *J. Biol. Chem.* 217:987–995 (1955).

Rosell, S., I. J. Kopin, and J. Axelrod. Fate of H^3-noradrenaline in skeletal muscle before and following sympathetic stimulation. *Am. J. Physiol.* 205:317–321 (1963).

Rosen, O. M. and E. G. Krebs, Eds. *Protein phosphorylation.* Cold Spring Harbor Laboratory, New York (1981).

Rosenberg, I. H. Intestinal absorption of folate. In *Physiology of the Gastrointestinal Tract,* Vol. 2, pp. 1221–1230, L. R. Johnson, Ed., Raven Press, New York (1981).

Rosenberg, I. H. and N. W. Solomons. Biological availability of minerals and trace elements: a nutritional overview. *Am. J. Clin. Nutr.* 35:781–782 (1982).

Rosenberg, I. H., R. R. Streiff, H. A. Godwin, and W. B. Castle. Absorption of polyglutamic folate: participation of deconjugating enzymes of the intestinal mucosa. *N. Engl. J. Med.* 280:985–988 (1969).

Rosenstreich, S. J., C. Rich, and W. Volwiler. Deposition in and release of vitamin

D₃ from body fat: evidence for a storage site in the rat. *J. Clin. Invest.* 50:679–687 (1971).

Rosensweig, N. S. and R. H. Herman. Control of jejunal sucrase and maltase activity by dietary sucrose or fructose in man. *J. Clin. Invest.* 47:2253–2262 (1968).

Rosenthal, H. L. and J. B. Allison. Some effects of caloric intake on nitrogen balance in dogs. *J. Nutr.* 44:423–431 (1951).

Ross, E. M. and A. G. Gilman. Biochemical properties of hormone-sensitive adenylate cyclase. *Ann. Rev. Biochem.* 49:533–564 (1980).

Ross Laboratories. *Assessment of Energy Metabolism in Health and Disease* (Report of the First Conference on Medical Research). Ross Laboratories, Columbus, Ohio (1980).

Ross, M. H. Length of life and caloric intake. *Am. J. Clin. Nutr.* 25:834–838 (1972).

Ross, R. Wound healing. *Sci. Am.* 220(6):40–50 (1969).

Rossmann, A. G., and P. Argos. Protein folding. *Ann. Rev. Biochem.* 50:497–532 (1981).

Rosso, P. Maternal malnutrition and placental transfer of α-amino isobutyric acid. *Science* 187:648–650 (1975).

Rosso, P., J. Hormazabal, and M. Winick. Changes in brain weight, cholesterol, phospholipid and DNA content in marasmic children. *Am. J. Clin. Nutr.* 23:1275–1279 (1970).

Roth, J., D. LeRoith, J. Shiloach, J. L. Rosenzweig, M. A. Lesniak, and J. Havrankova. The evolutionary origins of hormones, neurotransmitters, and other extracellular chemical messengers. Implications for mammalian biology. *N. Engl. J. Med.* 306:523–527 (1982).

Roth, R. A. and D. J. Cassell. Insulin receptor: evidence that it is a protein kinase. *Science* 219:299–301 (1983).

Rothenberg, S. P. Assay of serum vitamin B-12 concentration using $^{57}CoB_{12}$ and intrinsic factor. *Proc. Soc. Exp. Biol. Med.* 108:45–48 (1961).

Rothenberg, S. P. Identification of a macromolecular factor in the ileum which binds intrinsic factor and immunologic identification of intrinsic factor in ileal extracts. *J. Clin. Invest.* 47:913–923 (1968).

Rothman, J. E. and J. Lenard. Membrane asymmetry. *Science* 195:743–753 (1977).

Rothman, S. S. The digestive enzymes of the pancreas: a mixture of inconstant proportions. *Ann. Rev. Physiol.* 39:373–389 (1977).

Rothschild, J. The isolation of microsomal membranes. In *The Structure and Function of the Membranes and Surfaces of Cells*, pp. 4–31, (Biochemical Society Symposium 22) (1963).

Rothschild, M. A., M. Oratz, J. Mongelli, L. Fishman, and S. S. Schreiber. Amino acid regulation of albumin synthesis. *J. Nutr.* 98:395–403 (1969).

Roy, S., III, and B. S. Arant, Jr. Alkalosis from chloride-deficient neo-mull-soy. *N. Engl. J. Med.* 301:615 (1979).

Rubin, W. The epithelial "membrane" of the small intestine. *Am. J. Clin. Nutr.* 24:45–64 (1971).

Rubner, M. *Die Gesetze des Energieverbrauchs bei der Ernahrung.* Deuticke, Leipzig and Vienna (1902).

Rucker, R. B. and J. Murray. Cross-linking amino acids in collagen and elastin. *Am. J. Clin. Nutr.* 31:1221–1236 (1978).

Rude, R. K. and F. R. Singer. Magnesium deficiency and excess. *Ann. Rev. Med.* 32:245–249 (1981).

Rude, S., R. E. Coggeshall, and L. S. Van Orden. Chemical and ultrastructural identification of 5-hydroxytryptamine in an identified neuron. *J. Cell Biol.* 41:832–854 (1969).

Ruderman, N. B., M. N. Goodman, M. Berger, and S. Hagg. Effect of starvation on muscle glucose metabolism: studies with the isolated perfused rat hindquarter. *Fed. Proc.* 36:171–176 (1977).

Rudick, M. J. and H. D. Janowitz. Gastric physiology. In *Gastroenterology*, 3rd ed., Vol. 1, pp. 405–418, H. L. Bockus, Ed., W. B. Saunders Co., Philadelphia (1974).

Rupp, W. D. and P. Howard-Flanders. Discontinuities in the DNA synthesized in an excision-defective strain of *Escherichia coli* following ultraviolet irradiation. *J. Mol. Biol.* 31:291–304 (1968).

Rupp, W. D., C. E. Wilde, III, D. L. Reno, and P. Howard-Flanders. Exchanges between DNA strands in ultraviolet-irradiated *Escherichia coli. J. Mol. Biol.* 61:25–44 (1971).

Rushmer, R. F. *Cardiovascular Dynamics*, 2nd ed., W. B. Saunders Co., Philadelphia (1961).

Saarinen, U. M., M. A. Siimes, and P. R. Dallman. Iron absorption in infants: high bioavailability of breast milk iron as indicated by the extrinsic tag method of iron absorption and by the concentration of serum ferritin. *J. Pediatr.* 91:36–39 (1977).

Sabatini, D. D., K. Bensch, and R. J. Barnett. Cytochemistry and electron microscopy. The preservation of cellular ultrastucture and enzymatic activity by aldehyde fixation. *J. Cell Biol.* 17:19–58 (1963).

Sabatini, D. D., G. Blobel, Y. Nonomura, and M. R. Adelman. Ribosome-membrane interaction: structural aspects and functional implications. *Adv. Cytopharmacol.* 1:119–129 (1971).

Sabatini, D. D., Y. Tashiro, and G. E. Palade. On the attachment of ribosomes to microsomal membranes. *J. Mol. Biol.* 19:503–524 (1966).

Saffiotti, V., R. Montesano, R. Sellakumar, and S. A. Borg. Experimental cancer of the lung. Inhibition by vitamin A of tracheobronchial squamous metaplasia and squamous cell tumors. *Cancer* 20:857–864 (1967).

Said, A. K. and D. M. Hegsted. Evaluation of dietary protein quality in adult rats. *J. Nutr.* 99:474–480 (1969).

Salans, L. B., C. A. Bray, S. W. Cushman, E. Danforth, Jr., J. A. Glennon, E. S. Horton, and E. A. H. Sims. Glucose metabolism and the response to insulin by human adipose tissue in spontaneous and experimental obesity. Effects of dietary composition and adipose cell size. *J. Clin. Invest.* 53:848–856 (1974).

Salans, L. B., E. S. Horton, and E. A. H. Sims. Experimental obesity in man: cellular character of the adipose tissue. *J. Clin. Invest.* 50:1005–1011 (1971).

Salans, L. B., J. L. Knittle, and J. Hirsch. The role of adipose cell size and adipose tissue insulin sensitivity in the carbohydrate intolerance of human obesity. *J. Clin. Invest.* 47:153–165 (1968).

Salemme, F. R. Structure and function of cytochrome c. *Ann. Rev. Biochem.* 46:299–329 (1977).

Salyers, A. A. Energy sources of major intestinal fermentative anaerobes. *Am. J. Clin. Nutr.* 32:158–163 (1979).

Samonds, K. W. Computerization of nutrient data for dietary evaluation. In *Proceedings of the Symposium on Dietary Data Collection, Analysis and Significance*, pp. 50–58, V. A. Beal and M. J. Laus, Eds., Massachusetts Agri. Exp. Sta. Res. Bull. No. 675, Amherst (1982).

Sampson, H. W., J. L. Matthews, J. H. Martin, and A. S. Kunin. An electron microscopic localization of calcium in the small intestine of normal, rachitic and vitamin D-treated rats. *Calcif. Tissue Res.* 5:305–316 (1970).

Samuelsson, B., P. Borgeat, S. Hammarström, and R. C. Murphy. Leukotrienes: a new group of biologically active compounds. In *Advances in Prostaglandin and Thromboxane Research*, Vol. 6, pp. 1–18, B. Samuelsson, P. W. Ramswell, and R. Paoletti, Eds., Raven Press, New York (1980).

Samuelsson, B., M. Goldyne, E. Grandström, M. Hamberg, S. Hammarström, and C. Malmsten. Prostaglandins and thromboxanes. *Ann. Rev. Biochem.* 47:997–1029 (1978).

Samuelsson, B., E. Granström, K. Green, M. Hamberg, S. Hammarström, and C. Malmsten. Prostaglandins. *Ann. Rev. Biochem.* 44:669–695 (1975).

Sandell, E. B. *Colorimetric Determination of Traces of Metals.* Interscience, New York (1959).

Sander, J. E., S. Packman, and J. J. Townsend. Brain pyruvate carboxylase and the pathophysiology of biotin-dependent diseases. *Neurology (Minneap.)* 32:878–880 (1982).

Sandhu, J. S. and D. R. Fraser. Measurement of niacin metabolites in urine by high pressure liquid chromatography. A simple sensitive assay of niacin nutritional status. *Int. J. Nutr. Res.* 51:139–144 (1981).

Sandiford, I. and T. Wheeler. The basal metabolism before, during and after pregnancy. *J. Biol. Chem.* 62:329–352 (1924).

Sandstead, H. H. Zinc in human nutrition. In *Disorders of Mineral Metabolism,*

Vol. 1, pp.93–157, F. Bronner and J. Coburn, Eds., Academic Press, New York (1981).

Sandstead, H. H. Copper bioavailability and requirements. *Am. J. Clin. Nutr.*35:809–814 (1982).

Sandstead, H. H., R. F. Burk, G. H. Booth, and W. J. Darby. Current concepts on trace minerals. Clinical considerations. *Med. Clin. North Am.* 54:1509–1531 (1970).

Sandstead, H. H., K. P. Vo-Khactu, and N. Solomons. Conditioned zinc deficiency. In *Trace Elements in Human Health and Diseases*, Vol. 1, pp. 33–49, A. Prasad, Ed., Academic Press, New York (1976).

Sanghvi, R. S., R. M. Lemons, H. Baker, and J. G. Thoene. A simple method for determination of plasma and urinary biotin. *Clin. Chem. Acta* 124:85–90 (1982).

Santayana, G. *The Life Of Reason*, Vol. 1, Charles Scribner's Sons, New York (1905–1906).

Sarett, H. P. The metabolism of pantothenic acid and its lactone moiety in man. *J. Biol. Chem.* 159:321–325 (1945).

Sargent, F., II, and K. P. Weinman. Physiological individuality. *Ann N. Y. Acad. Sci.* 134:696–720 (1966).

Sarton, G. *The History of Science and the New Humanism*, George Braziller Inc., New York (1956).

Satterlee, L. D. *New concepts for the rapid development of protein quality*. University of Nebraska and National Science Foundation, Washington, D.C. (1977).

Satterlee, L. D., J. G. Kendrick, D. K. Jewell, and W. D. Brown. In *Protein Quality in Humans: Assessment and in Vitro Estimations*, pp. 316–338, C. E. Bodwell, J. S. Adkins and D. T. Hopkins, Eds., AVI Publishing Co., Westport, Conn. (1981).

Satterlee, L. D., H. F. Marshall, and J. M. Tennyson. Measuring protein quality. *J. Am. Oil Chem. Soc.* 56:103–109 (1979).

Sauberlich, H. E. Vitamin B_6 group. VIII. Active compounds and antagonists. In *The Vitamins*, Vol. 2, pp.33–44, W. H. Sebrell, Jr. and R. S. Harris, Eds., Academic Press, New York (1968).

Sauberlich, H. E. Ascorbic acid (vitamin C). *Clin. Lab. Med.* 1:673–684 (1981).

Sauberlich, H. E., J. E. Canham, E. M. Baker, N. Raica, Jr., and Y. F. Herman. Human vitamin B_6 nutriture. *J. Sci. Ind. Res.* 29:S28–S37 (1970).

Sauberlich, H. E., J. E. Canham, E. M. Baker, N. Raica, Jr., and Y. F. Herman. Biochemical assessment of the nutritional status of vitamin B_6 in the human. *Am. J. Clin. Nutr.* 25:629–642 (1972a).

Sauberlich, H. E., R. P. Dowdy, and J. H. Skala. *Laboratory Tests for the Assessment of Nutritional Status* (Critical Reviews in Clinical Laboratory Sciences, Vol. 4, Issue 3), CRC Press, Cleveland (1973).

Sauberlich, H. E., M. D. Green, and S. T. Omaye. Determination of ascorbic acid and dehydroascorbic acid. In *Ascorbic Acid: Chemistry, Metabolism, and*

Uses, pp. 199–221, P. A. Seib and B. M. Tolbert, Eds. (Advances in Chemistry Series 200), American Chemical Society, Washington, D.C. (1981).

Sauberlich, H. E., Y. F. Herman, C. O. Stevens, and R. H. Herman. Thiamin requirement of the adult human. *Am. J. Clin. Nutr.* 32:2237–2248 (1979).

Sauberlich, H. E., J. H. Judd, G. E. Nichoalds, H. P. Broquist, and W. J. Darby. Application of the erythrocyte glutathione reductase assay in evaluating riboflavin nutritional status in a high school student population. *Am. J. Clin. Nutr.* 25:756–762 (1972b).

Savin, M. A. and J. D. Cook. Mucosal iron transport by rat intestine. *Blood* 56:1029–1035 (1980).

Scanu, A. M., P. Lagocki, and J. Chung. Effect of apoprotein A-II on the structure of high density lipoproteins: relation to the activity of lecithin-cholesterol acyl transferase *in vitro*. *Ann. N. Y. Acad. Sci.* 348:160–171 (1980).

Scanu, A. M. and F. R. Landsberger, Eds., *Lipoprotein structure*. N. Y. Academy of Sciences, New York (1980).

Schachter, D., E. B. Dowdle, and H. Schanker. Active transport of calcium by the small intestine of the rat. *Am. J. Physiol.* 198:263–268 (1960).

Schachter, D., J. D. Finkelstein, and S. Kowarski. Metabolism of vitamin D. I. Preparation of radioactive vitamin D and its absorption in the rat. *J. Clin. Invest.* 43:787–796 (1964).

Schachter, D. and S. Kowarski. IMCal: Vitamin D-dependent membrane component of the intestinal calcium transport mechanism. In *Calcium and Phosphate Transport Across Biomembranes*, pp. 155–158, F. Bronner and M. Peterlik, Eds., Academic Press, New York (1981).

Schachter, D. and S. Kowarski. Isolation of the protein IMCal, a vitamin D-dependent membrane component of the intestinal transport mechanism for calcium. *Fed. Proc.* 41:84–87 (1982).

Schachter, D., S. Kowarski, and P. Reid. Molecular basis for vitamin D action in the small intestine. *J. Clin. Invest.* 46:1113–1114 (1967).

Schachter, D. and S. M. Rosen. Active transport of Ca^{45} by the small intestine and its dependence on vitamin D. *Am. J. Physiol.* 196:357–362 (1959).

Schade, S. G., R. J. Cohen, and M. E. Conrad. Effect of hydrochloric acid on iron absorption. *N. Engl. J. Med.* 279:672–674 (1968).

Schade, S. G., B. F. Felsher, G. M. Bernier, and M. E. Conrad. Interrelationship of cobalt and iron absorption. *J. Lab. Clin. Med.* 75:435–441 (1970).

Schaeffer, E. S. and M. Aaronson. Infant education research project: implementation and implication of a home tutoring program. In *The Preschool in Action: Exploring Early Childhood Programs*, pp. 410–434, R. K. Parker, Ed., Allyn & Bacon, Boston (1972).

Schatz, G. Biogenesis of mitochondria. In *Membranes of Mitochondria and Chloroplasts*, pp. 251–314, E. Racker, Ed., Van Nostrand Reinhold Co., New York (1970).

Scheib, D. Properties and role of acid hydrolases of the Mullerian ducts during sexual differentiation in the male chick embryo. In *Ciba Foundation Symposium on Lysosomes*, pp. 264–277, A. V. S. de Reuck and M. P. Cameron, Eds., Little, Brown & Co., Boston (1963).

Schekman, R., A. Weiner, and A. Kornberg. Multienzyme systems of DNA replication. *Science* 186:987–993 (1974).

Schemmel, R., O. Mickelsen, and J. L. Gill. Dietary obesity in rats: body weight and body fat accretion in seven strains of rats. *J. Nutr.* 100:1041–1048 (1970).

Schenk, R. K., D. Spiro, and J. Wiener. Cartilage resorption in the tibial epiphyseal plate of growing rats. *J. Cell. Biol.* 34:275–291 (1967).

Schepartz, B. *Regulation of amino acid metabolism in mammals.* W. B. Saunders Co., Philadelphia (1973).

Schiff, D., L. Stern, and L. Leduc. Chemical thermogenesis in newborn infants: catecholamine excretion and the plasma non-esterified fatty acid response to cold exposure. *Pediatr.* 37:577–582 (1966).

Schlaphoff, D. and F. A. Johnston. The iron requirement of six adolescent girls. *J. Nutr.* 39:67–82 (1949).

Schlenk, H. Odd numbered and new essential fatty acids. *Fed. Proc.* 31:1430–1435 (1972).

Schmidt, U., P. Grafer, K. Altland, and H. W. Goedde. Biochemistry and chemistry of lipoic acids. *Adv. Enzymol.* 32:423–469 (1969).

Schmitt, F. O., R. S. Bear, and G. L. Clark. X-ray diffraction studies on nerve. *Radiology* 25:131–151 (1935).

Schnaitman, C. and J. W. Greenawalt. Enzymatic properties of the inner and outer membranes of rat liver mitochondria. *J. Cell Biol.* 38:158–175 (1968).

Schneider, H., J. J. Lemasters, M. Höchli, and C. R. Hackenbrock. Liposome-mitochondrial inner membrane fusion. *J. Biol. Chem.* 255:3748–3756 (1980).

Schneider, W. C. and V. R. Potter. Intracellular distribution of enzymes. IV. The distribution of oxalacetic oxidase activity in rat liver and rat kidney fractions. *J. Biol. Chem.* 177:893–903 (1948).

Schnoes, H. K. and H. F. DeLuca. Recent progress in vitamin D metabolism and the chemistry of vitamin D metabolites. *Fed Proc.* 39:2723–2729 (1980).

Schoeller, D. A., E. van Santen, D. W. Peterson, W. Dietz, J. Jaspan, and P. D. Klein. Total body water measurement in humans with ^{18}O and ^{2}H labeled water. *Am. J. Clin. Nutr.* 33:2686–2693 (1980).

Schoenheimer, R. *The Dynamic State of Body Constituents.* Harvard University Press, Cambridge (1942).

Schoenheimer, R. and D. Rittenberg. Deuterium as an indicator in the study of intermediary metabolism. III. The role of the fat tissues. *J. Biol. Chem.* 111:175–181 (1935).

Scholler, J., T. M. Farley, and K. Folkers. Therapeutic activity of coenzyme Q for reproduction. *Int. Z. Vitaminforsch.* 38:362–368 (1968).

Schraer, H., A. S. Posner, R. Schraer, and I. Zipkin. Effect of fluoride on bone "crystallinity" in the growing rat. *Biochim. Biophys. Acta* 59:565–567 (1962).

Schraer, R., J. A. Elder, and H. Schraer. Aspects of mitochondrial function in calcium movement and calcification. *Fed Proc.* 32:1938–1943 (1973).

Schrauzer, G. Selenium and cancer: a review. *Bioinorg. Chem.* 5:275–281 (1976).

Schricker, B. R., D. D. Miller, R. R. Rasmussen, and D. Van Campen. A comparison of *in vivo* and *in vitro* methods for determining availability of iron from meals. *Am. J. Clin. Nutr.* 34:2257–2263 (1981).

Schrier, R. W. and T. Berl. Nonosmolar factors affecting renal water excretion. *N. Engl. J. Med.* 292:81–88; 141–145 (1975).

Schroeder, H. A. Chromium deficiency in rats: a syndrome simulating diabetes mellitus with retarded growth. *J. Nutr.* 88:439–445 (1966).

Schucker, R. E. Alternative approaches to classic food consumption measurement methods: telephone interviewing and market data bases. *Am. J. Clin. Nutr.* 35(5 Suppl.):1306–1309 (1982).

Schultz, G. E. and R. H. Schirmer. *Principles of Protein Structure*, Springer-Verlag, New York, Heidelberg, and Berlin (1978).

Schultz, J. and N. J. Smith. A quantitative study of the absorption of food iron in infants and children. *A.M.A. J. Dis. Child.* 95:109–119 (1958).

Schultz, S. G. Salt and water absorption by mammalian small intestine. In *Physiology of the Gastrointestinal Tract*, Vol. 2, pg. 983–989, L. R. Johnson, Ed., Raven Press, New York (1981a).

Schultz, S. G. Ion transport by mammalian large intestine. In *Physiology of the Gastrointestinal Tract*, Vol. 2, pp. 991–1002, L. R. Johnson, Ed., Raven Press, New York (1981b).

Schultz, S. G. and P. F. Curran. Intestinal absorption of sodium chloride and water. In *Handbook of Physiology*, Section 6: Alimentary Canal, Vol. 3, pp. 1245–1275, C. F. Code, Ed., American Physiological Society, Washington, D.C. (1968).

Schultz, S. G. and R. A. Frizzell. Amino acid transport by the small intestine. In *Intestinal Absorption and Malabsorption*, pp. 77–93, T. Z. Csaky, Ed., Raven Press, New York (1975).

Schultz, S. G., R. E. Fuisz, and P. F. Curran. Amino acid and sugar transport in rabbit ileum. *J. Gen. Physiol.* 49:849–866 (1966).

Schultze, H. E. and J. F. Heremans. *Molecular Biology of Human Proteins*, Vol. 1, Elsevier Publishing Co., Amsterdam (1966).

Schutte, J. E., J. C. Longhurst, F. A. Gaffney, B. C. Bastian, and C. G. Blomqvist. Total plasma creatinine: an accurate measure of total striated muscle mass. *J. Appl. Physiol.: Respirat. Environ. Exer. Physiol.* 51:762–766 (1981).

Schutz, Y., E. Ravussin, R. Diethelm, and E. Jeguier. Spontaneous physical activity measured by radar in obese and control subjects studied in a respiration chamber. *Int. J. Obesity* 6:23–28 (1982).

Schwartz, R. M. and M. D. Dayhoff. Origins of prokaryotes, eukaryotes, mitochondria and chloroplasts. *Science* 199:395–403 (1978).

Schwarz, K. and C. M. Foltz. Selenium as an integral part of factor 3 against dietary necrotic liver degeneration. *J. Am. Chem. Soc.* 79:3292–3293 (1957).

Schwarz, K. and W. Mertz. Chromium III and the glucose tolerance factor. *Arch. Biochem. Biophys.* 85:292–295 (1959).

Scott, B. L. The occurence of specific cytoplasmic granules in the osteoclast. *J. Ultrastruct. Res.* 19:417–431 (1967).

Scott, D. Clinical biotin deficiency ("egg white injury"). *Acta Med. Scand.* 162:69–70 (1958).

Scott, J. M. Thin-layer chromatography of pteroylmonoglutamates and related compounds. *Methods Enzymol.* 66:437–443 (1980).

Scott, M. L. Advances in our understanding of vitamin E. *Fed. Proc.* 39:2736–2739 (1980).

Scott, P. J., L. P. Vissentin, and J. M. Allen. the enzymatic characteristics of peroxisomes of amphibian and avian liver and kidney. *Ann. N. Y. Acad. Sci.* 168:244–264 (1969).

Scrimshaw, N. S. Analysis of past and present recommended dietary allowances for protein in health and disease, Parts I and II. *N. Engl. J. Med.* 294:136–142; 198–203 (1976).

Scrimshaw, N. S. and M. Behar. World-wide occurrence of protein malnutrition. *Fed. Proc.* 18:82–87 (1959).

Scrimshaw, N. S., M. Behar, G. Arroyave, F. Viteri, and C. Tejada. Characteristics of kwashiorkor (sindrome pluricarencial de la infancia). *Fed. Proc.* 15:977–985 (1956).

Scrimshaw, N. S., W. Davy, A. Perera, and V. R. Young. Protein requirements of men: obligatory urinary and fecal nitrogen losses in elderly women. *J. Nutr.* 106:665–670 (1976).

Scrimshaw, N. S., V. R. Young, R. Schwartz, M. Piche, and J. B. Das. Minimum dietary essential amino acid-to-total nitrogen ratio for whole egg protein fed to young men. *J. Nutr.* 89:9–18 (1966).

Scriver, C. R. and J. H. Hutchinson. The vitamin B_6 deficiency syndrome in human infancy: biochemical and clinical observations. *Pediatr.* 31:240–250 (1963).

Scriver, C. R. and L. E. Rosenberg. Amino acid metabolism and its disorders. In *Major Problems in Clinical Pediatrics*, Vol. 10, W. B. Saunders Co., Philadelphia (1973).

Sealock, R. and H. E. Silberstein. The control of experimental alcaptonuria by means of vitamin C. *Science* 90:517. (1939).

Seamarks, D. A., D. J. H. Trafford, and H. L. J. Makin. The estimation of vitamin D and metabolites in human plasma. *J. Steroid Biochem.* 14:111–123 (1981).

Second European Nutrition Conference. Reviews and views on recommended dietary intakes of different countries. *Nutr. Metab.* 21:215–279 (1977).

Sedvall, G. and I. J. Kopin. Acceleration of norepinephine synthesis in the rat submaxillary gland *in vivo* during sympathetic nerve stimulation. *Life Sci.* 6:45–51 (1967).

Segal, H. L. Enzymatic interconversion of active and inactive forms of enzymes. *Science* 180:25–32 (1973).

Seifter, S. and S. England. Energy Metabolism. In *The Liver: Biology and Pathobiology*, pp. 219–249, I. Arias, H. Popper, D. Schachter, and D. A. Shafrits, Eds., Raven Press, New York (1982).

Seljelid, R. Endocytosis in thyroid follicle cells. IV. On the acid phosphatase activity in the thyroid follicle cells, with special reference to the quantitive aspects. *J. Ultrastruct. Res.* 18:237–256 (1967).

Seltzer, C. C., R. F. Goldman, and J. Mayer. Triceps skinfold as predictive measure of body density and body fat in obese adolescent girls. *Pediatr.* 36:212–218 (1965).

Seltzer, C. C. and J. Mayer. Simple criterion of obesity. *Postgrad. Med.* 38:A101–A107 (1965).

Semenza, G., S. Auricchio, A. Rubino, A. Prader, and J. D. Welsh. Lack of some intestinal maltases in a human disease transmitted by a single genetic factor. *Biochim. Biophys. Acta* 105:386–389 (1965).

Setlow, R. B. and W. L. Carrier. The disappearance of thymine dimers from DNA: an error-correcting mechanism. *Proc. Nat. Acad. Sci. U. S.* 51:226–231 (1964).

Shah, B. G. and B. Belonje. Bioavailability of zinc in beef with and without plant protein. *Fed. Proc.* 40:855A (1981).

Shaik, B., N. J. Pontzer, S. S. Huang, and W. L. Zielinski. Determination of N^1-methylnicotinamide in urine by high-performance liquid chromatography. *J. Chromatogr. Sci.* 15:215–217 (1977).

Shambaugh, G. E., Jr., and J. Causse. Ten years experience with fluoride in otosclerotic (otospongiotic) patients. *Ann. Otol. Rhinol. Laryngol.* 83:635–642 (1974).

Shantz, E. M. Isolation of pure A_2. *Science* 108:417–419 (1948).

Shapira, J. F., I. Kircher, and R. J. Martin. Indices of skeletal muscle growth in lean and obese Zucker rats. *J. Nutr.* 110:1313–1318 (1980).

Shapiro, B., I. Chowers, and G. Rose. Fatty acid uptake and esterification in adipose tissue. *Biochim. Biophys. Acta.* 23:115–120 (1957).

Shapiro, B., M. Staffer, and G. Rose. Pathways of triglyceride formation in adipose tissue. *Biochim. Biophys. Acta* 44:373–375 (1960).

Share, L. Interrelations between vasopressin and the renin-angiotensin system. *Fed. Proc.* 38:2267–2271 (1979).

Shaw, J. C. L. Evidence for defective skeletal mineralization in low-birthweight infants: the absorption of calcium and fat. *Pediatr.* 57:16–25 (1976).

Shaw, J. H. and E. A. Sweeney. Nutrition in relation to dental medicine. In *Modern*

Nutrition in Health and Disease, 6th ed., pp. 855–891, R. S. Goodhart and M. E. Shils, Eds., Lea & Febiger, Philadelphia (1980).

Shearer, M. J., P. Barkhan, and G. R. Webster. Absorption and excretion of an oral dose of tritiated vitamin K_1 in man. *Br. J. Haematol.* 18:297–308 (1970).

Sheehan, R. G. Unidirectional uptake of iron across intestinal brush border. *Am. J. Physiol.* 231:1438–1444 (1977).

Sheehan, R. G. and R. P. Frenkel. The control of iron absorption by the gastrointestinal mucosal cell. *J. Clin. Invest.* 51:224–231 (1972).

Sheldon, W. Congenital pancreatic lipase deficiency. *Arch. Dis. Child.* 39:268–271 (1964).

Shelling, D. H. Calcium and phosphorus studies. III. The source of excess serum calcium in viosterol hypercalcemia. *J. Biol. Chem.* 96:229–243 (1932).

Sheppard, A. J. and W. D. Hubbard. Gas chromatography of vitamins D_2 and D_3. In *Methods in Enzymology*, Vol. 18, Part C, pp. 733–746, D. B. McCormick and L. D. Wright, Eds., Academic Press, New York (1971).

Sherman, H. C. Calcium requirement of maintenance in man. *J. Biol. Chem.* 44:21–27 (1920).

Sherwood, J. B. and E. Goldwasser. Extraction of erythropoietin from normal kidneys. *Endocrinology* 103:866–870 (1978).

Sheving, L. E., W. H. Harrison, P. Gordon, and J. E. Pauly. Daily fluctuation (circadian and ultradian) in biogenic amines of the rat brain. *Am. J. Physiol.* 214:166–173 (1968).

Shidoji, Y., W. Sasak, C. S. Silverman-Jones, and L. M. DeLuca. Recent studies on the involvement of retinyl phosphate as a carrier of mannose in biological membranes. *Ann. N. Y. Acad. Sci.* 359:345–357 (1981).

Shils, M. E. Experimental human magnesium depletion. I. Clinical observations and gland chemistry alterations. *Am. J. Clin. Nutr.* 15:133–143 (1964).

Shils, M. E. Magnesium. In *Modern Nutrition in Health and Diseases*, 6th ed., pp. 310–323, R. S. Goodhart and M. E. Shils, Eds., Lea & Febiger, Philadelphia (1980).

Shimazu, T. Central nervous system regulation of liver and adipose tissue metabolism. *Diabetologia* 20:343–356 (1981).

Shishiba, Y., D. H. Solomon, and G. N. Beall. Comparison of early effects of thyrotropin and long-acting thyroid stimulation on thyroidal secretion. *Endocrinology* 80:957–961 (1967).

Shnitka, T. K. Pinocytotic labelling of liver-cell lysosomes with colloidal gold: observations on the uptake of the marker, and its subsequent discharge into bile canaliculi. *Fed. Proc.* 24:556A (1965).

Shojania, A. M., G. Harnady, and G. H. Barnes. Oral contraceptives and serum-folate levels. *Lancet* 1:1376–1377 (1968).

Shorb, M. S. Activity of vitamin B_{12} for the growth of *Lactobacillus lactis*. *Science* 107:397–398 (1948).

Shrago, E., J. A. Glennon, and E. S. Gordon. Enzyme studies in human liver and adipose tissue. *Nature* 212:1263. (1966).

Shulman, R. G. NMR spectroscopy of living cells. *Sci. Am.* 248(1):86–93 (1983).

Siekevitz, P. Protoplasm: endoplasmic reticulum and microsomes and their properties. *Ann. Rev. Physiol.* 25:15–40 (1963).

Siekevitz, P. and G. E. Palade. A cytochemical study on the pancreas of the guinea pig. III. *In vivo* incorporation of leucine-l-C^{14} into the proteins of cell fractions. *J. Biophys. Biochem. Cytol.* 4:557–566 (1958).

Siekevitz, P. and G. E. Palade. A cytochemical study on the pancreas of the guinea pig. V. *In vivo* incorporation of leucine-l-C^{14} into the chymotrypsinogen of various cell fractions. *J. Biophys. Biochem. Cytol.* 7:619–630 (1960).

Silber, R. H. and K. Unna. Studies on the urinary excretion of pantothenic acid. *J. Biol. Chem.* 142:623–628 (1942).

Silbernagl, S., E. D. Foulkes, and P. Deetjen. Renal transport of amino acids. *Rev. Physiol. Biochem. Pharmacol.* 74:105–167 (1975).

Silk, D. B. A., Digestion and absorption of dietary protein in man. *Proc. Nutr. Soc.* 39:61–70 (1980).

Silk, D. B. A., P. D. Fairclough, N. J. Park, A. E. Lane, J. P. Webb, M. L. Clark, and A. M. Dawson. A study of relations between the absorption of amino acids, dipeptides, water and electrolytes in the normal human subject. *Clin. Sci. Mol. Med.* 49:401–408 (1975).

Silk, D. B. A., J. P. W. Webb, A. E. Lane, M. L. Clark, and A. M. Dawson. Functional differentiation of human jejunum and ileum: a comparison of the handling of glucose, peptides, and amino acids. *Gut* 15:444–449 (1974).

Silve, C. M., G. T. Hradek, A. L. Jones, and C. D. Arnaud. Parathyroid hormone receptor in intact embryonic chicken bone: characterization and cellular localization. *J. Cell Biol.* 94:379–386 (1982).

Silverman, M., F. Ebaugh, and R. C. Gardiner. The nature of labile citrovorum factor in human urine. *J. Biol. Chem.* 223:259–270 (1956).

Silverman, W. A., A. Zamelis, J. C. Sinclair, and F. J. Agate. Warm nape of the newborn. *Pediatr.* 33:984–987 (1964).

Simmonds, W. J. Fat absorption and chylomicron formation. In *Lipids and Lipoproteins*, pp. 705–743, G. J. Nelson, Ed., John Wiley & Sons, New York (1972).

Simon, E. J., A. Eisengart, L. Sundheim, and A. T. Milhorat. The metabolism of vitamin E. II. Purification and characterization of urinary metabolites of α-tocopherol. *J. Biol. Chem.* 221:807–817 (1956).

Simonson, E. The concept and definition of normality.. *Ann N. Y. Acad. Sci.* 134:541–558 (1966).

Simonson, M., J. K. Stephan, H. M. Hanson, and B. F. Chow. Open field studies in offspring of underfed mother rats. *J. Nutr.* 101:331–335 (1971).

Simoons, F. J. Geographic patterns of primary adult lactose malabsorption. A further interpretation of evidence for the Old World. In *Lactose Digestion,* pp. 23–48, D. M. Paige and T. M. Bayless, Eds., Johns Hopkins University Press, Baltimore (1981).

Simopoulos, A. and F. Bartter. The metabolic consequences of chloride deficiency. *Nutr. Rev.* 38:201–205 (1980).

Simpson, I., B. Rose, and W. R. Loewenstein. Size limit of molecules permeating the junctional membrane channels. *Science* 195:294–296 (1977).

Simpson, K. M., E. R. Morris, and J. D. Cook. The inhibitory effect of bran on iron absorption. *Am. J. Clin. Nutr.* 34:1469–1478 (1981).

Sims, E. A. H. Experimental obesity, dietary induced thermogenesis, and their clinical implications. *Clin. Endocrinol. Metab.* 5:377–395 (1976).

Singer, J. E., M. Westphal, and K. Niswander. Relationship of weight gain during pregnancy to birth weight and infant growth and development in the first year of life. *Obstet. Gynecol.* 31:417–423 (1968).

Singer, S. The properties and the endocrine control of the production of the steroid sulfotransferases. In *Biochemical Actions of Hormones,* Vol. 9, pp. 271–303, G. Litwack, Ed., Academic Press, New York (1982).

Singer, S. J. The molecular organization of biological membranes. In *Structure and Function of Biological Membranes,* pp. 145–222, L. I. Rothfield, Ed., Academic Press, New York (1971).

Singer, S. J. A fluid lipid-globular protein mosaic model of membrane structure. *Ann. N. Y. Acad. Sci.* 195:16–23 (1972).

Singer, S. J. and G. L. Nicolson. The fluid mosaic model of the structure of cell membranes. *Science* 175:720–731 (1972).

Singleton, J. W. and L. Laster. Biliverdin reductase of guinea pig liver. *J. Biol. Chem.* 240:4780–4789 (1965).

Sinning, W. E. Body composition, cardiovascular function and rule changes in women's basketball. *Res. Q. Ann. Assoc. Health Phys. Educ.* 44:313–321 (1973).

Sinning, W. E. Body composition assessment of college wrestlers. *Med. Sci. Sports* 4:139–145 (1974).

Sinsheimer, R. L. Is the nucleic acid message in a two-symbol code? *J. Mol. Biol.* 1:218–220 (1959).

Siperstein, M. D. and M. J. Guest. Studies on the site of the feedback control of cholesterol synthesis. *J. Clin. Invest.* 39:642–652 (1960).

Siri, W. E. Fat, water and lean tissue studies. *Fed. Proc.* 12:133A (1953).

Siri, W. E. The gross composition of the body. *Adv. Biol. Med. Phys.* 4:239–280 (1956).

Siri, W. E. Body composition from fluid spaces and density: analysis of methods. In *Techniques for Measuring Body Composition,* pp. 223–244, National Academy of Sciences, National Research Council, Washington, D.C. (1961).

Sjöstrand, F. S. *Biochemical Problems of Lipids,* Vol. 1, Elsevier, Amsterdam (1963).

Sjöstrand, F. S. The endoplasmic reticulum. In *Cytology and Cell Physiology,* 3rd ed., pp. 311–375, G. H. Bourne, Ed., Academic Press, New York (1964).

Sjöstrand, F. S. Ultrastructure and function of cellular membranes. In *The Membranes,* pp. 151–210, A. J. Dalton and F. Haguenau, Eds., Academic Press, New York (1968).

Sjöström, L., P. Björntorp, and J. Vrana. Microscopic fat cell size measurements on frozen-cut adipose tissue in comparison with automatic determination of osmium-fixed fat cells. *J. Lipid Res.* 12:521–530 (1971).

Skinner, S. L., J. W. McCubbin, and I. H. Page: Control of renin secretion. *Circ. Res.* 15:64–76 (1964).

Skou, J. C. Enzymatic basis for active transport of Na^+ and K^+ across cell membrane. *Physiol. Rev.* 45:596–617 (1965).

Slater, E. C., J. J. M. De Vijlder, and W. Boers. The binding of NAD^+ and NADH to glyceraldehydephosphate dehydrogenase. *Vitam. Horm.* 28:315–328 (1970).

Slater, T. F. Lysosomes and experimentally induced tissue injury. In *Lysosomes in Biology and Pathology,* Vol. 1, pp. 469–492, J. T. Dingle and H. B. Fell, Eds., Wiley-Interscience, New York (1969).

Slaughter, M. H. and T. G. Lohman. An objective method for measurement of musculo-skeletal size to characterize body physique with application to the athletic population. *Med. Sci. Sports Ex.* 12:170–174 (1980).

Slautterback, D. B. Mitochondria in cardiac muscle cells of the canary and some other birds. *J. Cell Biol.* 24:1–21 (1965).

Slavin, J. L. and J. A. Marlett. Influence of refined cellulose on human small bowel function and calcium and magnesium balance. *Am. J. Clin. Nutr.* 33:1932–1939 (1980).

Sleisenger, M. H., D. Pelling, D. Burston, and D. M. Matthews. Amino acid concentrations in portal venous plasma during absorption from the small intestine of the guinea pig of an amino acid mixture simulating casein and a partial enzymic hydrolysate of casein. *Clin. Sci. Mol. Med.* 52:259–267 (1977).

Sloan, A. W. Estimation of body fat in young men. *J. Appl. Physiol.* 23:311–315 (1967).

Smiciklas, H. A., R. L. Pike, and H. Schraer. Ultrastructure of adrenal glands in sodium-deficient pregnant rats. *J. Nutr.* 101:1045–1056 (1971a).

Smiciklas, H. A., D. G. Pohanka, and R. L. Pike. Progressive histochemical and ultrastructural changes in the zona glomerulosa induced by sodium deficiency during pregnancy in the rat. *J. Nutr.* 101:1439–1444 (1971b).

Smith, A. D. and H. Winkler. Lysosomes and chromaffin granules in the adrenal medulla. In *Lysosomes in Biology and Pathology,* Vol. 1, pp. 155–166, J. T. Dingle and H. B. Fell, Eds., Wiley-Interscience, New York (1969).

Smith, C. M. The effect of metabolic state on incorporation of [^{14}C]pantothenate into CoA in rat liver and heart. *J. Nutr.* 108:863–873 (1978).

Smith, C. M., M. L. Cano, and J. Potyraj. The relationship between metabolic state and total CoA content of rat liver and heart. *J. Nutr.* 108:854–862 (1978).

Smith, D. H. Introduction. In *Transport Across the Intestine*, pp. 1–12, W. L. Burland and P. D. Samuel, Eds., Churchill Livingstone, Edinburgh (1972).

Smith, D. S. The structure of flight muscle sarcosomes in the blowfly *Calliphora erythrocephala (diptera). J. Cell Biol.* 19:115–128 (1963).

Smith, D. S., U. Jarlfors, and R. Beranek. The organization of synaptic axoplasm in the lamprey (*Petromyzon marinus*) central nervous system. *J. Cell Biol.* 46:199–219 (1970).

Smith, E. L. and L. F. J. Parker. Purification of anti-pernicious anemia factor. *Biochem. J.* 43:viii–ix (1948).

Smith, F. R., and D. S. Goodman. The effect of diseases of the liver, thyroid, and kidneys on the transport of vitamin A in human plasma. *J. Clin. Invest.* 50:2426–2436 (1971).

Smith, F. R., D. S. Goodman, M. S. Zaklama, M. K. Gabr, S. El Maraghy, and V. N. Patwardhan. Serum vitamin A, retinol-binding protein, and prealbumin concentrations in protein-calorie malnutrition. I. A functional defect in hepatic retinol release. *Am. J. Clin. Nutr.* 26:973–981 (1973).

Smith, J. A., J. W. Drysdale, A. Goldberg, and H. N. Munro. The effect of enteral and parenteral iron on ferritin synthesis in the intestinal mucosa of the rat. *Br. J. Haematol.* 14:79–86 (1968).

Smith, J. C. and K. Schwartz. A controlled environment system for new trace element deficiencies. *J. Nutr.* 93:182–188 (1967).

Smith, J. E. and D. S. Goodman. Retinol-binding protein and the regulation of vitamin A transport. *Fed. Proc.* 38:2504–2509 (1979).

Smith, J. E., Y. Muto, and D. S. Goodman. Tissue distribution and subcellular localization of retinol-binding protein in normal and vitamin A-deficient rats. *J. Lipid Res.* 16:318–323 (1975).

Smith, K. T., R. J. Cousins, B. L. Silbon, and M. L. Failla. Zinc absorption and metabolism by isolated vascularly-perfused rat intestine. *J. Nutr.* 108:1849–1857 (1978).

Smith, L. C., H. J. Pownall, and A. M. Gotto, Jr. The plasma lipoproteins: structure and metabolism. *Ann. Rev. Biochem.* 47:751–777 (1978).

Smith, M. D. and I. M. Pannacciulli. Absorption of inorganic iron from graded doses. Its significance in relation to iron absorption tests and the "mucosal block" theory. *Br. J. Haematol.* 4:428–434 (1958).

Smith, R. and M. Dick. Total urinary hydroxyproline in osteomalacia and the effect upon it of treatment with vitamin D. *Clin. Sci.* 34:43–56 (1968).

Smith, R. E. Thermogenic activity of the hibernating gland in the cold-acclimated rat. *Physiologist* 4:113A (1961).

Smith, R. E. and M. G. Farquhar. Modulation in nucleoside diphosphatase activity of mammotrophic cells of the rat adenohypophysis during secretion. *J. Histochem. Cytochem.* 18:237–250 (1970).

Smith, R. E. and B. A. Horwitz. Brown fat and thermogenesis. *Physiol. Rev.* 49:330–425 (1969).

Smith, T., R. Hesp, and J. MacKenzie. Total body potassium calibrations for normal and obese subjects in two types of whole body counter. *Phys. Med. Biol.* 24:171–175 (1979).

Smith, U., D. S. Smith, H. Winkler, and J. W. Ryan. Exocytosis in the adrenal medulla demonstrated by freeze-etching. *Science* 179:79–82 (1973).

Smuts, D. B. The relation between the basal metabolism and the endogenous nitrogen metabolism with particular reference to the maintenance requirement of protein. *J. Nutr.* 9:403–433 (1935).

Snell, E. E. The vitamin B_6 group. *J. Biol. Chem.* 157:491–505 (1945).

Snell, E. E. and F. M. Strong. A microbiological assay for riboflavin. *Ind. Eng. Chem. Anal. Ed.* 11:346–350 (1939).

Snyder, D. S., C. S. Raine, M. Karooq, and W. T. Norton, The bulk isolation of oligodendroglia from whole rat forebrain: a new procedure using physiologic media. *J. Neurochem.* 34:1614–1621 (1980).

Snyder, S. H., S. P. Banerjee, H. I. Yamamura, and D. Greenberg. Drugs, neurotransmitters, and schizophrenia. *Science* 184:1243–1253 (1974).

Snyder, S. H., A. B. Young, J. P. Bennett, and A. H. Mulder. Synaptic biochemistry of amino acids. *Fed. Proc.* 32:2039–2047 (1973).

Snyderman, S. E., L. E. Holt, Jr., J. Dancis, E. Roitman, A. Boyer, and M. E. Balis. Unessential nitrogen: a limiting factor for human growth. *J. Nutr.* 78:57–72 (1962).

Soberon, G. and Q. Sanchez. Changes in effective enzyme concentration in the growing rat liver. I. Effects of fasting followed by repletion. *J. Biol. Chem.* 236:1602–1606 (1961).

Solomon, A. K. Pores in the cell membrane. *Sci. Am.* 203(6):146–156 (1960).

Solomons, N. W. Zinc and copper in hepatobiliary and pancreatic disorders. In *Zinc and Copper in Medicine*, pp. 317–346, K. A. Karcioglu and R. Sarper, Eds.; Charles C. Thomas, Springfield, Ill. (1980).

Solomons, N. W. Biological availability of zinc in humans. *Am. J. Clin. Nutr.* 35:1048–1075 (1982).

Solomons, N. W. and L. H. Allen. The functional assessment of nutritional status: Principles, practice and potential. *Nutr. Rev.* 42:33–50 (1983).

Solomons, N. W. and R. A. Jacob. Studies on the bioavailability of zinc in humans. IV. Effects of heme and nonheme iron on the absorption of zinc. *Am. J. Clin. Nutr.* 34:475–481 (1981).

Sommer, P. and M. Kofler. Physicochemical properties and methods of analysis of phylloquinones, menaquinones, ubiquinones, plastoquinones, menadione, and related compounds. *Vitam. Horm.* 24:349–400 (1966).

Somogyi, J. C. Antivitamins. In *Toxicants Occurring Naturally in Foods,* 2nd ed., National Academy of Sciences Press, Washington, D.C. (1973).

Soprano, D. R., J. E. Smith, and D. S. Goodman. Effect of retinol status on retinol-binding protein biosynthesis rate and translatable messenger RNA level in rat liver. *J. Biol. Chem.* 257:7693–7697 (1982).

Sottocasa, G. L., B. Kuylenstierna, and A. Bergstrand. Separation and some enzymatic properties of the outer and inner membranes of liver mitochondria. In *Methods in Enzymology,* Vol. 10, pp. 448–463, R. Estabrook and M. Pullman, Eds., Academic Press, New York (1967).

Sottocasa, G. L., G. Sandri, E. Panfill, and B. de Bernard. Glycoprotein in the mitochondrial compartments of rat liver. In *Biochemistry and Biophysics of Mitochondrial Membranes,* pp. 431–443, G. F. Azzone, E. Carafoli, A. L. Lehninger, E. Quagliariello, and N. Siliprandi, Eds., Academic Press, New York (1972).

Sourkes, T. L. Dopa decarboxylase: substrates, coenzyme, inhibitors. *Pharmacol. Rev.* 18:53–60 (1966).

Sourkes, T. L. Influence of specific nutrients on catecholamine synthesis and metabolism. *Pharmacol. Rev.* 24:349–359 (1972).

Sowers, A. E. and C. R. Hackenbrock. Alterations in size distributions of intra-membrane particles in the inner membrane of mitochondria from chloramphenicol-fed mice. *Eur. J. Cell Biol.* 24:101–107 (1981).

Spady, D. W. Total daily energy expenditure of healthy, free ranging school children. *Am. J. Clin. Nutr.* 33:766–775 (1980).

Speck, M. L. Interactions among lactobacilli and man. *J. Dairy Sci.* 59:338–343 (1976).

Spencer, H., L. Kramer, D. Osis, and C. Norris. Effect of a high protein (meat) intake on calcium metabolism in man. *Am. J. Clin. Nutr.* 31:2167–2180 (1978).

Spencer, H., J. Menczel, I. Lewin, and J. Samachson. Effect of high phosphorous intake on calcium and phosphorous metabolism in man. *J. Nutr.* 86:125–132 (1965).

Spencer, H., B. Rosoff, A. Feldstein, and S. Cohn. Metabolism of zinc-65 in man. *Radiat. Res.* 24:432–445 (1965).

Spencer, R., M. Charman, P. Wilson, and E. Lawson. Vitamin D-stimulated intestinal calcium absorption may not involve calcium-binding protein directly. *Nature* 263:161–163 (1976).

Spencer, R., M. Charman, P. Wilson, and E. Lawson. The relationship between vitamin D-stimulated calcium transport and intestinal calcium-binding protein in the chicken. *Biochem. J.* 170:93–101 (1978).

Spencer, R. P., S. Purdy, R. Hoerdtke, T. M. Bow, and M. A. Markulis. Studies on intestinal absorption of L-ascorbic acid-C^{14}. *Gastroenterol.* 44:768–773 (1963).

Spencer, R. P. and N. Zamchek. The intestinal absorption of riboflavin by the rat and hamster. *Gastroenterol.* 40:794–797 (1961).

Spies, T. D., C. Cooper, and M. A. Blankenhorn. The use of nicotinic acid in the treatment of pellagra. *JAMA* 110:622–627 (1938).

Spiller, G. A. and R. M. Kay, Eds., *Medical Aspects of Dietary Fiber,* Plenum, New York (1980).

Spinnler, E., E. Jeguier, R. Vavre, M. Dolivo, and A. Vannotti. Human calorimeter with a new type of gradient layer. *J. Appl. Physiol.* 35:158–165 (1973).

Spirichev, W. B. and N. V. Blazheievich. Mechanism of toxicity of vitamin D. *Int. Z. Vitaminforsch.* 39:30–36 (1969).

Spirin, A. S. and L. P. Gavrilova. *The Ribosome,* Springer-Verlag, New York (1969).

Sporn, M., N. M. Dunlop, D. L. Newton, and W. R. Henderson. Relationships between structure and activity of retinoids. *Nature* 263:110–113 (1976).

Sprynarova, S. and J. Pařízková. Functional capacity and body composition in top weightlifters, swimmers, runners and skiers. *Int. Z. Angew. Physiol.* 29:184–194 (1971).

Srere, P. A. The intrastructure of the mitochondrial matrix. *Trends Biochem. Sci.* 5:120–121 (1980).

Srivasta, U., M. L. Vu, and T. Goswami. Maternal dietary deficiency and cellular development of progeny in the rat. *J. Nutr.* 104:512–520 (1974).

Stadtman, T. C. Vitamin B_{12}. *Science* 171:859–867 (1971).

Stadtman, T. C. Selenium biochemistry. *Science* 183:915–922 (1974).

Staehlin, L. A. Structure and function of intercellular junctions. *Int. Rev. Cytol.* 39:191–283 (1974).

Stamler, J. Debate. The established relationship among diet, serum cholesterol and coronary heart disease. *Acta Med. Scand.* 207:433–446 (1980).

Stanbury, J. Familial goiter. In *The Metabolic Basis of Inherited Disease,* pp. 206–239, J. Stanbury, J. Wyngaarden, and D. Fredrickson, Eds., McGraw-Hill, New York (1978).

Stanfield, J. P., M. S. R. Hutt, and R. Tunnicliffe. Intestinal biopsy in Kwashiorkor. *Lancet* 2:519–523 (1965).

Stansell, M. J. and A. R. Hyder. Simplified body-composition analysis using deuterium dilution and deuteron photodisintegration. *Aviat. Space Environ. Med.* 47:839–845 (1976).

Starling, E. H. On the absorption of fluids from the connective tissue spaces. *J. Physiol. (London)* 19:312–326 (1896).

Stassen, F. L. H., G. J. Cardinale, and S. Udenfriend. Activation of prolyl hydroxylase in L-929 fibroblasts by ascorbic acid. *Proc. Nat. Acad. Sci. U. S.* 70:1090–1093 (1973).

Steele, R. Reflections on pools. *Fed. Proc.* 23:671–679 (1964).

Steenbock, H. The induction of growth promoting and calcifying properties in a ration by exposure to light. *Science* 60:224–225 (1924).

Stefanik, P. A. and M. F. Trulson. Determining the frequency intakes of foods in large group studies. *Am. J. Clin. Nutr.* 11:335–343 (1962).

Steggerda, F. R. and H. H. Mitchell. Further experiments on the calcium requirement of adult man and the utilization of the calcium in milk. *J. Nutr.* 21:577–588 (1941).

Steggerda, F. R. and H. H. Mitchell. Variability in the calcium metabolism and calcium requirement of adult human subjects. *J. Nutr.* 31: 407–422 (1946).

Steggerda, F. R. and H. H. Mitchell. The calcium balance of adult human subjects on high- and low-fat (butter) diets. *J. Nutr.* 45:201–211 (1951).

Stegink, L. D., J. B. Freeman, J. Wispe, and W. E. Connor. Absence of the biochemical symptoms of essential fatty acid deficiency in surgical patients undergoing protein-sparing therapy. *Am. J. Clin Nutr.* 30:388–393 (1977).

Stein, G. S. and R. Baserga. Cytoplasmic synthesis of acidic chromosomal proteins. *Biochem. Biophys. Res. Commun.* 44:218–223 (1971).

Stein, G. S., T. C. Spelsberg, and L. J. Kleinsmith. Nonhistone chromosomal proteins and gene regulation. *Science* 183:817–824 (1974).

Stein, O. and Y. Stein. Lecithin synthesis, intracellular transport and secretion in rat liver. IV. A radioautographic and biochemical study of choline-deficient rats injected with choline-^{3}H. *J. Cell Biol.* 40:461–483 (1969).

Stein, W. D., Y. Eilam, and W. R. Lieb. Active transport of cations across biological membranes. *Ann. N. Y. Acad. Sci.* 227:328–336 (1974).

Steinberg, D., M. Vaughan, and S. Margolis. Studies of triglyceride biosynthesis in homogenates of adipose tissue. *J. Biol. Chem.* 236:1631–1637 (1961).

Steinkamp, R., R. Dubach, and C. V. Moore. Studies in iron transportation and metabolism. VIII. Absorption of radioiron from iron-enriched bread. *Arch. Int. Med.* 95:181–193 (1955).

Stenflo, J., P. Fernlund, W. Egan, and P. Roepstorff. Vitamin K-dependent modifications of glutamic acid residues in prothrombin. *Proc. Nat. Acad. Sci. U. S.* 71:2730–2733 (1974).

Stephan, A. M. and J. H. Cummins. The microbial contribution to human faecal mass. *J. Med. Microbiol.* 13:45–56 (1980).

Stephens, R. E. Reassociation of microtubule protein. *J. Mol. Biol.* 33:517–519 (1968).

Stephenson, L. S. and M. C. Latham. Lactose intolerance and milk consumption: the relation of tolerance to symptoms. *Am. J. Clin. Nutr.* 27:296–303 (1974).

Sterling, K. and J. Lazarus. The thyroid and its control. *Ann. Rev. Physiol.* 39:349–371 (1977).

Stetten, M. R. Some aspects of the metabolism of hydroxyproline studied with the aid of isotopic nitrogen. *J. Biol. Chem.* 181:31–37 (1949).

Stetten, M. R. and R. Schoenheimer. The metabolism of *l*(-)-proline studied with the aid of deuterium and isotopic nitrogen. *J. Biol. Chem.* 153:113–132 (1944).

Stevens, V. J., C. A. Rouzer, V. M. Monnier, and A. Cerami. Diabetic cataract formation: potential role of glycosylation of lens crystallins. *Proc. Nat. Acad. Sci. U. S. 75:2918–2922 (1978).*

Stevenson, N. R. and M. K. Brush. Existence and characteristics of Na$^+$-dependent active transport of ascorbic acid in guinea pig. *Am. J. Clin. Nutr.* 22:318–326 (1969).

Stewart, R., N. Griffiths, C. Thomson, and M. Robinson. Quantitative selenium metabolism in normal New Zealand women. *Br. J. Nutr.* 40:45–54 (1978).

Steyn-Parvé, E. P. The mode of action of some thiamine analogues with antivitamin activity. In *Thiamine Deficiency: Biochemical Lesions and Their Clinical Significance,* pp. 26–42, (Ciba Foundation Study Group No. 28), G. E. W. Wolstenholme and M. O'Connor, Eds., Little, Brown & Co., Boston (1967).

Stiebeling, H. K. Food budget for nutrition and production programs (Miscellaneous Publication 183). U.S. Department of Agriculture, Washington, D.C. (1933).

Stiller, E. T., S. A. Harris, J. Finkelstein, J. C. Keresztesy, and K. Folkers. Pantothenic acid. VIII. The total synthesis of pure pantothenic acid. *J. Am. Chem. Soc.* 62:1785–1790 (1940).

Stirling, K., M. A. Brenner, and J. H. Lazarus. Thyroid hormone action: the mitochondrial pathway. *Science* 197:996–999 (1977).

Stirling, K., J. H. Lazarus, P. O. Milch, T. Sakurada, and M. A. Brenner. Mitochondrial thyroid hormone receptor: localization and physiological significance. *Science* 201:1126–1129 (1978).

Stoeckenius, W. Some observations on negatively stained mitochondria. *J. Cell Biol.* 17:443–454 (1963).

Stoeckenius, W. Morphological observations on mitochondria and related structures. *Ann. N. Y. Acad. Sci.* 137:641–642 (1966).

Stoffel, W. and H.-G. Schiefer. Biosynthesis and composition of phosphatides in outer and inner mitochondrial membranes. *Hoppe-Seyler's Z. Physiol. Chem.* 349:1017–1026 (1968).

Stohlman, F., Jr. Humoral regulation of erythropoiesis. XIV. A model for abnormal erythropoiesis in thalassemia. *Ann. N. Y. Acad. Sci.* 119:578–585 (1964).

Stohlman, F., Jr. Kinetics of erythropoiesis. In *Regulation of Hematopoiesis,* Vol. 1, pp. 317–326, A. S. Gordon, Ed., Appleton-Century-Crofts, New York (1970a).

Stohlman, F., Jr. Regulation of red cell production. In *Formation and Destruction of Blood Cells,* pp. 65–84, T. J. Greenwalt and G. A. Jamieson, Eds., J. B. Lippincott, Philadelphia (1970b).

Stohlman, F., Jr. Erythropoietin and erythroid cell kinetics. In *Kidney Hormones,* pp. 331–341, J. W. Fisher, Ed., Academic Press, London (1971).

Stohlman, F., Jr., S. Ebbe, B. Morse, D. Howard, and J. Donovan. Regulation of erythropoiesis. XX. Kinetics of red cell production. *Ann, N. Y. Acad. Sci.* 149:156–172 (1968).

Stohlman, F., Jr., D. Howard, and A. Beland. Humoral regulation of erythropoiesis. XII. Effect of erythropoietin and iron on cell size in iron deficiency anemia. *Proc. Soc. Exp. Biol. Med.* 113:986–988 (1963).

Stone, N. and A. Meister. Function of ascorbic acid in the conversion of proline to collagen hydroxyproline. *Nature* 194:555–557 (1962).

Straus, E and R. S. Yalow. Cholecystokinin in the brains of obese and nonobese mice. *Science* 203:68–69 (1979).

Straus, E. and R. S. Yalow. Gastrointestinal peptides in the brain. *Fed. Proc.* 38:2320–2324 (1979).

Straus, W. Lysosomes, phagosomes and related particles. In *Enzyme Cytology*, pp. 239–319, D. B. Roodyn, Ed., Academic Press, New York (1967).

Strauss, E. W. Absorption of fat from solutions of mixed bile salt micelles by hamster intestine *in vitro*. *J. Cell Biol.* 23:90A (1964).

Strauss, E. W. Electron microscopic study of intestinal fat absorption *in vitro* from mixed micelles containing linolenic acid, monolein, and bile salt. *J. Lipid Res.* 7:307–323 (1966).

Strauss, E. W. Morphological aspects of triglyceride absorption. In *Handbook of Physiology*, Section 6: Alimentary Canal, Vol. 3, pp. 1377–1406, C. F. Code, Ed., American Physiological Society, Washington, D.C. (1968).

Strauss, E. W. and S. Ito. Autoradiographic and biochemical study of linolenic acid-C^{14} absorption by hamster intestine from mixed micelles *in vitro*. *J. Cell Biol.* 27:101A (1965).

Streffer, C. and D. H. Williamson. The effect of calcium ions on the leakage of protein and enzymes from rat-liver slices. *Biochem. J.* 95:552–560 (1965).

Streiff, R. R. Folate deficiency and oral contraceptives. *JAMA* 214:105–108 (1970).

Strickler, A. J. Corn syrup selections in food applications. In *Food Carbohydrates*, pp. 12–24, D. R. Lineback and G. E. Inglett, Eds., AVI Publishing Co., Westport, Conn. (1982).

Stryer, L. Implications of x-ray crystallographic studies of protein structure. *Ann. Rev. Biochem.* 37:25–50 (1968).

Stryer, L., Ed., *Biochemistry,* 2nd ed. W. H. Freeman & Co., San Francisco (1981).

Subba Rao, K., S. Seshadri, and P. Ganguly. Studies on metabolism of vitamin A. 2. Enzymic synthesis and hydrolysis of phenolic sulphates in vitamin A-deficient rats. *Biochem. J.* 87:312–317 (1963).

Subba Rao, Y., A. B. Hastings, and M. Elkin. Chemistry of anti-pernicious anemia substances of liver. *Vitam. Horm.* 3:237–296 (1948).

Subramanian, N., B. K. Nandi, A. K. Majumder, and I. B. Chatterjee. Role of L-ascorbic acid on detoxification of histamine. *Biochem. Pharmocol.* 22:1671–1673 (1973).

Suda, T., H. F. DeLuca, H. K. Schnoes, Y. Tanaka, and M. F. Holick. 25,26-Dihydroxycholecalciferol, a metabolite of vitamin D_3 with intestinal calcium transport activity. *Biochem.* 9:4776–4780 (1970).

Sueoka, N. Compositional correlation between deoxyribonucleic acid and protein. *Cold Spring Harbor Symp. Quant. Biol.* 26:35–43 (1961b).

Sueoka, N. Correlation between base composition of deoxyribonucleic acid and amino acid composition of protein. *Proc. Nat. Acad. Sci. U.S.* 47:1141–1149 (1961a).

Sugimoto, K., T. Okazaki, and R. Okazaki. Mechanism of DNA chain growth. II. Accumulation of newly synthesized short chains in *E. coli* infected with ligase-defective T4 phages. *Proc. Nat. Acad. Sci. U.S.* 60:1356–1362 (1968).

Sulakhe, P. V. and N. S. Dhalla. Excitation-contraction coupling in heart. X. Further studies on the energy-linked calcium transport by subcellular particles in the failing heart of myopathic hamster. *Biochem. Med.* 8:18–27 (1973).

Sund, H. *The Pyridine Nucleotide Coenzymes,* Interscience, New York (1968).

Sunde, R. and W. Hoekstra. Structure, synthesis and function of glutathione peroxidase. *Nutr. Rev.* 38:265–273 (1980).

Sung, J. H., S. H. Park, A. R. Mastri, and W. J. Warwick. Axonal dystrophy in the gracil nucleus in congenital biliary atresia and cystic fibrosis (mucoviscidosis): beneficial effect of vitamin E therapy. *J. Neuropathol. Exp. Neurol.* 39:584–597 (1980).

Sutherland, E. W. Studies on the mechanism of hormone action. *Science* 177:401–408 (1972).

Sutherland, E. W., T. W. Rall, and T. Menon. Adenyl cyclase. I. Distribution, preparation, and properties. *J. Biol. Chem.* 237:1220–1227 (1962).

Sutherland, E. W. and G. A. Robison. The role of cyclic 3′,5′-AMP in responses to catecholamines and other hormones. *Pharmacol. Rev.* 18:145–161 (1966).

Suttie, J. W. Vitamin K. In *The Fat-Soluble Vitamins,* pp. 211–277, H. F. DeLuca, Ed., Plenum, New York (1978).

Suttie, J. W. The metabolic role of vitamin K. *Fed. Proc.* 39:2730–2735 (1980b).

Suttie, J. W. *Vitamin K Metabolism and Vitamin K-Dependent Proteins,* University Park Press, Baltimore (1980a).

Svirbely, J. L. and A. Szent-Györgyi. The chemical nature of vitamin C. *Biochem. J.* 26:865–870 (1932).

Swan, P. B. Food consumption by individuals in the United States: Two major studies. *Ann. Rev. Nutr.* 3:413–432 (1983).

Swedish National Food Administration. *Swedish nutrition recommendations.* Uppsala, Sweden (1981).

Sweeley, C. C. and B. Siddiqui. Chemistry of mammalian glycolipids. In *Mamalian Glycoproteins and Glycolipids,* Vol. 1, pp. 459–540, M. I. Horowitz and W. Pigman, Eds., Academic Press, New York and London (1977).

Swell, L., E. C. Trout, Jr., H. Field, Jr., and C. R. Treadwell. Absorption of H^3-B-sitosterol in the lymph fistula rat. *Proc. Soc. Exp. Biol. Med.* 100:140–142 (1959a).

Swell, L., E. C. Trout, Jr., H. Field, Jr., and C. R. Treadwell. Intestinal metabolism of C^{14}-phytosterols. *J. Biol. Chem.* 234:2286–2289 (1959b).

Swendseid, M. E., W. H. Griffith, and S. G. Tuttle. The effect of low protein diet on the ratio of essential to nonessential amino acids in blood plasma. *Metabolism* 12:96–97 (1963).

Swendseid, M. E., I. Williams, and M. S. Dunn. Amino acid requirements of young women based on nitrogen balance data. I. The sulfur-containing amino acids. *J. Nutr.* 58:495–505 (1956a).

Swendseid, M. E., I. Williams, and M. S. Dunn. Amino acid requirements of young women based on nitrogen balance data. II. Studies on isoleuscine and on minimum amounts of the eight amino acids fed simultaneously. *J. Nutr.* 58:507–517 (1956b).

Swift, R. W., G. P. Barron, Jr., K. H. Fisher, N. D. Magruder, A. Black, J. W. Bratzler, C. E. French, E. W. Hartsook, T. V. Hershberger, E. Keck, and F. P. Stiles. Relative dynamic effects of high versus low protein diets of equicaloric content. Penn. Agr. Exp. Sta. Bull. No. 618, U.S. Department of Agriculture, Washington, D.C. (1957).

Swift, R. W. and C. E. French. *Energy Metabolism and Nutrition,* Scarecrow Press, Washington, D.C. (1954).

Sydenstricker, V. P. The history of pellagra, its recognition as a disorder of nutrition and its conquest. *Am. J. Clin. Nutr.* 6:409–414 (1958).

Szent-Györgyi, A. Observations on the function of peroxidase systems and the chemistry of the adrenal cortex. *Biochem. J.* 22:1387–1409 (1928).

Szent-Györgyi, A. *Chemistry of Muscular Contraction*, Academic Press, New York (1947).

Szent-Györgyi, A. *Nature of Life,* Academic Press, New York (1948).

Szent-Györgyi, A. *Bioenergetics,* Academic Press, New York (1957).

Szent-Györgyi, A. Muscle research. *Science* 128:600–702 (1958).

Taheri, M. R., R. G. Wickremasinghe, B. F. A. Jackson, and A. V. Hoffbrand. The effect of folate analogues and vitamin B_{12} on provision of thymidine nucleotides for DNA synthesis in megaloblastic anemia. *Blood* 59:634–640 (1982).

Takagi, M. and K. Ogata. Direct evidence for albumin biosynthesis by membrane bound polysomes in rat liver. *Biochem. Biophys. Res. Commun.* 33:55–60 (1968).

Takagi, S., H. Masuda, and M. Tagawa. On some physical properties of the Golgi complex in the living cell as revealed by micro-operations under the phase microscope. *Okajimas Folia Anat. Jp.* 40:497–517 (1965).

Takaki, K. Health of the Japanese Navy. *Lancet* 2:86 (1887).

Talbot, J. M. Role of dietary fiber in diverticular disease and colon cancer. *Fed. Proc.* 40:2337–2342 (1981).

Tall, A. R. and D. M. Small. Body cholesterol removal: role of plasma high density lipoproteins. *Adv. Lipid Res.* 17:2–51 (1980).

Tanaka, Y. and H. F. DeLuca. The control of 25-hydroxyvitamin D metabolism by inorganic phosphate. *Arch. Biochem. Biophys.* 154:566–574 (1973).

Tanaka, Y., H. Frank, and H. F. DeLuca. Biological activity of 1,25-dihydroxyvitamin D_3 in the rat. *Endocrinology* 92:417–422 (1973).

Tandler, C. J. and J. L. Sirlin. Some observations on the nuclear pool of ribonucleic acid phosphorus. *Biochim. Biophys. Acta* 55:228–230 (1962).

Tao, M. Mechanism of activation of a rabbit reticulocyte protein kinase by adenosine 3′,5′-cyclic monophosphate. *Ann. N. Y. Acad. Sci.* 185:227–231 (1971).

Tao, S. and J. Suttie. Evidence for a lack of an effect of dietary fluoride level on reproduction in mice. *J. Nutr.* 106: 1115–1122 (1976).

Tappel, A. L. Lysosomal enzymes and other components. In *Lysosomes in Biology and Pathology,* Vol. 2, pp. 207–244, J. T. Dingle and H. B. Fell, Eds., Wiley-Interscience, New York (1969).

Tappel, A. L. Vitamin E and free radical peroxidation of lipids. *Ann. N. Y. Acad. Sci.* 203:12–28 (1972).

Tappel, A. L. Lipid peroxidation damage to cell components. *Fed. Proc.* 32:1870–1874 (1973).

Tappel, A. L. and C. J. Dillard. *In vivo* peroxidation: measurement via exhaled pentane and protection by vitamin E. *Fed. Proc.* 40:174–178 (1981).

Tappel, A. L., P. L. Sawant, and S. Shibko. Lysosomes: distribution in animals, hydrolytic capacity and other properties. In *Ciba Foundation Symposium on Lysosomes,* pp. 78–108, A. V. S. de Reuck and M. P. Cameron, Eds., Little, Brown & Co. Boston (1963).

Tappel, A. L. and H. Zalkin. Inhibition of lipide peroxidation in mitochondria by vitamin E. *Arch. Biochem. Biophys.* 80:333–336 (1959).

Tashiro, Y. and P. Siekevitz. Ultracentrifugal studies on the dissociation of hepatic ribosomes. *J. Mol. Biol.* 11:149–165 (1965).

Taton, R., Ed., *Ancient and Medieval Science,* p. 419, (trans. A. J. Pomerans), Basic Books, New York (1963).

Taussig, H. B. Possible injury to the cardiovascular system from vitamin D. *Ann. Intern. Med.* 65:1195–1200 (1966).

Taylor, A. E. Capillary fluid filtration. Starling forces and lymph flow. *Circ. Res.* 49:557–575 (1981).

Taylor, A. N. and R. H. Wasserman. Correlations between the vitamin D-induced calcium binding protein and intestinal absorption of calcium. *Fed. Proc.* 28:1834–1838 (1969).

Taylor, A. N. and R. H. Wasserman. Immunoflourescent localization of vitamin D-dependent calcium-binding protein. *J. Histochem. Cytochem.* 18:107–115 (1970).

Teitel, P. Basic principles of the "filterability test" and analysis of erythrocyte flow behavior. *Blood Cells* 3:55–70 (1977).

Temin, H. M. RNA-directed DNA synthesis. *Sci. Am.* 226(1):24–33 (1972).

Teng, C-S and T. H. Hamilton. Role of chromatin in estrogen action in the uterus. II. Hormone-induced synthesis of nonhistone acidic proteins which restore histone-inhibited DNA-dependent RNA synthesis. *Proc. Nat. Acad. Sci. U. S.* 63:465–472 (1969).

Tengerdy, R. P. Disease resistance: immune response. In *Vitamin E: A Compre-*

hensive Treatise., pp. 429–444, L. J. Machlin, Ed., Marcel Dekker Inc., New York (1980).

Tepperman, B. L. and M. D. Evered. Gastrin injected into the lateral hypothalamus stimulates secretion of gastric acid in rats. *Science* 209:1142–1143 (1980).

Tepperman, J. *Metabolic and Endocrine Physiology*, 2nd ed., Year Book Medical Publishers, Chicago, (1968).

Tepperman, J. *Metabolic and Endocrine Physiology*, 3rd ed., Year Book Medical Publishers, Chicago (1973).

Terroine, E. F. and R. Bonnet. Le méchanism de l'action dynamique spécifique. *Ann. Physiol.* 2:488–598 (1926).

Thach, R. E., K. F. Dewey, J. C. Brown, and P. Doty. Formylmethionine codon AUG as an initiator of polypeptide synthesis. *Science* 153:416–418 (1966).

Thedering, F. Pernicious anemia and its variants. *Vitam. Horm.* 26:539–546 (1968).

Theorell, H. Reindarstellung (Kristallisation) des gelben atmungsfermentes un die reversible Spaltung dessellen. *Biochem. Z.* 272:155–156 (1934).

Thoene, J., H. Baker, M. Yoshino, and L. Sweetman. Biotin-responsive carboxylase deficiency associated with subnormal plasma and urinary biotin. N. Engl. J. Med. 304:817–820 (1981).

Thoma, F., Th. Koller, and A. Klug. Involvement of histone H1 in the organization of the nucleosome and of the salt dependent superstructure of chromatin. *J. Cell. Biol.* 83:403–427 (1979).

Thomas, C. D. The precursors of hypertension and coronary artery disease: insights from studies of biological variation. *Ann. N. Y. Acad. Sci.* 134:1028–1040 (1966).

Thomas, L., R. T. McCluskey, J. L. Potter, and G. Weissmann. Comparison of the effects of papain and vitamin A on cartilage. *J. Exp. Med.* 111:705–718 (1960).

Thompson, G. R., B. Lewis, and C. C. Booth. The absorption of vitamin D_3-^{3}H in control subjects and in patients with intestinal malabsorption. *J. Clin. Invest.* 45:94–102 (1966a).

Thompson, G. R., B. Lewis, and C. C. Booth. Vitamin-D absorption after partial gastrectomy. *Lancet* 1:457–458 (1966b).

Thompson, G. R., B. Lewis, G. Neale, and C. C. Booth. Mechanisms of vitamin D deficiency in patients with lesions of the gastrointestinal tract. *Q. J. Med.* 34:486–487 (1965).

Thompson, J. N. and G. Hatina. Determination of tocopherols tocotrienols in foods and tissues by high performance liquid chromatography. *J. Liq. Chromatogr.* 2:327–329 (1979).

Thompson, J. N., J. McC. Howell, and G. A. J. Pitt. Vitamin A and reproduction in rats. *Proc. R. Soc. Lond.* B159:510–535 (1964).

Thompson, J. N. and M. L. Scott. Role of selenium in the nutrition of the chick. *J. Nutr.* 97:335–342 (1969).

Thompson, R. H. S. The function of a vitamin: the legacy of this concept to biochemistry. *Biochem. Pharmacol.* 20:513–517 (1971).

Thompson, S. A. and C. W. Weber. Influence of pH on the binding of copper, zinc, and iron in six fiber sources. *J. Food Sci.* 44:752–754 (1979).

Thomson, A. B. R. and J. M. Dietschy. Experimental demonstration of the effect of the unstirred water layer on the kinetic constants of the membrane transport of D-glucose in rabbit jejunum. *J. Membr. Biol.* 54:221–229 (1980).

Thomson, A. B. R. and J. M. Dietschy. Intestinal lipid absorption: major extracellular and intracellular events. In *Physiology of the Gastrointestinal Tract,* Vol. 2, pp. 1147–1220, L. R. Johnson, Ed., Raven Press, New York (1981).

Thomson, A. D., H. Baker, and C. M. Leevy. Pattern of ^{35}S-thiamine hydrochloride absorption in the malnourished alcoholic patient. *J. Lab. Clin. Med.* 76:34–45 (1970).

Thomson, A. D., O. Frank, H. Baker, and C. M. Leevy. Thiamine propyl disulfide: absorption and utilization. *Ann. Int. Med.* 74:529–534 (1971).

Thomson, A. D. and C. M. Leevy. Observations on the mechanism of thiamine hydrochloride absorption in man. *Clin. Sci.* 43:153–163 (1972).

Thomson, A. M. Diet in pregnancy. 1. Dietary survey technique and the nutritive value of diets taken by primigravidae. *Br. J. Nutr.* 12:446–461 (1958).

Thomson, A. M. Diet in pregnancy. 2. Assessment of the nutritive value of diets, especially in relation to differences between social classes. *Br. J. Nutr.* 13:190–204 (1959a).

Thomson, A. M. Diet in pregnancy. 3. Diet in relation to the course and outcome of pregnancy. *Br. J. Nutr.* 13:509–525 (1959b).

Thomson, C. and M. Robinson. Selenium in human health and disease with emphasis on those aspects peculiar to New Zealand. *Am. J. Clin. Nutr.* 33:303–323 (1980).

Thomson, R. Y., F. C. Heagy, W. C. Hutchinson, and J. N. Davidson. The deoxyribonucleic acid content of the rat cell nucleus and its use in expressing the results of tissue analysis, with particular reference to the composition of liver tissue. *Biochem. J.* 53:460–474 (1953).

Thrasher, T. N. Osmoreceptor mediation of thirst and vasopressin secretion in the dog. *Fed. Proc.* 41:2528–2532 (1982).

Tibbits, G. F., T. Nagatomo, M. Sasaki, and R. J. Barnard. Cardiac sarcolemma: compositional adaptation to exercise. *Science* 213:1271–1273 (1981).

Tillotson, J. A. and E. M. Baker. An enzymatic measurement of the riboflavin status in man. *Am. J. Clin. Nutr.* 25:425–431 (1972).

Tillotson, J. A., H. E. Sauberlich, E. M. Baker, and J. E. Canham. Use of carbon-14 labeled vitamins in human nutrition studies: pyridoxine. *Proc. 7th Int. Cong. Nutr. (Hamburg)* 5:554–557 (1968).

Timiras, P. S. *Developmental Physiology and Aging.* Macmillan Co., New York (1972).

Tissières, A. and J. D. Watson. Ribonucleoprotein particles from *Escherichia coli*. *Nature* 182:778–780 (1958).

Titani, K., P. Cohen, K. A. Walsh, and H. Neurath. Amino-terminal sequence of rabbit muscle phosphorylase. *FEBS Lett.* 55:120–123 (1975).

Todhunter, E. N. Development of knowledge in nutrition. I. Animal experiments. II. Human experiments. *J. Am. Diet. Assoc.* 41:328–334; 335–340 (1962).

Toepfer, E. W. and J. Lehmann. Procedure for chromatographic separation and microbiological assay of pyridoxine, pyridoxal and pyridoxamine in food extracts. *J. Ass. Offic. Agr. Chem.* 44:426–430 (1961).

Toepfer, E. W. and M. M. Polansky. Recent developments in the analysis for vitamin B_6 in foods. *Vitam. Horm.* 22:825–832 (1964).

Tolbert, N. E. Metabolic pathways in peroxisomes and glyoxysomes. *Ann. Rev. Biochem.* 50:133–157 (1981).

Tontisirin, K., V. R. Young, W. M. Rand, and N. W. Scrimshaw. Plasma threonine response curve and threonine requirements of young men and elderly women. *J. Nutr.* 104:495–505 (1974).

Torun, B., V. R. Young, and W. M. Rand, Eds., *Protein-energy requirements of developing countries: evaluation of new data,* WHTR-4/UNUP-295, UNU Tokyo, (1981).

Toskes, P. P. and J. Deren. The role of the pancreas in vitamin B_{12} absorption: studies of vitamin B_{12} absorption in partially pancreatectomized rats. *J. Clin. Invest.* 51:216–223 (1972).

Toskes P. P. and J. J. Deren. Vitamin B_{12} absorption and malabsorption. *Gastroenterol.* 65:662–683 (1973).

Toskes, P. P., J. Hansell, J. Cerda, and J. Deren. Vitamin B_{12} malabsorption in chronic pancreatic insufficiency. *N. Engl. J. Med.* 284:627–632 (1971).

Tower, D. B., S. A. Luse, and H. Grundfest. *Properties of Membranes*. Springer-Verlag, New York (1962).

Trams, E. G., L. E. Giuffrida, and A. Karmen. Gas chromatographic analysis of long-chain fatty acids in gangliosides. *Nature* 193:680–681 (1962).

Tranzer, J. P., H. Thoenen, R. L. Snipes, and J. G. Richards. Recent developments on the ultrastructural aspect of adrenergic nerve endings in various experimental conditions. In *Mechanisms of Synaptic Transmission,* K. Akert and P. G. Waser, Eds., *Prog. Brain Res.* 31:33–46 (1969).

Travis, S., M. M. Mathias, and J. Dupont. Effect of biotin deficiency on the catabolism of linoleate in the rat. *J. Nutr.* 102:767–771 (1972).

Treadwell, C. R., L. Swell, and G. V. Vahouny. Factors in sterol absorption. *Fed. Proc.* 21:903–908 (1962).

Treadwell, C. R. and G. V. Vahouny. Cholesterol absorption. In *Handbook of Physiology,* Section 6: Alimentary Canal, Vol. 3, pp. 1407–1438, C. F. Code, Ed., American Physiological Society, Washington, D.C. (1968).

Treble, D. H. and E. G. Ball. The occurrence of glycerolkinase in rat brown adipose tissue. *Fed. Proc.* 22:357A (1963).

Trebukina, R. V., Y. M. Ostrovsky, V. G. Petushok, M. G. Velichko, and V. N. Tumanov. Effect of thiamin deprivation on thiamin metabolism in mice. *J. Nutr.* 111:505–513 (1981).

Trenkle, A. Hormonal and nutritional interrelationships and their effects on skeletal muscle. *J. Anim. Sci.* 38:1142–1149 (1974).

Trier, J. S. and J. L. Madara. Functional morphology of the mucosa of the small intestine. In *Physiology of the Gastrointestinal Tract,* Vol. 2, pp. 925–961, L. R. Johnson, Ed., Raven Press, New York (1981).

Triner, L., G. G. Nahas, Y. Vulliemoz, N. I. A. Overweg, M. Verosky, D. V. Habif, and S. H. Ngai. Cyclic AMP and smooth muscle function. *Ann. N. Y. Acad. Sci.* 185:458–476 (1971).

Trowell, H. C., T. Moore, and I. M. Sharman. Vitamin E and carotenoids in the blood plasma in kwashiorkor. *Ann. N. Y. Acad. Sci.* 57:734–736 (1954).

Trulson, M. F. and M. B. McCann. Comparison of dietary survey methods. *J. Am. Diet. Assoc.* 35:672–676 (1959).

Truswell, A. S. A comparative look at recommended nutrient intakes. *Proc. Nutr. Soc.* 35:1–14 (1976).

Truswell, A. S., T. Konno, and J. D. L. Hansen. Thiamin deficiency in adult hospital patients. *S. Afri. Med. J.* 46:2079–2082 (1972).

Ts'o, P. O. P., J. Bonner, and J. Vinograd. Structure and properties of microsomal nucleoprotein particles from pea seedlings. *Biochim. Biophys. Acta* 30:570–582 (1958).

Tullis, I. G., V. Lawson, and R. Williams. The digital computer in calculating dietary data. *J. Am. Diet. Assoc.* 46:383–386 (1965).

Turnbull, A. Iron absorption. In *Iron in Biochemistry and Medicine,* pp. 369–403, A. Jacobs and M. Worwood, Eds., Academic Press, New York (1974).

Turnbull, A., F. Cleton, and C. A. Finch. Iron absorption. IV. The absorption of hemoglobin iron. *J. Clin. Invest.* 41:1897–1907 (1967).

Turner, J. B. and D. E. Hughes. The absorption of some B-group vitamins by surviving rat intestine preparations. *Q. J. Exp. Physiol.* 47:107–123 (1962).

Turpeinen, O., M. J. Karvonen, M. Pekkarinen, M. Miettinen, R. Elosuo, and E. Päävilainen. Dietary prevention of coronary heart disease: the Finnish mental hospital study. *Int. J. Epidemiol.* 8:99–118 (1979).

Tyor, M. P., J. T. Garbutt, and L. Lack. Metabolism and transport of bile acids in the intestine. *Am. J. Med.* 51:614–626 (1971).

Tzankoff, S. P. and A. H. Norris. Effect of muscle mass decrease on age-related BMR changes. *J. Appl. Physiol.: Respirat. Environ. Exer. Physiol.* 43:1001–1006 (1977).

Tzankoff, S. P. and A. H. Norris. Longitudinal changes in basal metabolism in man. *J. Appl. Physiol.: Respirat. Environ. Exer. Physiol.* 45:536–539 (1978).

Uber, F. M. *Biophysical Research Methods,* Wiley-Interscience, New York (1950).

Udenfriend, S. Tyrosine hydroxylase. *Pharmocal. Rev.* 18:43–51 (1966).

Ugolev. A. M. Membrane (contact) digestion. *Physiol. Rev.* 45:555–595 (1965).

Ugolev, A. M. Membrane (contact) digestion. In *Intestinal Absorption*, pp. 285–362, D. H. Smyth, Ed., *Biomembranes*, Vol. 4A, Plenum, New York (1974).

Ullrich, K. J. Sugar, amino acid, and Na^+ cotransport in the proximal tubule. *Ann. Rev. Physiol.* 41:181–195 (1979).

Ulrich, I. H., H-Y Lai, L. Vona, R. L. Reid, and M. J. Albrink. Alterations of fecal steroid composition induced by changes in dietary fiber consumption. *Am. J. Clin. Nutr.* 34:2054–2060 (1981).

Umbarger, H. E. Intracellular regulatory mechanisms. *Science* 145:674–679 (1964).

Umbreit, W. W. Vitamin B_6 antagonists. *Am. J. Clin. Nutr.* 3:291–297 (1955).

Umbreit, W. W. and I. C. Gunsalus. The function of pyridoxine derivatives: arginine and glutamic acid decarboxylases. *J. Biol. Chem.* 159:333–341 (1945).

Underwood, E. J. *Trace Elements in Human and Animal Nutrition*, 4th ed., pp. 170–195, Academic Press, New York (1977).

Unger, R. H. The milieu interieur and the islets of Langerhans. *Diabetologia* 20:1–11 (1981).

Unger, R. H. and L. Orci. Physiology and pathophysiology of glucagon. *Physiol. Rev.* 56:779–826 (1976).

Unglaub, W. G. and G. A. Goldsmith. Evaluation of vitamin adequacy; urinary excretion tests. In *Methods for Evaluation of Nutritional Adequacy and Status—Symposium*, pp. 69–81, Advisory Board on Quartermaster Research and Development, Committee on Foods, National Academy of Science, National Research Council, Washington, D.C. (1954).

Uri, N. Physico-chemical aspects of autoxidation. In *Autoxidation and Antioxidants*, Vol. 1, pp. 55–106, W. O. Lundberg, Ed., Interscience Publishers (1961).

Urist, M. R., R. J. DeLange and G. A. M. Finerman. Bone cell differentiation and growth factors. *Science* 220:680–686 (1983).

U.S. Department of Agriculture. *Food* (Home and Garden Bull. No. 228), Human Nutrition Center, Consumer and Food Economics Institute, Washington, D.C. (1980).

U.S. Department of Agriculture, U.S Department of Health, Education, and Welfare, *Nutrition and Your Health. Dietary Guidelines for Americans* (1980).

U.S. Department of Health, Education, and Welfare. *Ten-state nutrition survey 1968–1970. III. Clincal anthropometry dental* (DHEW Publication No. 72-8131), Washington, D.C., (n.d.).

U.S. Department of Health, Education, and Welfare. *Ten-state nutrition survey 1968–1970. V. Dietary* (DHEW Publication No. [HSM] 72-8133), Washington, D.C. (n.d.).

U.S. Department of Health, Education, and Welfare. *Preliminary Findings of the First Health and Nutrition Examination Survey, 1971–1972; Dietary and Biochemical Findings*, U.S. Government Printing Office. 731-289/120 (1974).

U.S. Department of Health, Education, and Welfare. *Dietary Intake Findings*

United States, 1971–1974 DHEW Publication No. [HRA] 77-1647, Washington, D.C. (1977a).

U.S. Department of Health, Education, and Welfare. *NCHS Growth Curves for Children Birth-18 Years United States* (DHEW Publication NO. [PHS] 78-1650), National Center for Health Statistics, Hyattsville, Md. (1977b).

U.S. Pharmocopeial Convention, Inc. *The Pharmacopeia of the U.S.A.,* XVI, Mack Publishing Co., Easton, Pa. (1960).

Uy, R. and F. Wold. Post-translational covalent modification of proteins. *Science* 198:890–896 (1977).

Vaes, G. Studies on bone enzymes. The activation and release of latent acid hydrolases and catalase in bone tissue homogenates. *Biochem. J.* 97:393–402 (1965).

Vaes, G. On the mechanisms of bone resorption. The action of parathyroid hormone on the excretion and synthesis of lysosomal enzymes and on the extracellular release of acid by bone cells. *J. Cell Biol.* 39:676–697 (1968).

Vaes, G. Lysosomes and the cellular physiology of bone resorption. In *Lysosomes in Biology and Pathology,* Vol. 1, pp. 217–253, J. T. Dingle and H. B. Fell, Eds., Wiley-Interscience, New York (1969).

Vaes, G. Collagenase, lysosomes and osteoclastic bone resorption. In *Collagenase, Lysosomes and Bone Resorption,* pp. 185–207, D. E. Wooley and J. M. Evanson, Eds., John Wiley & Sons, New York (1980).

Vaes, G. and P. Jacques. Studies on bone enzymes. The assay of acid hydrolases and other enzymes in bone tissue. *Biochem. J.* 97:380–386 (1965).

Vahlquist, A., P. A. Peterson, and L. Wibell. Metabolism of vitamin A transporting protein complex. I. Turnover studies in normal persons and in patients with chronic renal failure. *Eur. J. Clin. Invest.* 3:352–362 (1973).

Vahouny, G. V. Dietary fiber, lipid metabolism, and atherosclerosis. *Fed. Proc.* 41:2801–2806 (1982).

Valle, D., G. S. Pai, G. H. Thomas, and R. E. Pyeritz. Homocystinuria due to cystathionine β-synthase deficiency; clinical manifestations and therapy. *Johns Hopkins Med. J.* 146:110–117 (1980).

Vallee, B. and J. Coleman. Metal coordination and enzyme action. *Comp. Biochem. Physiol.* 12:165–235 (1964).

Van Baelen, H., R. Bouillon, and P. De Moor. Vitamin D-binding protein (Gc-globulin) binds actin. *J. Biol. Chem.* 255:2270–2272 (1980).

Van Berge Henegouwen, G. P., T. N. Tangedahl, A. F. Hofmann, T. C. Northfield, N. F. LaRusso, and J. T. McCall. Biliary secretion of copper in healthy man: quantitation by an intestinal perfusion technique. *Gastroenterol.* 72:1228–1232 (1977).

Van Bruggen, E. F. J., P. Borst, G. F. C. M. Ruttenberg, M. Gruber, and A. M. Kroon. Circular mitochondrial DNA. *Biochim. Biophys. Acta* 119:437–439 (1966).

Van Campen, D. Regulation of iron absorption. *Fed. Proc.* 33:100–105 (1974).

Vandenheuvel, F. A. Study of biological structure at the molecular level with stereomodel projections. I. The lipids in the myelin sheath of nerve. *J. Am. Oil Chem. Soc.* 40:455–471 (1963).

Vander, A. J. Control renin release. *Physiol. Rev.* 47:359–382 (1967).

Vander, A. J. *Renal Physiology*, 2d ed., McGraw-Hill, New York (1980).

Vander, A. J. and R. Miller. Control of renin secretion in the anaesthetized dog. *Am. J. Physiol.* 207:537–546 (1964).

Vanderkooi, G. Organization of proteins in membranes with special reference to the cytochrome oxidase system. *Biochim. Biophys. Acta* 344:307–345 (1974).

Vanderslice, J. T. and C. E. Maire. Liquid chromatographic separation and quantification of B_6 vitamins at plasma concentration levels. *J. Chromatogr.* 196:176–179 (1980).

Vanderslice, J. T., C. E. Maire, and G. R. Beecher. B_6 vitamer analysis in human plasma by high performance liquid chromatography: a preliminary report. *Am. J. Clin. Nutr.* 34:947–950 (1981).

Vanderslice, J. T., K. K. Stewart, and M. M. Yarmas. Liquid chromatographic separation and quantificaiton of B_6 vitamers and their metabolite, pyridoxic acid. *J. Chromatogr.* 176:280–285 (1979).

Van Dorp, D. A., R. K. Beerthuis, D. H. Nugsteren, and H. Vonkeman. The biosynthesis of prostaglandins. *Biochim. Biophys. Acta* 90:204–207 (1964).

Van Leersum, E. C. The discovery of vitamines. *Science*, 64:357–358 (1926).

van Os, C., W. Ghijsen, and H. de Jonge. High affinity Ca-ATPase in basolateral plasma membranes of rat duodenum and kidney cortex. In *Calcium and Phosphate Transport Across Biomembranes*, pp. 159–162, F. Bronner and M. Peterlik, Eds., Academic Press, New York (1981).

Van Rij, A., C. Thompson, J. McKenzie, and M. Robinson. Selenium deficiency in total parenteral nutrition. *Am. J. Clin. Nutr.* 32:2076–2085 (1979).

Vasington, F. D. and J. V. Murphy. Ca^{++} uptake by rat kidney mitochondria and its dependence on respiration and phosphorylation. *J. Biol. Chem.* 237:2670–2677 (1962).

Vaughan, M. Lipid metabolism. I. Introductory remarks. *Pharmacol. Rev.* 18:215–216 (1966).

Vaughan, M. The mechanism of the lipolytic action of catecholamines. *Ann. N. Y. Acad. Sci.* 139:841–848 (1967).

Vaughan, M., D. Steinberg, and R. Pittman. On the interpretation of studies measuring uptake and esterification of [I-^{14}C] palmitic acid by rat adipose tissue *in vitro. Biochim. Biophys. Acta* 84:154–166 (1964).

Vaughan, O. W. and L. J. Filer, Jr. The enhancing action of certain carbohydrates on the intestinal absorption of calcium in the rat. *J. Nutr.* 71:10–14 (1960).

Ventura, U. and G. Rindi. Transport of thiamine by the small intestine *in vitro. Experientia* 21:645–646 (1965).

Vergroesen, A. J., F. Ten Hoor, and G. Hornstra. Effects of dietary essential fatty acids on prostaglandin synthesis. In *Nutritional Factors: Modulating Effects on Metabolic Processes.* pp. 539–549, R. F. Beers, Jr., and E. G. Bassett, Eds., Raven Press, New York (1981).

Verney, E. B. The antidiuretic hormone and the factors which determine its release. *Proc. R. Soc., Ser.* B 135:25–106 (1947).

Verzar, F. and E. J. McDougall. *Absorption from the Intestine,* London: Longmans Green and Co. (1936).

Victor, M., R. D. Adams, and G. H. Collins. *The Wernicke-Korsakoff syndrome: a clinical and pathological study of 245 patients, 82 with post-mortem examination.* F. A. Davis Co., Philadelphia (1971).

Vidaver, G. A. Glycine transport by hemolyzed and restored pigeon red cells. *Biochemistry* 3:795–799 (1964a).

Vidaver, G. A. Mucate inhibition of glycine entry into pigeon red cells. *Biochemistry* 3:799–803 (1964b).

Vidaver, G. A. Some tests of the hypothesis that the sodium-ion gradient furnishes the energy for glycine-active transport by pigeon cells. *Biochemistry* 3:803–808 (1964c).

Villar-Palasi, J. Larner, and I. C. Shen. Glycogen metabolism and the mechanism of action of cyclic AMP. *Ann. N. Y. Acad. Sci.* 185:74–84 (1971).

Viveros, O. H., L. Arqueros, and N. Kirshener. Release of catecholamines and dopamine-β-oxidase from the adrenal medulla. *Life Sci.* 7:609–618 (1968).

Vivier, F. Observations ultrastructurales sur 1' enveloppe nucléaire et ses "pores" chez des sporozoaires. *J. Microscopie* 6:371–390 (1967).

Voit, C. Physiologie des allgemeinen Stoffwechsels und der ernahrung. In *Handbuch der Physiologie,* Vol. 6. Part 1, L. Hermann, Ed., (1881).

Volpe, J. J. and P. R. Vagelos. Mechanisms and regulation of biosynthesis of saturated fatty acids. *Physiol. Rev.* 56:339–417 (1976).

von Bezold, A. Untersuchungen uber die Vertheilung von Wasser, organischer Materie und anorganischen Verbindungen im Thierreiche. *Z. Wissensch. Zool.,* 8:487 (1857).

von der Decken, A. Peptidyl transferase activity in rat skeletal muscle ribosomes after protein restriction. *J. Nutr.* 107:1335–1339 (1977).

von Ehrenstein, G. Transfer RNA and amino acid activation. In *Aspects of Protein Biosynthesis,* Part A, pp. 139–214, C. B. Anfinsen, Jr., Ed., Academic Press, New York (1970).

von Euler, U. S. Zur Kenntnis der pharmakologischen Wirkungen von Nativsekreten und Extrackten mannlicher accessorischer Geschlechtsdrüsen. *Arch. Exp. Path. Pharmak.* 175:75–84 (1934).

von Euler, U. S. A depressor substance in the vesicular gland. *J. Physiol. (London)* 84:21p–22p (1935).

von Euler, U. S. Distribution and metabolism of catechol hormones in tissues and axones. *Rec. Prog. Horm. Res.* 14:483–512 (1958).

von Euler, U. S. Adrenergic neurotransmitter functions. *Science* 173:202–206 (1971).

Vorhees, C. V., R. J. Barrett, and S. Schenker. Increased muricide and decreased avoidance and discrimination learning in thiamine deficient rats. *Life Sci.* 16:1187–1199 (1975).

Vorhees, C. V., D. E. Schmidt, R. J. Barrett, and S. Schenker. Effects of thiamin deficiency on acetylcholine levels and utilization *in vivo* in rat brain. *J. Nutr.* 107:1902–1908 (1977).

Vos, J., I. Molenaar, M. Searle-vanLeeuwen, and F. A. Hommes. Mitochondrial and microsomal membranes from livers of vitamin D-deficient ducklings. *Ann. N. Y. Acad. Sci.* 203:74–80 (1972).

Wachstein, M. Evidence for a relative vitamine B_6 deficiency in pregnancy and some disease states. *Vitam. Horm.* 22:705–721 (1964).

Wacker, W. *Magnesium and Man,* pp. 11–51, Harvard University Press, Cambridge (1980).

Waddell, J. The provitamin D of cholesterol. I. The antirachitic efficacy of irradiated cholesterol. *J. Biol. Chem.* 105:711–739 (1934).

Waelsch, H., W. M. Sperry, and V. A. Stoyanoff. A study of the synthesis and deposition of lipids in brain and other tissues with deuterium as an indicator. *J. Biol. Chem.* 135:291–296 (1940a).

Waelsch, H., W. M. Sperry, and V. A. Stoyanoff. Lipid metabolism in brain during myelination. *J. Biol Chem.* 135:297–302 (1940b).

Waelsch, H., W. M. Sperry, and V. A. Stoyanoff. The influence of growth and myelination on the deposition and metabolism of lipids in the brain. *J. Biol. Chem.* 140:885–897 (1941).

Waite, L. C. Carbonic anhydrase inhibitors, parathyroid hormone and calcium metabolism. *Endocrinology* 91:1160–1165 (1972).

Wakil, S. J. A malonic acid derivative as an intermediate in fatty acid synthesis *J. Am. Chem. Soc.* 80:6465. (1958).

Wald, G. Vitamin A in the retina. *Nature* 132:316–317 (1933).

Wald, G. The biochemistry of vision. *Ann. Rev. Biochem.* 22:497–526 (1953).

Waldron, H. A. and D. Stöfen. *Subclinical Lead Poisoning,* Academic Press, London (1974).

Walker, A. R. P. Does low intake of calcium retard growth or conduce to stuntedness? *Am. J. Clin. Nutr.* 2:265–271 (1954).

Walker, A. R. P. and U. B. Arvidsson. Studies on human bone from South African Bantu subjects. I. Chemical composition of ribs from subjects habituated to diet low in calcium. *Metabolism* 3:385–391 (1954).

Walker, A. R. P. and U. B. Arvidsson. Iron overload in the South African Bantu. *Trans. R. Soc. Trop. Med. Hyg.* 47:536–548 (1973).

Walker, M. C., B. E. Carpenter, and E. L. Cooper. Simultaneous determination of niacinamide, pyridoxine, riboflavin and thiamine in multivitamin preparations by high-pressure liquid chromatography. *J. Pharm. Sci.* 70:99–101 (1981).

Walker, R. M. and H. M. Linkswiler. Calcium retention in the adult human male as affected by protein intake. *J. Nutr.* 102:1297–1302 (1972).

Wall, R. Overlapping genetic codes. *Nature* 193:1268–1270 (1962).

Wallace, W. M. Nitrogen content of the body and its relation to retention and loss of nitrogen. *Fed. Proc.* 18:1125–1136 (1959).

Walravens, P., K. M. Hambidge, K. Nelder, A. Silverman, W. Van Doorninck, G. Mierau, and B. Favara. Zinc metabolsim in acrodermatitis enteropathica. *J. Pediatr.* 93:71–73 (1978).

Walsh, J. H. Gastrointestinal hormones and peptides, In *Physiology of the Gastrointestinal Tract,* Vol. 1, pp. 59–144, L. R. Johnson, Ed., Raven Press, New York (1981).

Walton, A.G. *Polypeptides and Protein Structure.* Elsevier, New York (1981).

Warburg, O. and W. Christian. Über ein neues Oxydationsferment und sein Absorptionspektrum. *Biochem. Z.* 254:438–458 (1932).

Warburg, O. and W. Christian. Co-Fermentproblem. *Biochem. Z.* 275:112–113; (1935).

Ward, G. M., H. J. Krzywicki, D. P. Rahman, R. L. Quaas, R. A. Nelson, and C. F. Consolazio. Relationship of anthropometric measurements to body fat as determined by densitometry, potassium 40 and body water. *Am. J. Clin. Nutr.* 28:162–169 (1975).

Wardzala, L. J., S. W. Cushman, and L. B. Salans. Mechanism of insulin action on glucose transport in the isolated rat adipose cell. *J. Biol. Chem.* 253:8002–8005 (1978).

Warnock, L. G. A new approach to erythrocyte transketolase measurement. *J. Nutr.* 100:1057–1062 (1970).

Warnold, I., G. Carlgren, and .M. Krotkiewski. Energy expenditure and body composition during weight reduction in hyperplastic obese women. *Am. J. Clin. Nutr.* 31:750–763 (1978).

Warshawsky, H., D. Goltzman, M. F. Rouleau, and J. J. M. Bergeron. Direct *in vivo* demonstration by radioautography of specific binding sites for calcitonin in skeletal and renal tissues of the rat. *J. Cell Biol.* 85:682–702 (1980).

Wasserman, R. H. The vitamin D-dependent calcium-binding protein. In *The Fat-Soluble Vitamins,* pp. 21–37, H. F. DeLuca and J. W. Suttie, Eds., University of Wisconsin Press, Madison (1970).

Wasserman, R. H. Molecular aspects of the intestinal absorption of calcium and phosphorus. In *Pediatric Diseases Related to Calcium,* pp. 107–132, H. F. DeLuca and C. S. Anast, Eds., Elsevier North-Holland, New York (1980).

Wasserman, R. H., R. A. Corradino, and A. N. Taylor. Vitamin D-dependent calcium-binding protein. Purification and some properties. *J. Biol Chem.* 243:3978–3986 (1968a).

Wasserman, R. H. and C. S. Fullmer. Calcium transport proteins, calcium absorption, and vitamin D. *Ann. Rev. Physiol.* 45:375–390 (1983).

Wasserman, R. H. and A. N. Taylor. Vitamin D_3-induced calcium-binding protein in chick intestinal mucosa. *Science* 152:791–793 (1966).

Wasserman, R. H. and A. N. Taylor. Vitamin D-dependent calcium-binding protein. Response to some physiological and nutritional variables. *J. Biol. Chem.* 243:3987–3993 (1968).

Wasserman, R. H. and A. N. Taylor. Metabolic roles of fat-soluble vitamins D, E, and K. *Ann. Rev. Biochem.* 41:179–202 (1972).

Waterlow, J. C. Protein nutrition and enzyme changes in man. *Fed. Proc.* 18:19–31 (1959).

Waterlow, J. C. and G. A. O. Alleyne. Protein malnutrition in children: advances in knowledge in the last ten years. *Adv. Protein Chem.* 25:117–242 (1971).

Waterlow, J. C. and T. Weisz. The fat, protein and nucleic acid content of the liver in malnourished human infants. *J. Clin. Invest.* 35:346–354 (1956).

Watson, C. J. Gold from dross: the first century of the urobilinoids. *Ann. Int. Med.* 70:839–851 (1969).

Watson, J. D. *Molecular Biology of the Gene*, 2nd. ed., W. A. Benjamin, New York (1970).

Watson, J. D. and F. H. C. Crick. Molecular structure of nucleic acids: a structure for deoxypentose nucleic acids. *Nature* 171:737–738 (1953).

Watson, P. E., I. D. Watson, and R. D. Batt. Obesity indices. *Am. J. Clin. Nutr.* 31:736–737 (1979).

Watt, B. L. and A. L. Merrill. *Composition of Foods—Raw, Processed, Prepared* (Agriculture Handbook No. 8), Agricultural Research Service, U.S. Department of Agriculture. Revised (1963).

Waugh, W. A. and C. G. King. Isolation and identification of vitamin C. *J. Biol. Chem.* 97:325–331 (1932).

Waxman, S., J. J. Corcino, and V. Herbert. Drugs, toxins and dietary amino acids affecting vitamin B_{12} or folic acid absorption or utilization. *Am. J. Med.* 48:599–607 (1970).

Waxman, S. and C. Schrieber. Measurement of serum folate levels. Current status of the radioassay methodology. In *Folic Acid. Biochemistry and Physiology in Relation to the Human Nutrition Requirement*, pp 98–109, National Research Council, National Academy of Sciences Press, Washington, D.C. (1977).

Webb, P. Energy balance over a 45-hour period with a suit calorimeter. In Proceedings of the First Ross Conference on Medical Research, *Assessment of Energy Metabolism in Health and Disease*, pp. 24–31, Ross Laboratories, Columbus, Ohio (1980).

Webb, P., J. F. Annis, and S. J. Troutman. Human calorimetry with a water cooled garment. *J. Appl. Physiol.* 32:412–418 (1972).

Weber, A. L. and S. L. Miller. Reasons for the occurrence of the twenty coded protein amino acids. *J. Mol. Evol.* 17:273–284 (1981).

Weber, F. and O. Wiss. Über den Stoffwechsel des Vitamins E in der Ratte. *Helv. Physiol. Pharmacol. Acta* 21:131–141 (1963).

Weber, R. Behaviour and properties of acid hydrolases in regressing tails of tadpoles during spontaneous and induced metamorphosis *in vitro*. In *Ciba Foundation Symposium on Lysosomes*, pp. 282–300, A. V. S. de Reuck and M. P. Cameron, Eds., Little, Brown & Co., Boston (1963).

Weber, R. Tissue involution and lysosomal enzymes during anuran metamorphosis. In *Lysosomes in Biology and Pathology*, Vol. 2, pp. 437–461, J. T. Dingle and H. B. Fell, Eds., Wiley-Interscience, New York (1969).

Weibel, E. R., W. Stäubli, R. Gnägi, and F. A. Hess. Correlated morphometric and biochemical studies on the liver cell. I. Morphometric model, stereologic methods and normal morphometric data for rat liver. *J. Cell Biol.* 42:68–91 (1969).

Weigand, E. and M. Kirchgessner. Total true efficiency of zinc utilization: determination and homeostatic dependence upon the zinc supply status in young rats. *J. Nutr.* 110:469–480 (1980).

Weiner, N. Regulation of norepinephrine biosynthesis. *Ann. Rev. Pharmacol.* 10:273–290 (1970).

Weiner, N. and A. Alousi. Influence of nerve stimulation on rate of synthesis of norepinephrine. *Fed. Proc.* 25:259A (1967).

Weiner, N., G. Cloutier, R. Bjur, and R. I. Pfeffer. Modification of norepinephrine synthesis in intact tissue by drugs and during short-term adrenergic nerve stimulation. *Pharmacol. Rev.* 24:203–221 (1972).

Weinsier, R. Overview: salt and the development of essential hypertension. *Prev. Med.* 5:7–14 (1976).

Weinstock, I. M. and A. A. Iodice. Acid hydrolase activity in muscular dystrophy and denervation atrophy. In *Lysosomes in Biology and Pathology*, Vol. 1, pp. 450–468, J. T. Dingle and H. B. Fell, Eds., Wiley-Interscience, New York (1969).

Weinstock, M. and C. P. Leblond. Formation of collagen. *Fed. Proc.* 33:1205–1218 (1974).

Weintraub, L. R., M. E. Conrad, and W. H. Crosby. Absorption of hemoglobin by the rat. *Proc. Soc. Exp. Biol. Med.* 120:840–842 (1965).

Weintraub, L. R., M. B. Weinstein, H.-J. Huser, and S. Rafal. Absorption of hemoglobin iron: the role of a heme-splitting substance in the intestinal mucosa. *J. Clin. Invest.* 47:531–539 (1968).

Weiss, P. A. A cell is not an island entire of itself. *Perspect. Biol. Med.* 14:182–205 (1971).

Weiss, P. and H. B. Hiscoe. Experiments on the mechanism of nerve growth. *J. Exp. Zool.* 107:315–395 (1948).

Weissbach, H., J. Toohey, and H. A. Barker. Isolation and properties of B_{12} coenzymes containing benzimidazole or dimethylbenzimidazole. *Proc. Nat. Acad. Sci. U. S.* 45:521–525 (1959).

Weissmann, G. Lysosomal mechanisms of tissue injury in arthritis. *N. Engl. J. Med.* 286:141–147 (1972).

Weissmann, G. and L. Thomas. Studies on lysosomes. II. The effect of cortisone on the release of acid hydrolases from storage granule fraction of rabbit liver induced by an excess of vitamin A. *J. Clin. Invest.* 42:661–669 (1963).

Welham, W. C. and A. R. Behnke. The specific gravity of healthy men. *JAMA* 118:498–501 (1942).

Weller, M. Protein phosphorylation. Pion Ltd., London (1979).

Wells, I. C. Hemorrhagic kidney degeneration in choline deficiency. *Fed. Proc.* 30:151–154 (1971).

Welsh, S. O. and R. M. Marston. Zinc levels of the U.S. food supply—1909-1980. *Food Tech.* 29(1):70–76 (1982).

Wenger, R., B. Ziegler, W. Kruspl, B. Syre, G. Brubacker, and R. Pillat. Beziehungen zwischen dem vitaminstatus (Vitamin A, B1, B6, and C), Klinischen Befunden und den Ernährungsgewohnheiten in einer Gruppe von Alten Leuten in Wein (Relationships between the vitamin status, clinical findings and food habits in a group of old people in Vienna). *Wein. Klin. Wochenschr.* 91:557–563 (1979).

Wensel, R. H., C. Rich, A. C. Brown, and W. Volwiler. Absorption of calcium measured by intubation and perfusion of the intact human small intestine. *J. Clin. Invest.* 48:1768–1775 (1969).

Werner, S. and W. Neupert. Functional and biogenetical heterogeneity of the inner membrane of rat liver mitochondria. *Eur. J. Biochem.* 25:369–396 (1972).

Wessel, J. A., A. Ufer, W. D. Van Huss, and C. Cederquist. Age trends of various components of body composition and functional characteristics in women aged 20–69 years. *Ann. N. Y. Acad. Sci.* 110:608–622 (1963).

West, D. W. and E. C. Owen. The urinary excretion of metabolites of riboflavine by man. *Br. J. Nutr.* 23:889–898 (1969).

West, D. W. and E. C. Owen. Reduction of 7,8-dimethyl-10-(formylmethyl) isoalloxazine by an enzyme in liver. *Br. J. Nutr.* 29:43–50 (1973).

West, R. Activity of vitamin B_{12} in Addisonian pernicious anemia. *Science* 107:398. (1948).

West, W. Calmodulin-regulated enzymes: modifications by drugs and disease. *Fed. Proc.* 41:2251–2252 (1982).

Westergaard, H. and J. M. Dietschy. The mechanism whereby bile acid micelles increase the rate of fatty acid and cholesterol uptake into the intestinal mucosal cell. *J. Clin. Invest.* 58:97–108 (1976).

Westmoreland, N. Connective tissue alterations in zinc deficiency. *Fed. Proc.* 30:1001–1010 (1971).

Wetzel, B. K., S. S. Spicer, and S. H. Wollman. Changes in fine structure and acid phosphatase localization in rat thyroid cells following thyrotropin administration. *J. Cell Biol.* 25:593–618 (1965).

Whaley, W. G. Proposals concerning replication of the Golgi apparatus. In *Probleme der Biologischen Reduplication,* pp. 340–371, P. Sitte, Ed., Springer, Berlin-Heidelberg-New York (1966).

Whaley, W. G. The Golgi apparatus. In *The Biological Basis of Medicine,* Vol. 1, pp. 179–208, E. E. Bittar and N. Bittar, Eds., Academic Press, New York (1968).

Whaley, W. G. and M. Dauwalder. The Golgi apparatus, the plasma membrane, and functional integration. *Int. Rev. Cytol.* 58:199–245 (1979).

Whaley, W. G., M. Dauwalder, and J. E. Kephart. Assembly, continuity, and exchanges in certain cytoplasmic membrane systems. In *Origin and Continuity of Cell Organelles,* Vol. 2, pp. 1–45, J. Reinert and H. Ursprung, Eds., Springer-Verlag, New York (1971).

Whaley, W. G., M. Dauwalder, and J. E. Kephart. Golgi apparatus: influence on cell surfaces. *Science* 175:596–599 (1972).

Wheby, M. S. and W. H. Crosby. The gastrointestinal tract and iron absorption. *Blood* 22:416–428 (1963).

Whedon, G. D. Effects of high calcium intakes on bones, blood and soft tissue: relationship of calcium intake to balance in osteoporosis. *Fed. Proc.* 18:1112–1118 (1959).

Whitaker, J. R. Denaturation and renaturation of proteins. In *Food Proteins,* pp. 14–49, J. R. Whitaker and S. R. Tannenbaum, Eds., AVI Publishing Co., Westport, Conn.(1977).

White, A., P. Handler, and E. L. Smith. *Principles of Biochemistry,* 5th ed., McGraw-Hill, New York (1973).

White, A., P. Handler, E. L. Smith, R. L. Hill, and I. R. Lehman. *Principles of Biochemistry,* 6th ed., p. 573, McGraw-Hill, New York (1978).

Whitehead, R. G. and G. A. O. Alleyne. Pathophysiological factors of importance in protein-calorie malnutrition. *Br. Med. Bull.* 28:72–78 (1972).

Whitehead, R. G. and R. F. A. Dean. Serum amino acids in kwashiorkor. I. Relationship to clinical condition. *Am. J. Clin. Nutr.* 14:313–319 (1964).

Whitin, J. C., R. K. Gordon, L. M. Corwin, and E. R. Simons. The effect of vitamin E deficiency on some platelet membrane properties. *J. Lipid Res.* 23:276–282 (1982).

Whiting, M. G. and R. M. Leverton. Reliability of dietary appraisal: comparisons between laboratory analysis and calculation from tables of food values. *Am. J. Pub. Health* 50:815–823 (1960).

Whittaker, V. P. and M. N. Sheridan. The morphology and acetylcholine content of isolated cerebral cortical synaptic vesicles. *J. Neurochem.* 12:363–372 (1965).

Whittam, R. The molecular mechanisms of active transport. In *The Neurosciences,* pp. 313–325, G. C. Quarton, T. Melnechuk, and F. O. Schmitt, Eds., Rockefeller University Press, New York (1967).

Wickner, W. The assembly of proteins into biological membranes: the membrane trigger hypothesis. *Ann. Rev. Biochem.* 48:23–45 (1979).

Wicks, W. D. Regulation of hepatic enzyme synthesis by cyclic AMP. *Ann. N. Y. Acad. Sci.* 185:152–165 (1971).

Wicks, W. D., C. A. Barnett, and J. B. McKibbin. Interaction between hormones and cyclic AMP in regulating specific hepatic enzyme synthesis. *Fed. Proc.* 33:1105–1111 (1974).

Widdowson, E. M. Nutritional individuality. *Proc. Nutr. Soc.* 21:121–128 (1962).

Widdowson, E. M. Early nutrition and later development. In *Diet and Bodily Constitution,* pp. 3–10, G. E. W. Wolstenholme and M. O'Connor Eds., Little, Brown & Co., Boston (1963).

Widdowson, E. M. Chemical analysis of the body. In *Human Body Composition,* pp. 31–47, Josef Brozek, Ed., Pergamon Press, Oxford (1965).

Widdowson, E. M. Harmony of growth. *Lancet* 1:901–905 (1970).

Widdowson, E. M. and J. W. T. Dickerson. Chemical composition of the body. In *Mineral Metabolism,* Vol. 2, Part A, pp. 1–247, C. L. Comar and F. Bronner, Eds., Academic Press, New York (1964).

Widdowson, E. M., O. G. Edholm, and R. A. McCance. The food intake and energy expenditure of cadets in training. *Br. J. Nutr.* 8:147–155 (1954).

Widdowson, E. M. and R. A. McCance. Iron exchange of adults on white and brown bread diets. *Lancet* 1:588–591 (1942).

Widdowson, E. M. and R. A. McCance. *The composition of foods.* (Medical Research Council Special Report Series No. 297), H.M. Stationery Office, London (1960).

Widdowson, E. M. and R. A. McCance. The effect of finite periods of undernutrition at different ages on the composition and subsequent development of the rat. *Proc. R. Soc., Ser. B* 158:329–342 (1963).

Widdowson, E. M., R. A. McCance, and C. M. Spray. The chemical composition of the human body. *Clin. Sci.* 10:113–125 (1951).

Wiese, H. F., A. E. Hansen, and D. J. D. Adams. Essential fatty acids in infant nutrition. I. Linoleic acid requirement in terms of serum di, tri and tetraenoic acid levels. *J.Nutr.* 66:345–360 (1958).

Wikström, M., K. Krab, and M. Saraste. Proton-translocating cytochrome complexes. *Ann. Rev. Biochem.* 50:623–655 (1981).

Wildman, S. G., T. Hongladarom, and S. I. Honda. Chloroplasts and mitochondria in living plant cells. *Science* 138:434–435 (1962).

Wilhelmj, C. M., J. L. Bollman, and G. C. Mann. Studies on the physiology of the liver. XVII. The effect of the removal of the liver on the specific dynamic action of amino acids administered intravenously. *Am. J. Physiol.* 87:497–509 (1928).

Williams, C. D. A nutritional disease of childhood associated with a maize diet. *Arch. Dis. Child.* 8:423–433 (1933).

Williams, G. A., E. Bowser, W. J. Henderson, and F. Uzgiries. Effects of vitamin D and cortisone on intestinal absorption of calcium in the rat. *Proc. Soc. Exp. Biol. Med.* 106:664–666 (1961).

Williams, R. H., Ed., *Textbook of Endocrinology*, 5th ed., W. B. Saunders Co., Philadelphia and London (1974).

Williams, R. H., Ed., *Textbook of Endocrinology*, 6th ed., W. B. Saunders Co., Philadelphia and London (1981).

Williams, R. J. *Biochemical Individuality: The Basis for the Genotrophic Concept*, John Wiley & Sons, New York (1956).

Williams, R. J., J. H. Truesdail, H. H. Weinstock, E. Rohrmann, C. M. Lyman, and C. H. McBurney. Pantothenic acid. II. Its concentration and purification from liver. *J. Am. Chem. Soc.* 60:2719–2723 (1938).

Williams, R. R. *Toward the Conquest of Beriberi*. Harvard University Press, Cambridge (1961).

Williams, R. R. and J. K. Cline. Synthesis of Vitamin B_1. *J. Am. Chem. Soc.* 58:1504–1505 (1936).

Williams, R. R., H. L. Mason, B. F. Smith, and R. M. Wilder. Induced thiamine deficiency and the thiamine requirement of man. *Arch. Int. Med.* 69:721–738 (1942).

Willis, A. L. Nutritional and pharmacological factors in eicosanoid biology. *Nutr. Rev.* 39:289–301 (1981).

Willis, W. D. and R. G. Grossman. *Medical Neurobiology*, 2nd ed. C. V. Mosby, St. Louis (1977).

Wilmore, J. H. *Training for Sport and Activity*. 2nd ed., Allyn & Bacon, Boston (1982).

Wilmore, J. H. and A. R. Behnke. Predictability of lean body weight through anthropometric assessment in college men. *J. Appl. Physiol.* 25:349–355 (1968).

Wilmore, J. H. and C. H. Brown. Physiological profiles of women distance runners. *Med. Sci. Sports* 6:178–181 (1974).

Wills, L. The nature of the hemopoietic factor in marmite. *Lancet* 224:1283–1286 (1933).

Wills, V. G. and J. C. Waterlow. The death rate in the age group 1–14 years as an index of malnutrition. *J. Trop. Pediatr.* 3:167–170. (1958).

Wilson, C. S., A. E. Schaefer, W. J. Darby, E. B. Bridgeforth, W. N. Pearson, G. F. Combs, E. C. Letherwood, Jr., J. C. Greene, L. J. Teply, I. C. Plough, W. J. McGanity, D. B. Hand, Z. I. Kertesz, and C. W. Woodruff. A review of methods used in nutrition surveys conducted by the interdepartmental committee on nutrition for national defense (ICNND). *Am. J. Clin. Nutr.* 15:29–44 (1964).

Wilson, R. P. Absence of ascorbic acid synthesis in channel catfish, *ictalurus punctatus* and blue catfish, *ictalurus frucatus. Comp. Biochem. Physiol.* 46B:635–638 (1973).

Wilson, T. H. *Intestinal Absorption,* W. B. Saunders Co., Philadelphia (1962).

Wilson, T. H. Intestinal absorption of vitamin B_{12}. *Physiologist* 6:11–26 (1963).

Wilson, T. H. and B. R. Landau. Specificity of sugar transport by the intestine of the hamster. *Am. J. Physiol.* 198:99–102 (1960).

Wilson, T. H., E. C. C. Lin, B. R. Landau, and C. R. Jorgensen. Intestinal transport of sugars and amino acids. *Fed. Proc.* 19:870–875 (1960).

Wilson, T. H. and D. W. Wilson. Studies *in vitro* of digestion and absorption of pyrimidine nucleotides by the intestine. *J. Biol. Chem.* 233:1544–1547 (1958).

Wilson, T. H. and G. Wiseman. The use of sacs of everted small intestine for the study of the transference of substances from the mucosal to the serosal surface. *J. Physiol.* (London) 123:116–125 (1954).

Wingo, W. J. and J. Awapara. Decarboxylation of L-glutamic acid by brain. *J. Biol. Chem.* 187:267–271 (1950).

Winick, M. Cellular growth of the placenta as an indication of abnormal fetal growth. In *Diagnosis and Treatment of Fetal Disorders*, Proceedings of International Symposium on Diagnosis and Treatment of Disorders Affecting the Intrauterine Patient, pp. 83–101, K. Adamson, Ed., Springer-Verlag, New York (1968).

Winick, M. Nutrition and nerve cell growth. *Fed. Proc.* 29:1510–1515 (1970a).

Winick, M. Fetal malnutrition and growth processes. *Hosp. Pract.* 5:33–41 (1970b).

Winick, M. Malnutrition and mental development. In *Nutrition: Pre- and Postnatal Development,* pp. 41–60, M. Winick, Ed., Plenum, New York, (1979).

Winick, M., J. A. Brasel, and P. Rosso. Nutrition and cell growth. In *Nutrition and Development,* Vol. 1, pp. 49–97, M. Winick, Ed., John Wiley & Sons, New York (1972).

Winick, M., A. Coscia, and A. Noble. Cellular growth in human placenta. I. Normal placental growth. Pediatr. 39:248–251 (1967).

Winick, M., K. K. Meyer, and R. C. Harris. Malnutrition and environmental enrichment by early adoption. *Science* 190:1173–1175 (1975).

Winick, M. and A. Noble. Quantitative changes in DNA, RNA, and protein during prenatal and postnatal growth in the rat. *Dev. Biol.* 12:451–466 (1965).

Winick, M. and A. Noble. Cellular response in rats during malnutrition at various ages. *J. Nutr.* 89:300–306 (1966).

Winick, M. and P. Rosso. The effect of severe early malnutrition on cellular growth of human brain. *Pediatr. Res.* 3:181–184 (1969).

Winkler, H., A. D. Smith, F. DuBois, and H. van den Bosch. The positional specificity of lysosomal phospholipase A activities. *Biochem. J.* 105:38C–40C (1967).

Wischnitzer, S. The nuclear envelope: its ultrastructure and functional significance. *Endeavour* 33:137–142 (1974).

Wiseman, G. Active transport of amino acids by sacs of everted small intestine of the golden hamster (*Mesocricetus auratus*). *J. Physiol. (London)* 133:626–630 (1956).

Wiseman, G. Absorption of protein digestion products. In *Intestinal Absorption, Biomembranes*, Vol. 4A, pp. 363–481, D. H. Smyth, Ed., Plenum, London (1974).

Wiss, O. and H. Gloor. Absorption, distribution, storage, and metabolites of vitamins K and related quinones. *Vitam. Horm.* 24:575–586 (1966).

Wittwer, A. J. and C. Wagner. Identification of the folate-binding proteins of rat liver mitochondria as dimethylglycine dehydrogenase and sarcosine dehydrogenase. *J. Biol. Chem.* 256:4102–4108 (1981a).

Woese, C. R. *The Genetic Code. The Molecular Basis for Genetic Expression*, Harper & Row, New York (1967).

Wolf, S. *The Stomach*, Oxford University Press, New York (1965).

Wolf, S. and H. G. Wolff. *Human Gastric Function: An Experimental Study of a Man and His Stomach*, Oxford University Press, New York (1943).

Wolin, M. J. Fermentation in the rumen and human large intestine. *Science* 213:1463–1468 (1981).

Wolin, M. J. and T. L. Miller. Interactions of microbial populations in cellulose fermentation. *Fed. Proc.* 42:109–113 (1983).

Wollman, S. H. Secretion of thyroid hormones. In *Lysosomes in Biology and Pathology*, Vol. 2, pp. 483–512, J. T. Dingle and H. B. Fell, Eds., Wiley-Interscience, New York (1969).

Wood, P. D. and W. L. Haskell. The effect of exercise on plasma high density lipoprotein. *Lipids* 14:417–427 (1979).

Wood, P. D. and W. L. Haskell. Interrelation of physical activity and nutrition on lipid metabolism. In *Diet and Exercise. Synergism in Health Maintenance.* pp. 39–47, P. L. White and T. Mondeika, Eds., American Medical Association, Chicago (1982).

Woodrow, I. L. and J. M. de Man. Distribution of *trans*-unsaturated fatty acids in milk fat. *Biochim. Biophys. Acta* 152:472–478 (1968).

Woods, S. C., P. H. Smith, and D. Porte, Jr. Role of the nervous system in metabolic regulation and its effects on diabetes and obesity. In *Handbook of Diabetes Mellitus*, Vol. 3, pp. 209–271, M. Brownlee, Ed., Garland STPM Press, New York (1981).

Woodward, R. B. Recent advances in the chemistry of natural products. *Pure Appl. Chem.* 25:283–304 (1971).

Wool, I. G. The structure and function of eukaryotic ribosomes. *Ann. Rev. Biochem.* 48:719–754 (1979).

Woolley, D. W. Production of a scurvy-like condition of guinea pigs with glucoascorbic acid, and its prevention with ascorbic acid. *Fed. Proc.* 3:97A (1944).

Woolley, D. W. Some new aspects of the relationship of chemical structure to biological activity. *Science* 100:579–583 (1944a).

Woolley, D. W. Production of nicotinic acid deficiency with 3-acetyl-pyridine the ketone analogue of nicotinic acid. *J. Biol. Chem.* 157:445–459 (1945).

Woolley, D. W. *Metabolic Inhibitors,* Academic Press, New York (1963).

Woolley, D. W. and L. O. Krampitz. Production of a scurvy-like condition by feeding of a compound structurally related to ascorbic acid. *J. Exp. Med.* 78:333–339 (1943).

World Health Organization. Expert Committee on medical assessment of nutritional status (WHO Technical Report Series No. 258), WHO, Geneva (1963a).

Worthington, C. R. X-ray studies on nerve and photoreceptors. *Ann. N. Y. Acad. Sci.* 195:293–308 (1972).

Woteki, C. E., E. Weser, and E. A. Young. Lactose malabsorption in Mexican-American children. *Am. J. Clin. Nutr.* 29:19–24 (1976).

Wretlind, A. Introduction. General aspects on recommended dietary allowances. *Nutr. Metab.* 21:210–214 (1977).

Wretlind, A. Standards for nutritional adequacy of the diet: European and WHO/FAO viewpoints. *Am. J. Clin. Nutr.* 36:366–375 (1982).

Wright, F. S. Potassium transport by successive segments of the mammalian nephron. *Fed. Proc.* 40:2398–2402 (1981).

Wurtman, R. J. Nutrients that modify brain function. *Sci. Am.* 246(4)50–59 (1982).

Wurzberger, R. J. and J. M. Musacchio. Subcellular distribution and aggregation of bovine adrenal tyrosine hydroxylase. *J. Pharmacol. Exp. Ther.* 177:155–167 (1971).

Wuthier, R. E. A review of the primary mechanism of endochondral calcification with special emphasis on the role of cells, mitochondria and matrix vesicles. *Clin. Orthoped.* 169:219–242 (1982).

Wyse, B. W., C. Wittwer, and R. G. Hansen. Radioimmunoassay for pantothenic acid in blood and other tissues. *Clin. Chem.* 25:108–110 (1979).

Yagi, K., T. Nagatsu, I. Nagatsu-Ishibashi, and A. Ohashi. Migration of C^{14}-labelled riboflavin into rat-tissues. *J. Biochem. (Tokyo)* 59:313–315 (1966).

Yamada, T., A. Kajihara, Y. Takemura, and T. Onaya. Antithyroid compounds. In *Handbook of Physiology,* Section 7, Endocrinology, Vol. 3, pp. 345–357, Williams & Wilkins, Baltimore (1974).

Yamamoto, T. On the thickness of the unit membrane. *J. Cell Biol.* 17:413–421 (1963).

Yang, C. S. and D. B. McCormick. Degradation and excretion of riboflavin in the rat. *J. Nutr.* 93:445–453 (1967).

Yanofsky, C. Gene structure and protein structure. *Harvey Lect.* 61:145–168 (1967).

Ycas, M. *The Biological Code,* Frontiers of Biology, Vol. 12, North-Holland Publishing Co., Amsterdam (1969).

Young, C. M. A comparison of dietary study methods. 2. Dietary history vs. seven-day record vs. 24-hr. recall. *J. Am. Diet. Assoc.* 28:218–221 (1952a).

Young, C. M. Dietary Methodology. *In assessing food consumption patterns,* pp.

89–118, Committee on Food Consumption Patterns, Food and Nutrition Board, National Research Council, National Academy of Sciences Press, Washington, D.C. (1981).

Young, C. M., J. Blondin, R. Tensuan, and J. H. Fryer. Body composition studies of "older" women thirty to seventy years of age. *Ann. N. Y. Acad. Sci.* 110:589–607 (1963a).

Young, C. M., F. W. Chalmers, H. N. Church, M. M. Clayton, R. E. Tucker, A. W. Werts, and W. D. Foster. A comparison of dietary study methods. I. Dietary history vs. seven-day-record. *J. Am. Diet. Assoc.* 28:124–128 (1952).

Young, C. M., M. E. K. Martin, R. Tensuan, and J. Blondin. Predicting specific gravity and body fatness in young women. *J. Am. Diet. Assoc.* 40:102–107 (1962).

Young, C. M., R. S. Tensuan, F. Sault, and F. Holmes. Estimating body fat of normal young women. *J. Am. Diet. Assoc.* 42:409–413 (1963b).

Young, E. G. Dietary standards. In *Nutrition, an Advanced Treatise*, Vol. 2, pp. 299–350, G. H. Beaton and E. W. McHenry, Eds., Academic Press, New York (1964).

Young, H. B. Body composition, culture, and sex: two comments. In *Human Body Composition, Approaches and Applications*, pp. 139–159, J. Brozek, Ed., Pergamon Press, Oxford, Eng. (1965).

Young, J. R. *An Experimental Inquiry into Principles of Nutrition and the Digestive Process, 1803*. University of Illinois Press, Urbana (1959).

Young, V. R. Regulation of protein synthesis and skeletal muscle growth. *J. Anim. Sci.* 38:1054–1070 (1974).

Young, V. R. Dynamics of human whole body amino acid metabolism: use of stable isotope probes and relevance to nutritional requirements. *J. Nutr. Sci. Vitaminol. (Tokyo)* 27:395–413 (1981a).

Young, V. R. Protein metabolism and nutritional state in man. *Proc. Nutr. Soc.* 30:343–359 (1981).

Young, V. R., M. A. Hussein, E. Murray, and N. S. Scrimshaw. Plasma tryptophan response curve and its relation to tryptophan requirements in young adult men. *J. Nutr.* 101:45–60 (1971).

Young, V. R. and H. N. Munro. N$^\tau$-Methylhistidine (3-methylhistidine) and muscle protein turnover: an overview. *Fed Proc.* 37:2291–2300 (1978).

Young, V. R., A. Nahapetian, and M. Janghorbani. Selenium bioavailability with reference to human nutrition. *Am. J. Clin. Nutr.* 35:1074–1088 (1982).

Young, V. R., W. M. Rand, and N. S. Scrimshaw. Measuring protein quality in humans: a review and proposed method. *Cereal Chem.* 54:929 (1977).

Young, V. R. and N. S. Scrimshaw. Human protein and amino acid metabolism and requirements in relation to protein quality. In *Evaluation of Proteins for Humans*, pp. 11–54, C. E. Bodwell Ed., AVI Publishing Co., Westport, Conn. (1977).

Young, V. R. and N. S. Scrimshaw, Nutritional evaluation of proteins and protein requirements. In *Protein Resources and Technology*, pp. 136–173, M. Milner, N. S. Scrimshaw and D. I. C. Wang, Eds., AVI Publishing Co., Westport, Conn. (1978).

Young, V. R., K. Tontisirin, L. Ozalp, F. Lakshmanan, and N. S. Scrimshaw. Plasma amino acid response curve and amino acid requirements in young men: valine and lysine. *J. Nutr.* 102:1159–1169 (1972).

Yunghans, W. N., T. W. Keenan, and D. J. Morré. Isolation of a Golgi apparatus-rich fraction from rat liver. III. Lipid and protein composition. *Exp. Mol. Pathol.* 12:36–45 (1970).

Zakrzewski, S. F. Mechanism of reduction of folate and dihydrofolate. In *Biochemical Aspects of Antimetabolites and of Drug Hydroxylation* (Federation of European Biochemical Society Vol. 16), pp. 49–64, D. Shugar, Ed., Academic Press, New York (1969).

Zalkin, H. and A. L. Tappel. Studies of the mechanism of vitamin E action. IV. Lipide peroxidation in the vitamin E-deficient rabbit. *Arch. Biochem. Biophys.* 88:113–117 (1960).

Zamenhof, S., E. Van Marthens, and L. Grauel. DNA (cell number) and protein in neonatal rat brain: alteration by timing of maternal dietary protein restriction. *J. Nutr.* 101:1265–1270 (1971).

Zannoni, V. G., P. H. Sato, and L. E. Rikans. Ascorbic acid and drug metabolism. In *Nutrition and Drug Interrelations*, J. N. Hathcock and J. Coon, Eds., Academic Press, New York (1978).

Zeisel, S. H. Dietary choline: biochemistry, physiology, and pharmacology. *Ann. Rev. Nutr.* 1:95–121 (1981).

Zemmel, M. B. and H. M. Linkswiler. Calcium metabolism in the young adult male as affected by level and form of phosphorous intake and level of calcium intake. *J. Nutr.* 111:315–324 (1981).

Zile, M., R. J. Emerick, and H. F. DeLuca. Identification of 13-cis retinoic acid in tissue extracts and its biological activity in rats. *Biochim. Biophys. Acta* 141:639–641 (1967).

Zile, M. H., E. G. Bunce, and H. F. DeLuca. On the physiological basis of vitamin-A-stimulated growth. *Am. J. Clin. Nutr.* 109:1787–1796 (1979).

Zile, M. H. and M. E. Cullum. The function of vitamin A: current concepts. *Proc. Soc. Exp. Biol. Med.* 172:139–152 (1983).

Zipkin, I., S. Zucas, and B. Stillings. Biological availability of the fluoride of fish protein concentrate in the rat. *J. Nutr.* 100:293–299 (1970).

Ziporin, Z. Z., W. T. Nunes, R. C. Powell, P. P. Waring, and H. E. Sauberlich. Excretion of thiamine and its, metabolites in the urine of young adult males receiving restricted intakes of the vitamin. *J. Nutr.* 85:287–296 (1965).

Zucker, L. M. Some effects of caloric restriction and deprivation on the obese hyperlipemic rat. *J. Nutr.* 91:247–254 (1967).

Zull, J. E., E. Czarnowska-Misztal, and H. F. DeLuca. Actomycin D inhibition of vitamin D cation. *Science* 149:182–184 (1965).

Zurier, R. B., R. G. Campbell, S. A. Hashim, and T. Van Itallie. Enrichment of depot fat with odd and even numbered medium-chain fatty acids. *Am. J. Physiol.* 212:291–294 (1967).

Zweifach, B. W. *Functional Behavior of the Microcirculation.* Charles C. Thomas, Springfield, Ill. (1961).

index